Cajal on the Cerebral Cortex

HISTORY OF NEUROSCIENCE, No. 1

A series of books published by Oxford University Press
in cooperation with the Fidia Research Foundation.

Editors

Pietro Corsi, M.D.
Edward G. Jones, M.D., Ph.D.
Gordon M. Shepherd, M.D., Ph.D.

CAJAL
ON THE
CEREBRAL CORTEX
An Annotated Translation
of the Complete Writings

JAVIER DeFELIPE

Instituto Cajal, Madrid

and

EDWARD G. JONES

University of California, Irvine

New York   Oxford
OXFORD UNIVERSITY PRESS
1988

OXFORD UNIVERSITY PRESS

Oxford   New York   Toronto
Delhi   Bombay   Calcutta   Madras   Karachi
Petaling Jaya   Singapore   Hong Kong   Tokyo
Nairobi   Dar es Salaam   Cape Town
Melbourne   Auckland

and associated companies in
Berlin   Ibadan

LIBRARY OF CONGRESS
Library of Congress Cataloging-in-Publication Data

Ramón y Cajal, Santiago, 1852–1934.
Cajal on the cerebral cortex : an annotated translation of the
complete writings / [edited by] Javier DeFelipe and Edward G. Jones.
p.   cm. — (History of neuroscience ; no. 1)
Bibliography: p.   Includes index.   ISBN 978-0-19-505280-0
1. Cerebral cortex—Histology.   I. DeFelipe, Javier.   II. Jones,
Edward G., 1939–   .   III. Title.   IV. Series.
QM575.R29 1988   611'.81—dc19   87-23055   CIP (Rev.)

. . . that sort of unfathomable physiological sea, into which, on the one hand, were supposed to pour the streams arising from the sense organs and from which, on the other hand, the motor or centrifugal fibers were supposed to spring like rivers originating in mountain lakes.

Santiago Ramón y Cajal (1917)

Foreword

It is deeply satisfying to write the foreword to this attractive book by Javier DeFelipe and Edward G. Jones. I am very happy that a significant part of Santiago Ramón y Cajal's work will now be available to the international scientific community in English. Javier DeFelipe and Edward G. Jones are to be congratulated for their intelligent and opportune translation of Cajal's works on the cerebral cortex. Contemporary neuroscience would benefit from authoritative translations of other publications by Cajal, in particular the monumental *Textura del Sistema Nervioso del Hombre y de los Vertebrados* (3).

The appearance of this book in the centenary of Cajal's "peak" year is a fortunate coincidence. It was in 1888 that Cajal defined the "neuron doctrine" on the basis of his findings in the cerebellum, retina, spinal cord, and other regions by using the Golgi method. The present volume is a splendid way to celebrate this anniversary.

It is gratifying to acknowledge the high quality of the present translation. I am well aware of the difficulties in translating Cajal's writing. A man of his time, he used a luxuriant language, full of charm, that often contributes to the subtlety and profundity of his descriptions but complicates the task of the translator. Cajal's thinking can be attuned to modern conceptions easily enough, given his lasting scientific wisdom, but it is nonetheless an accomplishment to express his ideas in the streamlined language used in science nowadays. The editors of this volume have succeeded in preserving Cajal's special style and, at the same time, have made it easily accessible to neuroscientists in the last decades of the twentieth century.

An additional merit of this book is the incorporation of Cajal's own opinion of his works in the editors' introductions to the various periods they distinguish in his career. Cajal commented on his works in the *Historia de mi labor científica* (5), judging them from the perspective of old age. His remarks offer precious insights into the nature of his thinking.

The book fulfills the editors' objectives. The extent of Cajal's work on the cerebral cortex is clearly demonstrated, as well as the accuracy of his drawings in relation to the information present in his slides. The editors appropriately describe the evolution of Cajal's ideas on the morphology and function of cortical structures and provide evidence that his descriptions and interpretations are tenable today.

That Cajal's work has endured the passage of time is true not only for the cerebral cortex (7) but also for many other topics he studied. Let me quote Viktor Hamburger: "[I]ndeed, it is very difficult to be original in neurogenesis, *regeneration and plasticity,* with Cajal looking over one's shoulder" (8). I have often wondered how Cajal achieved so much without the technical and conceptual advantages of modern neuroscience. At least part of the answer lies in his being a tireless worker with the microscope, and in his meticulous description of the observations he made. He sensibly held that "the facts remain and theories slip away," and that "lasting fame only accompanies the truth." His perception of the truth, however, surpassed the actual evidence: it was his genius to generalize beyond the details of individual variations.

As is pointed out by DeFelipe and Jones (chapter 30), this ability enabled Cajal to see the basic similarities of nerve cells and neural structures, emphasize the differences in conformational models, and establish organizational units that accommodate the essential similarities and differences of their components. In addition, by viewing thousands of slides, he was able to define the connections of neural structures with an accuracy that was only surpassed with the introduction of modern axonal tracing techniques. It was on these bases of rigor and broad conceptions, with the conviction that "fortune is the muse of persevering and patient persons," that Cajal produced such an extensive, diverse, and lasting body of work. An exceptional devotion to science, a strong will and passion, together with great talent in planning experiments and interpreting the results, all contributed to the excellence of his work.

I would like to underscore the contemporary significance of Cajal's work by considering two topics that are not discussed in this book: plasticity and regeneration in the cerebral cortex. In the second volume of his work *Estudios sobre la Degeneración y Regeneración del Sistema Nervioso* (4) Cajal wrote that when the axon of a pyramidal neuron is sectioned below the emergence of its collaterals, this type of neuron "is a perfect reproduction of a cell with a short axon, except that the terminal arborization is composed of hypertrophic branches which involve an enormous part of the cortex." According to Cajal, "the genetic plans have been modified; we have transformed a neuron with a long axon into another with a short axon." He also described for the first time what is now known as a "pruning effect" (9) following partial transection of axonal branches. The conclusions that Cajal drew from these results are interesting in relation to the reorganization of the multidimensional intracortical circuitry. He pointed out that "the nerve impulse that reaches the mutilated neuron (or arciform pyramidal cell) is not absolutely lost, since it is now diverted, through the enlarged channel of the collaterals, towards other congenerous neurons." However, he added that "in order to accept faithfully this idea, it would be necessary to prove that the arciform pyramidal cells subsist indefinitely without becoming atrophied, and maintain their original connections" (4). He had previously arrived at similar findings and conclusions in the cerebellar cortex.

Cajal also described Tello's experiments on pyramidal axonal regeneration in implants of sciatic nerve within the subcortical white matter (4). He discussed the capacity for axonal growth of these neurons provided they are given an environment that is "favorable, eminently trophic, and conducive to the assimilation and growth of the newly formed axons." These assertions are very close to the conclusions reached recently by researchers in this field (1,2).

Cajal's posthumous work "¿Neuronismo o Reticularismo?" (6) can be considered his scientific testament. It offers the reader a unique panorama that helps us understand the persistence of Cajal's work. Since 1888, when he defined the neuron doctrine, his scientific life was devoted to its defense. Toward this end, he carried out a genuine multidisciplinary effort. He studied almost every neural structure in different species, used a wide variety of the methods available in his time, and devised new experimental tools to pursue his goals.

Long before he wrote his posthumous work, Cajal stated that "the superb complexity of the cerebral gray matter is so intricate that for many centuries it will constitute a major challenge to the curiosity of scientists" (5). In the last sentence on the cerebral cortex in "¿Neuronismo o Reticularismo?" he referred to the study of the intrinsic and extrinsic connections of the cerebral cortex as a captivating program for the future. Almost a century has passed since Cajal's early studies on the cerebral cortex first appeared, and only a few secrets of its "superb complexity" have been revealed by the powerful tools of modern neuroscience.

There is no doubt that the study of the cerebral cortex will remain a major challenge to neuroscientists for many years to come. This book will provide them with fundamental information to face the challenge.

Fernando Reinoso-Suárez
Departamento de Morfología
Facultad de Medicina
Universidad Autónoma de Madrid

References

(1) Aguayo, A. (1985). "Axonal Regeneration from Injured Neurons in the Adult Mammalian Central Nervous System." In *Synaptic Plasticity*. C. W. Cotman, ed. The Guilford Press, New York, pp. 457–84.

(2) Björklund, A., Gage, F. E., Dunnett, S. B. and Steveni, U. (1985). Regenerative Capacity of Central Neurons as Revealed by Intracerebral Grafting Experiments." In *Central Nervous System Plasticity and Repair*. A. Bignami, C. L. Bolis, F. E. Bloom, and A. Adeloya, eds. Raven Press, New York, pp. 57–62.

(3) Cajal, S. Ramón y (1899–1904). *Textura del Sistema Nervioso del Hombre y de los Vertebrados*. N. Moya, Madrid.

(4) Cajal, S. Ramón y (1913–14). *Estudios sobre la Degeneración y Regeneración del Sistema Nervioso*. N. Moya, Madrid.

(5) Cajal, S. Ramón y (1923). *Recuerdos de mi vida: Historia de mi labor científica*. 3rd edn. Juan Pueyo, Madrid.

(6) Cajal, S. Ramón y (1933). "¿Neuronismo o Reticularismo?" *Arch. Neurobiol.*, 13:1–144.

(7) Reinoso-Suárez, F. (1984). "Introduction." In *Cortical Integration*. F. Reinoso-Suárez and C. Ajmone-Marsan, eds. Raven Press, New York, pp. 1–11.

(8) Reinoso-Suárez, F. (1987). "Cajal's Concepts on Plasticity in the Central Nervous System Revisited: A Perspective." In *Neuroplasticity*. R. L. Masland, A. Portera and G. Toffano, eds. Liviana Press, Padua, pp. 31–37. Emphasis added.

(9) Schneider, G. E. (1973). "Early lesion of superior colliculus: factors affecting the formation of abnormal retinal projections." *Brain Behav. Evol.*, 8:73–109.

Preface

Santiago Ramón y Cajal stands prejudged as the greatest neurohistologist. But in the eyes of most contemporary neuroscientists, this assessment probably stems from the French work *Histologie du système nerveux de l'homme et des vertébrés,* a translation by Leon Azoulay of Cajal's great Spanish textbook, and first published in 1909–1911. The *Histologie* has been reprinted frequently up to the present day. To the large group of neuroscientists generally unfamiliar with Spanish, the original, more extensive works in Cajal's native language are essentially unknown. His major studies on the cerebral cortex total fifteen in number, cover several hundred pages, and contain nearly three hundred figures, many of the latter not reproduced in the *Histologie.* A number of the Spanish works were translated into German soon after their original publication, but only that of 1922 on the cat visual cortex, published in the *Journal für Psychologie und Neurologie,* is readily available. The extensive works on the human cortex originally published between 1899 and 1901 in the *Revista Trimestral Micrográfica* and its successor, the *Trabajos del Laboratorio de Investigaciones Biológicas,* as rendered into German by

J. Bressler, are, to the best of our knowledge, available in only one library in the United States and one in Britain. In any case, it is doubtful that more than a few English-speaking neuroscientists are any more familiar with German than they are with Spanish.

Among English translations, only that by Kraft (Cajal, 1955) of the three 1901–1902 papers on the olfactory cortex from the *Trabajos* has been published, but it has been long out of print. The English translation of Cajal's lectures given at the Clark University decennial celebrations is not in wide circulation and, in any case, is necessarily brief. Portions of Cajal's work on brain structures other than the cerebral cortex—mainly derived from the *Histologie,* from compilations of selected Cajal papers (such as Guth's *Studies in Neurogenesis*), or, secondarily, from the German translations by Bressler—have appeared at intervals. But there has been no direct translation of the extensive *Revista* and *Trabajos* papers on the human sensory-motor, visual, and auditory cortex, nor of the earlier and later works on the cortex of nonhuman mammals.

Our purpose in preparing the present annotated translations from the *Revista,* the *Tra-*

bajos, other Spanish sources, and an original work published in French in *La Cellule* has been fourfold. First, we wanted to demonstrate how much more extensive is Cajal's work on the cortex in comparison with that appearing in his books—the Spanish *Textura* and the French *Histologie.* Second, we wished to demonstrate by means of photomicrographs of Cajal's original preparations (still extant in the Museum of the Instituto Cajal) that these are as good as his drawings suggest and that the published drawings are by no means imaginative representations as is sometimes claimed. Third, we were determined to trace the development of Cajal's ideas on cortical structure and function, including his occasional vacillation over a particular point of interpretation. Finally, we were anxious to place his work in a modern context, not only because his descriptions have a remarkably modern flavor but also because the application of newer, more functionally oriented methods of cell identification to the cerebral cortex has led to a renewed interest in cortical circuitry. With the exception of Lorente de Nó's understandably superficial general account of 1938, virtually no Golgi study of significance was published on the neocortex for nearly fifty years after 1922, the year in which Lorente de Nó, Cajal's illustrious pupil, published his first— and the master himself published his last— paper on the cortex of rodents. The modern period of renewed interest in Golgi studies began in the early 1970s, but it is sad that the considerable advances in understanding that these have helped bring about, especially when allied with electron microscopy, intra-cellular physiology, and immunocytochemistry, have proceeded with little more than lip service being paid to the work of the great Spaniard. If our efforts prove that his descriptions and insights are still useful today, then we will have been successful.

We are particularly indebted to Professor Joaquín Del Río, director of the Instituto Cajal in Madrid, for granting us permission to reproduce all the illustrations from Cajal's works on the cortex and for providing us with access to Cajal's original preparations. We are also grateful to María Angustias Pérez de Tudela, librarian of the Instituto Cajal, for helping us obtain copies of many, largely inaccessible works. We could not have succeeded in preparing the translations without the dedicated secretarial assistance of Elizabeth Peck, the bibliographic help of Azucena Ortiz, and the photographic help of Patricia Callahan, Alberto Cobas, and Joaquín Sancho. We would also like to thank our colleagues, fellows, and students for their encouragement and advice, particularly Dr. Alfonso Fairén and Dr. Stewart Hendry. We wish to thank, too, Jeffrey House of Oxford University Press for his support in the early days of the project. Finally, we wish to acknowledge grants NS 10526 and NS 21377 and a Fogarty International Fellowship from the National Institutes of Health, United States Public Health Service, which supported our research, alluded to in the final chapter.

Madrid and Irvine   J. DeF.
June 1987   E.G.J.

A Note on the Translation

In producing this translation, we have resisted the temptation to "rewrite" Cajal in contemporary scientific English and have, instead, chosen an idiom appropriate for the period and for the language in which Cajal was writing. If our sentence structure is somewhat expansive, therefore, it is deliberate and done in an attempt to capture the cadences and some of the color of Cajal's prose. Cajal is often at his most personable when waxing eloquent over some new aspect of neuronal connectionism or when referring to the work of others, especially when expressing pique at their failure to recognize his contributions. We have sought to preserve this personal quality at all costs. Cajal's descriptions of his material are usually straightforward, and it is rare that one cannot immediately comprehend what he is describing. Generally, we have preserved his terminology except where equivalent English words of the period have gone completely out of fashion (e.g., *anfractuosities* for *sulci, nerve tubes* for *myelinated fibers,* or *axis cylinders* for *axons*) or where preservation of the original nomenclature would, in our estimation, have led to confusion. Some of Cajal's terms, however, such as *strangulations* for *nodes of Ran-*

vier, are too expressive to be lost, and we have chosen to retain them. Where, in the interest of clarity, we have occasionally introduced a rendering of an expression that is not completely literal, our phrase appears in square brackets. A number of additional explanations appear as editors' notes.

Our procedure has been to work primarily from the original Spanish writings, except in the case of chapter 5, which appeared only in French. However, we have followed older French and German translations in parallel with our own English version, and where new material was added or a point of interpretation modified we have included an English version of the relevant passage from the French or German. The primary translations from the Spanish were undertaken by J. DeF., those from the French and German by E.G.J. The definitive version is a joint effort.

All the figures appearing in the translations are taken from the original publications and are reproduced, in the majority of cases, without retouching. We have numbered them sequentially, our bracketed numbers appearing in italics in both text and figure captions. However, the figure numbers from the original publications have always been given in parallel in order to facilitate comparison with the original.

Cajal's method of referencing, like that of most of his contemporaries, is somewhat casual, with full names and bibliographic details rarely given. Apart from corrections of dates and obvious typographical errors, we have let the textual citations stand in the form in which they originally appeared. We have, however, identified and checked the vast majority of these and have listed all of them in full in the bibliography at the end of this volume.

Contents

PART I. THE EARLY PERIOD (1890–1894):
Studies on Small Mammals

1.   Introduction   3

2.   Texture of the cerebral gyri of the lower mammals (*Gaceta Médica Catalana,* 1890) 10

3.   Short Anatomical Communications II: On the existence of collaterals and bifurcations in the fibers of the white matter of the gray cerebral cortex (*Pequeñas Comunicaciones Anatómicas,* 1890)   17

4.   On the existence of special nerve cells in the first layer of the cerebral convolutions (*Gaceta Médica Catalana,* 1890)   20

5.   On the structure of the cerebral cortex of certain mammals (*La Cellule,* 1891)   23

6.   Structure of the inferior occipital cortex of the small mammals (*Anales de la Sociedad Española de Historia Natural,* 1893)   55

7.   *From:* A new concept of the histology of the nerve centers (*Revista de Ciencias Médicas de Barcelona,* 1892)   62

8.   *From:* The Croonian Lecture: The fine structure of the nerve centers (*Proceedings of the Royal Society of London,* 1894)   83

PART II. AN INTERLUDE (1896–1897):
Methylene Blue and the Special Cells of Layer I

9.   Introduction   91

10.   The collateral spines of the cells of the cerebrum stained with methylene blue (*Revista Trimestral Micrográfica,* 1896)   94

11. *From:* Methylene blue in the nerve centers (*Revista Trimestral Micrográfica,* 1896)
     104

12. The short-axon cells of the molecular layer of the cerebrum (*Revista Trimestral Micrográfica,* 1897)   113

PART III. THE MIDDLE PERIOD (1899–1902):
The Great Works on the Human Cortex

13. Introduction   131

14. Notes on a structural study of the visual cortex of the human cerebrum (*Revista Ibero-Americana de Ciencias Médicas,* 1899)   139

15. Studies on the human cerebral cortex [I]: Visual cortex (*Revista Trimestral Micrográfica,* 1899)   147

16. Studies on the human cerebral cortex II: Structure of the motor cortex of man and higher mammals (*Revista Trimestral Micrográfica,* 1899 and 1900)   188

17. Studies on the human cerebral cortex III: Structure of the acoustic cortex (*Revista Trimestral Micrográfica,* 1900)   251

18. *From:* Studies on the human cerebral cortex IV: Structure of the olfactory cerebral cortex of man and mammals (*Trabajos del Laboratorio de Investigaciones Biológicas de la Universidad de Madrid,* 1901–1902)   289

19. On a special ganglion of the spheno-occipital cortex (*Trabajos del Laboratorio de Investigaciones Biológicas de la Universidad de Madrid,* 1901–1902)   363

PART IV. THE YEARS OF CONSOLIDATION (1904–1911):
The *Textura* and the *Histologie*

20. Introduction   379

21. General plan of the structure of the cerebral cortex   382

22. *From:* Chapters 25–33 of *Histologie du Système Nerveux de l'Homme et des Vertébrés* (1911)   428

23. Comparative structure of the cerebral cortex   437

24. Histogenesis of the cerebral cortex   453

25. Anatomicophysiological considerations on the cerebrum   465

PART V. THE FINAL YEARS (1921–1935):
The Cat and the Rodents; the Return to the Neuron Doctrine

26. Introduction   493

27. Histology of the visual cortex of the cat (*Archivos de Neurobiología,* 1921)   495

28. Studies on the fine structure of the regional cortex of rodents (*Trabajos del Laboratorio de Investigaciones Biológicas de la Universidad de Madrid,* 1922)   524

29. The final view   547

PART VI. CONCLUSION: A MODERN VIEW

30.   The functional histology of the cerebral cortex and the continuing relevance of Cajal's observations   557

Bibliography   622

Index   643

PART I

The Early Period (1890–1894)

Studies on Small Mammals

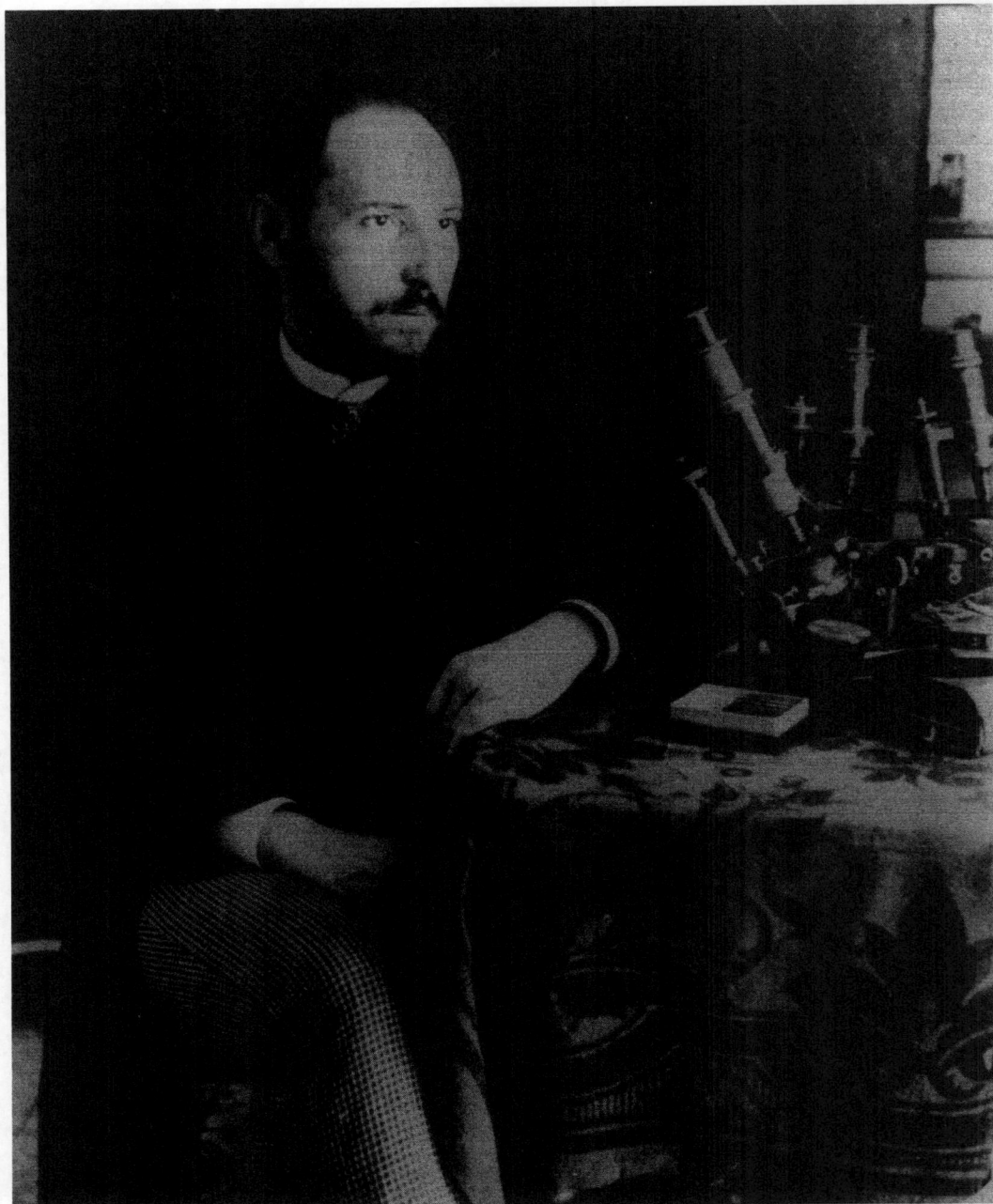

Santiago Ramón y Cajal, aged about thirty-five, in Valencia shortly before his move in 1887 to the chair of histology and pathological anatomv at the University of Barcelona. *From:* a photograph in the Cajal museum (Albarracín, 1982).

1

Introduction

In this section, we have translated a series of relatively short communications which represent Cajal's earliest publications on the cerebral cortex, together with a more extensive paper published in French in *La Cellule,* a part of his Croonian lecture of the Royal Society, and part of a series of lectures on the histology of the nervous system. This collection covers virtually all of Cajal's early works on the cerebral cortex and deals primarily with the cortex of what he called the small mammals, particularly the mouse, rat, and guinea pig.

Cajal commenced working on the peripheral nervous system around 1880, shortly before his accession to the chair of anatomy in the University of Valencia. He published his first major papers in 1886 with the help of Wilhelm Krause, then professor of anatomy at Göttingen University. In 1873, the Italian Camillo Golgi described the method that was to make both him and Cajal famous. He published his great works on the structure of the nervous system in 1883–1884 and 1886. Cajal initially made no attempt to use the Golgi method because, by his own account, it did not receive more than a somewhat disdainful

mention in the treatise of Ranvier, which Cajal then regarded as his technical bible.

In 1887, however, while on a visit to Madrid and shortly before transferring to the chair of histology and pathological anatomy in the University of Barcelona, he became acquainted with the Golgi method thanks to Luis Simarro, a young psychiatrist and neurologist, and thereafter he was hooked!

In his autobiography, Cajal recalls visiting the laboratory Simarro had set up in his home and seeing a Golgi preparation for the first time, "*de visu* the marvelous revealing capacity of the silver chromate reaction." At the time, he wondered why the method had not been used before, but, with the benefit of hindsight, he says, "Now that I know well the psychology of the experts, I find the thing very natural. In France as in Germany, and more in the latter than in the former, there reigns a strict scholastic discipline. Out of respect for the master, customarily no pupil uses methods of investigation that are not those of the Professor. In deference to the great investigators, they would believe it dishonorable to work with methods belonging to someone else."

3

After his first experience, Cajal began working tenaciously on the Golgi method, trying to correct its capriciousness and haphazard character. Later he says, "To my success of that time [1888], there contributed, without doubt, some of my improvements of the silver chromate method, especially the double impregnation procedure . . . and above all that of applying the method before axons become myelinated (an almost insurmountable obstacle to the reaction)." Then he adds, "The silver chromate reaction, incomplete and chancy in the adult, leads in embryos to splendid, singularly extensive, and consistent staining."

The use of neonatal or embryonic material was an important factor in Cajal's success, in comparison with that of other workers, including Golgi himself. The lack of consistency in staining at the hands of others undoubtedly contributed to the later decline in popularity of the method, something to which Cajal became increasingly sensitive in his later years (see chapters 26–29 in this volume).

Finally Cajal says, "Being conscious of having found a productive direction, I tried to take advantage of it, devoting myself to the work not only eagerly but with a fury. To the rhythm of each new fact emerging from my preparations, ideas were bubbling up and boiling over in my mind."

By 1890, he had thoroughly studied the fine structure of the cerebellum and had made extensive contributions on the retina, olfactory bulb, spinal cord, peripheral ganglia, and brainstem. These formed the basis of his elucidation of the neuron doctrine. So productive had he become that he found it necessary, in 1888, to found a new journal, the *Revista Trimestral de Histología Normal y Patológica*. As he says in his autobiography, "the vortex of publication entirely swallowed up my income." In 1889, he was ready to present himself at the Berlin meeting of the German Anatomical Society. He met Weigert and Ehrlich on the way, and his trip culminated in his "discovery" by Kölliker and the anatomical world.

By this time, as related in his autobiography, "devotion to the cerebral cortex, [that] enigma of enigmas, was old in me [and] the subject attracted me with singular force." Therefore, shortly before his transfer to the chair of normal histology and pathological anatomy in the University of Madrid, he set out—with what he later came to regard as misplaced optimism—to complete a study of the cortex as detailed as that which he had previously made on the cerebellum. He initially found this "cerebral jungle," even in nonmammals, almost inaccessible because of its great complexity and the lack of order and symmetry previously observed in the cerebellum and spinal cord. The confidence of youth, however, convinced him that "if I launched myself into that impenetrable thicket in which so many explorers had lost themselves, I would be permitted to capture, if not lions and tigers, as least some minor game neglected by the great hunters." Among these great hunters he listed Meynert, Golgi, Edinger, Flechsig, Kölliker, and Forel.

His first forays in the field were the subject of a series of short communications published in the *Gaceta Médica Catalana* and the *Anales de la Sociedad Española de Historia Natural* between 1890 and 1893. He was sufficiently confident of his work on lissencephalic mammals to publish an extensive article in French in the Belgian journal *La Cellule* (Cajal, 1891d). This paper is perhaps unique among Cajal's publications in languages other than Spanish, for it does not seem to have had a precursor published in Spanish. The style of the writing is unmistakably Cajal, but whether he wrote it in French himself or had it translated by a colleague (which is more likely) cannot be determined. The first identifiable translation of his works by Leon Azoulay was in 1894. The *La Cellule* paper is also of interest in that it is one of the few in which Cajal describes his methods of staining, including such novelties as painting the surface of the cortex with blood in order to promote staining of layer I and his method of drawing cells. In the latter case, he makes it clear that he used a Zeiss camera lucida, and we have been able to identify a Zeiss-made Abbé drawing apparatus from this era among Cajal's equipment, currently housed in the Museo Cajal [*fig. 1*]. The use of this particular camera lucida is illustrated in all editions of Cajal's elementary textbook of histology, starting in 1889 and ending in 1928 (Cajal and Tello, 1928), and here we reproduce illustrations [*fig. 2*] from a work of

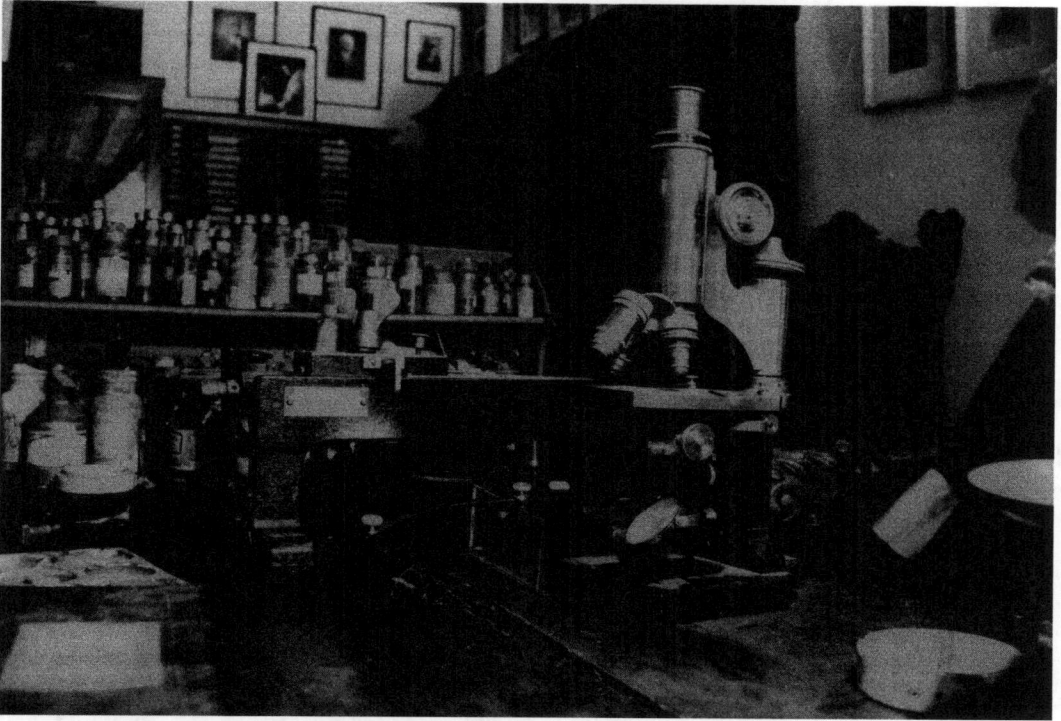

[*FIG. 1*] Photograph taken in the Museo Cajal in 1986, showing one of Cajal's favorite Zeiss microscopes, purchased after 1885; his Reichert sliding microtome; and, in the foreground, his Abbé camera lucida, also made by Zeiss. The lens fits over the monocular eyepiece of the microscope, and the image of pencil and paper is projected onto the mirror and into a side port (see *fig. 2*).

1893 (Stirling, 1893) showing the same Abbé apparatus and the other type of camera lucida then in use. The commonly heard myth, which probably owes its origins to Penfield's introductory note to the English translation of *¿Neuronismo o Reticularismo?* (Cajal, 1954), of Cajal drawing his cells from memory in bed while spattering the wall with ink and wiping his pen on the sheets should now be laid to rest.

In the early papers on the cortex, Cajal was primarily concerned with the presence of special, seemingly multiaxoned cells in layer I, with the laminar distributions of pyramidal and nonpyramidal ("sensory cells of Golgi") cells, the afferent fibers from the white matter, the collaterals of pyramidal cell axons, and the lack of anastomoses between any of the processes. Here, however, we should permit Cajal to speak for himself. The following excerpt is taken from pages 170 and 205 of the second volume of the *Recuerdos de mi vida* (Cajal, 1917).[A]

[Page 170, referring to his study of 1890:]

Cerebrum of the Mammals[1]

In a first work on the subject, these three interesting facts were pointed out:

a) Discovery, in the first cerebral layer of the mammals, of certain special nerve cells whose dendrites, very long and horizontal, run over an enormous extent of the cortical surface.

b) Finding, in the same layer, of several small cells with short axon, unknown to the authors.

c) Succinct description of the terminal arborization, in the molecular layer, of the [apical dendritic] shaft of the pyramidal cells, that is to say, of a ter-

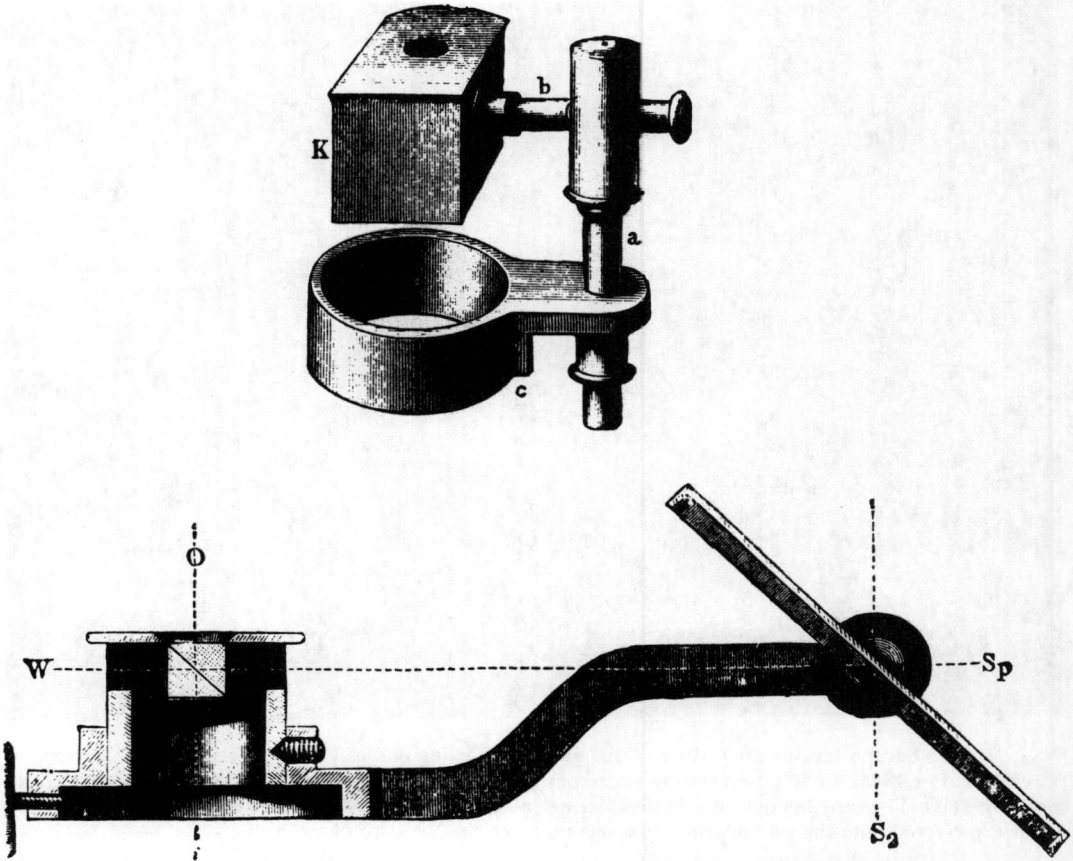

[*FIG. 2*] The two forms of camera lucida manufactured in the 1890s. *Above:* simple camera lucida in which a prism housed in K covers half the eyepiece of the monocular microscope, the other half serving to project the image onto a piece of paper. *Below:* Abbé camera lucida of the type used by Cajal, showing the prism and line of reflected light. *From:* Stirling, (1893).

minal frond or cup, that had escaped the sagacity of Golgi and his disciples.

These acquisitions were first confirmed by Retzius, who designated the special cells of the first layer (cells that he studied meticulously in the human cerebrum) *cells of Cajal.* Kölliker, van Gehuchten, Schaffer, Veratti, etc., have confirmed this, adding, naturally, new morphological features.

We will deal opportunely with a fundamental work about the cerebrum that appeared in 1892.

In a second, much more extensive [1890] communication,[2] the following data regarding the structure of the gray cortex of the cerebrum were added:

a) It is proven that the axons of the medium and large pyramids, as well as of the polymorphic cells,

penetrate the white matter, where sometimes they are bifurcated.

b) The spines of the [apical dendritic] shaft and the terminal [dendritic] tuft of the pyramids are mentioned.

c) It is stated that the corpus callosum consists of direct fibers and of collaterals of axons [belonging to] pyramids of projection or of association.

d) Collaterals and bifurcations are discovered on the fibers of the corpus callosum.

e) In embryos and young mammals, the existence of epithelial cells, extending from the ventricles to the cerebral surface, is confirmed, and the mistakes of Magini about the composition of these fibers are refuted.

f) It is proven that in the cerebrum, as in the spinal cord, many neuroglial cells are displaced and migrated epithelial elements.

g) With the method of Weigert, the strangulations of the myelinated cerebral nerve fibers, denied by many [authors], are revealed, etc., etc.

[On page 205, referring to his studies of 1891, he says:]

1) One of the features better appreciated then was the revelation of the constant presence in the cerebral cortex of the batrachians, reptiles, birds, and mammals of the *pyramidal cell,* which I dared to call, with an audacity of language of which at present I am somewhat ashamed, the *psychic cell.*[3] Its characteristics are: elongated shape more or less conical or pyramidal; radial orientation; a dendritic shaft constantly extended up to the molecular or tangential layer of the cerebrum; and an axon or nerve fiber process directed to the deep regions, where it forms pathways of intercortical or corticospinal association.

Fig. 36 [*fig. 34* in chapter 7] excuses me from entering into details about the said *psychic cell,* which was later the subject of exhaustive analysis by my brother and on which my pupil, Cl. Sala, initiated a good study in birds.

2) The finding in the molecular layer of the cerebrum of small mammals (in which only neuroglial cells and nerve fibers were supposed to exist) of numerous *neurons with short axons* ending in the thickness of that layer, and classifiable into two main varieties (fig. 37, *a, b*) [*fig. 3*].[B]

3) Description of *numerous fusiform neurons,* inhabiting all layers of the cerebral cortex and characterized by an axon with ascending direction that arborizes in the *layers of the small, medium, and large pyramids* (fig. 37, *c, e*) [*fig. 3*].

4) Following, for the first time, the course of projection fibers down through the corpus striatum and detecting their collaterals to the corpus striatum and to the callosal commissure (fig. 37, *g*) [*fig. 3*].

5) Discovery of certain thick fibers arriving from the corpus striatum and branching freely in the layers of the pyramids (fig. 37, *f*) [*fig. 3*]. Such fibers, confirmed by Kölliker, who called them fibers of Cajal,[C] probably represent the terminations of the central sensory pathway.

6) Demonstration of the free terminations of the collaterals of the axons of the pyramids and of the fine axon branches of the cells with short axon (fig. 37, *D*) [*fig. 3*].

7) Observation that the cells of Martinotti, or cells with ascending axon ramifying in the molecular layer, do not solely inhabit layers near the molecular layer, but all layers of the cortex (fig. 37, *d*) [*fig. 3*].

8) New obervations on the embryonic development of the pyramidal cells and neuroglial cells, etc. [Here he mentions that these findings became known thanks to his precaution of publishing them in French in *La Cellule.*][D]

By 1892, Cajal was arriving at a synthetic view of the cerebral cortex of lissencephalic mammals and of nonmammalian vertebrates. It seems apparent that he was also seriously contemplating a general work on the histology of the nervous system. In the penultimate translation of this section (Chapter 7), we present part of a work derived from a series of lectures that Cajal presented to the Academia y Laboratorio de Ciencias Médicas de Cataluña in March 1892 and which were published in Spanish (1892, 1893), German (1893),[E] and French (1894, 1895). An English translation of the original Spanish version of these lectures was undertaken by D. A. Rottenberg (Rottenberg and Hochberg, 1977). These lectures include several illustrations that do not appear elsewhere. In the lectures, we can see, in both text and figures, the germ of the *Textura.* Cajal says on page 212 of his autobiography that the success of the somewhat expanded French version actually gave him the idea for a larger work, even though it meant "working like a Benedictine." Significantly, Azoulay is acknowledged for the first time as a translator of Cajal's works in the French version of the lectures. It is evident from Cajal's comments on page 261 of his autobiography that Azoulay also played a significant role in improving Cajal's original French version of the Croonian lecture, published in 1894 in the *Proceedings of the Royal Society of London,* which concludes part I of this volume.

The Spanish version of the lectures of 1892 has a number of points of interest, not the least of which is the evidence that even in this early period preceding the great works on the human cortex, Cajal was groping for general principles of cerebral cortical organization. It is also interesting in that it contains his earliest speculations on the role of neurons and circuitry in higher cerebral functions, including the payment of lip service to the religious

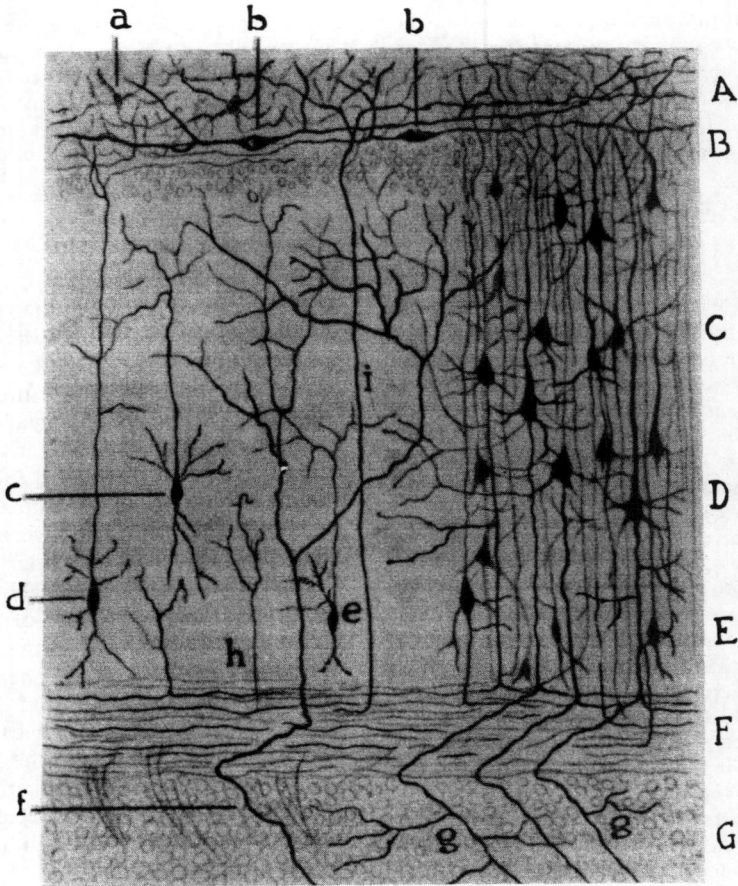

[*FIG. 3*]   FIG. 37. Scheme of a section of the cerebral cortex of a mammal of small size (rabbit, mouse, etc.). In this figure have been condensed some of my findings of 1890 and 1891. *a*, small stellate cells of the plexiform or superficial layer; *b*, horizontal, fusiform cell; *c*, cell with axon arborizing in the layer of the medium pyramids; *d*, neuron located at the level of the polymorphic cells, whose axon is arborized in the molecular layer; *h*, collateral of the white matter; *f*, terminal ramification of the sensory fibers; *g*, collaterals of the axons of pyramids, destined for the corpus striatum; *A*, plexiform layer; *B*, [layer] of the small pyramids; *C*, [layer] of the medium pyramids; *D*, [layer] of the giant pyramids; *E*, [layer] of the polymorphic cells; *F*, white matter; *G*, corpus striatum.

point of view—no doubt because his audience included many clerics.

Throughout the lectures, Cajal is particularly concerned to stress his belief in connections by contact and in van Gehuchten's generalization of the dynamic polarization of the nerve cell, namely that dendrites are receiving and axons transmitting elements. His considerations of cortical connectivity betray little finite knowledge of the sources of subcortical af-

ferents to the cortex, and he even includes the dorsal roots of the spinal cord as potential origins. This is not surprising for its time. Gudden and Monakow had gained the first intimations of thalamocortical connectivity in 1882, but Monakow's (1895) and Nissl's (1913) definitive works on the subject were still some years away. Use of the Marchi technique to demonstrate that ascending spinal and brainstem pathways all terminated in the thalamus and not in the cortex occurred only late in the 1890s (e.g., Mott, 1895; Ferrier and Turner, 1894; Monakow, 1895, 1897; Bechterew, 1895; Probst, 1898, 1900a, b; Wallenberg, 1900). Until then, it was still possible to believe that many ascending systems, such as the medial lemniscus, could bypass the thalamus (e.g., Meynert, 1884). Cajal's own first work on the thalamus and the pathways afferent to it only appeared in 1900.

Among other features of the 1892 publication is an uncharacteristically generous assessment of the initial contributions of Golgi on the cortex, though discounting the latter's classification of cortical cells into sensory and motor.[F] In place of the latter, Cajal substitutes his own categorization of cells with short axon and cells with long axon, which he says does not prejudice their functions. We also see him still convinced of the presence of multiple axons on the special cells of layer I, although he is less insistent on the multiple axons in the French version than in the Spanish. He here makes points about the comparative anatomy of the cortex, which can be seen as the basis for his later treatment of this subject in the *Textura* and the *Histologie*.

The period of early studies on the cerebral cortex culminated in 1894 with Cajal's presentation of the Croonian lecture of the Royal Society of London. In this lecture, delivered in French and published in Spanish and French (Cajal, 1894a, d), he dealt with three topics: the spinal cord, the cerebellum, and the cerebral cortex. His concern appears to have been not only to outline the fundamental principles of neuronal organization in each of these centers but also to use data derived from them to drive home the message of the neuron doctrine, namely communication by contact. The section on the cerebral cortex, which we translate here, generalized rather more than is usual with Cajal and presents an interesting schematic figure that, to the best of our knowledge, was not published elsewhere. The published French text of the Croonian lecture clearly betrays the hand of Azoulay. Contemporary reviews of the lecture can be found in the *Illustrated London News* for April 7, 1894, and in the *British Medical Journal* of the same month. In the former, the reviewer was particularly captivated by Cajal's ideas on dendritic plasticity and the establishment of new connections throughout life as a result of mental exercise.

Cajal's Notes

1. Sobre la existencia de células nerviosas especiales en la primera capa de las circunvoluciones cerebrales, *Gaceta Médica Catalana*, December 15, 1890.

2. *Textura de las circunvoluciones cerebrales de los mamíferos inferiores*, Barcelona, October 1890. With two figures.

3. Estructura de la corteza cerebral de batracios, reptiles y aves. August 1891.

Editors' Notes

A. Craigie, in his English translation of Cajal's autobiography (Cajal, 1937), omits the three pages devoted to this summary in the Spanish text.

B. The figure numbers are changed in Craigie's English version. Fig. 37 of the original is not reproduced there, nor is it reproduced elsewhere, except for Tello (1935).

C. Kölliker refers to them as "Ramón's fibers" in the 1896 edition of his *Handbuch der Gewebelehre des Menschen*.

D. Cajal (1891). "Sur la structure de l'écorce cérébrale de quelques mammifères." *La Cellule* 7:125–176. See chapter 5 in this volume.

E. The German translation appears to have been made by Hans Held, then assistant to Wilhelm His, professor of anatomy at the University of Leipzig, and later one of Cajal's chief adversaries in the battle over the neuron doctrine. In a footnote to the third edition (1923) of his autobiography, Cajal notes that the translation was rather inaccurate because of Held's unfamiliarity with Spanish. This comment does not appear in the equivalent footnote to the first edition (1917) on page 212.

F. Denied by Golgi in his Nobel lecture of 1906. See: Golgi C, pp. 189–217. In: *Nobel Lectures: Physiology or Medicine, 1901–1921;* 1967, Elsevier, Amsterdam.

2

Texture of the Cerebral Gyri of
the Lower Mammals

[*Gaceta Médica Catalana*, December 1890, pp. 22–31]

Preliminary Note

While we are finishing a special work, with illustrations, dealing with the subject which is the topic of this writing, allow us to expose here the most important positive data obtained from our observations.

Our experiments have been made in the cerebrum of newborn and 15-to-30-day-old mammals (rabbit, cat, rat, and mouse), either with the method of Golgi or with that of Weigert-Pal. The preferred region for the examination has been an intermediate transverse region that includes the corpus callosum and the gray matter of the hemispheres overlying it.

The gray cerebral cortex of the mouse, rabbit, and other small mammals shows the same layers and other elements as the human gyri. Hence, for the enumeration of the layers we will follow a nomenclature analogous to that of Meynert and Schwalbe.

1. Molecular Layer

Besides the neuroglial cells that lie in its external part and the innumerable dendritic arborizations of the underlying pyramidal cells that traverse it, [the molecular layer] contains a considerable number of branched medullated nerve fibers, with a course horizontal or parallel to the free surface and which were already described some time ago by Kölliker[1] and Exner.[2]

Where do these fibers come from? Martinotti[3] has recently proved that some of them are ascending axons originating in pyramidal cells of underlying layers. We have confirmed this finding, and we can add that such cells are little numerous and [that] they are situated especially in the deep third of the gray matter (fig. 2, *i*) [*fig. 5*]. A large proportion of these cells have a spindle shape and the vertical orientation of the pyramids; from their cell body, [which is] commonly small, arise long descending and ascending dendrites. The axon arises sometimes from the upper part of the cell body, but more frequently from an ascending dendritic branch; [the axon] ascends in an almost straight line, giving off numerous collaterals during its course, and, finally, it bifurcates [and] ends in the first cerebral layer by means of an infinity of very extensive horizontal freely terminating small branches.

10

But this origin of the superficial nerve fibers is the least important. The vast majority come from certain special nerve cells, situated in the molecular layer itself. Such cells are of two kinds: polyhedral and fusiform.

The said nerve [cells] are not stainable in the adult brain,[4] and without doubt for that [reason] the modern authors who have worked with the method of Golgi (Golgi, Kölliker, Martinotti, etc.) do not mention them. However, the histologists who used the method of carmine often mention in the first or molecular layer certain very scarce, polygonal nerve cells, with an unknown [morphology] and connections (Meynert, Schwalbe, Ranvier, Obersteiner, etc.).

The existence of these cells was for us an indubitable thing, even before we managed to impregnate them in the newborn and few-days-old rabbit, guinea pig, [and] cat. Here is our reasoning:

The large part of the medullated nerve fibers that course in the first layer (man, dog, etc.) are very thick and numerous, whereas the vast majority of the ones that ascend from the underlying gray layers are extraordinarily thin. We thought, how is it possible that thin and weakly myelinated fibers become superficially, that is to say, at their point of arborization, thicker and more heavily myelinated collaterals than the trunks of origin? If so, this would be the first known case in which the ramifications of a fiber are thicker than the fiber itself. Thus, we supposed, of course, that the thick fibers of the first cerebral layer were originating from cells existing in the same layer.

Polygonal Cells (fig. 1, B) [fig. 4]

They are large in size, at least larger than the small pyramids; they lie irregularly scattered among the nerve fibers, and possess four, five, or more short, varicose, divergent, and branched dendrites.

The axon commonly arises from a side of the cell body or from a dendritic branch (e, f, g); it travels horizontally among the fibers of the first layer, repeatedly branching until it loses its individuality. In such a way it gives rise to an infinity of fine parallel threads, situated underneath the cerebral surface and freely terminating by means of granular and varicose branches. Often, at the beginning, the axon is directed downward to turn back soon to the fibrillar layer where it bifurcates and gives rise to arborizations of large extent.

Fusiform Cells (fig. 1, F), [fig. 4]

The dominant form is that of a perfect spindle, with two very long dendrites directed par-

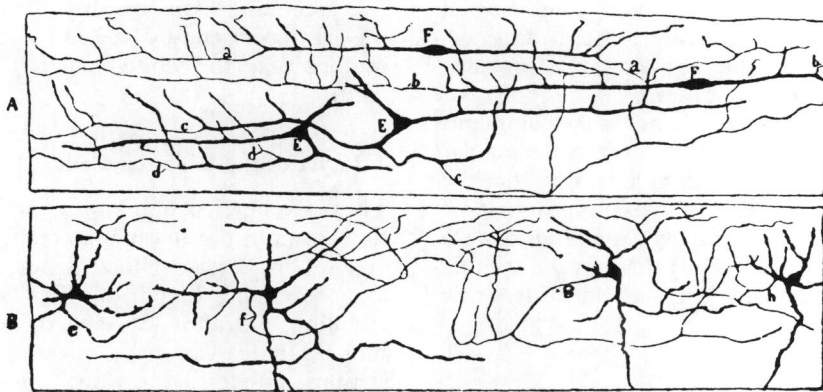

[FIG. 4] Fig. 1. Cells of the first cerebral layer (molecular layer). A, anteroposterior section of the molecular layer of the cerebrum of the rabbit of two days; F, fusiform cells; E, triangular cells; a,a, axons of a single fusiform cell; b,b, another pair of axons of a similar cell; d,d, axons emerging from a single dendritic shaft of a triangular cell; c,c, another pair of axons of a triangular cell. B, anteroposterior section of the same cerebral layer of the rabbit in which is shown some types of polygonal or stellate cells. The fusiform [cells] have not been drawn. e,f,g,h, axons of several cells ramifying in the first cerebral layer.

allel to the fibrillar layer and commonly with an anteroposterior orientation. Because of this orientation, study of them must be carried out preferably in anteroposterior sections. Each of the rectilinear dendrites gives off, almost at a right angle, small ascending branches that end near the free surface. After an almost always very long and horizontal course, the terminations of each polar dendritic shaft bend, getting lost near or at the [very] cerebral surface.

The axon is *at least double,* and concerning such a unique peculiarity, it must be clearly understood that we have tried to make ourselves secure. The emergence of these axons commonly takes place at the point at which the polar dendrites turn to ascend (fig. 1, *a, b*) [*fig. 4*]. The axons run in opposite directions and with an anteroposterior orientation, giving off at intervals fine, ascending, branched filaments that come to complicate notably the plexus of the superficial [sublayer].

Another form of the cited cells is the triangular, [which is] notably voluminous [*fig. 4, E*]. Two dendrites course in an anteroposterior orientation; the other often descends, later to ascend and branch repeatedly in the fibrillar layer. The axons usually emerge from the trajectory of two thick dendritic branches with opposite directions [*fig. 4, c, d*]. Frequently we have noticed that a single dendritic shaft gave off two or more axons (*d*). In any case, these are branched upward, and their small branches run horizontally through an enormous extent of the fibrillar layer, probably ending by free extremities.

For the present, we do not make comments about the significance of these very singular cells, limiting ourselves to affirming that the described axons have a clear appearance of such and that never is any axon seen to leave either from the cell body or from the starting point of the two or three thick dendritic branches.

2. Layer of the Small Pyramids

We will only add two details to the description given by Golgi: first, the peripheral arborization of the ascending shaft bristles with short spines ending in a small knob. The gulfs that

are between such collateral spines receive the impression of innumerable small fibers of the superficial layer. Exactly the same disposition is possessed by the terminal peripheral arborization of the large pyramids. Second, the descending axons of these cells terminate at different levels of the middle and deep third of the gray matter by free and varicose branches which lose their individuality as [main] axons. Never have we seen the arrival of an axon, not even in the smaller mammals such as the mouse and the bat, at the white matter or the corpus callosum (fig. 2, *O*) [*fig. 5*].

In the lower mammals (rabbit, rat, etc.), the most superficial rows of small pyramids consist, in fact, of spheroidal or polyhedral cells whose dendrites [are] mainly ascending. They lack a main dendritic shaft, but their axon is straight and descending like the true pyramids placed underneath.

3. Layer of the Large Pyramids

We will add to the known description[5] that in the small mammals we have been able to follow the axon with complete certainty to the white matter and corpus callosum (fig. 2, *a*) [*fig. 5*]. In the region studied by us in the mouse and rat, these fibers follow an anteroposterior direction in the white matter, giving off from time to time during their trajectory fine ascending filaments that, once arrived at the gray layer, end by free and varicose arborizations (like the white matter of the spinal cord).

4. Layer of the Globular Cells

These are small, ovoid or spheroidal, and form tight rows in the lower mammals. Almost all give off two basilar lateral dendrites and one long ascending [dendrite]. The axon is descending, and, after a variable trajectory, it terminates (at least in many cases) by free arborizations, either in the same layer or in the underlying [layer].

In this layer lie the majority of the fusiform cells with ascending axon, as well as certain large polyhedral or stellate cells whose axon, either ascending or lateral or descending, soon

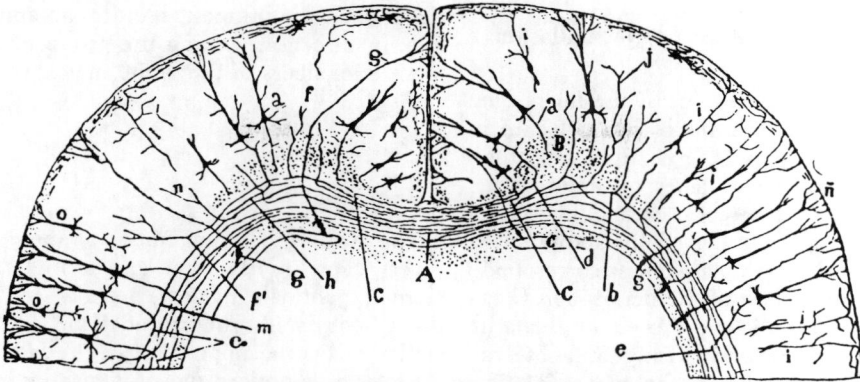

[FIG. 5]   Fig. 2. Transverse section of the superior part of the cerebral hemispheres and corpus callosum of a mouse of twenty days (semischematic figure). *A*, corpus callosum; *B*, anteroposterior fibers originating mainly from large pyramids; *C*, lateral ventricle; *a*, large pyramid with axon in the layer of anteroposterior fibers; *b*, callosal fiber bifurcating into a branch that is arborized in the gray matter and another that continues in the corpus callosum; *c*, callosal fiber that comes from an axon of the white matter running anteroposteriorly; *d*, callosal fiber that originates from a pyramidal cell; *e*, axons of lateral pyramidal cells which follow a descending course in the corpus callosum without forming part of the commissure; *f,f'*, the two final branches coming from a fiber of the corpus callosum and arborizing in the gray matter; *h*, fiber [coming from] a large pyramid, giving off a fine collateral to the corpus callosum; *g*, epithelial cells arborized at the cerebral surface (*ñ*); *i*, fusiform cells whose axons ascend to the molecular layer; *j*, terminal arborization of a callosal fiber originating on the opposite side.

terminates by a very extensive and complicated arborization (polyhedral cells and sensory [cells] of Golgi).

5. Layer of the Fusiform and Triangular Cells

Here there is a great variety of forms, pyramidal cells of greater or lesser size also being observed. The majority exhibit a fine *axon* that can be followed to the white matter, after having [given off] numerous collateral branches.

White Matter (fig. 2) [*fig. 5*]

The cerebral region studied by us, situated above the corpus callosum and lateral ventricles, exhibits two kinds of fibers: superior with an anteroposterior direction (*B*) and inferior with a transverse direction (*A*). The first are axons of association that relate the frontal lobe to the occipital (remember that we are referring only to the mouse, rat, and rabbit); the second represent callosal or commissural fibers with a much smaller diameter, destined to relate homologous parts of each hemisphere.

The transverse sections of the brain show well the course and termination of the corpus callosum, above all in the preparations stained with the procedure of Weigert-Pal. These same preparations show that the corpus callosum is reinforced in its lateral and descending portion by a group of transverse and descending fibers, originating from the large pyramids of the inferolateral gray cortex of the hemisphere (fig. 2, *e*) [*fig. 5*]. Such fibers, which form a bend when they reach the corpus callosum, do not participate in the formation of the commissure, since they do not supply any medially directed branch, probably representing [instead] vertical commissural fibers established between the high or parietal part of the hemispheres and the low or sphenoidal.

All of these fibers are perfectly stained with the method of Golgi, especially the callosal [ones], which possess a very delicate myelin sheath.

Origin of the Fibers of the Corpus Callosum

Examining the lateral ends of the fibers that constitute the center of the corpus callosum, it is observed that they bend at right or obtuse angles and in different planes, to penetrate the deep layers of the cerebral cortex. The place where the larger number of fibers enters is a delta or fan-shaped enlargement corresponding to the upper part of the hemispheres (fig. 2, B) [fig. 5]. How do these fibers originate in the gray matter? Summarizing our observations made especially in the mouse of one month, we can affirm that the callosal fibers, at least most of them, are, first, direct axons of the large and medium pyramidal cells and, second, medial collaterals of axons of association and of anteroposterior direction. In sum: axons of pyramids or small branches of these axons.

We have not confirmed the opinion of Monakow, who claims that the axons of the large pyramids go to the internal capsule and of the small [pyramids] to the corpus callosum and systems of association.[6]

With regard to the termination [of the callosal fibers], our observations are not entirely conclusive.

Examining carefully the arrival on the other side of certain callosal fibers of medium size, it is noticed that, in the corpus callosum itself and when they tend to ascend, they divide in two branches [that are] smaller than the trunk (which indicates that they are branches); one of them immediately penetrates and arborizes in the gray matter; and the other, after continuing the direction of the trunk for a variable distance, also gets lost in the gray matter of the hemispheres (fig. 2, b) [fig. 5]. At other times (j), there is no bifurcation, the fiber penetrating into the said cortex without losing its individuality, to arborize and terminate in an unknown manner, although it may be conjectured that the arborization will be free, and contacting the nerve cells of the associated region.[7]

To be complete, let us add that in some sections we have noticed in the final bifurcation of certain callosal fibers that one of the branches, the thinnest, acquires an anteroposterior direction, joining the group of anteroposterior fibers of the white matter (fig. 2, B) [fig. 5]..

Epithelial Cells

The form and arrangement of these appear very clear in newborns and term fetuses of small mammals (fig. 2, g) [fig. 5].

Choosing [for their study] the epithelium that covers the upper part of the lateral ventricles, it is noticed that it is made up of very long cells extending from the ependyma to the free cerebral surface (Magini, Falzacappa). These cells can be considered to have three portions: epithelial or internal, callosal or middle, and external or cerebral.

The internal is thick and offers the characteristic of a prismatic epithelium, possessing an ovoid enlargement that contains the nucleus; a thick and short expansion that extends to the ventricle, forming with its fellows a polygonal mosaic; and another external [that is] uneven and provided with fine and crinkly collateral processes.

The middle or callosal portion is thin and notably varicose, resembling a string of pearls.[8] It does not travel in isolation, but it associates with others, forming septa that separate the little round bundles of nerve fibers of the corpus callosum.

The external portion is formed by a fine fiber, a continuation of the previous portion, that radiates throughout the gray matter, terminating at the cerebral surface by a tuft of ascending threads ending in cones with a peripheral base (fig. 2 ñ) [fig. 5].

Fibers with Myelin

When a section of a gyrus stained by the procedure of Weigert is compared with another impregnated by the [method] of Golgi, similarities and differences are noticed. The deep half of the gray matter presents an equal aspect, since the preparations of Weigert and of Golgi both reveal little bundles of fibers that radiate through the white matter. From which, it is completely certain that the axons of the large pyramids and fusiform and triangular cells of the last layer possess a myelin sheath.

By contrast, the axons of the small pyramids, especially of the most superficial, probably lack the said sheath, because neither in the adult man nor in the adult dog, cat, and guinea pig in which we have preferentially studied [those cells] does the method of Weigert reveal those fine, divergent, and almost parallel nerve fibers in the layer of the small pyramids that the procedure of Golgi stains with complete precision. The greater part of the fibers stained with the hematoxylin have a transverse or oblique direction, and the few that have an ascending [direction] almost always reach the superficial fibrillar layer, revealing to us that they are probably ascending axons of fusiform nerve cells.

In the guinea pig and mouse, there are zones in the layer of the small pyramids that do not contain any medullated fibers or even fibers ascending to the molecular layer.

The axons of the cells of the first layer possess myelin, at least in their main trunks. In man, these medullated fibers are thick and very abundant, contrasting with the poverty and thinness of the ones that course in the subjacent layer. In the guinea pig and mouse, they are very scarce, with zones in which none is found; for that reason, we believe it very probable that almost all the fibers ending or originating in the molecular layer lack a myelin sheath.

When the medullated fibers of the gyri are examined carefully, it is noticed that, at intervals, they are interrupted and that, like the peripheral myelinated fibers, the length of the myelinated segments is in inverse ratio to the thickness of the fibers. Very rarely, we have been able to observe branchings of myelinated fibers like those indicated by Kölliker[9] in the cerebellum and by Flechsig in the cerebrum; because of that, it seems to us very probable that the branchings take place at the level of the strangulations [nodes of Ranvier], a fact that Flechsig has also proved with his particular staining procedure.[10]

Development

With regard to this particular, our studies are quite incomplete, since they have fallen on term fetuses and newborn mammals. Thus, rather than phases of development, we will indicate phases of growth.

At the time of birth, the nerve cells of some mammals such as the cat, guinea pig, and common rabbit are perfectly formed; only the small pyramids (rabbit, rat, dog) appear embryonic, with an ovoid or fusiform shape and with a short and thick external dendrite without terminal arborization and another thick, internal process without the very clear characteristics of an axon.

In general, the last to be formed in the cerebrum is the peripheral [dendritic] arborization of the large and small pyramids, from which it results that, at some time, the molecular layer, in large measure made up by the gathering together of the [peripheral dendritic arborizations], is proportionately narrower than in the adult. Likewise, the poverty of dendrites gives to the cerebral layers a character of epithelial tightness which is lacking in the adult.

With respect to the neuroglia, for the present we can say little that is not a repetition of that revealed in [our] previous works.[11]

Suffice it to indicate that we concur in the opinion that the neuroglia have two origins, one epithelial and the other vascular. The cells of an epithelial character are located especially in the corpus callosum, appearing because of their orientation and lengthening as though they are short and displaced epithelial cells of the ependyma. But regarding the submeningeal cells of the cortex and those that surround and are inserted into the vascular wall, we think that they are endothelial derivatives, because, before they make themselves into arachniform cells, they pass through a phase in which they resemble simple thickenings of the endothelium, either rounded and bare, as Lachi[12] has shown in the spinal cord, or provided with numerous divergent expansions, as we indicate.

Whatever it may be, the neuroglial cells are

shown almost completely formed at the time of birth (cat, rabbit, guinea pig, etc.) In the dog and mouse, the majority of them are in the process of development.

Cajal's Notes

1. Handbuch der Gewebelehre, 1852.
2. Zur Kenntnis vom feinern Bau der Grosshirnrinde, *Sitzungsber. d. Kais. Akad. d. Wiss. in Wien*, 1881.
3. Beitrag zum Studium der Hirnrinde und dem Centralursprung der Nerven, *Intern. Monatsch. f. Anat. u. Phys.*, Vol. VIII, Pt. 2., 1890.
4. Recently we have also been able to impregnate them in the adult rabbit.
5. See the work of Golgi: Sulla fina anatomia degli organi centrali del sistema nervoso, 1886.
6. Monakow, Rôle des diverses couches des cellules ganglionnaires dans le gyrus sigmoïde du chat, *Arch. d. Scien. Phys. et Nat.* XX, 10 October 1888.

7. According to very demonstrative preparations of my brother, who has also dealt with this interesting subject, the callosal fibers terminate in an arborization that [extends through] the whole thickness of the gray matter, their upper branches reaching to the first or fibrillar layer.
8. These varicosities have been seen by Magini in the fetuses of mammals; but instead of considering them as protoplasmic accumulations, he considers them as cells with nuclei [that are] inserted into the strings. We have not been able to confirm this assertion. See: Magini, Nouvelles recherches histologiques sur le cerveau du fetus, *Arch. Ital. de Biologie*, Vol. X, 1888.
9. Das Kleinhirn, *Zeitschr. f. Wissenschaftliche Zool.* XLIX, 4, 1890.
10. Ueber eine neue Färbungsmethode des centralen Nervensystems etc., *Berichte d.k. Sachs. Gesellsch. d. Wissen. Math. Phys. Clas.*, August 1889.
11. Especially see: Contribución al estudio de la médula espinal, *Rev. Trim. de Histol.*, numbers 3 and 4, 1889.
12. Contributo alla istogenesi della neuroglia nel midolo spinale del pollo. Pisa, 189[1].

3

Short Anatomical Communications
II. On the Existence of Collaterals and Bifurcations in the Fibers of the White Matter of the Gray Cerebral Cortex

[From *Pequeñas Comunicaciones Anatómicas,* December 1890, pp. 6–8.]

In a work that we have just published on the structure of the cerebrum of the small mammals,[A] we have indicated the presence of true collaterals in the white matter, on the whole comparable to the bundles of the spinal cord.

At the same time that that work was printed (3rd of December), we obtained preparations [that are] even more demonstrative of the said collaterals and which are shown not only in the layer of anteroposterior axons situated above the corpus callosum but also on the descending fibers coming from pyramids and which reinforce the corpus callosum in its inferolateral part, and even on the callosal or commissural fibers near their extremities (fig. 3, *a, b, c, g,* etc.) [*fig. 6*].

The best region for the study of the said collaterals is that closest to the interhemispheric fissure (fig. 3, *C*) [*fig. 6*], because in this place the cerebral gray cortex is thinner than in others, and thus the complete pursuit of the fibers is easier.

The said region is made up of anteroposterior fibers emanating from axons of large pyramids (mainly); medially it is narrow (fig. 3, *C*) [*fig. 6*], but laterally it thickens notably (fig. 3, *C²*) [*fig. 6*], forming a bundle which is semilu-

nar in transverse section, inferiorly concave, and among whose axons lie some fusiform nerve cells.

The collaterals emerge from these fibers at right angles, traveling in several directions but especially toward the gray cortex situated above. The ones that come from the vicinity of the interhemispheric fissure (fig. 3, *a, b, c*) [*fig. 6*] are repeatedly branched and can be easily followed to the molecular layer (n) where they form a varicose terminal arborization with branches oriented in several [directions]. The collaterals originating in the most external plane (fig. 3, *e, f*) [*fig. 6*] also ascend [following] the direction of the corresponding cerebral radius, branching and getting lost in the gray matter. Perhaps some of their branches also go to the first cerebral layer, but the notable thickness of the gray matter situated above the white matter almost always impedes an efficacious pursuit. A single nerve fiber of the white matter gives off several collaterals, but it is necessary to add that this is very rarely observed, because such branchings in the cerebrum are much less numerous than in the spinal cord.

The majority of the axons that arrive at the

17

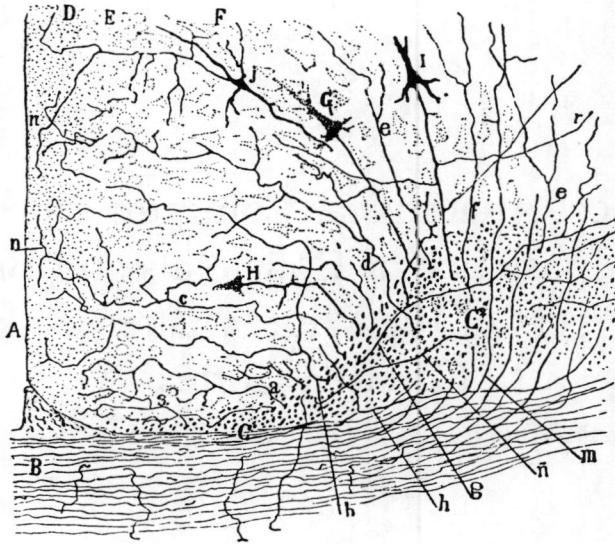

[*FIG. 6*]   Fig. 3. Piece of a transverse and vertical section of the brain of a mouse of ten days. *A*, inter-hemispheric fissure; *B*, corpus callosum; *C*, most internal portion of the white matter formed by anteroposterior fibers; C^2, lateral thicker portion; *a, b, c, g*, collaterals of the fibers of the white matter that are arborized in the gray [matter]; *j*, cell whose axon is arborized in the molecular layer; *I, G*, large pyramidal cells whose axons go to the white matter; *ñ*, nerve fiber that changes plane; *n*, final arborization of the collaterals.

white matter (mainly [from] medium and large pyramids) are continuous in it with a myelinated fiber at a simple bend, but occasionally, as in the spinal cord, there are noticed axons terminating in a Y, whose two branches are of equal thickness and of opposite direction in the white matter. In many cases, one of the branches of bifurcation is thinner than the other, representing a thick collateral (unequal bifurcation).

These divisions in Y notably abound in the white matter of the lateral part of the hemispheres, that is to say, in the white band that forms the roof of the lateral ventricles and which transverse sections show to be in continuity with the fibers of the corpus callosum. Therefore, we consider it likely that the medial branch of bifurcation of these axons, on occasions as thin as a collateral, is truly incorporated into the group of commissural fibers of the corpus [callosum].

The collaterals that the axons give off during their course in the gray matter in the mouse can be easily followed until their termination which constantly occurs by means of

a small swelling. In the gray matter, collaterals abound that are not branched during their trajectory, following an almost straight line until their termination (fig. 3, *r*) [*fig. 6*].

Corpus Callosum

Most of the callosal fibers are fine, varicose, almost parallel, and as thin as collateral branches or axons of small cells. The vast majority ascend in the gray matter, in an almost straight line, to terminate at the level of the medium pyramidal cells.

But there are also numerous fibers which, extending to the most lateral and inferior parts of the hemispheres, seem to be continuations of the branches of equal or unequal bifurcation of medium and even of large pyramids of the gray matter.

In summary, the fibers of the corpus callosum appear to be, first, direct axons of medium pyramids and perhaps of some other small cells of the gray cortex; second, fine internal branches that could be called collaterals of bifurcation (since at their starting points the axon changes direction) of axons of pyramidal cells of medium and large size; a few branches of bifurcation of axons of equal origin.

We give these origins, which modifies somewhat what was exposed in [our] recent work, not as a definitive matter but as a probable hypothesis, since the absolute demonstration could only be made by following the cited fibers to the midline or central part of the corpus callosum, a task [that is] at present unattainable even in the most fortunate preparations.

We will note the great analogy that exists between the corpus callosum and the anterior commissure of the spinal cord. In the latter are also interwoven direct axons and thick collaterals of other [axons] with robust diameter that are situated in the anteroposterior lateral bundle. The terminations are likely identical in the cerebrum and spinal cord, occurring preferentially as free arborizations in the thickness of the gray matter.

The corpus callosum contains also fine flexuous and vertical fibers that appear to come from anteroposterior fibers of the underlying fornix. These fibers, after ascending among the callosal fibers, suddenly take an anteroposterior direction, escaping from observation.

Editors' Note

A. He probably refers to the short paper of December 1890 on the texture of the cerebral gyri of the lower mammals. See chapter 2 in this volume.

4

On the Existence of Special Nerve Cells in the First Layer of the Cerebral Convolutions

[*Gaceta Médica Catalana* 13, 1890, pp. 737–739][A]

Of the five layers that Meynert indicates in the thickness of each gyrus, the most external, also called the molecular [layer], encloses in its upper part a very tight plexus of nerve fibers [that are] horizontal or parallel to the free surface. Most of these fibers possess a myelin sheath, as already indicated many years ago by Kölliker[1] and Exner,[2] who respectively relied on the revelations of the potash and osmic acid methods. Recently Obersteiner,[3] Edinger,[4] and Martinotti[5] have obtained analogous results, taking advantage of the Weigert-Pal hematoxylin method.

What is the origin of such fibers? The only author who has succeeded in determining the origins of some of them is Martinotti. In the opinion of this histologist, they would proceed from the branches of certain pyramidal axons (second and third layers), which, instead of descending as do others to the white matter, would go up to the cerebral surface to form a very rich mesh of a sensory nature.

Our experiments demonstrate the accuracy of the observations of Martinotti with regard to the cellular origin, except that, in the lower mammals, the cited cells are not pyramidal but fusiform, most of them lying in the deep third of the gray matter.

But the aforementioned origin is not sufficient to explain the origins of the infinite number of fibers that both the Weigert procedure and that of Golgi reveal in the first cerebral layer, all the more so when some of these fibers are thicker than those ascending from the underlying layers, for it is hard to believe that the ramifications of the nerve fibers would be larger in diameter than the [parent] fibers themselves.

Already the anatomists of the last decade, such as Meynert,[6] Krause,[7] Henle,[8] and Schwalbe,[9] and some modern [authors], such as Ranvier,[10] Kahler,[11] and Obersteiner,[12] mention in the first layer (*cell-poor* layer of Meynert) the existence of occasional stellate nerve cells; it is only the method of Golgi that might reveal their nature, but as they could not be stained with it, the authors who have worked with this method, such as Golgi,[13] Edinger,[14] and Martinotti,[15] do not pay attention to such cells, considering them as probable neuroglial cells.

Firmly persuaded about the existence of

such cells, and that it is among them that we have to search for the origins of the fibers of the molecular layer, we have devoted [our] attention to repeated experiments involving Golgi impregnations, choosing for that purpose newborn mammals (cat, rabbit, dog, rat), in which experience has taught us that the silver chromate reaction is obtained with much greater reliability than in adult mammals.

Success has crowned our efforts, justifying our foresight.

The nerve cells of the first layer are of two kinds: *polyhedral* and *fusiform*. They are irregularly scattered among the horizontal nerve fibers, usually with the fusiform occupying the most superficial plane.

1. The *polyhedral* are of medium size, and from their angles arise four or five thin, rough dendritic branches that branch and diverge, some of them customarily descending for some distance in the molecular layer. The axon usually arises from one side of the cell, and it is directed in the same orientation as the fibrillar layer, branching repeatedly and giving rise to an infinity of small horizontal fibers with a very long course. Often, the axon initially descends in the molecular layer, then traces an arch to go up again and to branch freely[B] in the most superficial part. These axons or their branches never go down to the white matter.

2. The *fusiform* cells are thinner, with a smooth contour, and are particularly elongated. In small mammals, they are anteroposteriorly extended, covering a large part of the hemisphere. They possess an ovoid soma and two almost straight polar dendrites. These processes give off ascending collaterals and, after bending to be directed upward, end freely.

The axon is double or triple, a very peculiar circumstance that does not occur in any [other] central [nervous system] cell. When there are two, a case that is very frequent, these leave from the extremity of the polar dendrites from the point at which these bend to become ascending. Then they are directed horizontally and in the opposite orientation, supplying an infinity of small ascending branches that, in the upper part of the first layer, turn horizontally.

Some cells of this kind are triangular, having, besides the two anteroposterior dendrites, another, either ascending or descending. The axons leave always from the course of the dendritic branches, with a horizontal direction, and end in free arborizations.

In summary, the fibers of the cerebral first or molecular layer come from, first, ascending axons of some fusiform cells of the fourth and fifth layers; second, polyhedral cells lying in the first layer itself; and third, fusiform special cells with several axons, also located in the first layer.

If it should be permissible to expound a hypothesis that would explain the physiological role that such cells perform, we would be inclined to think that their purpose is to link or associate the actions of the pyramidal cells situated at different [radial locations in the cortex]. To this end, all the pyramidal cells, either large or small, send to the first layer an [apical dendritic] shaft that is richly arborized among the mentioned fibers, ending by small free branches bristling with spines and gulfs of impression.[C]

The link would be established by contacts, as we have demonstrated in the cerebellum and in the spinal cord, between the arborizations of *nerve fibers* on the one hand and *dendritic branches* on the other.

For that [reason], we would willingly call the nerve cells just described *superficial cells of association.*

Cajal's Notes

1. Kölliker, *Handbuch der Gewebelehre*, 1852.
2. Exner, Zur Kenntnis vom feinerem Bau der Grosshirnrinde, *Sitzungsbericht d. Kais. Acad. d. Wissensch. in Wien*, 18[81].
3. Obersteiner, *Anleitung beim Studium des Baues der nervösen Centralorgane, etc.*, Wien, 1888.
4. Edinger, *Vorlesungen über nervösen Centralorgane*, 2nd ed., 1889.
5. Martinotti, Beitrag zum Studium der Hirnrinde und dem Centralursprung der Nerven, *Inter. Monat. f. Anat. u. Physiol.*, Vol. VII, pt. 2, 1890.
6. Meynert, Der Bau de Grosshirnrinde, etc. *Vierteljahrschr. f. Psychiat.*, 1867, 1868.
7. Krause, *Allgemeine u. mikroskopische Anatomie*, 1876.
8. Henle, *Handbuch der Nervenlehre des Menschen*, 1879.
9. Schwalbe, *Lehrbuch der Neurologie*, 1881.

10. Ranvier, *Traité technique d'Histologie*, 1875–1886.

11. Kahler and Toldt, *Lehrbuch der Gewebelehre*, 1888.

12. Obersteiner, loc. cit.

13. Golgi, *Sulla fina anatomia delgi organi centrali del sistema nervoso*, 1886.

14. Edinger, loc. cit.

15. Martinotti, loc. cit.

Editors' Notes

A. Reprinted (1924) in S. Ramón y Cajal, *Trabajos Escogidos*, Madrid, Jiménez and Molina, Printers, Vol. 1, pp. 625–628.

B. The word *freely* or *free* refers to the concept being strongly promulgated by Cajal at this time that the nerve cells are individual morphological entities, in contradistinction to the alternative view, current at that time, that the collaterals and terminal arborizations of nerve cells were joined to form a diffuse anastomosing mesh or reticulum. (See Cajal, *Neuron Theory or Reticular Theory? Objective Evidence of the Anatomical Unity of Nerve Cells*, trans. by M. Ubeda-Purkiss and C. A. Fox. [Madrid: C.S.I.C., 1954]. This is an English translation of *Neuronismo o Reticularismo?* first published in *Archivos de Neurobiología* 13:1–144, 1933.)

C. Cajal's words. We find it difficult to interpret this expression but feel that it may refer to elongated spines with bifurcated necks or the spaces enclosed by adjacent spines.

5

On the Structure of the Cerebral Cortex of Certain Mammals[1]

[*La Cellule* 7:125–176, 1891]

Among the anatomical problems that have captured the attention and exercised the wisdom of the authorities, in first place, without contradiction, is that of the structure of the mammalian cerebral cortex. But the difficulties one encounters in this study are so great that, despite the number of works devoted to it, one could affirm that our ignorance exceeds our science and that it will necessitate without doubt a long series of researches before we arrive at a complete understanding of the fine anatomy of the cerebral gyri and ganglia.

Our ignorance is such that, even today, to a question so important and yet so simple as the general connections of nerve cells, science does not have an answer for the more or less probable hypotheses. There are many causes for which this question of the interrelations of the cells, [already] resolved for the majority of tissues, resists repeated and multiple efforts. They are, on the one hand, the enormous size and extraordinary complexity of the [axonal and dendritic processes] and, on the other, the absence of an abundant [extracellular substance] separating clearly the cellular outlines. [This is] because the nerve cells, like other ectodermal derivatives, lack the property

of secreting amorphous matter; their cellular processes are in intimate contact and intertwined like the filaments of a woven felt.

One can readily understand how the complexity of the entanglement of thousands of filaments of great length imposes serious limitations and insufficient clarity on the examination of microscopic sections. A thin section of the gray matter stained by no matter which method always presents such an ill-formed mass of fiber trunks and fragments of cells that a comparison with those other sections of the same organ conveys to us scarcely any enlightenment on account of the uniformly granular aspect of the cellular processes and the unrelieved unmyelinated nerve fibers.

It is no great wonder, therefore, that those authorities who have exclusively applied imperfect methods have fallen into grave errors. It is not likely to be otherwise, and, instead of being critical, we express great admiration for the various important results obtained by dedication and by laborious investigations. The demonstration of the axon of the nerve cells, the discovery of the neuroglial cells, the arrangement of myelinated fibers, the form and laminar organization of the various nerve cells of the cortex are the fruits of this work which in the history of the science is inseparable from the names of Gerlach, Wagner, Schultze, Deiters, Stieda, Krause, Kölliker, Exner, etc.

The method of thin sections and above all that of dissociation have allowed us to reveal the details relating to the form and structure of nerve cells. However, we must recognize that the deeper understanding which we have acquired about the morphology of the nerve cells and neuroglial cells of the cerebrum and cerebellum dates solely from the use of the elective silver chromate staining method of M. Golgi.[2] The researches of this authority have led without discussion to the following general facts:

1. Free terminations of the processes of nerve cells and of those spidery or neuroglial cells.
2. Existence of collaterals branching off the axons.
3. Existence of two types of cells which on the basis of their axonal properties are: the cells in which this process loses its individuality through branching, without penetrating the white matter; and the cells whose axon, in spite of giving off numerous collaterals, preserves its individuality and is continuous with a myelinated fiber of the white matter.

The more recent works of Tartuferi,[3] Mondino,[4] Fusari,[5] Nansen,[6] Kölliker,[7] Toldt and Kahler,[8] Obersteiner,[9] Petrone,[10] Marchi,[11] Magini,[12] Falzacappa,[13] Flechsig,[14] Edinger,[15] His,[16] and ourselves[17] confirm and extend in certain ways the admirable discoveries of the Italian histologist.

Concerning the fine structure of the brain, Golgi has revealed to us the form of the cells and the disposition of their processes in the cortex; he has demonstrated the presence of axons arising from the pyramidal cells and revealed the considerable contribution that the axons make to the filamentous intercellular substance; he has finally led us to recognize the enormous length of the peripheral dendrites of the pyramids, most of which reach the molecular layer and which intertwine in a very tightly laced plexus and enter into connection with neuroglial filaments.

After Golgi, Flechsig[18] demonstrated with the aid of a special staining method that the branches of the cortical axons have a myelin sheath and that the divisions of the fibers occur at the level of the strangulations of the fibers, an opinion which we support on the basis of certain fiber branches in the cerebellum and tectum.

Most recently, Martinotti[19] has discovered how the myelinated fibers of the first layer of the cortex are branched and arise from various ascending axons coming from certain pyramidal cells situated in the deep layers.

In spite of these notable discoveries, the problem of the connections of the cells of the cortex remains without a satisfactory solution. One knows well the hypothesis conceived by Golgi to account for the functional relationships of those nerve cells. Between the latter, he discerns a very rich network made up, first, of the collaterals of the axons of cells of the first type *(motor cells);* second, of the terminal branches of axons of cells of the second type *(sensory cells);* and third, of the ramifications of nerve fibers coming from the white matter *(sensory nerves).* His views have been endorsed by certain authors, notably by Tartuferi, Fusari, and Martinotti. However, it is true to say, in spite of the great authority of Golgi, that the hypothesis of the intercellular network of the gray matter loses ground and every day seems more and more unlikely, while the opinion of the independence of the cells and of the terminations of the nerve fibers conversely becomes more general, as the result of the work of Forel,[20] His,[21] Kölliker,[22] and ourselves.[23] Retzius[24] has recently proved the cellular independence and the free termination of axonal arborizations in the ganglia of crustacea, that is to say, in the *Punktsubstanz* of Leydig, where the defenders of the network [theory] marshaled the arsenal of their arguments the most strongly. These facts are [therefore] the more interesting.

If we transfer the problem of the general connections of the nerve cells and nerve fibers to one of the relationships of the cells of the cortex either to one another or to association or commissural fibers, we will soon see that, apart from certain hypotheses based on the research of pathological anatomy or experimental pathology, there is virtually nothing more to say. And it is recognized that neither the embryologic method of Flechsig, nor those of Weigert and of Golgi can furnish in this respect any direct anatomical proof capable of definitely answering the question.

But if we are not able to overcome the imperfections of the methods or the inherent difficulties in staining or, above all, the complete pursuit of the nerve fibers of the cortex—the enormous length of the fibers hindering finding their entire length in a single section—we can to some extent alleviate the problems by resorting to more favorable conditions.

These conditions are, first, the use of very small mammals (mouse, rat, bat, etc.) in order to diminish as much as possible the distance of the fibers and the volume of the various layers of the cortex; and second, the preferential study of the embryonic brain, that which offers a very simple, almost schematic structure and in which the method of Golgi yields more complete and more consistent results, above all in regard to the staining of the axons.

It is clear that, in spite of the application of these rules, we remain very far off from resolving the weighty questions relating to the structure of the cerebral cortex because the difficulties one encounters are extraordinary. However, in the meantime, we have gathered certain details which enlarge a little our understanding of the morphology of the [cellular] elements of the brain and which may help perhaps to set out a little, for the future, the question of the reciprocal connections of the cells of the gyri.

Technique

As we have previously indicated elsewhere, we use for preference the rapid method of Golgi. For the particular case of the study of the corpus callosum and the cerebral cortex, we use, especially, small mammals a few days old—mice and rats, from birth up to one month of age—and similarly embryos of mammals close to term—rat, mouse, rabbit, guinea pig.

The period most favorable for obtaining staining of the nerve cells of the cortex is not the same for all small mammals. In the mouse, for example, the *optimum* time varies between the eighth and the twenty-fifth or thirtieth day. Within the first few days of birth, the cells are so embryonic that good impregnations of the cortex are very rare. In the rabbit, the favorable period is much closer to birth (from first to fifteenth day), at which time the cerebral cortex is more developed than in the mouse.

In embryos of the mouse, rat, and rabbit, the cells impregnate in a very uncertain fashion; in contrast to the epithelial elements, the vessels and nerve fibers are only constantly stained when the time dedicated to fixation does not exceed two or three days.

The length of fixation of pieces in the osmium-dichromate mixture may be extended over two, three, or five days, after which it depends on whether the newborn mammals have reached a certain size (rabbit, guinea pig, cat) and, a stronger reason, if they are aged eight to fifteen days.

The time varies for each animal and for each stage of development; one can say the same thing concerning the staining of certain elements to the exclusion of others. Thus, to obtain staining of the cells of the molecular layer of the rabbit, it is necessary to fix for five days or thereabouts (rabbit aged eight days), while staining of the collaterals of the white matter necessitates six or seven.

It is very important for assured results to operate always at an almost constant temperature. We choose during the wintertime 25°[C] to 26°[C], and for this we employ a drying oven equipped with a thermoregulator. At lower temperatures, fixation requires a longer time, which can be determined by trial and error.

The size of the blocks to be fixed is also of great importance: the thickness of the pieces cannot exceed a half-centimeter for a quantity of solution of 25 to 30 cc.

Sometimes one does not obtain the reaction, or it is very imperfect, possibly on account of exceeding the time necessary for the impregnation. In this case, after leaving the silver bath, we immerse the pieces again in a new mixture [of osmium dichromate] for twenty-four or thirty-six hours, and we repeat the reaction a second time. Often one obtains in this way very complete impregnations, including sometimes even the connective tissue, muscular, cartilaginous elements, etc.; one succeeds similarly in staining nerve cells which retain scarcely any [stain] under ordinary conditions.

Whenever you would stain the superficial cellular elements of the brain, it is very important to preserve the peripheral layers of the pieces from crystalline deposits of silver chromate; that is obtained in the manner indicated by Martinotti[25] and Sehrwald.[26] Sometimes, by leaving the pia mater and the arachnoid on the cortex before fixation, one avoids in large part these deposits, principally when working on the rabbit.[27] One obtains the same result by investing the surface of the pieces with a thin layer of fresh blood from the same animal; the layer adheres very well to the pieces as it coagulates and allows them to be cut more easily than with the coating of gelatine advised by Sehrwald. Moreover, the coating of blood—which needs, of course, to operate upon the fresh pieces before fixation—renders us equally good service in the impregnation of nerve fibers of the heart and the retina of small mammals.

As to the proportions of the substances which constitute both the osmium-dichromate mixture and the silver bath, we have not introduced any modifications; we ourselves follow in outline those that we have noted in other works.[28]

Regarding the preservation of the impregnated sections, notwithstanding the new modifications introduced by Greppin[29] and Obregia,[30] we follow faithfully, save certain details, the protocol of Golgi. According to our experience, the treatment of the deposit of silver chromate either by hydrobromic acid (Greppin) or by gold chloride (Obregia) fixes well, it is true, the dendrites and the large axons, but it always eats away at and often removes the thinnest collaterals.

Cerebral Cortex

Our observations have been carried out preferentially on the psychomotor region of the cortex; the other areas present a few different characteristics that we will have occasion to study in another work.

Frontal sections of the cortex of small mam-
mals (rat, mouse, rabbit, etc.) very distinctly demonstrate the cellular layers recognized by the authors in the human brain.

One feature about which the authorities are not in agreement is the number of layers of the cerebral cortex. Meynert[31] recognizes five; Stieda,[32] Henle,[33] Boll,[34] and Schwalbe[35] have fixed on four; and Krause[36] has described seven.

Golgi, not being able to agree with the fixed limits of the various layers described by the authors, takes the position of dividing the gray cortex into three equal layers, or into three tiers: *superficial, middle,* and *deep.*[37]

It is indubitable that the layers of the cortical gray matter are continuous by gradual transitions, except for the first or molecular layer, whose limits are quite precise. However, in spite of all, we find very convenient for study a division into four layers, accepted by various authors, notably Schwalbe; for, in reality, the fourth and fifth layers of Meynert do not stand alone, and the nervous plexus and layers fourth and sixth, which Krause considers to be special zones, [also] do not possess an obvious individuality, being made up of a mixture of nerve cells.

We have adopted the nomenclature of Meynert and Schwalbe, because, given the present state of the science, it would be difficult to replace it without causing regrettable confusions; besides, it does not presuppose anything about the nature and the physiological role of the cortical cells.

1. Layer Poor in Cells (First Layer of Meynert, Layer without Cells of Stieda, Molecular Layer of certain authors)

This layer, rather thick in small mammals, presents a finely granular, sometimes clearly reticular appearance in preparations stained by carmine or with the method of Weigert.

The most external part of this layer includes many neuroglial cells, according to what has been described by several authors, notably Golgi and Martinotti, who have given a good description of these cells.

However, the more important features and those which constitute the greater part of the first layer are the following: first, the nerve fibers; second, the special nerve cells; third, the dendritic processes of pyramids situated in subjacent layers.

a. Nerve Fibers (figs. 4, 6) [figs. 10, 12]

Whenever one examines a section of the cerebral cortex stained by the Weigert method, one sees the molecular layer traversed by a large number of varicose myelinated fibers, of variable thickness and directed horizontally or almost parallel to the cerebral surface. These fibers were discovered some time ago by Kölliker[38] with the aid of the potassium [chromate] procedure, and, more lately, Exner[39] has given a very good description based on the use of the osmic acid method. Recently also, Obersteiner,[40] Edinger,[41] and Martinotti,[42] employing the hematoxylin stain of Weigert-Pal, have studied and drawn these fibers.

However, these methods stain a very small proportion of the nerve fibers of the first layer, because the majority lack myelin. Now, for the demonstration of unmyelinated nerve fibers, it is necessary to use the rapid Golgi method, applying it, above all, to young mammals.

In good preparations, one observes an extraordinary multitude of very fine fibers (fig. 6, A) [fig. 12], often varicose and flexuous, seated above all in the very superficial portion of the molecular layer and oriented in all directions, but principally in the horizontal direction. In small animals, such as the mouse, rat, or rabbit, it is seen besides that the majority of fibers have an anteroposterior direction.

Many of these fibers are frankly branched, as recognized by Martinotti, who also observed certain of them descending into the subjacent layers, and their continuity with certain axons. We consider that our observations on this point confirm his exactly.

b. Nerve Cells

The descending axons that we have already mentioned are not furnished with branches that can be revealed in the first layer, either by the method of Weigert or by that of Golgi. Our observations demonstrate that some of these fibers have their origins from the special nerve cells, situated in the [first] layer, within the confines of the superficial nervous plexus (figs. 1, 2, 3) [figs. 7, 8, 9].

These cells have been mentioned by all the anatomists over the last twenty years, such as Meynert, Henle, Schwalbe, Krause, Ranvier, Toldt and Kahler, Obersteiner, etc. They have been considered as stellate or triangular cells, placed here and there, at considerable distances throughout the whole thickness of the first layer, which as a consequence receives the designation of the layer *poor in cells* (*zellenarme Schicht*). But, because of the ineffectiveness of the Golgi method in staining these cells, the authorities who have devoted attention to the study of the cortex [using the Golgi method], such as Golgi, Mondino, Edinger, and Martinotti, have ended up with [no more than] an approximation of these cells; they have considered them to be probably neuroglial cells.

Despite the [contrary] testimony of anatomists who made use of the older staining methods, a fact of which we are firmly convinced is the existence of nerve cells in the molecular layer. Behold. When one examines the aforesaid layer in the brain of man and higher mammals, after impregnation by the Weigert method, there are found, among the thin myelinated fibers, certain other extremely large fibers, much thicker than those which descend into subjacent layers of the gray matter (fig. 4, *b*) [fig. 10]. Now, if these robust fibers are the myelinated fibers reaching the molecular layer and if their branches become horizontal, it is to be supposed that one thin fiber is capable of giving rise to a large number of thicker myelinated fibers, a fact certainly a little strange and perhaps without precedent in the anatomy of the nerve centers. Let us add further that it is impossible to discern a continuity between the thick horizontal fibers and the other, thinner fibers which have an ascending course.

As a result of attempting impregnations in young mammals, we have succeeded in furnishing direct proof of the existence of special nerve cells, whose axons correspond in part to the large fibers that we have just mentioned. It is in the rabbit of a few days that we have had the more successful impregnations; however, one achieves staining, although less com-

Plate I

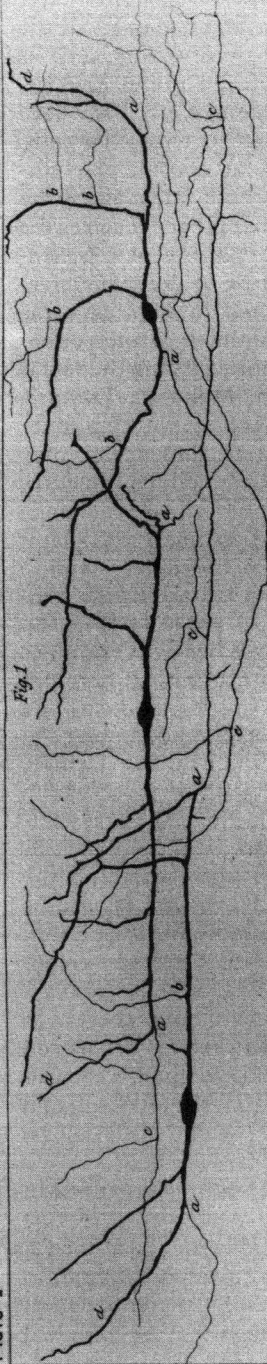
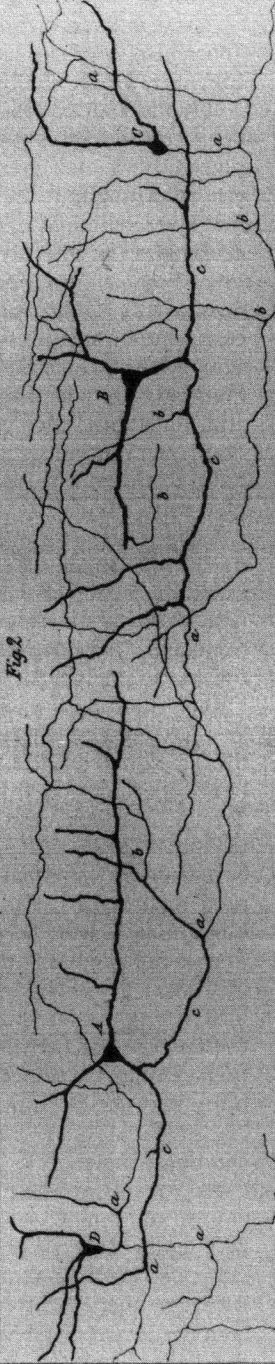
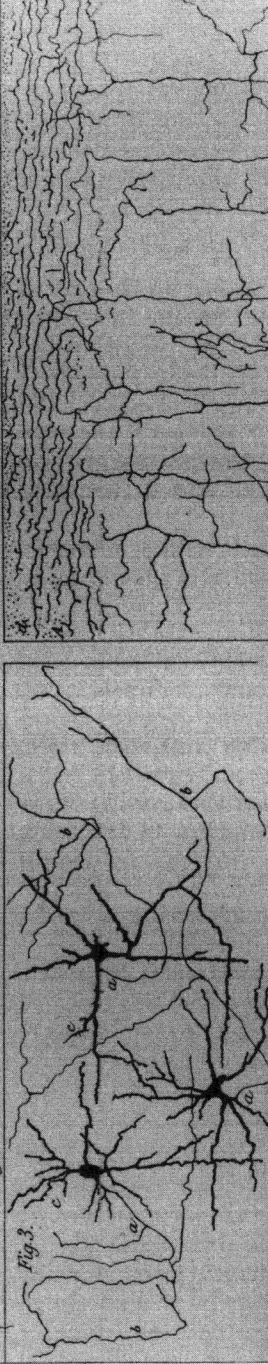
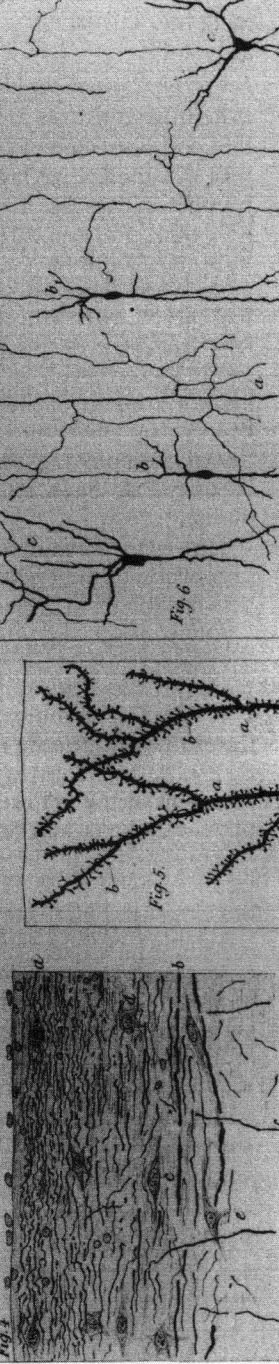
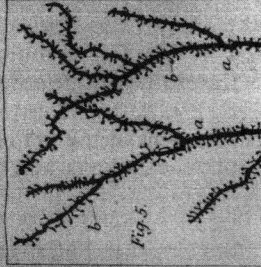
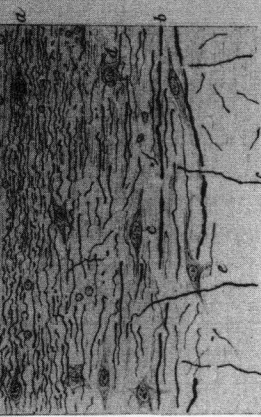

pletely, in the mouse and the cat of the same age.

The cells are of three types: first, the polygonal cells with a short axon; second, the fusiform, multipolar cells; third, the triangular or irregular, multipolar cells.

Polygonal Cells (fig. 3) [*fig. 9*]. These cells are few in number, dispersed without order through the whole thickness of the molecular layer. They are polygonal or stellate in form and provided with four, five, or an even larger number of divergent branched, varicose processes. These processes extend in all directions, reaching above to the free surface of the brain and below almost penetrating the layer of the small pyramids.

The axon ordinarily leaves from a lateral part of the cell and very rarely from the upper or lower part. It has either a horizontal or ascending direction, and it next branches and gives rise to a large number of fine, varicose fibers whose trajectory is variable but often parallel to the free surface. The branches do not have a tendency to descend to the subjacent layers; they remain always within the limits of the molecular layer, and there terminate freely.

Fusiform Cells (fig. 1) [*fig. 7*]. These cells are thin, with a smooth contour and enormously long. In the rabbit of eight days, in which they are stained very well, they appear perfectly fusiform, horizontal, and oriented in an anteroposterior direction, a circumstance which obliges us to study them in sections of the same orientation.

The processes, in number two, leave the poles of the cell accordingly in opposite directions; they are extended horizontally over a considerable distance—and it is because of this extreme length that one rarely finds complete cells in the sections—finally, after a variable and almost straight course, they bend at an ob-

---

Explanation of the plates: The majority of our figures have been made using the Zeiss camera lucida, with the objective C of that manufacturer, and employing sometimes the ocular 4, sometimes the ocular 2. Figs. 4 and 5 [*figs. 10 and 11*] have been made with the very powerful objectives E and Zeiss 1.30 apochromatic.

Plate I. [*FIG. 7*]   Fig. 1. Longitudinal section of the molecular layer of the cerebral cortex of the rabbit aged eight days. Impregnation by the rapid Golgi method. Three fusiform, multipolar, anteroposterior cells are drawn: *a*, polar or principal axons, traveling in opposite directions; *b*, supernumerary axons arising from various dendritic branches; *c*, branches of the axons.

[*FIG. 8*]   Fig. 2. Same section and same method as in the preceding figure. A and B, triangular multipolar cells in the molecular layer of a young rabbit (eight days); *a*, principal axons, whose direction is anteroposterior; *b*, supernumerary axons; C and D, smaller multipolar cells with an almost round shape; *a*, axons; *b*, their collaterals.

[*FIG. 9*]   Fig. 3. Part of an anteroposterior section of the cerebral cortex of the rabbit of eight days. Polygonal cells of the molecular layer; *a*, axons; *b*, collaterals; *c*, dendritic branches.

[*FIG. 10*]   Fig. 4. Fragment of an anteroposterior section of the cortex of an adult rabbit, Weigert-Pal method and carmine of Orth. *a*, very fine and flexuous myelinated fibers, placed in the external portion of the molecular layer; *b*, very large anteroposterior fibers, situated in the deep part of the same layer; *c*, fusiform cell; *d*, polygonal cell; *e*, triangular cell; *f*, ascending fibers coming from the deep layers of the cortex.

[*FIG. 11*]   Fig. 5. Portion of the terminal arborization of an [apical dendritic] shaft of a pyramidal cell of the adult mouse. 1.30 Zeiss apochromatic objective. *a*, shaft and dendritic branches; *b*, collateral spines.

[*FIG. 12*]   Fig. 6. Transverse section of the cortex of the mouse of twenty days. In it are drawn the cells which in various sections of the same region send their axons toward the surface. Zeiss objective C, ocular 2. *a*, axon arising from a large cell of the fourth layer; *b*, axons arising from less deep cells; *c*, ascending axons which terminate in extensive branches on arriving at the molecular layer; A, molecular layer; *d*, varicose terminal branches of fibers of this layer.

tuse angle and ascend almost to the cerebral surface, where they seem to end freely (fig. 1, d) [fig. 7]. During their horizontal trajectory, these processes give off collateral processes, which appear also to terminate in the uppermost part of the molecular layer. However, this termination is not always clearly seen, on account of the irregular deposits of silver chromate which often contaminate the external limit of the layer.

The axon does not arise from the cell body or from any of the very large processes; it is because of this that we were not able to identify it in our first preparations, which were also somewhat incomplete. However, on continuing our observations with the aid of better impregnations, we have been struck by the sight of double or even triple axons, which come off the [dendritic] branches at a large distance from the cell body.

When the axon is double, which often happens, each axon arises at an obtuse angle from the elongated processes which are destined to become ascending (fig. 1, a) [fig. 7]. Next, the branches run anteroposteriorly and in opposite directions, traveling over a considerable extent of the molecular layer; they ordinarily elude pursuit of their entire course. More or less at a right angle, the axons give rise to a large number of ascending collaterals, which seem to terminate in small varicose branches, after dividing to some extent. These small branches, which seem to us to end freely, always remain within the terrain of the first layer and give extreme complexity to the structure of this cerebral layer.

Sometimes, besides the two anteroposteriorly directed axons which we have already described, another is observed arising from the straight trajectory of the polar [dendritic] processes, and likewise from certain secondary dendritic branches. These supernumerary axons very often have an ascending direction and behave, otherwise, like the principal axon (fig. 1, b) [fig. 7].

The fusiform cells of the molecular layer are not very frequent. In an anteroposterior section of the cortex of a rabbit of eight days, which measured a half-centimeter in length, we have found six or seven. We think, however, that they are more abundant, if we make

allowance for their rarity and the difficulty of their impregnation. Very often the molecular layer does not give the reaction because of excessive fixation with the [fixative] mixture, or otherwise it is spoiled by irregular precipitates; in others, the small nerve fibers are exclusively stained, and it is impossible to determine their origin.

When one resorts to preparations simply stained with carmine or nigrosine, etc., these cells are revealed with a certain clarity. They are, in fact, little abundant, though in certain regions of the cortex they appear in reasonably large numbers. Their fusiform cell body is very pale and does not attract either carmine or osmic acid; they stand out clearly against a dark and granular background. The nucleus is elongated and oriented in the same direction as the cell (fig. 4, c) [fig. 10].

Triangular Cells (fig. 2, A, B) [fig. 8]. Here we deal with cells that are larger and more numerous than the preceding [cells] and most of which possess a triangular body and three large and very long dendrites, extending almost in a straight line and with few branches. Commonly, two are found either oblique or horizontal with a tendency to ascend within the molecular layer. The third is descending; it soon divides, giving rise to two very long branches, sometimes arciform and directed horizontally (fig. 2 c) [fig. 8]. Other cells show many variations in the shape, number, and direction of the processes.

The axons number two, three, four, or even more. They always come off the dendritic branches and commonly appear along the course of the anteroposterior processes (fig. 2, a) [fig. 8]. It is easy to detect the following facts: whatever its mode of origin and initial direction, the axon inclines constantly toward the top of the molecular layer and ramifies at intervals with the branches becoming more or less horizontal. Some small branches have the appearance of free terminations on short and varicose stems, but the great extent of the field over which the small branches spread hinders, even in good impregnations, the pursuit of the whole arborizations.

The cells shown in fig. 2 at *C* and *D* [fig. 8] can be considered as a cellular variety very similar to those which we have already described. These cells are smaller and possess a more or less rounded cell body. They are characterized above all by the fact that in addition to the processes originating from dendritic branches, there is found another process which arises from the soma, promptly divides, and also terminates in small ascending branches in the upper part of the molecular layer.

These nerve cells with multiple axons have certain features in common which it is appropriate to remark upon. They have a soma provided with a very limited number of dendrites in comparison with ordinary cells. The processes are of an enormous length, extending more or less horizontally and provided with the varicosities and spines characteristic of all the cells of the cortex, including the polygonal cells of the first layer. To appreciate fully these differences, it is sufficient to compare the cells of figs. 3 [*fig. 9*] (polygonal with one axon) and 6 [*fig. 12*] with those shown in figs. 1 and 2 [*figs. 7 and 8*].

Are the multiple axons that we have described in reality the true functional axons of these nerve cells? We think that doubt is impossible in this regard, unless the current ideas on the anatomical properties of axons are modified. We wish merely to say that all the axons shown in figs. 1 and 2 [*figs. 7 and 8*], arising from the dendrites of the bipolar and triangular cells, present the full range of characteristics usually associated with axons, namely an extreme thinness in comparison with dendrites, perfectly smooth contours with maintenance of their original diameter, an enormous length and with extraordinarily delicate right-angled branches, and finally their clear coffee color, by virtue of the thinness of the silver deposit, etc. Let us add also the impossibility of distinguishing these fibers from axons given off by other cells with which they are mixed.

We think, besides, that the axons of the bipolar cells and a few of those of the triangular cells are furnished with a myelin sheath. As we have frequently noticed, there is a perfect correlation between the course and length of the polar axons of the cells mentioned on the one hand and those of certain myelinated fibers in the molecular layer. These are, in particular, certain horizontal, anteroposteriorly oriented myelinated fibers larger in comparison with the others and placed in the deep part of the superficial nerve plexus (fig. 4, *b*) [*fig. 10*], which seems to us to represent these characteristics.[43]

In the rabbit, where we have frequently noted these correlations, we see that nearly all the fibers that possess myelin have an anteroposterior direction, the thinnest and most varicose being those most superficially placed. In man, the large fibers are more abundant still, but they do not have a regular orientation, nor are they gathered in a consistent manner at the deep level of the superficial nervous plexus.

c. Terminal Dendritic Branches of the Pyramids

The molecular layer is traversed, according to Golgi, who recognized it first, by the peripheral processes of the pyramidal nerve cells. These processes branch repeatedly in the thickness of the layer mentioned, and most of the branches, after a variable, commonly horizontal or oblique course, end near the free surface beneath the pia mater, as Martinotti has very well noticed. There are, however, oblique or arciform dendritic branches which terminate at different levels in the molecular layer, interweaving with the nerve fibers (fig. 7, A) [*fig. 13*]. We have not been able to find any special relationships between the dendritic branches and the blood vessels or neuroglial cells.

The small terminal dendritic branches of the pyramids do not have smooth contours, as the authors appear to represent them; they bristle with teeth given off more or less at a right angle (figs. 7, 5) [*figs. 13, 11*], and ending in a round and slightly thickened tip. These collateral spines are also found, although in smaller numbers, on the large ascending shafts of the medium and large pyramids, from the moment they begin emitting little branches in the deep layers of the cortex.

The terminal tufts of all of these radial dendritic branches in the molecular layer are intertwined at varying angles, like the interweaving of trees in a very dense forest. In the small spaces left between the branches, probably in the hollows separating two spines, are found the innumerable small nerve fibers of the aforementioned layer.

It is impossible to contemplate with indifference, as do certain authorities, this admirable relationship established between the nerve fibers of the first layer and the terminal parts of virtually all the pyramidal cells of the cortex. This connection, which constantly demonstrates the same appearance in all mammals in all regions of the cortex including Ammon's horn and the olfactory lobe, must have great importance in the functioning of the brain. Let us remember that a similar relationship is found in the molecular layer of the cerebellum—which represents the first layer of the [cerebral] cortex—where there also converge, as in the cerebrum, a multitude of dendritic branches of the Purkinje cells and an infinite number of small nerve fibers without myelin (parallel fibers originating from the granule cells). In short, it is a very general fact that the accumulation of dendritic branches occurs in places where small nerve fibers without myelin are found, or among the terminal arborizations of certain axons (olfactory bulb, retina, corpora quadrigemina, optic lobe of birds, etc.).

In our earlier works,[44] we have considered the dendrites of nerve cells, not so much as the *providers* of nutrition or absorption, following the opinion of Golgi, but rather as arrangements permitting the establishment, by multiple contacts, of the communications of nervous action either between neighboring cells or between cells at a distance. Whenever nervous transmission occurs over a great distance, we have to admit, in which we rely upon examples, that the propagation of the nervous excitation occurs between the dendritic arborizations on the one hand and the unmyelinated nerve fibers on the other.

In applying these principles to the interpretation of the structure of the molecular layer of the brain, we have first to consider that the superficial fusiform and triangular cells, by means of their multiple axons and their very long dendrites, are in contact and intermingled with a large number of terminal dendritic tufts of subjacent pyramidal cells. It does not seem unlikely, therefore, that the considerable

group of these latter, situated in remote regions and at various depths of the cerebral cortex, are brought into dynamic association by means of these multiple contacts. It is in supposing such a coordinating action that we have in another work[45] given these cellular elements of the molecular layer the name of *cells of association.*

Apart from this function of coordination, the cells of the first layer may also have some other dynamic roles which are impossible to determine, given the present state of the science.

2. Layer of the Small Pyramids (Second Layer of Meynert, Upper Layer of Golgi)

This layer is made up of an agglomeration in various rows of a considerable number of pyramidal cells of small stature, with the dimensions increasing as they occupy the deeper levels [of the layer]. The disposition and the properties of these cells in mammals are identical to those which Golgi describes in the human (fig. 7, B) [fig. 13].

The cells of this layer which are situated just beneath the molecular layer are not strictly pyramidal. In the small mammals they are rather polygonal or stellate. From the upper and lateral aspect of their cell body, often only some diverging dendrites which terminate in spiny branches in the molecular layer are seen to arise, while from the lower part comes the fine axon, almost straight, and descending like those of all the subjacent cells of the same layer (figs. 7, c; 14, j; 15, m) [figs. 13, 20, 21].

Whence goes the axon of the small pyramids? What is the arrangement of its collaterals? These are among the more obscure points in cerebral anatomy. Golgi, in his important work, observed the axons only over a short part of their course. Martinotti followed them over a much longer course and noted the presence of collateral branches. But it seems to me that in no case did these authors succeed in following the axons to the white matter; this is understandable in view of the great length and extreme fineness that these fibers present in higher mammals.

Our first tentative efforts at impregnation for following the complete course of these axons were not crowned with success. However, in choosing as regular objects of study newborn small mammals, we have succeeded in pursuing them as far as the white matter, from which, depending on the cerebral region, they passed into the corpus striatum (anterior and lateral region of the [frontal] lobe). However, in the cortical regions placed on top of the lateral ventricles, the axons probably participate, as previously suggested by Monakow, in the formation of the corpus callosum. We will return to the latter point.

During their descending trajectory through the gray matter, the axons of small and medium pyramids emit fine collaterals, given off at a right angle, or nearly so, and which terminate in a little nodule, after an almost straight course, either transverse or oblique.

This free termination can be observed only in brains which are more or less embryonic, such as the mouse of eight to twelve days, for example; in adult animals, it is impossible, because of the enormous length acquired by the collaterals and the frequent branchings that they present.

It is noticeable that the collaterals arise invariably in the upper part of the course of the axon; the lower part, thinner and paler, descends flexuously without giving off branches up to the moment that it penetrates the white matter (fig. 14, *j*) [*fig. 20*].

We have occasionally seen the axon to end in the middle layers of the cortex by dichotomizing, after which its individuality and original direction are lost (fig. 15, *a*) [*fig. 21*]; nevertheless, one cannot rule out the possibility that one of the branches may attain the white matter after a more or less oblique course.

In summary, the great majority, perhaps all, of the axons of the small pyramids reach the white matter and continue on as myelinated fibers.

3. Layer of Large Pyramids (Third Layer *or* Ammon's Horn Formation *of Meynert,* Middle Layer of Nerve Cells *of Stieda,* Middle Layer *of Golgi*).

Joined by insensible transitions with the previous layer, this layer presents in the small mammals the same characteristics as in man; the differences that exist are secondary and entirely [those of] detail. The cell bodies are less frankly pyramidal and are almost ovoid; their volume is less large than in man, in keeping proportionately with the size of the animal; the basilar dendrites are shorter and less numerous than in man; it is from these same cells that the large external or radial [dendritic] shaft arises (fig. 7) [*fig. 13*].

The axon is thick; it descends partly in a straight line toward the white matter, where it continues either as an association fiber or as a myelinated fiber of the corona radiata. Upon this point, we have no doubt, because we have often been fortunate in having had the opportunity to follow the whole course of the axon through the cortex and over a considerable length into the white matter. For the rest, Golgi claims to have seen the arrival of the same axons at the white matter; however, in man, tracing them naturally presents very great difficulties.

The collaterals of the axons of the large pyramids are very numerous; they come off at a right angle or at an obtuse angle. On many of them, we have counted seven to eight collaterals, but most frequently the number is reduced to four or five, especially in the deeper pyramids. At deep levels, the axon is usually flexuous and not generally furnished with collaterals (fig. 14, *a*) [*fig. 20*].

The direction of the collaterals is usually horizontal or oblique; they commonly maintain their direction, and they branch one or two times. It is not rare to observe that the uppermost ones have an ascending course, and they branch and extend their small ramifications toward the molecular layer; in certain cases, one notices that two or three collaterals arise from a small, short stem.

In considering their terminations, [it is noted that] they always end in a free granular or thickened tip, without terminal branching. As we have indicated above, this circumstance can only be observed in the cortex of young small mammals. In the rat and mouse of four to eight days, for example, one notices that almost all the collaterals terminate at the same distance and in the same manner, that is to say, in a small thickening (figs. 14, *j*; 15, *m*) [*figs.*

Plate II

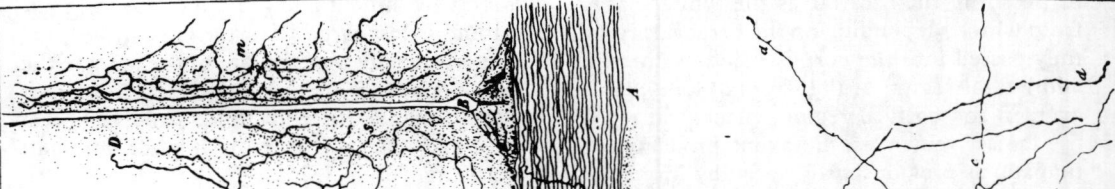

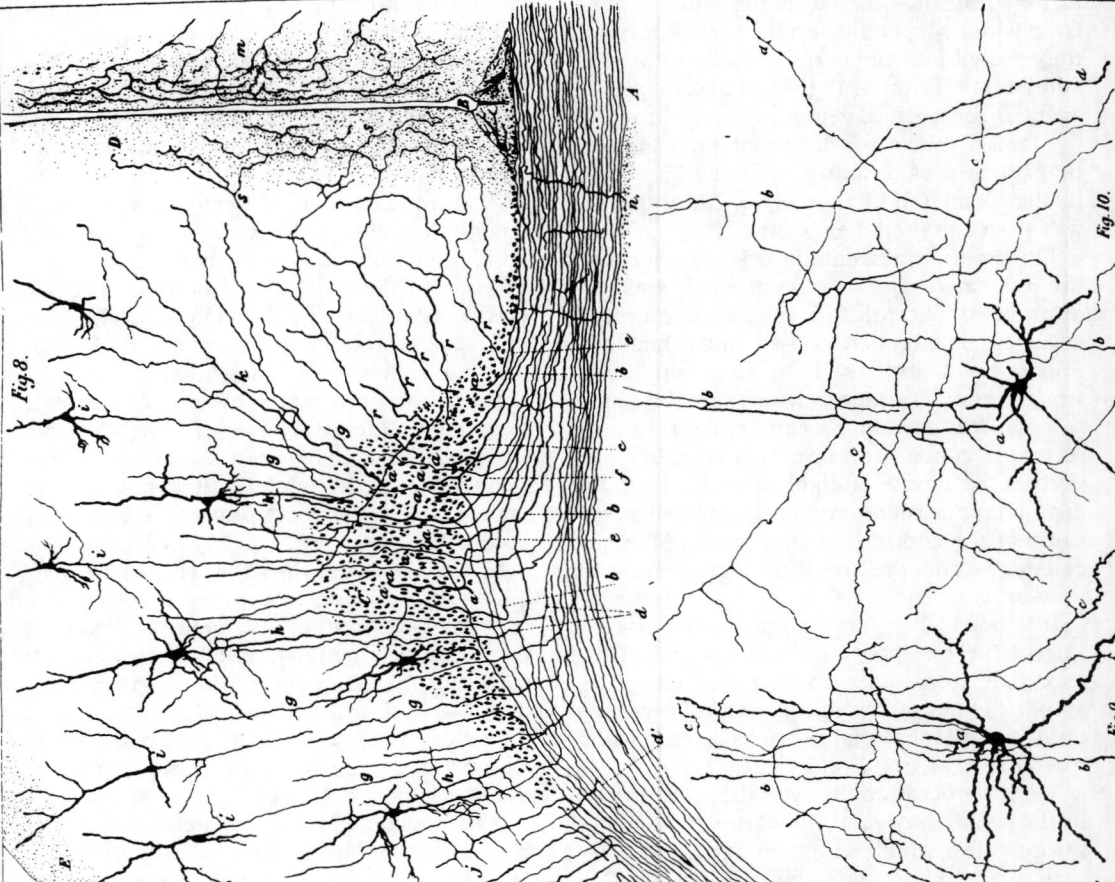

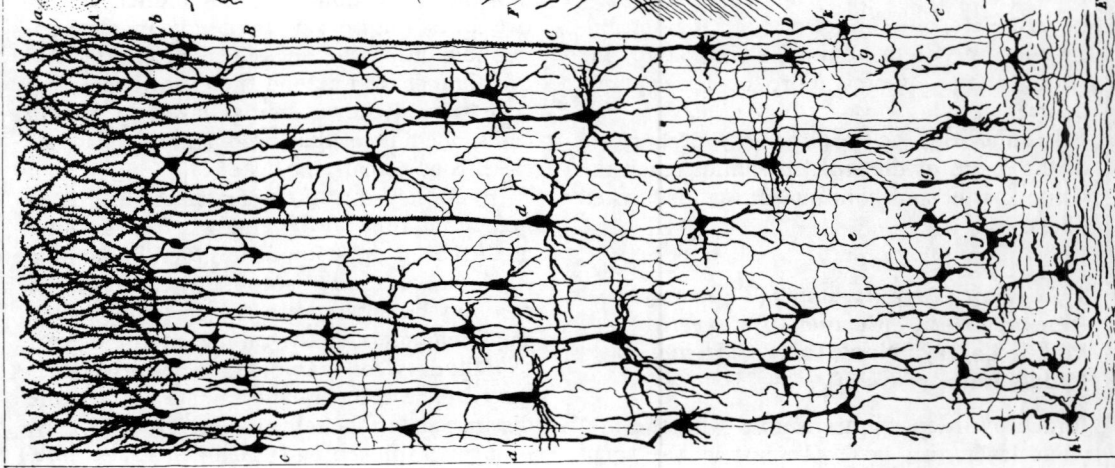

34

20, 21]. The adult brain presents collaterals that are longer and branched, but essentially identical, in regard to their behavior to the cells of the young brain; however, following their entire course is very difficult and frequently absolutely impossible.

4. Layer of the Polymorphic Cells (Third and Fourth Layer of Meynert, Layer of the Small Nerve Cells of Schwalbe, Deep Layer of Golgi, etc.)

This layer presents a great variety of forms and sizes of cells. In general, the cells of which it is composed are more or less globular and much inferior in size to the large pyramid (fig. 7, g, j, h) [fig. 13]. But it is also possible to see, as did Golgi, who has recognized them before in man and higher mammals, a great number of fusiform cells and also true pyramids oriented in the same manner as the cells of the second and third layers. The majority of these cells, whatever their shape, are furnished with ascending and descending dendrites, but with an orientation less rigorous than that of the pyramids. The ascending [dendrites] which often are represented by a very thick shaft can reach beyond the middle layers of the cortex, but we have never seen them attain the molecular layer. The descending [dendrites] pass more or less obliquely toward the white matter, into which they sometimes penetrate. From the sides of the cell body also arise some slender processes [that are] shorter, more flexuous, and more varicose than the others (figs. 7, 15) [figs. 13, 21].

The greater part of the axon descends and describes large sinuosities, in order to adapt to the curves of the globular cells dominating this layer. Along its course, [the axon] is furnished with various fine collaterals, very flexuous and with an irregular course, and finally, now very much thinned, it is continuous with a very delicate fiber of the white matter. This continuation has been definitely observed by us in many cells: globular, fusiform, and triangular cells of this layer, also in the cells placed near the large pyramids and, finally,

---

Plate II. [FIG. 13] Fig. 7. Transverse sections of the cortex of a mouse of one month (supraventricular region) objective C, ocular 3. A, molecular layer; B, layer of small pyramids; C, layer of large pyramids; D, layer of polymorphic cells; E, white matter; a, spiny tufts of the pyramids; b, more superficial small pyramids; c, axon of a small pyramid; d, large pyramid; e, its axon; f, cell with ascending axon; g, similar but smaller cells; h, cells situated in the white matter, i, round cell, whose axon is directed toward the white matter; j, sensory cell of Golgi.

[FIG. 14] Fig. 8. Transverse section of the cortex and corpus callosum of a mouse of eight days. It shows the dispositions of the more common callosal fibers, the arcuate fasiculus, and its collaterals that return to the gray matter. Zeiss objective C, ocular 2. The fibers indicated by a have an anteroposterior direction; A, middle region of the corpus callosum; B, interhemispheric fissure; C, arcuate fascicle cut transversely; D, molecular layer of the internal face of the hemisphere; E, superior part of the latter; b, callosal fibers continuous with a fiber of the arcuate fascicle; c, identical callosal fibers but giving off a collateral that turns laterally; d, ascending collateral fibers of the callosal fibers; e, callosal fiber representing a collateral of the arcuate fascicle; f, callosal fiber coming from the bifurcation of an association fiber and giving off a collateral laterally; g, callosal fibers ascending to near the middle layer of the cortex; h, axons forming the fibers of the arcuate fascicle; i, descending and very fine axons of small and medium pyramids; j, axons coursing laterally with the callosal fibers; k, terminal arborization of an association fiber; r, collateral fibers of the arcuate fasciculus; s, varicose arborizations of certain collaterals in the molecular layer on the internal surface of the hemisphere; m, arborizations of ascending axons; n, vertical fibers that transverse the corpus callosum and become converted into anteroposterior fibers.

[FIG. 15] Fig. 9. Sensory cell of Golgi in the fourth layer of the cortex of the newborn rabbit. a, ascending axon; b, straight and vertical small branches; c, varicose terminal branches.

[FIG. 16] Fig. 10. Sensory cell of Golgi taken from the middle region of the cortex of a rabbit aged two months. a, axon; b, small radial branches; c, very long horizontal branches; d, free varicose tip.

upon cells situated in the vicinity of the white matter.

The mode of termination in the white matter takes place either by a bifurcation (division in Y or in T) or, most frequently, after a simple bend. In the latter case, the axon becomes horizontal, directed either medially or laterally, and appears to go to different regions of the cortex.

In the small mammals (mouse, bat, rat, etc.), the deep layer, that is to say, the layer of polymorphic cells, extends below into the thickness of the white matter. In effect, among the fascicles of this, there are observed certain generally fusiform or stellate cells, whose dendrites run in all directions but principally in the direction of the fibers of the white matter. A certain number of these cells give rise to an axon that is continuous with a [myelinated fiber] of the white matter; nevertheless, it is observed that the axon of many of the cells affects an ascending direction and thus behaves like that of the sensory cells of Golgi.

5. Cells with Short Axon

Among the cells of the diverse layers of the cerebral cortex, two types of cells are observed scattered, here and there, and without order: the sensory cells of Golgi and the cells whose axons ascend to the molecular layer.

a. Sensory Cells of Golgi

These cells, discovered by Golgi and rediscovered by Martinotti, are little abundant; they can be recognized in all the cerebral layers but especially in that of the polymorphic cells (figs. 7, j; 9; 10) [figs. 13, 15, 16].

They are large and stellate, sometimes elongated in a radial direction; their dendrites diverge in all directions, branch and dichotomize successively without attaining great length and without reaching the molecular layer.

The axon, well described by Golgi and Martinotti, is characterized by not having a fixed orientation. Sometimes it descends, while at others it ascends, or it is directed more or less horizontally. It is distinguished above all by the fact that, after a short and sinuous course, it terminates in an ample arborization [that is]

very complicated and completely free (fig. 9, c) [fig. 15].

According to Golgi, these axonal ramifications would form by their union with other fiber branches a diffuse and extraordinarily complicated network, in the interior of which all the nerve cells would communicate, in an indirect manner, either with one another or with the fibers of the white matter (sensory fibers). Martinotti[46] also holds this opinion, and in addition he claims the existence of anastomotic branches uniting the descending axons of the pyramids (cells of the first [Golgi] type);[47] but the existence of the nerve net in the gray matter, according to what we have had occasion to indicate above, is no more than an anatomical hypothesis which has not been confirmed. The same can be said in regard to the imagined anastomotic branches described by Martinotti.

What led [Martinotti] to suppose the existence of anastomoses is a relatively frequent peculiarity of the sensory cells of Golgi, namely the presence on the terminal arborizations of their axons of straight and long nerve branches, either ascending or descending, and with a resemblance to the axons of the pyramids (figs. 9; 10, b) [figs. 15, 16].

But a careful examination demonstrates, first, that the mentioned vertical branches are always very thin and that they rarely give off collaterals at right angles, which is the usual manner for the true axons of pyramids; second, that after a variable course they little by little become thinner and end with a varicosity or in a number of granular branches (fig. 9, b) [fig. 15]; and third, that these never terminate in nerve cell [bodies].

For the rest, all the ramifications of the axons of the sensory cells behave the same; after a flexuous course during which they embrace the bodies of the nerve cells, they end freely, after giving rise to small, short, and varicose collateral branches (fig. 9, c) [fig. 15].

For demonstrating the free endings of these arborizations, one must avoid making observations only in adult animals, because with these, even those that are very small—the mouse, for example—the arborization is so extensive and complicated that it is impossible to trace the branches completely. By contrast, it is easy to follow the terminal branches in the brain of the mouse a few days old, and also in the newborn cat and rabbit (fig.9) [*fig. 15*].

If we were to advance an opinion about the significance of the sensory cells of Golgi, we would not hesitate, in view of the disposition of their axonal arborization and the number of cells with which they establish contacts, to consider them *association cells*. In addition to other functions yet unknown, these cells could exist for the purpose of bringing the joint action of a group of nerve cells more or less together.

b. Cells with Ascending Axon (fig. 6) [*fig. 12*]

Golgi has previously mentioned in the deep layer of the cerebral cortex cells with an axon which, instead of descending, ascends toward the [surface]; but it is Martinotti who deserves the credit for having stated that in at least a certain number of these cells the axon arborizes in the molecular layer.

The cell illustrated by Martinotti in his paper lies in the layer of medium or small pyramids and affects a triangular shape. In our preparations of the cortex of the mouse, rat, and rabbit, these cells are for the most part fusiform or globular and are positioned in the deeper layers of the cortex; in the layer of medium or small pyramids, they are much rarer. Fig. 6 [*fig. 12*] shows the more common cells of this type that are encountered in our preparations.

The fusiform cells (fig. 6, *b,b*) [*fig. 12*] are oriented like the pyramids and present an elongated body that gives off one or two descending dendrites and one ascending, less long and soon branching. The axon commonly leaves from the upper part of the cell body or from the ascending dendritic branch; it ascends almost vertically, giving off [a certain number of] collaterals, and finally reaches the molecular layer. There it decomposes into an arborization of nearly horizontal branches of great extent. Frequently, the axon, on arriving at the [molecular] layer, bifurcates and sends branches in opposite directions; others make a simple bend, proceed horizontally, and give off sundry branches at an acute angle. Finally, sometimes also the axon, having bent or bifurcated in the upper part of the molecular layer, emits horizontal collaterals, lying in the lowermost part of the layer.

The great extent traveled by these fibers in the first layer presents an obstacle to observing the entire arborization of the axon. Nevertheless, horizontal sections of this layer demonstrate the enormous extent of the terminal ramifications and the great variety of directions which these last pursue, which, like all the nervous ramifications, seem to end freely in varicose extremities. The very fine terminal branches are characterized by their very flexuous course, and also by the peculiarity of giving off little spines or short branchlets [that are] granular, arising at a right angle or an obtuse angle and ending in a varicosity.

All of the cells with an ascending axon do not dispatch their axons to the molecular layer. Cells are also observed (fig. 6, *c*) [*fig. 12*] whose axon, after running for a time toward the [surface], decomposes, in either the second or the third layer, in extensive branches, among which those with a course [that is] horizontal or parallel to the cerebral surface predominate. These cells differ from the sensory cells of Golgi in that their terminal axonal arborization is relatively weak, and thus they preserve over a considerable extent the individuality of the [parent] axon.

6. Fibers of the White Matter Arborizing in the Gray Matter

All authors since Gerlach admit the branching within the gray matter of sensory nerve fibers coming from other regions of the nervous system, perhaps [from] the sensory nerves. Golgi also supported this opinion; he supposed that the branches of these fibers, probably sensory [in character], contributed to the formation of the diffuse network of the gray matter. Other authors—Monakow,[48] for example—admit not only that the branching fibers coming from other nervous compartments penetrate the gray matter, but also that all the cerebral regions are points of origin of association fibers and the point of termination [in paintbrushlike configurations] of fibers of the same nature arriving from other sorts of centers.

But the indications of these authors are very vague; it seems that they are led to admit the existence of these fibers rather from deductive theories than from direct anatomical observations. Golgi, who undoubtedly saw them in the cerebellum, the evidence of which can be seen in his drawings, does not illustrate them or give a special description of them in the cerebral cortex; in the general description of his views on the origins of the nerves, he is uncertain if he has really seen them in the cortex or whether they are nothing more than the axons of incompletely impregnated pyramidal cells.

The preceding doubts arise on account of the very great difficulty with which staining of these fibers is obtained. Always in the brains of adults, it has been impossible for us to impregnate them using the three Golgi impregnation procedures. Previously, we despaired of providing a demonstration of their existence, but, recently, in the brain of the mouse of eight days and in that of the newborn rabbit, they have been revealed to our view with perfect clarity.

At first we will say that we possess a criterion sufficiently certain for their identification. They are ordinarily among the largest fibers which cross the gray matter of the cerebral cortex; their thickness surpasses by far that of the axons of the giant pyramids; furthermore, they are differentiated from these latter in that their course is sometimes oblique, sometimes horizontal or zigzag (fig. 16, *a, b*) [*fig. 22*].

These fibers come from the white matter, from which we have followed them for some distance. They are bent at a right angle or at an obtuse [angle] upon penetrating the cortex, and, after a variable trajectory, but almost always oblique, they divide into two or three large divergent branches. These branches ascend obliquely and extend over a large distance; then they branch many times, and, finally, their very fine terminal branches end in ample free and varicose arborizations, lying preferentially in the vicinity of the small and medium pyramids.

During its ascending course, the parent trunk gives off some large collaterals which pass almost horizontally in a straight line (fig. 16, *d*) [*fig. 22*] through an enormous extent of the gray matter. At other times [it is seen] that one of these same branches of bifurcation has

a horizontal or slightly oblique trajectory that can exceed a half-millimeter. Finally, it sometimes occurs that the [parent] nerve trunk changes direction: at first horizontal or oblique, it soon deviates vertically and commences its branching.

The vast plexus produced by the branches of the said fibers embraces the second and third layers and a part of the fourth. Sometimes we have also had occasion to follow some fine branches to the molecular layer, where they would form varicose arborizations (fig. 16, *c*) [*fig. 22*].

The fibers which we have described are never anastomosed to other fibers of the white matter and do not end in nerve cells, either. Their abundance varies among the preparations, but as judged from several sections, in which they are preferentially stained, one cannot doubt that they constitute a factor of great importance for the cerebral cortex.

A comparison of preparations made with the Golgi method with those obtained with the Weigert-Pal method demonstrates, very conclusively, that all of these fibers and their principal branches possess a particularly thick myelin sheath. On account of the great thickness of the myelin, and above all because of the irregular trajectory—sometimes horizontal, sometimes oblique—they are distinguishable from the axons of the pyramids, whose course, as is known, is virtually straight and descending (radial fasciculi of myelinated fibers).

After having observed them in the small mammals, it is not difficult to recognize them in sections of the gyri of man, stained by the Weigert-Pal method. In our opinion, all the extraordinarily large fibers with an oblique or horizontal course which cross the gray matter in the middle and deep cortical layers belong to this type. One can easily reveal the true strangulations [nodes of Ranvier] of the myelin, [between which are] very long interannular segments.

7. Myelinated and Unmyelinated Fibers of the Cortex

In many preceding paragraphs, we have already indicated that there are fibers that have a myelin sheath; but it seems to us advantageous to examine this point in a more detailed fashion.

The first question which presents itself is whether all the collaterals and all the nerve fibers are provided with a myelin sheath. When one compares a section of the cortex of a rabbit or rat after staining with the Weigert-Pal procedure with another well impregnated by the Golgi method, one notices similarities and differences.

The deep half of the gray matter presents a similar aspect; with the help of the two methods of preparation, the radial fasciculi of axons described by the authors are observed and a very compact interfascicular plexus corresponding to the accumulation of the small collateral fibers. Naturally, the plexus is much less rich in the Weigert preparations because the last branches of the collaterals lack myelin. One can immediately infer from these observations that the axons of the medium and large pyramids, and probably also those of the polymorphic cells, possess a myelin sheath.

A comparative study of this kind proves the same for the ascending axons destined for the molecular layer, as well as for their principal terminal branches of arborization.

The axons of the small pyramids seem to us to lack the [myelin] sheath, unless the myelin commences a long way from their point of origin. In effect, the rare myelinated fibers that cross the lower parts of [the layer of] the small pyramids are oblique and short and resemble the collaterals coming from very deep parts; moreover, the small number among them which are ascending appear to end in the molecular layer, coinciding with the ascending axons previously mentioned.

With regard to the collaterals of the pyramids, we believe that all those of medium size or larger are furnished with a myelin sheath; this has previously been stated by Flechsig, aided by his method of staining. This author has also remarked on a point that we have previously indicated in our preceding works, namely that the divisions are given off, as in the peripheral myelinated fibers, from the strangulations. If this peculiarity [is unlike that] in the peripheral nerve terminations, [then] there are myelin-free strangulations so elongated in the central fibers that several segments of the same nerve fiber will be taken for different myelinated fibers.

8. Nerve Plexuses of the Gray Matter

The intervals which occur between the nerve cells are filled up with a plexus of small varicose fibers. This plexus is made up of the following elements: first, collaterals of pyramids and of polymorphic cells; second, terminal arborizations of the sensory cells of Golgi; third, small collateral and terminal branches of certain cells with ascending axon; fourth, small collateral fibers arising from association fibers of the white matter; fifth, terminal arborizations of the association fibers and probably of other nerve fibers from more remote central nervous organs; sixth, collaterals and terminal arborizations of the fibers of the corpus callosum.

One can easily understand the enormous complexity of the intercellular nervous plexus of the gray matter and the absolute impossibility of being able to determine for every type of fiber the details of its terminations, that is to say, the number and nature of the nerve cells with which it is related. It is for this reason that we are obliged to envisage the plexus as an ensemble, in which we are bound to indicate which nerve fibers seem to predominate in each portion or layer of the cortex.

The first nervous plexus, extraordinarily rich, corresponds to the molecular layer. It includes, first, the axons of the multipolar and polygonal cells; second, the ascending axons arising from deep cells of the cortex; third, the small collateral fibers of the white matter.

The second plexus is poorer in fibers than the preceding and corresponds to the [layer of the] small pyramids. It contains, first, the ascending collaterals of the axons of the medium and small pyramids (perhaps also the ascending collaterals of the large pyramids); second, the collateral branches of ascending axons; third, the terminal arborizations of fiber branches coming from the white matter.

The third plexus (*external stria* of Baillarger) is very dense and very rich in myelinated fibers. It corresponds to the level of the large and medium pyramids and it is composed principally, first, of the gathering together of a great number of collaterals arising from axons of small and medium pyramids; second, of many ascending collaterals of the axons of the large pyramids.

The fourth plexus encloses the layer of the polymorphic cells and is made up of, first, the collaterals of the axons of the giant cells; second, the collaterals of the polymorphic cells (particularly in the deepest part); third, the terminal arborizations of the axons of the sensory cells of Golgi.

In certain regions of the cortex, the middle portion of this plexus, where it is probably coextensive with the greater part of the collaterals of the giant pyramids, shows itself to be formed by a great number of relatively thick myelinated fibers (*second stria* of Baillarger, *internal nervous plexus* of Krause).

Apart from the first, the various plexuses are not perfectly delimited either in the human cortex or in that of lower mammals; that is certainly true in the case of the small collateral branches, of which the plexuses are principally composed, [for these] do not occupy at all a fixed and separate place, those which are coming from one cellular layer being mixed up with those coming from other layers.

The Weigert preparations give a very incomplete idea of the plexuses of collaterals, because the innumerable varicose and terminal branches which surround the cells of the cortex lack myelin. The second plexus is weakly represented by delicate, oblique myelinated fibers in sections stained with Weigert's hematoxylin.

In small mammals—guinea pig, rat, mouse—the number of collaterals carrying a myelin sheath is much smaller than in man and the higher mammals, because the molecular layer and the [layers] of the small and medium pyramids do not possess certain myelinated fibers corresponding probably to the ascending axons and to those of the multipolar cells. Accordingly, therefore, it can be suggested that the less developed the cerebral cortex of a mammal, the less proportionately are the number of myelinated fibers.

We may be permitted to ask ourselves at this moment what purpose is served by the plexuses of collaterals. Basing our point of view on the hypothesis of transmission by contact, expounded above, we can conjecture that it is their purpose to establish a communication either between the cells of the same layer or between cells of different layers. The connection between the cells of the same layer may be established by contact with the parts of collaterals that are deprived of myelin. But the communication between the pyramidal cells of different layers is probably established by contact between the [cell] body and the larger dendritic branches, on the one hand, and the last small collateral branches arising from superimposed cells, on the other hand.[49]

Nevertheless, for communication at short distance, the intervention of reciprocal contacts between the basilar dendritic branches and the lateral branches of the [apical dendritic] shafts of the pyramids are, we think, equally probable.

White Matter

The upper region of the cerebral cortex of the mammals studied (psychomotor region) contains two very distinct layers of white matter, especially in the vicinity of the interhemispheric fissure: the superficial one, situated beneath the gray matter, is formed mainly by the *intrinsic*[A] *or association fibers* of the cortex; the other, deeper one is none other than the *corpus callosum.*

9. Intrinsic Fibers of the Cortex

We have studied these particularly in the white matter situated over the lateral ventricles.

These are the myelinated nerve fibers of different sizes which, in large part, come from the large and medium pyramids and the polymorphic cells.

As in man, the *intrinsic fibers* do not all travel in the same direction. In the vicinity of the interhemispheric fissure corresponding to the upper prominent angle of the hemispheres, there exists a large anteroposterior fascicle [that is] semilunar in section and with an inferior concavity. This fascicle thins progressively medially until it arrives adjacent to the fissure, at which point it contains few fibers (fig. 8, *c*) [*fig. 14*].

From its situation and direction, this fascicle of nerve fibers corresponds to that which is called in the human brain the *fasciculus arcuatus,* because just as in [the human], the fibers that form it commence in the frontal lobe and appear to terminate in the occipital lobe, traveling in an anteroposterior direction.

The axons of cells in the cortex become continuous with myelinated fibers in the fascicle, by means of a simple right-angled bend; but sometimes it happens that a fiber divides in the white matter in a T or a Y, and the branches of bifurcation travel in opposite directions.

The arcuate fascicle must be considered as an accumulation of arciform fibers which, after a certain anteroposterior trajectory, reascend to the cortex, in order to terminate in a free and extensive arborization. Fig. 8, *k* [*fig. 14*] shows one of these terminal fibers, which goes up bent at a right angle in order to enter the superimposed gray matter, and it arborizes in the vicinity of the interhemispheric fissure. It is, however, possible that there may also be in the said fascicle fibers extending over the whole length of the latter. In no case have we observed terminations *en pinceau,*[B] which Monakow supposes exist.

In the lateral parts of the hemispheres, the fibers of the white matter change direction and are for the most part disposed in a broad transverse and descending band, which further on goes through the top of the corpus callosum (fig. 15, *A*) [*fig. 21*]. This band, which we have designated by the name *transverse fascicle,* probably represents a system of association between the middle or parietal part of the cortex and the spheroidal[C] or inferior lobe. It can also contain some descending fibers that are going to the corona radiata.

The fibers which make up this fascicle arise from the large and medium pyramids, but also from certain cortical, polymorphic cells located in the underlying cortex. We do not know if the [axons of the] small pyramids also enter into its formation.

Also confirmed are the dispositions mentioned above concerning the continuation of the myelinated association fibers with the descending axons of the cortex. These are found with those fibers which are divided in a T and with those others which simply bend. Among the latter, it is seen that the descending fiber deviates horizontally to travel sometimes medially, sometimes laterally; this leads us to think that the transverse fascicle—and perhaps all the association fascicles—include fibers traveling in opposite directions, and whose endings can be made in very remote parts of the cortex.

When the axons descending from the cortex divide in a Y or a T in the transverse fascicle, one of the branches is directed medially and upward, to become confused with the fibers of the corpus callosum. Fig. 15 [*fig. 21*] represents a fragment of the lateral region of the cortex, in which the tracks of the callosal fibers and of the transverse fascicle are mingled. In fig. 7, *E* [*fig. 13*], we reproduce the axons that go to form the transverse fascicle, as can be demonstrated in successful sections.

Collaterals of the White Matter

The association fibers are furnished with very fine collaterals, which arise at a right angle and ascend to the cortex, where they end in free arborizations; they behave, therefore, on the whole like the collaterals of the white matter of the spinal cord.

These collaterals come from all regions of the white matter, but there are places in which they appear to be more abundant, or at least to be stained more constantly. This is so, for example, in the cortex bounding the interhemispheric fissure, where, as a result of the thinness of the cellular layers, it is easier to follow the complete course of the fibers (fig. 8, *r, s*) [*fig. 14*].

The [collaterals] arise here at a right angle from the myelinated fibers of the arcuate fasciculus, are directed upward, either obliquely or in a radial direction, toward the superficial part of the cortex; then they are resolved into various divergent branches [that are] varicose and particularly flexuous, and certain of which ramify and terminate in the molecular layer, while others remain in the subjacent gray layers. There exist collaterals which, upon arriving in the gray matter, divide into two or a larger number of divergent branches, whose zones of termination are very widespread (fig. 8, *r*) [*fig. 14*]. Finally, there are observed collaterals which, instead of ascending [into the overlying cortex], are directed laterally, crossing a part of the white matter to penetrate and be dispersed in the gray matter, but in more remote regions of the cortex.

In the other cerebral regions, we have not been able to follow the collaterals to the first layer, or even to the middle layers of the cortex; this probably results from the enormous thickness of the [cortex] and the extreme length of the course traveled. However, we have also noted the same ascending or oblique course of the collaterals and their tendency to ramify in the superimposed gray matter.

Sometimes certain very delicate collaterals appear to terminate, after a more or less horizontal course, in the white matter itself, in which, according to what we have said above, some nerve cells are always observed.

The existence of collaterals on the fibers of the white matter is a general feature of the structure of the brain. They are very abundant in the lateral stria of the *olfactory tract,* the long fibers of the cerebral peduncles, in their passage beneath the *thalamus,* also on the long projection fibers which cross the corpus striatum, the branches of bifurcation of the sensory roots of the trigeminal [nerve], the glossopharyngeal [nerve], and perhaps on all the mixed cerebral nerves,[50] finally on certain fibers of the anterior commissure and corpus callosum. We will return to this point in a later work.

Let us comment, in passing, on the remarkable analogy that exists between the association fibers of the brain and those of the white matter of the spinal cord. These are also composed of arciform fibers destined to unite distant compartments of the gray matter, and to establish equally, during their course, a communication by means of collaterals with the adjacent nerve cells. In addition, the fascicles of the spinal cord include, as in the white matter of the brain, the long fibers which serve to effect communication between very distant nervous centers.

10. Corpus Callosum (fig. 8) [fig. 14]

Transverse sections of the brain of the mouse, the rat, etc., demonstrate very convincingly the course of the callosal fibers, both in preparations made with the Golgi method and in those stained by the Weigert method.

In sections stained by the latter method, it is noticed that the callosal fibers are thin, medullated, and varicose; they run horizontally in the midline region, but they are descending and curvilinear in the lateral parts of the hemispheres.

In adult mammals, the callosal fibers are rarely impregnated with the silver chromate [method]; the good impregnations are obtained only in mice and rats of eight to ten days, that is to say, before the appearance of the myelin sheath. These fibers are very fine, varicose, and stained a light coffee color. With respect to their thickness, they are comparable to those of the collateral fibers of the axons of the large pyramids. Nevertheless, there are noticed among them some fibers [that are] a little larger, comparable to direct axons.

On examining the course of the callosal fibers in their passage at the level of the interhemispheric fissure, it is noticed that all conserve their parallel [arrangement], without generating branches or penetrating the gray matter bordering the said fissure. But when the callosal fibers arrive beneath the arcuate fascicle of the white matter (fig. 8, *g*) [*fig. 14*], it can be seen that some of them are curved to become ascending and penetrate the overlying gray matter. The great majority of these small fibers become detached at the level of the thickest part of the said fascicle.

In more lateral regions of the cortex beneath the transverse fascicle of the white matter, the thickness of the corpus callosum is reduced, [and its fibers are] mixed with the fibers of the [transverse fascicle], because [the latter] have the same direction and the same position as the small callosal fibers. During their whole course, the callosal fibers continue always to turn upward into the cortex, but in smaller numbers than in the region of the arcuate fasciculus. It is very interesting to note that the corpus callosum sends a far greater number of small fibers to where the gray cortex is thicker.

One fact that is clothed with a certain importance is that the callosal fibers give off collaterals that ascend in the gray matter and there terminate in free arborizations. The point where the collaterals are seen relatively frequently is the callosal region beneath the arcuate fascicle (fig. 8, *d'*) [*fig. 14*]. Frequently, the collateral branch and the parent trunk which follows the original transverse direction appear, because of their equal diameters, to result from a bifurcation (fig. 8, *d*) [*fig. 14*]. Given the hypothesis that the principal trunk arises from a cortical cell situated on the opposite side, it results that the callosal fibers probably enter into a relationship not only with a [homotopic] point, but also with various distant regions of the cerebral hemisphere of the opposite side.

The number of collaterals is very limited. Possibly each small callosal fiber is furnished with not more than two; commonly they have only one, which has frequently the significance of a branch of bifurcation. Overall, the precise number cannot be established, because of the impossibility, even with the aid of the best preparations, of following the complete course of one fiber.

Where are the sites of origin and termination of the callosal fibers? Are they direct axons or collateral fibers?

These questions are very difficult to resolve. In spite of all our efforts to obviate the difficulties of the problem, that is to say, in working for preference on very small and very young animals, we have not been able to fulfill our desideratum, namely to identify at the same time the origin and the termination of a single callosal fiber in a single well-impregnated thick section. Most of the preparations, particularly in the most lateral regions of the corpus callosum, do not permit one fiber to be followed over more than a very limited part of its trajectory; besides, one is faced rather frequently with the impossibility of determining if a fiber, traveling in the direction and in the plane of the corpus callosum, represents a true commissural fiber or an association fiber having the same course.

Nevertheless, we are going to reveal certain observed facts which have allowed us to form an opinion about the origin and termination of the callosal fibers.

Origin

At first, let us say that the origin appears to be double. There exist callosal fibers that are sim-

ple continuations of axons (direct callosals); then there are others which either represent collateral branches of projection or association axons, or bifurcated branches of the latter.

a. Direct Callosals. When the region of the arcuate fasciculus and contiguous parts in the cortex of the mouse of a few days are examined in good preparations, there can be observed a great number of callosal fibers which are bent at a right angle in order to ascend into the gray matter along a relatively straight course, and which terminate at the level of the [layers of] the medium or small pyramids. This termination is not very distinct; it is due to defective impregnation, because the ends of the fibers always appear as though cleanly cut. During their ascending trajectory and in the upper part of the cortex, these fibers give off various collaterals similar to those given off by the axons of pyramids (fig. 8, *g*) [*fig. 14*].

[Despite] the absence of a final arborization and the fact that the impregnation never goes beyond the level just mentioned, we still suppose that the similar callosal fibers are the direct axons of small pyramids and, possibly, in part of the medium [pyramids]. Let us add that the thickness of the axons of these latter cells coincides exactly with that of the ascending callosal fibers.

Meanwhile, we hasten to declare that, in spite of all our attempts, we have not been able to prove an actual continuity between the said cells and the callosal fibers, because, unfortunately, whenever the latter are well stained, the small and medium pyramids are not impregnated. It is a defect of the Golgi method, to stain in the superficial layers of the [blocks], on account of very severe fixation, fibers and cells different from those which are impregnated in the deeper layers.

In the lateral regions of the cortex, the same is observed, in that certain callosal fibers are led up to near the small pyramids; but it is noticed also that the very thin axons of certain polymorphic cells (coming off at a right angle) pass among the subjacent, small callosal fibers, in which they bear the same direction as the latter (fig. 15, *e*) [*fig. 21*].

Besides these direct origins, there is reason to suppose that certain callosal fibers may also contribute to the formation of the association bundles, leading to endings on nerve cells. It is near the arcuate fasciculus that we have noticed these arrangements, which are reproduced in fig. 8 [fig. 14]. Thus, the ascending callosal fibers, b,b, are continuous with an anteroposterior fiber of the said fasciculus. The fibers designated by c, besides being continuous with anteroposterior large association fibers, also emit a fine collateral, which descends directly and is reunited with the callosal fibers. This arrangement shows us that an axon can not only seek, by means of a commissural fiber, a communication with cells of the opposite hemisphere, but also can establish a relationship with distant cells of its own hemisphere.

b. Collateral Callosal Fibers. In all the regions of the supracallosal gray matter, but especially toward the lateral parts of the hemispheres, it is noticed that certain axons arising either from medium and large pyramids or from the polymorphic cells of the fourth layer divide into two fibers on arriving at the corpus callosum; a fine internal [fiber] is directed medially and is continuous with a fiber of the corpus callosum, and another external [fiber], usually larger, is continuous [laterally] sometimes with an association fiber, sometimes with a projection fiber.

The projection fibers are found represented in fig. 14 [fig. 20]. There it is seen that at the level where these fibers are traversing the anterior and lateral part of the corpus callosum, they give off a collateral to the latter, which cannot be distinguished either by its direction or by its thinness from the true callosal fibers. The collaterals and the fine branches of bifurcation arising from the axons of association cells have been represented in fig. 15, d [fig. 21]. This figure reproduces a very lateral [part of a] transverse section from the cortex of a mouse of a few days.

We cannot vouch in an absolute manner that all these collaterals or branches of bifurcation arrive, when mixed with callosal fibers, at the middle region of the commissure. [This is] because the enormous distance which exists between this part and the point of origin of the fibers is an insurmountable obstacle to their pursuit. But the double fact that these collaterals are directed medially among the callosal fibers and that they show the course and the varicose appearance [similar to] the latter makes their participation in the commissure probable.

It is very certain that we can regard as callosals the collaterals of certain axons of the arcuate fasciculus (fig. 8, e) [fig. 14], because there, fortunately, the proximity of the midline region permits [us] to follow them easily from their place of origin to or beyond the interhemispheric fissure. These collaterals arising from the anteroposterior fibers soon descend to the surface of the corpus callosum, and there they are bent and directed medially among the fibers of this structure.

Sometimes these callosal collaterals give off from their point of bending a very fine branch which is directed laterally, to become mixed up with the callosal fibers originating more laterally. A more complicated case is shown in fig. 8, f [fig. 14]; an axon of the cortex (probably [from] a large pyramid) descends, bifurcates within the arcuate fasciculus, and gives rise to a fiber of [the fasciculus] and to another, descending and destined for the corpus callosum; this latter, before it deviates horizontally, gives off a fine collateral directed laterally, losing itself in the peripheral portions of the callosal fibers.

Termination of Callosal Fibers

The termination of these fibers is more difficult to study than their origin. We think, however, that it may be reasonable to consider as their terminal fibers certain fine ascending fibers, distributed throughout the cerebral cortex and branching freely in its middle and deep layers.

The situation that the branches of arborization are in large part ascending and the fact that the parent fiber decreases in thickness from deep to superficial permit [us] to distinguish terminal callosal fibers from callosal fibers originating [in the same area].

We confess, nevertheless, that we must raise a few reservations about the termination of the callosal fibers, because we have only been able to find a small number which clearly show branches in the cortex; moreover, in certain cases, it is difficult to distinguish a badly impregnated callosal fiber of origin from another that is ending.

In summary, the callosal commissure seems to contain, first, the direct axons of cells probably belonging to all layers of the cortex, except the giant cells and cells of the superficial layer; second, the collateral branches or the branches of bifurcation of axons of the cells of projection or of association.

We think that only some of the cells of each cortical layer send collaterals or [direct] axons to the corpus callosum; these cells which warrant the name *callosals,* are mixed everywhere with cells that, from [the nature of] the terminations of their axons, may be designated by the name of *cells of association* or of *projection.*

If our point of view is confirmed by subsequent research, there will exist a striking analogy between the corpus callosum and the anterior commissure of the spinal cord; this includes, like the corpus callosum, direct axons arising from cells situated in all [parts of] the gray matter of the spinal cord, and the collaterals of fibers of the white matter, representing for the spinal cord the association and projection fibers of the brain.

The corpus callosum contains also certain fine, vertical, flexuous fibers, which appear to be continuous with certain anteroposterior fibers of the cerebral trigone situated below; after a variable course in the thickness of the corpus callosum, these fibers become anteroposterior, positioned among the upper layer of commissural fibers, and escape all observation (fig. 8, *n*) [*fig. 14*].

Callosal Cells

The upper surface of the corpus callosum contains nerve cells described by several authors, notably Golgi,[51] Giacomini,[52] and Blumenau.[53]

Our observations on this point are as yet very incomplete. We have succeeded only in staining certain cells and fibers of the internal longitudinal striae or nerves of Lancisi, the only striae that appear well developed in the small mammals (mouse, rat, rabbit, etc.). The lateral striae[D] are extremely rudimentary in these animals; they are mixed in with the gray matter of the hemispheres, as already observed by Blumenau.

In mice, rats, etc., the nerves of Lancisi are triangular in section, with the base of the triangle covering entirely the upper surface of the corpus callosum (fig. 13) [*fig. 19*]. In sections well impregnated with silver chromate, and also in those stained with the Weigert method, the nerves of Lancisi present three layers: a *superficial* or molecular, *c*; a *middle* or cellular, *d*;[E] and a *deep* or white matter, *b, e.*

The cells of the middle layer are ovoid or fusiform and oriented toward the surface. As in the second and third layers of the brain, their size increases with depth. The axon leaves from the internal or deep part of the cell body, while from the superficial part arise certain dendritic processes that branch repeatedly, and their varicose and flexuous branches extend over the whole thickness of the molecular layer. This arrangement is like the pyramidal cells of the brain, as pointed out by Giacomini and Blumenau. The axon runs in a descending direction; after a short course, it becomes anteroposterior and is continuous with a myelinated fiber of the deep layer of white matter. Sometimes the arriving axon is divided in a Y, giving off one fiber directed anteriorly and another directed posteriorly (figs. 13, *e*; 11, *e*) [*figs. 19, 17*].

The deep layer of nerve fibers is formed by the gathering together of multiple axons of cells situated above. The anteroposterior sections, when well impregnated, show that the fibers give off collateral fibers, which turn up to the molecular layer, where they terminate, also in the middle layer, in very rich and extremely varicose arborizations. In the deep and middle layers of the striae of Lancisi, besides the anteroposterior axons, there are found others [that are] more strongly varicose and flexuous (fig. 12, *c*) [*fig. 18*], and whose excessive number of small collateral branches quickly exhaust them. We believe that these fibers end freely in the thickness of the nerves [of Lancisi], in the [same] manner as the final branches of the axons of the sensory cells of Golgi. About the origin of these fibers we cannot say anything truly positive.

The molecular layer is the point of convergence of virtually all of the dendrites; it contains, like the molecular layer of the cortex, a great number of small fibers [that are] very del-

46

icate, flexuous, branched, and with a longitudinal or anteroposterior course. The rare nerve cells situated in this layer are fusiform and oriented in an anteroposterior direction (fig. 11, *g*) [*fig. 17*]. Regarding the origin and the course of the axons of these cells, which

resemble in their morphology the cells of the molecular layer of the cortex, our observations are not yet sufficient for us to give a firm opinion.

From what we have exposed, it follows, as remarked by Blumenau, that the longitudinal

---

Plate III. [*FIG. 17*] Fig. 11. Transverse section of the supracallosal gray [matter] in the brain of a newborn rabbit. The longitudinal striae appear united as a mass of gray matter. *a*, fibers of the corpus callosum; *b*, large anteroposterior fibers of the nerves of Lancisi; *c*, large cells of the deep region; *d*, molecular or superficial layer; *f*, axon of a superficial cell; *e*, that of a deep cell; *h*, fundus of the interhemispheric fissure.

[*FIG. 18*] Fig. 12. Longitudinal section of a nerve of Lancisi in a rat of fifteen days. [*a*] Large and deep cells continuous at *b* with anteroposterior fibers; *c*, anteroposterior fiber [that is] notably varicose and very rich in ascending collaterals; *d*, fine anteroposterior fibers in the molecular layer.

[*FIG. 19*] Fig. 13. Transverse section of the nerves of Lancisi of the brain of a mouse of fifteen days. *a*, callosal fibers; *b*, layer of the deep, anteroposterior fibers; *c*, molecular layer; *d*, elongated deep cell; *e*, descending axon terminating in a T in the white matter; *f*, collaterals of the fibers of the deep layer.

[*FIG. 20*] Fig. 14. Frontal section of the cortex of a mouse of eight days. Projection fibers going to the corpus striatum, after having traversed the corpus callosum. The collaterals of the axons of the pyramids are seen over their whole extent. *a*, fine projection fibers coming from the medium pyramids; *b*, other very thick fibers arising from giant pyramids; *c*, short projection fibers coming from the polymorphic cells of the fourth layer; *d*, callosal collateral arising from the thick projection fibers; *e*, branch of bifurcation for the corpus callosum, produced by a thin projection fiber; *g*, *f*, collaterals of projection fibers and of callosal fibers; *i*, fascicles traversing the corpus striatum; *h*, collaterals for the corpus striatum leaving the fine projection fibers; *s*, small, more superficial pyramids.

[*FIG. 21*] Fig. 15. Frontal section of the supraventricular region of the cortex in a mouse aged fifteen days. The layer of white matter shows the ensemble of callosal and projection fibers (transverse fascicle). The arrow indicates the direction of the corpus callosum or midline. *a*, axon of a small pyramid; *b*, another continuous with an association fiber; *c*, axon of a giant pyramid, directed laterally [and] probably constituting an association fiber; *d*, globular cells of the fourth layer terminating in a T in the white matter, the finer branch directed medially, like the fibers of the corpus callosum; *e*, association or callosal fiber (?) passing medially; *f*, another directed laterally; *g*, collaterals of the white matter; *h*, epithelial cells; *i*, external tuft of these cells; *j*, perivascular neuroglial cells; *k*, displaced epithelial cell; *n*, neuroglial cells of the molecular layer.

[*FIG. 22*] Fig. 16. Transverse section of the supraventricular region of the brain of a mouse aged fifteen days. In it are shown the large fibers coming from the white matter and arborizing in the gray matter. *a*, ascending fibers bifurcating at *b*; *c*, final varicose branches; *d*, very long collaterals of the said fibers; *e*, large pyramids; *f*, globular cells; *A*, white matter; *B*, molecular layer.

[*FIG. 23*] Fig. 17. Frontal section of the cortex of a mouse embryo close to term. *A*, white matter; *B*, molecular layer; *a*, giant pyramids; *b*, medium pyramids; *c*, small pyramids; *d*, rudimentary collaterals; *e*, axons without collaterals; *f*, fusiform cell of the molecular layer.

[*FIG. 24*] Fig. 18. A pyramid of the cortex of a newborn mouse. *a*, basilar dendritic branches in the course of development; *b*, embryonic collaterals of the axon; *c*, terminal nodule of the collaterals.

[*FIG. 25*] Fig. 19. Anteroposterior section of the cortex of a rabbit aged eight days. In it are found the epithelial cells and some embryonic neuroglial cells. *a*, [cell] body of the epithelial cells; *b*, bundle of callosal fibers cut in cross-section; *c*, radial varicose fibers; *d*, conical terminal branches at the free surface; *e*, displaced epithelial cells; *f*, embryonic neuroglial cells furnished with very varicose filaments.

striae are nothing other than a prolongation of the cortex, which have fundamentally the same structure but in which the various layers are shown to be simplified and reduced.

11. Projection Fibers

From all of the regions of the frontal lobe situated in front of and above the borders of the corpus callosum, and also from a part of the cortex covering the latter, descend nerve fibers that penetrate the corpus striatum and reunite in small fascicles (fig. 14, i) [fig. 20].

The origin of many of these fibers is easily determined in the mouse embryo or in the mouse of a few days, as shown in fig. 14 [fig. 20]. These fibers are none other than the direct axons of the pyramids (small, medium, and large) and of the polymorphic cells. We have not been able to determine if the most superficial row of small pyramids is involved; for the medium and the deeper small pyramids, we are certain, because we have succeeded frequently in following their axons to the corpus striatum itself.

All of the projection fibers during their trajectory through the cortex give off a large number of collaterals terminating in varicose tips in the thickness of the gray matter. When these fibers arrive in the plane of the corpus callosum, they change their course, tracing a kind of step laterally (fig. 14, m) [fig. 20] to descend soon after into the corpus striatum, with others coming sometimes from somewhat distant points of the cortex. In the thickness of the corpus striatum, some of them are seen giving off fine collaterals, terminating in varicose and very complicated arborizations, situated among the intrinsic [cellular] elements of this ganglion (fig. 14, h) [fig. 20].

From the point of view of their thickness, the projection fibers are divided into thick and thin [types], the latter coming generally from the medium pyramids, a, and certain polymorphic cells, while the former, b, arise from the large pyramids. We have many times been able to confirm de visu this double origin; it is why we cannot accept the opinion of Monakow, who claimed that it is only the large pyramids that give off projection fibers.

At the level of the corpus callosum, a great number of projection fibers, but not all of them, give off a thin collateral in this structure (fig. 14, d) [fig. 20]. When the axon is rather thin, this branch represents a branch of bifurcation, e.

Anterior Commissure

We have not been able to stain this commissure in a complete manner. However, in partial impregnations, we have verified that it is composed of fibers [that are] fine, parallel, and varicose, with an appearance and properties similar to the callosal fibers. Among the thin fibers, which are the more numerous, are found certain larger axons provided, near the gray cortex of the sphenoidal lobe, with some collaterals.

Growth of the [Cellular] Elements of the Cortex

We do not have the intention of embarking here on a study of the early phases of histogenesis of nervous tissue; this question has been the object of numerous works, among which may be cited those of Boll,[54] Eichorst,[55] Besser,[56] Kölliker,[57] Löwe,[58] Vignal,[59] and the more recent ones of His[60] and of Lenhossék.[61] We ourselves[62] have devoted a number of pages to the study of this interesting question. Here, we will limit ourselves to some observations on the subject of the growth and transformations in the cells of the cortex [that occur] after the differentiation of the nerve and epithelial cells is accomplished.

Epithelial Cells

Our researches confirm those of Golgi, Magini, and Falzacappa.

The epithelial cells belonging to the lateral regions of the hemispheres first extend laterally on traversing the corpus callosum; then they assume a radial direction and terminate at the cerebral surface (fig. 15, i) [fig. 21]. These changes in course are also very distinct in the cells that are situated at the medial surface (interhemispheric fissure) of the hemispheres. At first they are carried laterally, traversing the corpus callosum obliquely; then they turn medially and terminate with their tufts at the free surface of the median fissure.

surface in conical thickenings (fig. 29, *d*) [*fig. 25*].

The varicosities along the course of these radial fibers have received the attention of Magini,[63] who considers them to be superimposed nuclei. We are inclined to regard them instead as protoplasmic thickenings, because if they were nuclei, they would be more regular in their dimensions, and the silver chromate would not stain them any better than it stains the nuclei of the embryonic epithelial cells.

At any rate, therefore, the presence of these varicosities with the absence of branches of the radial fibers are precise characteristics, which permit [us] to draw a distinction between these epithelial processes and the axons of the pyramidal cells.

Toward the eighth day after birth, the epithelial fibers become noticeably thinner and the varicosities are partially effaced. After the twentieth day, the remaining part of the radial fiber becomes no more than a weak filament, almost devoid of granules. From this fact, we suppose that the external process of the epithelial cells disappears through atrophy; it, in effect, becomes no more than a short and branched appendage, not passing beyond the deeper layers of the corpus callosum. We have observed an analogous type of atrophy in the epithelial cells of the spinal cord.

The course and the disposition of the epithelial cells vary following the different radii of the brain. In the corpus callosum of the newborn animal, they are gathered together in little flexuous fascicles (fig. 19, *b, c*) [*fig. 25*], tending to separate in an arc to leave cylindrical transverse spaces, in which the large fascicles of the callosal fibers are positioned. The lower part of the fibers bristles with spines [that are] irregular, varicose, and extremely complicated.

The epithelial cells belonging to the lateral regions of the hemispheres first extend laterally on traversing the corpus callosum; then they assume a radial direction and terminate at the cerebral surface (fig. 15, *i*) [*fig. 21*]. These changes in course are also very distinct in the cells that are situated at the medial surface (interhemispheric fissure) of the hemispheres. At first they are carried laterally, traversing the corpus callosum obliquely; then

they turn medially and terminate with their tufts at the free surface of the median fissure.

It is not easy to determine the role fulfilled by these embryonic epithelial cells. We cannot share the opinion of Magini, who considers them to be the points of origin of the nerve cells. In effect, after the important work of His on the histogenesis of the spinal cord, it is very probable that all the nerve cells arise from *neuroblasts,* which this authority calls the piriform cells arising by the division of certain primitive spheroidal cells.[64]

We think very more likely a hypothesis which suggests that the radial cells represent a support or provisional scaffolding, destined to maintain the shape of the [nervous] centers during the development of the nerve cells.

With regard to the supposition of His that the epithelial cells serve to direct and to orient the development of the axons, this seems to us little probable insofar as it concerns the brain, because, in that organ, the radial fibers are finer than in the [spinal] cord, and they leave between themselves large spaces, which would permit the embryonic nerve fibers to travel without hindrance and in all directions. Besides, the question of why the axons in the course of their maturation are carried in a particular direction rather than in another is one of the more difficult and more obscure [questions] that histogenesis presents.

Neuroglia

The majority of authors who have recently studied the origin of the neuroglia, such as Duval,[65] Unger,[66] Löwe,[67] Ranvier,[68] Kölliker,[69] Gierke,[70] Merk,[71] Golgi,[72] Rauber,[73] Burckhardt,[74] Vignal,[75] Lahousse,[76] Magini,[77] Falzacappa,[78] Lachi,[79] and Lenhossék,[80] are unanimous in regarding the [neuroglial] cells as having an ectodermal derivation. Some, such as Vignal, Cajal, and Lachi, are inclined to think that certain neuroglial cells are none other than the epithelial cells of the ependyma, having migrated toward the periphery.

This migration is observed in its diverse phases, in studying the cortex of the fetus of the mouse or rat. Before the time of birth, it is recognized that all the epithelial cells are waiting at the medial aspect of the ventricular cavity; but some days after birth, it is already observed that some among them move away from the epithelium, their somata appearing at various levels of the corpus callosum and also in the thickness of the cortex (fig. 19, *e*) [*fig. 25*]. This would imply that by their ameboid contractions they go toward the periphery. We believe that these displaced cells are transformed, by a mechanism identical to that which transforms the epithelial cells of the embryonic [spinal] cord, into the cells of Deiters [neuroglial cells]. In effect, their bodies are shortened; from the periphery of the latter, as well as from the surfaces of the radial processes, arise varicose appendages, which come off at a right angle and go in all directions. Little by little, the radial shaft atrophies; it is transformed into a delicate filament, but more robust than the others and conserving the initial orientation; sometimes a process converging internally, representing the old epithelial [cell] body, is also observed. These converging processes show the origin and also the primitive orientation of the epithelial cells.

Regarding the cells lacking the radial orientation that are found in relation to the vessels in the adult brain, we think that they do not come from the epithelium but rather from the endothelial cells of the vessels, or from the connective [tissue] cells, which flatten when they penetrate the thickness of the cerebral cortex with the capillaries.

In fig. 15, *j* [*fig. 21*], we show that the first phase of the cells is spidery; the simple perivascular nipples blackened by the silver chromate are seen and are continuous, to all appearances, with the endothelial walls. The following phase, *o*, consists of one in which the swellings mentioned are successively stretched, becoming piriform and acquiring a degree of independence. This, however, is never complete, because a more or less thin and elongated bridge is always seen joining the spidery cell to the vascular wall. The neuroglial filaments, at first thick and varicose, become more and more thin and elongated, until they reach the adult form, easily recognized from the descriptions of Golgi and of Petrone.

It is impossible to expose in the first phases of the process a clear-cut border between the vascular endothelium and the neuroglial nipples. The use of other methods of staining does not furnish us with sufficiently clean results for determining the nature of the said swellings; it is because of this that we will not hazard to advance a supposition on this subject.

Apart from the two species of neuroglial cells mentioned, we remain doubtful about the question of whether knowledge exists regarding certain spidery cellular elements originating from the connective tissue of the pia mater, which are dispersed, for preference, throughout the white matter, according to what Lachi has supposed. Perhaps this relates, as indicated by Kölliker,[81] to certain undifferentiated ectodermal cells commencing their development after the differentiation of the neuroblasts and epithelial cells.

In summary, in the thickness of the gray and white matter of the cerebral cortex there exist two types of neuroglial or supporting cells. Those of epithelial origin are seen to be more or less radial and independent of the vessels; the others, of uncertain origin, appear around the vessels, into which they are inserted by means of a thick filament, as previously recognized by Golgi.

Nerve Cells

Fig. 17 [*fig. 23*] depicts a vertical transverse section of the cortex of a mouse embryo, two or three days before birth. It can be seen that the nerve cells are already completely identifiable in almost all the layers of the cortex, and that they show a very characteristic radial orientation.

Let us remark that, in the majority of the cells, the basal dendrites are absent, or are represented by large spines, while the radial or external dendrite is already very robust, flexuous, carrying the hollows for lodging the neighboring elements, and ending in the molecular layer in a tuft of thick branches [that are] short and strongly varicose. The cell body is ovoid, like that of the small cells of Ammon's horn, as already noted by Magini. In certain cells, frequently the more superficial of the pyramids, it appears fusiform and provided with two larger dendrites, the one which is descending providing the point of origin of the axon (fig. 17, *c*) [*fig. 23*].

The axons are relatively thick, more or less straight, possessing certain varicosities as indicated by Magini. Those of the medium and large pyramids can be followed easily to the white matter. However, what is very interesting about these axons is the absence of collaterals, or, if they are present, they are reduced to simple, short spines, arising at a right angle and ending in a varicosity (fig. 17, *d*) [*fig. 23*].

The pyramidal cells of the newborn mouse are always large (fig. 18) [*fig. 24*], and begin to be furnished with basilar dendrites, *a*, of some length, but rarely branches. The axon carries somewhat longer collaterals ending in a protoplasmic thickening. Let us observe, in fig. 18, *b*, *c* [*fig. 24*], that each collateral also arises from a swelling of the axon.

Finally, the mouse of eight to ten days shows already well-developed collaterals; they are at that time very favorable for the study of their course and their manner of termination (figs. 14, 15) [*figs. 20, 21*]. At this stage, the dendrites of the pyramids are already well developed; only those of the more superficial small pyramids preserve a certain fusiform and, therefore, somewhat embryonic appearance; they still possess more ascending branches [that are] very varicose and thickly branched.

Our experiences relative to the nerve cells of the first layer are still very incomplete. We can only say that these elements are already in large part differentiated in the cortex of the mouse embryo near to term (fig. 17, *f*) [*fig. 23*]; they are often fusiform and oriented anteroposteriorly.

In the brain of the newborn rat, there are also found in the molecular layer certain fusiform cells, with one of the horizontal processes having the appearance of an axon; but the very embryonic appearance of these cells does not allow [us] to establish conclusively their identity with those of the adult or nearly adult cortex.

General Conclusions

1. The cerebral cortex of small mammals possesses the same fundamental structure as that of the human brain.
2. The first cerebral layer possesses special nerve cells, characterized principally in that they present more than one axon.
3. To the first cerebral layer come to be arborized, first, the axons of the special

cells situated in its thickness; second, the axons of deep cells of the cortex; third, the collateral fibers coming from myelinated axons of the white matter.

4. The axons of pyramids and those of spheroidal cells of the fourth layer give rise, in certain regions of the brain, to the projection fibers (pyramidal tracts and fibers of the corona radiata); in certain other regions, they are continuous with association fibers.
5. The callosal fibers are either the collaterals of association and projection fibers or the direct axons of the small cells of the cortex. These cells seem to us to be scattered through diverse parts of the gray matter, and commissural and projection cells are mixed without order.
6. It is not possible to distinguish, either by their positions or by their special morphological characteristics, the cells with an axon forming an association fiber [from] the cells with an axon deviating either as a projection fiber or as a commissural fiber. The direction and the distinct termination of each axon appear to depend especially on the region of the cortex in which the cell of origin is located. Thus, there are regions in which the majority of the cells seem to belong to the class of association cells and callosal cells, while certain other regions contain for preference the projection cells.
7. All the axons coming from association cells and callosal cells, as well as their collaterals, terminate in the gray matter, by means of small branches or arborizations [that are] free and intercellular. The collaterals of the axons of the pyramids terminate in varicose, nonbranched ends.
8. The white matter of the brain (corpus callosum, association fibers, etc.) possesses just as in the spinal cord, collateral fibers which ascend into the cortex and there terminate freely in varicose arborizations.
9. In the cortex, there exist nerve fibers, sometimes large, sometimes of medium thickness, coming from the white matter and branching freely in the gray matter. The fibers of medium thickness seem to

be the terminations of association fibers. But, in regard to the thicker ones, we do not know their origin; perhaps they are axons coming from the cerebellum or from other distant components of the nervous system.

10. In the brain, as in the spinal cord, axons are found dividing in a Y or in a T on their arrival in the white matter. An identical disposition is also observed in the sensory fibers of the trigeminal [nerve], [vagus nerve], etc., where the ascending and descending branches resulting from the bifurcation also give off numerous collaterals.

11. It results from our researches on the connections of the nerve cells of the brain that neither in the embryo nor in the adult do anastomoses exist between nerve fibers of the gray matter. It is thus very likely that the transmission of the nervous excitation between the cells of different layers of the cortex is made by contact either between the dendrites alone or between these and the final branches or collaterals of the axons.

12. The cortex of lower animals appears to be particularly distinguished from the cerebral cortex of man, first, in that its cells are less large, less numerous, and less rich in primary and secondary dendritic branches; second, in that its axons present more rare collaterals; third, in that these in general lack myelin, are more limited in length, and have less abundant branches.

13. The more remote in the ontogeny of the brain of mammals, the more the dendrites and the collaterals of axons in the cortex become rare and short. The same fact is seen on descending the animal scale. To be convinced of this, it is sufficient to compare the Purkinje cells of the cerebellum in man, mouse, bird, and fish. There will be seen a successive diminution in the number of secondary branches of the dendrites and in the collateral branches of the axons. As much can be said, with certain differences, about all the other nervous organs: cerebral cortex, optic lobe, retina, etc.

As a final synthesis, it can be affirmed that the human brain [must] owe the superiority of its actions, in large part, not only to the considerable number of its cells but above all to the extraordinary richness of its means of association, that is to say, the collaterals of the axons, the dendritic branches, etc.

Cajal's Notes

1. A part of this work was published in Spanish: Textura de las circunvoluciones cerebrales de los mamiferos inferiores, 10 December 1890. And: Sobre la existencia de colaterales y bifurcaciones en las fibras de la sustancia blanca del cerebro, 20 December 1890.

2. Golgi, Sulla fina anatomia degli organi centrali del sistema nervoso, Milano, 1885.

3. Tartuferi, Sull'anatomia microscopica delle eminenze bigemine dell'uomo e degli altri mammiferi, Gazzetta Med. Italiana, Ser. VIII, Vol. III, 1877.

4. Mondino, Ricerche macro-microscopische sul centri nervosi, Torino, 1887.

5. Fusari, Untersuchungen über die feinere Anatomie des Gehirnes der Teleostier, Intern. Monatsschrift f. Anat. u. Physiol., 1887.

6. Nansen, The Structure and Combination of the Histological Elements of the Central Nervous System, Bergen, 1887.

7. Kölliker, Die Untersuchungen von Golgi über den feineren Bau des centralen Nervensystems, Anatom. Anz. II, p. 480, 1887.

8. Toldt and Kahler, Lehrbuch der Gewebelehre, 3rd edition, 1888.

9. Obersteiner, Anleitung beim Studium des Baues der nervösen Centralorganen, Wien, 1888.

10. Petrone, Intorno allo studio della struttura della nevroglia dei centri nervosi cerebrospinali, Preliminary note, Gaz. degli Ospitali, 1887.

11. Marchi, Sulla fina struttura dei corpi striati e dei talami ottici, Rev. Speriment. di Frenatr. XII, 1887.

12. Magini, Nevroglia e cellule nervose cerebrali nei feti, Atti dell XII. Congresso Medico, Pavia, 1888.

13. Falzacappa, Genesi della cellula specifica nervosa e intima struttura del sistema centrale nervoso degli uccelli, Bolet della Societa di Naturalist in Napoli, Ser. I, Vol. II, 1888.

14. Flechsig, Ueber eine neue Farbungsmethode des centraler Nervensystems, etc., Arch. f. Anat. u Physiol. (Physiol. Abtheilung, 5 and 6, 1889).

15. Edinger, Zwölf Vorlesungen über den Bau der nervösen Centralorgane, etc., 2nd edition, Leipzig, 1889.

16. His, Histogenese und Zusammenhang der Nervenelemente, Ref. in der Anat. Section des Internat. Med. Congresses zu Berlin, Session of 7 August 1890.

17. Ramón y Cajal, Estructura de los centros nerviosos de las aves, Rev. Trim. de Histología, No. 1, 1888. Sobre las fibras nerviosas de la capa molecular del cerebelo, Rev. Trim. de Histología, no. 2, 1888.

18. Flechsig, Ueber eine neue Farbungsmethode des centralen Nervensystems, etc., *Bericht d. Kais. Sachs. Gesellsch. d. Wissensch. Math. Phys. Clas.,* Stuttgart, 1889.

19. Martinotti, Beitrag zum Studium der Hirnrinde und dem centralen Ursprung der Nerven, *Interna. Monats. f. Anat. u. Physiol.,* Vol. VII, 1890.

20. Forel, Einige hirnanatomische Betrachtungen und Ergebnisse, *Arch f. Psychiatr.,* [1887] Vol. XVIII.

21. Loc. cit., and Zur Geschichte des menschlichen Rückenmarkes u. der Nervenwurzeln, *Abhandl d. Math. Phys. Class. d. Königl. Sächsischen Gesellsch. d. Wissensch.,* Vol. XIII, no. VI, 1886.

22. Kölliker, Zur Anatomie des centralen Nervensystems, Das Rückenmark, *Zeitschrift f. Wissenschaf. Zool.,* 1890.

23. Ramón y Cajal, Sur la morphologie et les connexions des éléments de la rétine des oiseaux, *Anat. Anz.,* no. 4, 18[89]. And also: Sur l'origine et la direction des prolongations nerveuses de la couche moléculaire du cervelet, *Intern. Monatssch. f. Anat. u. Physiol.,* Vol. VI, 1889.

24. Retzius, Zur Kenntnis des Nervensystems der Crustaceen, *Biol. Unters., Neue Folge* I, Stockholm, 1890.

25. Martinotti, Su alcuni migloramenti della tecnica della reazione al nitrato d'argento, etc., *Ann. di Freniatria,* Vol. I, 188[7].

26. Sehrwald, Zur Technik der Golgischen Färbung, *Zeitschr. f. Wiss. Mikroskopie,* Vol. VI, 1889, p. 443.

27. The addition to the mixture of one or two drops of a concentrated solution of chromic acid has often given us very good results concerning the staining of small collateral fibers. In the spinal cord this modification is advantageous, above all when cutting sections of the cord with the vertebral column (small mammals); in effect, the inorganic material of the bone is dissolved by the chromic acid. Otherwise, the acid accelerates the fixation.

28. Sur l'origine et la direction des prolongations nerveuses de la couche moléculaire du cervelet, *Intern. Monatsschr. f. Anat. u. Phys.,* Vol. VI, 1889. And: Sur l'origine et les ramifications des fibres nerveuses de la moelle embryonnaire, *Anat. Anz.,* nos. 3 and 4, 1890.

29. Greppin, Weiterer Beitrag zur Kenntniss der Golgischen Untersuchungsmethode des centralen Nervensystems, *Archiv. f. Anat. u. Physiol.; Suppl. Bd,,* 1889, p. 55.

30. Obregia, Fixirungsmethode der Golgi'schen Präparate des centralen Nervensystems, *Virch. Archiv.* CXXII, 1890, p. 387.

31. Meynert, Vom Gehirne der Säugethiere, *Strickers Handbuch der Lehre von den Geweben,* [1872] Vol. 2, pp. 694, 808. And also: Skizze des menschlichen Grosshirnstammes nach seiner Aussenform und seinen innern Bau, *Arch. f. Psychiatr.,* Vol. IV, 1874.

32. Stieda, Studien über das centrale Nervensystem der Vögel und Säugethiere, *Zeitschr. f. Wiss. Zool.,* XIX, 1868.

33. Henle, *Handbuch der Nervenlehre des Menschen,* 1879.

34. Boll, Die Histiologie und Histiogenese der nervösen Centralorgane, *Archiv. f. Psychiat.* (Westphal), Vol. IV, 1874.

35. Schwalbe, *Lehrbuch der Neurologie,* 1881.

36. Krause, *Allgemeine u. mikroscopische Anatomie,* 1876.

37. Golgi, Sulla fina anatomia degli organi centrali del sistema nervoso, Milano, 1886.

38. Kölliker, *Handbuch der Gewebelehre,* 1852.

39. Exner, Zur Kenntniss vom feineren Bau der Grosshirnrinde, *Sitzungsber. d. Kais. Akad. der Wissensch. in Wien,* 1881.

40. Obersteiner, *Anleitung beim Studium des Baues der nervösen Centralorgane,* etc., Wien, 1888.

41. Edinger, *Zwölf Vorlesungen über den Bau der nervösen Centralogane,* etc., 2nd edition, 1889.

42. Martinotti, Beitrag zum Studium der Hirnrinde, etc., *Intern. Monatschr. f. Anatom. u. Physiol.,* Vol. VII, 1890.

43. The existence of supernumerary axons is not an isolated fact in science. We have found these, although less commonly, on certain cells of large size in the optic lobe of birds. These cellular processes have the same significance as those recently mentioned by Retzius in the ganglia of invertebrates.

44. Ramón y Cajal, Conexión general de los elementos nerviosos, *La Medicina Práctica,* 1889. A propos de certains éléments bipolaires du cervelet avec quelques détails nouveaux sur l'évolution des fibres cérébelleuses, *Intern. Monatsschr. f. Anat. u. Physiol.,* Vol. VII, 1890.

45. Ramón y Cajal, Sobre la existencia de células nerviosas especiales en la primera capa de la corteza cerebral, *Gac. Méd. Catalana,* December 1890.

46. Martinotti, Su alcuni migloramenti della tecnica della reazione al nitrato d'argento, etc., *Annali di Freniatria,* Vol. I, 188[7], p. 34.

47. Mondino is also inclined to accept these anastomoses. See: Richerche macro e microscopiche sui centri nervosi, Torino, 1887.

48. Monakow, Rôle des diverses couches des cellules ganglionnaires dans le gyrus sigmoïde du chat, *Arch. des Scien. Phys. et Nat.* XX, 10 October 1888.

49. According to the ideas of His, the contacts could take place by means of a conductive material. This is no other than the granular and varicose-appearing layer which seems to surround the last small nerve branches, giving a greater thickness to them.

50. See our work: Sobre la existencia de bifurcaciones y colaterales en los nervios sensitivos craneales y substancia blanca del cerebro, *Gaz. San.,* 10 April 1891.

51. Loc. cit. p. [132].

52. Giacomini, *Giornale della R. Accademia de Medicina di Torino,* November and December 1883.

53. Blumenau, Zur Entwicklungsgeschichte und feineren Anatomie des Hirnbalkens, *Arch. f. Mikroskop. Anat.,* Vol. XXXVII, 189[1].

54. Boll, Die Histologie und Histiogenese der nervösen Centralorgane, *Arch. f. Psychiatr.* (Westphal), Vol. IV, 1874.

55. Eichorst, Ueber die Entwickelung des menschlichen Rückenmarkes und seiner Formelemente, *Virchows Archiv.,* Vol. LXIV, 1875.

56. Besser, Zur Histogenese der nervösen Elementantheile in den Cerebralorganen des neugeborenen Menschen, *Virchows Archiv.*, Vol. XXXVI, 1866.

57. Kölliker, *Embryologie*, etc., Paris, 1882.

58. Löwe, *Beiträge zur Anatomie und zur Entwickelungsgeschichte des Nervensystems, etc.*, Vol. I. *Die Morphogenesis des centralen Nervensystems*, Berlin, 1880.

59. Vignal, Sur le développement des éléments de la moelle des mammifères, *Archives d. Physiol.* 7, 188[4]. And: Recherches sur le développement de la substance corticale du cerveau et du cervelet, *Archives d. Physiologie*, etc., 1888.

60. His, loc. cit. Also see: Die Neuroblasten und deren Entstehung in embryonalen Mark, Vol. XV, *Abhandl. d. Mathem. Phys. Class. d. Königl. Sach. Gesellsch. d. Wissensch*, Leipzig, 1889.

61. Lenhossék, Zur ersten Entstehung der Nervenzellen und Nervenfasern beim Vögelembryo, *Mittheilungen a. dem Anat. Institut im Vesalianum in Basel*, 189[1]. And: Die Entwickelung der Ganglienanlagen bei dem menschlichen Embryo, *Arch. f. Anat. u. Physiol. Anat. Abtheilung*, 1891.

62. Ramón y Cajal, A quelle époque apparaissent les expansions des cellules nerveuses de la moelle épinière du poulet? *Anat. Anzeiger*, nos. 21 and 22, 1890.

63. Loc. cit.

64. After we had seen in the embryonic [spinal] cord of the chicken certain nerve cells having the form and situation of epithelial cells, we had thought that the epithelium enclosing the central canal, in certain cases, could give rise to true nerve cells. However, we now admit that one is dealing there with certain neuroblasts which, being placed among the epithelial cells, from the time of their transformation into nerve cells, had kept a certain radial orientation and an elongated [cell] body, bordering the spinal canal with its base.

65. Duval, Sur le sinus rhomboïdal des oiseaux, *Gaz. Méd. de Paris*, no. 34. And also: Recherches sur le sinus rhomboïdal des oiseaux et sur la névroglie périépendymaire, *Journ. de l'Anat. et de la Physiol.*, 1877.

66. Unger, Untersuchungen über die Entwickelung des cerebralen Nervengewebe, *Sitzungsb. d. Kais. Akad. d. Wissensch. zu Wien*, Vol. LXXX, 18[80].

67. Loc. cit.

68. Ranvier, De la névroglie, *Arch. de Physiol. Norm. et Pathol.*, Series III, Vol. I, no. 2, 1883.

69. Kölliker, loc. cit. And also: Das Rückenmark, *Zeitschr. f. Wissensch. Zool.*, LI, I, 1890.

70. Gierke, Die Stützsubstanz des Centralnervensystems, *Arch. f. Mikros. Anat.*, Vols. XXV and XXVI, 1885.

71. Merk, Die Mitosen im Centralnervensystem, *Denkschriften d. Wiener Akad.*, Vol. LIII, 1887.

72. Op. cit.

73. Rauber, Die Kerntheilungsfiguren im Medullarrohr der Wirbelthiere, *Arch. f. Mik. Anat.*, Vol. XXVI, 1886.

74. Burckhardt, Histologische Untersuchungen am Rückenmark der Tritonen, *Arch. f. Mik. Anat.*, Vol. XXXIV, Pt. I, 1889.

75. Op. cit.

76. Lahousse, La cellule nerveuse et la névroglie, *Anat. Anzeiger*, 1886, p. 5.

77. Op. cit.

78. Op. cit.

79. Lachi, Contributo alla istogenesi della nevroglia nel midollo spinale del pollo, Pisa, 189[1].

80. Lenhossék, Zur Kenntniss der ersten Entstehung der Nervenzellen und Nervenfasern beim Vogelembryo, *Archiv. f. Anat. und Physiologie, Anat. Abtheilung*, 189[1].

81. Kölliker, Zur feineren Anatomie des centralen Nervensystems, Das Rückenmark, *Zeitschr. f. Wissensch. Zool.*, Vol. LI, Pt. I, 1890.

Editors' Notes

A. Cajal says "fibres propres."

B. i.e., like a paintbrush.

C. Probably sphenoidal.

D. Presumably, some of the longitudinal association bundles of the cerebral hemisphere.

E. The text incorrectly says *j*.

6

Structure of the Inferior Occipital Cortex of the Small Mammals

[*Anales de la Sociedad Española de Historia Natural* 22:115–125, 1893]

As is well known, not all [areas] of the cerebral cortex exhibit exactly the same structure. It was some time ago that neurologists first mentioned in the brains of the higher mammals certain regions in which [there are] considerable variations, either in the number of layers or in the volume and abundance of cells and nerve fibers.

Such cortical territories, in the mammals of large size, would be joined together by means of gentle structural transitions, whereas in the rabbit and the rest of the mammals with smooth cerebral cortex, if we are to believe Bevan Lewis,[1] they would be accurately and rigidly separated.

Among the cortical territories whose texture differs from that of the psychomotor region [is] the gray matter of the cuneus and the surroundings of the *calcarine fissure*, where, as already indicated by Gennari and Vicq d'Azyr, the cortex appears striped with concentric white lines. Broca[2] has confirmed the presence of the intermediate white layer, and has shown that it is a constant feature of the inferior plane of the occipital lobule.

In the mammals of small size, such as the rabbit, guinea pig, and rat (on which our observations have preferentially fallen), the said region is extremely long and extensive, extending through almost the whole inferior occipital cortex, that is to say, through the extensive band of gray matter situated behind the subiculum. The white line of Vicq d'Azyr is observed with the naked eye, showing up distinctly in the sections impregnated with the hematoxylin of Weigert-Pal.

In man, Meynert,[3] Schwalbe,[4] and Obersteiner,[5] among others, have carefully described this cortical region. Meynert, for example, mentions eight concentric layers, among which are included his five classic layers of the cortex, which are increased by a new layer of giant pyramidal cells (sixth layer or [layer] of solitary large cells) and by two layers of nuclei or small cells.

The description of Meynert, accepted by Hugenin, Obersteiner, etc., is so difficult to harmonize with the results of our recent investigations in the small mammals that we are obliged for the present to dispense with it until we have been able to study in detail the said region in brains with gyri and especially in the human brain. It is, anyway, undoubted that the imperfect methods used by the mentioned authorities have led them into grave mistakes. Thus, [according] to Obersteiner, the molecular layer is extremely thin [in man] but when it occurs in the rabbit and guinea pig it is much thicker than any other part of the cortex. The intermediate white layer, in the opinion of Meynert, corresponds to layer fourth, of the rare giant cells, fifth, of the nuclei, and sixth of the neuroglia and solitary giant cells, [but] according to our observations, it lies at the level of the third, that is to say, in the layer of the small pyramids.

The most notable changes that the inferior occipital region shows in comparison with the typical cortex [are found] in the molecular layer and in the second and third layers.

The molecular layer stands out for its great thickness and because among its cells the multipolar fusiform and triangular [cells] notably abound. Such cells are also impregnated easier than in other regions of the cortex, which has allowed us to extend, with some new data, the story of such enigmatic cells.

The second layer (or [layer] of the small pyramids in other regions of the cortex) appears substituted by several strata of very tiny fusiform cells that as far as we know are not found in any other cortical region.

Here are the layers of the occipital cortical region: first, molecular; second, layer of the vertical fusiform cells; third, middle fibrillar layer or layer of small pyramids; fourth, layer of large pyramids; fifth, layer of polymorphic cells.

1. Molecular Layer

As we have already said, it is very thick and contains an extraordinary amount of small nerve fibers. It is possible to establish in it a subdivision in two sublayers: external, poor in medullated fibers and rich in polygonal cells; internal, abundant in medullated fibers and provided with numerous fusiform cells.

Internal Sublayer

a. Cells

Almost all are of the multipolar fusiform type, lying horizontally in proximity to the layer of the vertical fusiform [cells]. The polar branches are of great length and have the notable peculiarity of giving off, in the manner of collaterals, very fine horizontally directed threads, ramified at right angles and with all the characteristics of axons. The thick shafts, with the appearance of dendrites, after a very long trajectory also end up by transforming into fibers with the appearance of axons (figs. 1, 2) [*figs. 26, 27*].

To expose briefly what our new investigations show with regard to the multipolar cells of the cerebrum, [we can do] nothing better than copy here the main propositions of the work read last December before the Spanish Natural History Society. To sum up the modifications made of our old opinion, it is sufficient to remember that we had been able previously to follow only the fine fibers, with the appearance of axons, of the multipolar cells, to their termination; the thick polar appendages were not possible [to follow] except for a relatively short distance, on account of which we had not succeeded in revealing all of their characteristics.[A]

1. If the thick, more or less horizontal processes that emerge either from the poles or from the angles of these cells are followed to their ends, it is observed that they gradually acquire the characteristics of axons, because they become notably thin, varicose, and give off fine collaterals at a right angle. The horizontal extent of such processes is in many cases not less than a millimeter, so that it is very difficult for a single section to show the complete arborizations of the polar processes and of their fine collaterals. On occasion, the ascending branches originating at right angles from the main shafts are divided and subdivided, acquiring in turn the appearance of small axonal fibers, with the secondary and tertiary small branches running in a more or less horizontal direction. Some ascending collateral processes seem to terminate at the very cerebral surface by two or three short little branches. We cannot be sure, however, that such a disposition is not due to an incomplete impregnation (fig. 2, *d*) [*fig. 27*].

2. The form of the special cells of the first cerebral layer is often elongated and spindle-shaped, but those of a triangular or starlike configuration also abound; [these have] several

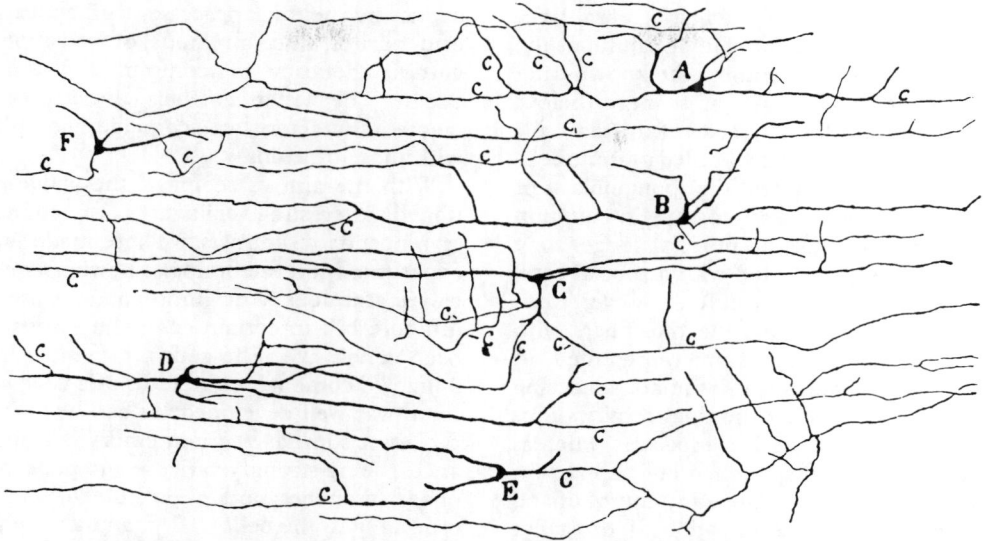

[*FIG. 26*]   Fig. 1. Several cells of the first or molecular layer of the cortex of the rabbit of eight days, found in different regions of the cerebrum. *A*, cells whose two polar branches acquire an appearance of axons at a certain distance from their origins; *B, C, D, E*, analogous cells although with somewhat different forms. Note: the letter *c* labels the small branches whose characteristics coincide completely with axons. Toward the upper part of the figure is the cerebral surface.

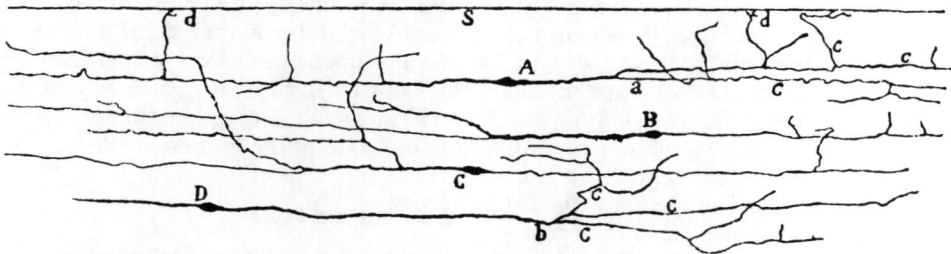

[*FIG. 27*]   Fig. 2. Horizontal fusiform cells of the first cerebral layer of the rabbit of eight days. Method of Golgi, double [impregnation]. *A*, cell whose polar processes gradually acquire the appearance of axons; *B, C, D*, other cellular types. The letter *c* labels the processes that showed all the characteristics of axons, it being probable that the other processes, if they could have been followed sufficiently, would have also shown analogous characteristics at their ends.

radial [branches] which are directed more or less parallel to the free surface.

3. The cells about which we are talking lie in all [cortical] regions. The region of the olfactory lobule, the gyrus of Ammon's horn (*subiculum*), the occipital lobule, etc., contain them in variable proportions, as well as the psychomotor region of the frontal lobe. In the cortex of the mammals of small size (rabbit, guinea pig), the mentioned fusiform cells not only adopt an anteroposterior orientation but all other orientations except that perpendicular to the cortex. Hence the extreme difficulty of obtaining complete cells in vertical sections.

4. In the embryonic period, the contrast between the thick and fine processes is little noticeable, as all of them appear varicose and have the appearance of thick axons (fetal brain of cow, dog, rabbit).

5. From [what has been] exposed, it follows

that the special cells of the first cerebral layer constitute an original type [that cannot at the moment be classified among] the known categories of nerve cells. We must, nevertheless, declare that the characteristics of the said cells approach somewhat the so-called granule cells of the olfactory bulb and the spongioblasts of the retina, since all of them have in common the lack of a fine [axonal process], longer than the others and connected with a special category of nerve cells. They differ, however, in an important characteristic: the fine fibers with the appearance of axons are represented, in certain spongioblasts (our radiate amacrine cells of the retina), by the final ramifications of one or several [dendritic] processes, whereas in the cerebral cells, such pseudaxonal filaments sometimes arise along the course of and at others from the termination of the polar [dendritic] shafts.

6. What is interesting, however, is the observation that all these cells (special cells of the cerebral first layer, spongioblasts, etc.) are ramified precisely among the dendritic shafts of the underlying cells and at the level of the plexiform layers (molecular layers of the authors), in which there exists an [axodendritic] connection or articulation.[B]

Figs. 1 and 2 [figs. 26, 27] show some special cells of the molecular layer found in the [brain] of the rabbit of four to fifteen days. In fig. 2 [fig. 27], we have represented the ones that have a spindle shape, and in fig. 1 [fig. 26] those that have other shapes, such as triangular and stellate. In some of these cells, it is seen that there does not exist an exact separation between the fine processes with appearance of axons and the thick processes with appearance of dendrites, since all [kinds] of transitions regarding delicacy of contour and thinness occur. The letter c labels those processes whose characteristics coincide completely with those of axons.

With the aim of seeing if the above-mentioned interesting cells are also found in [gyrencephalic] animals, we have made several experiments on the brains of newborn or fetal calves and dogs. The impregnations are very difficult, but in certain cases the results have been conclusive. The cells represented in fig. 3 [fig. 28] come from the fetus of a cow whose brain was well developed. As can be seen, the processes still have certain embryonic appearances, being strongly varicose and poor in secondary branches; but it is possible to recognize, especially in the cells a, b, g, and e,[C] the types described in the common rabbit. Undoubtedly, Retzius has also seen some of these cells in the human brain.[6]

b. Fibers

The internal sublayer is the point of termination of numerous ascending fibers which, in ramifying, form a very dense plexus around the multipolar cells. Many of these fibers are thick, run horizontally, and possess a thick myelin sheath. Later we will see what is the main origin of these fibers.

External Sublayer

It also contains numerous small ramified nerve fibers which constitute a dense felt in whose meshes are lodged some sensory nerve cells of

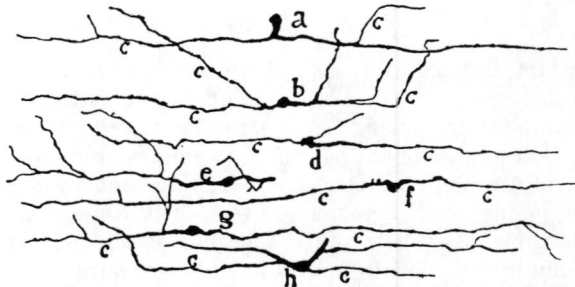

[FIG. 28] Fig. 3. Special cells of the first cerebral layer of the fetus of a cow. The pseudaxonal or fine processes are labeled with a c.

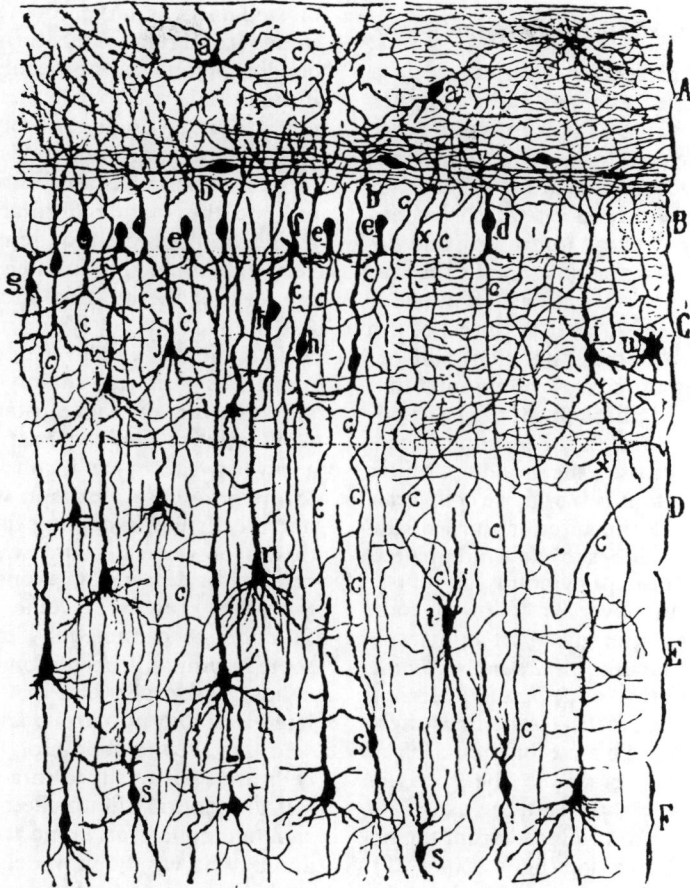

[*FIG. 29*]   Fig. 4. Section of the inferior occipital cortex of the rabbit of eight days. Method of Golgi, double [impregnation]. *A*, molecular layer; *B*, layer of the fusiform cells; *C*, layer of the middle medullated fibers; *D*, layer of the medium pyramids; *E*, layer of the large pyramids; *F*, layer of the polymorphic cells; *a*, stellate cells of the first cerebral layer; *b*, fusiform or special cells of the cortex; *d*, vertical fusiform [cells]; *f*, small pyramid; *e*, piriform cell; *g*, cell with ascending axon; *h*, vertical fusiform [cell] of the third layer; *j*, small pyramid; *r*, giant pyramid; *s*, cells with ascending axon.

Golgi (second type of the cells of the molecular layer). These cells are stellate and are irregularly scattered in the thickness of the external sublayer; their dendrites are repeatedly divided and subdivided, showing a toothed and irregular appearance that contrasts with the smoothness of the processes of the multipolar cells; their axons run parallel to the cortex, and at a short distance each is resolved into a complicated terminal arborization (fig. 4, *a*) [*fig. 29*], whose little varicose branches do not go beyond the frontiers of the molecular layer.

Some multipolar cells can also be found in this sublayer, although only occasionally. In the brain of rabbit, rat, and guinea pig, the said sublayer is almost bereft of medullated fibers.

In summary, the molecular layer of the occipital region exhibits the fundamental features of the typical cortex. In it are found sensory cells of Golgi, multipolar cells, the terminal tufts of the pyramids, and an infinite number of small nerve fibers originating either from intrinsic ganglion cells or from ascending axons.

[2.] Layer of the Vertical Fusiform Cells

Underneath the molecular layer, there is a band of diminutive cells very close together [and] arranged in three or four irregular rows. These cells are characterized by their vertically elongated ovoid somata from whose poles arise two dendrites: *ascending,* which reaches the molecular layer where it ramifies; and *descending,* which forms a horizontal arborization of three or four branches at the moment that it reaches the third layer or [layer] of the middle medullated fibers. The axon is of extraordinary thinness (perhaps the thinnest that is known), and it originates from the descending dendrite at the level of the terminal arborization; [it then] crosses the middle fibrillar layer, in which it leaves two or three collaterals and goes down into the inferior third of the cortex. Perhaps it reaches to the white matter, like the axon of the small pyramids, but in our preparations it can never be followed completely. Sometimes, after giving off a thick collateral, it seems to change direction, becoming noticeably oblique (fig. 4, *d*) [*fig. 29*]. Among the vertical fusiform [cells], sometimes there are found cells that, because of their lack of ascending dendrites, resemble the spongioblasts of the retina. For the rest, the axon is of great thinness and also originates from the inferior dendritic arborization (fig. 4, *e*) [*fig. 29*].

[3.] Layer of the Middle Medullated Fibers (*External Stria* of Baillarger, *Line* of Gennari)

It contains nerve cells and numerous medullated and unmedullated fibers.

The cells are of three kinds: small pyramids that behave like those of the same name in the typical cortex (fig. 4, *j*) [*fig. 29*]; vertical fusiform [cells] analogous to those of the preceding layer (fig. 4, *h*) [*fig. 29*]; thicker triangular or fusiform [cells], characterized by their ascending axon terminating by an extensive arborization in the molecular layer (fig. 4, *i*) [*fig. 29*]. This axon always gives off, before reaching the layer of the fusiform cells, some collaterals that branch and run horizontally in the middle fibrillar layer.

In this fibrillar layer or in the subsequent [layer] are also found certain ovoid, triangular,

or stellate cells larger than the [above]-mentioned [triangular or fusiform cells], whose ascending axon has the peculiarity of running, in its initial trajectory, either downward, tracing a rounded angle, or more or less horizontally. These axons are very robust and emit a large number of extensive and robust collaterals to the middle fibrillar layer. The final aborization, directed to the molecular layer, is very extensive and situated preferentially at the level of the multipolar cells (fig. 4, *u*) [*fig. 29*].

The fibers of the layer under study are very numerous and run mainly horizontally, extending over very large distances. The method of Weigert reveals that many of them possess a myelin sheath and run in all directions, forming a dense plexus in whose hollows the nerve cells lie. Excepting the fibers that cross this layer vertically and which represent ascending or descending axons of nerve cells, all the others represent collaterals of axons, although one cannot deny the possibility that some terminal arborizations of cells with ascending axon also end in the layer. The collaterals are so numerous and so richly arborized that, in the good Golgi preparations, the cells are seen wrapped in a very tight fibrillar felt. In general, the thickest and most prolixly ramified collaterals come from the ascending axons, whereas the most delicate threads come from the trajectory of the axons of the vertical fusiform [cells] and small pyramids.

From what [has been] exposed, it can be seen how the authors W. Krause and Schwalbe have much reason to consider the stria of Vicq d'Azyr as a plexus of medullated nerve fibers. Equally, it is possible to maintain [in agreement] with Krause that this stria does not represent more than the exaggeration of a nerve plexus (*external plexus* of Krause lying in the cerebral fourth layer) which would already exist in a rudimentary form in the whole cortex. However, the layer of the superficial fusiform [cells] must be considered as a completely new organizational feature.

[4.] Layer of the Large Pyramids

They do not seem very numerous and behave like those of the typical cortex. They are robust ovoid or pyramidal cells (fig. 4, *r*) [*fig. 29*], whose [dendritic] shaft goes up to form in the molecular layer a spiny dendritic tuft and whose descending axon can be followed to the white matter.

As happens in the typical cortex, above the large pyramids there lies a band of transition whose cells gradually decrease in size until they become equal to the small pyramids.

[5.] Layer of the Polymorphic Cells

In it abound the small pyramids whose radial [dendritic] shaft does not appear to reach the molecular layer, and there are also seen not a few fusiform or triangular cells. Among the fusiform cells, those provided with an ascending axon (fig. 4, s) [fig. 29] call for special attention.

This axon ends in the molecular layer, according to the arrangement well known since the works of Martinotti, Retzius, and ourselves, and gives off numerous collaterals in the intermediate fibrillar layer.

It is undoubted that in the construction of the cited layers there are also involved [direct] axons and numerous collaterals arriving from the white matter, but our studies do not allow us yet to detail the behavior of these factors [of construction].

Cajal's Notes

1. Lewis (Bevan), Researches on the Comparative Structure of the Cortex Cerebri (*Phil. Trans.*, 1880, and *Textbook of Mental Diseases*, 1889).

2. Broca, *Bulletin de la Société d'Anthropologie*, Vol. II, 1861, p. 313.

3. Meynert, *Vom Gehirne der Säugethiere, Strickers Handbuch*, 1872, p. 710).

4. Schwalbe, *Lehrbuch der Neurologie*, 1881.

5. Obersteiner, *Anleitung beim Studium des Baues der nervösen Centralorgane*, etc., 1892 edition.

6. He tells us so in a letter that he very kindly sent to us.

Editors' Notes

A. What follows is an exact duplication of a short paper entitled "Anatomical Observations on the Cerebral Cortex and Ammon's Horn I. Cerebral Cortex," published in the *Anales de la Sociedad Española de Historia Natural (Actas)*, Vol. 21 (second series. Vol. I), December 1892, pp. 1–3.

B. The text of the 1892 paper ends here.

C. The text incorrectly says *c*.

7

From: A New Concept of the Histology of the Nerve Centers[A] [Conference] II
III. Gray Cortex of the Cerebrum

[From: *Revista de Ciencias Médicas de Barcelona* 18:457–476, 1892; and *Les nouvelles ideés sur la structure du système nerveux chez l'homme et chez les vertébrés*, trans. by L. Azoulay (Paris: Reinwald, 1894)]

The structure of the cerebral cortex of mammals has been a preferred object of investigation by the neurologists, among whom deserve to be cited, for their elucidation of and progress toward knowledge on this very difficult theme, Gerlach, Wagner, Schültze, Deiters, Stieda, Krause, Kölliker, Exner, Meynert, Edinger, Betz, Golgi, Martinotti, Flechsig, and Retzius.

Before the appearance of the famous book of Golgi (*Sulla fina anatomia degli organi centrali del sistema nervoso*, 1885), all that was known about the structure of the cortical gray matter can be summarized as follows:

1. The existence in the gray matter of pyramidal cells provided with a branched dendritic shaft, directed toward the cerebral surface, and with a descending axon that was supposed not to branch. The presence of an axonal process was determined only on the giant cells.

2. The recognition of a certain number of layers made up, apparently, of cells with different characteristics. In the description of Meynert, blindly followed by Hugenin and many others, the following layers were counted from top to bottom: first layer, made up of neuroglia, nerve fibers, and a few fusi-form or triangular ganglionic cells; second layer, or layer of small pyramids; third layer, or ammonic formation, which consists of large pyramidal cells, like those seen in Ammon's horn; fourth layer, or layer of the small spherical and triangular cells; fifth layer, or layer of the fusiform cells.

About the cells of all these layers, the little that was known concerned the form of the cell body and thickest processes, but there was the most absolute ignorance regarding the disposition of the thinner dendritic branches and the existence and course of the majority of the axonal processes. In order to explain the functional connections of the cells of the cortex, the doctrine of the protoplasmic network of Gerlach, which we reviewed at the previous conference, was accepted.

3. The knowledge of the existence of numerous myelinated fibers, arranged in little bundles that converge in the deep layers and form an irregular plexus in the middle [layers]. These fibers would be continuous above with the axons or basal processes of the pyramids and below would form the nerve fibers of the corona radiata.

The fine structure of the cerebral cortex was

in such a state when Golgi appeared on the scene armed with his valuable method for staining the nerve cells.

The investigations of this authority put the following facts outside discussion:

1. Discovery of the total complex arborization of the dendritic processes of the pyramids and demonstration of the absence of anastomoses.

2. Demonstration that the descending axons of almost all the cortical pyramids are furnished with branched collaterals.

3. Existence in the gray matter of two kinds of cells based on the characteristics of the axon: cells whose axon, after numerous branches, loses its individuality; and cells whose axon, in spite of numerous collaterals, maintains its individuality, to become continuous with a fiber of the white matter. To the former cells, [Golgi] attributed, as we have already expounded at the previous conference, a sensory role and to the others a motor function.

4. Demonstration of the true structure of the neuroglia, showing the whole connective weft of the [nerve] centers to be formed by the interlacing (without anastomosis) of the innumerable, fine processes radiating from the spidery cells (cells of Deiters).

Except for some rather risky physiological assertions such as the distinction already mentioned about the motor and sensory cells, the ideas of Golgi were more or less completely confirmed by Tartuferi, Mondino, Fusari, Nansen, Kölliker, Toldt and Kahler, Obersteiner, Edinger, Retzius, and ourselves.

After Golgi, and in spite of the six years that have passed since the publication of his important work, our knowledge of cerebral histology has scarcely expanded. Let us mention, however, Flechsig, who has been able to prove, aided by a special method of staining, the existence of myelin on the collaterals of the nerve fibers of the cortex (1890), and Martinotti, who recently (1891) has demonstrated that a proportion of the fibers of the first cerebral layer comes from certain pyramids with an ascending axon.

In spite of the very persistent labor of so many investigators and despite analytical methods newly introduced into science, the problems awaiting solution, with regard to the structure and function of the cerebral cortex, are as numerous as they are transcendental.

What are the properties of the nerve cells of the first cerebral layer? Do the collaterals of the axons form a network, or do they terminate freely like those of the white matter of the spinal cord? From which kind of cells do the fibers forming the corpus callosum arise? Are the [parent] cells of the association, projection, and commissural fibers positioned in different cortical layers, or are they mixed, as happens in the spinal cord? In which part of the pyramidal cell does the excitation begin, and what is the significance of that singular [dendritic] tuft that such cells send to the cerebral surface in all vertebrates? Are there motor and sensory cells in the cortex? Does the law of intercellular connection by means of [axodendritic] contacts, which we find in the cerebellum, spinal cord, olfactory bulb, etc., govern also the relationships of the cells of the cerebrum?

It is clear that the anatomists and physiologists in the last two decades had already provided more or less ingenious solutions to many of these questions. But these solutions rested on imperfect observations or on data from pathological anatomy capable of several interpretations, on account of which the complete reexamination of the subject has become indispensable, submitting, with serene impartiality, the structure of the cerebral cortex to the analytical methods that have provided us with such excellent lessons in the spinal cord and cerebellum.

The cerebral cortex is a very difficult theme, perhaps the most difficult study presented to any anatomist; the supreme dignity of the organ and the inextricable complexity of its functions would demand a corresponding fabric of immense complexity, whose threads the most sagacious investigators will be able to disentangle only partially, and in which will constantly become entangled and lost all those who imagine that nature is capable of developing multifarious and highly elevated functions by means of simple mechanisms and schematic formulae. But let us also admit that the method followed up till now by Golgi and his disciples, although excellent for revealing certain details of cellular morphology, is not the most appropriate for arriving at knowledge of the general connections of the cells of the cortex. These authorities, and almost all those who have applied modern methods to the subject, have preferentially attacked the human cerebrum and that of large mammals, in which it is almost impossible, because of the enormous distances and the intricate and labyrinthine nature of the fabric, to pursue an axon or a collateral from its starting point to its termination.

By contrast, in using the smallest mammals,

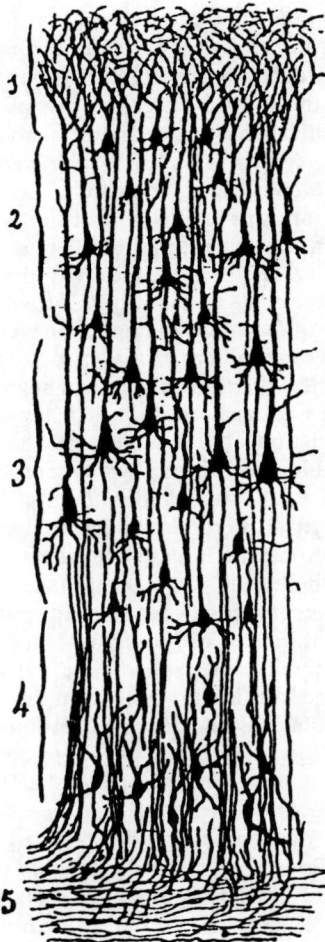

[*FIG. 30*] Fig. 7. Perpendicular section of the gray matter of a gyrus. *1,* molecular layer; *2,* layer of the small pyramids; *3,* layer of the large pyramids; *4,* layer of the polymorphic cells; [*5,* white matter]

and preferably newborns and even embryos (rat, mouse, bat, guinea pig, etc.), the layers become thinner, the distances shortened, the staining of the fibers more constant, and it is not impossible to determine the origin, course, and termination of certain nerve fibers. Such has been our method, and to the preferential use of it we owe the discovery of certain facts which, if they do not solve all the outstanding questions (because this, given the difficulty of the task, is more than an impossible undertaking for us), enlarge somewhat our knowledge and perhaps serve to raise questions that in the future will come close to solution.

The results of this method of investigation must not inspire in us any distrust in their capacity to be generalized to man and higher mammals, given that the cerebrum is substantially identical in all the mammals, varying only in macroscopic form and relative volume of its structural elements.

Let us pass now to the particular study of the cerebral cortex, paying attention to those arrangements of structure that are not lacking in any mammal and which, therefore, can be considered as fundamental structural elements.

In it we will distinguish four layers: first, or *molecular layer;* second, or *layer of the small pyramids;* third, or *layer of the large [pyramids];* fourth, or *layer of the polymorphic cells.* The first and fourth layers are clearly distinguished from their bordering [layers]; but this does not occur with the second and third [layers], which merge by smooth transitions (fig. 7) [*fig. 30*].

Molecular Layer

When this layer is examined in sections of cerebrum simply stained with carmine or with aniline dyes, it exhibits a finely granular or reticulated appearance. Here and there are observed some small nuclei, corresponding to neuroglial cells, especially abundant near the pia mater; and other extremely scarce, large nuclei, surrounded by a triangular or fusiform cell body that probably correspond to nerve cells.

In the most superficial part of the molecular layer, Kölliker discovered a stratum of hori-

zontal myelinated fibers that later was confirmed by Exner with his osmic acid and ammonia method, and by Edinger, Obersteiner,
Toldt, Martinotti, etc., with the more valuable
Weigert-Pal procedure (fig. 9, A) [fig. 33].

Little or nothing was known regarding the
origin of these nerve fibers, of which only
some appear to descend to deeper layers of the
cortex, until two years ago when Martinotti,
using the method of Golgi, demonstrated two
important facts: that some of these fibers bend
to become vertical and continuous with ascending axons coming from certain pyramids,
and that the majority of the horizontal fibers
of the first layer are repeatedly branched as if
they were terminal axonal arborizations.

But the problem of the origin of the majority of the said nerve fibers remained to be
solved. We considered that the superficial
layer contained intrinsic [varicose] fibers,
much thicker and more numerous than those
that descend to the underlying layers, and we
suspected that perhaps all the thick fibers and
a good portion of the fine [fibers] would come
from those intrinsic cells of the first layer,
which are still not well known and which the
authors, having not been able to impregnate
them with the method of Golgi, were inclined
to consider neuroglial cells. Our suspicions
were confirmed, and our investigations in
young and small-sized mammals revealed the
existence of four[B] different cell types.

1. Polygonal Cells

They are of medium size (fig. 8, C) [figs. 31, 32,
D],[C] and from their angles arise four or
six rough dendritic branches, repeatedly
branched and more or less divergent. Some of
the dendritic branches usually descend to the
layer of the small pyramids. The axon is thin,
usually arises from one side of the cell or from
a thick dendritic branch, and runs either
obliquely or horizontally through the thickness of the molecular layer, branching several
times and decomposing in a mass of thin and
very long varicose branches with a course parallel to the surface of the cortex. These axons,
unlike those of the pyramids, never go down
toward the white matter.

Special Cells of the Molecular Layer[D]

We have described in our previous works two
types of horizontal cells: first, the *fusiform cells*
[fig. 32, A, C] provided with two polar dendritic
processes that bend at a certain distance from
their origin to become directed toward the surface of the cerebrum; second, the *triangular or
stellate cells* [fig. 32, B] whose dendritic
branches also run in a more or less horizontal
direction, furnishing during their course little
ascending branches that arise at right angles.
The characteristic of these two cell types is the
peculiarity of possessing not one but two or
more axonal processes horizontally extending
through the thickness of the molecular layer
in which they divide repeatedly at a right
angle, thus traversing a truly enormous space.

Not having been able to follow completely
the course of the thick branches with the appearance of dendrites, and suspecting that perhaps they also have, near their termination,
the thinness, smooth appearance, and mode of
branching of axonal processes, we have made

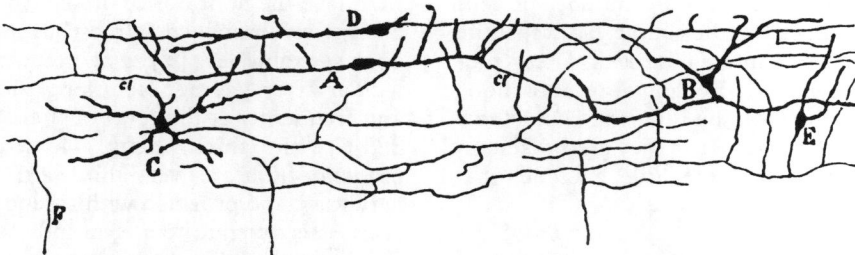

[FIG. 31] Fig. 8. Nerve cells of the first cerebral layer. A, fusiform cells with two horizontal axons; B,
triangular cells; C, polygonal cells with a single axon; D, fusiform cell with a horizontal axon; E, small cell
with a bifurcated axon.

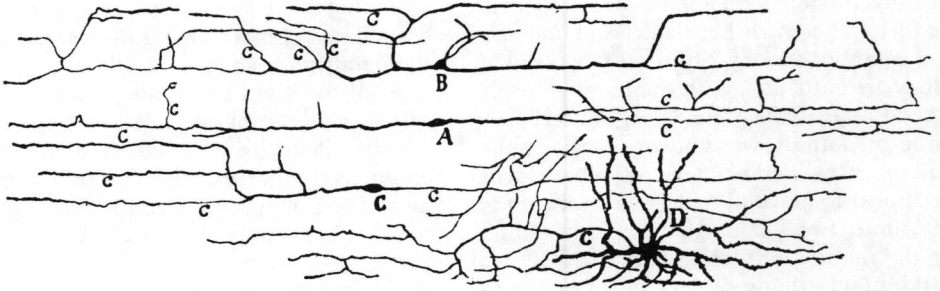

[*FIG. 32*] [Fig. 11 of the French version.] Special cells of the molecular layer of the cerebral cortex of a dog aged one day. *A*, fusiform cell; *B*, triangular or stellate cell; *C*, another fusiform cell; *D*, polygonal cell furnished with numerous dendritic prolongations and an axon subdivided a large number of times; *c* indicates the axonal fibers. [When this figure was republished as fig. 845 of the *Textura* and as fig. 529 of the *Histologie*, the legend read: Elements of the plexiform layer of a rabbit aged a few days. Method of Golgi, double impregnation. *A, B, C*, large horizontal or special cells, also called cells of Cajal (Retzius). (All of the processes marked with a *c* on the cells *A* and *B* are fine and appear to be the axons; it is probable, however, that that is incorrect and that only one among them [is the axon.]) *D*, cells with a short, more or less horizontal axon resolved into a large arborization in the plexiform layer.]

new investigations in the rabbit and guinea pig, choosing as the subject of study the occipital region of the cortex (stria of Gennari or of Vicq d'Azyr). Here the molecular layer reaches a notable thickness, and the cells in question are remarkably abundant. The success of these investigations was difficult, not only because the other nerve fibers of the molecular layer are almost always impregnated at the same time as the cellular subjects of our particular study, giving rise to possible confusions, but also because the irregular orientation and enormous extent of the processes with a dendritic appearance (they sometimes reach 0.7 mm) frequently prevents observation of their totality in a single section.

However, by dint of trying, we have been able to impregnate a certain number of cells [see *fig. 32*] in which [the characteristics] of the thick processes can be observed. These processes, after either a horizontal or an oblique course, acquire little by little the characteristics of axons [*fig. 32, A*] or they are broken up into two, three, or more little branches that have the same appearance as axons.

As a consequence, the *special cells* of the molecular layer of the cerebral cortex must be considered a category of nerve cells which would show no differences between axons and

dendrites or, rather, in which all the processes have the status of axons, if we adhere to morphological criteria.

Thus, our first description must be modified in the following manner.

2. Fusiform Cells[E]

These are ovoid or fusiform cells, oriented in the horizontal plane [*figs. 32, A, C, 31, A*], and possess two thick polar and almost straight [dendritic] shafts. These shafts, whose contours are more or less smooth, furnish more or less at right angles some little ascending branches, which soon bend to approach the surface of the cerebrum and break up into two, three, or several very long, varicose filaments that have the appearance of axons.[F] These filaments are branched (almost always at right angles) exclusively in the territory of the molecular layer [*fig. 31, ci*]. Along their course, and frequently at the level of their bends [*fig. 32, C*], the thick shafts give rise to thin branches [that are] very thin, horizontal, and very long, and provided with ascending collaterals. It is not rare to see, as indicated in [*fig. 32, A*], polar shafts that, without changing direction and gradually becoming thinner, are transformed into a single or double axon.

3. Triangular or Stellate Type [figs. 32, B; 31, B]

It is distinguished from the previous [type] in that, instead of two polar shafts, the cell body is furnished with three or several; these, whatever their initial course, do not delay in running horizontally over a very long trajectory, and little by little they become filaments with the appearance of axons.[G]

During their course, the thick [dendritic] shafts of the cells of this type, like those of the bipolar cells of the fusiform type, generally give rise to fine collaterals that are impossible to distinguish from the axons of the molecular layer.

Many other types of cells of this kind exist, but all of them resemble one another in regard to the characteristics of their processes.

4. Unipolar Fusiform Cells[H] (fig. 8, D) [fig. 31]

In some newborn or embryonic mammals (rat, cat, dog), elongated, fusiform cells are very often observed, more or less evenly distributed, wtih a cell body lying horizontally in the molecular layer, and continued at one pole by a thick horizontal dendritic process that soon becomes branched. From the other pole arises a long horizontal axon that gives rise at right angles to collaterals and terminates by extensive horizontal arborizations.

We do not know if these cells, which so far we have found only in newborn or term fetuses of mammals, correspond to a developmental phase of the fusiform cells previously described or if they are special cells persisting in the adult.

[These special cells inhabit the molecular layer of all areas of the cortex; but their habitual location is in the deep or internal half of this layer, by contrast with the ordinary stellate cells (furnished with a single axon) that are preferentially found in the external half. This, at least, appears clearly in the inferior occipital region of the cerebrum of the rabbit.

[Analogous or very similar cells are also found in the large mammals. In the fetus of the cow or dog, in which we have sometimes

been able to impregnate them, although appearing somewhat embryonic, they are furnished with strongly varicose processes that soon acquire the appearance of axons. We do not doubt that these cells also exist in the human cerebrum, because the figures that illustrate the work of Retzius on the cerebral cortex of the human fetus prove that this authority has been able to impregnate them without, however, being able to study all their characteristics.

[Additionally, Retzius now admits that certain cells of the molecular layer, which he thought to be neuroglial in nature, probably correspond to the multipolar cells that we have described.

[It results from this exposition that the above-mentioned cells represent a specific cellular type. There is no need, however, to ignore the analogy of this cellular type with certain spongioblasts of the retina (spongioblasts with radiated and very thin fibers), whose varicose and horizontal processes also resemble axons. The most characteristic characteristic differentiating these spongioblasts from the special cells of the cortex is that the latter furnish little pseudaxonal branches not only from the ends of their dendritic shafts but also along the course of these same shafts. Let us note also the peculiarity shared by the retinal spongioblasts and the special cells of the cortex: that they inhabit only the molecular layers, that is to say, the regions in which are found the terminations of the dendritic tufts coming from the underlying ganglion cells.

[Retzius, in a recent work (June 1893), has studied in his turn these singular cells, observing them in embryos of man and mammals. For him, confirming our opinion, they are special cells provided with several processes having an axonal appearance. But he adds a detail that rarely appears in our preparations, namely that the little ascending collateral branches end at the very surface of the cerebrum by means of a thick nodularity. The observations of Retzius having been made on embryos, that is to say, under conditions in which the cells may not present their complete development, we are inclined to consider these little submeningeal ascending branches as a developmental peculiarity comparable to those that are displayed to us by many other cells during their development, for example, the granule cells of the cerebellum and the bipolar cells of the spinal ganglia.][1]

The assemblage of all of these intrinsic nerve fibers, together with those that ascend from the underlying layers, forms in the first cerebral layer a very tight plexus amongst whose meshes pass the terminal branches of the ascending [dendritic] tufts of the pyramids (fig. 9, A) [fig. 33]. It is impossible not to consider this singular arrangement, which, by the way, is found with the same characteristics in all vertebrates, as an important example of neural transmission by contact, comparable to that occurring in the cerebellum between the tiny parallel fibers and the dendritic arboriza-

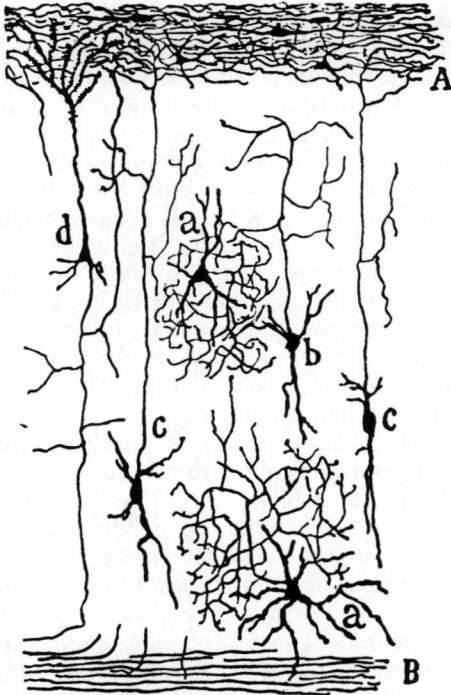

[FIG. 33] Fig. 9. Section of the cortical gray matter of the cerebrum. A, molecular layer; B, white matter; a, cells with short axon forming an extensive arborization; b, cell with ascending axon that does not reach the molecular layer; c, cell with ascending axon branching in the molecular layer; d, small pyramidal cell.

tions of the Purkinje cells. This contact would be transverse or oblique, on account of which the terminal [dendritic] branches of the pyramids possess short collateral spines, in the gaps between which the thinnest small axonal fibers bereft of myelin seem to be tightly caught.

Before proceeding to the particular examination of each of the following layers, it is convenient to describe the general morphological characteristics possessed by all the pyramidal cells of the cortex, irrespective of the layer to which they belong.

General Morphological Characteristics of the Pyramidal Cells[1]

The cell body is conical or pyramidal with an inferior base from which the axon always arises. The dendritic processes are very numerous and can be distinguished by their origin as *ascending shaft or primordial process; collaterals of this shaft;* and *basal processes or those arising from the cell body* (figs. 7; 10, D) [figs. 30, 34].

The [apical dendritic] *shaft* is thick and is directed toward the surfce of the cerebrum parallel to those of the other pyramids, and when it reaches the molecular layer, it breaks up into a splendid tuft of dendritic branches, freely terminating among the small nerve fibers of the said layer. The assemblage of all the peripheral [dendritic] tufts gives rise to a very dense dendritic plexus, to which this part of the cortex owes its finely reticulated appearance in ordinary carmine preparations.

According to Golgi and Martinotti, these dendritic branches would enter into relationship with the blood vessels or with neuroglial cells; but, in fact, they show no such preference, being distributed and terminating throughout the whole thickness of the molecular layer, that is to say, in all the places in which terminal axonal arborizations exist. Retzius has also confirmed this arrangement in human fetuses.[1]

We call the [apical] dendritic shaft primordial because, in the development of the nerve cell, it appears before all the other dendritic branches, as can be seen in the developmental scheme of fig. 10 [fig. 34].

The *lateral processes* of the [apical dendritic]

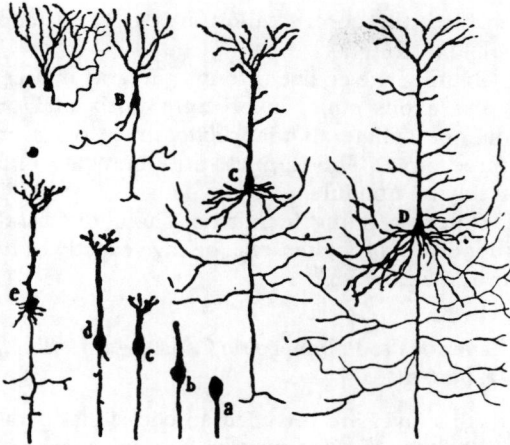

[FIG. 34] Fig. 10. Scheme of the evolution of the pyramidal cells in the animal series. [The preceding sentence was added to the French version.] In the upper part is shown the psychic cell in different vertebrates: A, frog; B, wall lizard; C, mouse ["rat" in the French version]; D, man. In the lower part are shown the phases of development traversed by the psychic cell or cerebral pyramid: a, neuroblast without dendritic shaft; b, beginning of the [dendritic] shaft and terminal tuft; c, more developed [dendritic] shaft; d, appearance of the collaterals of the axon; e, formation of the dendritic processes of the cell body and [dendritic] shaft.

ning either horizontally or obliquely, end by two or three extremely delicate, little branches.

Such is the disposition of the mammalian pyramidal cell, which we could call the *psychic cell,* invoking its special morphology and its exclusive location in the cerebral cortex, the *substratum* of the highest nervous activities.

Descending in the [phylogenetic] scale of the vertebrates, the form of the *psychic cell* is simplified, correspondingly decreasing in length and volume.

In the batrachians (fig. 10, A) [*fig. 34*], all the dendritic processes are reduced to the terminal tuft branching in the molecular layer, a layer that appears notably developed in these animals. Lacking, therefore, are the collaterals of the [dendritic] shaft and the basal [dendritic] processes.

In reptiles (fig. 10, B) [*fig. 34*], the peripheral [dendritic] shaft is already initiated, but collaterals still do not arise from it; from the cell body, as a representative of the basal [dendritic] processes of the mammals, a single descending, more or less branched process is seen.

Second Layer or [Layer] of the Small Pyramids

It consists of many polyhedral or pyramidal cells of small or medium size (from 10 to 12 μm).

The general disposition of the pyramids being already known, little remains to be added with respect to the pyramids that make up the second layer of the cerebrum (fig. 7) [*fig. 30*].

The size of these cells, as well as the length of the peripheral [dendritic] shaft increases from superficial to deep. The latter, frequently dichotomized near the cell body, ends in a rather ample tuft, which, interlacing with the tufts of the adjacent pyramids, occupies most of the thickness of the molecular layer. The basal [dendritic] processes are quite numerous and branched.

With regard to the axon, it is only fitting to say that it is very thin, descending, and gives rise at some distance from its starting point to four or five thin collaterals that dichotomize

shaft arise at right or acute angles at the level of a thickening and are directed toward the sides, freely ending after a number of dichotomous branchings.

The *basal processes* arise from the cell body and are directed either toward the sides or downward, successively branching and getting lost in the vicinity.

The *axon* of the pyramids comes, as we have said, from the base of the cell or from the origin of a basal dendritic process; it is directed downward, crosses all the cerebral layers, and terminates in the white matter by becoming continuous with a nerve fiber. The authors thought that this continuation always took place at a bend; but we have demonstrated that, often, it takes place at a bifurcation, giving rise, thus, to two fibers of the white matter. During its course through the gray matter, the axon emits thin collaterals in number six to ten, which originating at right angles and runonce or twice. In some cases, we have seen the upper collaterals of the said axons ascend to the very molecular layer (fig. 9, *d*) [*fig. 33*].

How do the collaterals terminate? Golgi, who discovered them, supposed that after several branchings they become anastomosed to one another, collaborating in the formation of that continuous interstitial network he recognized in the gray matter.

This is one of the very many problems whose elucidation can only be looked for in ontogeny and comparative anatomy. The [axonal] collaterals of man and of mammals of larger size are of extraordinary length, and there is no section, no matter how thick, that allows us to examine the complete course of one of these fibers.

By contrast, in embryos and in newborn mammals of small size, the collaterals are extremely short, and it is very easy to see that they terminate in a varicosity without any terminal branching. We should even be able to witness, if we make the examination in sufficiently young fetuses, the whole process of growth of the collaterals, since they are no more than simple warty appendages of the axon until the moment at which their terminal divisions are developed (fig. 10, *d, e*) [*fig. 34*].

In adult small mammals, such as the mouse, bat, and white rat, it is easy to confirm such an arrangement, although the distances are already much longer than in embryos (fig. 10, *C*) [*fig. 34*].

Third Layer or [Layer] of the Large Pyramids (Ammonic Layer of Meynert)

It is distinguished from the previous layer only by the large size of its cells (from 20 to 30 μm) and by the greater length and thickness of their peripheral [dendritic] shafts. Superficially, this layer merges with the preceding by smooth gradations of cell size; deeply, it appears better delimited, although it is not rare to see large pyramids scattered in the broad layer of the polymorphic cells (fig. 7, *3*) [*fig. 30*].

The axon is very thick, descends almost in a straight line, and, on reaching the white matter, it generally continues as a fiber of projection. On occasions, it bifurcates or gives rise to a thick collateral, which seems to be destined

to form the corpus callosum (fig. 13, *B* [and *G*][K]) [*fig. 37*].

During the course through the gray matter, these axons emit six or eight horizontal or oblique collaterals that dichotomize twice or three times. The thinnest little branches end freely in a nodule.

The ascending [dendritic] shaft, the basal [dendritic] processes, etc., behave exactly as in the small pyramids.

Layer of the Polymorphic Cells (figs. 7, *4*; 13, *D*) [*figs. 30, 37*]

In this layer are included an occasional pyramid either of giant or medium size, whose peripheral [dendritic] shaft is directed toward the molecular layer; but the majority of the cells that lie here are ovoid, fusiform, triangular, or polygonal. Two items characterize almost all these cells: the lack of a strict orientation of the peripheral [dendritic] shaft (there are exceptions), and the circumstance that, no matter how great its length, it never reaches the plexiform layer, the meeting point of the [dendritic] tufts of all the pyramids. In not a few cases, the peripheral [dendritic] shaft is lacking, being represented by two or more short and oblique processes, and it is not rare to find cells with three thick dendritic processes, two of which reach the white matter.

The axon is thin and descending, gives rise to three or four collaterals that branch several times, and is continuous, either at a bend or at a T-shaped division, with one or two fibers of the white matter (fig. 13, *G*) [*fig. 37*].

Cells with Short Axon (fig. 9) [*fig. 33*]

Mixed with the cells of the last three layers of the cortex, although in small numbers, there are found two cellular types characterized by the peculiarity that their axons terminate by arborizing in the gray matter itself.

These two types are the *sensory cells* of Golgi [and] the *cells with ascending axon* of Martinotti.

The former (fig. 9, *a*) [*fig. 33*] are usually robust and polygonal, radiating dendritic processes in all directions. The axon, coming from either the superficial, deep, or lateral part of the cell body, runs in a variable direction and is broken down, at a short distance, into a free, varicose arborization whose tiny branches envelop the somata of adjacent cells.

Golgi, the discoverer of these cells, thought that, because their axons soon lose their individuality, the cells would have a sensory function; but, as we will show later, there is insufficient basis for such a deduction. The [sensory cells are] cells with short axon, which seem to be destined to interrelate several adjacent cells, but it is impossible to guess anything about the nature of the actions that they perform (fig. 9, a) [fig. 33].

The cells with ascending axon were first mentioned by Martinotti (fig. 9, C) [fig. 33]. We, who have studied them in mammals of small size, have found them in the three lower layers but, above all, in the layer of the polymorphic cells. They are either fusiform or triangular, with ascending and descending dendritic processes. The axon, which it is not rare to see leave from an ascending dendritic shaft, goes up almost in a straight line to the molecular layer, where it divides into two or three thick branches, which, extending and branching horizontally, make up a final arborization of very large extent. Sometimes it has seemed to us that the terminal arborization was extended not through the first layer but in that of the small pyramids (fig. 9, b) [fig. 33].

White Matter

It consists of four kinds of fibers: first, *projection fibers;* second, *callosal or commissural fibers;* third, *fibers of association;* and fourth, *centripetal or terminal fibers.* All of these fibers appear mixed up in the white matter of the mammals of large size (dog, sheep, cow, man, etc.), it being absolutely impossible to determine by direct observation either their origins or their terminations. Fortunately, in the small mammals, the analytical difficulties are diminished, so that it is feasible to pursue many of these fibers over a quite considerable distance.

Projection Fibers (fig. 12, a [and C]^{L}) [fig. 36]

These fibers come from all regions of the cortex, converging in the corpus striatum in order to enter the cerebral peduncles. In the small mammals, on arriving at the level of the cor-

pus callosum, they emit a thick collateral to this; then they descend in little bundles separated by septa of gray matter, to which they provide very thin collaterals. Axons of projection also exist, which on passing through the plane of the callosal fibers, do not give rise to any collaterals, keeping their individuality and their lack of branches through the whole thickness of the corpus striatum.

From which cells come the fibers of projection? Certain authors, Monakow among others, suppose that the said fibers are exclusively continuations of the giant pyramids, while the fibers of association and the callosal would have their origins in small pyramids.

The observations that we have made with regard to this point, although very far from complete, seem to us to establish in an unequivocal manner that the fibers of projection arise from both large and small pyramids, even without excluding some polymorphic cells; and this origin from cells of variable size could serve to explain why the little bundles of projection fibers that descend through the corpus striatum contain mixed thick and thin axons.

With regard to the terminations of these fibers at lower levels, direct observation by means of the anatomical methods can tell us nothing. But pathological anatomy and the method of Flechsig show us that a good proportion of them make up the *pyramidal pathway,* the descending route of the voluntary motor excitations.

Fibers of Association (fig. 11) [fig. 35]

These fibers probably have their origins in the three layers of cerebral cells (small and large pyramids and polymorphic cells); but up to the present, we have only been able to observe, *de visu,* their union with polymorphic cells and with an occasional giant pyramid, which could depend on the relative ease of pursuing the axons of these cells, since they are so close to the white matter.

The continuity of these axons with the fibers of association takes place, in the majority of cases, at a simple bend; nevertheless, T-shaped divisions are also found, with equal or unequal branches (fig. 11, c) [fig. 35]. In the latter case, the medial branch of bifurcation may be insinuated among the callosal fibers. Any-

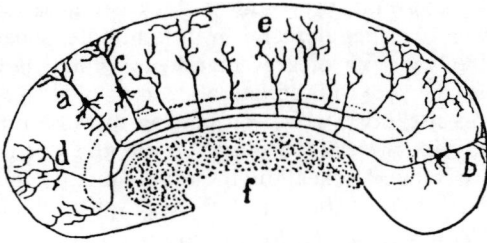

[*FIG. 35*] Fig. 11. Scheme of an anteroposterior section of the cerebrum, to show the arrangement of the fibers of association between the anterior and posterior lobes. *a,* medium pyramid; *d,* terminal axonal arborization; *e,* ascending [axonal] arborizations of the collaterals [of the fibers of association (in the French version)]; *f,* corpus callosum cut in cross-section.

way, it is convenient to point out that many fibers of association, as a consequence of the variable direction and connections of their two branches of bifurcation, can bring a cell at a given point of the cortex into relation with many cells lying in different territories and perhaps in different lobes of the same hemisphere.

The fibers of association increase in number in proportion to the mass of gray matter; so that in man and large mammals, in which the [gray matter] is folded in gyri, the fibers of association form by their abundance the main mass of white matter. The extraordinary number and length of such fibers, and their intimate mixture with projection and callosal fibers, make the anatomical pursuit of a single fiber completely impossible; because of that, it is absolutely essential to study them in small cerebra (mouse, bat, rat, etc.), not only for the relative shortness of the distances, but because the systems of association, commissural, and projection fibers appear perfectly demarcated in certain regions.

Collaterals of the Fibers of Association

The application of the Golgi method to small and newborn mammals has allowed us to discover a fact of some importance: the existence on many fibers of association of very thin, ascending collaterals that branch in several layers of the superimposed gray cortex (fig. 11, *e*) [*fig. 35*]. Choosing for examination certain fa-

vorable regions—for example, the medial surface of the hemispheres—it is observed that some collaterals reach the very molecular layer, in which they terminate in extensive free arborizations, an arrangement that appears also very evident in the cerebral cortex of reptiles. Besides these radiating collaterals destined for the gray matter, one discovers others that seem to terminate in the white matter or at the deep border of the gray matter; their orientation is less regular than the radiating fibers, and they seem destined to establish connections with the numerous descending dendritic processes located and terminating in the broad white matter. These collaterals of the *white matter* must be similar to the peripheral collaterals that are seen in the batrachians and reptiles, and which arborize among the branches of a perimedullary dendritic plexus.

With regard to the termination of the fibers of association, this takes place in the same manner as in the fibers of the white matter of the spinal cord, that is to say, by means of free and varicose arborizations, so extensive that they embrace almost the whole thickness of the cortex, including the molecular layer (fig. 11, *a*) [*fig. 35*].

Callosal Fibers (fig. 12, A) [*fig. 36*]

They lie underneath the fibers of association, and in the small mammals form a well-delimited transverse plane that serves as a cover for the lateral ventricles. In the good impregnations [with silver chromate],[M] the corpus callosum naturally attracts attention because of the extreme delicacy of its fibers: it could be said that they are simple axon collaterals. In preparations stained by the method of Weigert-Pal, they also present a singularly thin myelin sheath. The callosal fibers arise from all parts of the cortex of one side and terminate in all parts of the other, except in the sphenoidal regions of the hemispheres, where the commissural fibers run separately, forming the anterior commissure (fig. 12, B) [*fig. 36*].

When transverse sections of the cerebrum of a newborn mouse are examined, and in cases in which the silver chromate had been fixed with a certain exclusiveness in the callosal fibers, it is observed that many of these emit,

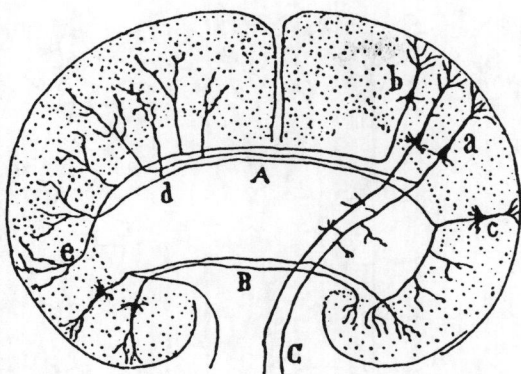

[FIG. 36] Fig. 12. Scheme of a transverse section of the cerebrum, to show the probable arrangement of the commissural and projection fibers. A, corpus callosum; B, anterior commissure; C, pyramidal pathway formed by fibers of projection.

preferentially at certain places, very thin collaterals that behave like those arising from the fibers of association. Generally, each callosal fiber gives rise to two or at most three such collaterals, which, ascending almost at a right angle, get lost in the superimposed gray matter, in which they end freely. There are divisions that seem to be true bifurcations, the commissural fiber being resolved into one fiber that follows the original horizontal course and another that enters the gray matter (fig. 12, d) [fig. 36].

How do the callosal fibers originate? Do they represent the continuation of direct axons, or do they instead correspond to collaterals of the white matter? Could it not happen that the corpus callosum, like the anterior commissure of the spinal cord, would contain both direct axons and collateral fibers of the white matter?

The latter opinion is the one that better harmonizes with our observations. There are observed, in effect, in many parts of the white matter certain axons, either association or projection, that emit a thin collateral that enters the corpus callosum. Sometimes more than simply a collateral branch, the fiber to the corpus callosum seems to be a branch of bifurcation.

In addition, it is not rare to notice that certain fibers originating from several levels of the gray matter, but mainly from the level

of the small pyramids, descend to the plane of the corpus callosum, continuing by means of an inflection with the true fibers of this. Therefore, such fibers, which resemble [main] axons, could represent the direct continuation of certain axons of small cells of the cortex. However, let us hasten to say that we have not yet been able to confirm directly this interpretation.

How do the callosal fibers terminate? This is a very obscure point that we have not yet been able to clarify in spite of very persistent investigations. Sometimes we have succeeded in observing that certain tiny callosal fibers ascend through the gray matter and branch in it; but, unfortunately, we have not been able to follow their complete arborization and, thus, to ascertain the connections of the final little branches (fig. 12, e) [fig. 36]. Hence, it is necessary to undertake new investigations on this theme.

In summary, in our opinion, the callosal fiber does not represent, as once thought, a junctional link between two symmetrical regions of each hemisphere, but a very complex system of transverse association, in which the fiber originating, for example, at one point in a hemisphere can enter into contact relationships not only with symmetrical cells of the opposite point, but also (by means of collaterals) with many other cells of different radii and layers of the cortex.

Fibers Branching in the Gray Matter (fig. 13, E) [fig. 37]

We have already said above that fibers of association coming from more or less remote territories of the same hemisphere penetrate the gray cortex and that these fibers are extensively arborized in the gray matter. But there also exist other much thicker fibers coming perhaps from the spinal cord, cerebellum, etc., which, running commonly obliquely or horizontally through the thickness of the gray matter, form throughout the full thickness of this, including the molecular layer, an axonal arborization of enormous extent. The last branches form varicose arborizations that seem preferentially to surround the small pyramids. Do such fibers represent by chance the cerebral terminations of the sensory nerves, or at least the terminations of the axons coming from cells connected with the final little branches of the sensory nerves? It seems probable but cannot be confirmed. For the rest, such fibers are very easily impregnated in the reptiles, where the main arborizations are concentrated in the molecular layer.

Having set down the fundamentals of the histology of the cerebral cortex, we are now going to expound some considerations about the connections of the nerve cells that constitute it.

Connections of the Cells of the First Cerebral Layer

We have previously seen that all the pyramids send a dendritic tuft to the molecular layer, the common point of gathering of an infinity of terminal nerve fibers. Thanks to this axodendritic connection, whose importance must be great because it is not lacking in the cortex of any vertebrate, the pyramids can receive the activity of many [cellular] elements. Let us declare, of course, that, in our opinion, the connections take place by contact, between the terminal axonal arborizations and collaterals of the axons on the one hand and the cell body and dendritic processes on the other. The direction of the [impulse] is *cellulifugal* in the axon and *cellulipetal* in the cell body and dendritic processes (Cajal, van Gehuchten), or, in other words, the dendritic processes and cell body always receive, and the terminal branches of the axons and their little collateral branches transmit.

With this background, we will now be able to try out the interpretation of the connections of the first cerebral layer. At the level of this layer, the [dendritic] tufts of the pyramids can receive [impulses from], first, the intrinsic cells of the molecular layer, thanks to the axonal arborizations of these [cells]; second, vertical fusiform cells of the cortex by means of the upper arborization of the ascending axon of the same; third, pyramidal cells of association, inhabitants of more or less remote radii of the cortex, by means of ascending collaterals and terminal arborizations of the axons of the same; fourth, cells perhaps of the cerebellum, spinal cord, etc., by means of extensive nerve arborizations that form in the whole gray mat-

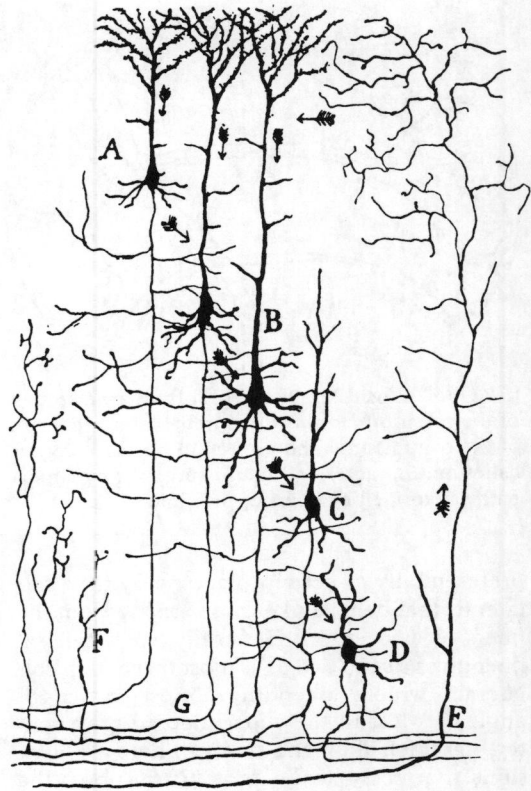

[*FIG. 37*]   Fig. 13. Scheme designed to show the probable course of the [impulses] and the axodendritic connections in the cells of the cortex. *A*, small pyramid; *B*, giant pyramid; *C* and *D*, polymorphic cells; *E*, terminal fiber arriving from other centers; *F*, [axonal] collaterals of the white matter; *G*, axon bifurcating in the white matter.

ter certain thick fibers arriving from the white matter; fifth, perhaps cells of the opposite hemisphere, thanks to the terminal branches of callosal fibers.

Connections at the Level of the Layers of the Pyramids and Polymorphic Cells

These connections are of enormous complexity and take place between the cell body, dendritic shaft, and processes of the cells, on the one hand, and five kinds of nerve fibers, on the other, namely collaterals of the white matter; collaterals of the corpus callosum; terminals of interlobar association fibers and [of subcortical fibers], axonal arborizations of the cells of Golgi (sensory), and, finally, an infinite number of tiny collateral fibers emitted along the intracortical course of the axons of the cells of the three deep strata of the gray matter. The plexus formed around these cells by so many filaments is so complicated that it would be a hasty presumption to specify all the individual connections of a pyramid.

We will only say by way of probable conjecture that, thanks to this fibrillar plexus, the pyramids can receive the action, first, of cells with short axon (cells of Golgi) located in the same layer; second, of cells of association, inhabitants of several lobes of the same hemisphere; third, of cells inhabiting the opposite [hemisphere] (by means of the callosal fibers or those of the anterior commissure); fourth, of cells of the [subcortical] sensory regions; fifth, of cells lying in the superimposed layers of the same cortical region (fig. 13) [fig. 37].

The last connection is surely one of the most important, and seems to be established by the following elements: first, little collateral branches of the axons of superimposed pyramids; second, cell bodies, dendritic shafts, and basal dendrites of pyramids located in underlying layers. Each collateral, thanks to its great length, branches, and more or less horizontal course, can contact transversely the [dendritic] shafts and cell bodies of hundreds of cells, in such a way that a single small pyramid, by virtue of its axonal collaterals, can influence several series of medium and small pyramids situated below it. And in its turn, each large pyramid, as a consequence of the considerable surface of contact presented by its [dendritic] shaft, its dendritic collaterals, and the descending basilar [dendritic] processes, can receive [impulses] from a large number of superimposed pyramids (fig. 13, A, B, C, D) [fig. 37].

In the already mentioned hypothesis of dynamic polarization of the cell processes, the [impulses] in the gray matter must go from the small pyramids to the large pyramids and from these to the polymorphic cells. In fig. 13 [fig. 37], the arrows indicate the direction of the impulses.

If we knew positively the point of termination of the sensory nerve fibers, coming from the spinal cord or from more rostral brain nuclei, it would be possible to establish, with some element of certainty, where the [impulses] to voluntary movement begin in the cells of projection. In spite of our ignorance about this interesting point, there is no lack of data on which to base a hypothesis. Thus, for example, the [afferent] nerve fibers, comparable from more than one point of view to sensory fibers, are observed to terminate always by free arborizations in the molecular layer of the cerebrum or in the equivalent layer of other nerve centers (cortical layer of the optic lobe of birds), entering into relationships with the peripheral dendritic tufts of elongated cells. This disposition is perfectly demonstrable in the olfactory lobe of the mammals, in which a good portion of the fibers coming from the olfactory bulb sends collateral and terminal branches to a superficial layer, the point of assemblage of the [dendritic] tufts of pyramids, and the perfect facsimile of the molecular layer of the cortex. In the cerebral cortex of the reptiles, not only the olfactory fibers but all the deep axons, among which must probably be included the sensory fibers arriving from the spinal cord, are arborized preferentially in the superficial or molecular layer of the cortex.

These and other reasons incline us to think that the incitement to voluntary movement begins in the [dendritic] tuft of the pyramids and that it is engendered in the thickness of the molecular layer. This would explain why the physiologists, who have subjected the cerebral cortex to the action of mechanical, chemical, and electrical stimuli, have provoked movements in certain groups of muscles: the excitation diffusing through the molecular layer would act preferentially either directly on the [dendritic] tuft of the pyramids or indirectly on the little nerve fibers of the said layer [that are] intimately connected with the dendritic tufts; in such a way, the stimulus would have its effect at the same place in volition as in the experimental animal.

Morphological Types of Cerebral Cells

A question that has always been given special attention by the anatomists is to deduce from the morphological characteristics of a nerve cell the nature of the function it performs. In this way, Golgi has supposed that in the nerve centers there exist two morphologically and physiologically different types: (1) cells whose axons soon lose their individuality by dint of branching; (2) cells whose axons maintain their individuality until the white matter, not before having given rise to collaterals in the gray matter. The former type would be sensory because the branches of its axon are linked with networks emanating from little centripetal fibers; the second type would have a motor character because its axon is continuous with the motor roots.

This classification of Golgi cannot be maintained (as Kölliker, His, Waldeyer, van Gehuchten, etc., have recognized) in either the morphological or physiological arena.

Morphologically, the cells of the former or sensory type only differ from the second or motor type in the length of the axon. In the former, the axon is short and does not leave the gray matter, in which it ends very close [to the parent cell] in a free arborization; in the second, the axon is long, runs to the white matter, and sends its terminal arborization to other nerve centers or to extracentral organs. For this reason, we have designated the two types of Golgi with the names of *cells with short axon* and *cells with long axon,* a nomenclature which, because it does not prejudge anything in relation to cellular physiology, has been accepted by several authors.

Physiologically, it is also not possible to maintain the distinction of the two types of Golgi, because, first, organs [that are] evidently sensory, such as the retina, the olfactory bulb, the olfactory mucosa, etc., include a large number of cells with long axon (motor cells of Golgi); second, organs [that are] evidently devoted to motor function, such as the cerebellum or the psychomotor area of the cerebral cortex, include a large number of cells with short axon.

In fact, the morphological types of the cerebral cortex correspond to three kinds: first, *cells with short axon* (sensory cells of Golgi, polygonal cells, and some fusiform cells of the first cerebral layer); second, *cells with long axon* (pyramids, polymorphic cells, etc.); third, *cells*

with multiple axons (the bipolar and triangular cells of the first[N] layer). The latter also exist in the batrachians and reptiles, showing the peculiarity that all their processes, at their commencement somewhat thick, acquire gradually and as they branch the appearance of nerve fibers. If it were possible to demonstrate also in the mammals (something that, so far, we have not achieved) that any process with the dendritic appearance of the fusiform and triangular cells of the cerebral first layer ends by thin fibers, like little axonal branches, then the cerebrum would resemble the retina and olfactory bulb, in which, in addition to the two main types of cells, there is found another characterized by the lack of distinction between the dendritic and axonal processes.

In summary, in the present state of the science, it is not possible to link a particular functional modality (afferent, motor, sensory, commissural, association, etc.) to a special morphology of nerve cells. And the same affirmation could be made, although with certain restrictions, to the layers of the cortex; that is to say, the commissural, association, and projection cells are not placed in a particular layer, but they seem to inhabit all the layers, being intermingled in an intimate manner. This is a disposition that perhaps explains the extreme rarity of intellectual alterations confined to a particular sphere of activity and the maintenance of cerebral functions in cases of grave lesion of a particular cerebral region.

The Cerebral Cortex of Lower Vertebrates[o]

Reptiles

Among the lower vertebrates (birds, reptiles, batrachians, fishes), the reptiles are the only ones, as Edinger has noted, that possess a cerebral cortex comparable to that of the mammals. Here are the layers presented by the anterior vesicle of *Lacerta agilis* (fig. 17) [*fig. 38*] as an example of a reptile.

First, Molecular Layer

Its structure bears three elements, as in the mammals: (a) the terminal [dendritic] tufts of the pyramidal cells; (b) the horizontal processes of certain fusiform or globular cells

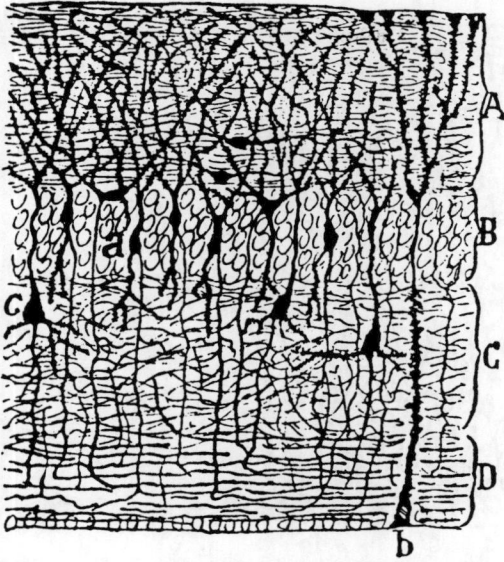

[FIG. 38]   Fig. 17. Section of the cerebral cortex of *Lacerta agilis. A,* molecular layer or superficial plexiform [layer]; *B,* layer of the pyramidal cells; *C,* molecular layer or deep or lower plexiform [layer]; *a,* pyramidal cell; *b,* epithelial cell; *c,* pyramidal cell of the lower plexiform layer.

comparable to the special cells of the same layer in the mammals; (c) the terminal arborizations of an infinity of nerve fibers, some of which are the collaterals or terminal axonal fibers of the white matter and some the ascending collaterals of the axons originating from cells of the gray matter.

Second, Layer of the Pyramidal Cells

It consists of several compact series of cells with either a fusiform, triangular, or pyramidal appearance. The dendritic processes of these cells get lost in the molecular layer; their axons go to the white matter.

Third, Plexiform Layer

It contains some large pyramidal cells that behave like the preceding ones and are only a little different. But what predominates in this layer is the considerable number of nerve fibers arranged in a tight plexus. The vast majority of these fibers represent collaterals coming from the white matter and from the descending course of the axons of the pyramidal cells.

Fourth, Layer of the White Matter

In it are distinguished the callosal fibers, fibers of projection, and there could also be fibers of association. The neuroglia are represented here, as P. Ramón first indicated, by the radial epithelial cells, which, starting at the ventricle, terminate by means of a tuft of spiny filaments at the very surface of the cerebrum.

Batrachians

The investigations of Oyarzum, Edinger, and ourselves in the batrachians proved that, if the cerebral cortex resembles that of the mammals in relation to the morphology of the cells, it is not in relation to the number of layers and course of the nerve fibers (fig. 18) [*fig. 39*].

In the frog, for example, there exist only two well-delimited nerve layers: first, the *molecular layer* or superficial layer, having as elements of its structure, as in the reptiles and mammals, the assemblage of spiny [dendritic] tufts of pyramidal cells, the processes of horizontal nerve cells, not differentiated into dendritic and axonal processes, and, finally, the terminal arborizations of a countless number of ascending axonal fibers; second, the *layer of the pyramidal cells* which occupies the whole deep half of the cortex and whose axonal processes, the vast majority of which are ascending, are distributed and branched in the molecular layer.

Oyarzum has also observed pyramidal cells whose axons are directed downward; they would probably represent the fibers of projection. But these cells are not found in all regions of the anterior vesicle; they are lacking in the superior regions of the hemispheres.

Calleja has also recently seen in the cortex of *Pleurodeles waltii,* besides pyramidal cells with ascending axon, cells of the sensory type of Golgi, whose short arborization forms a plexus among the cell bodies of the pyramidal cells and in a portion of the molecular layer situated above them.

To which cells of the cortex of mammals do the pyramidal cells of the frog correspond? We believe that they should be considered as the cells of association whose axon, instead of running horizontally over a long trajectory in the

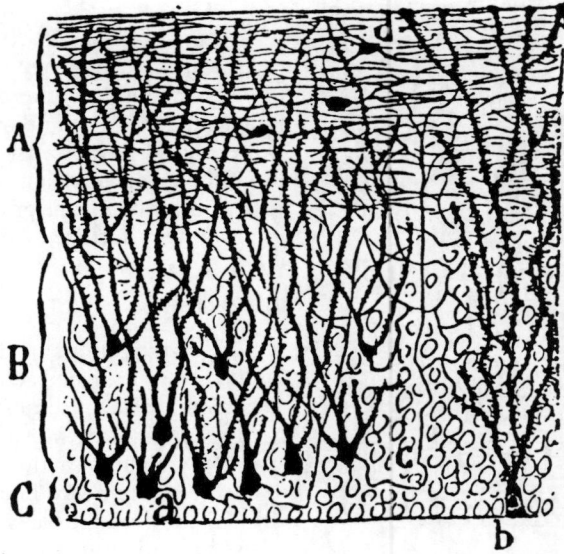

[*FIG. 39*]   Fig. 18. Section of the cerebral cortex of the frog. *A*, molecular layer; *B*, layer of the pyramidal cells; *C*, epithelial layer; *a*, cell body of a pyramidal cell giving rise to an ascending axon (*c*); *d*, cell of the molecular layer; *b*, epithelial cell with branches going up to beneath the pia mater.

regions adjacent to the ventricular cavities, would ascend rapidly, at a short distance from their origins, toward the molecular layer to enter into relationship with a considerable number of pyramidal cells by means of the very extensive arborizations they emit in this layer. The commissural cells would be completely lacking in the cerebral cortex of the frog, and the cells of projection would only exist in the inferior region of the anterior vesicle.

With regard to the neuroglia, which have been described in detail by Oyarzum, they are represented, as in the reptiles, by epithelial cells whose large tufts of peripheral branches terminate underneath the pia mater by means of conical dilations (fig. 18, *b*) [*fig. 39*].

Birds

The cerebral cortex of the birds (subventricular region), according to the recent studies of Cl. Sala, does not show any very real advance in comparison with the cortex of the reptiles. Because of the lack of a layer of white matter, the predominance of the cells with ascending axons, and the lack of commissural cells, this cortex seems to be closer to the cortex of batrachians than to the cortex of reptiles. The number of its layers is three: first, or molecular; second, or layer of small and large pyramidal cells; third, or layer of the stellate cells (fig. 19) [*fig. 40*].

The *molecular layer* has the same structure as in the reptiles and batrachians; it is formed by the interweaving of the ascending nerve fibers, dendritic processes of the pyramidal cells, and the pseudaxonal processes of certain globular or fusiform, special cells.

The *layer of the pyramidal cells* consists of several rows of more or less elongated cells with ascending and descending dendritic processes; the ascending processes reach the molecular layer, whereas the descending processes branch in the third layer. The axons of these cells either terminate at a short distance [from the parent soma] by free arborizations among the somata of the pyramidal cells, or they go up to the molecular layer in which they branch in a luxuriant manner. Among these cells are seen some whose axon runs in a vertical direction toward the interhemispheric portion of the cortex to form, with a large number of other axons, a deep and anteropos-

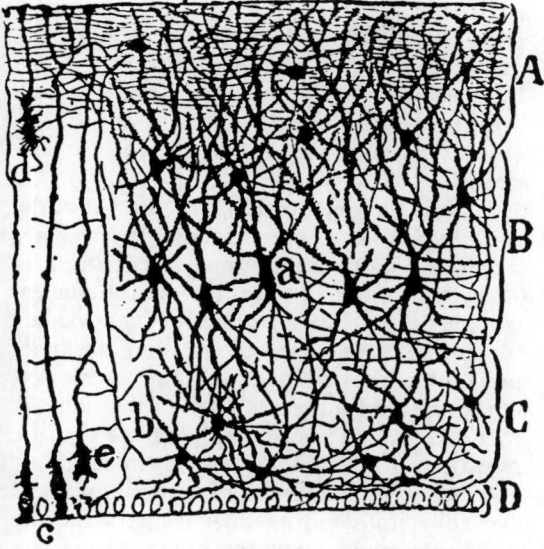

[*FIG. 40*] Fig. 19. Section of the cerebral cortex of a chicken a few days old, at the level of the supraventricular region; taken from a preparation of Cl. Sala. *A*, molecular layer; *B*, layer of the pyramidal cells; *C*, layer of the stellate cells (corresponding to the [layer] of the polymorphic cells of mammals); *D*, epithelium; *a*, pyramidal cell; *b*, stellate cell giving rise to an ascending axon; *c*, epithelial cells; *d, e*, epithelial cells [that are] displaced or migrating, in the process of transformation into spidery cells.

terior fascicle that would probably represent a system of projection, which is the *fascicle of the septum of the longitudinal fissure* (*Bündeln der sagittalen Scherdewand* of the Germans).

The *layer of the stellate cells* is found very close to the [ependymal] epithelium; the dendritic processes of these cells run in all directions but do not reach the molecular layer; their axons correspond or at least are very similar to the axons of the sensory cells of Golgi; they branch among the adjacent cell bodies of the pyramidal and stellate cells. In some cases, the nerve branches or axons can reach the molecular layer.

Anatomicophysiological Conclusions

After this already long excursion through the anatomy of the centers, it is now time to end, before I lose your patience and benevolent at-tention, by expounding some considerations of a physiopsychological nature, which legitimately and simply follow from what I said above in relation to the disposition of the psychic cells.

1. The external morphology of the psychic cells, or their manner of relationship among themselves, cannot explain to us, in the present state of the science, the supreme dignity of cerebral functions. Their morphology presents but little modification of the common nerve cell type, so [their function] is explained by the great richness of relationships that any psychic cell can maintain. In effect, nerve cells, whatever their functional category, appear to be built according to the same model, and even seem to exhibit the same fine structure and chemical composition. The motor cells of the anterior horn of the spinal cord, the ganglion cells of the retina, the cells of the sympathetic [nervous system] of vertebrates, etc., possess the same axon, the same dendritic processes, the same manner of relationship [with other cells] and transmission of [impulses], in short, all the characteristics of the psychic cell to which, nevertheless, we attribute the highest activities of life (association [of ideas],[p] memory, intelligence, etc.). From the point of view of the complexity of the connections and the variety of morphological types, the cerebral cortex cannot even compete with the marvelous fabric of the cerebellum and retina, whose activities, although important, are coarse tasks in comparison with the unique functions of the cerebral cortex. Science, therefore, in order that one does not become discouraged in this perpetual and very tough struggle in search of the mechanistic explanation of thought, must imagine that *that* something which separates the cerebral cell from the cell of the spinal cord or ganglion cell [of the retina] is not the external form but the structure and chemical content, and that the active phenomena that occur in the dendritic fabric of the psychic cell are nowhere near the same as those that occur in the nerve cells of inferior category.

2. Another conclusion that must derive from the anatomicophysiological study of the cortex (a conclusion that has been reached by many anatomists and has also been brilliantly

defended by Letamendi) is that the cerebrum does not contain [a unique]^Q receptive center for all the afferent and sensory fibers, nor is it [a unique] source of all motor fibers; but the whole cortex can be considered as a series of centers, each of which receives one type of afferent or sensory fiber and is attached to a certain order of motor fiber. These regions are gathered together with the aim of attaining all kinds of mental associations (sensory-motor, conscious, and unconscious) by means of the systems of association and commissural fibers. These special zones of the cortex do not possess a specific texture that explains their particular function; rather, according to what Golgi has indicated, what is specific about the function derives from the special peripheral connections (with sensible parts [of the body], muscles, etc.) of the fibers appended to these cortical centers.

3. With some reservations, it can be affirmed that psychic functions in the animal series are related to the presence of the pyramidal cells (psychic cells). In the fish, where the anterior cerebral vesicle still does not contain true pyramids, intellectual manifestations in the strict sense do not exist, as Edinger has recently indicated.

The pyramid or psychic cell possesses specific characteristics that are never absent (batrachians, reptiles, birds, and mammals), among which there deserve to be cited the presence of a dendritic shaft and tuft directed toward the cerebral surface; the existence of collateral spines on the dendritic processes; and the connection of all [the spines],^{R} at the level of the molecular layer, with a tight plexus of little terminal nerve fibers (see fig. 10) [*fig. 34*].

4. The elongated form of the pyramids, with their diversity of processes, exists for the purpose of making it possible for a cell to receive the influence of many elements of different categories. In the same way as the cell of Purkinje of the cerebellum acquires an enormous development and each of its parts (cell body, main [dendritic] shaft, and dendritic processes) enters into relationship with nerve fibers of different origins, so also the pyramids acquire an extreme length in order to receive on the cell body, basal [dendritic] processes, [dendritic] shaft, and terminal [dendritic] tuft the influence of nerve fibers of different origins. The extent and degree of differentiation reached by a cell's dendritic arborization can thus be a measure of the number of elements of different categories with which the cell is connected.

5. Since, as one ascends the animal scale, the psychic cell correspondingly becomes larger and more complicated, it is natural to attribute to this progressive morphological complexity at least a portion of its advanced functional state. This progression does not pertain, perhaps, to the essence of psychic acts but to the amplitude and form of the same.

It can thus be considered probable that the psychic cell performs its activity more amply and usefully the larger the number of somatic and collateral dendrites that it offers and the more numerous, long, and branched the collaterals emitted by its axon. The degree of development of the nerve cell sometimes goes together with its size, but it is often independent of this. In general, the volume seems to be related to the size of the animal; in this way, the hen and the [common] lizard have bigger pyramidal cells than the sparrow and wall lizard, respectively, but not more differentiated and, consequently, unable to engender superior intellectual activities. [It can also be claimed that the dimensions of the cell body are related to the extent and richness of the little branches of the terminal arborization of the axonal process. In other words, the more voluminous the cell, the larger the number of cells (nerve cells, glandular cells, muscular cells, etc.) with which it forms connections. It is not the length of the axon nor the extent of the dendritic arborization that seems to influence, at least in a constant manner, the size of the cell body.]^S

6. The psychic cell begins its ontogenic development as a simple neuroblast, that is to say, as a piriform cell furnished with a single process: the axon. Then it becomes more complicated by the appearance of the [dendritic] shaft or peripheral primordial process, and finally, the lateral branches of the [dendritic] shaft, cell body, and axon appear.

7.^{T} From the fact that the gaps that separate the psychic cells are filled with axonal and dendritic arborizations, there can also be deduced a means of measuring the degree of differentiation of these psychic cells by the gaps that exist between them. In this way, in the batrachians and reptiles, the cell bodies of the psychic cells are in many places almost in contact, whereas in man they are found at the maximum separation.

The doctrine that we have just expounded regarding the relationship that exists between the functional level of cells and the number of their collaterals could perhaps explain two facts that are very difficult to interpret by the generally accepted hypothesis that intelligence bears a relation to the number of cerebral cells, whether these represent a simple instrument of the mind or are considered as an exclusive condition of psychic activity. These facts are the remarkable intellectual increase that is observed in men devoted to deep and continuous mental exercise, and the coexistence of marked talent and even of true genius with brains of medium size or of smaller size and weight than normal.

In the former case, since the production of new cells is not possible (the nerve cells do not multiply as do the muscular cells), it could be supposed that cerebral gymnastics leads to a little beyond ordinary development of dendritic processes and axonal collaterals, forcing the establishment of new and more extensive intercortical connections. In this process, in order to explain the maintenance of the same cerebral volume, there can be imagined a correlative decrease in the [size] of the cell body of the nerve cells or a decrease in the neuroglial network.

In the second case, nothing exists that would impede us from accepting that certain cerebra, whether by inheritance of previous adaptations or for other reasons, offer, as compensation for the smaller number of cells, a remarkable development of all kinds of collaterals.

These interpretations rest naturally on a very rational hypothesis regarding the role played by the cells and their processes. It is necessary to suppose that each psychic [cell] in a state of activity contains, in some [mechanical]^U or chemical form at present unknown, a simple image of each of the impressions received either from the external world

or from the fabric of our organs (muscular sense).

Now then, whatever the nature of that superior function that associates, judges, compares, etc., the way its actions are mediated cannot be other than by the axonal and dendritic processes.

If understanding is, as Bain says, the perception of similarities or differences between ideas, the richness and amplitude of judgment will be greater the larger the number of acquisitions or images that serve as its material and the more extensive the system of relations between the cells that allows them to establish the cellular *substratum* of the cerebrum.

The preceding considerations refer only to certain conditions of the psychic act, not to its nature which at present no hypothesis can elucidate. Neither materialism nor spiritualism explains to us how a phenomenon of excitation arriving at the first cerebral layer is converted there into such a different thing as an act of consciousness.

From the point of view of the link and continuity between the sensory-afferent and motor spheres, both hypotheses give a relatively satisfactory explanation; in spiritual doctrine, the soul would act as a receptor [organ]^V at a given point of the cerebrum and as a driving [organ]^W at another point, coming to be something akin to the telegraphist who, situated at a central station, is capable of receiving and transmitting orders over all the concurrent lines. The system of material relationships established between the motor and sensory pathways would only explain automatic behavior; in conscious behavior, the linking arc would be the soul itself.

In the materialistic hypothesis, things would occur in the same manner, except that consciousness occurring in the loop between centripetal and centrifugal activity, instead of being represented by an immaterial substance [that is] the annihilator and generator of the activity, would be [represented] by a very special activity [that is] a transformation of the sensory excitation and a producer of the motor excitation. There would thus be no interruption of the current [flowing] between the two ends of the conscious arc, but [conscious phenomena would] simply be a reflection of the same, under different conditions. The nature, extent, and complexity of the motor reaction caused by the reception of a sensory excitation, as well as the awareness of it by way of a representation or an idea, would result inevitably from the anatomical construction of the receptive cortical region, because each of these regions possesses, probably, its own group of associated cells for the retention of impressions and its subordinate system of projection or excitomotor cells.

Cajal's Note

1. We have made the same observations on the cortex of the occipital gyri of the child—Azoulay. [This footnote is added to the French version of the text.]

Editors' Notes

A. We have translated only the part referring to the cerebral cortex from the original Spanish version, with additions from the more extended French version.

B. Three in the French version.

C. Fig. 8 of the Spanish version does not appear in the German and French versions, being replaced by fig. 845 of the later *Textura*. The legend to the figure in 1894 says "dog one day old," but in the *Textura* (1904) and the *Histologie* (1911) it says "rabbit of a few days."

D. This title and the accompanying text appear only in the French version.

E. We have translated the description of this type of cell and that of the following (triangular or stellate type) from the French version since it is more detailed. To this has been added the corresponding fig. 8 that Cajal used to illustrate these types of cells in the Spanish version.

F. The Spanish version says categorically that the axon is double and sometimes triple.

G. The Spanish version says the following with regard to the axons of these cells: "[T]he multiple axons come from either the cell body or from the several dendritic branches, and all of them extend more or less horizontally inside the molecular layer, resolving themselves into broad and varicose arborizations, which, like the [axonal arborizations] of the other cells of this layer, seem to be connected with the peripheral [dendritic] shafts of the pyramids."

H. This title and the accompanying text appear only in the Spanish version.

I. The five paragraphs in square brackets appear only in the French version.

J. This title appears only in the French version.

K. Added in the French version.

L. Added in the French version.

M. The phrase in square brackets is added in the French version.

N. Both Spanish and French texts incorrectly say second instead of first.

O. This title and the accompanying text are only in the French version.

P. Added in the French version.

Q. Added in the French version.

R. Added in the French version.

S. The passage in square brackets is not in the Spanish version.

T. The text accompanying this point is only in the French version.

U. Here and elsewhere, Cajal says "resonant."

V. Added in the French version.

W. Added in the French version.

8

From: The Croonian Lecture[A]
The Fine Structure of the Nerve Centers

[*Proceedings of the Royal Society of London* 55:444–468, 1894]

The last subject, which we have deliberately left to the end of this lecture because of its fundamental importance and the psychophysiological deductions that can be drawn [from it], deals with the *connections of the cerebral cortex* (fig. 6) [*fig. 41*]. In order that you may envisage the cerebral cortex in a clearer manner, we will divide it schematically into three fundamental layers that, from the outside in, are a molecular layer, a layer of large and small pyramidal cells, and finally a layer of polymorphic cells.

The *molecular layer*, which is never lacking in the brain of the vertebrates, is formed by a very complicated plexus whose main [components] are the peripheral [dendritic] tufts of the pyramidal cells, which, in short, we will call pyramids; the terminal nerve arborizations of certain cells of the layer of the pyramids whose axons are ascending; and the ramifications of certain intrinsic cells. The last mentioned cells, which lie in the thickness of the molecular layer, have a spindle or triangular shape, and the majority of their processes become horizontal, resolving themselves into a considerable number of small branches with the appearance of axons. These cells can be compared to the spongioblasts of the retina and the granule cells of the olfactory bulb because they also lack a distinction between dendritic and axonal processes.

The *layer of the pyramids,* the thickest of the cortex, includes numerous rows of elongated cells with a pyramidal shape, whose sizes increase as they move away from the surface. The main characteristics of these cells are that they possess a radial dendritic shaft, terminating in the molecular layer by a tuft of fibers more or less horizontal and bristling with spiny appendages; they emit several lateral and descending dendrites [that are] repeatedly branched; and, finally, they give rise to a descending axon continuing in the white matter either as a fiber of projection, as a fiber of association, or as a callosal or transverse commissural fiber.

The last layer, or [layer] *of the polymorphic cells,* includes cells with a variety of shapes, generally elongated, sometimes triangular or fusiform, but one of their processes is very often directed toward the cerebral surface. However, this external or radial process does not resolve itself into a tuft like the shaft of the pyramidal cells and does not reach the molec-

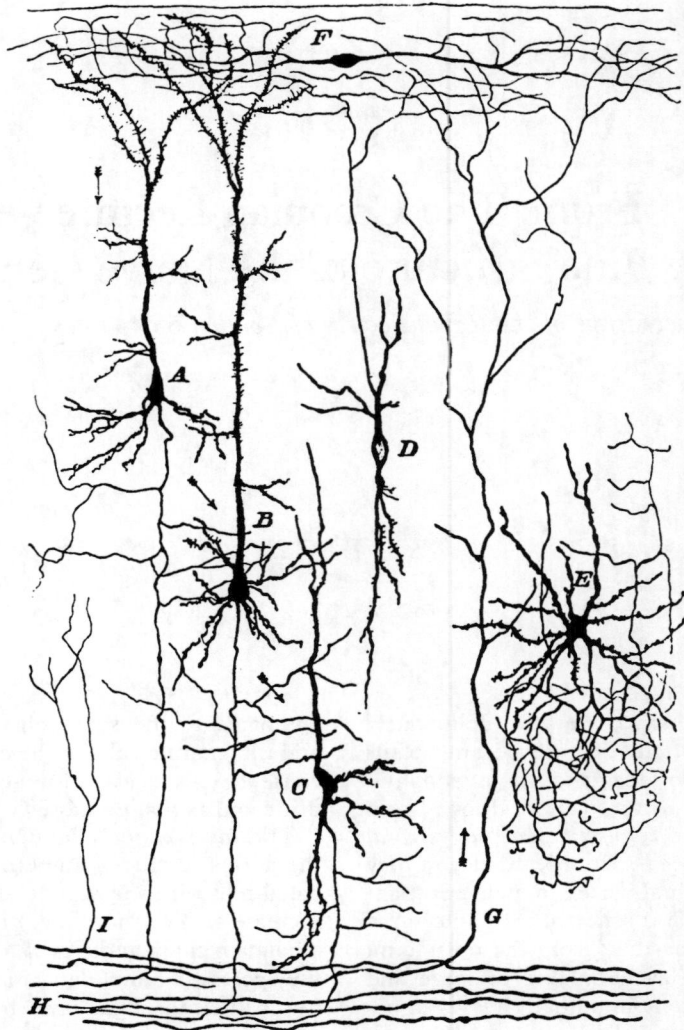

[*FIG. 41*]   Fig. 6. The principal cellular types of the cerebral cortex of mammals. *A*, pyramidal cell of medium size; *B*, giant pyramidal cell; *C*, polymorphic cell; *D*, cell whose axon is ascending; *E*, cell of Golgi; *F*, special cell of the molecular layer; *G*, fiber that terminates freely in the thickness of the cortex; *H*, white matter; *I*, collateral of the white matter.

ular layer. With regard to the axon, it penetrates into the white matter, where it behaves like those of the pyramidal cells.

During their course in the gray matter, all the axons of the pyramids and polymorphic cells give rise to a large number of branched collaterals, which freely terminate around the nerve cells, as we have observed in newborn small mammals. The accumulation of the col-

lateral ramifications engenders in the gray matter and around the cells a plexus of an extreme complexity. This plexus also receives the ramifications of the small collateral branches coming from the fibers of the white matter and those of the terminal arborizations of the callosal and association fibers.

You will understand from this inextricable complexity of the cerebral cortex that darkness still enshrouds our knowledge of its intercellular connections. The considerable spread of the terminal nerve arborizations and the lack of precise separation of the nerve connections corresponding to each cellular layer are the cause of all the difficulties. We will be thus very sober about this point, and we will limit ourselves to indicating only those connections that appear to be the best determined or the most probable.

The connections of the pyramidal cells of the cortex can be distinguished as *superficial* or in the molecular layer, and as *deep* or in the underlying layers.

At the level of the molecular layer, each dendritic tuft of the pyramids enters into contact with an almost infinite number of small terminal nerve fibers. These small fibers belong to the following categories: the terminal arborizations of the fibers of association, that is to say, of the fibers whose cells of origin lie either in the same hemisphere or in the opposite hemisphere; the nerve arborizations originating in special cells situated in the underlying layers, the cells with ascending axon which have been described by Martinotti, Retzius, and by he who has the honor of addressing you; the terminal arborizations of certain special cells lying in the first cerebral layer itself; the terminal ramifications of the small collateral fibers coming from the white matter, or from deep layers of the gray matter and from many other terminal arborizations whose enumeration would cost us too much time.

It is seen, therefore, that at the level of this molecular layer, each pyramid can be affected not only by the cells that inhabit the same region of the cortex—cells with ascending axon, ascending collaterals, etc.—but also by cells that reside in other lobes, either of the same side or on the opposite side. It is also probable, as we revealed when we studied the relationships of the olfactory nerve fibers, that the first cerebral layer receives the final ramifications of the sensory fibers. In this way, the peripheral tuft of the pyramids would be the point from which the voluntary motor excitation would commence; from there, it would be transmitted to the pyramidal cell body and to the fibers of projection forming the pyramidal tract.

It can be admitted, besides, that when the cerebral cortex of an animal is electrically stimulated, the muscular contractions are generated because the *stimulus* acts either on the tuft of the pyramids or on the nerve fibers of the molecular layer, whose role, in my opinion, would be to bring impulses to the tufts.

With regard to the deep connections, that is to say, those that take place in the very thickness of the layer of the pyramids and of the polymorphic cells, they seem to have the aim of linking the actions of cells of one row with those of underlying rows. The elements of this nerve articulation are, on the one hand, the [cell] body, the radial [dendritic] shaft, and the basilar branches of the pyramids of a deeper row and, on the other, the innumerable nerve collaterals originating from the axons of the pyramids of an upper row. Each one of these collaterals, thanks to their numerous branches and their considerable extent, can touch and affect hundreds of underlying pyramids.

We do not want to prolong further this tedious exposition of the intercellular connections of the cerebral cortex, and we will conclude this talk with some general considerations that follow from the totality of our investigations on the nervous centers.

Synthetically, it can be said that all the nervous centers are formed by the association of the following four elements: the nerve cells with short axon, that is to say, with axons ramified in the gray matter itself; the terminal nerve fibers arriving from other centers or from distant regions of the same center; the nerve cells with long axon, that is to say, prolonged into the white matter; the collaterals originating either along the course of the axons of the cells with long axons in the gray matter, or along the course of the fibers in the white matter. In certain systems, such as the retina, the olfactory bulb, and the first cerebral layer, it remains to add a fifth structural feature: the cells characterized by lacking differentiation [between] axonal and dendritic processes, those we call the granule cells of the cerebellum, the spongioblasts of the retina, and the special cells of the cerebral cortex.

Any nerve fiber is the continuation of the axon of a nerve cell. This law is also observed in the sympathetic ganglia whose cells, according to our observations, confirmed by Retzius, van Gehuchten, [Cl.] Sala, and von Lenhossék, show two kinds of processes: the branched appendages or dendrites that freely terminate in the same ganglion, and the axonal process that continues as a fiber of Remak.

The nerve cells constitute the units, the *neurons* of Waldeyer, whose reciprocal relationships consist of true articulations. The elements of each contact are, on the one hand, the somata and the dendrites of the cells and, on the other, the terminal arborizations of the nerve fibers.

In the systems where the origin of the [nervous] excitation is well established, it is recognized that the cells are polarized, that is to say, that the nervous impulse arrives always by the dendritic apparatus or the cell body and that it leaves by the axon which transmits it to a new dendritic apparatus.

The complicated differentiation of the dendritic apparatus, basilar dendrites, radial dendritic shaft, terminal [dendritic] tufts, etc., that the pyramids of the brain show us, and in part also the cells of Purkinje of the cerebellum, appears to have the aim of permitting each of the cells of this type to establish different contacts with several kinds of nerve fibers.

Those cells, such as the spongioblasts of the retina or the cells of the spinal ganglia, which lack a dendritic apparatus, enter into relationship with a single kind of nerve fiber. In these cells, the apparatus of reception is represented only by the cell body.

One can conclude that the more numerous, branched, and differentiated the dendrites of a cell, the greater the number of [other] cells by which it is influenced. In the same way, the greater the extent of the axon and its collateral and terminal branches, the greater the number of cells to which it will be able to send its impulses. From this dual point of view—differentiation and abundance of dendrites, enormous quantity of small collateral and terminal axonal branches—no [other] nerve cell appears to approach, even remotely, the cerebral pyramid of the mammals.

The result of our comparative investigations on the characteristics of the cerebral pyramid is that as one descends the [phylogenetic] scale of the vertebrates, the dendritic apparatus appears to be less differentiated, and the collaterals of the axons less numerous, less long, and less branched. Thus, in the birds, the pyramid lacks a radial [dendritic] shaft and a true external [dendritic] tuft; in the reptiles, the [dendritic] shaft and the peripheral [dendritic] tuft exist, but the basilar and lateral processes are absent or reduced to only one or two descending processes; in the fishes, the pyramidal cell is absent. A similar gradation can also be observed in the several classes of vertebrates in relation to the number and ramifications of the axon collaterals.

However, it is not necessary to leave the class of mammals in order to observe the differences, sometimes very considerable, in the richness of the dendrites and axonal collaterals of the pyramids. So, where in the mouse the basilar processes are short and little branched, in man they become very numerous, long, and highly branched; furthermore, the axonal collaterals in the mouse, as well as in the cells of the rat, rabbit, etc., are divided only once or twice, whereas in man these same collaterals, much more numerous, are divided four or five times, forming small branches so long that one cannot obtain them complete in a single section.

On the other hand, our research on the development of the embryonic nerve cells or neuroblasts of His has shown us that as the cerebral cortex increases [in size], the dendrites and the collaterals of the axons of the pyramids become proportionately longer and more branched. Initially, the axonal process of the [pyramids] lacks branches and terminates by means of a spiky enlargement that we have called the *growth cone;* then, along the course of the axon arise short little collateral branches similar to spines, which, by growing and dividing successively, establish contacts with a more and more considerable number of nerve cells. In fetuses close to term, as well as in infants of a few months, the basilar dendrites and the axonal collaterals are still very short and simple, and it is probable that the process of extension of these cellular processes continues into adulthood.

The facts of observation that we have succinctly exposed, and which are of considerable significance per se, have suggested to us a hypothesis capable of being better understood than all the others, as to why intelligence is acquired after a well-directed mental education, why intelligence is hereditary, why professional cerebral adaptations arise, and why certain artistic aptitudes are created.[B]

Cerebral gymnastics are not capable of improving the organization of the brain by increasing the number of cells, because it is known that the nerve cells after the embryonic period have lost the property of proliferation; but it can be admitted as very probable that mental exercise leads to a greater development of the dendritic apparatus and of the system of axonal collaterals in the most utilized cerebral regions. In this way, associations already established among certain groups of cells would be notably reinforced by means of the multiplication of the small terminal branches of the dendritic appendages and axonal collaterals; but, in addition, completely new intercellular connections could be established thanks to the new formation of [axonal] collaterals and dendrites.

An objection is raised immediately in your minds: how, you will say, can the volume of the brain be maintained if there is a multiplication and a new formation of small terminal branches of dendrites and axonal collaterals?

To answer this objection, nothing prevents us from claiming a correlative decrease of the cell bodies or a porportional compression of the regions of the brain whose functions are not directly related to the exercise of the intelligence.

The capacity of a family for the hereditary transmission [of intelligence] to immediate or distant (by atavism) descendants could be explained by this superior organization of the connections of the pyramidal cells.

Many other deductions are possible; thus, in men whose talents, as in the example furnished by Gambetta, coincide with a brain of small dimensions, the nerve cells could be less numerous, or they could be simply smaller, but in return they would present a very complicated system of axodendritic associations. By contrast, excessively voluminous brains,

which are often associated with an inferior intelligence and also imbecility, could contain a larger number of cells, but the connections of these cells would be very imperfect. This could happen in the large brains of the whale and elephant.

This anatomicophysiological hypothesis is not original in principle, because there is no lack of physiologists and psychologists who have searched for the morphological correlate of intelligence in the richness of cellular associations, but it is now based on the positive facts of structure and not on pure suppositions concerning the disposition and relationships of the nerve cells.

A propos of the reticular theory, the capacity for increase in the free arborizations of the cellular processes appears not only more probable but also more encouraging. A preestablished continuous network, a kind of system of telegraphic wires in which it is not possible to create either new stations or new lines, is something rigid, immutable, immodifiable, which runs counter to the opinion shared by all of us that the organ of thought is, within certain limits, malleable and capable of perfection, above all during its period of development, by means of well-directed mental gymnastics. If we did not fear to abuse a comparison, we would uphold our conception by saying that the cerebral cortex is similar to a garden filled with trees, the pyramidal cells, which, thanks to an intelligent culture, can multiply their branches, sending their roots deeper and producing more and more varied and exquisite flowers and fruits.

Furthermore, we are very far from thinking that the hypothesis we have just outlined could explain by itself the great quantitative and qualitative differences that brain functioning displays in diverse animals and in the same animal species. The morphology of the pyramidal cells is only one of the anatomical conditions of thought. This special morphology will never be sufficient for us to explain the enormous differences that exist from the functional point of view either between the pyramidal cell of a rabbit and that of man or between the pyramidal cell of the cerebral cortex and the stellate cell of the spinal cord or sympathetic nervous system. Also in our opinion, it is very probable that besides the complexity of their relationships, the pyramidal cells possess a very special intraprotoplasmic structure, also perfected in the intelligences of the elite, a structure that would not exist in the cells of the spinal cord or ganglia.

Editors' Notes

A. We have translated only pages 461–468. The remainder of the text deals with the spinal cord, olfactory system, retina, and cerebellum.

B. It is this part of Cajal's lecture that particularly attracted the reviewer for *The Illustrated London News* (Wilson, 1894).

PART II

An Interlude (1896–1897)

Methylene Blue and the Special Cells of Layer I

9

Introduction

In 1896, Cajal spent several months experimenting with various forms of nonneurological stains on tumors and blood cells. In the course of this work, he appears to have become familiar with methylene blue as a vital stain, one that had potential for neurohistological studies.

Paul Ehrlich first used methylene blue as a bacteriological stain in 1881. By 1886, he discovered that peripheral nerves could be stained by injecting the dye into blood vessels of living animals. In the next ten years, the method acquired considerable popularity, particularly for staining the peripheral nervous system, and there were several attempts to apply it to the central nervous system. The main problem was that the stain only became fully developed in nerve cells and their processes when subjected to oxygenation. Peripheral tissues could easily be exposed to air during application of the stain, but the CNS presented serious difficulties. Added to these difficulties was the problem of the solubility of the stain in dehydrating and clearing agents and its fading with time. The Russian histologist Dogiel (1896), with whom Cajal takes issue in one of the papers included in this section, introduced a number of practical modifications to the method, enabling it to be applied to rather thin, freshly cut slices of CNS tissue. To these, Bethe (1895) added fixation in ammonium molybdate, which served to preserve the stain somewhat through sectioning and dehydration and rendered it more or less permanent. Cajal himself suggests other modifications designed to make this fixation even more effective. In an effort to improve CNS staining, S. Meyer (1895, 1896), whose paper is attacked by Cajal, further adopted the practice of injecting large amounts of the dye into the living animal until it died, later exposing slices of the brain or peripheral tissues to the air. He thus introduced the method called supravital staining. A modern version of his technique is to perfuse oxygenated methylene blue through the vasculature (Boyd, 1958).

The papers included in this section are the most complete exposition of Cajal's experiences with vital staining using methylene blue. The first paper is interesting not only because it gives a detailed account of his methods but also because it shows Cajal at his most typical—concerned, as always, with priority,[A] rising to real or imagined insults, and defending to the end his beloved Golgi method. Apart from the technical procedures outlined, the major thrust of these papers is directed toward convincing even those with mild reservations, such as Kölliker, that dendritic spines are true entities and that the methylene blue method, even when used supravitally, usually gives very incomplete and often artifactual staining of nerve cells and their processes. If, in the course of this discussion, he also demonstrates that his methylene blue preparations are better than those of most of his critics, so much the better. A third paper (Cajal, 1896), not included here, is a more general work dealing with the collateral branching and terminations of various forms of axons in the cerebellum, medulla oblongata, and spinal cord and serving to reinforce the doctrine of connection by contact. A fourth (Cajal and Olóriz, 1897) deals with the structure of sensory ganglia.

Following our usual practice of permitting Cajal to speak for himself about what he saw as the more significant of his contributions, we here translate pages 297–304 of the *Recuerdos de mi vida* (1917), which deal with his methylene blue studies on the cerebral cortex.

[On pages 297–304, in referring to the controversy about the dendritic spines and the use of methylene blue, Cajal says:]

Even the correct Kölliker, a fervent believer in the miracles of the admirable tool brought forward by Italian science, had reservations about the existence of certain features exclusively revealed in the Golgi preparations: I refer especially to the *collateral spines,* indicated by me on the neuronal dendrites (cerebrum, cerebellum, Ammon's horn, etc.). To the scholar of Wurzburg, we could have been dealing, perhaps, with a superficial precipitate, like a crystallization of needles, fortuitously deposited on the dendritic surface. For the rest, similar doubts had been expressed by Golgi himself about the reality of these appendages, which, with the passing of time, have been the subject of many physiopathological investigations.

It is clear that I did not participate in such suspicions. My widening experience with the method brought to me the deep conviction that the said downiness, as well as the dispositions that appear in good silver chromate preparations (that is, in those obtained from fresh pieces rapidly fixed and whose very fine and uniform impregnation lacks irregular precipitates), corresponds strictly to reality.[B] Needless to say, however, my confidence, justified by fifteen years of incessant labor using several methods, could not be sanctioned by authorities little fond of techniques not invented by themselves or inexperienced observers without a formed opinion on the subject. It was thus absolutely necessary to show to everybody clear and unequivocal images, both of the spines and of the other morphological dispositions discovered by me, using for this technical tools radically different from the Golgi [method].

This purpose mainly governed my tenacious campaign at the end of 1896 and almost the whole year of 1897, during which time I used almost exclusively the methylene blue method of Ehrlich. My attempts, crowned with the best success, were several, one on the controversial *collateral spines.*

In the first communication,[1] published in June 1896, it is demonstrated dramatically, by means of a modified method of Ehrlich, that the said spines exist on the [apical dendritic] shaft and terminal tuft of the pyramids of the cerebrum (rabbit and cat), where they are exhibited stained a clear blue and provided with a certain, intensely impregnated terminal swelling (the *piriform* tumefactions, later studied by Demoor, Stefanowska, Manoumelian, Deyber, etc.) (fig. 60, *b, d*) [*fig. 43*].

The third monograph, based on the revelations of the methylene blue, was devoted to the *cerebral cortex* of the small mammals (cat, rabbit, etc.), illustrating mainly the structure of the *first or plexiform layer* in which, besides confirming completely the results of the Golgi method, [we] described numerous new types of cells with short axon,[2] for example:

a) Small cells with very short and promptly ramified axon.

b) Cells with horizontal short axon distributed over a larger extent inside the first layer (fig. 65, A) [*fig. 53*].

c) Large cells, with long dendrites, provided with a very long horizontal axon, whose destination could not be revealed.

d) Cell with descending axon, arborized in the second and third layers.

e) It is proved that the special cells of the first layer (cells of Cajal, according to Retzius) possess true dendrites, which are recognized by their varicosities in the presence of the methylene blue.

f) Very long horizontal medullated fibers which, often dichotomized, were discovered in the molecular layer.

g) It was conjectured that the cells of Golgi or those with short axon are generators of nervous current, etc., etc.

later better investigated by Golgi, Donagio, Held, Bethe, etc., was the starting point of great controversies. Such is the *pericellular reticulum*, so called by Golgi, and exactly and meticulously described by this authority in 1898 (fig. 66, A, a)[C] [*fig. 42*].

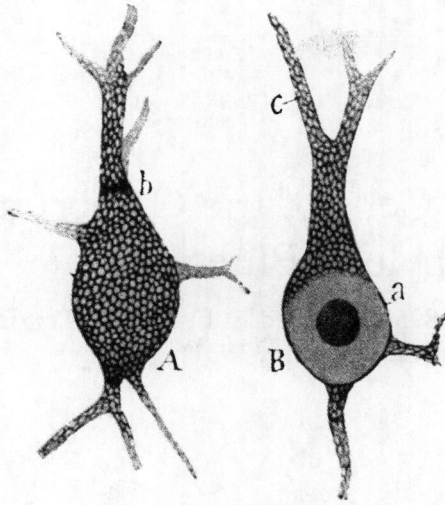

[*FIG. 42*] Fig. 66. Cells with short axon of the cerebral cortex. *a*, superficial mesh situated on the protoplasmic membrane (Ehrlich methylene blue).

h) A special nonnervous mesh is indicated around the nerve cells with short axon; [this], when

Cajal's Notes

1. Las espinas colaterales de las células del cerebro teñidas con el azul de metileno, *Revista Trimestral Micrográfica*, no. 2, June 1896. With 8 illustrations.
2. Las células de cilindro-eje corto de la capa molecular del cerebro. *Revista Trimestral Micrográfica*, June 1897. With 7 figures.

Editors' Notes

A. Written in Cajal's hand on the reprint of a paper by Meyer (1897), presently in the Cajal Library, are the words "He completely ignores my recent works."
B. See *fig. 48*.
C. Not reproduced by Craigie.

10

The Collateral Spines of the Cells of the Cerebrum Stained with Methylene Blue

[*Revista Trimestral Micrográfica*, I:123–136, 1896; reprinted in French in *Revista Trimestral Micrográfica*, reimpresión I:5–19, 1931]

In several of our monographs on the cerebrum and cerebellum,[1] we have called [attention] to the existence, along the dendritic processes of nerve cells, of an infinity of spiny appendages, arising at right angles and terminating in varicosities. Several authors, such as Retzius,[2] Schaffer,[3] Edinger,[4] Azoulay,[5] Berkley,[6] and Monti,[7] have confirmed and illustrated this interesting disposition, whose physiological significance is possibly of great importance for the function of the terminal dendritic processes.

Other authors, however, are quite reserved about the existence of such spines. Kölliker,[8] in his last book, affirms that the varicosities described on the dendrites of nerve cells represent embryonic dispositions, not visible in the adult; and [to him] the spines indicated by us would be simply, at least in the majority of cases, artifacts, perhaps irregular crystallizations or deposits of silver chromate.

To accept the above-mentioned appendages as real [entities], we had taken into account many reasons: first, that they appear both in preparations stained by the method of Golgi and in those impregnated by the method of Cox; second, that they are presented constantly by the same parts of the dendritic arborization, no matter what animal is studied, [and are] always lacking at certain levels, [such as] the axon, cell body, and origins of the thick dendrites; third, that they are also seen in the large ganglion cells of the retina of certain animals (for example, the frog) treated with the method of Ehrlich; fourth, that on examining them with apochromatic objectives, they do not possess the appearance of irregular crystals or deposits, but of very fine appendages, either simple or branched, substantially continuous with the mass of the dendrites, etc.

Recently, S. Meyer[9] has again questioned the objectivity of these spines, claiming that they are artificial products of the Golgi method. He bases this conclusion on the fact that he has never been able to stain them with methylene blue, either on the cells of Purkinje or on the cerebral pyramids of the rabbit. The method used by this author is not precisely the Ehrlich-Dogiel method but a special procedure that consists of injecting a rabbit, subcutaneously and at intervals of some hours, with 8 or 10 cc of a concentrated solution of methylene blue until that animal dies of poisoning. The brain, which acquires an intense blue color, is rapidly removed and is cut into small pieces that are fixed in the solution of ammonium molybdate recommended by Bethe.[10] This new fixing reagent has the advantage over ammonium picrate of forming a complex with the methylene blue that is almost insoluble in alcohol; therefore, once the color is fixed, the pieces can be hardened in this reagent, cut in paraffin or celloidin, and mounted with balsam, as if they were an ordinary preparation. Proceeding in this way, S. Meyer claims to have achieved, although with a certain inconsistency, quite complete staining of either the cerebral pyramids, the cells of Purkinje, or the nerve fibers. In the plate that illustrates the work of this author, in fact, a cerebral pyramid and a cell of Purkinje, both quite rich in processes and completely devoid of collateral spines, are seen en face. It is to be noted that the blue color in both drawings is extremely pale, which seems to indicate an extremely weak impregnation.[11]

Following the recommendations of Meyer, we tried this method of staining in a guinea pig and a common rabbit which died in twenty-four hours, after having received, in three or four injections, more than 30 cc of the solution of the methylene blue. But the preparations obtained showed only a few cellular bodies, so weakly stained that they did not reveal any morphological detail. On my advice, one of the histology students, Mr. Cutanda, repeated the experiments with several rabbits and guinea pigs, but without more brilliant results. It is true that in some cases a few cells and certain bundles of nerve fibers were seen stained either in the cerebellum or in the cerebrum, but the dendrites were so pale that it was impossible to pursue them completely. Under such conditions, it will be understood that observations of the very fine collateral spines could not be made. The method of Meyer thus is not appropriate, because of its inconsistency and paleness of the staining, for deciding the question of the existence of the above-mentioned appendages. And, in any case, and even supposing that the methylene blue were unable to reveal the collateral spines whatever the conditions of application, it seems to us there is little reason to deny the existence of the same, when two methods so different as those of Cox and Golgi reveal them clearly and with absolute constancy. Besides, in good scientific logic, negative facts of observation do not invalidate positive observations. When a method does not allow us to confirm a fact easily demonstrable with other methods, the only fact that we can legitimately claim is the insufficiency of the resources used to make the verification, unless it is proven in an unimpeachable manner (and this nobody has done up to now) that the procedures revealing such morphological detail lead to artificial alterations in the cells.

In our case, we have never doubted either the existence of the mentioned spines or the capacity of the methylene blue to reveal them, and this by virtue of a quite simple argument, because we have seen them many times perfectly stained with the method of Ehrlich in the retina of the frog and of other vertebrates, although only in the impregnations of great intensity and before the appearance of the varicose coagulation.

In spite of the denials of S. Meyer and the reservations of Kölliker, we had suspected that the method of Ehrlich, appropriately applied, would also confirm the existence of the spiny appendages, under conditions in which a great intensity of staining of the dendrites is achieved. Experience has led us to justify this reasonable foresight, and even though the preparations obtained with the methylene blue in the cerebrum, cerebellum, and spinal cord are always fragmentary and somewhat inconsistent, they are sufficient to resolve the debated question. Besides, these preparations have a positive value, as S. Meyer himself has already noted, because they confirm many of the morphological data gained with the method of silver chromate, and if all points are not confirmed, it is because of the incapacity of the procedure of Ehrlich to stain the fine axons and nerve collaterals.

Methylene blue can be applied in the cerebrum, cerebellum, medulla, etc., in three ways: first, by the method of the subcutaneous injections in vivo (method of S. Meyer), with which only palely impregnated cells, inappropriate for a detailed study of their processes, are obtained, at least in my experience; second, by the method of Ehrlich-Dogiel, which consists of infiltrating thin pieces of cerebrum, cerebellum, etc., exposed to the open air, with a solution of a tenth of a gram per 100 [cc] [of methylene blue]; third, by a method that we will call *staining by propagation or diffusion,* and in which it is not necessary to have the help of the air, and the stain, either in powder form or in a saturated solution, is deposited on the surfaces of pieces of nervous tissue, pieces whose thickness must not exceed two or three millimeters. The fixation of the stain is achieved with Bethe's fluid, a 10 percent solution of ammonium molybdate to which a few drops of chlorhydric acid are added.

The effects obtained with the latter two procedures are very diverse. By means of the Ehrlich-Dogiel method, the superficial cells of the molecular layer of the cerebrum and cerebellum, as well as a multitude of small peripheral nerve fibers, are stained exclusively. Thus, in the cerebellum of birds and mammals, the method succeeded in impregnating the small stellate cells of the molecular layer, which are shown provided with strongly varicose dendrites (a very frequent alteration in methylene blue preparations), and odd fibers of the granule cell layer. In the cerebrum of mammals, some multipolar cells are observed, generally with only their cell bodies and thick [dendritic] processes impregnated and some small nerve fibers of the white matter with an occasional cell of Golgi and a polymorphic cell. The cerebral pyramids are rarely stained, and when they are, they appear always very incomplete. In the olfactory bulb, a peripheral tufted process and some olfactory fibers are occasionally stained. In the medulla and spinal cord, usually the method is successful in impregnating the fibers of the white matter. The spines of the dendrites lack stain completely.

In the *procedure by diffusion or propagation of the stain* deposited on the surfaces of freshly cut pieces [of nervous tissue], the effects are diverse and, from the point of view of the staining of the deeply situated cells, better than with the method of Ehrlich-Dogiel. Unfortunately, this procedure is also very inconsistent and requires making a large number of trials [in order] to obtain cerebral pyramids completely and intensely stained.

It is in the cerebrum that the results obtained with this procedure are most beautiful and instructive. When thin slices of cortex are cut and coated on both sides with stain, there are observed underneath the surface, if the impregnation went off well, several alternating zones with a blue color, and immediately underneath an occasional or entire group of pyramidal cells strongly stained and with all the morphological details, including the spines, revealed by the silver chromate. The most expressive preparations are those in which the intercellular substance is little stained or remains totally colorless.

As seen in fig. 1 [*fig. 43*], the body, as well as the [dendritic] shaft and [other] dendritic processes, takes an intense blue stain, almost perfectly homogeneous, that is to say, without those dark clots and granules that are observed in preparations stained by the procedure of Ehrlich-Dogiel when, by virtue of some post-mortem effect on the protoplasm and with the help of the air, the methylene blue is deposited in the nerve cells. The nucleus commonly shows up clearly on a darker background of the protoplasm and exhibits a granular appearance.[12] In some parts of the [dendritic] shaft, the 1.40 Zeiss apochromatic [lens] reveals certain clear places resembling longitudinal angular vacuoles, as though a tight spongioplasm whose trabeculae have a mainly longitudinal orientation were stained. The whole cell body and the initial portion of the [dendritic] shaft lack spines, nor are these seen in the extremely pale dendritic processes, but when the staining is intense, such appendages are presented with absolute clarity on the upper portion of the radial [dendritic] shaft and on all [other] dendrites, whether they be basilar (fig. 1 *d*) [*fig. 43*] or collaterals of the [apical] shaft. The spines show up exactly the same as in the good preparations of Golgi, that is to say, pale in the pedicles and strongly stained in their terminal granules or varicosities.

The axon of the pyramids leaves from an elongated cone (fig. 1, *c*) [*fig. 43*], where the methylene blue is particularly concentrated; then it decreases in thickness, forming a fine fiber, progressively paler, so that it can only be followed for a certain distance, perhaps to the point at which the myelin sheath begins. We have not been able to stain its collaterals.

If the thin dendrites are followed as far as possible, it is observed that they become very unequal in contour and that they terminate freely. Frequently, the cessation of impregnation does not allow us to reach the last branches. In any case, the dendrites, unless one is dealing with very superficial and modi-fied cells, lack varicosities. Neither are these shown in good preparations of the method of Golgi.

The Purkinje cells of the cerebellum are also shown with the diffusion procedure and have the same characteristics as those in Golgi preparations. The cell body and thick dendrites lack [spines], but the final dendritic branches exhibit the collateral spines very clearly. The axon can often be followed to the

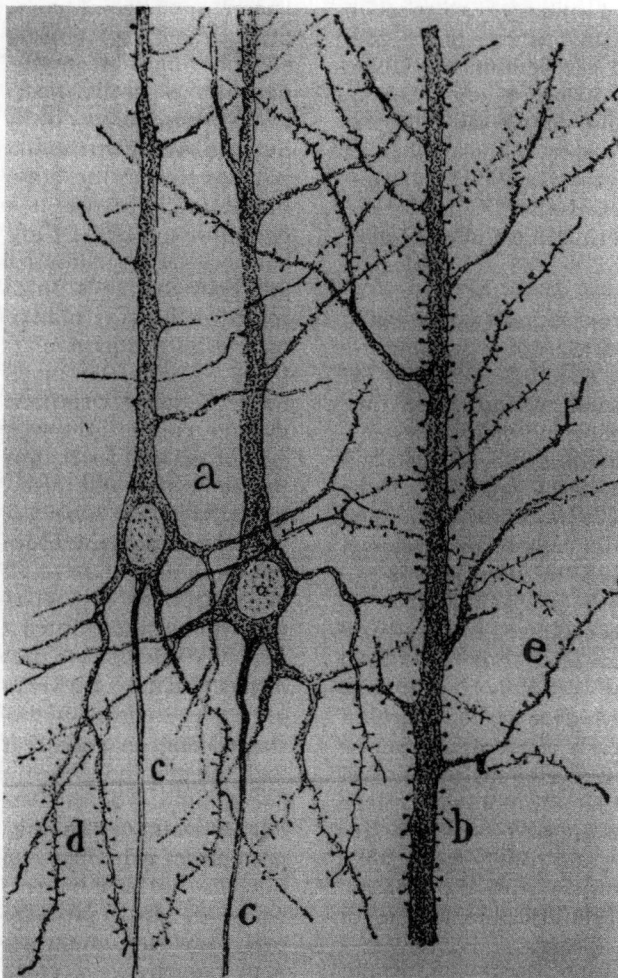

[*FIG. 43*]   Fig. 1. Pyramidal cells of the cerebrum of an adult common rabbit. Staining with methylene blue. Impregnation by propagation. 1.40 apochr[omatic] Zeiss objective. *a*, two medium pyramids; *b*, collateral spines of a radial [dendritic] shaft belonging to a giant pyramid; *c*, axons; *d*, spines on basilar dendrites; *e*, spines on collateral dendrites of the [apical] shaft.

white matter. Unfortunately, the intense staining of the secondary and tertiary ramifications of the dendritic arborization is very infrequent and fragmentary, since generally it is only the thick processes and branches of bifurcation of the said cells that are impregnated. Meyer must have stained the Purkinje cells in this way, so it is not surprising that he was not able to observe the spiny appendages.

We consider, therefore, that the question of the spines of the dendritic processes is definitely closed. Three methods reveal them in an absolutely concordant manner in the cells of the cerebrum and cerebellum: the Golgi, the Cox, and the methylene blue. This concordance will serve also for showing the extraordinary analytic power of the method of Golgi [when] properly used, as well as how unfounded are the criticisms that Dogiel, Meyer, and some other authorities have made regarding the reality of some of the morphological details revealed with the silver chromate.

The method of propagation (which would probably also work with other staining reagents, since we got excellent although extraordinarily inconsistent results some time ago with Turnbull's blue[A] on blocks fixed in a mixture of bichromate and red prussiate[B]) is capable of staining the rods and cones of the retina, the epithelial cells of the same, and above all the epithelial cells of the brains of reptiles and batrachians. In the frog, this epithelium is stained with great constancy, provided that the stain is deposited in the ventricles. The ependymal cells show an almost colorless nucleus; the cell body is pale blue; the shaft and its peripheral branches are intensely stained. It clearly confirms a detail already known from the revelations of the silver chromate, namely: that the contours of the shaft and its branches are covered with an infinity of short, warty, and rough appendages, which come into contact with the adjacent processes, outlining cylindrical containers for the passage of nerve fibers.

Also in the cerebellum, the method of diffusion sometimes impregnates, more or less fragmentally, the elongated neuroglial cells, that is to say, those producing the fibers of Bergmann. Here is verified once more the admirable fidelity with which the method of Golgi stains all kinds of cellular processes. As is known, the silver chromate reveals around the adult fibers of Bergmann an infinity of rough, short, and warty appendages, and they are so irregular that the majority of the authors have not even mentioned them, undoubtedly because they consider them to be amorphous deposits of silver salt; well then, these deformed clots are shown exactly the same in preparations stained with methylene blue and in which we have sometimes seen that the collateral appendages come into contact with those emanating from adjacent epithelial cells, engendering horizontal containers for that part of the parallel fibers extending between two flattened masses of Purkinje cell branches. Such an arrangement, like that which we have just revealed in the brain of the frog, is very interesting, because it makes probable the opinion expressed by my brother and me regarding the insulator role of the neuroglial and epithelial cells. In our opinion, the neuroglia of the gray matter has the aim of protecting all the parts of the medullated nerve fibers, exempt from myelin, and those parts of the terminal nerve arborizations in which contacts or connections with dendritic branches do not exist. The reasons on which we base this conjecture will form, with some newly observed facts, the subject of other work.

When methylene blue is used according to the usual procedure of Ehrlich-Dogiel (pieces of cerebral or cerebellar cortex coated with methylene blue diluted 0.1 per 100 and exposed for one hour to the action of the air), the effects obtained are very different from those of the preceding method.[13] Nerve cells are stained only in regions in immediate contact with the air, and they show up blue on a clear background. The nucleus is almost always intensely stained, and the more or less bluish protoplasm exhibits a clearer halo around the nucleus. We have never been able to see a cell whose dendritic processes could be followed over their full extent as in good silver chromate preparations; commonly, after one or two dichotomies, the dendrites become progressively paler until the stain disappears. The same thing happens with the axon; it is possible to follow it for a certain distance and even in some cases to distinguish collaterals, as seen

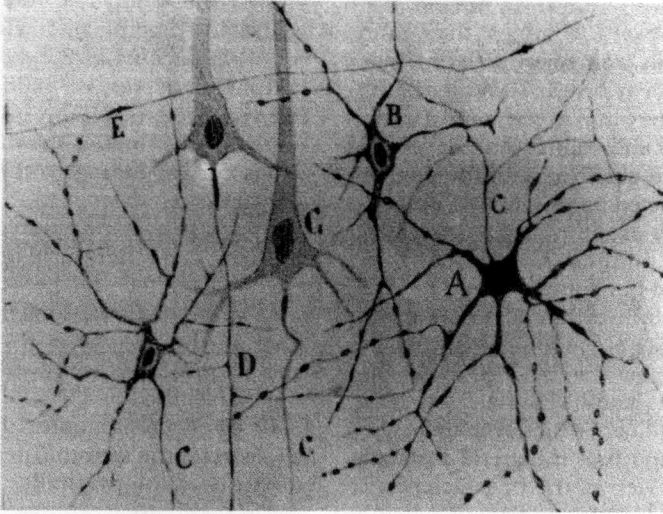

[*FIG. 44*]   Fig. 2. Cells of the deep third of the cerebral cortex of a rabbit. Method of methylene blue (procedure of Ehrlich-Dogiel). A, Golgi cell; B, Martinotti cell; C, pale and incompletely stained pyramids; D, collaterals of the axon of a pyramid; E, oblique nerve fiber provided with cruciform thickenings. The letter c indicates the axon.

at c [and D], fig. 2 [*fig. 44*]; but in most of the cells, the axon is only well stained near its starting point and vanishes without exhibiting any collaterals.

Among the cells of the cortex, the best stained are the polymorphic cells of the deep layers, the cells of Golgi, and the special cells of the molecular layer. The pyramids reject in a selective manner the methylene blue, showing at most a pale staining of the cell body and an almost colorless peripheral [dendritic] shaft (fig. 2, C) [*fig. 44*]. The starting point of the axon often possesses a strong accumulation of stain, a peculiarity that we have also noticed many times in the retina.

In fig. 2 A [*fig. 44*], we reproduce an intensely stained Golgi cell, which lay in the deep third of the cortex. Its cell body is so dark that the nucleus is hardly seen, and the dendritic processes that run in all directions often divide once or twice and rapidly become varicose. The fine and slightly varicose axon could only be followed to its thick branches.

The polymorphic cells are often stained, but always incompletely; the dendritic processes are lost to sight after some divisions (fig. 2) [*fig. 44*]. The descending axon does not display col-

laterals, nor is it possible to follow it to the white matter. In this same fig. 2 [*fig. 44*], we reproduce a cell that, because of the shape of the cell body and the ascending direction of the axon, identifies itself with the cells of Martinotti. It is not rare either to find small branched nerve fibers among the pyramids and an occasional myelinated fiber en passage, obliquely oriented and provided with robust thickenings at the level of the strangulations [nodes of Ranvier] (fig. 2, E) [*fig. 44*].

In the thickness of the molecular layer, the method of Ehrlich-Dogiel demonstrates clearly, although very inconsistently, the special cells or *Cajal'sche Zellen* of Retzius, the ascending tiny nerve fibers, and the peripheral [dendritic] tufts of the pyramids.

We have only been able to impregnate the cell body and the thickest part of the branched processes of the special cells of the molecular layer. But, although the staining is incomplete, it is possible to recognize easily the main multipolar types, namely fusiform, triangular, and polygonal (fig. 3, a, b) [*fig. 45*]. In the fusiform [type], the polar processes could be followed to the first collaterals; in the polygonals, the processes appear so thin that after the first division, and even before, they avoid observation. Anyway, however incomplete the figures of the referred cells stained with the method of Ehrlich-Dogiel may be, they have a positive interest because they affirm the neural character of these cells and confirm in essence the morphological data obtained with the method of Golgi and collected by us and by Retzius.

The nerve fibers of the molecular layer are easily recognized by their smoothness, thinness, very long and horizontal course, and frequent divisions; however, branches are much rarer than in Golgi preparations, and we attribute this to the fact that most of the collaterals fail to impregnate. At some points, it is observed that the fiber is smoothly bent, becoming vertical, and that it penetrates deeply into the cortex. In view of their characteristics, it is undoubted that many of these fibers correspond to the ascending fibers of the cells of Martinotti. An interesting detail captures attention when the horizontal trajectory of the thickest fibers of the molecular layer is studied with a powerful objective; each 200 or 300 microns, the smoothness of the axon is interrupted (fig. 3, f) [fig. 45] by the appearance of either a fusiform thickening or a double thickening divided into two halves by a pale bridge of normal caliber. At the level of such thick-

enings, the methylene blue is intensely concentrated. Judging by analogy, and considering what occurs at the strangulations of the peripheral nerves, in which the stain is also fixed vigorously, we must consider the mentioned thickenings as the naked portion of the axons corresponding to the strangulations of Ranvier.

As we first demonstrated and as Flechsig, Kölliker, and others have confirmed, the nerve fibers of the [central nervous system] possess true strangulations, longer and less regular than on the peripheral myelinated fibers and characterized, above all, by the absence of a transverse disc.

In some preparations, the methylene blue also reveals the terminal dendritic processes of the tufts of the pyramids. The appearance of such branches is so different from that shown by the Golgi method that it is hard to recognize the nature of the same. Instead of that magnificent tuft of small dendritic branches of unequal contour and bristling with very fine spines, we find branched fibers, so strongly varicose that they look like strings of pearls. Many varicosities display an empty cavity; that is to say, they consist of a crust of cyanophilic matter with a colorless central vacuole. This same varicose appearance is also displayed by

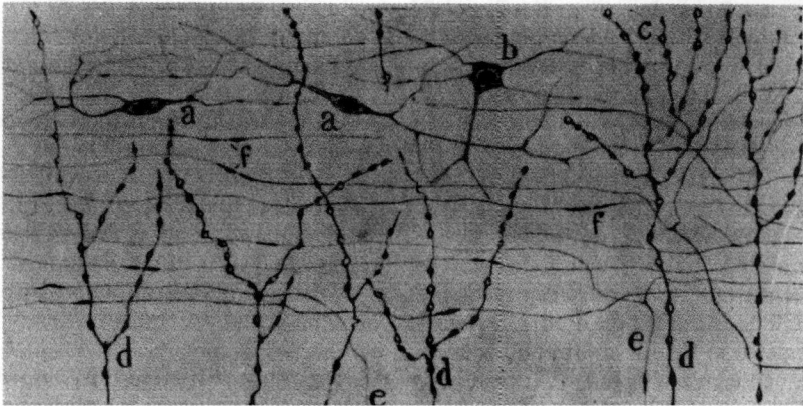

[FIG. 45] Fig. 3. Molecular layer of the cerebral cortex of a guinea pig. Staining with methylene blue (procedure of Ehrlich-Dogiel). a, b, special cells of the molecular layer; c, varicose processes of the [dendritic] shafts of the pyramids; e, nerve fiber that enters the molecular layer; d, [dendritic] shafts of the pyramids; f, thickenings of the nerve fibers.

the stellate cells of the molecular layer of the cerebellum and the superficial cells of the cerebrum of birds.

For us, it is indubitable that these varicosities are postmortem alterations, a kind of phenomenon of coagulation that both the dendrites and axons undergo, and which is perhaps exaggerated by the action of the air, indispensable, as is known, for staining with the method of Ehrlich-Dogiel. The observation, already mentioned above, speaks in favor of this opinion; that is, the said varicosities are not displayed by the deep cells stained by the diffusion procedure, which, even though reached by the stain, are not so easily reached by the oxygen of the air. Perhaps this better preservation also depends on the normal way in which death reaches the deep cells much later than the superficial cells. In some cases, when cells stained by the diffusion procedure have been well exposed to the air, the varicosities, sometimes of enormous size, are even formed on the thick [dendritic] shafts of the pyramids. Let us add that the method of Golgi does not reveal the referred varicosities in the adult period, which may be attributed to the rapid fixation that occurs in nervous tissue by [means of] the osmium-bichromate mixture; however, even the silver chromate is able to exhibit the above-mentioned thickenings, but under conditions of late fixation of the pieces, that is to say, at a time in which the spontaneous varicose alteration is well advanced.

In conclusion, the methylene blue, used by infiltration (method of Ehrlich-Dogiel), can still render some service in the study of the structure of the [central nervous system], especially by way of contrast to or in confirmation of the revelations of the Golgi [method]; but its analytical power is very inferior to the latter, not only because of the inconsistency of its effects in the cerebrum, cerebellum, and spinal cord, but also because of these three grave defects: first, the impossibility of obtaining cells with completely stained dendrites; second, the rarity and the extreme paleness with which the [axonal] collaterals are stained and, in general, all small fibers of great delicacy; and third, the impregnation of the processes as a late, postmortem phenomenon that

occurs when, after some time of exposure to the air, the cells have suffered varicose coagulations and other grave alterations (preternatural slimmings and widenings of fibers, coalescence, etc.) [that are] completely absent in preparations obtained by those methods in which the action of a fixer reagent (osmic acid, potassium bichromate, etc.) intervenes, in vivo.[14]

Cajal's Notes

1. S. Ramón y Cajal, Sur la structure de l'écorce cérébrale de quelques mammifères, *La Cellule*, Volume VII, 1891.

2. Retzius, Ueber den Bau der Oberflächenschichte der Grosshirnrinde beim Menschen und bei den Säugethiere, *Biologiska Foreningens Forhandlingar*, 1891.

3. Schaffer, Beitrag zur Histologie des Ammonshornformation, *Arch. f. Mickros. Anat.*, Vol. 39, Part I, 1892.

4. Edinger, Vergleichend—entwickelungsgeschichtliche und anatomische Studien im Bereiche der Hirnanatomie, *Anat. Anzeiger.*, nos. 10 and 11, 1893.

5. See, in the work of Dejerine, *Anatomie des centres nerveux*, Vol. I [1895], various figures of cerebral pyramids prepared and drawn by Dr. Azoulay.

6. J. Berkley, Studies on the Lesions Produced by the Action of Certain Poisons on the Nerve-Cell, *The Medical News*, 1895.

7. Monti, Sur l'anatomie pathologique des éléments nerveux dans les processus provenant d'embolisme cérébral, *Arch. Ital. de Biol.*, Vol. XXIV, 1895.

8. A. Kölliker, *Handbuch der Gewebelehre des Menschen*, 6th edition, Vol. 2, part 2, 1896, p. 647.

9. S. Meyer, Die Subcutane Methylenblauinjection, ein Mittel zur Darstellung der Elemente des Centralnervensystems, etc., *Arch. f. Mikros. Anat.*, Vol. 46, 1895.

10. Bethe, Studien ueber das Centralnervensystem von Carcinus maenas nebst Angaben über ein neues Verfahren der Methylenblaufixation, *Arch. f. Mikros. Anat.*, Vol. 44, 1895.

11. During the printing of this work, Semi Meyer has published another communication (Ueber eine Verbindungweise der Neuronen, etc., *Arch. f. Mikros. Anat.*, Vol. 47, 1896), assuring himself of the incapacity of the methylene blue to stain the spines and adding some improvements to his method of injection. These essentially lie in injecting saturated solutions of methylene blue BX (saturated at body temperature). He chooses for preference the newborn guinea pig, and injects subcutaneously 2 cc of stain each quarter- to half-hour.

12. It will not be superfluous to reveal here some details of the modus operandi. [Once] the brain of the rabbit is exposed to view, we begin by making in the cortex

serial parallel cuts no more than two or three millimeters apart, using a very sharp clasp knife, and immediately we cut the sheets of gray matter obtained in
this way into anteroposterior or transverse sections. By
means of a paintbrush wetted by a saturated solution of
methylene blue BB (Grübler brand), we soak all surfaces of previously cut sections, or we deposit on them
(which in many cases we find preferable) fine powder
of the mentioned stain. The pieces of gray matter may
remain in their natural situation, again covered by the
cranial vault, for half to three-quarters of an hour; then
they are removed carefully to be washed rapidly in a
normal solution of common salt, and they are fixed for
two or three hours in the solution of Bethe, namely ammonium molybdate 10 g; water 100 cc; hydrochloric
acid 10 drops. Bethe still adds a certain amount of hydrogen peroxide to this fluid, but we have not found
any advantage with such an addition, and we omit it.

The pieces being removed from the fixative solution,
they should be washed several times in water for some
minutes in order to remove excess of molybdate salt,
and they should be hardened for three or four hours in
the following fluid: formol 40 cc; water 60 cc; platinum
chloride 5 cc.

The platinum chloride, besides its fixing action, has
the aim of reinforcing the insolubility of the molybde-
num combination with the methylene blue. The platinic salt, which also forms an insoluble combination
with methylene blue, cannot be used as an initial fixative because it produces precipitates of a coarse color;
but in return it has the valuable property of giving any
liquid—water, formol, alcohol, glycerin, etc.—an absolute incapacity to attack the methylene blue.

Finally, the pieces are rapidly washed in order to remove the formol; [then] they are put for some minutes
in an alcoholic solution of platinum chloride at 1 part
per 300, and either after routine embedding in paraffin
or after a superficial embedding of the pieces in this
material (mounting on a block of paraffin and forming,
by means of a hot scalpel, a crust that holds the piece
to be cut securely), relatively thick sections are cut and
dehydrated in absolute alcohol [to which] platinum
chloride (1 part per 300) has been added; [then] they are
cleared in xylene or bergamot and mounted in balsam.

The decoloration produced by alcohol is prevented
by the alcoholic solution of the platinum chloride, because [alcohol], even when [cooled with] ice, as recommended by Bethe and Meyer, always separates out
the methylene blue, especially during dehydration of
the sections. The last change of dehydration can be
made without inconvenience in pure absolute alcohol,
provided it is carried out rapidly.

When working with small objects such as retina,
nerve ganglia, brain of frog, etc., complete embedding
in paraffin is made. To this end, and after washing out
the excess molybdate, the pieces are dehydrated in the
platinic-absolute alcohol and cleared in xylene; [then]
they are brought to a solution of paraffin in xylene and,
finally, mounted, by means of a hot scalpel, upon a
block of hard paraffin, upon which a crust will be
formed that surrounds the piece destined for
sectioning.

13. To apply the method of Ehrlich-Dogiel to the
cerebral cortex, it is necessary to cut fine horizontal or
vertical sections (1 to 2 mm) of the fresh cerebrum by
means of a well-sharpened clasp knife wet either with
blood plasma or with a weak solution of methylene
blue. It must be borne in mind that the reaction is only
achieved near the surface of the pieces and over a
thickness that is usually not more than a third of a
millimeter.

Once the sections are prepared, it is necessary to
leave them for three-quarters of an hour to one hour in
a humid chamber, in such a way that they will be
bathed with air over their whole superficial extent. To
this end, we keep [the sections] in a small frame of tulle
or of any very fine net with wide meshes. These small
frames, which can be of wire and resemble sieves, can
be superimposed without bringing the pieces in contact. From time to time, and over both sides of the sections, a paintbrush loaded with methylene blue is
stroked. On occasions, we have obtained better results
by placing the humid chamber in the oven at 38°[C]
and making a current of humid air pass among the
frames that hold the pieces, as in the procedure of
Roux for the culture of the diphtheria bacillus. For
lack of a pump joined to a water pipe, a bellows could
be used. It is clear that to work in such a way, the
humid chamber must have two openings situated in
front of the interstices of the frames, through which
the current of air will pass. However thin the piece may
be, it will be impossible to observe it [in its] entirety;
thus, it will be necessary to reduce it to sections that
can be mounted in balsam. The fixing, hardening, etc.,
is as in the previous procedure.

14. During the printing of this work, there has appeared a monograph of Dogiel (Die Nervenelemente
in Kleinhirn der Vogel und Säugethiere, Arch. f. Mikros. Anat., Vol. 47, 1896), in which [he] describes the
effects obtained with methylene blue in the cerebellum
of birds (procedure of Ehrlich-Dogiel, applied to thin
sections of fresh tissue). This author confirms the details discovered by us in the [axonal] processes of the
small stellate cells of the molecular layer (terminal baskets, etc.) and in the mossy fibers of the granular layer,
except that instead of the free arborizations indicated
by us on the mossy excrescences (see our first work on
the cerebellum of birds, Revista Trimestral de Histología, No. 1, 1888), he talks of terminal tangles, that is to
say, of complicated, pericellular nerve arborizations, interpreting the figures of free small branches shown by
me, van Gehuchten, Retzius, etc., as defects of irregular deposits of silver chromate, which would transform
the fine meshes of the terminal tangle into thick
masses. Dogiel does not know a fact that we had already demonstrated many years ago, namely that the
mossy fibers of birds possess richer, more complicated,
and tighter arborizations than the corresponding fibers
of mammals; and it is clear, on comparing his preparations of the cerebellum of birds with the drawings
that the authors have published on the mossy fibers of
mammals, that he must have found a discrepancy that
he arbitrarily attributes, and according to his deep-
seated custom, to defects of the Golgi staining method.

Very recently we have again applied the method of Dogiel to the cerebellum of birds, finding from the preparations obtained that the ramifications of the mossy fibers stained by the methylene blue are completely equal to those shown with the silver chromate. It is clear that the anastomoses in the tangles, drawn by Dogiel, are mere preconceptions of this expert, since they do not appear either in the Golgi preparations or in those of Ehrlich, if you make your observations with a powerful apochromatic objective (Zeiss 1.40). For the rest, the mistakes that can be made in the retina and other [systems] with the method of Ehrlich have been completely demonstrated by us in a work that will soon appear in the *Journal de l'Anatomie et de la Physiologie* [Cajal, 1896 b].

Editors' Notes

A. A commercial form of Prussian blue.
B. Potassium ferricyanide.

11

From: Methylene Blue in the Nerve Centers[A]

[*Revista Trimestral Micrográfica* I:151–203, 1896; reprinted in French in *Revista Trimestral Micrográfica*, reimpresión I:21–82, 1931]

As is known, Bethe has found[1] a method of fixing the blue staining of nerve cells that occurs with the method of Ehrlich by treatment with ammonium molybdate. The advantage of this fixation, which resists alcohol and formol quite well, is that it is easy to fix [the tissue] and cut thin sections [that are] preservable in balsam, not only of the retina but also of the cerebrum, spinal cord, and cerebellum, obtaining in this way preparations that, as we have demonstrated in other works,[2] completely confirm the revelations of the Golgi method.

We will not dwell here on the technique used, since it has been exposed in detail in previous monographs. We will indicate, however, those technical details that have allowed us to obtain staining with methylene blue of dorsal roots and collaterals [of the white matter] of the spinal cord, of cells of Ammon's horn, and of many fibers and cells of the cerebellum and cerebrum.

I. Technical Indications

Our experiments began with the procedure of coating of Dogiel, obtaining intensive impreg-

nation by depositing the methylene blue [either] pure or in a saturated solution [directly] on the fresh nervous tissue; but this procedure, excellent in certain cases, does not constitute a general analytic method. After many trials, we have convinced ourselves that the most reliable procedure, applicable, if not to all, certainly to the majority of cases, is the old Ehrlich method, somewhat modified, namely vascular injection of concentrated solutions of methylene blue, until the nervous system is intensely stained, and exposure of the tissue to air in an oven over three-quarters of an hour to two hours, after previously reducing the tissue to macroscopic sections with an extensive surface.

The time of exposure to air will vary with the results desired; in this way, after half or three-quarters of an hour of exposure to the air, there will be obtained preferential staining of the nonmedullated nerve fibers and of the dendritic processes, whereas the impregnation of the medullated fibers, and particularly of the axonal bifurcations and collaterals, requires one to two hours of aeration. Often the still air of the oven is sufficient; sometimes,

104

however, better results can be achieved with renewed aeration (continuous current of humid air with the apparatus of Roux).

One of the conditions for success is the concentration of the solution of the staining reagent. Experience has convinced me that in order to avoid direct application (method of Dogiel), it is convenient to use cold concentrated or saturated solutions, and make the injection through the aorta or carotids until the nervous centers acquire an intense blue color. In order to avoid vascular ruptures by excess of injected liquid, we make two or three injections, with an interval of some minutes between them; in this way, a portion of the methylene blue arriving early at the tissues has had time to disperse when a new amount of reagent arrives. It is not desirable, however, to force excessively the injection, because we could alter the chemical character of the nerve cell so rapidly that the reaction of Ehrlich would be impossible. Furthermore, an excess of methylene blue in the neuropil always gives rise, in the presence of the fixative, to crystalline precipitates. There is thus in this an end point that only practice will determine, and which will vary, of course, for each animal subject to experimentation. In general, it can be expected that the [nervous] centers have received a good dose of reagent when the conjunctiva and the tongue show a blue tone of regular intensity. As the reagent is rapidly reduced in the gray matter, it often happens that when the skull is opened the cerebrum and cerebellum are found to be pale or slightly stained, but exposure to air soon restores the blue [color] that must stain with a clear shade the surface of the newly cut pieces.

Another item that must not be forgotten is the size of the animal under study. In general, vertebrates of small size, such as frogs, lizards, mice, and guinea pigs, are to be preferred, the reason being that because the reaction is only achieved on the surface of the pieces (commonly to half a millimeter of thickness), we will have more probability of staining the relatively deep [cellular] elements. Here we refer, especially, to the systems that can be exposed intact to the action of the air; but it is also possible, as Dogiel[3] has indicated with reference to the cerebellum of the young pigeon, to impregnate very deep zones, on condition that the pieces are rapidly and cleanly cut, and to aerate one or both sides of these, for which we advise pads of tulle or any arrangement that impedes the contact of the nervous tissue with the surface of the receptacle used as a humid chamber. In spite of everything, in the spinal cord, the sectioning procedure gives worse results than the exposure of the entire organ; this can also be affirmed for all of those nervous parts that can hardly be sectioned fresh. However, the section procedure is efficacious and absolutely indispensable in the cerebrum, cerebellum, Ammon's horn, and medulla. For this, the clasp knife to make the cuts must be perfectly sharp, and to avoid adherence, it should be lubricated either with aqueous humor or with methylened blood plasma (with some methylene blue in the plasma solution) or also, although less innocuously, with an aqueous solution of the staining reagent.

Only when the injection has been incomplete and it is observed that under the action of the air the parts are not blue enough do we paint the denuded surfaces with the methylene blue. The water that carries the added methylene blue to the pieces is very far from being innocuous in all cases; in general, the incorporation of the methylene blue into the cellular elements and especially the achievement of colorless backgrounds on which the fibers show up perfectly are much better when the reagent has been supplied intravenously and, therefore, mixed with blood plasma.

In the adult animals, it is a difficult task to obtain completely stained cells. Among the cells [that are] more refractory to the staining are the cerebral pyramids and the Purkinje cells. However, nothing is easier than to obtain quite good impregnated Golgi cells or cells with short axon in the cerebrum, and particularly the small stellate cells of the molecular layer of the cerebellum. The insensitivity to staining is only relative, since sometimes, for unknown reasons, pyramids and especially portions of the dendritic arborizations of Purkinje cells are found to be intensely stained.

The staining of nerve cells and fibers, whatever their kind, is much more constant in young and newborn animals. Thus, in the cat of eight days, magnificent impregnations of the dorsal roots and collaterals of the white matter of the spinal cord (especially in the dorsal spinal cord, where it is the thinnest) are achieved that are only accomplished from time to time in adult animals. Ammon's horn of the rabbit of fifteen to twenty days is also shown to be much more propitious to the method of Ehrlich than that of the adult rabbit. The cerebellum of the young pigeon is likewise better than that of the adult pigeon. These observations have led us to try out the stain in the fetuses of large and medium-sized mammals, having noted that the newly formed nerve cells, that is to say, those close to term in their development, are impregnated more consistently than the adult cells, and that in their turn the nonmedullated nerve fibers and, even better, the newly medullated fibers (newborn dog, cat, etc.) possess a greater avidity for the methylene blue than the thick, already developed myelinated fibers.

Another advantage of young animals or of fetuses of advanced development is the thinness of the masses of white matter and the resulting shortness of the distance that the fibers must traverse, a very important consideration when dealing with a method that only stains thin peripheral zones. Thus, by virtue of this favorable condition, we have been able to follow in the cat of a few days the course and termination of some collaterals of the [substantia gelatinosa] of Rolando.

In special cases, we also use the procedure discovered by Meyer. As is known, this author has shown that if a certain amount of methylene blue is supplied to the nervous centers of a living animal by subcutaneous injection, the cells and fibers are stained with intensity, although not sufficiently to allow one to follow the last dendritic branches or to demonstrate the [dendritic] spines or the axonal collaterals and terminals. Because of this deficiency, the method of Meyer is much less revealing than that of Ehrlich. At the most, it could serve to determine the topography and general morphology of certain cells and groups of medullated fibers. At least, we have not been able to

observe with it a single collateral of the white matter or a single terminal arborization of the cerebrum or cerebellum. Only the acoustic baskets of Held, in the nucleus of the trapezoid body, are satisfactorily impregnated with this method, as Meyer[4] himself has recently shown. But, in order to obtain the reaction of Meyer, it is not necessary to poison the animals with subcutaneous injections; the common method of Ehrlich is more than sufficient, on condition that, by means of arterial injections made in newly sacrificed animals, the nervous centers be oversaturated with methylene blue (which is achieved using very concentrated solutions and leaving a pause of five to ten minutes between injections) and a wait of one or two hours be observed before removing the centers and subjecting them to the fixer of Bethe. Proceeding in this way, the cited reaction is absolutely constant, and the results are much better than with the method of [Meyer], since all the motor cells, interstitial [cells], etc., of the medulla, the cerebral pyramids, etc., are always found stained a quite intense blue. In spite of the fact that Meyer believes that his reaction is *vital*, we think that it is a postmortem chemical phenomenon that occurs without the help of the air, hence being only obtained in the deep parts of the pieces. Oxygen seems to impede the reaction; thus, we have never found, even in the medulla, where the method of Meyer gives the best staining, a cell or a nest of Held in superficial parts of the pieces which exhibit average impregnation.

Because the reaction of Ehrlich acts in the superficial parts and that of Meyer in the deep parts, the possibility of combining both in the same preparation can be perfectly feasible. We achieve it by subjecting the pieces overinjected with methylene blue to the action of the air. The staining of Meyer gives the general background and the topography of the deep cells (a circumstance that allows us to recognize the general structure of the organ), and that of Ehrlich shows the superficial fibers and cells intensely and selectively impregnated. To distinguish the two reactions, we will call that of Ehrlich *aereal staining* or reaction and that of Meyer, which can also be obtained (and even better, as we have proven in other works) by surface coating with concentrated solutions of methylene blue, *anaereal staining*, that is to say, without the help of the air.

Both reactions are postmortem phenomena. Whatever one may say in defense of the pretended *vital reaction* of Ehrlich, this is only obtained after the cells have suffered for at least one hour the deleterious action of the air, and when numerous phenomena of alteration and of true disorganization have occurred in the dendritic processes (formation of varicosities, thinning and paleness of their connecting [cytoplasmic] bridges, vacuolation of the [varicosities], disappearance or absorption of the spines, etc.), alterations erroneously considered as normal dispositions by Dogiel and other authors.[5] To expect that a nerve cell is normal when it is cold, altered, without nutritious circulation, when subjected for one hour to the action of the atmosphere, and this after the animal has been sacrificed by chloroform (which, after all, must provoke some alteration incompatible with life in the nervous protoplasm) or by hemorrhage (which kills, above all, because the nerve cells lose their normal nutritious stimulant), seems to me the height of good faith. I will not at all deny that the reaction can be initiated in living or almost living cells or fibers, but I cannot accept that these elements still possess vital properties during the phase of intense and complete staining, which is just when they reveal to us certain details of their morphology and structure. To accept the views of Ehrlich and Dogiel is as much as to affirm that the nerve cell which the pathologists and physiologists describe to us as the most vulnerable that is known possesses a resistance to suspension of nutrition, cold, influence of the air, action of water (solutions of methylene blue), and poisons (the methylene blue is a true poison, as is proven by the experiments of S. Meyer), and that this resistance is much greater than that of such other cells as epithelial cells, muscle cells, and blood cells, for which we know that any of the cited conditions is sufficient within some minutes to suspend vitality definitively.

Regarding the procedure of fixing, sectioning, etc., we adopt the procedure described in previous monographs, that is to say, we fix the pieces in the solution of Bethe[6] with or without hydrogen peroxide (water, 100 parts; ammonium molybdate, 10 parts; hydrochloric acid, 10 drops; hydrogen peroxide, some drops), in which [the pieces] remain from four to twenty-four hours; then we wash [the pieces] with water for half an hour to one hour; we fix them for six to twelve hours in formol (formol, 40 parts; water, 100 parts; solution of platinum chloride at 1 per 100, some drops); we section them, previously mounted on a block of paraffin; and, finally, we dehydrate the sections with platinic alcohol (1 per 300), or, what is almost the same (and thus prevents in part opaqueness of the sections), with alcohol that contains some drops of an aqueous solution of platinum chloride. In this way, we avoid the action of the pure alcohol, [which] always somewhat alters the stain. We make the last dehydration with pure absolute alcohol, that is to say, without platinum.

In order to impede the decomposition of the platinic salt in the presence of alcohol, this solution should be recently made. The most practical method is to add two or three drops of the aqueous platinic solution to the same porcelain well full of alcohol in which the sections are collected. In this way, we avoid the use of ice, which Bethe and Meyer recommend to exclude the deleterious action of the alcohol.

Mounting in paraffin should be made with a hot scalpel; it is not thus an embedding but a means of keeping the block steady. Given the superficiality of the reaction, it is convenient not to waste the superficial sections which are the only ones in which stained cells will be found. In general, the first section is always the best, then the second is usually also useful, but the third rarely contains stained cells, unless one is dealing with cylindrical blocks such as the spinal cord, in which, if it is thin and was kept completely surrounded with air, all the sections may present a superficial, quite well-stained zone.[B]

V. Cerebral Cortex

Our previous studies with methylene blue on this subject oblige us to brevity. Here we will show only some details relative to the fibers and cells that were not presented with complete evidence in our preceding observations.

Of course, we have confirmed in the adult cat, dog, and rabbit the great resistance to the methylene blue possessed by the pyramids. Nevertheless, this resistance is somewhat less in young animals (cat of eight to fifteen days), in which we have been able to see many very well-stained pyramids, particularly those of the small type.

These cells show us three phases of staining: one, the most common, reveals perfectly outlined branches of the terminal [dendritic] tuft, a part of the radial [dendritic] shaft, and the collaterals emerging from it, but without the cell body and axon appearing stained; in another, only the [main] axons but not the [axonal] collaterals appear impregnated, a disposition [that is] very common when the aeration of the sectioned nerve pieces has been prolonged for more than one hour; and the third which is extremely rare, shows everything stained, although with respect to the axon the impregnation is usually less intense. As a variant of the latter phase can be counted the complete impregnation of the cell body, [dendritic] shaft, and branches, but without obvious staining of the axon, a disposition [that is] more common than the preceding.

However, more consistent stainings of the cells of the molecular layer, of the cells of Martinotti, and of the several kinds of cells of the layer of the polymorphic cells are achieved.

The cells of the molecular layer, already indicated in previous works, can be studied quite well in parallel sections of the cortex (in the first section corresponding to the part bathed with air). Their form is ovoid, triangular, or stellate; the protoplasm of the cell body [is] relatively scarce, and from its angles arise horizontal processes that are divided several times, reaching such an enormous extent that the termination of the last small branches cannot be observed. The study of these cells, as well as of the medullated fibers of the molecular layer, is improved in superficial and tangential sections of the molecular layer not subjected to the decoloring action of alcohol, rather than in pieces fixed and sectioned by the usual method

of Bethe. With this purpose, we separate with the help of scissors a thin little slice of the fresh and methylene-blue-impregnated cerebrum; we put it on a slide, where it is fixed with molybdate; we cover it with a coverslip; and, finally, we replace the solution of molybdate with a drop of glycerin that contains ammonium molybdate. The preparations made in this way do not last a long time, but, on the other hand, once cleared in glycerin, they reveal better the fine dendritic and axonal ramifications.

Examining such preparations, we have convinced ourselves that the long horizontal processes of the special cells of the cortex lack myelin and have the characteristics of the undifferentiated processes of the amacrine [cells] of the retina. The ascending branches, well described by Retzius in the embryonic cerebrum, are not clearly shown in preparations [made by] the method of Ehrlich. Another fact easily appreciable is the enormous length in the adult of certain medullated fibers of the molecular layer, corresponding probably to the ascending axons of [the cells of] Martinotti. There are fibers of this [kind] in the cerebrum of the adult cat, which have been followed over more than two millimeters, without inclination to terminate and showing in their trajectory several collaterals and some dichotomous branching. This greater length of the superficial nerve fibers in comparison with that seen in the Golgi preparations is well explained by accepting that in the cat of eight days or in the rabbit of fifteen, where the silver chromate has given the best results, the cited fibers have not reached the complete development they will have in the adult.

We have nothing new to add to that said concerning the pyramids and polymorphic cells. To show the appearance that the cerebral cells exhibit in the adult cat, when they are well stained, we represent fig. 8, A [fig. 46] a cell of the layer of the polymorphic cells. As we already know by the teachings of the Golgi method, in these cells the ascending dendritic process does not quite reach the molecular layer, becoming rapidly varicose. The collaterals of the axon arise from this cell at the level of a triangular thickening, deeply blue stained (b); sometimes, when the axon gives rise to a collateral, it traces a little angle, although less marked than with the fibers of the spinal cord (e). For the rest, there is also often observed in these cells the pale [axon hillock] and the more or less cyanophilic region of the [axon] situated above the commencement of the myelin (a). The exposure of the sections of the adult brains of cat, rabbit, or guinea pig to the air for an hour and a half reveals the nerve fibers and their collaterals almost exclusively stained. In these preparations (fig. 8) [fig. 46],

there is seen, both in the layer of the large pyramids and in that of the polymorphic cells, a plexus of small fibers almost as rich as the one revealed in good Golgi preparations.

Three kinds of fibers are distinguished at a glance: axons of pyramids arranged in little vertical bundles (fig. 8, B) [fig. 46]; small collateral fibers of several calibers which run in all directions but preferentially in the horizontal direction (fig. 8, e) [fig. 46]; and centripetal fibers, that is to say, those arriving from the

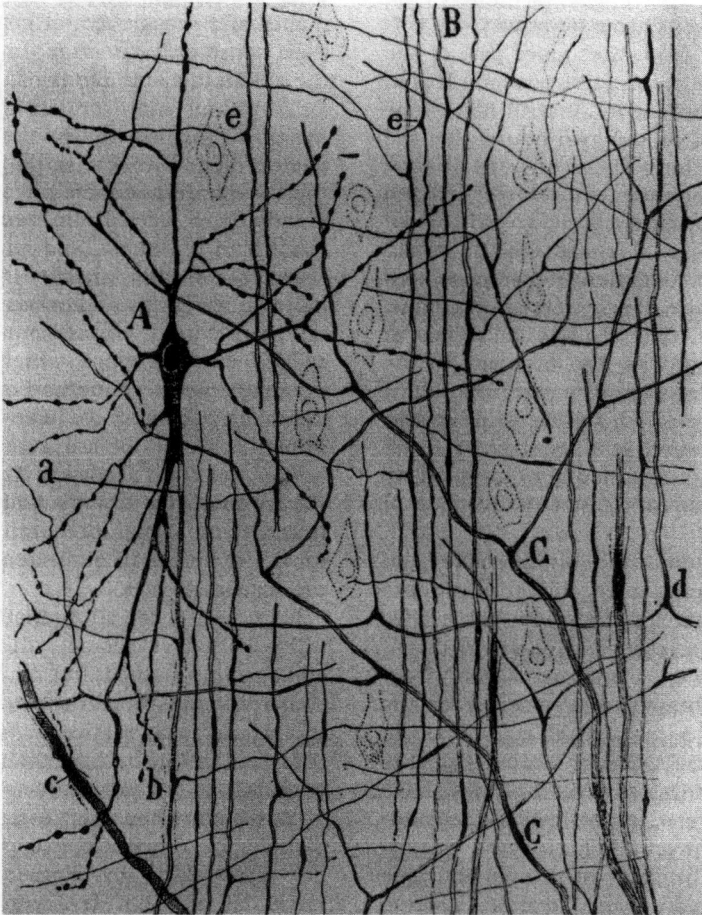

[FIG. 46]   Fig. 8. Cerebral cortex of the adult cat. Method of Ehrlich. Nerve fibers of the layer of the polymorphic cells. A, fusiform cell with long axon; B, bundles of axons of pyramidal cells; C, thick fiber coming from the white matter and repeatedly bifurcated; a, axon of a polymorphic cell; b, collaterals of this; c, short strangulation of a robust [myelinated] fiber; e, collaterals of axons of pyramids; d, early bifurcation of an axon.

white matter and ramifying in the gray [matter] (C).

(a) The axons of the pyramids offer an arrangement that resembles that in the preparations of Weigert. They are arranged in vertical bundles, loose in the upper part [and] more compact at the level of the layer of the polymorphic cells, and in which are found fine, medium, and thick fibers. The latter correspond to the axons of the giant pyramids. In its course, each of these fibers exhibits intensely stained strangulations [nodes of Ranvier]; some (the majority) are bereft of collaterals; others are provided with them. Commonly, as the silver chromate proves, the collaterals originate from the upper part of the axon and number three, four, or more. It is in the prolonged impregnations with methylene blue (aeration for one or two hours) that the collaterals appear best; [these] arise, as we have said, from a triangular thickening, beneath which they often trace a little arc with a superior concavity (fig. 8, e) [fig. 46]. In certain preparations, the methylene blue stains well the trajectory of the fibers, either thin or fine, but do not allow us to see any collaterals. A similar circumstance is also observed in the spinal cord, where suddenly a region can show us a great richness of collaterals, while in others none can be found. It is necessary, in order to avoid falling into lamentable mistakes, to bear in mind these caprices of the reaction of Ehrlich.

(b) The collaterals are innumerable, and when they are well stained, they form a dense and inextricable plexus among the nerve cells. The absence of varicosities allows us to distinguish, at first glance, a small nerve fiber from a fine dendritic branch. If the course of any robust collateral is pursued, it is common to see it dichotomize once or even twice, the branchings occurring, as we and Flechsig have already demonstrated, at the level of the strangulations of the myelin. The longest collaterals are seen in the layer of the polymorphic cells and deeper part of the [layer] of the large pyramids; most of them have an oblique or horizontal course and can be followed over very long trajectories.

With respect to the final small branches of the collaterals, that is to say, those devoid of a myelin sheath, so far, and in spite of our repeated attempts at staining, they have escaped our examination.

For the rest, in the adult cat, the course of collaterals is much longer than that which the silver chromate allows us to recognize in young animals, which depends, undoubtedly, on the greater development of [the collaterals] in the adult.

Branched Fibers in the Gray Matter

They are robust fibers arriving from the white matter and recognized, of course, not only by their commonly superior thickness to that of the collaterals and axons of the pyramids but also by their more or less oblique trajectory (fig. 8, C) [fig. 46] and by the right- or acute-angled dichotomies that they present during their ascending course in the gray matter. Generally, the resulting branches of each division run obliquely, and when they are followed for a long distance, three, four, and more successive dichotomies can be observed on them. The divisions occur at the intensely stained strangulations which are easily impregnated with the method of Ehrlich. So far, in our preparations, we have only been able to impregnate the diffuse myelinated ramification of the cited arborized fibers. This ramification coincides exactly with that which we traced from Golgi preparations and showed for the first time in our extensive memoire on the cerebral cortex.[7]

Commonly, the strangulations of the medullated fibers reveal only the axon thickened and strongly stained; but on occasion, the periphery of the myelin sheath near to or bordering the strangulation acquires a light blue color, and so around the axon and joining the two ends of myelin there is observed a blue crust which, when short (fig. 8, c) [fig. 46], has all the appearances of the cement or transverse disc discovered by Ranvier in peripheral [myelinated] fibers.[C] In a word, in certain cerebral fibers and under peculiar conditions of the staining, the methylene blue reveals in the cerebrum true crosses of Ranvier.[D] When the crust of cement is long (most of the cases), the appearance of a cross disappears, and the cement only serves to reinforce the axon at its bare portion.

As in the white matter of the spinal cord, in some fibers, the cyanophilic segment appears separated in two by a clear intermediate band.

White Matter

The axons of the white matter are very well stained, forming a dense plexus in which are revealed fine, medium, and thick medullated fibers. On them, the strangulations are clearly outlined, and, often, also the sheathing of cement is deeply stained. In general, the giant [myelinated] fibers present a thick and short sheathing of cement, almost as narrow as in the peripheral nerve fibers, whereas the fine [myelinated] fibers show it long and thin.

In any gyrus, it is necessary to separate two regions of white matter: the central or axial, and that bordering or at the frontier of the gray matter.

The [myelinated] fibers of the *axial region,* and in general those of all zones very distant from the gray cortex, do not allow us to see collaterals or bifurcations. If they exist, they must be rare, since they have completely escaped our examination.

By contrast, the [myelinated] fibers of the *frontier region* show quite frequent collateral fibers and dichotomies, although not as often as in the white matter of the spinal cord.

The collaterals are recognized not only by their thinness but also because at the level of their origin, the parent [myelinated] fiber does not change direction; such small fibers run in several orientations, and sometimes it is possible to follow them to the very gray matter; more often, the distance they have to travel in order to reach the cortex is such that it is not possible to observe their destination.

The bifurcations occur commonly on the robust [myelinated] fibers provided with thick sheathings of cement. They are distinguished as two kinds: first, division at an acute angle and into equal branches, which run more or less divergently toward the cortex, penetrating it at different radii—such bifurcations seem to correspond to centripetal [myelinated] fibers

coming from other gray areas; second, division in a T, in which a [myelinated] fiber, which seems to come from the gray matter, engenders two fibers of the same or similar thickness, which separate at a right angle and run in opposite directions. Probably, these dichotomies correspond to the divisions that, as we indicated in other work, are presented by certain axons of the pyramids as soon as they reach the white matter. For the rest, these bifurcations are much rarer in the cerebrum than in the spinal cord and medulla oblongata.[E]

Cajal's Notes

1. Bethe, Studien ueber des Centralnervensystem von Carcinus maenas nebst Angaben ein neues Verfahren der Methylenblaufixation, *Arch. f. Mikros. Anat.,* Vol. 46, 1895.
2. S. R. Cajal, Las espinas colaterales de las células del cerebro teñidas por el azul de metileno. *Revista Trimestral Micrográfica,* August 1896, parts 2, 3. Las colaterales y bifurcaciones de las raices posteriores de la médula espinal demostradas con el método de Ehrlich, *Revista de Clínica, etc.,* 10 October 1896. Nouvelles contributions à l'étude histologique de la rétine et à la question des anastomoses des prolongements protoplasmiques. *Journ. de l'Anat. et de la Physiol.,* no. 5, Sept.–Oct. 1896. Actas de la Sociedad Española de Historia Natural, October 1896 [Cajal, 1896c].
3. Dogiel, Die Nervenelemente im Kleinhirn der Vögel und Säugethiere, *Archiv. f. Mikroskop. Anat.,* Vol. 46, 1896.
4. Semi Meyer, Ueber eine Verbindungsweise der Neuronen, *Arch. f. mikros. Anat. u. Entwicklungsgeschichte.,* Vol. 47, 1896. In this work, Meyer claims to have been able to stain the collaterals and bifurcations of nerve fibers in the cerebrum, cerebellum, and spinal cord. I have never achieved this, not even using the new modification that this author has introduced in his methylene blue method. We do not deny that this procedure is able to stain the collaterals, peculiarly the thick ones, but we doubt much that it stains the point of union of the collateral with the parent trunk. In my opinion, this method obscures the staining of the strangulations at the division of fibers, as well as of any nonmedullated and very thin small nerve fibers.
5. See our short work, Nouvelles contributions à l'étude [histologique] de la rétine et à la question des anastomoses des prolongements protoplasmiques, *Journ. de l'Anatomie et de la Physiol. et Pathol,* Vol. XXXIII, Sept.–Oct. 1896, pp. 481–543.
6. Bethe, in a recent work (*Anatomischer Anzeiger,* Vol, XII, 1896), insists on the usefulness of the hydrogen peroxide. It is positive that a fixative solution con-

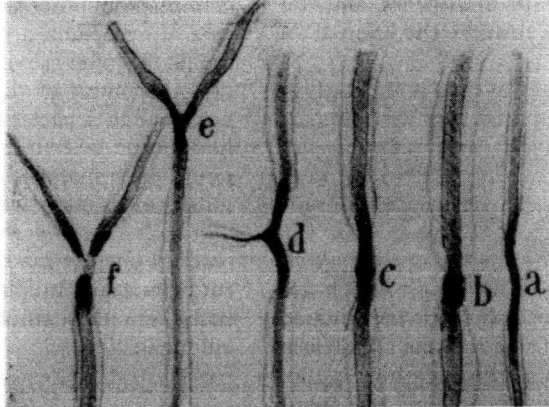

[*FIG. 47*]   Fig. 95. Nerve fibers of the deep gray matter of the cerebral cortex of the cat. Ehrlich-Bethe or methylene blue method. *a*, strangulation of a fine fiber; *b*, strangulation with a junctional disc on a thick fiber; *c*, strangulation with biconical swelling; *d*, strangulation with a collateral; *e*, *f*, strangulations with fiber bifurcations. The Schwann membrane is drawn in the form of a pale line.

taining hydrogen peroxide attacks less the blue color of the pieces, but the effects of preparations mounted in balsam are not so obvious. The majority of our better preparations were achieved without adding the said reagent, but that does not mean that it is absolutely unnecessary. In order to pronounce on this point, new and patient comparative trials would be necessary.

7. Cajal, Structure de l'écorce cérébrale de quelques mammifères, *La Cellule*, 189[1].

Editors' Notes

A. We have translated the introduction (page 151), part I (pages 151–157), and part V (pages 188–193). The remaining parts deal with subjects other than the cerebral cortex.

B. Here follow descriptions of the results of Cajal's methylene blue studies on the dorsal roots and white matter of the spinal cord, on the cerebellum of mammals and birds, and on Ammon's horn and the fascia dentata. Our translation recommences on page 188.

C. Where the two myelin internodes come together at the node.

D. A cross formed by the axon and the material lying in the space between the two internodes. The appearances described by Cajal can be seen in figs. 93, 95, and 96 of Vol. I of the *Histologie du système nerveux*. Fig. 95 is also reproduced as fig. 63 of the *Recuerdos* (1917), and we reproduce it here as *fig. 47*.

E. The paper continues with a description of methylene blue staining of the calyces of Held in the nucleus of the trapezoid body, plus a description of neuroglial and dendritic spine staining with the method. In the course of this discussion, one more figure of cortical spines (fig. 13, *A*) [*fig. 48*] is inserted.

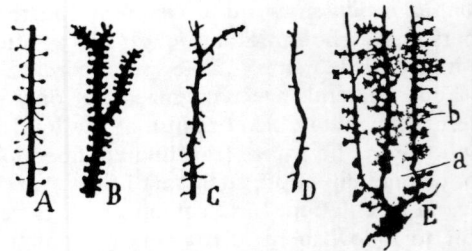

[*FIG. 48*]   Fig. 13. Varieties of spines that are seen on the cells of the molecular layer of the cerebellum of the mouse. Silver chromate. *A*, spines of a cerebral pyramid; *B*, spines of the Purkinje cells; *C*, spines of a basket cell; *D*, spines of a Golgi cell; *E*, excrescences on a neuroglial cell of the cerebellum; *a*, large space for the stellate cells; *b*, small gaps for the parallel fibers.

12

The Short-Axon Cells of the Molecular Layer of the Cerebrum

[*Revista Trimestral Micrográfica* 2:105–127, 1897]

In our extensive work on the cerebral cortex,[1] we noted the existence, within the molecular layer of the cerebrum, of two classes of cells: bipolar or multipolar special cells, horizontally oriented and characterized by the axonal appearance of many of their processes; and stellate cells with short axon, on the whole comparable to the Golgi [type II] cells of the cerebrum and cerebellum.

The latter cells, whose existence has recently been confirmed by Schaffer,[2] are much more abundant than we had initially thought. Our recent observations, made on the cerebrum of the adult cat and dog with the aid of methylene blue, authorize us to affirm that the cells of Golgi in the molecular layer of the cerebrum are at least as numerous as the residents of the molecular layer in the cerebellum and Ammon's horn.

The examination of the main forms of these cells, plus some other details revealed by the methylene blue, in relation to the fine structure of the molecular layer, will form the subject of this pamphlet.

Before starting with the study of the Golgi cells, let us remember that the molecular layer of the cerebrum is composed of the following

elements: first, small and medium cells with short axon; second, giant horizontal cells with robust axon; third, special cells of the cortex (*Cajal'sche Zellen* of Retzius); fourth, thin ascending fibers of Martinotti; fifth, horizontal robust myelinated axons; sixth, terminal [dendritic] tufts of the pyramids; seventh, ascending collaterals arising either from the axons of pyramids or from the fibers of the white matter.

Small and Medium Cells with Short Axon

These are spherical, triangular, or polygonal cells, whose size ranges between 10 and 20 [microns], and which lie in the whole thickness of the molecular layer excluding the external neuroglial rim that is made up exclusively, as demonstrated by Martinotti and confirmed by Weigert, of fibers and neuroglial cells.

The method of Golgi applied to the cerebral cortex of the cat and dog of fifteen to twenty-five days stains these cells quite well; however, in the young rabbit and mouse, on which our first observations had preferentially fallen, they are rarely impregnated; hence we had

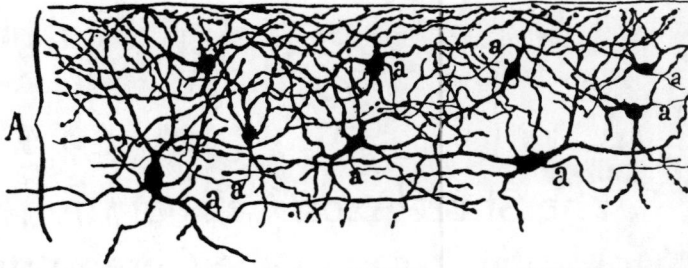

[*FIG. 49*] Fig. 1. Cells of the molecular layer of the cerebrum of the adult cat. Perpendicular section of a gyrus. Method of Ehrlich. *A*, molecular layer; *a*, axons stained only in their initial portion.

[previously] only observed a few cells of this kind. But to estimate the abundance of such cells, it is necessary to have recourse to the method of Ehrlich, with which it is not rare to see them completely stained over a rather considerable extent of the molecular layer. The [methylene] blue stains intensely and homogenously the thick or initial portion and the main branches of each dendrite, whereas in the thin branches the stain is concentrated almost exclusively at the level of the thick varicosities [which are] commonly provided with a clear vacuole.

In fig. 1, [*fig. 49*], we show the richness in cells of this class that the methylene blue reveals in transverse sections, and in fig. 2 [*fig. 50*], [we show] the principal forms of these cells exactly as they are observed in tangential sections of the cortex. Examination of these figures shows, of course, the great variety of forms and sizes, as well as the lack of a precise orientation of such cells. In general, it is possible to affirm that the diameter of these cells decreases as they occupy more superficial planes, and that the dominant form is stellate with dendrites oriented in all directions, but especially concentrated at the cerebral surface, where they form a very dense and more or less horizontal plexus. For the rest, the [methylene] blue stains the soma so intensely that it is almost never possible to distinguish the nucleus, and when the staining has not been excessive, it is not rare to observe on the soma and on some thick process an occasional delicate, collateral spine. The spines are entirely lacking from the more diminutive cells (fig. 2, *F, G*) [*fig. 50*], which are also characterized by the delicacy and shortness of their dendritic processes.

The axon can be observed in the majority of these cells. In the most voluminous, the [methylene] blue impregnates it well at its commencement and [over its] initial portion, it being possible, in the most fortunate cases, to observe some bifurcations. But in the smaller cells, the method of Ehrlich is impotent in demonstrating the axon. In no case is this method able to stain the entire terminal axonal arborization, a defect that places the methylene blue, from the point of view of its analytic capacity, much beneath that of silver chromate.

It is necessary thus to use the method of Golgi (double impregnation) to obtain staining of the complete course of the axon of such cells. As is observed in figs. 3 and 4 [*figs. 51, 52*], the direction, length, and robustness of these processes are extremely diverse. The presence of types of transition, in regard to the extent or to the plane or the height at which the axon is ramified, makes it difficult to draw distinctions among the cells; however, we believe that they can be classified in three groups: first, cells with a long horizontal axon, [i.e., cells] of association at large distances; second, cells with very short axon or [cells] of association at short distances; third, cells with ascending or oblique [axon] or [cells] of vertical association.

(1) The cells *A* and *B*, fig. 3 [*fig. 51*], are examples of the first type[A] or [type with] axon quickly ramifying in the immediate surroundings. The soma is smooth or poor in spines, and the dendritic processes rapidly become varicose, running either downward to the layer of the pyramids or upward and sideways. The axon, which arises sometimes from the soma and at others from a dendrite, runs in a diver-

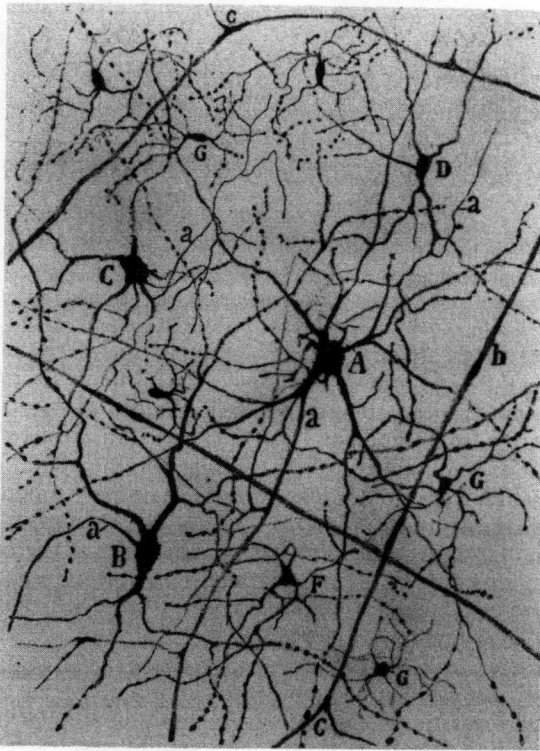

[FIG. 50] Fig. 2. Surface of a cerebral gyrus of the adult cat. Method of Ehrlich. *A*, giant multipolar cell with a robust horizontal axon (*a*); *B*, cell of the same kind, but less voluminous; *C*, *D*, cells of medium size; *F*, *G*, smaller cells; *a*, axons; *b*, strangulations of robust medullated fibers; *c*, collaterals.

sity of directions, often horizontally, and, at a short distance, it resolves itself into an extensive arborization whose small branches run in all directions, although predominantly horizontal. Each small branch is dichotomized several times, and after presenting a somewhat varicose appearance, [the branches] end freely in little, rough branches, sometimes adorned with very short collateral branches.

(2) The cells with horizontal (fig. 4) [*fig. 52*] and relatively long axon[B] customarily reside in the middle or deep third of the molecular layer. Neither their somata nor their appendages offer anything special. With regard to the

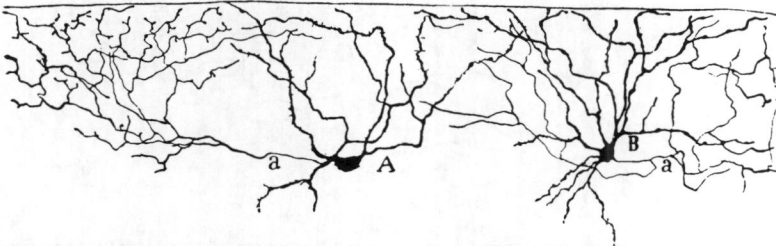

[FIG. 51] Fig. 3. Two small cells with short axon of the molecular layer of the cerebrum of the cat of twenty-four days. *a*, axon (method of Golgi).

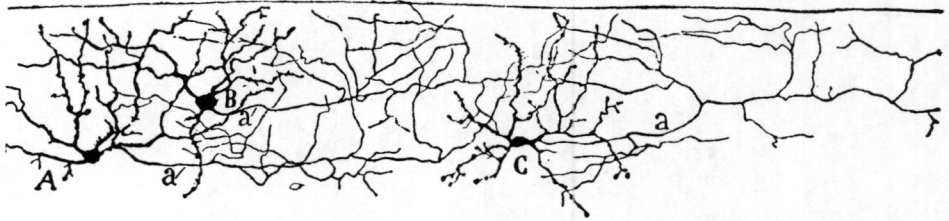

[*FIG. 52*] Fig. 4. Small cells with horizontal axon. Molecular layer of the cerebrum of the cat of twenty days. *a,* horizontal axon [Golgi method].

axon, which usually arises from a lateral dendrite, it runs resolutely in the same orientation as the molecular layer, that is to say, tangentially, giving off, naturally, some collaterals with a variable but often ascending direction, and after becoming very thin, it ends up by losing its individuality, giving rise to a complex arborization of thin, small, largely ascending branches.

This cellular type includes two varieties: one with a very long axon, extending for more than a tenth of a millimeter, and another variety with a shorter and thinner axon, which also has a relatively small soma.

(3) The type with ascending or oblique axon commonly resides in the middle and upper thirds of the molecular layer. Fig. 5, A [*fig. 53*] offers us an example of this cell, whose volume was rather moderate, and in which the axon, originating from an ascending dendrite, runs toward the cerebral surface, giving off on its way numerous small branches which are largely directed horizontally.

There also exist very minute cellular types whose somatic dimension does not exceed that of the granule cells of the cerebellum. Some

of them are pear-shaped, and generally the axon is difficult to impregnate (fig. 5, *C*) [*fig. 53*]. When it is stained, it can be noticed that it is very thin, with a very weak and nearby terminal ramification. Such dwarf cells, which usually lie very superficially (there are exceptions), can be compared to the diminutive superficial cells of the cerebellum or to the residents in the external half of the molecular layer of the fascia dentata.

Giant Cells with Short Axon

In the tangential sections from the cat, dog, and rabbit, processed by the method of Ehrlich, there are also found, associated with the medium and small cells described above, giant cells with a triangular or stellate shape, and notable both for the robustness of the horizontal axon and for the length of the dendritic processes (fig. 2, *A, B*) [*fig. 50*]. Both the cell body and the emerging thick [dendritic] shafts show, at intervals, collateral spines. Such dendritic shafts number three, four, or more and run more or less tangentially, and in some cases they reach such a length that, including

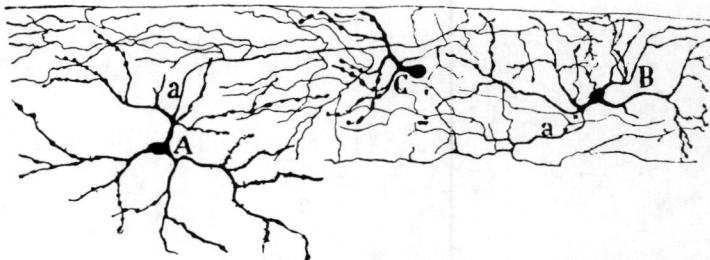

[*FIG. 53*] Fig. 5. Small cells with short axon of the molecular layer. *A,* cell with ascending axon; *B,* cell with oblique and descending axon; *C,* cell with poorly ramified axon [Golgi method].

their terminal branches, they can be followed for about one-tenth of a millimeter; in their course, they repeatedly dichotomize and become varicose, when the diameter of the secondary branches reaches about 1½ to 2 µm. The varicosities are very robust, and it is not rare to find them broken, that is to say, with the stained [cell membrane] torn and the interior [of the varicosity] flattened and empty. As a consequence of this tearing of the outer layer of the cytoplasm (tearing that is also very common in the branches of the terminal tufts of the pyramids), the cyanophilic substance leaves the varicosity and stains blue a more or less extensive and generally spherical area of the [neuropil]. Such a phenomenon, which for shortness we will henceforth call *cyanophilorrhage*, proves two things: first, that around the dendritic process there exists a thin elastic, dilatable membrane able to be broken when the tension of the cyanophilic matter in the varicosity reaches a certain level; second, that the cyanophilic matter, that is to say, the substance of the nervous protoplasm that attracts the methylene blue, is in the beginning dissolved in the cellular sap, and therefore it is capable of pouring out and being soaked up in the interstices of the [neuropil]. Examination of the cyanophilic spots or spillings with an immersion objective (Zeiss, 1.40 apochromatic) shows us the said matter stained an inhomogenous blue and exclusively or almost exclusively located in the intercellular cement.

For the rest, it will be unnecessary to say that cyanophilorrhage, a phenomenon that is very common in the molecular layer of the cerebrum subjected for more than one hour to the action of the air, is a postmortem transformation, an alteration produced by the method of Ehrlich, and as artificial as the actual production of varicosities or accumulations of cyanophilic material along the length of the thinner dendrites.

The axon of these cells is quite well stained with the [methylene] blue. As is seen in fig. 2, A [*fig. 50*], this process is thick, it is intensely stained at the starting cone,[c] then turns pale to recover later a staining never so intense as that of the dendrites and, finally, after giving off at right angles some thick collaterals, this axon turns pale, [and it becomes] impossible to de-

termine its destination. The preparations of Ehrlich give, as we have just seen, very incomplete revelations; they are, however, instructive, as they demonstrate, thanks to those concentrations of stain characteristic of the points of branching of the medullated fibers, the existence on the said axons of true strangulations [nodes of Ranvier] and, therefore, of a myelin sheath.

The preparations of Golgi complement to a large extent the fragmentary revelations of the method of Ehrlich. Although impregnation with the silver chromate is difficult, by dint of trying, we have been able to stain two or three of the [relevant] cells in the cerebral cortex of the cat twenty days old (fig. 6, A) [*fig. 54*]. The soma, which lies in the deep third of the molecular layer, is voluminous, triangular, fusiform, or stellate, and its dendrites, somewhat downy, run largely horizontally (there is no lack either of oblique and descending dendrites); and, finally, the axon, of great robustness, arising sometimes from the soma, at others from a thick dendrite, runs always horizontally, it being possible to follow it over a long trajectory, in which it gives off numerous collaterals, ramifying in several planes of the molecular layer. Some of these branches follow a recurrent course, being distributed in territories situated on the other side of the cell. We do not know the definitive destination of the axon, because in no preparation did it present itself completely impregnated; we think it likely, however, that it is distributed over a very extensive area of the molecular layer, bringing it into connection with the tufts of pyramids located in extremely remote regions.

The cells with short axon are very abundant at the deep limits of the molecular layer, between this and the tufts of the pyramids, and especially among the most superficial pyramidal cells. Schaffer has called attention to the richness in cells of this intermediate zone, which he names the *zone of the superficial polymorphic cells,* by allusion to the varied form of its cells. In it he indicates, from the point of view of the direction and relationships of the axon, three types of neurons: first, cells with short axon of the kind called Golgi [cells], in which the axon breaks up either immediately or after a variable, often horizontal, trajectory

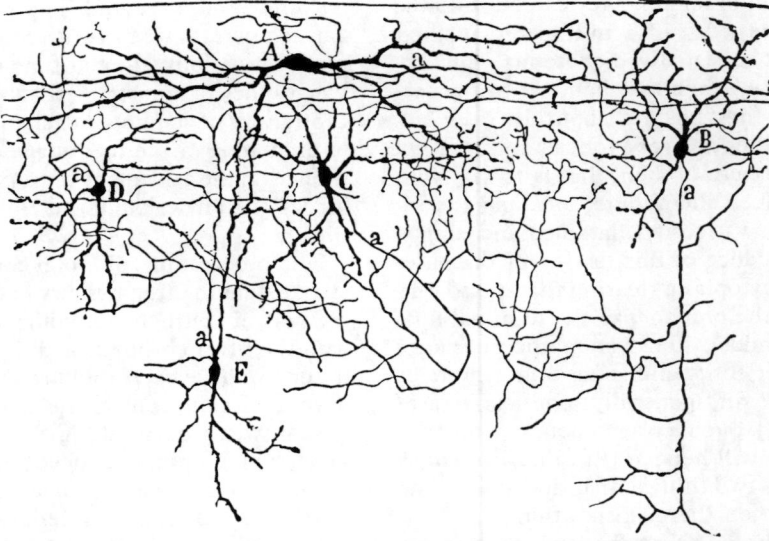

[*FIG. 54*] Fig. 6. Cells of the molecular layer of the cat of twenty days. *A*, robust horizontal cell of the molecular layer with a long and thick tangential axon; *B, D, C,* cells with short axon situated in the zone of transition between the molecular layer and the layer of the small pyramids; *E*, cell of Martinotti; *a*, axon [Golgi method].

into a terminal arborization either scattered or concentrated—many of the ascending collaterals of these axons would be distributed in the molecular layer; second, cells with descending axon, ramifying either at the level of the small or at the level of the large pyramids, where it would resolve itself into long, thin branches often with a horizontal course; third, cells of the same type but with a longer descending axon, which would disseminate little terminal branches in the layer of the polymorphic cells—its initial collaterals would be recurrent, and often they would reach the molecular layer.

It seems to us that the layer of the *superficial polymorphic cells* of Schaffer does not have a well-marked individuality. Between its constituent cells and those located in the different planes of the true molecular layer, there does not exist any rigorous frontier. In our opinion, some of the cells described by Schaffer correspond evidently to the cells with short axon that we had denoted as intrinsic to the molecular layer (deep portion of this). However, it is definite that the cells with descending axon ramifying in the very layer of the pyramids

(some types of which were already announced by us, although not without doubts about the subsequent course of the axon) have their habitual residence in the territory of transition from the molecular [layer] to the layer of the small pyramids and even in the thickness of the latter. Such are the cells that Schaffer has described very exactly, unraveling their connections, according to which they could be named *cells of vertical association.* By contrast with the cells of Martinotti, such cells, whose dendritic processes probably receive impulses of the molecular layer, would carry the impulse by the axon to groups of pyramids more or less deeply located. In fig. 6, *D, C* [*fig. 54*], we have presented some of the types of this class found in our preparations: in *A*, the axon was oblique, and its little terminal branches were scattered among the small pyramids, some of them ascending to the molecular layer; in *B*, the axon had a greater length, and after an almost straight descent, it traced an arc of external concavity to go up and be distributed among the small and medium pyramids; from the arc arose a thin process that could be followed to the giant pyramids. As

Schaffer says, the upper collaterals definitely reach the molecular layer. But anyway, the existence in the superficial portion of the layer of the small pyramids, of the cells with short and descending axon, is not sufficient to establish a new cerebral layer. The abundance of such cells appears very variable in the different regions of the cortex, and again, the Nissl method does not reveal clearly any separate stratum containing cells of special morphology between the molecular layer and [the layer] of the pyramids. The confusion about the superficial limits is also similar in regard to the deep limits because of the existence in all the cerebral layers, although not so abundant as in the said zone of transition, of cells with short axon and several orientations, as already mentioned by Golgi and confirmed by Mondino and ourselves. For all of these reasons, we find it more prudent to consider the cells with descending or oblique axon, described by Schaffer, as cellular elements of the layer of the small pyramids, among which they very often lie, although exceptionally they can be displaced up to the frontier and perhaps even into the very thickness of the molecular layer.

Special Cells of the Molecular Layer

These singular cells, discovered by us in the cerebral cortex of the rabbit[3] and well studied by Retzius in the human fetal cerebrum,[4] are characterized by their horizontal orientation, their considerable size, and the peculiarity of showing several tangential, smooth or almost smooth processes of an enormous length, and on the whole comparable, when they reach a certain thinness, to axons. Initially, we drew a distinction between dendrites and axons, because we thought that certain thin little branches prolifically ramified at right angles, and arising either from the soma or from the course of the robust polar dendrites, had the characteristics of axons; but having managed later to follow the very long tangential processes to their ends, and having recognized that their final branches also have the appearance of axons, we modified our first opinion and considered it likely that the special cells of the molecular layer, like the spongioblasts of

the retina, lack a differentiation of processes [into axons and dendrites], that is to say, that all the tangential processes of such cells had the same morphological significance.

Retzius, after having observed and carefully drawn the said cells, in human fetuses, revealing the several phases of their development and the richness and extreme length of the tangential branches (whose [further] ascending branches arose at right angles and ended under the pia by means of a varicosity), reserved judgment about the significance of the diverse cellular processes. Nevertheless, he was inclined to regard such cells as a special category of Golgi cells or cells with short axon, in which there would sometimes exist a single axon and in other cases many. For the rest, such a plurality of axons could be found also, according to Retzius, in the large cells of the granular layer of the cerebellum.

In subsequent work, Retzius[5] appeared still more undecided about the character of such cells. In it, he publishes new observations made on the human fetus from the fifth to the ninth month. The more important features following from these investigations are the enormous length that the tangential processes have in the human fetus (they literally fill the molecular layer with parallel fibers) and the sprouting off, over the whole itinerary of these, of an infinity of ascending branches, ending at the cerebral surface by means of a thick varicosity. This mode of termination by the ascending collaterals of the tangential fibers would be maintained, according to Retzius, during the whole development of the special cells, and probably also in the adult state, even though his attempts at impregnation met with success only in the fetal cerebrum. The somewhat special properties that such cells exhibit in man have been the motive by which Kölliker, in his recent book, calls the cells of the molecular layer of the human fetal cerebrum *cells of Retzius,* reserving the name *Cajal'sche Zellen* for those of mammals.[6] For the rest, [Kölliker] has also confirmed the existence of the special cells in the molecular layer (rabbit, mouse, and human fetus), although he remains uncertain about their significance.

In our opinion, all the observations made so far on the special cells of the molecular layer have revealed no more than the initial or little-advanced stages of their development. The adult phase is completely unknown, because the only method[D] so far useful for the purpose does not stain these cells in the adult cerebrum. From the examination of the preparations corresponding to different developmental periods, one is persuaded that once they finish their development, they may experience large morphological modifications. As we already indicated in our second paper on the subject,[7] the earlier the developmental phase under study, the shorter are the tangential branches and the more numerous the secondary branches that arise at right angles, ascend vertically to the cerebral surface, and terminate in a knotty thickening. Then, in the newborn rabbit, many of the vertical branches tend to become oblique, losing their submeningeal spheres, and in [the rabbit] of eight to fifteen days, almost all the branches originating from the thick tangential shafts finally lose their verticality and parallelism, running in several directions and prolixly ramifying in the superficial planes of the molecular layer. Although not so accentuated as in the rabbit of a few days old, the same process of transformation is also observed in the human fetus, as revealed in the drawings of Retzius, which seem to us to show a progressive decrease in the ascending fibers and of their terminal spheres as development proceeds. In the cells that this author shows from the ninth month of fetal life, forms completely analogous to the ones that we had described in the rabbit of eight days can be seen.

In our opinion, the original radial orientation of the ascending collaterals of the tangential shafts is an embryonic disposition destined to disappear, because in these early phases of cerebral development, they are merely the consequence of the existence of the system of radial fibers represented by the embryonic epithelial cells.

[It is] precisely in the embryonic molecular layer that the peripheral tufts of the cells of the ependyma constitute a very tight fence, and under such mechanical conditions, the process originating from a horizontally oriented cell have no other resort than to be directed vertically, that is to say, in the orientation of lesser resistance. For us, therefore, the terminal spheres are none other than deposits of primordial protoplasm, that is to say, a kind of rudimentary growth cone destined to disappear when the tight epithelial fence is absorbed and the ascending processes recover their freedom for growing and branching.

Even the limited number of descending processes arising from the tangential shafts could be explained by mechanical conditions; for this, it should be sufficient to remember the obstacle formed immediately beneath the special cells by the multiple arches traced by the very numerous bifurcations situated at the starting point of the terminal tufts of the epithelial cells.

In favor of this interpretation are the examples of cells of other centers, which exhibit, in the first phases of their development, a radial orientation of the processes, destined to be modified in the adult state. Thus, the Golgi cells and the basket cells of the cerebellum, according to what has been demonstrated by the investigations of Athias[8] and Terrazas,[9] have radial or ascending [dendritic] branches that maintain on their course to the molecular layer a parallelism that is not preserved later. Sometimes, the said ascending processes penetrate the layer of superficial granule cells or [cells] of Vignal, to end in a spherical thickening at the cerebellar surface. Here, as in the cerebrum, the initial dendrites must suffer many metamorphoses in the course of their development.

In general, it is possible to affirm that the production of the first dendrites depends principally on the mechanical conditions of the environment (disposition of the neuroglial or epithelial cavities of which His has spoken); whereas the rectification and absorption of the useless processes and the appearance of the definitive ones are late phenomena related to the appearance of the terminal axonal arborization, which represents, in our opinion, the definitive vector or differentiating agent of the secondary and tertiary dendritic branches. Such should occur with the radial processes of the special cells of the molecular layer: before the terminal nerve fibers ramifying in this territory appear, the dendritic processes blindly grow toward the surface, surrendering to the fatalism of the law of least resistance; but when the [axonal] arborizations are formed, the processes change direction, entering into contact with the terminal fibers, perhaps impelled by positive chemotaxia.

The special cells of the molecular layer have been recently observed by Veratti,[10] an author who has chosen, as the subject of study, the newborn or few-days-old rabbit, an age during which, as we have already indicated, Golgi impregnations of the said cells are achieved fairly constantly. This author recognizes the unique properties by which such cells are differentiated from others of the cortex, particularly that relating to the existence of several processes with the appearance of axons (*pseudaxons* of this author); but he affirms, in spite of all, that only one such axiform process represents the axon; this would be a thin process originating either from the soma or from a horizontal dendrite, which would more or less descend and engender, in the deepest planes of the molecular layer, a vast terminal arborization.

In support of this opinion, according to Veratti, would be the existence in the earliest phases of development of the special cells (embryos of pig) of an axon [that is] differentiated and sufficiently different from the dendritic processes. And the thin pseudaxonic fibers would be nothing more than embryonic or developmentally transitional forms of genuine dendritic branches.

Figures similar to the ones Veratti includes in his paper, corresponding to the earliest phases of development of the special cells, were seen and drawn some time ago by us[11] and by Retzius.[12] In effect, there are cases in which a process is shown thinner than others and resembles an axon, but even more frequently cells are observed in which all the processes have the same appearance, it being impossible to distinguish which of them is the axon; finally, not a few times, there appear two or more processes with the appearance of axons.

On the other hand, the existence of a process thinner than others in the first stages of development of a cell is not a secure criterion for recognizing the axon. Let us remember, in support of this, the embryonic granule cells of

the cerebellum, which in their phase of primordial bipolarity commonly possess one branch thinner than the other, but, nevertheless, both represent axonal branches, because both will subsequently form the terminal branches of the axon.

There exists also a source of error that does not appear to have been suspected by Veratti. In the molecular layer of the cerebrum, there also reside numerous cells with short axon, some of them of large size (as we have previously demonstrated), whose embryonic phases correspond to those presented by the cells of the molecular layer of the cerebellum, according to the observations of Athias and Terrazas. The Golgi cells of the molecular layer of the cerebrum exhibit, in effect, a bipolar primordial form, a certain horizontality of direction, and the marked contrast indicated by Veratti between the primordial dendritic shaft and the axon; because of this, it would not be strange if the embryonic cells represented by this Italian worker would correspond to the earliest phases of these [short-axon] cells.

In spite of all the exposed reasons, we do not consider the discussion about the nature of the special cells of the cortex (*Cajal'sche Zellen* of Retzius) to be completely closed. All the observations, even those of Veratti, have had their origins in the embryonic phases, because of the impossibility of staining such cells with the Golgi method in the adult cerebrum; and it could very well happen that, with development ended, they would offer a morphology quite different from the embryonic, exhibiting a greater contrast among their processes and revealing themselves, therefore, in such a manner that there would be no doubt about the existence of an axon.

These doubts relating to the nature of the [special] cells of the cortex have motivated us to undetake new investigations with the method of Ehrlich in the cerebrum of the adult mammals (cat, dog, and rabbit).

Unfortunately, this method does not give such brilliant results in the cerebrum as in the retina and ganglia. It stains the dendrites with intensity and constancy so that they can be followed to their thinner little branches, but it is shown to be very unfaithful with respect to the axons, which only show up sufficiently well to

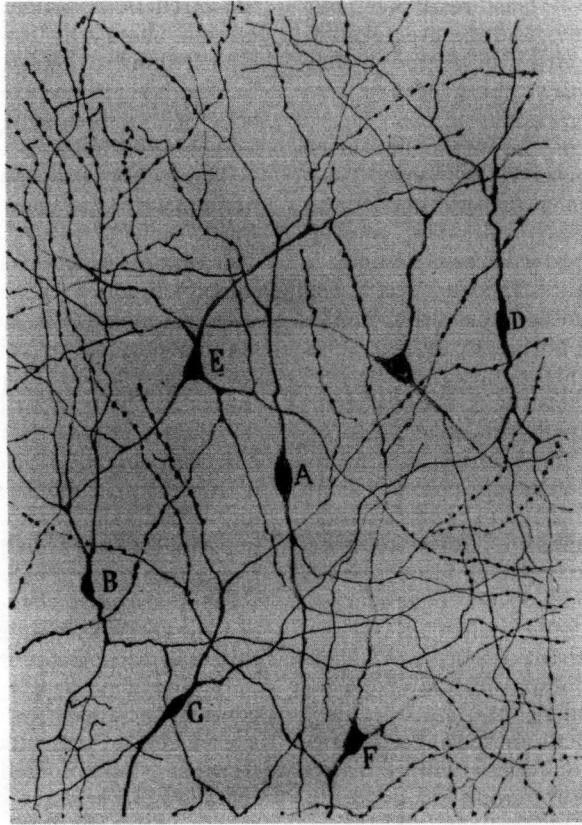

[*FIG. 55*] Fig. 7. Fusiform and triangular cells of the molecular layer of the adult cat. Method of Ehrlich. *A, B, D, C,* fusiform cells; *E, F,* triangular cells.

be recognized on the more voluminous cells of the cerebral cortex. We have not been able, therefore, to dispel at all the shadows that envelop this problem, and newer observations will be necessary to close definitively the discussion. In whatever way that may be, here are the obtained results.

When tangential sections of the cerebrum of the cat, impregnated with the method of Ehrlich, are examined facing up and properly cleared (mounted in balsam, previous fixation by the procedure of Bethe), very variable effects are observed, depending on the particular case. Sometimes, the medullated fibers and the terminal tufts of the pyramids appear exclusively stained; at others, the cells with short axon are presented perfectly impregnated; only in some cases is it possible to see the special cells regularly stained. However, by dint of [many] attempts at impregnation, quite complete staining of a good number of these cells is always achieved, [although they] are, without doubt, the most difficult to stain of all the residents of the molecular layer.

It is observed, of course, that they lie, commonly, in the deepest portion of the molecular layer, and this depth, without doubt, is the principal obstacle to their staining.

Their more common form is fusiform, but they can also be triangular and, less frequently, stellate (fig. 7) [*fig. 55*]. The cell body is presented in certain cases stained uniformly and intensely blue, it not being possible to recognize the nucleus; in other cases, it exhibits that disposition so many times represented by Dogiel, that is to say, the existence of a perinuclear ring [that is] less stained than the rest of the protoplasm. The nucleus can, on occasions, show a rosy color, a peculiarity that is also observed in many other cells.

From the poles of the cell arise the thick tangential processes [that are] generally smooth (sometimes, we have been able to see scarce but very distinct spines), straight or almost straight, and extended parallel to the cerebral surface over very long trajectories. In some cases, we have been able to follow tangential fibers over more than twenty-five hundredths of a millimeter. The horizontality of the [dendritic] shafts usually ceases near their terminations, and it is very frequent to see that the collateral branches of the shafts, as well as those resulting from their last dichotomies, ascend to the upper plane of the molecular layer, where they engender a very dense plexus. The parallel ascending branches originating at a right angle (embryonic disposition) do not exist or are very rare; commonly, such collaterals go up more or less obliquely, they dichotomize several times, and never terminate by means of thickenings or [clublike endings][E] underneath the pia, but preferentially as delicate and varicose threads, situated at several planes of the molecular layer. This appears to confirm the previously defended opinion, namely that the ascending collaterals terminating in [clublike endings], discovered by Retzius in the fetal cerebrum, represent an embryonic disposition.

The staining is homogenous in the thick processes, but when the branches acquire a dimension near a thousandth [of a millimeter], the varicosities appear, exhibiting the same characteristics seen in the dendrites of the ordinary cells. However, it has seemed to us that spines are lacking completely from the most delicate branches, a circumstance that establishes a capital distinction between the dendritic branches of the special cells and those of the cerebral pyramids.

In fig. 7 [fig. 55], we reproduce some of the special cells of the molecular layer of the adult or almost-adult cat. On them appear only the dendritic processes, which possess a large diversity of orientations, those originating from one cell interlacing with those originating from others. The little space available for the figure does not allow one to judge well the enormous extent of the tangential processes. To appreciate this fully, it would have been necessary to reduce exceedingly the soma of the cells or to reproduce them in a large lithographic drawing.

With respect to the axon, it has been impossible for us to stain it. If it exists, it must be very refractory to the methylene blue, and, of course, it does not appear to arise from the cell body. The question, then, about the nature of the special cells remains unresolved. If new attempts at staining with the [methylene] blue would allow [us] to demonstrate an axon, the problem would be definitively resolved; in such a case, all the radial or tangential processes, as well as their terminal branches, would possess, in spite of their thinness and smoothness, which make them resemble axons, the significance of dendrites, representing thus, together with the soma, the apparatus of reception of the cell.

Anyway, the intense and more or less homogenous staining that the tangential processes acquire by the method of Ehrlich prove, at least, that they do not have to do with multiple axons; because, if such processes should represent medullated axons, the [methylene] blue would reveal on them, by means of concentrations of stain, the strangulations of Ranvier, and if they should correspond to nonmedullated axons, the blue would not stain them, or it would stain them very lightly, since we must bear in mind that the nonmedullated fibers of the adult cerebrospinal axis are never or almost never impregnated with the method of Ehrlich. The existence of [true] varicosities also speaks against an axonal nature, because, although a varicose degeneration can happen in true axons or in fibers without myelin, the phenomenon appears very late, and the spheres of cyanophilic matter are not accustomed to acquire a large size or intense staining (fibers of Remak of the sympathetic ganglia).

In summary, although it is not possible to exclude the opinion presented in other papers (in which it is declared that the special cells of the cortex are analogous to certain types of retinal spongioblasts), we must confess that, with time, we are less reluctant to accept the old dictum of Retzius, who regarded the referred cells as a special category of Golgi cells or cells with short axon, provided in certain cases with one axon, in others with two or more.

Perhaps, finally, as Veratti proposes, the presence of a single axon might be the rule. Anyway, until new data appear that allow us to resolve the problem definitively, it cannot be doubted that the special cells of the molecular layer are morphologically distinguished from the ordinary Golgi cells by the enormous length of the principal [dendritic] processes and by the smoothness, thinness, and mode of ramification of the finer dendritic branches, which possess in the Golgi preparations an appearance like that of axons.

That the soma and thick processes of these cells constitute an apparatus of reception is proved by the intimate connections that they show with terminal nerve fibers. In many preparations in which fibers of Martinotti were well impregnated, we have seen that each soma of the special cells lies in a nest or bed of thin little nerve branches, among which were, besides the terminal arborizations of the ascending axons of Martinotti, no small number of little recurrent collateral branches of [the axons of] pyramids and, without doubt, also [axon] threads belonging to Golgi cells of the same molecular layer.

Tangential Thick Fibers

All the tangential sections of the molecular layer show an extremely rich plexus formed by medullated nerve fibers oriented in all directions, and either robust or of medium size. In certain preparations, the [methylene] blue stains exclusively those fibers on which the strangulations of Ranvier and numerous branches are shown with great clarity.

The medium and thin fibers are repeatedly divided and subdivided, and their branches are likewise provided with a myelin sheath; they seem to us to correspond to the ascending fibers of Martinotti. Their area of distribution usually does not exceed one or two millimeters. Anyway, the area outlined by the ramification as a whole is enormously larger than

that exhibited by the same fibers in the embryonic cerebrum in [our] previous Golgi [studies].

But there exist other myelinated fibers [that are] much thicker, commonly situated in the deeper half of the molecular layer, and whose horizontal course is so long that in some cases we have been able to follow them for more than four millimeters. Such fibers often run straight over a long trajectory to curve further on and change direction; not a few times, they bifurcate, and the two branches, separating in a V, go through vast territories without losing their horizontality. Finally, the said thick fibers give off at many of their strangulations long, medullated collaterals (fig. 2, c)[F] [fig. 50].

Whence come such robust fibers? Attending to [the fact] that some of them, followed [backward], appear to have a parent shaft that sinks into the cortex, and, in addition, considering their large diameter, which can only be compared to the axons of the giant pyramids and [which is] very superior to that of the cells of Martinotti, we are inclined to consider them as fibers arriving from the white matter that would be ramified over enormous extents of the molecular layer, entering into relationship, by means of their unmyelinated branches (which the methylene blue does not stain), with innumerable [dendritic] tufts of pyramids. It would not be strange if some such fibers should correspond also to the giant Golgi cells that exist in the molecular layer. In our opinion, then, the molecular layer contains, besides its special cells, long association fibers, completely analogous to those of the white matter, which makes the cortex of the mammals closer to that of the batrachians, where, as is known, almost all the cells of association send their axons directly to the molecular layer in which they spread over extensive regions. [The brain] would have, then, two planes of long association fibers: [those] of the molecular layer, [which would be] phylogenetically the oldest, and those of the white matter, which would have appeared more recently.

[Dendritic] Tufts of Pyramids

They are very well stained with the method of Ehrlich, showing branches of a very accentuated varicose appearance and a marked tendency to be concentrated in the more superficial planes of the molecular layer. From the point of view of the extent of the terminal ramification, it is possible to distinguish the tufts as *diffuse tufts* and as *compact or dense tufts.*

The diffuse tufts correspond in the main to the more superficial pyramids (there are exceptions); their very numerous dendritic tufts are extended over a considerable area of the molecular layer, entering, therefore, into relationship with innumerable nerve fibers. The tufts [with a] moderate [number of] branches are very frequent on the thick and medium pyramids, although they can also exist on the small [pyramids], and they are characterized both by the poverty of the terminal branches and by the small extent [of the molecular layer] that they customarily embrace.

The variable extent and richness of branching of the tufts of the pyramids is due, without doubt, to the variable number of impulses that each of these must receive and, consequently, to the position and quantity of the little terminal [nerve] fibers with which the tufts establish connections.

From all that has been said, it follows that the molecular layer of the cerebrum, as well as that of the cerebellum, contains in its bosom a large number of cells with short axon, destined probably to carry nerve impulses to specific groups of cells. This system of multiple relationships, this profusion of intercalated conductors in the chains of the central sensory and voluntary motor neurons, is related to the extraordinary complexity of the dynamic associations that the cerebrum reveals to us. But from the moment that one wants to specify these connections, doubts arise from all sides. [Regarding] the cells of short axon of the molecular layer, do they receive by their somata and dendrites the excitations carried exclusively by the fibers of Martinotti, or do they establish besides relations with the terminal arborizations and collaterals of the association fibers? Might it not be possible to suppose that the terminal axonal ramifications of certain Golgi cells propagate the excitation to the somata and dendrites of cells of the same kind, generating in this way true chains of cells in-

tercalated between the terminal fibers [coming from] the white matter and the [dendritic] tufts of the pyramids? It is impossible to resolve these questions. In the absence of data from direct observation, there is no other recourse than conjecture by analogy.

Observing what occurs with the cells of short axon in regions such as Ammon's horn, fascia dentata, and cerebellum, one tends to think that the cells of this class resident in the cerebrum will be obligatory intermediaries between the arborizations of long axons and the somata or dendritic tufts of cells of the motor type. The connections of the large Golgi cells of the cerebellum and of the basket cells of this same organ speak in favor of this opinion. In Ammon's horn, cells are often found in which axonal arborizations are disposed around the [dendritic] shafts or somata of cells of the Golgi motor type, whereas their [other] dendrites appear to be connected with little terminal [axonal] branches or collaterals of the white matter. However, as probable as this conjecture may seem, it will not be able to reach a stage of reasonable persuasiveness if we cannot in the meantime discover in all cases the axonal ramifications connected with the somata and dendrites of the cells with short axon. It is necessary to confess that such demonstrations have yet to be made for many cells of this category, since, although in some cases (dendrites of the basket cells, dendrites of the large Golgi cells of the cerebellum) it has been possible to observe little terminal axon branches in contact with dendrites of cells with short axon, in no case have true perisomatic arborizations been observed. Only in the spongioblasts associated with the retina (Cajal) and in the cells of the second type (Dogiel) in the dorsal root ganglia have such arborizations been found; but the morphological differences that separate these cells from the central Golgi [type II] cells are too great to allow a complete identification.

Another reason for delay in the definitive appreciation of the functional significance of the Golgi cells is the extreme smallness shown by the terminal axonal arborizations in some of these. In the superficial or molecular layer of the fascia dentata and in the layer of the same name of the cerebrum are found dimin-

utive cells whose axons embrace with their little terminal branches an area less extensive
than that made up by the dendritic ramification; the terminal territory of the axon is
moreover found so close to the soma and to
the dendrites that it is not easy to see this cell
operating as an intermediary or association
cell.

This peculiarity raises doubts that the role
of connection or of association would be the
only role performed by the mentioned cells.
Might they not also perform the role of condensers or producers of the energy necessary
for transmission over large distances and to
many cells? This necessity for summing many
generators of current in the path of conduction would account for the well-known fact
that the propagation of the sensory wave to the
cerebral cortex occurs by means of a chain of
[only] two neurons.

In conclusion, the Golgi cells probably represent intermediary links of association between axonal arborizations of cells with long
axon and somata or dendrites of cells of this
same kind. By means of the axonal arborization, they would carry to many, more or less
distant cells the impulses brought to the soma
or to the dendrite by a single fiber or by a small
number of fibers. They would constitute, then,
an apparatus of dissemination or divergence of
nervous excitation. But, in addition, they
would serve to reinforce the proper conduction, adding to the afferent flow a new contingent of energy.

Technical Indications

The methylene blue is somewhat unfaithful in
the cerebral cortex, much more so than in the
staining of peripheral [nerve fiber] terminations. Quite good preparations can be
achieved, however, by observing the following
rules.

The preparation of the methylene blue can
be made by injection, but this means is insufficient to stain the cells. Mere injection, with
exposure to the air for one to two hours, only
stains well the medullated nerve fibers of the
molecular layer and the terminal [dendritic]
tufts of the pyramids. The impregnation of the
Golgi cells of this layer requires the procedure

of impregnation of Dogiel. To that end, the
cerebrum is exposed, and after cutting it into
large pieces, they should be put with their
meningeal surface face up in the oven protected in a humid container. There, by means
of a smooth brush, the molecular layer is wetted with methylene blue from time to time
(every ten or twelve minutes), taking care not
to remove the pia mater in order to avoid al-
tering the tissue too much. After an hour and
a half, and when the cerebrum appears intensely blue, the fixative is applied. If the picrate of Dogiel is used, it should only act for
four or six hours, in order to avoid as much as
possible the softening of the cerebrum; then
the pieces should be immersed for twelve
hours in the molybdate, and finally they are
hardened in formol (see later for the technique for ganglia). In order to preserve the
spines well, one should have recourse to the
molybdate, taking care not to prolong the exposure to air for more than three-quarters of
an hour to an hour. The sections should be
made tangentially and by hand, and it is convenient that they should be rather thick and
include the entire molecular layer. Before sectioning, one should remove the pia. Preferably, the areas of the said layer that present intense staining should be chosen; only in such
territories will the special cells and many cells
with short axon be stained. It should be unnecessary to say that after mounting in balsam
or dammar (as in the Golgi preparations), the
cerebral surface must be facing up.

Perpendicular sections will also be useful,
especially for determining the positions of
cells visible in the tangential sections. In no
case does the impregnation go beyond the
deep limit of the molecular layer; the pyramids, therefore, will not be visible. The dye
stains intensely the somata of the Golgi cells
and of the special cells, as well as the medullated nerve fibers. Sometimes, [methylene]
blue is deposited only on the surface (fixative
of Bethe) of the cells, appearing as a blue
membrane sprinkled with clear vacuoles. This
reticular aspect is frequently very beautiful on
the somata of the pyramids stained thanks to
the infiltration of [dye into the] fresh perpendicular sections. We do not dare, however, to
proclaim without further studies the fibrillar

and reticular structure of this thin covering of the nerve cells.

Cajal's Notes

1. Cajal, Sur la structure de l'écorce cérébrale de quelques mammifères, *La Celulle,* Vol. VII, Pt. 1, 1891.
2. K. Schaffer, Zur feineren Struktur der Hirnrinde und über die funktionelle Bedeutung der Nervenzellenfortsätze, *Arch. f. Mikros. Anat.,* Vol. 48, Pt. IV, 1897.
3. S. Ramón y Cajal, Textura de las circunvoluciones cerebrales en los mamíferos pequeños, 10 December 1890. Sur la structure de l'écorce cérébrale de quelques mammifères, *La Cellule,* Vol. VII, Pt. 1 [1891].
4. G. Retzius, Die Cajal'sche Zellen der Grosshirnrinde beim Menschen und bei Säugethieren, *Biol. Unters. Neue Folge.,* Vol. V, 1893.
5. Retzius, Weitere Beitrage zur Kenntnis der Cajal'sche Zellen der Grosshirnrinde des Menschen, *Biolog. Untersuchungen Neue Folge,* 1894.
6. A. Kölliker, *Handbuch der Gewebelehre des Menschen,* 6th edition, Vol. 2, 1896. [See pages 659 to 663 of that work.]
7. S. Ramón y Cajal, Estructura de la corteza occipital inferior de los pequeños mamíferos, *Anal. de la Socied. Españ. de Historia Natural* XXII, 1893. Transla-

tion of this mémoir in *Zeitschrift f. Wissensch. Zool,* Vol. 56, Pt. 4, 1893.
8. Athias, Recherches sur l'histogenèse de l'écorce du cervelet, *Journal de l'Anatomie et de la Physiol. Norm. et Pathol.,* Vol. XXXIII, 1897.
9. Terrazas, Notas sobre la neuroglia del cerebro y el crecimiento de los elementos cerebelosos, *This Revista,* Pt. II, 1897.
10. E. Veratti, Ueber einige Struktureigenthumlichkeiten der Hirnrinde bei den Säugethieren, *Anat. Anzeiger.,* no. 14, April 1897.
11. S. Ramón y Cajal, Beiträge zur feineren Anatomie des grossen Hirns., etc., *Zeitschrift. f. Wiss. Zool.,* Vol. 56, Pt. 4, 1893 [loc. cit.].
12. Retzius, *Biol. Unter. Neue Folge,* Vol. V. Plate I [1893].

Editors' Notes

A. The first type mentioned here actually refers to the second type of the preceding paragraph.
B. These are the first type mentioned earlier.
C. Axon hillock.
D. Undoubtedly the Golgi method.
E. Cajal says "like a mace."
F. The original incorrectly says 2, *B.*

PART III

The Middle Period (1899–1902)

The Great Works on the Human Cortex

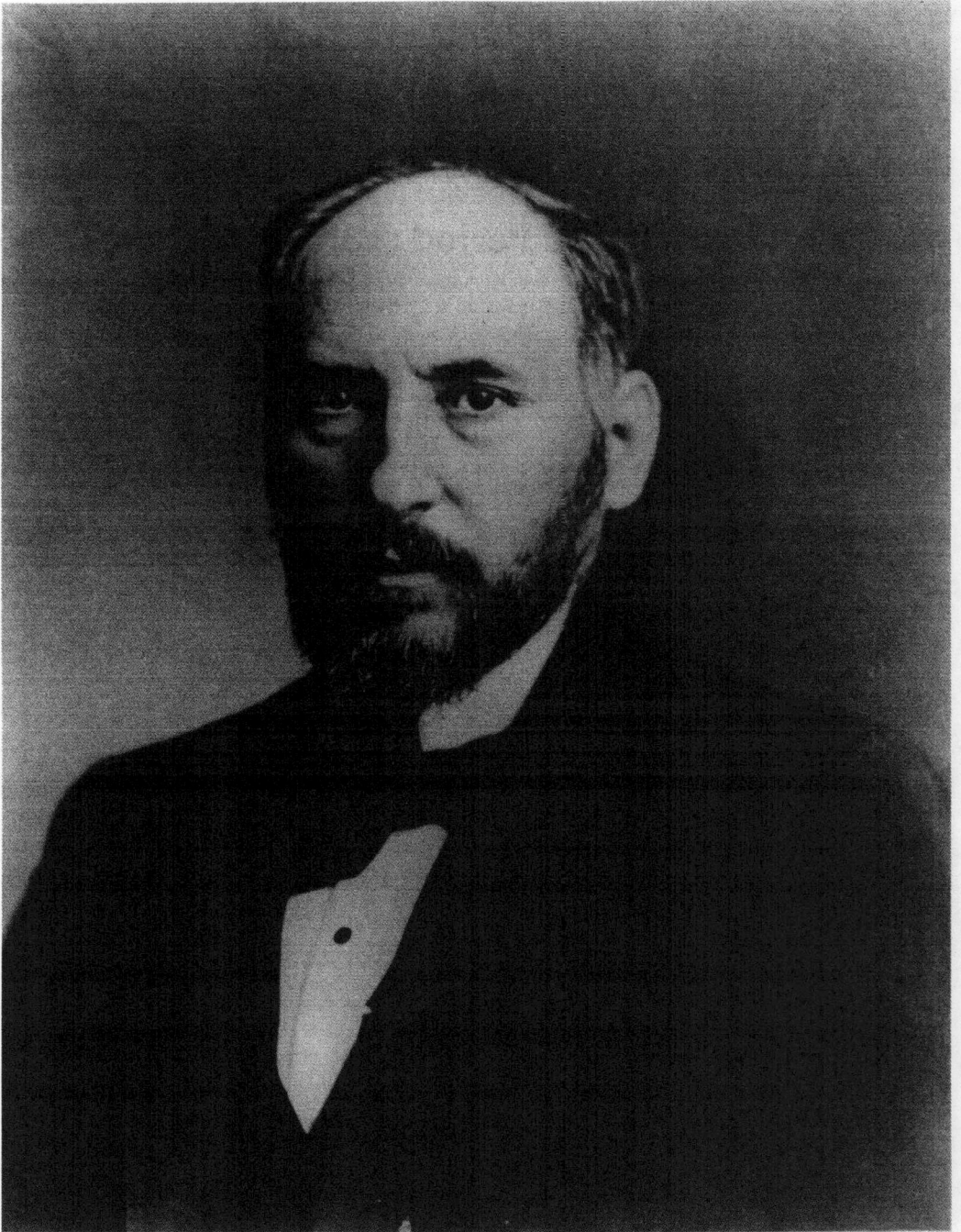

Photograph of Santiago Ramón y Cajal, aged forty-seven, published in 1899 in the volume containing the translated text of his three lectures delivered at the decennial celebrations of Clark University (Cajal, 1899c). Reproduced by permission of the President of Clark University.

13

Introduction

In 1899, after a series of successful studies on the retina, brainstem, thalamus, basal ganglia, pineal, pituitary, and peripheral ganglia, Cajal was ready to return to the cerebral cortex and to attack that of man, "the masterpiece of life." Perhaps he had been stimulated to do so by his experimentation in 1896 with the methylene blue method, which he had used to reinforce his earlier studies on layer I cells and to emphasize his observations that dendritic spines were real entities. From his studies with methylene blue, he may also have developed a new conviction concerning the usefulness of the Golgi method.

The first publication in what was to become a series of enormous depth was an extended short communication that appeared in March 1899 and was entitled "Notes on a Structural Study of the Visual Cortex of the Human Cerebrum." Virtually contemporaneous with this, the definitive paper on the visual cortex appeared in the fourth volume of the *Revista Trimestral Micrográfica,* and by December of the same year, the first of a two-part article on the motor cortex had also been published. In 1900, the conclusion of the motor cortex study and the study of the acoustic cortex appeared.

The series concluded early in 1902 with the publication of an extensive work on the olfactory cortex in the successor journal to the *Revista,* the *Trabajos del Laboratorio de Investigaciones Biológicas de la Universidad de Madrid.* Why Cajal never extended the series to include the association cortex remains something of a mystery, although he later confessed in the *Textura,* his great histological textbook, that he had few satisfactory preparations from these areas of cortex (see chapter 22 in this volume).

Even before publication was completed, Cajal reviewed his studies of the human visual and sensory-motor areas in a series of three lectures given at Worcester, Massachusetts, in July 1899 to celebrate the tenth anniversary of the founding of Clark University. Cajal was one of five distinguished foreign scientists invited to speak on this occasion. The other neuroscientist was August Forel. The lectures appear to have been given in Spanish but were translated into English by the faculty of Clark University and published as part of the volume commemorating the decenary.

The lectures commence with a brief introduction that is remarkably similar to that used in the opening to his "Notes on a Structural Study of the Visual Cortex of the Human Cerebrum" (see chapter 14). They then present a layer-by-layer account of the visual and Rolandic areas which, in the case of the visual cortex, is virtually identical to the description in the *Revista* article published in March of the same year (see chapter 15). The description of the Rolandic areas is somewhat abbreviated in comparison with the *Revista* article published later in 1899 (see chapter 16), but in both accounts all the figures are taken from the *Revista* articles. The Clark lectures make only brief mention of Cajal's ongoing studies of the acoustic and olfactory areas, but they conclude with a series of summarizing statements that were to dominate Cajal's ideas on the human cerebral cortex for years to come. They are virtually identical to the statements on the same theme in many of his subsequent works and clearly have their basis in many of his comments made in the course of his series of lectures before the Academy of Medical Sciences in Barcelona (see chapter 7). However, because they appear to represent Cajal's first systematic presentation of these points, we reproduce them here in full, by kind permission of the President of Clark University:

My work upon the topographical structure of the cortex has been fragmentary and leaves much to be desired. Many things, in fact, are still undiscovered. But, despite the very incomplete state of my researches and the narrow limits of the field they cover, I may draw a few anatomicophysiological conclusions, of which the chief are the following:

And first, as to the hierarchy of centres in the cortex of the human brain, comparing it with the mammalian brain, we may call to mind that, while it does not contain wholly new elements, it presents very distinctive characteristics, to wit:

1. The enormous development of the horizontal cells of the plexiform layer and the considerable length of their so-called tangential fibres.

2. The great abundance of cells with short axons scattered throughout the whole cortex, cells which form special varieties by reason of differences in their forms and the directions of their axons.

3. The presence of cells with short axons, very slender (bipanicled spider cells), with terminal arborizations whose delicacy is not approached by anything found in any animal.

4. The considerable development of basilar dendrites of the pyramidal cells.

5. The presence among the mid-layers of the cortex of a formation of so-called granular cells, a kind of focus occupied by enormous numbers of pyramids with short axons descending, arched, and ascending. This granular formation is present in gyrencephalous mammals, but in them it is very poor in cells with short axons and in small pyramids. In the smooth-brained animals it is almost wholly lacking.

The human cortex has evolved, accordingly, along three different lines: by multiplying cells with long axons and, above all, those with short axons; by decreasing the volume of cells and the diameter of certain fibres in order to make possible within the limits of space a delicate and greatly improved organization; finally, by varying and infinitely complicating the external morphology of the nerve elements, undoubtedly with the purpose of multiplying, in correspondence with their complexity, functional associations of all kinds.

As to differences and analogies in regional structure, the following propositions may be regarded as established:

1. The sensory as well as the so-called associational areas are made up by a combination of two orders of structural factors. The first order consists of common factors, which show very little modification. They are represented by the plexiform layers and the layers of pyramidal and polymorphic cells. The second order comprises special factors, structures peculiar to each cortical area. Their chief anatomical feature resides especially in the granular layer and is related mainly to the presence of particular centripetal fibres and of special types of cells with long axons (stellate cells of different kinds).

2. It seems probable that the common factors perform functions of a general order concerned, possibly, with ideas of representations of all kinds of movements related to the special sensations of which the cortical region is the seat. It seems also probable that the special anatomical factors of the sensory areas perform the function of elaborating specific sensations (sensation of seeing, hearing, etc.) and also of conveying sensory residues to the so-called association centres, where they may be transformed into latent images.

3. Each sensory cortical centre receives a special category of nerve fibres (fibres of central sensory tracts). Their cells of origin, as has been shown by the researches of v. Monakow, Flechsig, v. Bechterew, and many others, reside in the particular nuclei of the medulla, corpora quadrigemina, and optic thalami. It is precisely the presence of

these sensory fibres of the second order that constitutes the prime anatomical characteristic of the centres of sensation or projection.

4. The absence of these sensory fibres, which come from the corona radiata, may be used in all mammals to distinguish the so-called association centres. These centres, which exist even in the mouse, also have a nerve fibre plexus distributed among their median layers (layer of granules in the association areas in man). The fibres, however, which constitute them are very fine and appear to come from sensory centres of the brain. Possibly the cells about which these sensorio-ideational fibres terminate represent the substratum or, at any rate, the first link in the chain of nerve elements whose function is the representation of ideas.

5. Since we have seen that each afferent fibre in the sensory cortex comes into contact with an extraordinary number of nerve cells apparently scattered without any order, we must suspect that these relations conform to the preconceived design of a well-determined and constant organization.

As, at present, it seems to be impossible to discover these relations, we may surmise that each sensory fibre comes into contact, directly or through other cells, solely with those pyramids whose stimulation is necessary in order to effect, after the manner of the reflex arc, movements coordinated and intentional. We may also surmise (supposing that the stellate cells of the tactile and visual cortex form the link between the sensory and ideational centres) that each sensory afferent fibre, bringing a unit of sensation (the impression received by a cone of the retina or by the terminal arborization of any peripheral nerve fibre), enters into relation exclusively with the group of nerve cells entrusted with the function of conveying this impression to a particular point in the associational cortex.

Many other hypotheses are possible, but I must conclude for fear of tiring your kind and sympathetic attention and exhausting your patience. I fear that I have already made too free use of hypotheses and have pretended to fill the gaps of possible observations with arbitrary suppositions.

It is a rule of wisdom, and of nice scientific prudence as well, not to theorize before completing the observation of facts. But who is so master of himself as to be able to wait calmly in the midst of darkness until the break of dawn? Who can tarry prudently until the epoch of the perfection of truth (unhappily as yet very far off) shall come? Such impatience may find its justification in the shortness of human life and also in the supreme necessity of dominating, as soon as possible, the phenomena of the external and internal worlds. But reality is infinite and our intel-ligence finite. Nature and especially the phenomena of life show us everywhere complications, which we pretend to remove by the false mirage of our simple formulae, heedless of the fact that the simplicity is not in nature but in ourselves.

It is this limitation of our faculties that impels us continually to forge simple hypotheses made to fit, by mutilating it, the infinite universe into the narrow mould of the human skull—and this, despite the warnings of experience, which daily calls to our minds the weakness, the childishness, and the extreme mutability of our theories. But this is a matter of fate, unavoidable because the brain is only a savings-bank machine for picking and choosing among external realities. It cannot preserve impressions of the external world except by continually simplifying them, by interrupting their serial and continuous flow, and by ignoring all those whose intensities are too great or too small.

On looking back in 1917 at this exceptionally fruitful period, Cajal felt that he could highlight a large number of significant contributions. He speaks for himself in the following translation of pages 350–360 from the second volume of the *Recuerdos de mi vida.*

About the papers of 1899–1901,[A] Cajal says:

In figure 75[B] [*fig. 56*], I present the specific neuronal types that I found in almost all the cerebral [cortical] regions of man. There are: (1) a certain diminutive bitufted cell (fig. 75, *A*) [*fig. 56*] whose axon resolves itself into very tight plexuses of fine threads oriented in a radial direction; (2) a tiny cell, also with short axon and very short, delicate dendrites, whose axonal arborization, almost imperceptible because of its extreme thinness, forms a very tight web (fig. 75, *B, B¹*) [*fig. 56*]; (3) another cell (fig. 75, *C*) [*fig. 56*] provided with a more robust soma and whose axon forms baskets that surround the somata of the pyramids; (4) a certain [kind of] small pyramid (fig. 75, *E*) [*fig. 56*] characterized by exhibiting an axon that is almost completely exhausted in giving rise to very long arciform and recurrent collaterals; (5) a certain [kind of] cell of exiguous size whose ascending axon is arborized in the shape of a bramble patch within the confines of the molecular layer (fig. 75, *D*), [*fig. 56*]; (6) finally, numerous relatively robust neuronal varieties with ascending axons giving rise at several levels of the cortex to very long horizontal branches[C] (fig. 75, *F*) [*fig. 56*].

These cellular elements, particularly the first, second, fourth, and sixth, are extremely numerous and can be considered unique to the cerebrum of

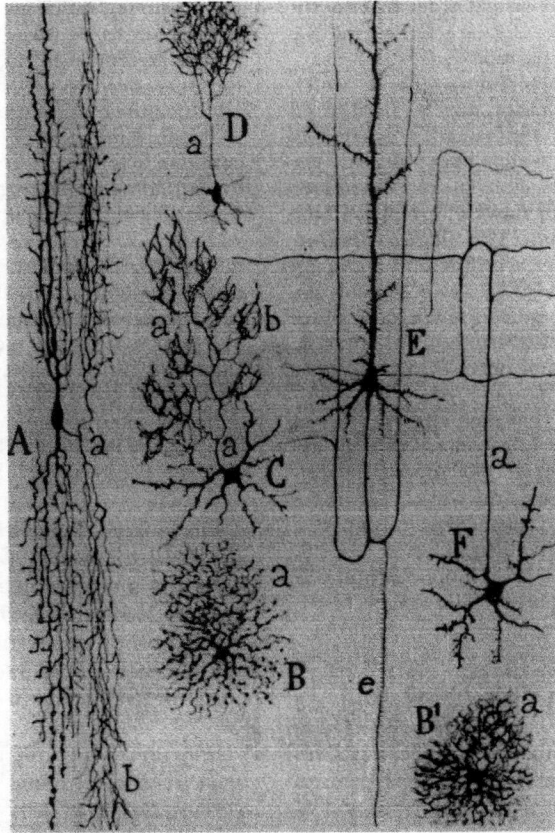

[*FIG. 56*]   Fig. 75. Several types of neurons with short axon found in the cerebral cortex of the child of a few months. *A*, bitufted cell; *B*, dwarf cell with short axon; *C*, basket cell; *E*, pyramid with arciform collateral branches; *D*, dwarf cell with axon resolving into a tuft; *F*, cell with ascending axon dividing into very long horizontal branches.

man. By this, I do not wish to exclude at all the possibility that some of them become apparent, though with ruder forms and sizes, in the cortex of higher mammals, especially in [that of] the dog and the monkey. In any case, my investigations showed that *the functional superiority of the human brain is intimately bound up with the prodigious abundance and unusual wealth of forms of the so-called neurons with short axons.* . . .

Visual Area

(a) Discovery of the terminal arborizations of the fibers of the central visual pathway (which arrive from the *lateral geniculate body*). In figure 76^D, *b, d* [*fig. 57*], we show a representation of the terminal plexus as a whole.

(b) The finding, in the layer in which the sensory fibers end, of certain special cells, devoid of an [apical dendritic] shaft and with a stellate shape. The axon of such cells goes to the white matter after giving off robust ascending collaterals (fig. 76, *C*) [*fig. 57*].

(c) The finding, in the deep layers of the visual cortex, of certain minute cells (deep granule cells), whose descending axon suddenly bends [upward], forming an arch to be distributed in the superimposed layers (figs. 76, *F*; 75, *E*) [*figs. 57, 56*].

(d) The discovery of a very minute type of cell with short axon (*bitufted cells*) whose very delicate axon resolves itself into small radial bundles of threads that are applied to the shafts and somata of the pyramids (figs. 76, *C*; 75, *A*) [*figs. 57, 56*].

[Closer pursuit of the problem of the structure of the visual cortex led us to add:]

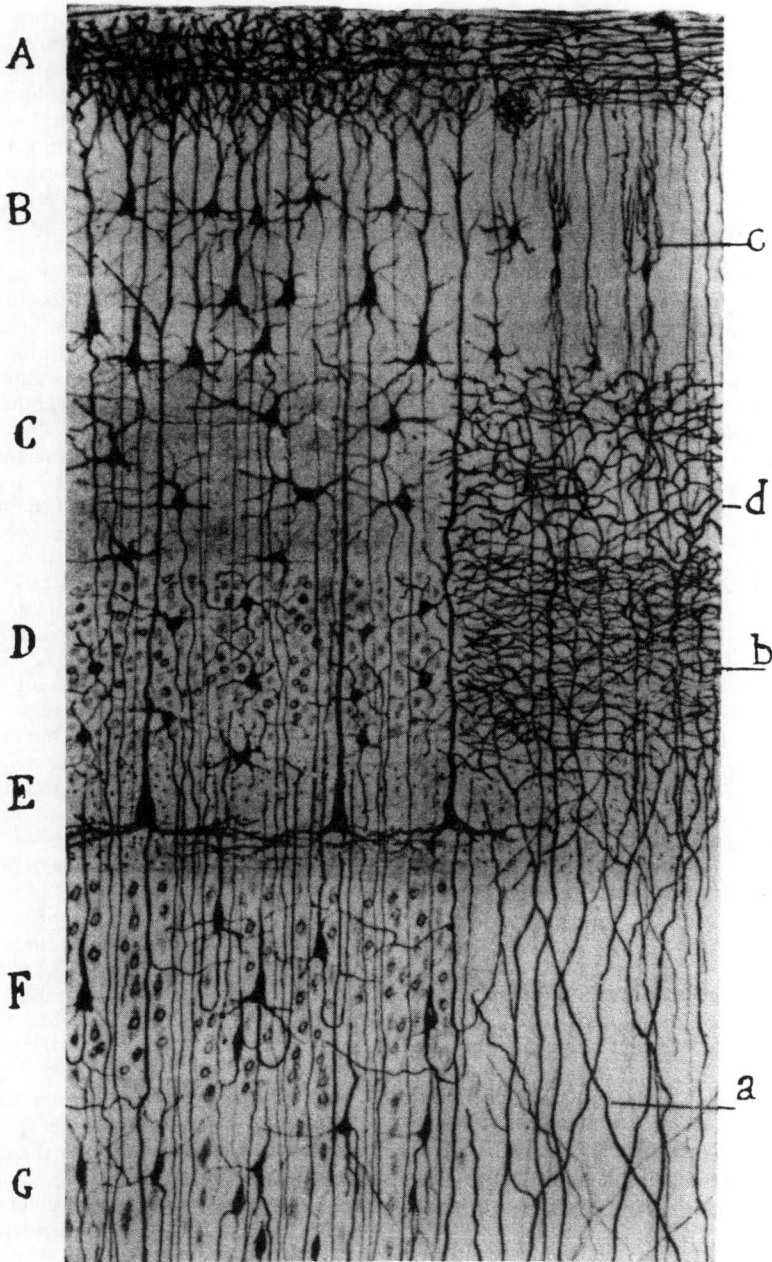

[*FIG. 57*] Fig. 76. Scheme of the main cells and layers of the visual cortex of man (calcarine fissure). *A*, molecular layer; *B*, layer of the small and medium pyramids; *C*, layer of the large stellate cells; *D*, layer of the granule cells or of the minute star-shaped cells; *E*, layer of the giant cells; *F*, layer of the pyramids with arciform axon; *G*, layer of the polymorphic cells; *a*, *b*, *d*, terminal arborizations of the centripetal visual fibers.

(a) A rational nomenclature and division of the layers of the cerebral gray matter.

(b) The detailed study of the horizontal cells (*Cajal'sche Zellen* of Retzius) of the *plexiform layer* (fig. 76, A) [*fig. 57*].

(c) The demonstration of the existence in this layer of numerous cells with short axon.

(d) The finding in the second and third layers of several types of cell with short axon peculiar to the human cerebrum (cells of short-range vertical and horizontal association, etc.). We give schemes of them in fig. 75 [*fig. 56*].

(e) The indication that certain cells with thin ascending axons give rise to very dense pericellular plexuses in the second layer.

(f) The detailed analysis of the *stria of Gennari* and layer of the *stellate cells* and the demonstration that this layer is inhabitated by several cellular types with long or short axon. (*External sublayer or layer of the giant stellate cells; internal sublayer or layer of the tiny stellate cells; cells with short ascending axon; cells with axon resolving into very delicate arborization close to the cell body*, etc., etc.)

(g) The discovery of the pericellular or basket arborizations, similar to those that surround the Purkinje cells of the cerebellum, on the cell bodies of the pyramids of the motor and visual cortex.

(h) The detailed analysis of the behavior of the component fibers of the plexus or *stria of Gennari* into whose formation the following contribute: (a) a plexus in which is revealed the existence of several kinds of terminal or visual fibers; (b) axons of the granule cells of the layer of the small stellate cells; (c) ascending axons of the cells with arciform axon of the underlying layers, etc. . . .

Motor Cortex

(a) A detailed analysis, with the Nissl method, of the central gyri, with determination of their analogies and differences and the exposition of a rational nomenclature of their layers. It was demonstrated, contrary to general opinion, that the postcentral gyrus lacks motor function and structurally belongs to the association system (a dictum confirmed by all modern authors) (fig. 78E) [*fig. 88*].

(b) The affirmation that the thick medullated tangential fibers represent the axons of the horizontal cells.

(c) The demonstration of the phenomenon of atrophy occurring in the ascending dendrites of the latter cells after birth.

(d) The finding of several types of cells with short axon that inhabit both the plexiform and the second and third layers, and the description of a very minute nerve cell, similar to the neuroglial cells, from

which it is distinguished by having a very delicate axon arborizing at a short distance.

(e) The demonstration that all the pyramids and cells with an [apical dendritic] shaft, even if they are located in the deepest layers, send a dendritic tuft or a single dendrite to the plexiform layer.

(f) The finding of several cells whose axons form terminal axonal nests around the pyramids.

(g) The detailed description of the morphology of the giant pyramids.

(h) The finding in the motor cortex of granule cells or small cellular elements similar to those characteristic of the visual area.

(i) The discovery of the terminal sensory fibers whose arborizations form a very tight plexus located in the layer of the medium pyramids (fig. 77F) [*fig. 115*].

(j) The indication of these same terminal fibers in the cortex of mammals of small size and the demonstration of the continuity [of the fibers] with myelinated fibers perforating the corpus striatum.

(k) The adoption of a new criterion for the delineation of the sensory areas of the cortex: the characteristic [feature] of these would not be, as hitherto considered, the presence of projection fibers but the existence of plexuses made up of exogenous fibers, arriving from the corpus striatum and continuous with second-order sensory fibers.

(l) A critique was made of the known classifications of the gyri into *association areas and projection areas,* and the existence of *association* areas and areas of [*memory function*] was defined in small mammals. . . .

As a special feature of the *auditory cortex,* we will indicate besides the existence of structural details impossible to summarize, (a) the constant presence of a certain [kind of] giant stellate cell with long axon (fig. 79G) [*fig. 130*]; and (b) the specific forms of the pyramids (fusiform, bitufted, etc.) (fig. 80H) [*fig. 136*]. . . .

Olfactory Cortex

1. Confirmation and extension of some findings made before in the frontal olfactory cortex (region underlying the *external root* of the olfactory nerve), particularly with respect to the manner of termination of the olfactory fibers of second order inside the *molecular layer* of the cerebrum. In fig. 83, A [*fig. 58*], which reproduces a section of the *external olfactory root* of the cat and of the underlying gray matter, this interesting terminal plexus appears in contact with the peripheral tufts of the pyramidal cells (fig. 83, D) [*fig. 58*].

2. The demonstration of the existence of characteristic pyramidal cell types (provided with a tuft

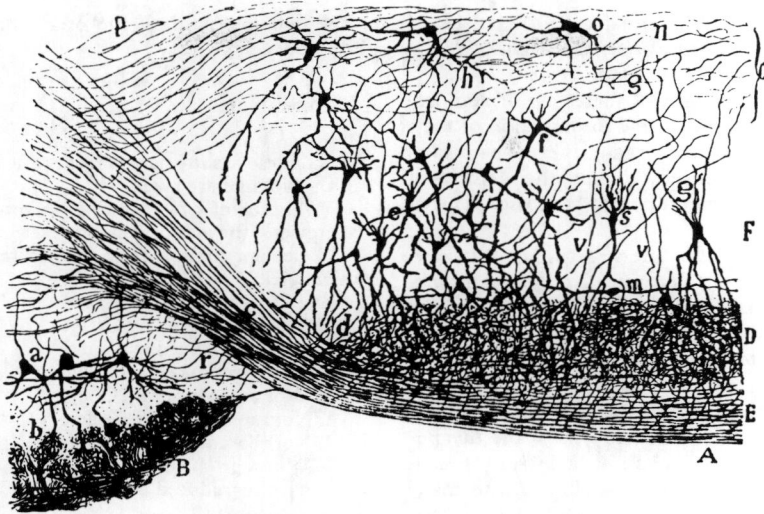

[*FIG. 58*]   Fig. 83. Anteroposterior section of the olfactory bulb and tract of the cerebrum of the mouse of fifteen days. Method of Golgi. *A*, external root of the olfactory nerve; *B*, olfactory bulb; *D*, molecular layer of the gray matter underlying the root; *F*, layer of the pyramids; *C*, layer of the polymorphic cells; *a*, mitral cells of the bulb; *b*, olfactory glomerulus; *c*, axon of the tufted cell constituents of the external root; *d*, collaterals of the root distributed in the molecular layer; *e, f*, pyramids; *g*, thick stellate cell; *h*, axon of a triangular cell; *o*, polymorphic cell; *n*, nerve fibers of the layer of the polymorphic cells; *v*, ascending axons; *m*, a horizontal fusiform cell; *v*, collaterals of the external root of the bulb. (Taken from Calleja). [This figure is fig. 747 of the *Textura*, and we have taken the legend from there since it is greatly expanded over that in the *Recuerdos*.]

or descending tassel) in the hippocampal gyrus and piriform lobe of man (fig. 81¹, *G*) [*fig. 152*], and the indication in other regions of the [hippocampal] gyrus of several specific neuronal types as well as the peculiar systems of grouping in which dwarf pyramids alternate with giant star-shaped cells (fig. 82ʲ*A*) [*fig. 148*].

3. Discovering, in the upper part of the *olfactory* or piriform *lobe* of the *lissencephalic* and *gyrencephalic* mammals of a special focus (fig. 84ᴷ) [*fig. 198*], with a singular structure, to which comes an important olfactory pathway and from which emanates the principal pathway of exogenous fibers destined for Ammon's horn. By virtue of this finding, there was established the existence of three sequential olfactory foci: the *primary olfactory focus* or *inferior sphenoidal cortex* (fig. 83, *A*) [*fig. 58*], in which terminate the fibers of the *external root* of the olfactory bulb; the *secondary olfactory focus* (which we have called *angular or spheno-occipital*), in which terminate the fibers originating in the preceding [focus]; and the *tertiary olfactory focus*, represented by Ammon's horn and the fascia dentata, the point of final arborization of the fibers emanating from the cited angular [focus].

4. It is recognized that the important route arising from the latter focus and ending in Ammon's horn consists of several pathways but mainly of these two:

(a) *Crossed spheno-ammonic bundle* or *dorsal psalterium* of the authors, which, being directed toward the raphe beneath the corpus callosum, is arborized in Ammon's horn and the fascia dentata of the contralateral side, after supplying not a few fibers to the presubiculum.

(b) The *direct spheno-ammonic bundle or perforant pathway,* whose axons, arranged in little bundles stepped from up down, cross the subiculum and are distributed in the molecular layers of the ipsilateral Ammon's horn and fascia dentata, entering, respectively, into contact with the tufts of the pyramids and the granule cells of these centers. In fig. 85ᴸ [*fig. 181*], we show a transverse section of the *spheno-occipital or angular* focus (*A*) and of the adjacent region of Ammon's horn and subiculum. Notice in *B*, *D*, *E* the very important flow of fibers that links that ganglion with the molecular layer of Ammon's horn and of the fascia dentata.

5. Differentiation of several regions of the sphenoidal cortex endowed with a peculiar structure and in connection with particular systems of fibers. Such

are the *presubicular focus* situated on the outside of the subiculum, the *central or principal sphenoidal region,* and the *external sphenoidal region.*

6. Description in each of these foci of very numerous types of neurons, and examination of their specific plexuses and afferent and efferent pathways. Many of these studies refer to man, the methods of Nissl, Golgi, and Weigert having been used for that purpose.

7. Description of the fine structure of the *interhemispheric cortex* or that near the corpus callosum, a region whose structure contrasts with that of the rest of the fissural region.

8. Precise determination of the origin of the fibers of the *cingulum,* a pathway of anteroposterior projection, provided with collaterals of association.

9. Finally, the structural analysis of the *longitudinal and supracallosal striae,* of *the nerves* of Lancisi, and of the *fornix longus* of Forel, with many new details regarding the origin and trajectory of the fibers. . . .

Editors' Notes

A. These are the papers from which chapters 15–18 in this volume are taken.

B. Fig. 68 of Craigie's English version, but Craigie abbreviates the accompanying description.

C. See our comments on the nature of the cell types in chapter 30.

D. Not reproduced by Craigie.

E. Not reproduced by Craigie.

F. Not reproduced by Craigie.

G. Not reproduced by Craigie.

H. Not reproduced by Craigie.

I. Not reproduced by Craigie.

J. Not reproduced by Craigie.

K. Not reproduced by Craigie.

L. Not reproduced by Craigie.

14

Notes on a Structural Study of the Visual Cortex of the Human Cerebrum

[*Revista Ibero-Americana de Ciencias Médicas* 1:1–14, 1899]

The important physiological investigations of Munk have proven that the region of the cerebral cortex to which retinal images are projected and in which the visual sensation is produced is the internal face of the occipital lobe, particularly in the territory of the *cuneus* and the *calcarine fissure.* The study of this cortical region has a considerable theoretical interest.

In science at present, with regard to structural concepts of the cerebral cortex, there are two trends: the *unitary,* initiated by Meynert and supported by the many who defend the structural unity of the gyri and explain the functional diversity [of the cortex] by the different peripheral connections of the cerebral cells; and the *particularist* (dualist or pluralist), whose most distinguished representatives at present are Flechsig and Nissl, and which claims that the special function of each cortical area implicates either a structural specialization or a diversity of connections of the cortical cells.

With the aim of taking a firm position in these discussions, we have undertaken a series of investigations about the comparative structure, region by region, of the human cerebral cortex, having used preferentially the cerebrum of the newborn child and [of the child] of fifteen, twenty, and thirty days. To that effect, we have utilized the methods of Nissl, Weigert, and Golgi; with the latter, we have added some new details that we are going to summarize briefly in this note. Let us, however, leave for later, when our works shall have covered all the territories of the cortex and when we shall have collected a greater amount of data, the formulation of a precise opinion about the question stated [above].

The occipital gray matter, particularly that corresponding to the calcarine fissure, is distinguished from the cortex of other cortical regions by presenting, as pointed out by Meynert, Lewis, Hammarberg, Botazzi, Schlapp, etc., a layer of granules or of small cells between the layers of the medium and large pyramids. It is also characterized by a stria or layer of intermediary white matter, visible with the naked eye in man, monkey, and dog, and located in the center of the cortex, more or less, beneath the [layer of] medium pyramids (*stria of Gennari, line of Vicq d'Azyr, internal and external medullary laminae of Kölliker,* etc.).

As a whole, and omitting for the present all discussion regarding [previous accounts of] the number of layers of this cerebral region, we will distinguish in the human visual cortex the following stratification:

1. *Molecular layer* or [layer] of the tufts of the pyramids.
2. *Layer of the small pyramids.*
3. *Layer of the medium pyramids.*
4. *Layer of the stellate cells* or stria of Gennari.
5. *Layer of the small spheroidal cells (granules* of the authors).
6. *Layer of the giant pyramids.*
7. *Layer of the polymorphic cells.*
8. *Layer of the white matter.*

The brevity that we have imposed on ourselves obliges us to omit from this succinct description the first three layers, which, however, offer nothing particularly characteristic of the visual cortex. The unique characteristic of this cerebral region is in the layer of the stellate cells, in which resides the medullated nervous plexus or stria of Gennari. About this layer, as well as about the underlying layers, we are therefore going to expose some data from [our] observations.

The layer of Gennari or layer of the stellate cells possesses a very complicated structure, as it results from the mixture and interweaving of many elements, namely (1) stellate and intrinsic spheroidal nerve cells; (2) ramifications of robust nerve fibers, arriving from the white matter; (3) ramifications of ascending axons arising from cells of the underlying layers (layer of the granules, layer of the giant pyramids, and layer of the polymorphic cells); (4) collateral ramifications of axons from the several cells located in superimposed layers (layers of the small and medium pyramids).

Intrinsic Cells or Stellate [Cells] of the Stria of Gennari

As can be seen in fig. 1 [*fig. 59*], the stria of Gennari consists of special cells, [which are] very numerous and of variable form, although predominating is the stellate [type], with several commonly divergent processes, ramifying exclusively inside the above-mentioned nervous plexus. Among the general stellate type, semilunar, fusiform, triangular, and sphe-

roidal variants are also observed, but these only refer to the soma, as, in reality, all of these cells give off several dendrites. We have not been able to find pyramids in the strict sense in this region. Attending to the size of the soma and to the behavior of the axon, it is possible to distinguish two [stellate] cell categories.

1. Giant Stellate Type and with Long Axon

Under this designation, we include certain quite numerous cells, with stellate, sometimes mitral or semilunar shapes (fig. 1 *A, C*), [*fig. 59*], whose dendrites, arising from all sides of the cell body, are repeatedly branched, extending in all directions, but especially horizontally, throughout a considerable area of the plexus. The axon is robust, descending; gives off two, three, or four thick collaterals ramifying in the nervous plexus; and continues its course through the underlying layers down to the white matter. Several morphological variants of this type exist, as well as differences in the size of the cells. The thickest cells have seemed to us to reside in the external frontier of the plexus, although sometimes they are also found in other regions of the same (fig. 1, *A, B*) [*fig. 59*].

In some cells, the axon becomes much thinner after the emergence of the collaterals, some of which, because of their robustness, appear to represent the continuation of the [primary axon] trunk. Generally, this thick collateral has a recurrent course and can arise even from the trajectory of the axon in the underlying layer (fig. 1, *b, c*) [*fig. 59*].

2. Small Type and with Short Axon

Commonly with a spherical shape, but sometimes with a triangular or polygonal [form], this cell lies in the whole thickness of the plexus, and it is characterized by the thinness, shortness, and varicose aspect of its dendrites, which, as in the previous type, come from all sides of the soma and are ramified exclusively inside the plexus. The axon is very thin and can arise from several points of the cell body, sometimes ascending, sometimes descending, and sometimes running horizontally to resolve

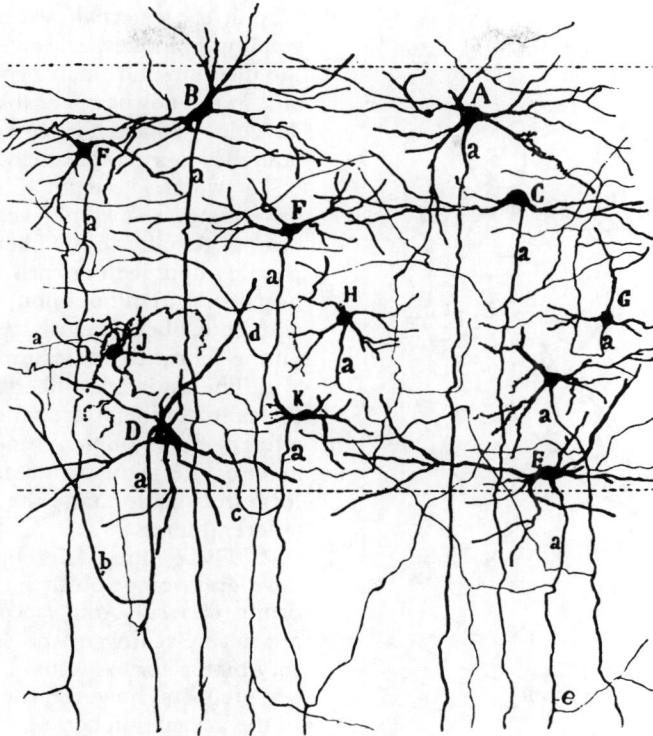

[FIG. 59]   Fig. 1. Cells of the stria of Gennari or of the layer of the stellate cells. Adult cerebrum. A, B, C, D, giant stellate cells; F, K, medium stellate cells; G, H, J, small cells with short axon; a, axon; b, d, ascending thick collaterals; e, collaterals to the deep layers.

finally into a terminal nerve arborization, confined to the territory of the stria. So far, neither in the newborn child nor in the adult man have we been able to observe these axon branches leaving the region in which the cell of origin lies (fig. 1, J, H, G) [fig. 59].

Ascending Robust Nerve Fibers Emanating from the White Matter

This is one of the most characteristic features of the visual region. Certainly, in other cerebral regions, particularly in the motor, robust centrifugal fibers demonstrated by us some time ago are not lacking; but we have to recognize that in no cerebral region are they so abundant as in the visual cortex. Another very interesting feature consists [of the fact] that the cited fibers are ramified and terminate preferentially in the stria of Gennari or of

Vicq d'Azyr. In fact, the white color of this band comes from the abundance of these fibers, which maintain their myelin sheaths up to their primary and secondary branches.

In fig. 2 [fig. 60], we reproduce some of these fibers, taken from the cerebrum of the child of three and of twenty-seven days. In general, such fibers, on arriving in the gray matter, do not usually run in the radial direction but obliquely, sometimes tracing large bends, until they reach the stria of Gennari or layer of the stellate cells, in which they usually become horizontal, going in this direction for enormous distances and giving off an infinity of small branches engendering a very dense plexus, which surrounds and touches in a thousand places the somata and dendrites of the intrinsic cells, as well as the [apical dendritic] shafts of the pyramids and of cells located in the underlying layers. In many

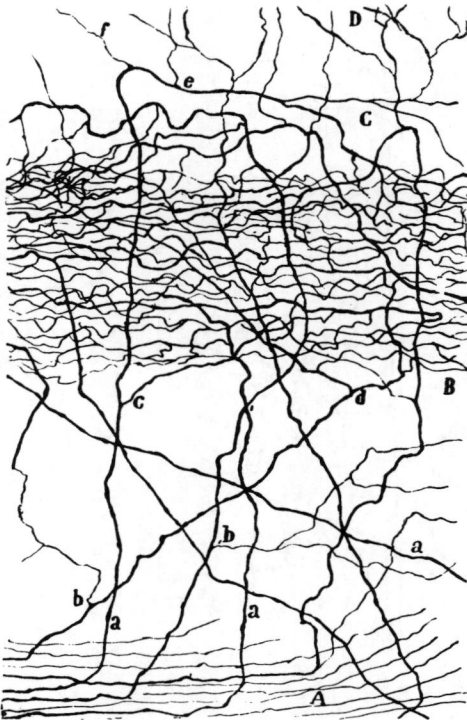

[FIG. 60] Fig. 2. Thick fibers arriving from the white matter and ramifying in the stria of Gennari. Cerebrum of the child of three days. A, white matter; B, layer of the stellate cells; C, arciform fibers; D, layer of the medium pyramids; a, trunk of the fiber; b, collateral to the deep layers; e, ascending collateral to the upper layers.

cases, the fibers cross the plexus vertically or obliquely up to its external limit or into the thickness of the layer of medium pyramids, then suddenly bend downward or go flexuously for a long distance (fig. 2, C) [fig. 60] and finally resolve themselves in descending collaterals and terminals that are consumed in the layer of the stellate cells. It is thus seen that the area of distribution of a fiber of this kind is enormous, it being possible to affirm that its small branches enter into contact with hundreds of nerve cells of the layer of the stellate cells and with not a few large, small, and medium pyramids.

It is very frequent to see that the cited fibers, after crossing the plexus and running horizon-

tally in the external part of this, give off ascending branches, arborizing in the layers of the medium and small pyramids (fig. 2, e) [fig. 60]. In the newborn child and [child] of a few days old, we have not been able to follow these branches to the molecular layer.

To which kind of fibers do the thick [myelinated axons] that we have just described belong? Are they optic fibers coming from the primary optic centers or intercortical association fibers? In our opinion, we are dealing here with optic fibers, and we base this presumption on the following indications:

1. The association fibers, and even more so the callosal [fibers], are much thinner than the afferent fibers of the visual region. Even the axon of the giant pyramids of the cortex has less thickness than the majority of the [afferent] fibers.

2. These thick afferent fibers, which we have discovered in other regions of the cerebrum (fibers of Cajal, according to Kölliker), are never lacking in the sensory cortex (sensory-motor cortex, visual cortex, acoustic cortex, etc.), but, however, they seem to be absent in the association cortex.

3. Physiology and anatomy jointly tell us that the visual region must receive a considerable flow of optic fibers; it is, then, natural to consider as such the innumerable thick fibers distributed in the layer of the stellate cells, [leading to the conclusion] that the dense plexuses engendered in this layer constitutes the new factor, almost specific for the visual sphere.

Thin Ascending Fibers Coming from the Layers of the Granules and of the Polymorphic Cells

[Among the] other specializations of the visual cortex is the enormous number of cells with ascending axons resident in the layer of the granule cells and the layer of the polymorphic cells. These axons, after giving off some collaterals to the deeper cortical layers, enter the optic plexus or stria of Gennari and ramify among the stellate cells, serving to complicate enormously the dense nervous arborization resident there. See fig. 3 [fig. 61].

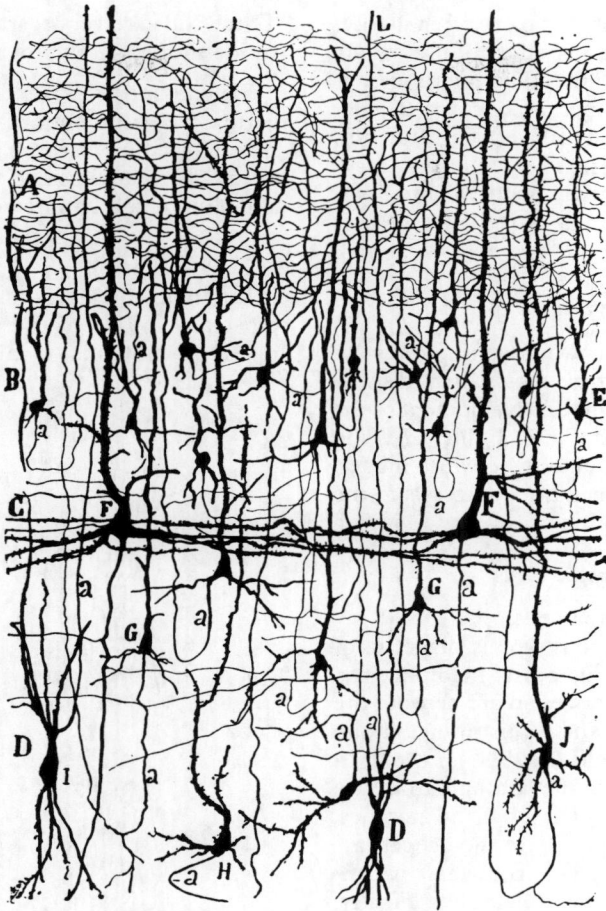

[*FIG. 61*]   Fig. 3. Deep layers of the visual cortex of the cerebrum of the child of twenty-seven days. *A*, layer of the stellate cells; *B*, layer of the granules; *C*, layer of the giant cells; *D*, layer of the polymorphic cells; *E*, granule cell with ascending axon; *F*, giant pyramid; *G*, small pyramid with ascending axon; *H*, *J*, other cells with similar axon; *I*, giant cell with axon destined for the molecular layer; *a*, axon.

Finally, let us add also, in order to conclude the examination of the layer of the stellate cells, that in this are distributed also the collaterals originating from the course of the ascending axons destined for the molecular layer (fig. 3, *I*) [*fig. 61*]; collaterals of superimposed medium pyramids; collaterals and probably terminals of axons belonging to ovoid or fusiform small cells, placed above the plexus (external granules). Finally, let us not forget either that the said layer is crossed by the [apical dendritic] shafts of the giant pyramids

and polymorphic cells, the ascending dendrites of the granule cells, and the small bundles of descending axons of the medium and small pyramids.

Layer of Granules (fig. 3, *B*) [*fig. 61*]

The granules are ovoid, small cells, provided with descending or lateral short dendrites and one or several ascending thin [dendritic] shafts directed to the layer of the stellate cells. The axon, [which is] very thin, can arise from the upper part of the soma; but more often it arises from the deeper part, goes down for a certain distance in a vertical direction, and traces, finally, an arc with a superior concavity to enter finally the superimposed layer (fig. 3, *E*) [*fig. 61*], where it arborizes and ends.

This layer also contains some medium pyramids and cells of Golgi or [cells] with short axon.

Layer of the Giant Pyramids

It is formed by one or two discontinuous rows of robust pyramids whose most salient distinction rests on the enormous development of the lateral basal dendrites (fig. 3, *F*) [*fig. 61*]. The axon, which is thick, enters the white matter, after supplying two or more collaterals to the layer of the polymorphic cells.

Layer of the Polymorphic Cells

It contains four kinds of cells:
1. The most numerous type is made up of fusiform, ovoid, or triangular, medium-sized cells, whose axon describes an arc beneath the soma, to ascend later and be distributed in the layer of the stellate cells (fig. 3, *G*) [*fig. 61*]. In some cells, both from the arc and from the course of the axon in the layer of the granules, some collaterals that ramify in the deeper layers are given off. The dendritic shaft is consumed in the layer of the stellate cells. Finally, the axon of some cells of this kind, at a certain distance along its descending course, is bifurcated into a thin branch, which is prolonged to the white matter, and which seems from its direction to be the continuation of [the parent axon], and another thick arciform branch that goes up to be consumed by ramifying in the layer of the stellate cells.
2. Robust fusiform or triangular cells, sometimes of giant size (fig. 3, *I*) [*fig. 61*], whose ascending axon crosses the whole cortex and reaches the molecular layer of the cerebrum, not before giving rise to some collaterals destined for the plexus of Gennari and for other layers.
3. Cells of Golgi or [cells] with short axons, scattered in the layer of the polymorphic cells.
4. Triangular or fusiform cells, radially oriented, whose axon enters the white matter.

These cells are very scarce, and many of them reside in the very white matter.

To conclude this brief study of the cerebral cortex, we will mention here two new cellular types found in several regions of the cerebrum. These are a small fusiform bitufted cell and a giant cell with horizontal axon.

First Type

It lies in all the layers of the cortex, but more especially in that of the medium pyramids. It is very possible that it inhabits all the gyri, al-

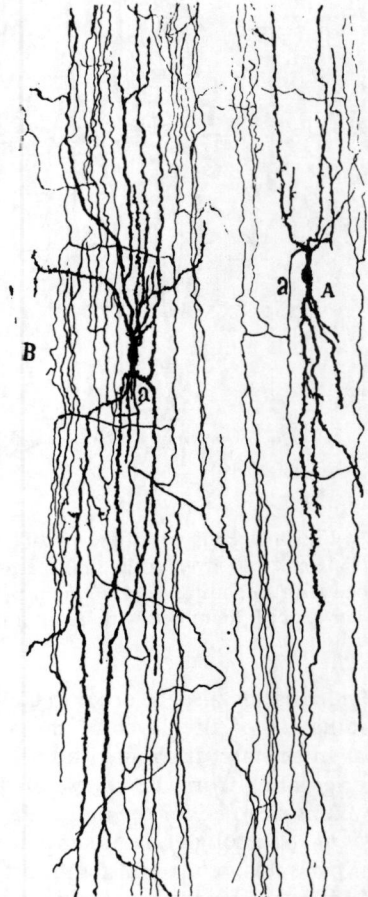

[*FIG. 62*] Fig. 4. Small cells inhabiting several layers. Acoustic cortex of the child of twenty-seven days. *A*, cell with descending moderately branched axon; *B*, cell with axon resolving itself into many very long, ascending and descending small bundles; *a*, axon.

though so far we have only found it in the visual, motor, and acoustic [gyri]. In the last, it exists in considerable numbers. As fig. 4 [fig. 62] shows, the form of the said cells is elongated, with two polar processes, rapidly resolving into tufts of great length, one ascending and the other descending. The branches of the latter, [which are] thin and varicose, can go up to reach the layer of the polymorphic cells. Besides a fusiform shape, such cells can have a triangular or stellate form, but in all cases the dendrites engender the said bundles. But what is really special about these cells rests on the behavior of the axon, which is very thin, arises either from the upper or from the deeper part of the soma, and resolves itself rapidly into an infinity of vertical threads, so abundant that they engender truly small bundles, comparable to locks of hair, and so long that they extend through almost the whole thickness of the gray matter.

In the cortex of the child of twenty-five to thirty days, the delicacy of these vertical threads is so great that they cannot be studied well except with a Zeiss 1.30 apochromatic

[lens], which reveals them to be flexuous, with a yellowish color, and thinly varicose. Because of their extreme length, the cells A and B of fig. 4 [fig. 62] have been reproduced over scarcely a third of their vertical trajectory. In some places, it is observed that the small bundles of threads are applied to the [apical dendrites] and somata of a vertical series of pyramids, from which we think it very probable that the referred cells are a special category of cells with short axon whose role would be to associate in the vertical direction pyramids resident in different layers.

It is noteworthy that such cells have never been seen by us in the cerebral cortex of the dog, cat, and rabbit. In that of man, they are so abundant that in the acoustic region, where they have been very completely impregnated [in our preparations], the small bundles of nerve threads belonging to adjacent cells are almost in longitudinal contact.

Second Type (fig. 5) [fig. 63]

It is a giant cell with soma almost as thick as that of a large pyramid. Its shape is stellate or

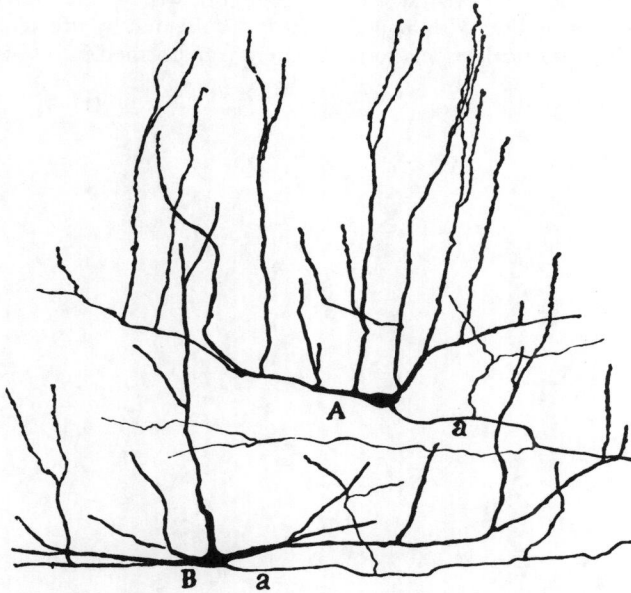

[FIG. 63] Fig. 5. Large horizontal thick cells of the acoustic cortex of the child of twenty-seven days. A, cell that resided in the layer of the small pyramids; B, another taken from the layer of the polymorphic cells beneath the giant pyramids; a, axon.

triangular, but in the perpendicular sections it appears fusiform because of the impossibility of discovering the processes of the opposite side. From the contour of the soma, [which is] flattened from above down, arise three or more horizontal primary dendrites of large length, from which arise successively divided ascending branches, the totality of which embrace a large extent of the cortex. Spines do not appear on its contour; the thin dendrites are strongly varicose. The axon is robust, its course is generally either oblique or horizontal, and it gives off in its trajectory a multitude of collaterals.

In cell *A* [of *fig. 63*], which inhabited the layer of the medium pyramids, the axon could not be followed completely; but in cell *B*, which resided beneath the [layer of] giant pyramids, the axon was horizontally extended for more than two-tenths of a millimeter, and it still did not end; nor did it show a tendency to descend to the white matter.

It is not possible to give a definite opinion about the significance of these cells while the termination of the axon is not completely elucidated. However, attending to the orientation of this and to other characteristics, we judge it probable that here we are dealing with a special variety of cell of intracortical association, a cell whose role would be to establish, over a large distance, connections between groups of widely separated pyramids although resident in the same layer or very close to it. In a word, and without prejudicing the opportunity of rectification in the presence of better information, such cells would be to the thickness of the cortex what the special cells of the molecular layer (*Cajal'sche Zellen* of Retzius) are to the surface part.

Our works on the other regions of the cortex are in too preliminary a stage for us to be able to give a precise idea about them.

With respect to the sensory-motor cortex, we can affirm, however, that it also contains certain thick fibers, probably continuous with the central sensory pathway, and ending preferentially in an intermediate layer of the gray matter, in which also reside special stellate cells, but in smaller numbers than in the visual cortex. And if these facts should be confirmed in all the sensory areas of the cortex (excluding the areas called by Flechsig *areas of association*), it could be considered that this particular layer is the specific anatomical factor of the sensory cortex, as well as the preferred place on which the image of the external world collected by the senses is projected and there transformed into sensation.

15

Studies on the Human Cerebral Cortex [I]:
Visual Cortex[1]

[*Revista Trimestral Micrográfica* 4:1–63, 1899]

The structure of the visual cortex is a fascinating object of study. The doctrine of cortical localization introduced by Fritsch, Hitzig, and Ferrier; the cortical regions on which are projected the images of the senses as discovered by Munk, Monakow, etc.; and Flechsig's published theory that divides the cerebral cortex into projection or sensory-motor centers and association or ideational centers all make it essential to undertake a comparative histological examination of all of these regions to see if it is possible to explain the functional specialization by a specialization of structure. In the case of a lack of distinct anatomical differences among these diverse cortical spheres, [it may be necessary] to turn to the theory of Meynert, nowadays defended by Golgi and Kölliker, which states that the above-mentioned functional plurality is a natural consequence of the diversity of nervous connections.

Of particular interest to these inquiries is the point that if, as suspected by many authors, the structural plan of the cortex undergoes important changes in each region, then it may be possible to determine the physiological significance of each anatomical element in the gray matter. Thus, for example, if an organizational detail is found exclusively in or is particularly exaggerated in the visual cortex, we will be justified in suspecting that it has something to do with cerebral visual function; conversely, if an anatomical detail is repeated equally in all cortical regions, we will be justified in assuming that it is devoid of specific functional significance and instead is of more general significance.

Similar considerations and the natural desire to widen the horizons of our knowledge of cortical structure have led us to study methodically all the sensory regions of the cortex, starting with the visual. [This is a subject that] is still enveloped in darkness, despite the contributions of Golgi, Martinotti, ourselves, Retzius, Kölliker, etc.

For better performance of this task, we have chosen man and gyrencephalic mammals as the objects of study. The reason for this preference is that in these animals the anatomist has a secure guide in the physiology, which, as illustrated by experimentation and by human pathological anatomy, has permitted the positions and extents of the sensory and motor cortical areas to be localized with reasonable accuracy. The uncertainty that still prevails

147

regarding the positions of these areas in smooth-brained mammals has obliged us to delay for the time being the completion of our studies of 1892 on the visual cortex of the mouse, guinea pig, and rabbit. Perhaps someday we will recommence that study, making a comparative structural analysis of the homonymous cortical regions in both categories of animals; for that task, we hope that the results obtained in the human brain will serve us as a key.

The present paper is thus the first of a series that will cover the whole cortex; none will dispute that if such studies are to have any physiological value, they must be comparative. General concepts of cortical structure will be the legitimate results derived from a comparative exploration of the whole cortex. From another point of view, this regional analysis can also illustrate the organization of the psychomotor region, so far hardly explored with the Golgi method; it is a matter of experience that in all anatomical explorations, only characteristics that are abundant and highly differentiated are the most clearly appreciated; conversely, characteristics that are rare and only barely manifest commonly pass unnoticed. In confirmation of this assertion of simple good sense, we will cite an example from our studies. The elements that in the course of this work we will call stellate cells and sensory fibers are recognizable in several cortical regions, particularly in the motor area, but we had not learned to recognize them until they appeared in great number and abundantly manifest in the human visual area. Similar examples of inattention, induced by insufficient differentiation of the explored tissue, show once again that even continuing arduous and watchful observation, in order to lead to a new [understanding], often needs the impact of an explosive impression.

Our preference for the human cortex also represents a methodological end point. When the subject of investigation is the fundamental plan of the brain, it is appropriate to turn to small mammals . and to early evolutionary stages; but once we wish to indicate the structural diversity of the cortical areas, it is necessary to choose man, in whom these topographic differentiations reach maximum

development and advancement. For the same reason, we prefer, instead of the human embryo, the infant and even the adult, for it is clear that the topographic differentiation will only appear distinctly in the period during which sensation and other higher psychic activities have emerged.

The particular demands of the Golgi method have obliged us to choose preferentially brains from infants fifteen to twenty-five days old, the age during which the Golgi reaction is very consistent and reliable; we have had, however, the good fortune to obtain some good preparations in the adult brain as well.

Among the gyrencephalic mammals that are the subjects of our analysis, most are cats and dogs of twenty to thirty days old, i.e., a period in which the organs of the senses are in full activity.

We have also put to work all the [other] more valuable methods of study: Nissl for staining the protoplasm, Weigert-Pal for impregnation of the myelin sheath, Ehrlich for staining the superficial [cortical] nerve cells and medullated axons, [Golgi-] Cox for the slow impregnation of the cortex of the dog and cat.

Historical Notes about the Structure of the Visual Cortex

That the visual cortex has a special anatomical character is an observation already made in the first part of this century by several scholars, among them Gennari, Vicq d'Azyr, Baillarger, and Broca, who pointed out in this region and visible to the naked eye the existence of an intermediate white line. But the first more or less precise histological analysis was that of Meynert, who, in the human visual cortex, recognized the following layers: first, molecular layer; second, layer of small pyramids; third, layer of nuclei or grains (equivalent to the fourth layer of the typical cortex); fourth, layer of large pyramids or solitary cells; fifth, layer of grains or medium nuclei; sixth, layer analogous to the fourth, composed of nuclei of neuroglia and scattered large cells; seventh, layer of nuclei or deep grains; eighth, layer of fusiform cells (analogous to the fifth layer of the typical cortex).[2]

W. Krause,[3] who has carefully studied the cortical layers, distinguishes in the motor region, first, the marginal layer, made up of medullated fibers; second, the molecular layer, with few nerve cells but rich in neuroglia; third, [the layer] of small pyramids; fourth, the layer of the external nervous plexus in which nuclei correspond to the sheaths of the axons that cross it; fifth, [the layer] of large pyramids; sixth, [the layer] of the internal nervous plexus in which nuclei correspond exclusively to the sheaths of the fibers; seventh, [the layer] of grains or small cells (in which W. Krause includes the grains and fusiform cells of the typical cortex of Meynert).

Regarding the visual cortex, it is characterized, in terms of Krause's classification, by a robust fourth layer or external nervous plexus (stria of Gennari and Vicq d'Azyr) formed by myelinated axons. Furthermore, the fifth and sixth layers would be extremely thin, particularly the fifth, which would contain only a few large pyramidal cells (the solitary cells of Meynert).

Schwalbe[4] accepts without reservation the description of Meynert and follows Krause in considering the stria of Vicq d'Azyr as a horizontal plexus of medullated nerve fibers.

According to Betz,[5] the occipital cortex is composed of the following strata: first, neuroglial (molecular) layer; second, layer of small pyramids; third, first layer of grains; fourth, layer of nerve fibers; fifth, second layer of grains; sixth, second layer of nerve fibers; seventh, layer of sparse, scattered pyramids; eighth, layer of fusiform cells.

In the opinion of Golgi,[6] the worker who first applied the method named after him to the study of the brain, the visual cortex (superior occipital convolution) is characterized by its very small number of giant pyramids. Let us remember, of course, that Golgi describes only three layers in the typical cortex; the *external, middle,* and *internal* thirds of the thickness of the gray matter. Now, the first two strata would exhibit similar characteristics in the motor and visual cortex; but at the level of the deep stratum, there should be a larger number of small cells (globular, pyramidal, or fusiform). Likewise, at the border between this zone and the middle layer, there should be some giant pyramids (solitary cells of Meynert).

In view of the little structural variation [that he sees] between the visual and motor cortex, Golgi declares that the specificity of function in the various cerebral regions derives not from their particular organization but from the specific peripheral apparatuses in which nerve fibers terminating in them arise. This doctrine, already defended by Meynert, is correct in essence, but Golgi exaggerates it in the case of the cortex, because, as we shall see below, the visual cortex displays unique organizational characteristics and a structural complexity far greater than that which the simplistic descriptions and schematic drawings of the sage of Pavia would presuppose. Furthermore, it is very doubtful that the region examined by Golgi has much relationship to visual function; we have not in the least found it to possess the particular structure of the cuneus and the borders of the calcarine fissure. In our opinion, this unique structure in man and mammals is characteristic only of the internal surface of the occipital lobule.

Hammarberg,[7] that unfortunate researcher who made an excellent comparative study of the histology of the human brain convolutions by the Nissl method, distinguished two types of cortical structure: the *motor* and the *sensory,* to [the latter of] which the visual cortex belongs.

[In Hammarberg's scheme,] the visual cortex would be distinguished by the lack of giant cells in the fourth layer, in which they are replaced by a broad stratum of grains or small cells divided into three substrata between which are two bands of molecular aspect, poor in nerve cells. Between the stratum of grains and the layer of fusiform cells would be a row of large pyramids (solitary cells of Meynert).

The Golgi method[8] was applied by us to the visual cortex of small mammals, particularly the rabbit, in which we obtained results scarcely comparable to those of the authors cited above. The most distinctive and original features of our still incomplete analysis were the discovery of a row of vertical, fusiform cells under the molecular or first layer and the demonstration that the plexus or band of Vicq d'Azyr is composed primarily of the collateral ramifications and terminals of numerous cells with ascending axons located in this band and in the deeper layers.

In regard to the typical cortex, in a prior study relating to the small mammals, we had distinguished the following layers: first, molecular layer; second, layer of small pyramids; third, layer of large pyramids; fourth, layer of polymorphic cells. For the remainder, a similar division into four layers is not applicable, either to the typical human cortex, where at least five strata exist, or to the visual cortex of mammals.[9]

From the point of view of the distribution of myelinated axons, Botazzi[10] has published a good study of the structure of the cortex, making use of the method of Weigert and a large number of vertebrates. According to this authority, the cortex of the mammals (rabbit, monkey, etc.) includes two classes of fibers: the *horizontal* and the *radial.*

The horizontal form several groups: the *internal horizontal fibers* are found at the levels of the layers crossed by radial bundles and corresponding in the occipital region to the line of Gennari; the *intermediate horizontal* fibers are residents of the layers of medium and small pyramids; the *tangential* or *external horizontal fibers* are located in the molecular layer. Corresponding to the intermediate fibers would be the stria of Bechterew, described by Kaes at the level of the small pyramids and not far from the tangential fibers.

Among the radial fibers, he includes the radial vertical bundles formed by the axons of pyramidal cells; isolated radial fibers that pass from one bundle to another, forming a plexus; loose radially ascending fibers extending up to the molecular layer and representing in part the vertical fibers of Martinotti; finally, radially ascending bundles representing prolongations of the white matter towards the molecular layer. These last bundles were suspected by Vulpian in the human cortex, noted by Botazzi in mammals, and demonstrated by us in the mouse cortex.[11]

In regard to the visual cortex of the cercopithecus [monkey], Botazzi pointed out the great development of the stria of Gennari, which consisted of oblique or horizontal medullated fibers of medium thickness. Within the layers of small and medium pyramids, there

would also exist plexuses of thin fibers increasing with age (supraradial network), which, because they only appear in the higher mammals and man, are considered to be one of the indicative signs of higher mental activity (quantity of associations). The so-called stria of Bechterew appears well developed in the visual cortex.

M. Schlapp,[12] who has recently studied the structure of the cerebral cortex of the monkey with the aid of the Nissl method, recognizes three types of gray matter: first, *frontal lobe type,* made up of five strata (first, molecular, of tangential fibers; second, small polymorphic cells; third, small pyramids; fourth, large pyramids or motor cells; fifth, polymorphic cells); second, the *second, parietal, and sphenoidal lobe type,* typically characterized by an intermediate band of small cells or grains in the interior of the fourth stratum; and third, the *visual type,* easily recognizable by its almost total lack of pyramids, with most of its cells spherical or irregular in form, except for the large-sized solitary cells of Meynert. The full complement of layers of the visual cortex of the monkey is as follows:

1. Layer of tangential fibers.
2. Layer of external polymorphic cells.
3. Layer of parapygnomorphic pyramidal cells (rather than pyramidal, the cells are of oval form).
4. Layer of the grains.
5. Layer of the small solitary cells.
6. Another layer of grains.
7. Layer poor in cells.
8. Layer of internal polymorphic cells.

In addition, Kölliker[13] notes in his classic book on histology some data concerning the human visual region. According to this authority, the stria of Vicq d'Azyr or of Gennari comprises a large quantity of horizontal fibers of medium and small caliber, mixed with some robust myelinated fibers. On occasion, within the stria, another, thinner stria, also composed of horizontal fibers, appears.

In regard to the cells, [Kölliker] calls attention to the numerous and densely compacted small pyramids, the more voluminous of them corresponding to the stria of Vicq d' Azyr which also contains an infinity of minute cells (grains), already illustrated by Hammarberg.

Not far from the white matter, above the polymorphic cells, as already illustrated by Golgi, [there] are some giant pyramids that escaped the attention of Hammarberg (solitary cells of Meynert).

As we can see from the preceding brief historical review, the data we possess regarding the human occipital cortex and that of the gyrencephalic mammals are quite incomplete and in part contradictory. The little knowledge that we have refers to the number of layers and to the gross morphology of the neuronal somata; but the fundamental point, the target to which we must look in any anatomical investigation, must lie in the gray matter, that is to say, in the fine morphology, distribution, and connections of the neuronal processes; this has still not been touched by anybody. To fill in, to the best of our ability, this important lacuna is the goal pursued in the present work.

Numbers of Layers of the Visual Cortex:

When a section of the adult visual cortex stained by the Nissl method is examined (fig. 1) [*fig. 64*], numerous stratifications are visible in it, as already pointed out by Meynert, who, despite his impoverished methods, has been the one who has best comprehended the special stratification of this region of the brain.

Here are the layers that are distinguishable at first sight: first, molecular or first plexiform; second, that of the small pyramids; third, that of the medium pyramids; fourth, second plexiform, composed of large stellate cells; fifth, composed of small cells or granules with a few larger cells; sixth, formed of small elongated elements; seventh, third plexiform, where there are some giant pyramidal cells (solitary cells of Meynert); eighth, built up of medium pyramids, very closely spaced; ninth, where reside fusiform and triangular cells separated by bundles of myelinated fibers.

Still more layers could be distinguished, but those already cited appear to us to be sufficiently indicative of [the area's] individuality; also, they correspond, as we shall see below, to groups of neurons with quite special morphological properties. There exist, however, transitions that on occasion make the delimitation of the layers difficult, above all in certain regions of each gyrus in which some [layers] ap-

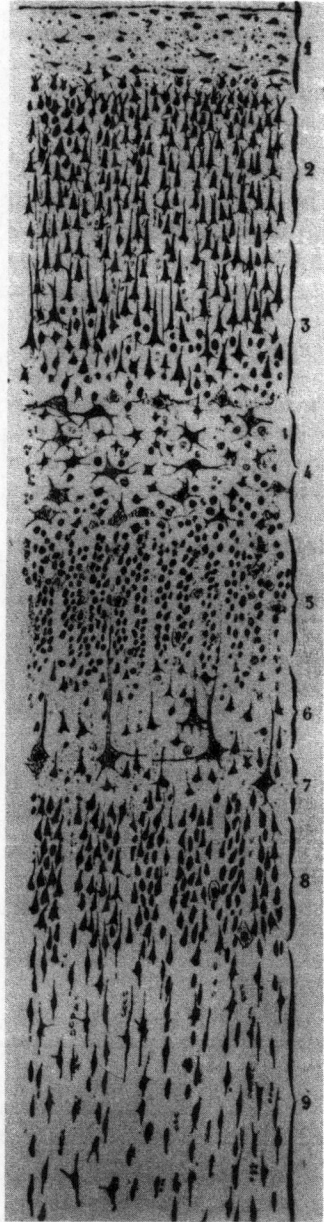

[*FIG. 64*] Fig. 1. Section from the visual cerebral cortex (borders of the calcarine fissure) of a man thirty years old. Method of Nissl. *1*, plexiform layer; *2*, layer of the small pyramids; *3*, layer of the medium pyramids; *4*, layer of the large stellate cells; *5*, layer of the small stellate cells; *6*, plexiform layer or layer of the small pyramids with ascending axon; *7*, layer of giant pyramids; *8*, layer of the pyramids with arched ascending axons; *9*, fusiform cells.

pear to be interrupted, change their height, or undergo considerable transformation, only to reappear further on. The changes in height are particularly frequent in layers 6 and 7.

Nomenclature of the Layers

[Those] who created the names of the cortical strata were [working] in an era when the methods of study were very imperfect and necessarily had to refer only to the gross appearance of the nervous fabric (sections stained with carmine, hematoxylin, or basic aniline [dyes]). Thus, they could not avoid two inconveniences: to christen with the same or similar names layers formed by cells of very different morphology, and to propose designations that give no idea of the internal structure of the strata.

Actually, because the texture of the protoplasm does not yield enough specific data, the nomenclature of the layers must be found in the fine morphology of the cells and in the course and connections of the axons, properties that can only be revealed with the silver chromate method. Accordingly, we propose the following designations:

1. Plexiform layer or [layer] of horizontal cells (molecular [layer] of the authors).
2. Layer of the small pyramids.
3. Layer of the medium pyramids.
4. Layer of the large stellate cells (part of the grains of the authors).
5. Layer of the small stellate cells (grains of the authors).
6. Layer of the small cells with arched axons.
7. Layer of the giant pyramids (solitary cells of Meynert).
8. Layer of the large cells with arched and ascending axons (deep grains of Meynert).
9. Layer of the triangular and fusiform cells (fusiforms of Meynert).

Because residing in each cortical layer there are cells of different morphology, it has been necessary to choose for the division and naming of the strata the predominant cellular form. It would still have been preferable to adopt for this purpose the criterion of the *termination of the axon*, as used by us in the classification of neurons in the spinal cord; unfor-

tunately, however, the incompleteness of the results obtained in the visual cortex do not permit us to adopt it for the time being.

I. Plexiform Layer (Molecular [Layer] of the Authors)

The plexiform layer of the visual cortex is, as already recognized by Meynert, thinner than in other cortical regions. This thinness can be attributed to the decrease in the number of medium and giant pyramids, which, as is known since our first works on the cerebral cortex, send a vast tuft of dendrites to the molecular layer.

On examining this layer with the method of Nissl, it displays a general granular or pale plexiform background, in which one can detect, here and there, the nuclei of neuroglia and of nerve cells.

The neurons detectable with this staining method are few and very small, and they extend without order throughout the thickness of the layer. Their protoplasm is lacking or very poor in [Nissl] granules, a circumstance that prevents determination of the morphology of the soma in Nissl preparations. Only in some elements is [the soma] appreciated as a spindle-shaped or triangular figure with processes arising from its angles.

If, instead of the adult visual cortex, that of a child a few days old is studied, the plexiform layer it presents is thinner, and one is able to note that while the nerve cells appear closer [to one another], the nuclei of neuroglia [appear] more abundant than in the adult. This last is caused by the fact that many displaced epithelial cells, destined to transform into neuroglial cells, have still to reach the plexiform layer. At the outer limit of this layer, immediately under the pia, can be recognized some relatively voluminous polygonal or triangular cells, with protoplasm quite rich in chromatin, which are not found in the adult cortex. Similar marginal elements correspond to certain border cells that the Golgi method stains well (see below); without doubt, these will occupy a deeper position in the adult cortex because of the growth and successive intercalation of fibers and tufts of pyramids among them. However, even in the adult, there are, from time to time, some nerve cells not very far away from the outer limit [of layer I].

But the true morphology of the cells of the plexiform layer can only be revealed with the methods of Golgi and Ehrlich. These methods reveal the following features: first, special neurons with long radiations; second, small or medium neurons with short axons; third, the tufts of pyramids; fourth, the ascending fibers of Martinotti; fifth, the ascending fibers of the white matter; sixth, various types of neuroglial cells.

We will not describe in detail all the features of the construction of the plexiform layer. We have already spoken about them in several papers,[14] to which we refer the reader. For now, it suffices to say that the cells mentioned thus far are very comparable in the visual cortex to those in other cortical regions and so do not warrant an individual description. Only in regard to the special cells with long radiations are we going to reveal some data.

As Retzius has recorded,[15] our *horizontal or special cells* (*Cajal'sche Zellen* of Retzius) have a quite extraordinary development in the human fetal brain. In fetuses of six, seven, and eight months, they appear throughout the thickness of the molecular layer in the form of fusiform, triangular, or stellate cells with very long horizontal, parallel, varicose processes from which, at right angles, emerge an infinity of small ascending branches; [these] end under the pia in a thick varicosity. The more superficially placed cells (marginal cells) are conical, having an external base adherent to the pia and a central pedicle from which also emerge very numerous and enormously long processes (fig. 2, *A, B*) [*fig. 65*]. The more deeply situated cells are more often spindle-shaped or triangular, and we can see that the ascending branches arise both as polar expansions and from the external surface of the soma. In fig. 2, *A, B, C* [*fig. 65*], which reproduces these cells as they appear in the newborn child, it can be seen that it is impossible to distinguish among the various elongated processes any with the characteristics of axons or the [typical] properties of dendrites. Retzius tends, however, to accept that some of them possess indications of a short axon; and Ver-

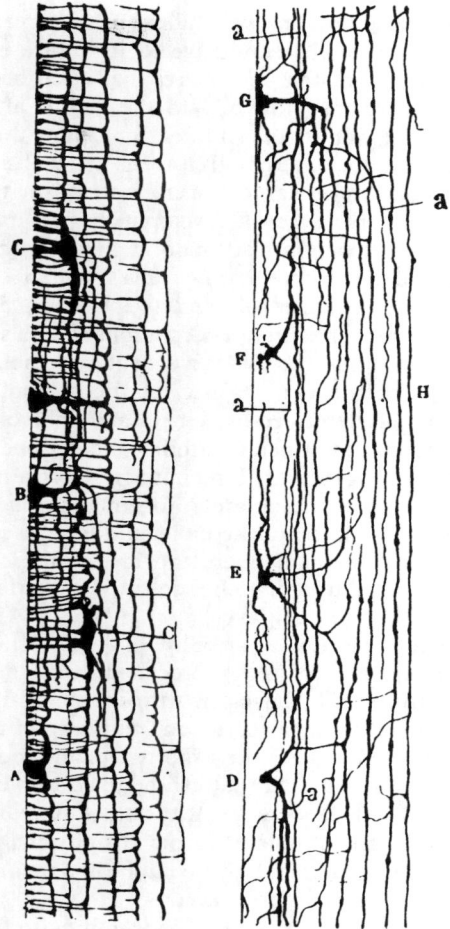

[*FIG. 65*] Fig. 2. Cells of the first or plexiform layer. *A, B, C*, horizontal cells of the visual cortex of the newborn child or the fetus close to birth; *D, E, F, G*, cells of the visual cortex of the child of twenty days; *H*, horizontal or tangential fibers from horizontal cells located far away in the same, first layer; *a*, fine processes with the morphological appearance of axons.

atti,[16] who has recently studied these cells in the cortex of the rabbit, assumes that, in spite of the axonlike appearance of the majority of the cellular processes (*pseudaxons* of this author), only one distributes and behaves like a legitimate nerve fiber.

Our recent observations in the cerebrum of the newborn and fifteen-to-thirty-day-old child, even if they do not permit us to answer the question definitively, allow us to contribute some details conducive to its future enlightenment. Retzius declares that it has been impossible for him to stain these cells after birth and admits that he does not know their definitive form, although it is his belief that it does not suffer large transformations in the subsequent course of development. We have been a little more fortunate in that we have succeeded in impregnating a few of the special cells on the fifteenth and twenty-third day after birth. These new observations allow us to confirm fully two of our recent statements: first, that the vast majority of the ascending collaterals described by Retzius are embryonic dispositions destined to atrophy and disappear; second, that the very long horizontal processes are preserved indefinitely, forming, throughout the thickness of the molecular layer, a system of horizontal fibers provided with scattered, thin, short branches destined for various levels of the same [layer].

The progressive atrophy of the vertical branches can be well appreciated in the days following birth. It begins with disappearance of the terminal varicosity and thinning of the parent shaft; this is then shortened, and it disappears in a period that can be fixed between twenty and thirty days. At the same time, the few collaterals protected from atrophy change direction and branch in a complicated manner high in the plexiform layer.

Concerning the axon, if indeed it exists, we can provide little that is new. In the stained cells from brains of eight, fifteen, and twenty days, all the processes seemed equal; only in two marginal cells (fig. 2, F, D, a) [fig. 65], at a time when almost all the vertical appendages had disappeared, have we been able to distinguish a process finer and thinner than the rest that might signify an axon. The long tangential fibers present in the first part of their course a roughened contour and numerous spines, factors that speak in favor of their dendritic nature.

Finally, the special cells cease to be stained definitively in the brain of twenty-five days and beyond. Around this date, the most successful impregnations only exhibit good staining of the robust and very long horizontal processes, some of which reach lengths of two- or three-tenths of a millimeter and are perhaps much longer, because their ends almost always appear cut and without indications of terminations. We ignore whether by chance, but for all the fibers of this class found in the sulci ran in parallel and seemed to join two neighboring gyri.

When the molecular layer of the adult cat is examined in horizontal sections stained by the method of Ehrlich from the visual or any other area, very long myelinated fibers are observed running horizontally and bifurcating several times. Some of these fibers probably correspond to fibers ascending from the white matter, but others originate, as we have shown, from robust cells located in the plexiform or first layer. The method of Weigert-Pal lends support to this interpretation, since it reveals in the plexiform layer, in addition to numerous thin fibers in the depths of this layer, a plane of tangential and horizontally directed robust fibers. The notable robustness of such fibers is greater than that of the ascending fibers of Martinotti; this and evidence of Botazzi that in the fetal brain they develop completely independently of the myelinated fibers of the white matter speak also in favor of the opinion that they arise in the robust cells of the plexiform layer. These cells could very well be the special cells with long horizontal processes.

In sum, the special cells of the cortex seem to represent association cells with enormous extensions by means of which they would bring association fibers of layer I into dynamic relationships with tufts of pyramids located in neighboring gyri.

As illustrated in fig. 7, G, F [fig. 70], the first layer in man also contains many short-axon stellate cells similar to those described by us in the cat and other small mammals. There is also no lack of arachniform nerve cells, with a very dense nervous arborization; of them, we will speak later (fig. 7, E) [fig. 70].

Lastly, in the infant ten to fifteen days old, we have found also some piriform cells very similar to neuroblasts, some horizontally, others vertically oriented, and with the soma close to the pia. We are uncertain of the significance of these elements, which are absent from numerous preparations (fig. 5, *H, I*) [*fig. 68*].

II. Layer of the Small Pyramids

These have in the visual cortex characteristics identical to those in the rest of the cerebral cortex. With a stellate or triangular form and lacking a radial shaft at the border of the plexiform layer, they lengthen and acquire progressively a pyramidal or conical shape as they occupy deeper planes. All of them send into the plexiform layer a tuft of spiny dendritic ramifications that comes in contact with the nervous plexuses of the plexiform layer; to the white matter, they send a very long, thin axon which in the upper part of its course gives rise to collaterals distributing in the layer of medium and small pyramids. In the human cerebral cortex, these pyramidal cells seem to us to be much more numerous and smaller than in the cat and dog.

According to Schaffer, the initial collaterals of the small pyramids should have a recurrent course, and they should arborize in the molecular layer. We have also confirmed this disposition, which, incidentally, was already mentioned by Martinotti; however, it must be recognized that in man, as in the cat and dog, the vast majority of these recurrent collaterals ramify in the external portion of the layer of small pyramids, without assaulting the frontier of the plexiform layer. In our opinion, the so-called initial collaterals are almost always distributed in regions of cells congeneric to the element from which they arise, with the object of carrying to these part of the excitation received, so as to provoke discharges that increase the energy of the impulse and the number of [cellular] elements affected. About this point, we will have more to say later.

When the layer is examined with the method of Nissl, attention is drawn to the large crowd of contained cells, particularly at the frontier of the molecular layer, where it is not unusual to note a quite well-demarcated row of small elongated cell bodies. A careful examination with the 1.30 apochromatic [lens] reveals that in this limiting zone not all the elements are pyramidal; some adopt spindle,

ovoid, and even stellate shapes, which justifies to some extent the designation of a *layer of superficial polymorphic cells,* given by Schaffer[17] and Schlapp to this zone of transition. But the pyramidal cells predominate (or at least those that, with respect to the destination of the axon, behave as pyramids), and the cells of short axon, not being privileged residents of this territory (since they are present also, although in less abundance, in the subjacent layers), do not give us sufficient reason to divide the second layer into two layers with different names.

Among the small pyramids and diminutive ovoid, fusiform, or stellate cell bodies demonstrated by the Nissl method, there are also some thick, ovoid, semilunar, or polygonal elements, whose angles extend into robust, divergent dendrites (fig. 6, *D, C*) [*fig. 69*]. Such cells, few in number and scattered without order in the whole layer of small pyramids, correspond probably to giant cells with more or less vertical short axons (see below).

III. Layer of the Medium Pyramids

In this stratum, the Nissl method reveals cells similar to those in the preceding stratum: pyramidal cells, somewhat larger and more widely separated than those above, and the same large polygonal cells with divergent dendrites. The deeper plane of the layer of the medium pyramids, from time to time, contains pyramids of large size, almost giants, and appears, moreover, infiltrated with small cells, similar in aspect to the inhabitants of the fifth layer, or [layer] of small stellate elements.

[When] stained by the Golgi method, the pyramids of the layer we are studying show the well-known shape, orientation, and connections (fig. 3, *C*) [*fig. 66*]. The very long and downy radial [dendritic] shaft ascends up to the plexiform layer, where it extends its terminal tuft, while the axon descends to the white matter, not before giving rise in the first part of its trajectory to collaterals destined for the very same level of the third layer and the upper part of the fourth layer. As they cross the fifth, sixth, and subsequent layers, the descending axons aggregate in small bundles and

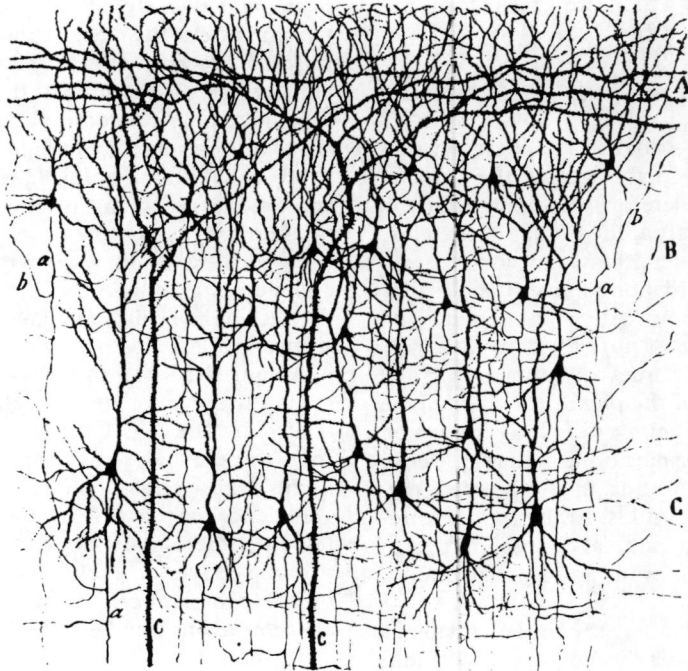

[*FIG. 66*] Fig. 3. Small and medium pyramids of the visual cortex of a child of twenty days (calcarine fissure). *A,* plexiform layer; *B,* layer of the small pyramids; *C,* layer of the medium pyramids; *a,* descending axon; *b,* recurrent collaterals; *c,* shafts of giant pyramids.

do not give off any collateral branches, an interesting circumstance which points to the relative independence of the upper pyramidal cells from the stellate cells of the fifth and sixth layers and from the deep or giant pyramids.

Short Axon Cells of the Layers of the Small and Medium Pyramids

We have seen that in the layers already mentioned the Nissl method reveals, besides pyramidal cell bodies, other cells, some of which are fusiform or stellate, while others are of large size, polygonal in shape, and with thick proximal processes. The Golgi method emphasizes the cells of small or medium size, among which we can so far count three different types: (a) fusiform or stellate, whose axon engenders a wide arborization; (b) very small cells with short axons ending in very tight proximal ramifications; (c) bitufted fusiform

cells, provided with an axonal arborization that devolves into little vertical bundles.

a. First Type

It inhabits the whole visual cortex, but it has a predilection for the layer of the small pyramids; some cells lie on the frontiers of the first layer, a place where they were already mentioned, although with reference to the cortex in general, by us and by Schaffer.

In fig. 4 [*fig. 67*], we show the principal cells of this type, stained in the visual region of a cat of twenty-five days. Notice that those situated at the external boundary of the layer of the small pyramids are minute and possess a spindle or pear shape (fig. 4, *a, b*) [*fig. 67*]; the ones lying somewhat deeper have a spindle, triangular, or stellate shape and have a slightly larger stature. In general, the dendrites run in all directions, but primarily in the radial direction; they are thin and varicose, ending at no great distance. The most numerous dendrites

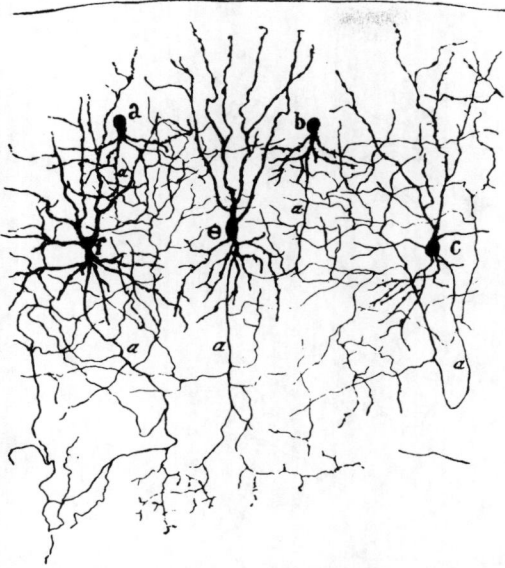

[FIG. 67] Fig. 4. Cells with short axon in the layer of the small pyramids of the visual cortex of a cat of twenty-eight days. *a, b,* piriform cells with short descending axon; *c,* cell with arched axon; *e, f,* cells with descending axon ramifying in the layer of the medium pyramids.

are the ascending, which often send a ramified tuft into the plexiform layer.

In man, these cells are also very numerous, although more difficult to stain than in the cat. In fig. 5 [*fig. 68*], we show the principal examples of this type impregnated in a child of fifteen to thirty days. There is no lack of the vertical fusiform type with minute soma, situated at the boundary of the plexiform layer (fig. 5, *G*) [*fig. 68*], but certain horizontally lying ovoid or triangular types are more abundant (fig. 5, *A, B*) [*fig. 68*]; they are provided with long polar dendrites from which arise ascending and descending branches. In the deep planes of the layer of the small and medium pyramids, the cells of short axon are somewhat larger, less abundant, and have a predominantly stellate shape.

All of these cells with short axon(s) are of small or medium size; but in the thickness of the second and third layers are also found, albeit rarely, certain large stellate cells provided with multiple, robust dendrites among which

those ascending and descending predominate. Such cells, whose size is at least twice as large as that of a small pyramid of the human cortex, correspond convincingly to the large stellate elements shown in these layers in Nissl preparations. A similar type is also found in the acoustic and motor cortex.

With respect to the course of the axon, all the aforementioned cells can be classified in three groups: first, cells whose axon runs horizontally, arborizing in territories situated in the same or a similar plane (fig. 5, *A, B, F*) [*fig. 68*]; second, cells whose axon arborizes indifferently, but always in the vicinity of the cell and at no great distance (fig. 5, *C, E*) [*fig. 68*]; third, cells whose axon ascends or descends, distributing in a different plane from that inhabited by the cell. Some of these axons can reach down to the depths of the layer of the medium pyramids, where they bifurcate and give off their last ramifications (fig. 4) [*fig. 67*]. Finally, no small number, as seen in figs. 5, *C*, and 6, *B* [*figs. 68, 69*], after a descending trajectory, trace an ascending arch to return and end in territories situated at the level of or above that occupied by the cell of origin. The axons of the giant stellate cells (fig. 6, *A, C*) [*fig. 69*] are robust, run vertically for a certain distance, and then resolve themselves into an arborization that is extremely extensive, [made up] of very long horizontal or oblique branches and related to a multitude of pyramids situated within its confines. Finally, there are cells, like those represented in fig. 6, *F* [*fig. 69*], whose axon, arched and ascending, resolves itself into an extremely complex arborization of relatively short branches.

b. Second Type

Throughout the thickness of the visual cortex, although in little abundance, there are minute cell bodies, provided with numerous radiated dendrites that are thin, tight, delicately varicose, and ending at no great distance from their origin. At first sight, these cells would be taken for neuroglial cells with short processes, but the absence of ramifying appendages on the dendrites and the presence of an axon promptly announce their nervous nature. The axon is very thin, and it resolves itself at a very short distance from its origin into a very tight

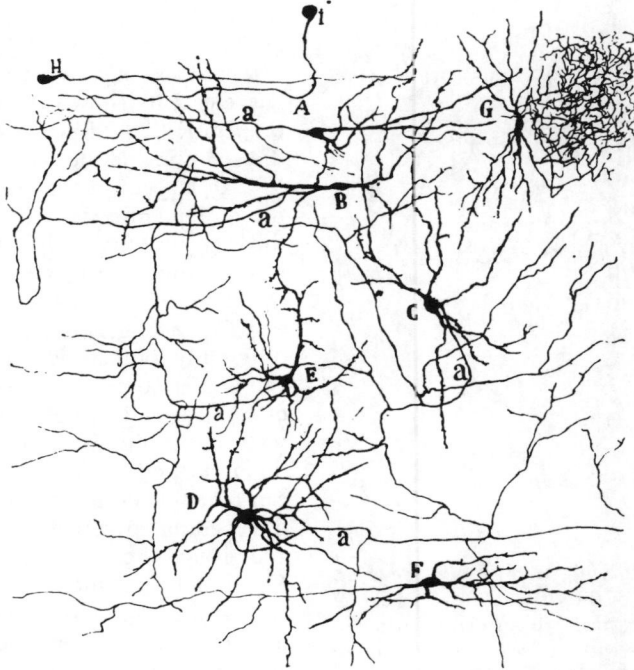

[*FIG. 68*]   Fig. 5. Cells with more or less horizontal short axons in the layers of the small and medium pyramids of the human visual cortex. Child of twenty days. *A, B,* cells with horizontal axon of the second layer; *C, E,* cells with axon ramifying in the second and third layers; *D, F,* cells with horizontal axon of the layer of the medium pyramids; *G,* small cell with very short axon arborizing among the small pyramids at the frontier of the first layer; *H, I,* piriform cells of the first layer.

arborization, whose delicate and varicose tiny branches demand, for a good examination, an apochromatic objective (fig. 7, *E*) [*fig. 70*]. On occasion, such tight arborizations are impregnated in isolation, that is, without the cell of origin, and this singularly facilitates their examination.

Possibly, the [axonal] arborizations of this class are certain very dense ramifications disposed in the form of small islands in the upper part of the layer of small pyramids. These ramifications, which we reproduce in fig. 7, *A, B, C* [*fig. 70*], enclose numerous hollows corresponding to a pleiad of minute pyramids. The extent of the ramification decreases from top to bottom, and on examining the preparation with good objectives (1.30 Zeiss), one observes that the whole arborization comes from two or three thin small branches (thinner than

in the arborization itself), which in turn originate from a vertical shaft that cannot be followed beyond the frontier of the medium pyramids. Although we have not been able to impregnate the cell of origin, judging by the form, fineness, and tightness of this arborization, we tend to regard it as the terminal nerve arborization of minute and fusiform cells with short axons that have not bound the silver chromate. Finally, we have found very tight arborizations of this same kind in the plexiform layer itself, and here sometimes the cell of origin appears (fig. 7, *E*) [*fig. 70*].

For the rest, the above-mentioned cells with short axon are also found in the cerebral cortex of the cat and dog, where they are somewhat larger and possess a less delicate axon.[18] In fig. 15, *E* [*fig. 78*], we reproduce one taken from the lower part of the layer of the medium

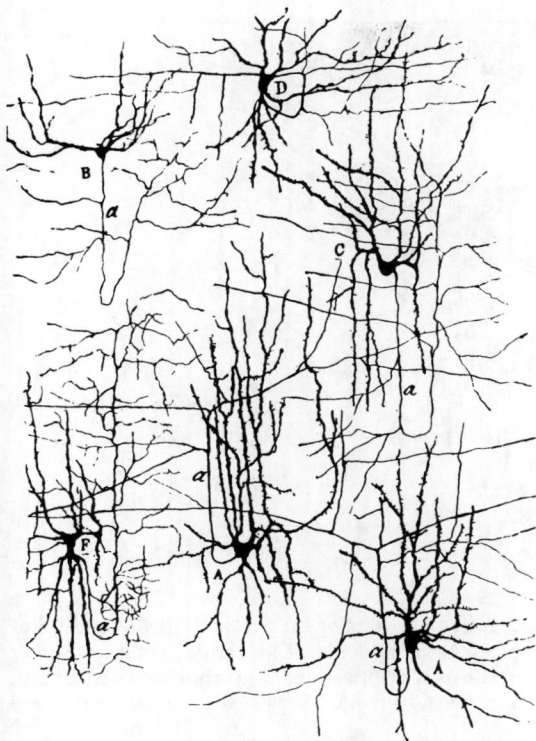

[*FIG. 69*] Fig. 6. Large cells with short ascending axons in the visual cortex of a child of fifteen days (second and third layers). *A,* large cells of the third layer, whose axon engenders very long horizontal or oblique branches; *C,* large cell with arciform axon; *D,* large cell at the border of the first layer; *B,* little cell with arciform axon in the layer of the small pyramids; *F,* medium-sized cell with thin ascending axon and complicated ramification.

pyramids. In fig. 13, *E* [*fig. 76*], we show two more that inhabited the layer of stellate cells in the brain of a child.

c. Third Type: Bitufted Fusiform Cell

Among the elements recently discovered by us in the human cortex are some small fusiform cells whose external and internal poles resolve themselves into a bundle of very thin varicose dendrites almost in parallel, with the descending ones, in particular, extending over a long distance. After the first and second branchings of these dendrites, they become so delicate that the silver chromate colors them a very

clear brown, so that in order to differentiate them from nerve fibers it is necessary to use the 1.30 Zeiss apochromatic objective. This is made even more necessary by the singular fact that in such cells the dendrites follow the same course and often occupy the same situation as the ramifications of the axon. There are some cells, however, whose dendrites are somewhat thicker and comparable to those originating from the cells with short axon.

Although the dominant type is bipolar, with a double tuft of dendrites, other forms are also found: triangular or stellate with not very long descending or ascending dendrites and one or two horizontal dendrites generally bifurcated at a short distance; and piriform, bearing only one tuft of ascending dendrites (fig. 11, *E*) [*fig. 74*].

But the more interesting peculiarity of this cellular species is the form of the axonal arborization. As we can see in fig. 8 [*fig. 71*], this axon is very delicate, and, arising from the soma or a dendrite, it follows an ascending or descending longitudinal course and resolves itself, generally at a large distance from the cell of origin, into a paintbrush of very thin longitudinal threads. During its long course, the axon gives off at right angles numerous collaterals that very quickly give rise also to parallel and sinuous bundles of yellowish varicose threads, ascending and descending over such a long distance that they can span almost the full thickness of the cortex. The axon is thin, and for its proper analysis the 1.30 Zeiss objective is absolutely essential. In the brain of the newborn or few-days-old child, these arborizations are still somewhat thick and not very extensive; to reveal them at their full development and to find out about the extreme delicacy of their threads, it is necessary to study them in the cortex of the child of twenty to thirty days. Fig. 8 [*fig. 71*] gives an incomplete idea of their delicacy, since the photozincographic procedure has significantly thickened the lines of the drawing.

Examining attentively each of the small [axonal] bundles, they are observed to enclose a vertical hollow which, judging by its size, seems to correspond to the shaft of a large or medium pyramid. And as each cell engenders

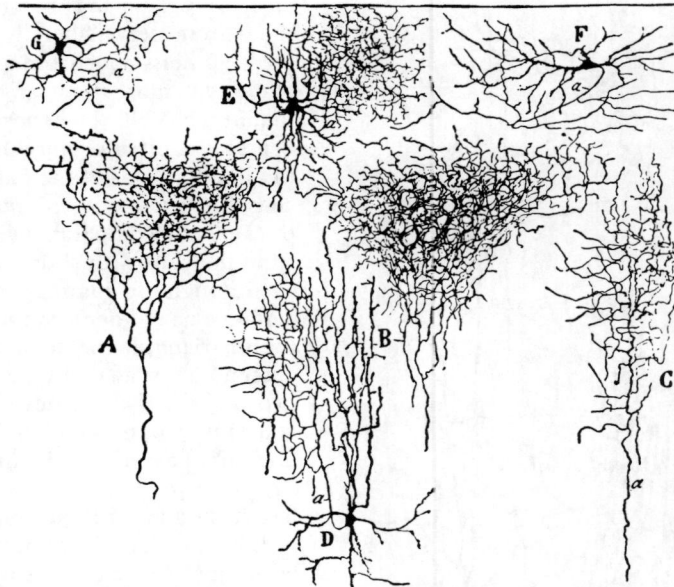

[*FIG. 70*]   Fig. 7. Fine nerve arborizations of the first and second layers of the visual cortex of a child of fifteen days. *A, B,* very dense nerve plexuses of the layer of the small pyramids; *C,* an arborization less dense; *D,* small cell with ascending axon resolving itself into an analogous arborization; *E,* arachniform stellate cell, whose axon generated a very dense plexus in the first layer; *F, G,* small cells with short, poorly arborized axons.

or can engender several bundles, it can be said that it could be related to several pyramids. Attending, then, to such singular connections, we said in our preliminary note about the visual cortex that such cells could fulfill the role of associating in the vertical direction pyramids resident in different layers.

The cells mentioned were first found by us in the acoustic cortex of the child of twenty-seven days; after that, we succeeded in impregnating them in the motor and visual cortex, and today we believe that they constitute an essential element of cortical structure. They inhabit all layers, but their preferred localization, if we can judge by the impregnations obtained so far, is the layer of small and medium pyramids. In some preparations of the motor and acoustic cortex, they are so abundant that the nervous arborizations or paintbrushes originating from some cells almost touch those formed by others, giving rise to a series of very long vertical fringes of a yellow color due to the unprecedented thinness of their constituent threads.

Recently, we have also found these cells in the visual cortex of the cat; but here they are deficient in small nerve branches, and these do not exhibit the extreme thinness and the enormous length of those of man (fig. 16, *d*)^A [*fig. 79*].

IV. Layer of the Large Stellate Cells

[This layer] is very characteristic of the visual cortex and easily recognized as much in Nissl as in Golgi preparations, because of the greater spaciousness of the intercellular plexuses (molecular substance) at its level and because of the large volume and lack of orientation of its cells, which, instead of affecting the radial direction characteristic of the pyramids, extend their dendrites in all directions, though horizontally for preference.

Even in Nissl preparations, the existence in

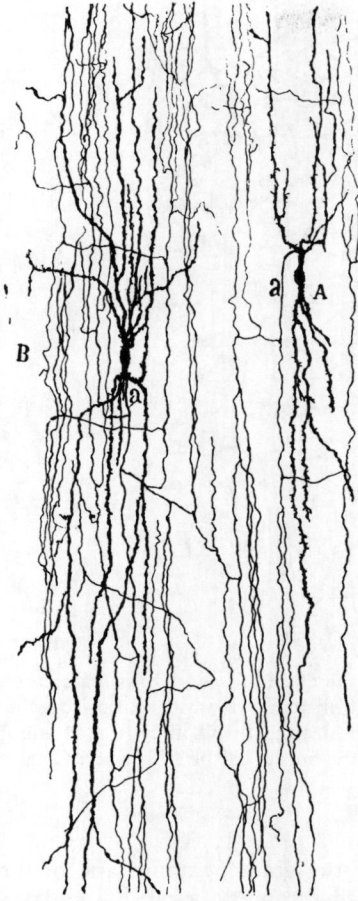

[FIG. 71]   Fig. 8. Small cells inhabiting several layers. Acoustic cortex of a child of twenty-seven days. A, cell with descending axon moderately ramified; B, cell with an axon that gives rise to many very long ascending and descending small bundles; a, axon.

this layer of two cellular types can be clearly revealed: large semilunar, triangular, or stellate elements, distributed irregularly and provided with a soma rich in reticulated protoplasm; and small ovoid or fusiform elements with dendrites preferentially ascending or descending. But the true morphology of all of these cells can only be fully appreciated in silver chromate preparations in which the following varieties can be clearly distinguished: first, giant or medium-sized stellate cell provided with a long descending axon; second, fu-

siform or ovoid cell with ascending short axon; third, some small stellate elements with short axon; fourth, medium or large displaced pyramid.

Giant Stellate Type

This constitutes the characteristic element and probably the most abundant of those that inhabit this layer (fig. 9, A) [fig. 72]. Its shape appears stellate if it is seen horizontally, but because of a certain flattening of the soma in vertical sections, it sometimes appears elongated and in the form of a spindle. There is no lack either of triangular, ovoid cells and even of mitral [cells], as can be seen in fig. 9, a, b [fig. 72].

Such cells occupy without order the various levels of the layer that we are studying, although it seems to us that they are found especially in the external part, where they are sometimes arranged in a discontinuous row.

The dendrites are robust, they run horizontally, they dichotomize several times, and they extend over a long distance. However, descending and even ascending dendrites are not rare, but in no case do the latter form a shaft that reaches the plexiform layer, an important negative feature by which, immediately, the stellate cell differs from the pyramid. In fig. 9 [fig. 72], we show the principal shapes of stellate cells in the cerebral cortex of the child of fifteen days. One observes the dominant spindle or semilunar shape of the soma and the horizontal direction of the dendrites. Comparing these cells with the ones of the adult brain, in which we have also obtained excellent impregnations (fig. 10) [fig. 73], one observes that the size has increased with age, with the most voluminous cells reaching almost twice the size. On the other hand, the orientation and position of the dendritic arborization is still maintained.

The axon is robust, arises from the inferior face of the soma or from the proximal part of a dendrite, and comes down almost in a straight line through the underlying layers, until it enters the white matter, where it is continued as a medullated nerve fiber. On its way through the layer we are studying, it gives

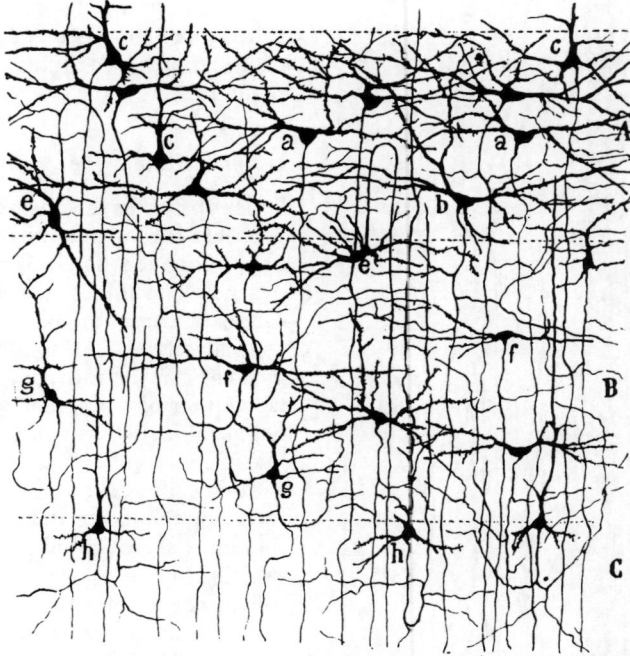

[*FIG. 72*] Fig. 9. Layers of stellate cells of the visual cortex of the child of twenty days (calcarine fissure). *A,* layer of large stellate cells; *a,* semilunar cells; *c,* cells with a thin radial dendrite; *b,* horizontal fusiform cell; *e,* cell with arched axon; *B,* layer of small stellate cells; *f,* horizontal fusiform cells; *g,* triangular cells with robust arched collaterals; *h,* pyramids with arched axon, at the border of the fifth layer; *C,* layer of the small pyramids with arched axon.

rise to a collateral ramifying among the cells of the same type; but the most robust and numerous collaterals arise during its passage through the layer of the small stellate cells in the interstices of which it engenders by successive branching a loose plexus, whose trabeculae have a mainly horizontal orientation and can be followed for a very long distance.

In some cells, the first collateral is so robust that it in fact represents the real continuation of the main axon, tracing an arch with an external concavity and ramifying in the external portion of the layer of the small stellate cells. Other cells exhibit two or more thick arciform and recurrent collaterals beyond which the primary axon becomes noticeably thinner; but in all cases, if the impregnation is complete, it is [still] possible to follow it as far as the white matter. It is not rare to see the axon give rise to some collaterals when it runs through the

layer of the giant pyramids and of the small cells with ascending axon; the collaterals are distributed in these regions or, what has seemed even more common to us, are directed in a recurrent direction up to the layer of the small stellate cells, where they arborize.

Finally, among the large stellate elements, there are some (fig. 9, *e*) [*fig. 72*], generally deeply situated, whose axon before going down goes up, tracing an arc within upper regions of the layer we are studying; here, it gives off several profusely ramifying collaterals.

Cells with Ascending Short Axons

They are quite numerous, located without order throughout the thickness of this layer. In man, as we show in fig. 11, *A, B, C* [*fig. 74*], the shape of these cells is ovoid, without a definite

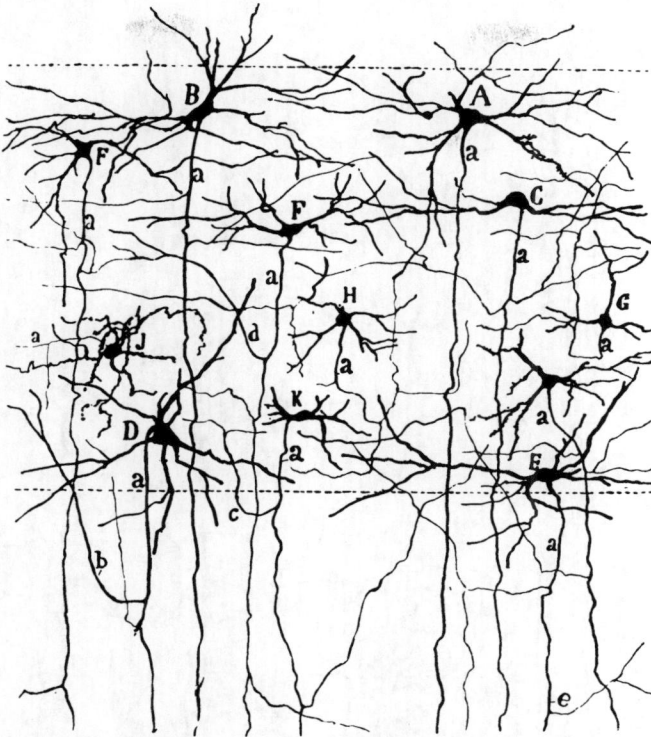

[FIG. 73] Fig. 10. Large stellate cells of the fourth and fifth layers. Adult cerebrum. *A, B, C, D,* giant stellate cells; *F, K,* medium stellate cells; *G, H, J,* small cells with short axon; *a,* axon; *b, d,* thick ascending collaterals; *e,* collateral to the lower layers.

orientation; the dendrites, thin, varicose, and with few spines, run in all directions, but generally without going beyond the layer in which the cell of origin is located. With regard to the axon, it usually arises from the upper part of the soma, goes almost in a straight line up to the external portion of the fourth layer, resolving into a wide terminal ramification whose mainly horizontal small branches contribute to the complexity of the nerve plexus located among the large stellate cells.

On the basis of the length of the axon, one may distinguish two varieties of this cell type: cells whose axon ramifies exclusively in the thickness of the layer of large stellate cells (fig. 11, *A*) [*fig. 74*]; and cells whose axon often gives rise to two or three collaterals to this stratum and then continues upward to reach the upper limit of the layer of the medium pyra-

mids or somewhat further, engendering an extensive terminal arborization (fig. 11, *B*) [*fig. 74*]. Lastly, in some cells of this class, one observes one or several collaterals that descend to the layer of the small stellate [cells]. In the cell of fig. 11, *C* [*fig. 74*], a collateral descended to near the lower limit of the latter layer, and it may have continued as a [myelinated] axon of the white matter.

Stellate Cells with Short Axon

The tiny stellate cell type with very short axon is here represented by some cells, not so delicate as those located in other layers, and characterized by the large number of their dendrites and by the bent and tangled aspect of these, something that reminds one of the dendrites of the cells of the bulbar olive. The very

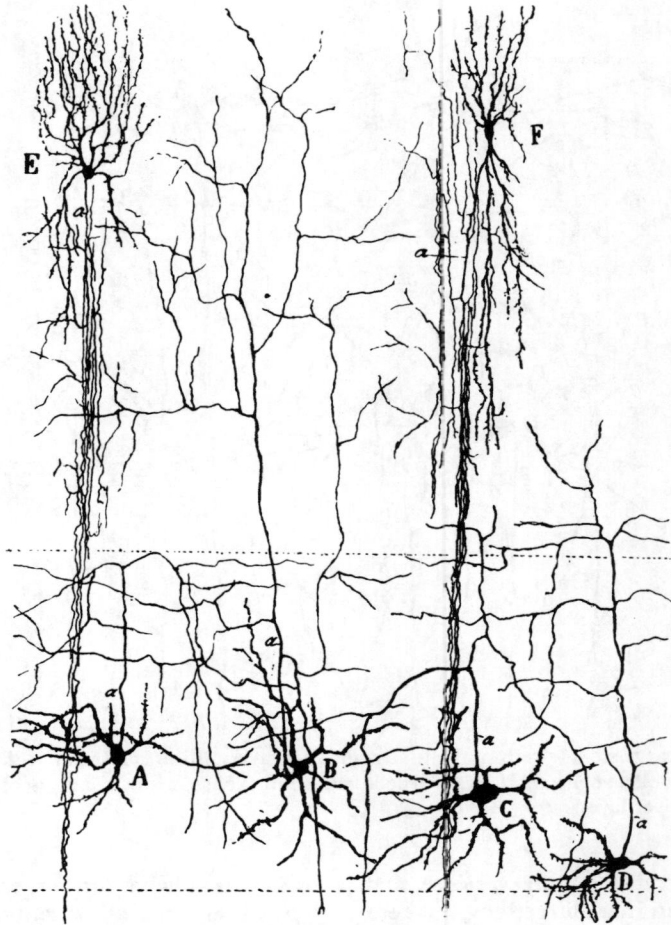

[*FIG. 74*]   Fig. 11. Cells of the visual cortex of a child of fifteen days (fourth layer). *A*, cell whose axon was distributed in the upper part of the fourth layer; *B*, cell whose axon spread into the fourth and third layers; *C*, cell that gave off nerve branches to the third, fourth, and fifth layers; *D*, cell whose ascending axon arborized in the fourth layer and at the border of the third; *E*, *F*, bitufted, minute cells of the layer of the medium pyramids; *a*, axon.

thin axon very close to its origin resolves itself into a tight terminal arborization of short extent.

Medium Pyramids

In some parts of the visual cortex, and particularly in the external portion of the layer we are studying, an occasional displaced pyramidal cell can be observed; its radial shaft is generally thin in comparison with that of homonymous cells and goes up to the molecular layer; the basilar dendrites run more or less horizontally, and the axon often gives off an occasional collateral to the subjacent layers before it disappears into the white matter (fig. 9, *C*) [*fig. 72*].

V. Layer of the Small Stellate Cells

This layer, equivalent to the layer of grains of others, in Nissl preparations is made up of a multitude of small, tightly packed nuclei, commonly arranged in pleiades or irregular small vertical islands separated by radial bundles of nerve fibers and by the dendritic shafts of underlying cells. The protoplasmic halo that surrounds such nuclei is thin and hardly perceptible; there is no lack, however, of cells provided with more abundant cytoplasm, which, because of their size and stellate shape, can be compared with the cells of medium size in the preceding stratum.

With the advantage of the Golgi method, one is easily persuaded that the grains of the authors are definite nerve cells, although belonging to different morphological types, among which we will mention the stellate cell with long descending axon, the stellate cell with ascending short axon, and the tiny arachniform cell with short and very thin axon.

Stellate Cells with Long Axon

These form the majority of the elements resident in the fifth layer, and they are noticeably similar to those located in the fourth, but differ from them in being of much smaller size and by the thinness and lack of ramifications of their dendrites. There are found, nevertheless, from time to time, cells almost as large as those of the preceding layer, as one can see in fig. 10 [fig. 73], taken from the adult human cortex.

Among the medium and small cells, the most common form is polygonal or ovoid, with three, four, or more thin, divergent dendrites ramifying within the same layer and ending at no great distance. The largest cells frequently exhibit a spindle or semilunar shape and long robust dendrites, preferentially extended in a horizontal direction (fig. 9, f) [fig. 72].

The axon essentially appears as the stellate cells of the preceding layer; it arises from the deeper part of the soma or from a dendrite, goes down, commonly becoming noticeably thinner as it reaches the sixth layer, and finally invades the white matter in which it continues as a thin or medium myelinated fiber. It is not rare to see the axon first ascend and then later go down, tracing an arc above the cell.

The collaterals generated in the initial course of the axon number three, four, or more, and are so robust that they could be considered in many cases the true termination of the functional axon. Some of them, given off at the level of the sixth layer, after that go backward to describe an arc up to the fifth, where they distribute; others that come off from the initial trajectory of the axon ascend near the fourth layer, [or layer] of the large stellate cells. All of these fibers ramify in a complicated manner in the thickness of the layer under study, engendering a complicated plexus, whose trabeculae run preferentially in the horizontal direction.

[Considering] the totality of the small, medium, and large stellate cells, have they the same behavior, [namely that of] sending the axon to the white matter?

In the adult visual cortex, it is confirmed, in fact, that the axons of the immense majority of these stellate cells, even those of medium size, after having formed a complicated collateral arborization, provide a more or less thin branch to the white matter; but one must confess that in the smaller cells of the visual cortex of infants of five, fifteen, and twenty days, demonstration of this is not always possible. As can be seen in fig. 12, a, b, c [fig. 75], there are minute stellate cells, whose very thin axons descend or ascend in the fifth layer; at a short distance, the axon bifurcates, and its branches successively become divided and scattered in diverse planes of this layer; they seem to end freely without sending any branches beyond the frontiers of the layer (fig. 12) [fig. 75]. In view of these data, one could suppose that one is dealing here with cells of short axon, characterized by the poverty, smoothness, and thinness of their dendrites; but it is impossible to discard a potential source of error when one works in a layer with a structure as thin and labyrinthine as that of the small stellate cells; one could, in effect, suppose that, given the thinness of the ultimate trunk of the axon, in comparison with the robustness of the initial collaterals, there has been a defect of impregnation or of development of the axon so that it presents itself to us as the only nerve arborization. [This is a] mistake all the more easy to commit, considering that in several small stellate cells, the final trunk of the axon does not always go down in a straight line but ascends

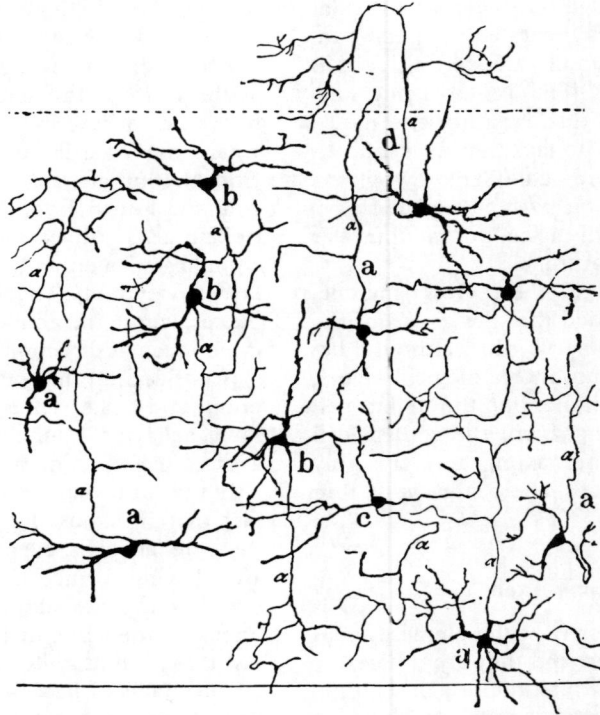

[*FIG. 75*]   Fig. 12. Small cells with short, moderately arborized axons in the layer of the small stellate cells. *a*, cells with thin ascending axon; *b*, *c*, cells with descending axon; *d*, cell somewhat larger, whose axon was distributed in the fourth layer; *a*, axon.

or runs more or less obliquely, tracing large bends that make it difficult to follow; [this is a] difficulty that become greater when, as frequently occurs, the plexus of small nerve fibers of the fifth layer is well impregnated. In any case, with the critical reservations necessary in so difficult a subject, we feel inclined to estimate that, if not all, [then] the majority of the minute elements represented in fig. 12, *a*, *b*, *c* [*fig. 75*] are cells with short axons, oriented in many diverse ways, and which, by contrast with the cells we are going to describe, do not leave the thickness of the fifth layer. Such cells could [thus] be classified as *cells with short axon, poor in dendrites*.

Cells with Ascending Axon

In this manner, we designate certain cells [that are] fusiform in the cat and dog but ovoid or stellate in man, whose axon, originating from the upper part of the soma, goes vertically upward to the layer of the large stellate cells, where it ends in a loose, horizontal arborization of large extent (fig. 13, *A*, *B*) [*fig. 76*].

In its ascending course, this process also provides collaterals to the layer under study. In some cases, as shown in fig. 13, *B* [*fig. 76*], the axon, after ascending to the fourth layer, descends to be distributed in the fifth, not before having given off in its arciform trajectory numerous collaterals to the layer of the large stellate cells. Finally, in a few cells, the terminal arborization to the fourth layer can give off small ascending branches distributed among the medium pyramids (fig. 13, *C*) [*fig. 76*]. In short, considering the collaterals and terminals of the axon as a whole, these cells may be considered as a variety of cells of short axon, destined to bring impulses preferentially to the fourth and fifth strata.

For the rest, the dendrites of these cells are

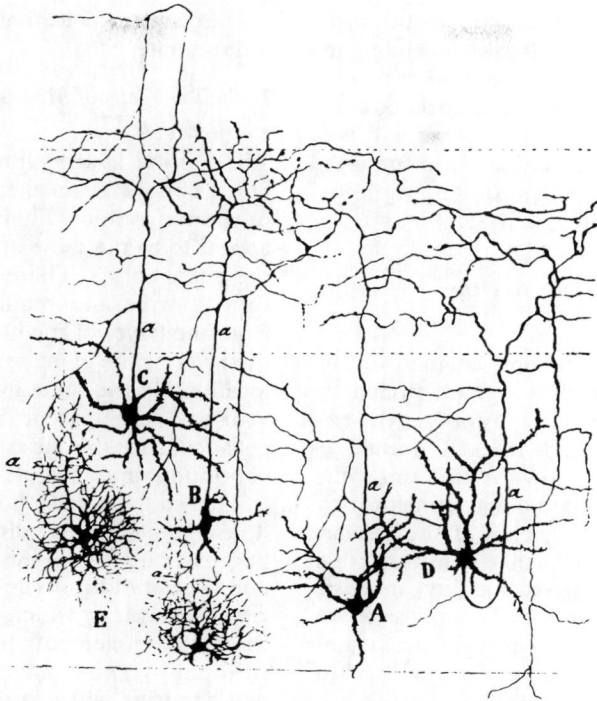

[*FIG. 76*]   Fig. 13. Cells with ascending axon of the fifth layer of the visual cortex. Child of fifteen days. *A, B,* cells whose axon is distributed in the layer of the large stellate cells; *C,* cell whose axon gave further branches to the layer of the medium pyramids; *D,* cell whose axon, which was arciform in its initial portion, gave branches to the fourth, fifth, and even sixth layers; *E,* very small cells with short ascending axon; *a* indicates the axon.

not numerous, run in all directions, although preferably in an ascending direction, and, as with the soma, present the peculiarity of exhibiting abundant spines or downiness. This downy appearance distinguishes them immediately from the medium or small stellate cells, whose somata and dendrites are smooth or almost smooth.

Stellate Cells with Short Axon

These can be recognized [to form] two morphological types: first, cells of medium size, provided with numerous, divergent varicose dendrites and with a thin ascending, descending, or horizontal axon, loosely ramified in the thickness of the fifth layer (fig. 10, *f*) [*fig. 73*]; and second, very minute arachniform cells, so exiguous that only the 1.30 Zeiss objective can show us clearly the character of their pro-

cesses. In fig. 13, *E* [*fig. 76*], we reproduce two cells of this latter class taken from the visual [cortex] of a child of fifteen days. Notice the extraordinary thinness and the considerable abundance of the dendrites, whose branches appear replete with very small, thin grains, and which engender a very tight plexus, marked by clear hollows that correspond to included cell [somata]. With respect to the axon, it is of unparalleled delicacy, runs in an ascending direction, and forms, at no great distance, a very complicated arborization, disposed around a pleiad of stellate cell [bodies]. The arachniform cells lie in the whole thickness of the fifth layer, and they are rather abundant, as judged by our later impregnations in the brain of the child. In summary, the fifth layer shelters an enormous number of [cellular] elements with short axon (type with thick varicose expansions, type with thin and scarce dendrites indicated above, arachniform type, thick stellate type with axon ascending to the fourth layer), thanks to which there should be established a vast system of connections between the optic fibers, which, as we will see later, are distributed preferentially in the fifth layer, and the stellate cells with long axon inhabiting this and the fourth [layers].

Layer of the Stellate Cells in Other Gyrencephalic Mammals

The excellent impregnations obtained in the brains of young cats and dogs (of fifteen to thirty days) have allowed us to confirm the existence of a very extensive layer of granule or stellate cells situated below the medium pyramids, but in which we could not define the two strata of large and small cells of the human cortex; the diverse cells that constitute this layer show up with mixed [quality] in Nissl and in Golgi stains, [and it is] only possible to affirm that the large stellate cells are somewhat more numerous in the external half to two-thirds of the layer.

Here are the cells that we have been able to differentiate.

1. Stellate Cells of Medium to Large Size (fig. 14, a, b) [fig. 77]

They reside in the whole layer under study, but are more abundant in the vicinity of the medium pyramids. Their distribution does not appear to be the same in the diverse regions of the visual cortex. There are places where they form a wide and regular stratum that goes from the [layer of medium pyramids] as far as the layer of the giant pyramids; while in other locations of the same gyrus, the pyramids invade to a large extent the field of the stellate cells, causing the latter to be reduced to discontinuous and irregular clusters.

The stellate cells possess numerous long downy dendrites, which run in all directions, but particularly in the horizontal direction, but the ramifications do not go beyond the territory or layer in which they reside. However, the frontier elements [near the layer of] the medium pyramids sometimes bear a thick radial dendrite, whose branches may invade the

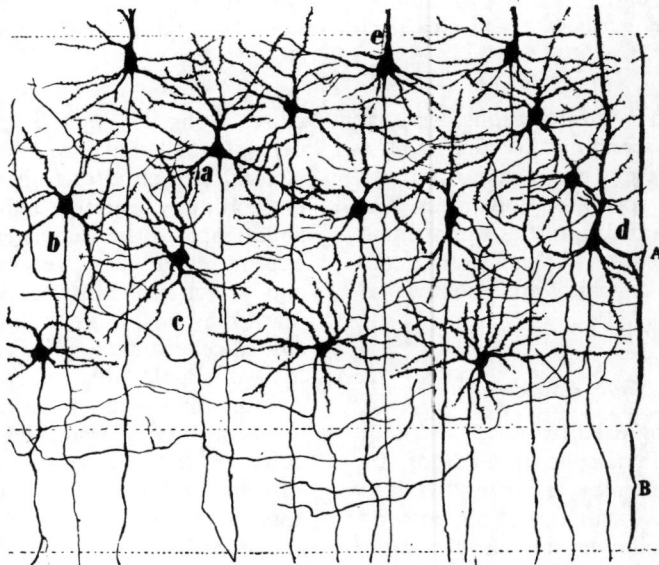

[FIG. 77] Fig. 14. Stellate cells of the visual region of a cat of twenty-eight days. A, layer of the stellate cells (fourth and fifth layers in man); B, layer of the giant pyramids; a, b, c, stellate cells with long descending axon; d, e, medium pyramids intermingled with stellate cells.

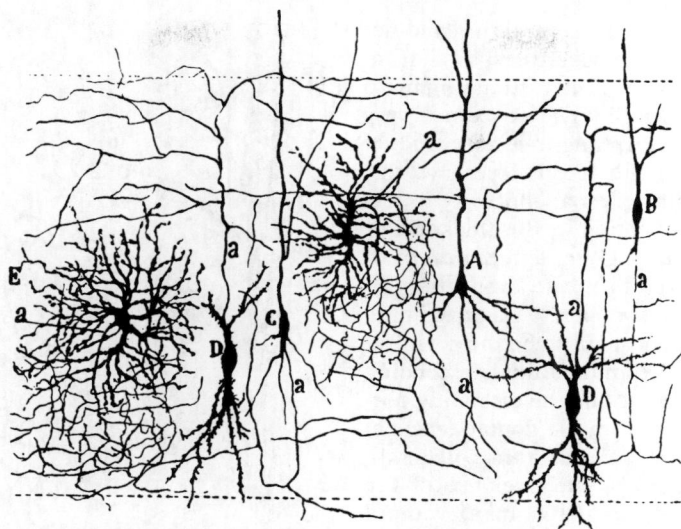

[*FIG. 78*]   Fig. 15. Diverse cellular elements taken from the layer of the stellate cells of the visual cortex of the cat of twenty-eight days. *A, B, C*, small pyramids and fusiform cells with arched ascending axon; *D*, thick fusiform cells with ascending axon; *E*, arachniform cells with short axon; *a*, axon.

overlying layer. This external dendrite soon bifurcates and does not appear to reach the plexiform layer; it represents, judging by all appearances, the atrophied radial shaft of a pyramid.

The axon is robust, descends almost vertically across the underlying layers, and enters the white matter. During its initial trajectory, it gives off three or four horizontal or ascending collaterals exclusively arborized in the layer under study.

In some cases, the fact pointed out above can be verified, [namely] that the initial collaterals are so thick that they represent the principal termination of the functional axon (fig. 14, *b, c*) [*fig. 77*].

2. Large Fusiform Cell with Ascending Axon (fig. 15, D) [*fig. 78*]

It is a vertically elongated cell [which is] quite abundant, and from whose poles arise two dendritic tufts, ascending and descending. All of these dendrites, as well as the soma, are covered with spines, like the homologous elements in man (cells with ascending axon of the layer of the small stellate cells).

With respect to the axon, it is quite thick, arises from the soma or from an ascending dendrite, goes up at once to the upper part of the layer under study, and resolves itself into a wide arborization, whose major branches are very long and horizontal and contact the stellate cells at many points.

3. Fusiform Cell or Small Pyramid with Short Axon

These reside [throughout] the whole layer of stellate cells, but prefer the inferior part of the layer where they appear predominant. Their small size and their abundance give to the fourth layer of the cortex of the cat and dog stained with the common methods its predominant appearance of granularity, as already noticed by the authors. In fig. 15, *A, B, C* [*fig. 78*], we reproduce the most typical elements of this class taken from the cerebrum of a cat of twenty-eight days. As one can see at [*B* and *C*][B] in fig. 15 [*fig. 78*], some can have a bipolar shape with a long external process, and a shorter, rapidly dividing basilar dendrite, from which the axon arises; but the majority of these cells possess the form of small pyramids, from whose base emanate several thin and not very long descending dendrites and from whose apex arises a thin shaft extending up to the first or plexiform layer. The axon is very thin, has a brief descending trajectory, and, at different depths in the fourth layer, returns, tracing an arc with external concavity to terminate in an arborization in the thickness of the layer under study. Other axons, instead of describing the arc, bifurcate, and the two branches more or less return to arborize in the same way. This seems to us to be the most frequent disposition. From the initial descending trajectory, from the arc and the ascending portion of the axon, or from the double terminal branch are born several very thin collaterals; these are distributed in the thickness of the fourth layer (fourth and fifth of man), without going beyond their superficial borders.

The more deeply located cells possess shorter axons than the others, and their extremely long collaterals and terminals run horizontally in the layer of the giant pyramids, with which they must maintain an intimate relationship.

4. Stellate Cells with Extensively Arborized Short Axons

Some stellate cells of medium size resident in the deeper third of the layer under study possess a descending axon that appears to be distributed in the thickness of the layer without extending to the white matter (fig. 16, a) [fig. 79].

5. Arachniform Cells with Very Short Axon

They are similar to the homonymous cells of the human cortex, differing from them only in having somewhat thicker and more strongly varicose dendrites. The axon decomposes rapidly into an arborization distributed in the different tiers of the layer of the stellate cells (fig. 16, b) [fig. 79].

6. Medium or Large Pyramids of Common Type

Usually, there is no lack, even in the better-differentiated visual areas of some cells of this class, irregularly distributed between the stellate cells, and well recognizable because of the length of the radial shaft and the direction and

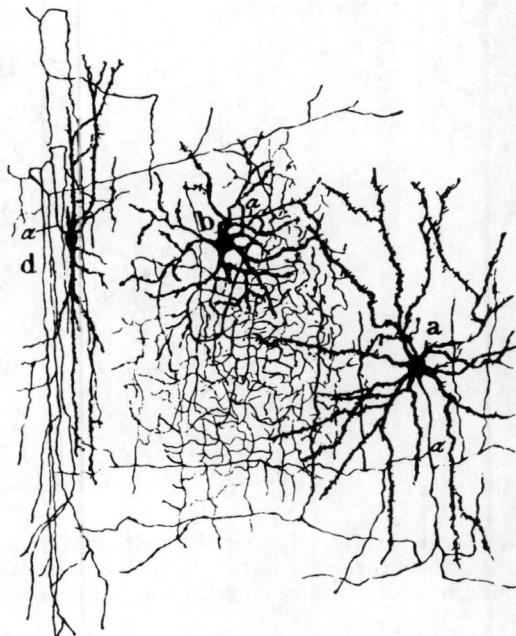

[FIG. 79] Fig. 16. Cells with short axon of the layer of the stellate cells of the visual cortex of a cat of twenty-eight days. a, large stellate cell with descending axon ramified in the deeper portion of the fourth layer (fourth and fifth layers of man); b, minute arachniform cell with tightly ramified axon; d, fusiform cell with axon ramified in tufts of threads.

destination of the axon. Their presence and the great facility with which they can be impregnated attract the attention, making it difficult in certain cases to determine the position and limits of the fourth layer, particularly when, as occurs quite frequently, the above-mentioned stellate cells do not retain the silver chromate. The pyramidal cells are very abundant in the external face of the pole of the occipital lobe; for that reason, one must always choose for the study of the visual cortex the internal face of this lobe, where the layer of the stellate cells reaches its maximum differentiation.

VI. Layer of the Small Pyramids with Ascending Axon

Below the stratum of the small stellate cells, the Nissl method reveals the existence of a

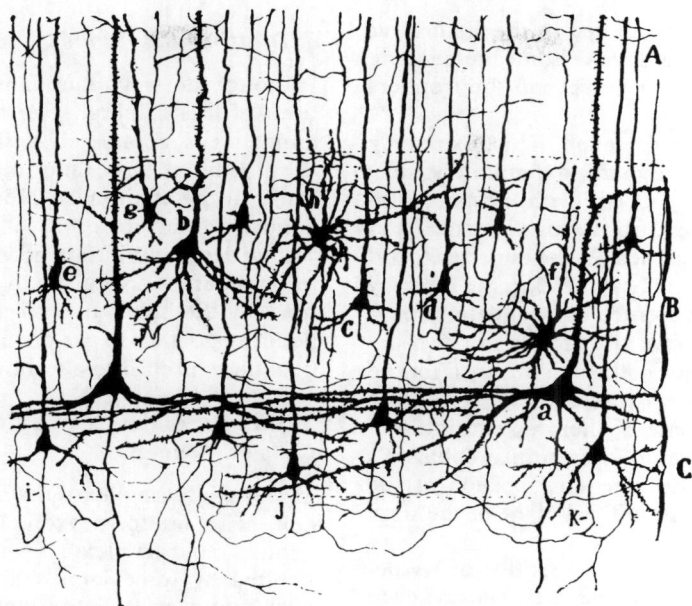

[*FIG. 80*]   Fig. 17. Cellular elements of the sixth and seventh layers of the human visual cortex (child of fifteen days). *A*, fifth layer; *B*, sixth layer; *C*, seventh layer; *a*, giant pyramid; *b*, medium pyramid with long descending axon; *c*, small pyramid with ascending arched axon; *d*, pyramid whose axon engenders two arches; *e*, pyramid whose axon forms several arched ascending fibers; *h, f, g*, stellate cells with ascending axons ramifying in the fifth and sixth layers; *i, j, k*, pyramidal cells with ascending arched axon ramifying in the seventh and eighth layers.

band with a plexiform appearance not very rich in [cellular] elements, [and these] become even more scarce in proximity to the row of giant pyramids. Although the deep border of the sixth layer is not easy to delimit, since it is masked by a smooth transition to the giant pyramids, the small volume and the special morphology of the cells that inhabit [the layer] permit its separate identification.

As we show in fig. 17, *B* [*fig. 80*], these [cellular] elements are of three kinds: first, pyramidal or ovoid cells with arched axon; second, large stellate cells with ascending axon; third, medium or large pyramidal cells of the common type.

1. Small Pyramidal or Ovoid Cells with Arched and Ascending Axon

They constitute the more numerous cells of this layer, and it is due to them that an ap-

pearance of disseminated small granules shows up in Nissl preparations.

Such cells have an exiguous size and a shape comparable to that of the small pyramids, although spindle and ovoid shapes are not rare; they can be recognized as superficial or frontier cells and as deep cells.

The superficial ones (fig. 19, *c*)[c] [*fig. 82*] constitute a discontinuous row set at the inferior border of the layer of the small stellate cells, and they are overall the more voluminous (there are exceptions) and the ones that reproduce better the pyramidal form. The ones located in the other planes of the sixth layer, although often showing the pyramidal type, also have ovoid or fusiform shapes.

All of these superficial and deep [cellular] elements possess the same properties: their size is minute; from the external part of the soma arises a radial [dendritic] shaft extending up to the first layer and from which short collateral branches distributed in the sixth layer arise; from the base arise some descending dendrites that do not go beyond the frontiers of this layer.

With respect to the axon, [it is] extremely thin and first descends for a certain distance; after that, it traces an arc with concavity uppermost and goes up across the fifth and fourth layers, to get lost in the superficial layers of the cortex, where the extreme delicacy of the fiber has prevented us from determining its destination. From the arc, one or two descending or oblique collaterals destined for the sixth layer arise; [these are] repeatedly branched, and some of them extend into the interior of the seventh layer; similar collaterals engendered by the ascending portion of the arc ramify in the superficial plane of the sixth layer.

On occasions, the axon divides in its descending trajectory, engendering two and even three arciform branches (fig. 17, *d*) [*fig. 80*], from which arise thin collaterals to the sixth layer; such branches seem to behave as the undivided axon of the congeneric cells; that is to say, they go up through the overlying layers, becoming lost, perhaps in the plexiform or first layer.

2. Stellate Cells with Ascending Axon

Though less abundant than the preceding cells, there is no lack of these cells in the sixth layer, in which they occupy all levels. One recognizes two types: first, small or medium stellate cell, provided with numerous divergent dendrites, extending in the sixth and seventh layers (fig. 17, *f, g, h*) [*fig. 80*]; the axon which arises from the upper part of the soma ascends to ramify and terminate in the layer of the small stellate cells, not before providing some collaterals to the sixth layer; and second, robust stellate cells, scarce in number, moderate in dendrites, whose larger axon traverses the superimposed layers to reach the first, where it arborizes and terminates. In some cases, this axon has seemed to us bereft of collaterals; but in others, when [the axon] passed the fifth and sixth layers, it gave off collaterals distributed in these and providing them [up] to the level of the medium and small pyramids.

3. Legitimate Pyramids

Although not very abundant, good impregnations of this cerebral layer always reveal pyramidal cells, completely analogous to those of the medium type, and distributed without order in the sixth layer. Nor is the giant pyramidal cell lacking.

The descending axon goes to the white matter, not before giving rise to collaterals distributed in the seventh layer; the robust radial dendrite goes up to the plexiform layer, where it resolves itself into a terminal tuft.

VII. Layer of the Giant Pyramids (Solitary Cells of Meynert)

Underneath the plexus that contains the small cells with arciform axon, Nissl preparations show a band or plexus of no great width, inhabited by some large cells with triangular, oval, and even stellate shape, and whose very abundant protoplasm exhibits very clear [Nissl bodies].

The placement of these giant cells shows great irregularity; in fact, they can occupy all the planes of the seventh layer and even the lower part of the sixth. However, in the majority of cases, their residence is at the upper border of the layer under study, forming there a row, not always clearly visible in Nissl preparations because of the distance, sometimes considerable, that separates the cell somata; but [the row is] clearly perceptible in Golgi preparations.

Golgi preparations establish much better the limits and characteristics of the seventh layer. Of course, they reveal that the giant cells are somewhat modified voluminous pyramids and that the more or less well-defined plexus in which they reside results from the transverse interlacing of their very long, basal dendrites (fig. 17) [*fig. 80*].

This plexus of long horizontal dendrites, thanks to which very [widely] separated giant cells are joined through the cortex, constitutes one of the characteristics of the visual cortex and an excellent reference point for determining in Golgi preparations the position of the layers and bordering cells. Generally, the lateral, concave portions of the visual gyri exhibit only a [single] row of giant cells, and therefore only one plexiform band; but at the level of the convex portions, the giant pyramids lose in thickness what they gain in length, and are arranged in two, three, or more irregular rows, proportionately thickening the [dendritic] plexus that links them. Furthermore, there is no lack of irregularities of situation and shape of the plexus, [these] being often noticeable with changes of plane in the same cortical territory, especially at the transition of the convexity to the flat and concave portions of the gyri.

For each pyramidal cell, [we] have to consider three things: the radial dendrite, the basilar dendrites, and the axon.

The radial dendrite is proportionately thinner than that of the giant pyramids of other regions of the cortex; it goes toward the surface (sometimes after an arched bend); it provides branches to the sixth layer, crosses without branching the layers of the stellate cells and pyramids, and lastly reaches the first or plexiform layer, where it generates an extensive and robust tuft. The branches of this tuft are outlined against those that belong to the medium and small pyramids because of their thickness, and they commonly occupy the lower part of the first layer, running horizontally over very long distances (fig. 3, c) [fig. 66].

The basilar dendrites are thick and very nu-

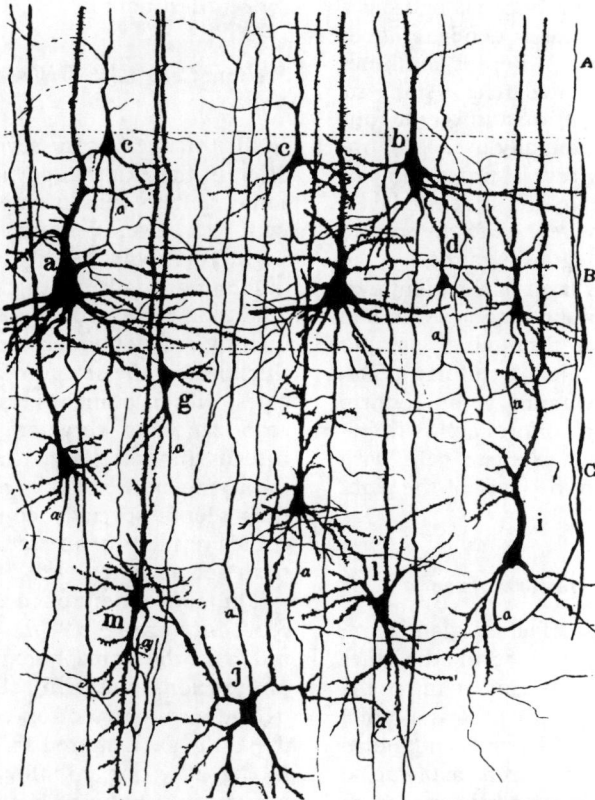

[FIG. 81] Fig. 18. Deep layers of the visual cortex of a cat of twenty days. A, lower portion of the layer of the stellate cells; B, layer of giant pyramids; C, layer of medium pyramids with arched axon; a, giant pyramids; b, medium pyramid with descending axon; c, d, pyramids with descending axon bifurcating and ramifying in the layer of the giant cells; g, triangular cell with arched axon and descending collateral; i, pyramid with arched ascending axon; l, triangular cell with descending axon; m, fusiform cell with descending axon; l, j, cells of the layer of the fusiform cells, one stellate with ascending axon, the other triangular with descending axon; a, axon.

merous. In some pyramids, they reach a greater thickness than the [apical dendrite] itself. Such robust processes present an interesting peculiarity that allows us to distinguish them, even on very superficial examination, from the homonymous ones at any other location in the cortex; their course is almost exclusively horizontal, creating at the level of the giant cells parallel bundles of dendrites, which are so long that they frequently exceed three-tenths of a millimeter. It has seemed to us that basilar appendages even longer than the apical shaft may exist. Such horizontal dendrites are rough and downy, repeatedly branched, and, with slight variations, keep to their initial plane.

The axon, arising from the soma or from a somewhat descending basal dendrite, goes down to the white matter, where it continues as a voluminous myelinated fiber. Along its course in the eighth layer arise three or four collaterals that run horizontally over long trajectories, dichotomizing several times; some of these branches ascend to the seventh layer, where they appear to be related to the somata and dendrites of homologous pyramids.

The seventh layer, or layer of the giant pyramids, usually also contains other pyramidal cells of the same kind, although of smaller stature, and three additional cellular types, namely, first, small pyramids with arciform axon; second, stellate or fusiform cells with ascending axon; and third, stellate cells with short axon arborizing in the layer of the giant pyramids.

Small Pyramids with Arciform Axon

They inhabit the whole layer of giant pyramids, and they exhibit the shape and the other properties of the cells of the same name in the sixth layer; that is to say, they possess a radial dendrite prolonged up to the first layer, and an arched descending and recurrent axon up to the fifth layer or perhaps even higher. As one saw in fig. 17, *J, K* [*fig. 80*], instead of one, they can form two arches with two ascending fibers, from whose lower parts arise collaterals ramifying in the thickness of the seventh and eighth layers. Certain axons resolve themselves into a still larger number of branches,

some ascending and others descending; but we have not been able to follow any of them down to the white matter. Anyway, the majority of the axonal arborizations of these small pyramids appear to be destined to make contact with the large pyramids of the seventh layer.

Stellate Cells with Ascending Axon

Few in number and of medium size, these elements possess divergent dendrites installed in the seventh layer and an ascending axon that crosses the sixth layer, to which it supplies collaterals, and it extends, perhaps up to the first or plexiform layer. The enormous distance traveled has not allowed us to determine *de visu* its destination.

Stellate Cells with Diffusely Ramified Short Axon

In the thickness of the seventh layer, and more often in the external portion of the eighth, lie some stellate cells of medium size provided with four, five, or more long divergent, only slightly downy, varicose, and repeatedly branching dendrites (fig. 19, *A, B*) [*fig. 82*]. The axon can ascend or descend, but more frequently runs obliquely or horizontally in the thickness of the seventh layer, where it bifurcates, with its branches resolving into terminal arborization of very long, mostly horizontal threads that trace large turns and terminate by ramifying between the giant cells, to which they seem especially consigned. In no case could we identify an ascending branch to the sixth and seventh layers.

The above-mentioned elements, which we reproduce in fig. 19 [*fig. 82*], are similar, as much for their morphology as for the behavior of the axon, to certain cells recently found by us in the motor cortex of the child. But in these, the axon offered an interesting peculiarity (fig. 20, *a*) [*fig. 83*]: the terminal [axonal] arborization, composed of very long horizontal or oblique branches, engendered at intervals nests of delicate and tortuous threads, situated around the pyramids or stellate cells, whose soma they outlined perfectly. On occasions, such little pericellular plexuses run onto the dendrites, marking with precision the direc-

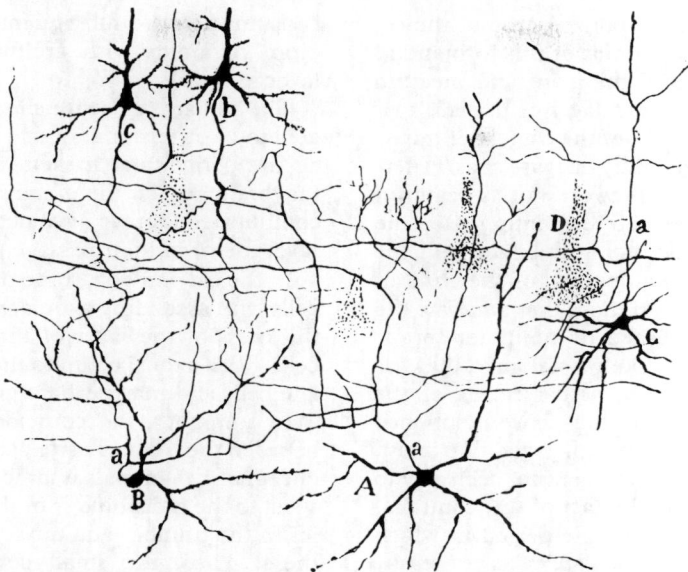

[*FIG. 82*] Fig. 19. *A, B*, stellate cells with ascending axon distributed in the layer of the large pyramids; *C*, cells with long ascending, ramified axon; *D*, pyramid of the seventh layer; *a*, axon; *c, b*, axons of small pyramidal cells of the sixth layer (child of twenty days). (Visual cortex.)

tion and the contour of the initial portions of these. One can see, then, that the cerebral cortex also contains pericellular baskets comparable to the ones discovered by us on the Purkinje cells of the cerebellum, red nucleus, and nucleus of Deiters,[19] similar to the ones iden-

tified by Held in the nucleus of the trapezoid body[20] and to the ones described by Lavilla in the heart of the superior accessory olive.[21] Similar cells exist also, according to our findings,[22] beneath the layer of the large pyramids in the inferior portion of Ammon's horn (stel-

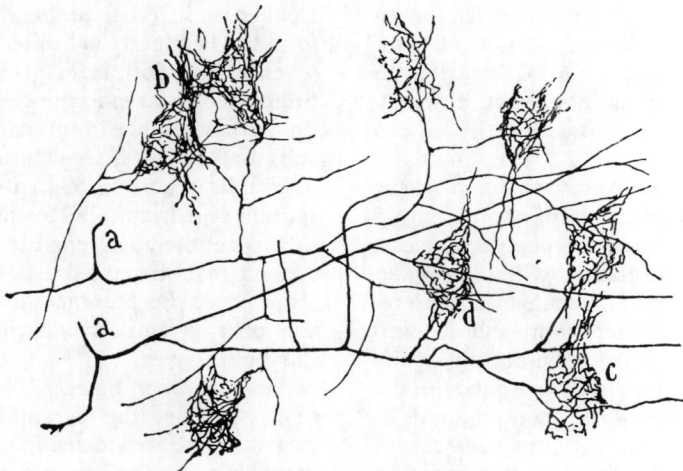

[*FIG. 83*] Fig. 20. Pericellular arborizations of the layer of the medium and deep giant pyramids of the motor cortex of a child of twenty-five days. *a*, axons dividing in long horizontal branches; *b, c, d*, pericellular baskets.

late cells with axon arborized around the somata of the large pyramids of this formation).

Now then, around the giant and medium pyramids of the seventh layer of the adult visual cortex of man and of the cat (cat of thirty-four days), [there] exist, likewise, basket terminations, although they are not as beautiful and dense as those before mentioned in the motor [cortex]. Associating this fact with the presence in the visual [cortex] of the child of stellate cells similar to those that generate the above-mentioned baskets in the motor cortex, one can admit, as a likely possibility, that the nests mentioned in the visual cortex of the adult are produced by the above-mentioned stellate cells of the seventh layer. We must, however, confess that we have not been able to demonstrate directly the fact of this continuation, perhaps because in the period in which the above-mentioned stellate cells are easily impregnated (cerebrum of the child of fifteen to twenty days), the nests are not yet sufficiently differentiated. This point needs, however, new and more precise investigations.

Layer of the Giant Pyramids in Other Mammals

In fig. 18, B [fig. 81], we reproduce this and the adjacent layers, taken from the visual cortex of the cat. One notices that the giant pyramids constitute, as in man, a fairly regular formation, it being not rare to find rows of cells provided with long, horizontal basal dendrites. In the cat and dog, they do not reach, however, the thickness and length [seen] in the human cortex.

The interior of this layer is inhabited also by numerous cells with arciform axon. Fig. 18 [fig. 81] shows the principal types of such cells, which essentially coincide with those described before in man. Notice that the axon resolves itself in two, three, four, and an even larger number of arched terminal fibers, the majority of which seem to us to arborize in the thickness of the layer of the giant pyramids itself. There is no lack, however, of arciform axons or ascending collaterals distributed in the deeper plane of the layer of the stellate cells or of other descending collaterals that arise from the arches and which seem to be

consumed in the subsequent layer of the medium pyramids with arciform axon (eighth layer in man).

The stellate type with short axon that is the generator of terminal nests exists in the cat, as do the pericellular baskets; but the course of the branches of the final arborization is so complicated that we have not [been able to unravel them] in their passage to the nests.

In the cat and dog, some fusiform or stellate cells with ascending axon are also found in the thickness of the layer of the giant pyramidal cells. [The axons] go up to the layer of the stellate cells and may perhaps go farther on.

In summary, the coincidence of structure between the human cortex and that of the gyrencephalic mammals is almost perfect with respect to the morphology of the cells, but it varies in the number and mode of distribution of these. Thus, the small cells with arciform axon, which in man constitute a special layer beneath that of the small stellates, are disseminated in the cat in the layer of the stellate cells and in that of the giant pyramids. [The cat], therefore, lacks a legitimate sixth layer, and it is not possible to recognize a fifth layer, [i.e.] a layer of small stellate elements, either.

VIII. Layer of the Medium Pyramids with Arciform Axon

Looked at in Nissl preparations, this layer is found to be clearly delimited by the bordering seventh and ninth layers, from which it is distinguished by its extreme cellular richness and the virtual absence of interstitial plexuses. The cells that inhabit it are cells of medium size, of pyramidal type (although there is no lack of spindle and triangular forms), often disposed in vertical pleiades separated by parallel bundles of [myelinated axons]. The Nissl method also reveals the presence of certain large stellate cells, irregularly distributed throughout the eighth layer.

As we show in fig. 18, C [fig. 81], the dominant types are the pyramidal, whose size is larger than those located in the sixth layer, and the triangular; the fusiform is the rarest of all. These diverse types possess long radial [dendritic] shafts prolonged up to the first or plexiform layer and lateral and descending somatic dendrites. The disposition and orientation of these somatic dendrites vary in the diverse types: in the pyramidal, which is the most common, the base of the cell body gives off several divergent dendrites from two, three, or more initial shafts; in the triangular, there exist two shafts generating [dendritic] branches, one lateral and the other descending (fig. 18, *l, g*) [*fig. 81*]; in the fusiform, the descending shaft is robust, going down to the ninth layer and giving off at acute angles several oblique dendrites.

But the true characteristic of the majority of the cells of the eighth layer resides in the axon, which, arising usually from the inferior portion of the soma and descending a certain distance, then describes an arc with an upward concavity and goes up to the layer of the large stellate cells, where it bifurcates and engenders a terminal aborization of very long horizontal branches (fig. 18, *i, g*) [*fig. 81*]. On its way, it supplies collaterals to the eighth layer and to the seventh layer.

On the basis of the behavior of the branches of the arched axon, one can differentiate two cell types: first, a cell whose axonal arch does not appear to give off collaterals, or, if it does so, they are short, and ramified among the cells of the eighth layer (fig. 18, *i*) [*fig. 81*]; and second, cells from whose arch a long descending collateral arises [and is] elongated to the white matter, where it reliably continues as a myelinated axon (fig. 18, *g*) [*fig. 81*].

The cells whose axons are incorporated directly into the white matter must be very rare in the human cortex; but in the visual region of the cat, where the above-mentioned type with arciform axon is less abundant, we have still been able to discern cells such as the fusiform or stellate type, whose axon can be followed into the white matter (fig. 18, *m, l*) [*fig. 81*]. The axon collaterals of such elements are ascending and thin, and seem to be exhausted in the thickness of the eighth and ninth layers.

Let us add that the eighth layer contains, although in short supply, these other cells: first, giant stellate cells provided with divergent and downy dendrites and with a robust ascending axon that reaches the first layer, after giving off collaterals along its course in the eighth and fifth layers (fig. 18, *j*) [*fig. 81*]; second, stel-

late cells with short axon, some small belonging to the arachniform type, and other large stellates with an axon ramifying diffusely in the surroundings of the cell of origin. This latter cell, which also inhabits other locations in the visual cortex, is none other than the famous sensory cell of Golgi, seen by this scientist, as well as by Mondino, Martinotti, and us, in diverse territories of the typical cortex.

IX. Layer of the Fusiform and Triangular Cells

This layer, which corresponds to the eighth [layer] of Meynert and to that of the deep polymorphic cells of Schlapp, is characterized by the predominance of the bundles of medullated axons and by the scarcity of nerve cells which are arranged in longitudinal interfascicular series. The majority of the cells of this layer have an ovoid, elongated, or fusiform shape. From the upper portion of the soma arises a strong [dendritic] shaft, often curved close to its origin, which is directed toward the surface, crossing the eighth and seventh layers; its turns and changes of plane are so many that it is impossible in the majority of cases to follow it beyond the sixth layer. However, in the cat, where the distances are shorter, we have been able to trace an [apical] shaft from some of the more superficial cells of the ninth layer to the first layer, by which time it is very thin, and this could well happen in all the similar cells of the [ninth] layer. From the deeper portion of the soma arise either a thick descending [dendritic] shaft ramified among the bundles of myelinated axons or two or three thin and divergent dendrites.

The cells of triangular form possess a thick and very long radial dendrite penetrating the superimposed layers; others, almost as long, are descending and ramified among the bundles of the white matter; and several [others are] lateral somatics, among which can show up a short transverse shaft, soon decomposing into ascending or descending oblique dendrites.

The cells situated close to the white matter, at the level of the concavity of the gyri, exhibit a large variety of forms and orientations. It is very common to find ovoid or fusiform cells extending long polar dendrites parallel to the plane of the white matter, one [large one] of which, after a long roundabout route, penetrates the overlying layers to reach, probably, the plexiform or first layer.

Lastly, the interior of the white matter also possesses a large number of elongated fusiform cells poor in basilar dendrites and provided with a very long radial [dendritic] shaft whose end is impossible to determine exactly.

With respect to the behavior of the axon, all the above-mentioned cellular types are similar. The axon arises from the deep part of the soma or from a thick basal dendrite (triangular and fusiform cells) and enters the white matter directly, where it continues as a myelinated fiber. From the first part of its trajectory arise two, three, or more collaterals, which commonly run recurrently to ramify in the interior of the ninth layer and even in the deeper portion of the eighth. In the fusiform cells [lying] parallel to the white matter (concave portions of the gyri), the axon often runs in the direction of the polar dendrites, following the plane of the white matter, at whose borders it describes several turns, until it turns radially, continuing as a myelinated nerve fiber.

Finally, the ninth layer also contains, although rarely, cells with an ascending, commonly arciform axon and an occasional cell with a short axon.

White Matter

Examining carefully the fibers of the white matter, it is observed that they are in large part different from those [beneath] other regions of the cortex, [being] of a medium or thin caliber. There exist, however, two kinds of thick myelinated axons: first, those continuous with the axons of the giant pyramids; second, more numerous terminal fibers ramifying and terminating in the fourth and fifth layers (optic fibers).

From the white matter arise collaterals distributed in the gray matter, in which they end in an unknown manner.

Furthermore, the method of Ehrlich reveals very well in the white matter of the cat and dog (visual region) not only collaterals but branches of thick myelinated axons which enter and diverge in the gray matter. At the level of origin of the branches, the parent fiber presents constantly, in accord with what we have noted,[23] a strangulation [node of Ranvier].

Nerve Plexuses of the Gray Matter

When sections of the human visual cortex stained by the method of Weigert-Pal are examined, all the layers of the gray matter are found to contain nerve plexuses formed by myelinated fibers of very diverse thickness.

The fibers that give rise to them adopt a variety of directions from which it is often possible to deduce their origin. Thus, the fibers disposed in vertical bundles extending from the white matter to well into the layer of the medium pyramids represent axons of small, medium, and giant pyramids as well as of stellate cells of the fourth and fifth layers. Moreover, the majority of the horizontal and oblique fibers dispersed through the diverse cortical layers (except for those given off in the fourth and fifth layers) are no other than the collaterals of axons of pyramids and terminal branches or collaterals of cells with ascending or descending short axon.

The medullated nerve plexuses of the cerebral cortex have been well described by the authors who have used the method of Weigert, particularly by Kölliker, Kaes, and Bottazzi. But this method only reveals a minimal proportion of the constituent fibers of the gray matter, as the majority lack a myelin sheath. Already, in our paper of 1892, we had called attention to the unusual richness of these plexuses and to the variety of their constituent fibers. We will not repeat here the revelations of that time, all the more because we will take up the question of the composition of the plexuses of the gray matter in our next paper on the motor cortex; here we will study only the most distinctive plexus of the visual cortex, that is to say, the one located at the level of the fourth and fifth layers and whose richness in medullated fibers is such that it constitutes a white stria visible to the naked eye (*stria of Gennari* or *of Vicq d'Azyr*).

Optic Plexus or Stria of Gennari

We have just seen that the thickness of the fourth and fifth layers encloses a plexus of medullated fibers that can be revealed in Weigert preparations, but the true composition and richness of this plexus can only be fully appreciated in preparations of silver chromate obtained in the cerebrum of the newborn child or [of the child] of a few days. In the good preparations of this type, at the level of the fourth and fifth layers, a very tight felt of threads is observed which shows up from all the other plexuses of the gray matter because of its density, and in which clear hollows appear that correspond to the stellate cells. As the cells of both the fourth and fifth strata possess a diverse size, the interstitial plexuses that surround them have different characteristics: at the level of the large stellate cells, the warp is more loose, being composed commonly of thicker threads that leave relatively considerable spaces; whereas at the level of the fifth layer, the framework is extremely tight, showing small fibers of great fineness and enclosing much more minute hollows.

What are the components of this plexus? The careful analysis to which we have submitted hundreds of well-impregnated sections has allowed us to separate in it five classes of nerve fibers: first, optic fibers; second, ascending fibers of neurons of the underlying layers; third, axon collaterals of stellate cells; fourth, bundles of axons of overlying pyramids; fifth, terminal arborizations of intrinsic cells with short axons.

Optic Fibers

With this name we will designate certain robust myelinated fibers coming from the white matter and arborizing in the layers of the large and small stellate cells. To these fibers, which dominate by their number and robustness those arborizing in the fourth and fifth layers, the intermediate region of the cortex owes its already mentioned white stria.

It would be difficult in the visual cortex of the child of fifteen to thirty days to distinguish the arborization formed by these robust visual fibers from those engendered by other nerve fibers, given that by this time all the elements composing the plexus of Gennari are frequently and simultaneously impregnated, but, fortunately, the precocity of the development of the optic fibers gives us the means to recognize them easily. These fibers appear al-

ready formed in the human fetus of eight months and especially in newborn children at an age when the other components of the plexus are not completely differentiated or lack affinity for the silver chromate. Accordingly, it is not rare to obtain preparations, such as the one reproduced in fig. 21 [*fig. 84*], where only the fibers coming from the optic radiation are stained.

These fibers are recognized by a group of characters: by their greater robustness compared with the axons of the large pyramids and obviously greater than the axons of the medium pyramids; by their course, which is more or less oblique, sometimes complicated by turns and changes of direction as they cross

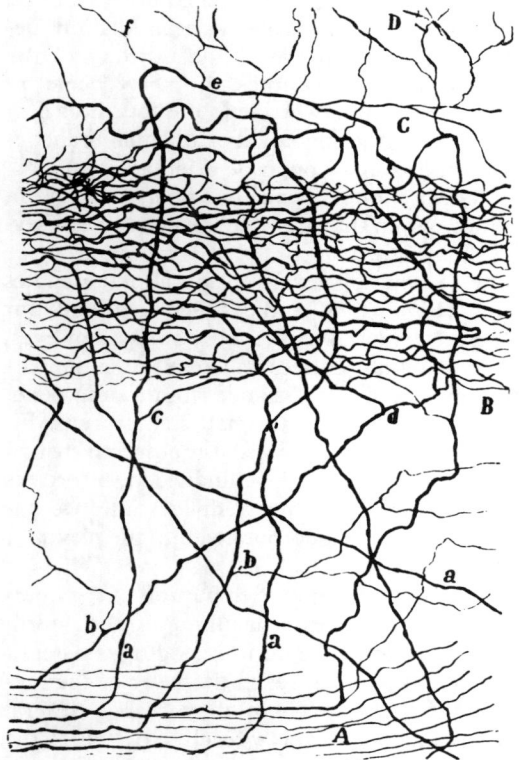

[*FIG. 84*] Fig. 21. Thick fibers coming from the white matter and ramifying in the stria of Gennari. Cerebrum of the child of three days. *A*, white matter; *B*, layer of the small stellate cells; *C*, arciform fibers and fourth layer; *D*, frontier of the layer of the medium pyramids; *a*, trunk of the fiber; *b*, collateral to the deep layers; *c*, ascending collateral to the upper layers.

the ninth, eighth, seventh, and sixth layers; and by the presence of branches at an acute angle, with the formation of ascending branches destined for the fourth and fifth layers. Once arrived at the layer of the small stellate cells, the optic fibers have diverse modes of behavior. Some suddenly bend in any of the planes of this layer, running horizontally for a very long distance and repeatedly bifurcating; others arrive high in the fourth layer, trace a bend and on occasion an arch with its concavity downward, then run horizontally and with bending along the outer limit or in the thickness of the layer; [after] describing an enormous itinerary, they lose themselves in the plexus that surrounds the large stellate cells.

The arcades [of the axons] go up in some cases to the layer of the medium pyramids, among which they trace wide undulations before later descending to the territory of the fourth layer. Sometimes, the nerve fibers bifurcate when they arrive in the fourth or fifth layer, engendering equal or unequal branches with the same or opposite orientations.

The branches of the optic fibers are very copious. When they traverse the deep layers (seventh, eighth, and ninth), it is common to see one or two collaterals arising at acute angles (fig. 21, b) [fig. 84] and destined apparently for these layers in which they arborize; however, in certain cases, these collaterals, like the parent axon and at a distance from it, also penetrate the layer of the small stellate cells. Finally, on some occasions, it is observed that an optic fiber, up till then undivided, bifurcates beneath the fifth layer or divides into two unequal branches incorporated into the plexus of the [fifth layer].

From the upper arched portion of the fibers arriving at the external limit of the fourth layer, one or two oblique ascending collaterals often arise; [these] reach the layer of the medium pyramids, where they branch several times, and possibly they reach in part up to the second and third layers (fig. 21, e) [fig. 84].

But the majority of the collaterals arising from the optic fibers come off the horizontal course of these through the fourth and fifth layers; such collaterals arising at a diversity of angles run in all directions, but more especially in a direction parallel to the [surface of]

the cortex; [after] branching repeatedly, they give rise to a very tight nerve plexus in whose hollows lie the stellate cells of the two layers. *Therefore, the immense majority of the branches arising from the optic fibers are distributed in the layers of the stellate cells; it becomes possible, therefore, to consider these strata as the main region of the gray matter to which the visual image is projected and in which the optic sensation is produced.* Each visual fiber establishes contacts not with one but with a huge number of small and large stellate cells situated over a wide cortical radius, which confirms once more the law of the *avalanche of conduction*, a law that seems to prevail especially in the neurons of the sensory pathways.[24]

A careful examination of the cortex of the newborn child allows one to observe also the existence of some nerve collaterals arising from the optic plexus which ascend to ramify in the layers of the medium and small pyramids. In two or three cases, these collaterals coming from the horizontal fibers of the stria of Gennari were very robust and were prolonged into the first or plexiform layer, where they were lost after running horizontally for some distance. But in any case, such ascending fibers, destined for other layers, represent an insignificant contingent in comparison with the extraordinary number of optic fibers distributed and terminating in the layers of the stellate cells.

But do these fibers definitely come from the primary optic centers? Might they not also be intracerebral association connections? It is necessary to confess that it is not possible at the present time to demonstrate completely the optic nature of the fibers, but very strong indications of that exist. Here are the facts that speak in favor of the visual origin of the thick fibers ramifying in the plexus of Gennari.

1. The stellate cells of the fourth and fifth layers, by contrast with the normal, appear very atrophic in men and animals that have lived blind for a long time. Cramer[25] has also noticed that fact in the calcarine fissure of the one-eyed human. This atrophy could be explained by the cessation or very notable diminution (in the case of blindness in one eye) of the luminous excitation brought by the secondary optic pathways, that is to say, by those

arising in the primary optic centers, the places of arborization and termination of the retinal fibers.

2. The fibers arriving at the stria of Gennari from the white matter are much thicker than the association fibers and thicker than the axons of the giant pyramids, at least in the newborn and neonatal child. This circumstance speaks in favor of their extracortical origin.

3. The axons of the cells resident in the lateral geniculate body and pulvinar, the foci of origin of the central optic pathway, are commonly extremely robust. So also, although somewhat less, are those arising in the superior colliculus.

4. The existence of thick myelinated afferent fibers (fibers of Cajal, according to Kölliker), discovered first by us in the sensory-motor cortex,[26] seems to be a characteristic of the sensory areas of the cerebrum. Until the present time, at least, we have not been able to find them in the gyri that Flechsig designates as centers of association.

5. The thick myelinated fibers arising from giant pyramids resident in the psychomotor region never penetrate other cerebral lobules, but go down across the striatum to constitute the pyramidal tract. This demonstration is easy in the cerebrum of the fetal mouse.

6. Physiology and anatomy together tell us that the visual region must receive a considerable volume of optic fibers; thus, it is natural to consider as such innumerable thick fibers distributed in the layer of the stellate cells, given that the dense plexuses originating from them constitute a new factor virtually specific for the visual area.

7. Given the dynamic scheme now in vogue about the centers of association and of projection and assuming that the foci of projection or of sensation do not represent the anatomical substratum of ideas but of sensations, it may be presumed that the majority of the association fibers of the visual cortex is formed by outgoing axons, not by incoming axons. We do not deny the existence of fibers other than those of optic conduction coming from other cortical provinces (centrifugal or moderator fibers of association of Flechsig), but we affirm that in the visual region these are less numerous than in

other cerebral areas and that consequently most of the fibers entering it must be regarded as optic in nature.

The optic fibers and plexus of Gennari show up very well in the visual area of the cat of a few days. As shown in fig. 23, B [fig. 86], many of them bifurcate or give off collaterals at acute angles, not far from the white matter or in the thickness of the deep layers, and reach the layer of the stellate cells, where they terminate as an arborization weaker than that described in the human visual cortex. Many fibers ascend obliquely to the heights of the layer, resolving themselves into tufts of varicose branches, some of which are prolonged into the layer of medium pyramids. In short, in the cat, the layer of the stellate cells is also the place of termination of the optic fibers or thick afferents; even the branches arising from these in deeper layers seem to us to be destined to contact the stellate cells.

Fibers Arising from the Cells with Ascending Axon

As can be seen in Fig. 22, B [fig. 85], besides the plexus of optic fibers, the fourth and fifth layers contain another, more delicate plexus engendered by the terminal arborizations of the multitude of arched axons of the pyramidal cells of the seventh and eighth layers, and by other ascending axons arising from stellate cells resident in the sixth, seventh, and eighth layers. This plexus is stained in the adult human relatively independently of the optic plexus, and in it are observed from time to time condensed parts that seem to correspond to arborizations situated around the stellate cells.

Still not having been able to determine the special connections received by the cells with arciform axons, both at the level of the first layer (tuft of [apical dendritic] shaft) and in the thickness of the sixth, seventh, and eighth layers (soma and descending dendrites), it is not permissible for one to make pronouncements about the physiological significance of such singular elements; it is possible only to affirm that by means of their axonal arborizations some actions collected in the first cortical layer are brought to the layer of the stellate cells and to the layer of giant pyramidal cells.

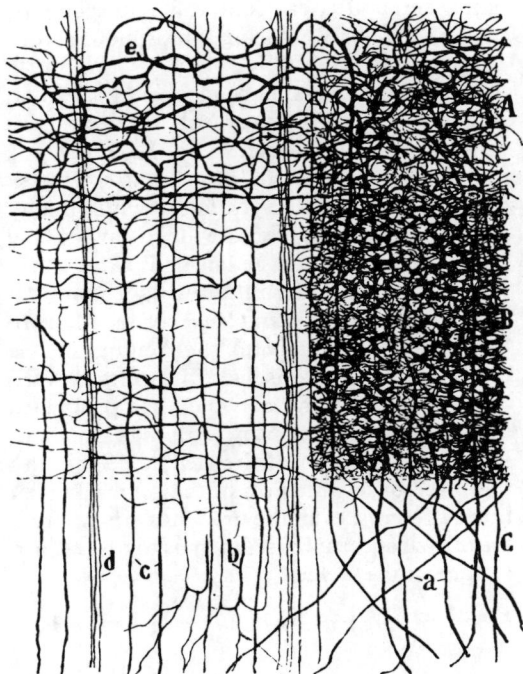

[*FIG. 85*] Fig. 22. Nerve plexuses of the fourth and fifth layers of the visual cortex of a child of twenty days. *A*, fourth layer; *B*, fifth layer; *C*, sixth layer; *a*, optic fibers; *b*, axons of the cells of the sixth layer; *c*, ascending axons of pyramidal cells of the eighth layer; *d*, bundles of axons of medium and small pyramids; *e*, arcades of optic fibers with ascending collaterals.

Collaterals of the Stellate Cells

We have already seen, when we dealt with these cells, that their collaterals, often more robust than the [parent axon], arborize in the thickness of the fourth and fifth layers, engendering a complicated plexus of long, preferentially horizontal trabeculae. According to the law of dynamic polarization of neurons, we must suppose that such collaterals have the aim of propagating to other neighboring stellate cells a part of the impulses received by the soma and dendrites; but it is necessary to confess that the frequent predominance in thickness of the initial collaterals over the [main] axon of the stellate cells creates a true difficulty with the theory, leading to not a few doubts.

A great darkness likewise reigns with respect to the role played by the axonal arborizations of so many cells with short axons resident in the thickness of the fourth and fifth layers. Are these cells obligatory links interposed between the optic fibers and the stellate cells with long axon? With such a supposition, one might consider them as generators of nervous energy, something like accumulators destined to increase the force of the luminous excitation with the aim of producing intense corticovisual reflexes, and to facilitate the recognition in other areas of the cerebrum of the sensorial image. Monakow[27] also represented in his schemes of the visual pathways cells with short axon intercalated in the communications between processes of the primary optic foci (cells of propagation or of intercalation); but the drawings of this author do not correspond with reality, since, as demonstrated first by my brother[28] and confirmed by us and by Kölliker, in the superior colliculus and lateral geniculate body, the optic arborizations contact immediately the soma and dendrites of robust cells with long axon. Anyway, and although our recent observations do not allow us to resolve definitely this question, we must declare that we are not opposed to the idea of considering the innumerable cells with short axon of the fourth and fifth layers as the first point of connection or of arrival of the optic fibers. From the cells with short axon, the visual current, more or less increased in intensity, is propagated to diverse cells, but with a preference for the large and medium stellate cells with which the axons of the [short-axon] cells establish intimate contacts.

Bundles of [Apical Dendritic] Shafts of Pyramids and of Cells with Arched Axon

Since such dendrites cross the fourth and fifth layers, where the optic fibers are principally distributed, it is natural to suppose that the pyramids are also capable of collecting the optic excitation [and then of conveying] it, perhaps to the nervous foci governing ocular reflexes.

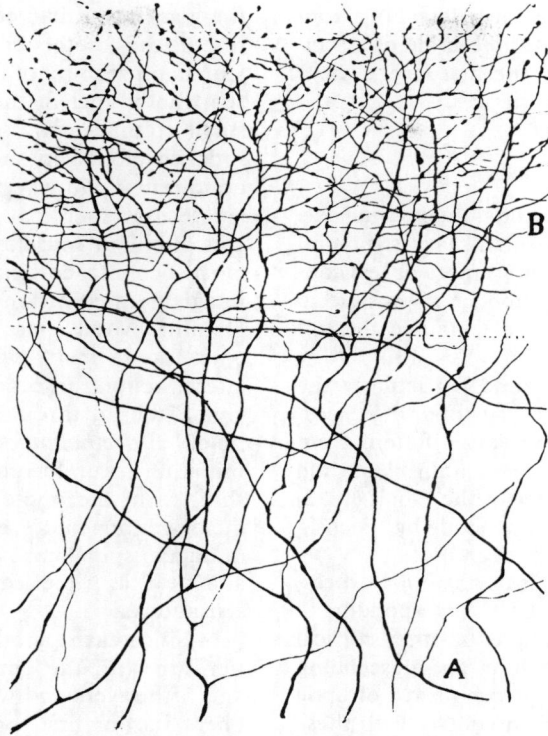

[*FIG. 86*] Fig. 23. Optic fibers of the visual cortex of the cat of five days. *A*, fibers with bifurcations coming from the white matter; *B*, optic nervous plexus of the layer of the stellate cells (fourth and fifth layers of man).

The peripheral tuft might receive other excitations, coming perhaps from the association fibers (*moderator fibers* of Flechsig).

About the other nervous plexuses of the visual cortex we have not yet made sufficient study. We believe, however, that with slight differences such plexuses (plexuses of the molecular layer, of the small and medium pyramids, of the layer of the giant cells, etc.) are composed of the same elements as the corresponding plexus in the other cortical regions. About that we will speak when we study the motor cortex and other areas of the gray matter of the human cerebrum. Here we will anticipate only that the plexiform or first layer, like the layers of pyramids, seem to us to contain ramifications originating from fibers thinner than the optic [fibers] and thinner than those arriving directly from the white matter. Perhaps these

myelinated fibers would belong to those called by Flechsig fibers of *centrifugal association*, that is to say, to those arising in regions of association and destined to act in a depressive manner on the sensory areas. More than moderators of sensation, such as Flechsig wants, we would prefer to give to such fibers a tonic or dynamic action, perhaps in relation to the process of attention and the regulation of physical-chemical conditions necessary for memory. But let us hasten to say that all of this is conjectural and without substance. For the rest, in favor of the associative nature of the fibers terminating in the first layer speaks a fact of analogy, demonstrated some time ago by us. The fact is that in the gray cortex of the internal face of the cerebrum of the mouse and rabbit, a region where the shortness of the distances facilitates following of the fibers, it is common to reveal nerve fibers detaching from the anteroposterior arciform bundle of association and distributed in the first layer, where they run for very long distances.

Summary and Conclusions

Although our studies on the human visual cortex are not ended and we still lack structural data relating to other regions more or less concerned with visual function, it is possible to take from the results so far obtained the following conclusions.

1. The visual region, and particularly the calcarine fissure and its surroundings, possesses a special structure very different from the rest of the cortex, which confirms our old works on the visual cortex of the rabbit (1892) and the predictions recently made by Flechsig and others.

2. This structure has as its anatomic expression the presence in the layer corresponding to the so-called layer of grains of other cortical areas stellate cells with long and descending axons; the creation of a dense plexus of optic fibers (stria of Gennari) in contact with these cellular elements; the existence of special layers composed of cells with arched ascending axons (sixth and eighth layers); and the scarcity, already noted by many, of giant and even of medium pyramidal cells.

3. Since the layers of small and large stellate cells represent the principal point of termination of the optic fibers, it is permissible to suppose that they are also the site of visual sensation.

4. It is also reasonable to assume that the *principal or memory impulse,* that is to say, that destined to be registered in the form of memories or latent visual images in the association cortex, leaves via the axons of the stellate cells. According to the theory of binocular vision, [equivalent parts of] each visual cortical area must receive fibers from identical points of both retinas; thus, a stellate cell will be related to both right and left optic arborizations; nevertheless, from what we have said in our work about the [optic] chiasm, this double communication might happen only in the primary optic centers.

5. It also seems reasonable to suppose that

the giant pyramidal cells and their axons represent the motor or reflex optic pathway, which, on account of the existence of other visual motor foci in the motor cortex and the small volume of muscle governed, would be little developed in the occipital cortex. This optic-reflex pathway would explain the conjugate movements of the eyeball, the eyelid, and pupillary muscle produced by excitation of the occipital cortex, as revealed in the physiological investigations of Schaffer, Unvericht, Danillo, Munk, etc. The above-mentioned optic-motor fibers, [which are] capable of bilateral action, descend, as affirmed by Munk and Flechsig, through the radiation of Gratiolet (*corticothalamic bundle* of Flechsig), terminating in or forming an indirect relationship with the motor foci of the corpora quadrigemina and even with those of the medulla and spinal cord (movements of the neck and head as a consequence of visual cortical sensations).

6. Since each pyramid is brought into relationship with the optic plexus in the fourth and fifth layers and with probable association fibers in the first, one thinks that the discharges provoked in them can have diverse origins; sometimes the optic excitation, [sometimes] other impulses generated in centers of association.

7. The innumerable cells with short axon in the central layers of the visual cortex could perform two roles: increase the energy of the optic impulse to create the sensation, and propagate this impulse to the pyramidal or stellate cells resident in different layers and [at different horizontal distances].

8. In the visual cortex and in the other cortical regions, there are common factors of organization [that are] little modified in spite of [different] functional localizations and correlated structural adaptations; hence, the first or plexiform layer is composed constantly of the same cells and nerve fibers, as are the layers of small and medium pyramids and that of the fusiform or polymorphic cells, layers that obey in their construction an identical plan. It is permissible, therefore, to imagine that this common anatomical *substratum* performs similar activities in the cortex as a whole.

If we could know with certainty that the

molecular layer receives the terminal arborizations of the intercortical association fibers (we have already seen that there is some indication of that), we could attribute to each of the two factors or mechanisms of construction of the sensory cortex a unique significance: the specific factor (stellate cells), preferential point of termination of the sensory fibers, would be the anatomical site of the sensation; and the [other] common factor (molecular layer, small and large pyramids, etc.) would represent the ideomotor mechanism, that is to say, the place where the special motor action (movements of the eyes, head, etc.), provoked in the first or plexiform layer by the action of the ideomotor fibers coming from the centers of association, would be elaborated. In addition to these ideomotor fibers, there could exist the moderator fibers of the sensation that Flechsig is talking about.

General Overview of the Construction of the Other Sensory Regions of the Cortex

Although our studies on the acoustic, motor, olfactory, and association cortex are not completed, we will bring forward here some data that can easily be linked with what we have said about the visual region.

1. Not only the visual cortex but the other sensory areas of the cortex possess their own characteristics, by which they are recognizable at first sight in good silver chromate preparations. For example, the olfactory or limbic cortex, as demonstrated by C. Calleja[29] and confirmed by Kölliker[30] and us, [is recognized] by the great thickness of the molecular layer, where, in a rare case, the sensory fibers are seen distributed (fibers coming from the lateral olfactory stria); by the absence of small pyramids, which are replaced by large triangular and fusiform cells; by the appearance of a descending tassel or tuft presented by the dendrites of the medium and giant pyramids; etc. The acoustic cortex is recognized by the existence of large, fusiform or horizontal, triangular cells, distributed in the middle cortical layers; by the extraordinary number and notable delicacy of the bitufted cells with axons ramified in paintbrushes; by the thinness of the fibers of the sensory plexus situated in the layer of the granule or small cells. Finally, the motor cortex is recognized by its great thickness; by the notable robustness of the plexiform layer, by the extraordinary numbers of medium and giant pyramids; by the existence of a very wide sensory plexus concentrated in the layer of the granule cells and extending into the layer of the giant and medium pyramids; [in this] plexus the myelinated axons are very robust, run in oblique directions, and display numerous branches.

2. The association cortex, like the motor and acoustic, consists of six layers, namely, first, plexiform; second, of the small pyramids; third, large pyramids; fourth, granule cells or small pyramids mixed with minute stellate cells; fifth, medium and deep giant pyramids; sixth, fusiform and polymorphic cells. The olfactory lacks the layer of the granule cells, but the other strata can be distinguished.

3. The so-called layer of the granule cells in the association cortex, as in the projection or sensory cortex, is the principal place of distribution of the fibers coming from other centers. Thanks to the presence of this intermediate layer, the large pyramids are separated into two strata: one supragranular, generally very rich in voluminous cells, and the other infragranular, poorer in these elements but more copious in medium pyramids. Often, the giant cells reach a still larger size in the infragranular stratum or fifth layer, a thing that occurs especially in the association cortex (anterior frontal and posterior parietal region), [the cells] being arranged in concentric rows joined by robust horizontal dendrites, reminding [one of] the typical disposition in the visual cortex.

Such a layer of granule cells encloses two classes of small cells: first, minute pyramidal cells with a long descending axon provided with thick initial collaterals [which are] sometimes arciform or recurrent; second, stellate or fusiform cells with short axon. Among these latter are recognized several types, namely (a) downy, fusiform, or stellate cells, provided with an ascending short axon, ramifying in the different levels of the fourth layer and even in the adjacent parts of the third layer; (b) fusiform and stellate cells, whose axon goes up to the first layer; (c) stellate cells with robust ascending axon, promptly dividing into very long and thick horizontal or oblique branches (these cells lie also in the fifth layer or [layer] of the deep giant pyramidal cells); (d) very small arachniform cells with very short and very thin axon, densely arborized in the thickness of the fourth layer; etc. In short, the fourth layer consists of an extraordinary number of cells with short, generally ascending axon, thanks to which the primary or secondary sensory excitation (secondary perhaps in the association areas) can be propagated to a large number of cells situated in a different stratum and [at different distances]. Let us note that almost all of these [cellular] elements of the layer of the granule cells in the motor and the association cortex are also present but are more or less modified in the layer of the small stellate cells of the visual cortex; the difference is that in the latter, such a granular stratum is subdivided and differentiated into three or four secondary layers and complicated by the appearance of the stellate cells with long descending axons.

Cajal's Notes

1. A brief preliminary communication, containing our principal results on the human visual cortex, was published in *Revista Ibero-Americana de Ciencias Médicas*, March 1899.

2. Th. Meynert; Der Bau des Grosshirnrinde und seine örtlichen Verchiedenheiten, etc. *Vierteljahrschrift für Psychiatrie*, etc., 1872.
Also see article: Vom Gehirne der Säugethiere in *Handbook der Lehre von den Geweben*, by S. Stricker, Vol. 2, 1872, Leipzig; and the book of Huguenin in which are summarized the ideas of Meynert: *Allgemeine Pathologie der Krankheiten des Nervensystems*, *Anat. Einleitung*, Zürich, 1873.

3. W. Krause, *Allgemeine und mikroskopische Anatomie*, Hannover, 1876.

4. Schwalbe, *Lehrbuch des Neurologie*, Erlangen, 1881.

5. Betz, *Centralbl. f. d. Mediz. Wissensch.*, nos. 11–13, 1881.

6. Golgi, Sulla fina anatomia degli organi centrali del sistema nervoso, Milano, 1886.

7. C. Hammarberg, *Studien über Klinik und Pathologie der Idiotie*, etc. (published after the death of the author by Professor S. E. Henschen), Upsala, 1895.

8. S. R. Cajal, Estructura del asta de Ammon, etc., II: Estructura de la corteza occipital inferior de los pequeños mamíferos. Work read before the Spanish Society of Natural History in the session of April 5, 1893.

Anal. de la Sociedad Esp. de Hist. Nat., Vol. XXII, 1893.

9. S. R. Cajal, Sur la structure de l'écorce cérébrale de quelques mammifères. *La Cellule*, Vol. III, part 1, 1891.

10. F. Bottazzi, Intorno alla corteccia cerebrale e specialmente intorno alle fibre nervose intracorticali dei vertebrati, 1893.

11. S. R. Cajal, *Beitrag zur Studium der Medulla oblongata, etc.*, Leipzig, 1896, p. 132.

12. M. Schlapp, Der Zellenbau der Grosshirnrinde des Affen, Macacus gynomolgus, *Arch. f. Psychiatrie*, Vol. 30, Part 2 [1898].

13. Kölliker, *Handbuch der Gewebelehre des Menschen*, Vol. 2., Leipzig, 1896.

14. S. Ramón Cajal, Sur la structure de l'écorce cérébrale de quelques mammifères, *La Cellule*, Vol. VII, 1891.

——, Textura de las circunvoluciones cerebrales en los mamíferos inferiores, 10 December 1890, Barcelona.

——, Sobre la existencia de colaterales y bifurcaciones en las fibras de la sustancia blanca del cerebro, 20 December 1890.

——, El azul de metileno en los centros nerviosos, *Revista Trimestral Micrográfica*. Vol. II, 1896.

——, Las células de cilindro-eje corto de la capa molecular del cerebro, *Revista Trimestral Micrográfica*, Vol. II, 1897.

15. G. Retzius, Die Cajal'sche Zellen der Grosshirnrinde beim Menschen und bei Säugetieren, *Bio. Unters.*, Neue Folge, Vol. V, 1893.

——, Weitere Beiträge zur Kenntnis der Cajal'sche Zellen der Grosshirnrinde des Menschen, *Biol. Unters.*, Neue Folge, 1894.

16. E. Veratti, Ueber einige Struktureigenthümlichkeiten der Hirnrinde bei den Säugetieren, *Anat. Anzeiger*, no. 14, 1897.

17. K. Schaffer, Zur feinere Struktur der Hirnrinde und über die funktionelle Bedeutung der Nervenzellenfortsätze, *Arch. f. Mikros. Anat.*, Bd. 48, [Pt.] IV, 1897.

18. Very small elements with short axon were also mentioned by Cl. Sala, in the cerebral basal ganglia of birds (*La corteza cerebral de les aves*, Barcelona, 1893), and by my brother in the cerebral cortex of reptiles and batrachians (Estructura del encéfalo del camaleón, *Rev. Trim. Micro.*, Vol. I, 1896).

19. S. R. Cajal, Beitrag zur Studium der Medulla oblongata, etc., Leipzig, 1896.

20. H. Held, Die centralen Bahnen des Nervus acusticus bei der Kätze: Die centralen Gehörleitung, *Arch. f. Anat. u. Physiol.*, Anat. Abth., 1891 and 1893.

21. J. Lavilla, Algunos detalles concernientes a la oliva superior y focos acústicos. *Rev. Trim. Microgr.*, Vol. III, 1898.

22. S. R. Cajal, Estructura del asta de Ammon y fascia dentata, etc., *Anal. de la Socied. Esp. de Historia Nat.*, Vol. XXII, 1893, p. 68.

23. Cajal, El azul de metileno en los centros nerviosos, *Rev. Trim. Micrográfica*, Vol. I, 1896.

24. S. Ramón y Cajal, Algunas conjeturas sobre el mecanismo anatómico de la ideación, asociación y atención, etc., Madrid, 1895.

25. A. Cramer, Beitrag zur Kenntnis der Optikus-kreuzung zur Chiasma, etc., Wiesbaden, 1898.

26. Cajal, Sur la structure de l'écorce cérébrale de quelques mammifères, *La Cellule,* 189[1].

27. Monakow, Experimentelle u. pathol. anatom. Untersuchungen über die optischen Centren und Bahnen, *Arch. f. Psych.* XXI, 1889.

28. P. Ramón, Investigaciones de histología comparada en los centros ópticos, etc., Zaragoza, 1890.

29. C. Calleja, La región olfatoria del cerebro, Madrid, 1893.

30. Kölliker, *Handbuch der Gewebelehre,* Vol. 2, 1896, p. 723.

Editors' Notes

A. The text incorrectly states fig. 15, *d.*

B. The text incorrectly states *A.*

C. The text incorrectly states *h.*

16

Studies on the Human Cerebral Cortex II: Structure of the Motor Cortex of Man and Higher Mammals

[*Revista Trimestral Micrográfica* 4:117–200, 1899, and 5:1–11, 1900]

It can be well affirmed that no cortical region has been studied more carefully than the motor, both in man and in [other] gyrencephalic mammals. Such preference is easily explained, considering that, of all the functional localizations in the cerebrum, the first and best delineated has been that of voluntary movements. In general, in these difficult domains of biology, the physiologist must precede the anatomist. It will be impossible for the latter to understand the functional significance of a certain structure if the physiology has not previously illustrated for him the role performed by the organ under examination. Knowing the physiological topography, histological analysis does not have to grope its way; its mission [then] consists not only of defining the fine anatomical details but also of resolving the gross, dynamic regional localizations into more precise and intimate localizations, that is to say, to determine the cells and fibers that carry out each of the elemental activities [included in] the integrative or collective functioning of the nervous organ.

Such has been the progression followed in the study of cortical functions. Thus, Hitzig, Fritsch, Ferrier, and others determined the cortical site [of representation] of voluntary movements; and then Betz, Bevan Lewis, etc., tried to assign the principal role in this functional mode to certain cells that were estimated as the starting points of the motor excitation. Finally, the existence of such cells and of other special structural arrangements will permit [us] to determine which are the genuine motor [cortical areas] in man and higher mammals, and in due course, when the analysis has revealed completely the connections of the diverse elements of the [motor] center, it will permit the elucidation of the physical-chemical mechanisms of voluntary movements. Through this, it is seen that the true understanding of cerebral activity will not be achieved until *organ physiology* has been transformed into *histophysiology,* changing the study of organic resultants[A] into [that of] the elemental components.

When we undertook the present work, we were inspired by one doctrine, more or less explicitly accepted by all the neurologists who have dedicated themselves to the histological analysis of the gyri, and openly proclaimed recently by Flechsig and Nissl: that of the organic plurality of the cerebrum, with its obligatory corollary, the diversity of structural topography.

In effect, if the gray cerebral cortex is an aggregation of organs with diverse functions, each of them must possess a special structure, within a [fundamental] plan whose general lines are appropriate for the whole cortex.

It is totally unreasonable to accept that the association areas have a structure identical to that of the areas of sensation, and among the latter it seems very little credible that all possess the same anatomy: those related to the chemical senses (taste and smell); those linked with apparatuses of wave [perception] (hearing and vision); and those connected with the skin, mucous membranes, and tendons, [i.e.] collector organs of nonperiodic stimuli and of thermal and painful stimuli.

For our part, we confess to be a confirmed supporter of the pluralist doctrine, so that we judge it [to be] applicable not only to the two orders of sensory and of association areas but also to the parts or functional subdivisions differentiated from each of them. So far, the examination of the above-mentioned anatomical diversities has only dealt with the sensory areas; at some future date, however, the peculiar anatomical adaptations of each association area will also be discovered. But in order that the anatomical analysis of the latter be fruitful, it is necessary that the histologist should have as a guide a physiology able to localize categories of ideas or of representations [just] as we already have a localist physiology of sensations and movements.

Nobody will contest that between a visual idea and a tactile or acoustic idea or memory, considering them as phenomena of consciousness, there are great differences that depend, in our opinion, not only on the specific nature of the peripheral receptor apparatus but also on the peculiar structures of the corresponding centers of sensation and association.

And omitting the centers of association, it is exceedingly probable that inside each sensory or projection area, there exist also zones endowed with some peculiarities of structure, which, without interfering with the general anatomical plan of the specific area, could be considered representations, either of some more or less exquisitely sensitive region of the receptor surface or of some particular quality of the sensation.

We have repeatedly observed this intra-areal topographic diversity, in the visual region and in the motor and olfactory regions. In reality, the point is not new, since in regard to the motor area, several authors, among them Betz, have already noticed that the giant cells are not disseminated equally but have a preferred location in the upper part of the said region and in front of the Rolandic fissure. The contradictions of the authors about the number of [cortical] layers have, in our opinion, a similar origin; that is to say, they have each analyzed different parts of the same sensory area.

Our observations relevant to this intra-areal variability are not sufficient to make a detailed exposition. At the present time, we must be content with noting some features that seem peculiar to each sensory area, considered as an anatomicophysiological unit. And, as we shall see, even in this modest venture, the results of our labor are very incomplete.

It is certainly not the lack of investigators or of zeal for analytic work that is the cause of our delay regarding the structure of the cerebral sensory areas, and particularly of the sensory-motor, but the irremediable deficiencies of the methods, which give only fragmentary revelations that can hardly [be] integrated into an anatomical synthesis. The Weigert [method], for example, shows only the course and position of the medullated fibers, that is to say, a minimal part of the [total population of the] nerve fibers. The Nissl [method] only reveals to us the gross shape and situation of the cell body. The Ehrlich [method], although [giving] more complete [staining], is not applicable to man, and when it is used in the cerebrum of animals, it is unable to stain all the cells or to impregnate the terminal axonal arborizations; besides, the interpretation of its results is sometimes very difficult, which explains the errors made in recent years by Dogiel, Meyer, Bethe, and Nissl. Finally, the Golgi method, even though it is the most expressive, has against it its limited applicability to the adult human cerebrum, which obliges us to use it in embryos and newborn animals, running the risk of accepting as definitive arrangements transitory phases in the development of the neurons. Only by using all of these methods, and particularly the latter, with great perseverance and patience, is it feasible to advance a little the knowledge of the structure of the human cerebral cortex.

This is what we have attempted to do in the present work, where, as the reader will see, if we have collected some new details on a certain number of points, we have unfortunately also left outstanding many very important questions regarding the [anatomy] and physiology of the motor cortex.

Our observations have been made primarily on the cerebrum of the child from fifteen days to two months, a period during which the silver chromate impregnation is very constant.

We have used for that very fresh cerebra in which decomposition had not begun.[1] It is possible, however, to obtain good impregnations also in cerebra of twenty-four and even of thirty-six hours, on condition that the gray matter keeps its turgor, a phenomenon that seems to us to depend on the illness that preceded death, even more than on the time after death. In general, the first [region] that is altered so as to prevent the reaction is the first or plexiform layer, especially at the level of the protuberant parts of the gyri; the concave parts of these, as well the deep layers, maintain their impregnability for a much longer time.

The following description[2] refers almost exclusively to the two Rolandic convolutions, precentral and postcentral. The motor parts of the adjacent regions have not been sufficiently explored by us.

Finally, to give our study a wider base, we have also carefully examined the same gyri of the adult human, with the methods of Nissl, Golgi, and Weigert, as well as the motor areas of some mammals (dog, cat, horse, rabbit, and mouse).

Historical Notes About the Structure of the Motor Cortex

The first more or less precise description of this cortical region in man is that of Meynert,[3] who attributed to almost the whole cortex, except the insula, the pole of the occipital lobe, and Ammon's horn, a structural type [consisting] of five layers, namely first layer, or layer of scarce, small cells; second layer, or layer of the tight-packed small pyramids; third layer, or layer of the large pyramids (Ammon's formation); fourth layer, or layer of the small and tight-packed cells (granular formation); and fifth, the layer of the fusiform cells.

The drawing corresponding to the third frontal convolution that Meynert presents in support of this division is very expressive; it lacks, however, the deep giant cells; perhaps they escaped the shrewdness of this expert. Anyway, the description of Meynert, even with the doubt about whether he really refers strictly to the motor region, is sufficiently exact and can be [made] applicable with some additions to the Rolandic gyri.

With slight variations, the ideas of Meynert about the stratification of the motor region and of the association areas (at that time not distinguished) have been accepted and confirmed by Schwalbe, Krause, Henle, Obersteiner, etc.

In reality, our knowledge of the structure of the motor region did not advance much until the publication of the work of Betz,[4] who noted, as characteristic of the motor region, the existence of giant pyramids at the level of the fourth layer of Meynert; [these are] absent from the rest of the cortex. Such cells, whose preferred location is the area extending in front of the Rolandic fissure, should possess motor function, while the inhabitants of the posterior portion of the hemispheres should have sensory or receptive functions. In such a manner, the cerebrum becomes reduced to two poles, motor and sensory, like the gray matter of the spinal cord, where, according to the belief of Betz, the anterior horn is motor and the posterior sensory.

The mentioned large cells were confirmed by Bevan Lewis,[5] for whom these elements in the motor cortex replace the granular formation of Meynert. In the remaining regions of the cortex, there is no lack of Betz cells, but they are more reduced (*ganglionic cells* of Lewis) and reside at the level of the fourth layer or deeper.

The appearance of a new method in the arena of investigation and of an observer as perspicacious as Golgi markedly advanced knowledge of the structure of the gray matter. As is well known, Golgi made in his fundamental work[6] an important study of the structure of the motor cortex (precentral gyrus). In this description, after noting the existence of three types of nerve cells scattered in the gray matter (pyramidal, fusiform, and globular cells), he divides the cortex into three zones or *superficial, middle,* and *deep* thirds. The first two are composed of pyramidal cells and the last of globular, polygonal, and irregular cells disposed in several orientations. The cells of the middle and external thirds send to the surface a dendritic shaft, while those of the deep third possess generally less radial processes that are never prolonged up to the submeningeal stratum. Concerning the destination of the axon, Golgi gives little information; beyond the fundamental discovery of the axonal collaterals, the savant of Pavia tells us only that the axons of many pyramids are directed either toward the white matter or toward the surface; but neither in the text nor in the appended plates is the continuity of such axons shown with fibers of the white matter. With regard to the special characteristics of the motor cortex, Golgi, deeply imbued with the unitary theory, seems to deny them, having not confirmed either the existence of special giant cells (cells of Betz) or that of the minute cells of Meynert (fourth layer of this author).

Between the motor and the occipital cortex (superior occipital convolution which corresponds probably to the association cortex), [Golgi] does not find more difference than the presence, in the deep stratum (inferior third) of the latter, of a larger number of small globular cells.

From an examination of the figures that illustrate the work of Golgi, it is clear that the deepest strata of the gray matter, particularly the layer of the deep giant pyramidal cells and that of the fusiform cells (fifth layer of Meynert), have escaped the attention of this author, perhaps because of defective impregnation. He was no more fortunate either in failing to observe the cells of the fourth layer or layer of the deep small pyramids, although this can be attributed to the notable variations in number that such cells undergo in certain motor areas.

The attractiveness and exceptional interest offered by the study of the cerebral cortex and the routinely satisfactory results that we have obtained in the histological analysis of the spinal cord and cerebellum[7] led us in 1890 to investigate the motor cortex of small mammals (mouse, guinea pig, and rabbit). It was then our purpose to fill as far as possible the lacunae that Golgi had left in his seminal exploration, particularly in relation to the course and terminations of the axons. To overcome better the large difficulties inherent in [making] such observations, we chose fetuses of small mammals or newborn animals. Fruits of our labor at that time were the demonstration, first, of the nerve cells of the molecular layer, and their diverse types; second, of the continuity of many axons of small, medium, and large pyramids with fibers of the white matter; third, of the free termination of the axon collaterals in the gray matter; fourth, of the bifurcation of many axons when they arrive in the white matter; fifth, of the origin of many callosal fibers; sixth, of the penetration of the corpus striatum by the axons of the pyramids; seventh, of the existence of thick centrifugal fibers ramifying in the gray matter; eighth, of the tuftlike disposition presented by the [apical dendritic] shafts of the pyramids when they arrive at the molecular layer; ninth, of the existence of cells with ascending axon, similar to the so-called cells of Martinotti, but whose terminal arborization does not reach the molecular layer; tenth, finally, of the morphology and development of several types of nerve and neuroglial cells, etc.

In regard to the number of layers, we fixed on four, namely first, molecular layer; second, layer of the small pyramids; third, layer of the large pyramids; fourth, layer of the polymorphic cells. We must not forget that in the referenced studies, we alluded at that time to the cortex of smooth-brained mammals; in the gyrencephalic mammals and particularly in man, the number of layers is larger.

For his part, Retzius[8] had the merit of confirming and extending in the human cortex many of [our] cited findings, adding very interesting facts, especially in regard to the unique cells of the first layer and to the disposition and development of the neuroglia.

Furthermore, in referring to special points on the structure of the layers of cortex in general, the later investigations of [K.] Schaffer,[9] Bevan Lewis,[10] and Veratti,[11] performed with the Golgi method, also deserve mention and confirm, at least in part, the facts discovered by Golgi, us, and Retzius.

[E.] A. Schäfer[12] adopted for the cortex in general the five layered division of Meynert, with the only variation being to call the fourth or granular layer the *layer of the polymorphic cells,* a designation that causes confusion because it has already been used for other layers (the second and the last) by us, [K.] Schaffer, and Schlapp.

With regard to the motor cortex, Schafer affirms, confirming the ideas of Betz and of Bevan Lewis, that its anatomic uniqueness rests on the presence of large pyramids arranged in clusters; and [he] copies from Lewis a figure that reproduces a section of the motor cortex, in which the fourth or granular layer is lacking.

Hammarberg,[13] whose important work we have already mentioned in our study on the visual cortex, distinguishes in the human cortex a sensory type and a motor type. He assures [us], moreover, that the motor cortex is characterized by lacking completely or almost completely the grains or the fourth layer of Meynert, being here replaced by the giant cells of Betz. However, in his drawings (consult [his] plate 1, fig. 2, which corresponds to the precentral gyrus), this authority illustrates some grains in the fourth layer of Meynert, and he places beneath these the giant cells of Betz; thus, implicitly, he recognizes in the motor cortex the existence of six layers, since he subdivides the fifth layer of Meynert into two strata or planes: *superficial,* where the Betz cells are located, and *deep* or [stratum] of the fusiform cells of Meynert. That the granule cells exist even in the motor cortex is something that, in spite of his reservations, Hammarberg himself also recognizes in some passages of his work. In short, from the descriptions and figures of Hammarberg, it is deduced that the motor cortex has the same layers as the association cortex, namely, first, molecular; second, of the small pyramids; third, of the large and medium pyramids; fourth, of the granule cells; fifth, of the cells of Betz and medium pyramids; and sixth, of

the fusiform cells. In addition, Hammarberg seemed to ignore the earlier investigators who used the Golgi method, [namely] Golgi, Martinotti, ourselves, and Retzius, since he neither mentions them nor tries to reconcile the revelations of this method with those of the methylene blue [method] of Nissl, the only method used by this unfortunate Swedish histologist.

Very worthy of esteem is the study that Kölliker[14] in his book of histology dedicated to the structure of the cerebral cortex of man and mammals. This expert has applied primarily the methods of Golgi and Weigert, confirming not a few of the facts discovered by Golgi, Martinotti, ourselves, and Retzius, and revealing some new details that it will be opportune to mention.

Kölliker adopts, for the cortex in general, a division into four layers, namely, first, white layer poor in cells; second, layer of the small pyramids; third, layer of the large and medium pyramids; fourth, layer of the polymorphic cells. But, like Hammarberg, he recognizes also the existence, in some regions of the cortex, of two other layers intercalated between the layer of the giant pyramidal cells and [the layer of] the polymorphic cells; these are the fourth layer or the second layer of the small pyramids, and the fifth layer of the large and deep medium pyramids. These two additional layers appear in a figure in which Kölliker illustrates a section of a parietal gyrus stained by the method of Golgi. The motor region does not seem to have been identified in it. With regard to the details of the cells and fibers revealed by [Kölliker], we will deal with them in the course of this work.

Like Kölliker, Edinger[15] divides the motor region of the human cerebral cortex into four layers: first, tangential fibers; second, layer of the small pyramids; third, layer of the large pyramids; and fourth, layer of the small cells (corresponding to the polymorphic cells of other authors). In the latter layer, Edinger includes the layers of the granule cells, of the deep pyramids, and of the fusiform cells of Hammarberg. Moreover, although he does not describe it, Edinger reproduces the fourth or granular layer in an illustration of a section of a gyrus stained by the Nissl method.

Schlapp,[16] who has made a comparative

study of the monkey cerebral cortex, by the Nissl method recognizes in the motor region of this animal the following layers: first, of the tangential fibers; second, of the external polymorphic cells; third, of the parapygnomorphic pyramids (medium pyramids); fourth, of the pygnomorphic giant pyramids (large pyramids); [fifth], of the deep polymorphic cells. The layers of the granule cells and of the deep giant cells are therefore lacking in the description of this author.

Finally, although they do not refer particularly to the motor region but to the cortex as a whole, or to special points of view on cerebral structure, we must also cite, for completeness, Tuczek,[17] Zacher,[18] Bechterew,[19] Vulpius,[20] and Kaes,[21] who have examined the distribution and development of the myelinated fibers of the human cerebral cortex; Bottazzi,[22] who has made [the same] examination in several species of vertebrates; Nissl,[23] who has investigated with his own method the structure of the several kinds of cortical cells; Azoulay,[24] who has drawn very nicely the pyramidal cells of the adult human; Van Gehuchten,[25] who has confirmed in mammals many of the recent observations; Flechsig,[26] Sax, Righetti, Dejerine, and Siemerling,[27] who, with the degeneration method or with that of Flechsig, have examined the successive myelination of the nerve fibers, in order to determine the origin and course of the projection and association fibers of the several cortical territories; Ballet and Faure,[28] Dotto and Pusatteri,[29] and Marinesco,[30] who have tried to determine the origin of the pyramidal tract in the cortex by using the method of Gudden's atrophy or that of Nissl based on the cellular chromatolysis [occurring] secondary to section of the axon, etc.

As already recognized by Hammarberg, the motor gyri do not possess exactly the same structure. Omitting slight topographic differences, it can be said that two anatomical types exist in the motor area: that of the postcentral gyrus and that of the precentral gyrus.

Structural Type of the Postcentral Gyrus

When a transverse section of this human gyrus previously stained by the Nissl method is examined, depending on the place examined, the following layers are more or less clearly distinguished:

1. *Plexiform layer or layer of the horizontal cells.*
2. *Layer of the small pyramids* (superficial polymorphic cells of Schaffer and Schlapp).
3. *Layer of the medium pyramids.*
4. *Layer of the external large pyramids.*
5. *Layer of the small pyramids and stellate cells* (fourth layer of Meynert or granular formation).
6. *Layer of the giant and deep medium pyramids* (cells of Betz, ganglionic cells of Lewis).
7. *Layer of the fusiform and triangular cells.*

In certain parts of the motor cortex, especially at the level of the protuberant portions of the gyri (fig. 1) [*fig. 87*], the seventh layer thickens noticeably, [and one is] able to divide it into two substrata: one superficial, formed by pyramids of medium size and by triangular cells (fig. 1, 7) [*fig. 87*]; the other deep, poorer in cells, made up of vertical series of fusiform cells separated by wide radial bundles of nerve fibers. These appear in fig. 1 [*fig. 87*], which reproduces somewhat schematically a section of the middle segment of the postcentral gyrus of a man thirty years old; the last cells of this substratum extend in the axis of the gyrus down to the very commencement of the white matter.

The abundance of cells, or, what is the same, the relative development of the axonal and dendritic plexuses that separate them, is different in each layer. The packing of cells, and the [concomitant] poverty of plexuses, reaches its maximum in the second layer; these plexuses are quite developed in the third, but only in the fourth and sixth do they reach a large size, the cells being separated by wide spaces.

In the vertical or radial direction, the cells are much less separated, often forming radial series that are already evident in the second layer, being very accentuated from the fourth [layer] up. At certain points, pyramids are seen [which are] so close that one could say they are in longitudinal contact.

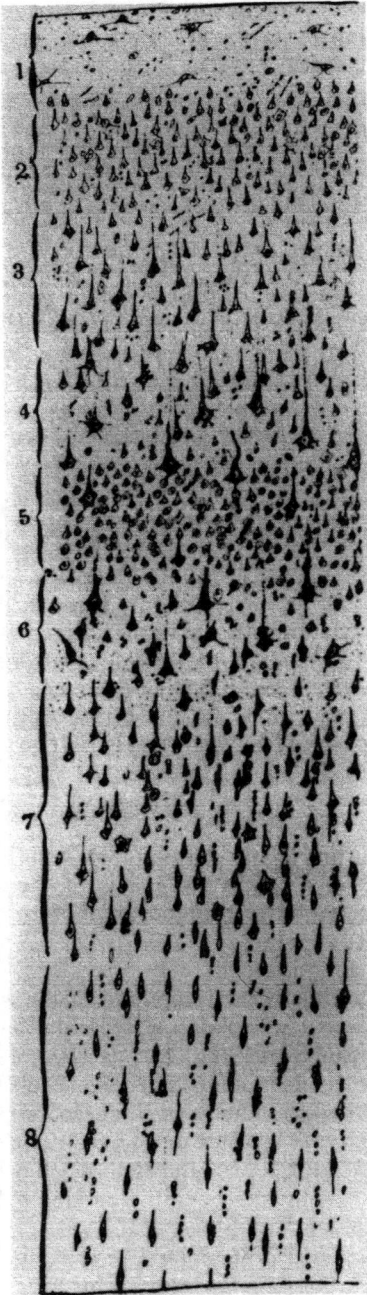

The richness of the intercalated plexuses is one of the characteristics of the human cerebral cortex; in the cat, rabbit, and mouse, the intercellular spaces are much more narrow. Moreover, these interesting plexuses consist principally, as we shall see later, of arborizations of endogenous and exogenous nerve fibers and of the ramifications of numerous basal dendrites. The latter factor is so important that, with some exceptions, it could be said that the transverse separation of the pyramids of a layer is in direct proportion to the number, length, and ramifications of their somatic dendrites. And since the length of these is related to the volume of the soma, it is also possible to affirm that the magnitude of the intercellular plexuses is in direct proportion to the diameters of the cell bodies. This law, applicable to all nervous centers, would be absolutely constant if the gray matter were to possess exclusively intrinsic elements; but the presence in many places of nerve plexuses of exogenous origin provides some [degree of] exception; [it also] leaves aside the fact that the intercellular spaces of the deep layers also undergo a notable enlargement as a consequence of the increase in long axons close to the white matter and independent of the volume of the somata.

With regard to the mode of distribution of the cells in the different radial [directions] of the gyrus, it is possible to see that all layers, except the first, increase their thickness in the convex portions [of the gyrus], and in particular the layers of large pyramids and of fusiform cells. It is recognized also that in the said convex regions, the transverse dimensions of the pyramids decrease, while, to the contrary, in the lateral and concave portions, these cells gain in thickness and decrease in height. Anyway, the cellular richness is more considerable in the convex portions than in the flat and concave regions.

The considerable thickness of the first layer in the funduses of the sulci is likely to be due to geometrical and mechanical conditions; on

[FIG. 87] Fig. 1. Section of the postcentral gyrus. Convex portion. Method of Nissl. 1, plexiform layer; 2, small pyramids; 3, medium pyramids; 4, external large pyramids; 5, layer of the small pyramids and stellate cells; 6, deep large pyramids; 7, layer of the fusiform and triangular cells; 8, deep portion of this layer, visible especially in the convex portions of the gyrus.

the one hand, to the convergent direction of the pyramids whose terminal tufts, because of the difference of radii between the superficial and deep limits, are concentrated in a reduced field of the first layer; and on the other hand, to the compression in the radial direction that such concentration seems to imply, and by which the tufts of the pyramids would gain in height what they lose in superficial extent. This compression of the gray matter at the level of the concave portions would perhaps explain, as proposed by Lugaro[31] for the cerebellar convolutions, the slight developmental retardation presented by the pyramids of the concave portions. It goes without saying that the contrary conditions (dilation of the cortex and difference in the opposite direction of the radii of the exposed surfaces) explain the thinness of the plexiform layer in the convex portions of the gyri.

Structural Type of the Precentral Gyrus

The precentral gyrus, the posterior extremity of the first and second frontal gyri, the superior contour or edge of the hemispheres (the upper end of the precentral gyrus), and, in part, the paracentral lobule possess, as we have already said, a stratification quite different from that which we have just seen in the postcentral gyrus. This explains the large differences in regard to the number and extent of the layers that we notice in the descriptions of the authors. In effect, in describing the motor cortex as a whole, some have taken as a base for their studies the postcentral gyrus, and others the precentral, believing, no doubt, that the structural plan did not undergo significant variations in the rest of the sensory-motor area.

For example, it is probable that Meynert, when he distinguished a true granular layer, alluded to the postcentral gyrus; while Golgi, Edinger, Kölliker, and other authors who do not mention that layer must have chosen as a base for their studies the precentral gyrus. We ourselves, in our first essays about the human motor cortex, focused principally on the postcentral gyrus,[32] presupposing an anatomical texture quite analogous in both central gyri. But, having later made a systematic study by the Nissl method of all the sensory-motor regions of the cortex, we have been convinced that the Rolandic fissure actually separates two motor areas with diverse structures, although this diversity does not go so far as to imply a special anatomical plan for each central gyrus.

To evaluate fully such deviations of structure, it is very convenient to examine, with the Nissl method, anteroposterior sections containing both central gyri; in this way, it will be easy to see in them the relative thickness of the layers and the disposition of the cells. If a comparison were to be made between gyri belonging to different individuals, the contrast would be less pronounced, and, in any case, differences relative to sex, age, and the unequal development of the cerebrum will perturb the results.

As can be appreciated in fig. 2 [fig. 88], in which we reproduce a transverse section of both central gyri of a woman twenty-five years old, the structural contrast affects especially the thickness and degree of development of some layers and the proportionate numbers of the cells. Let us indicate the principal differences layer by layer.

Plexiform Layer

It presents the same aspect in both gyri, but in the precentral it is rather thicker, by one-third or even by twice as much. Measurements made in several brains (convex parts of the gyri) give between nine and fourteen hundredths of a millimeter for the postcentral and between eighteen and twenty-four for the precentral. In the lateral portions of the gyri, the thickness increases, becoming double or even treble in the bottom of the fissures but maintaining always the differential thickness between the gyri.

The greater development of this layer in the precentral gyrus depends, according to what Bevan Lewis has suggested, on the distinctive contingent of pyramids of the underlying layers, all of which are represented in the first layer by a terminal [dendritic] tuft.

Layer of the Small Pyramids

It is somewhat thicker in the precentral gyrus, as shown in fig. 2 [fig. 88].

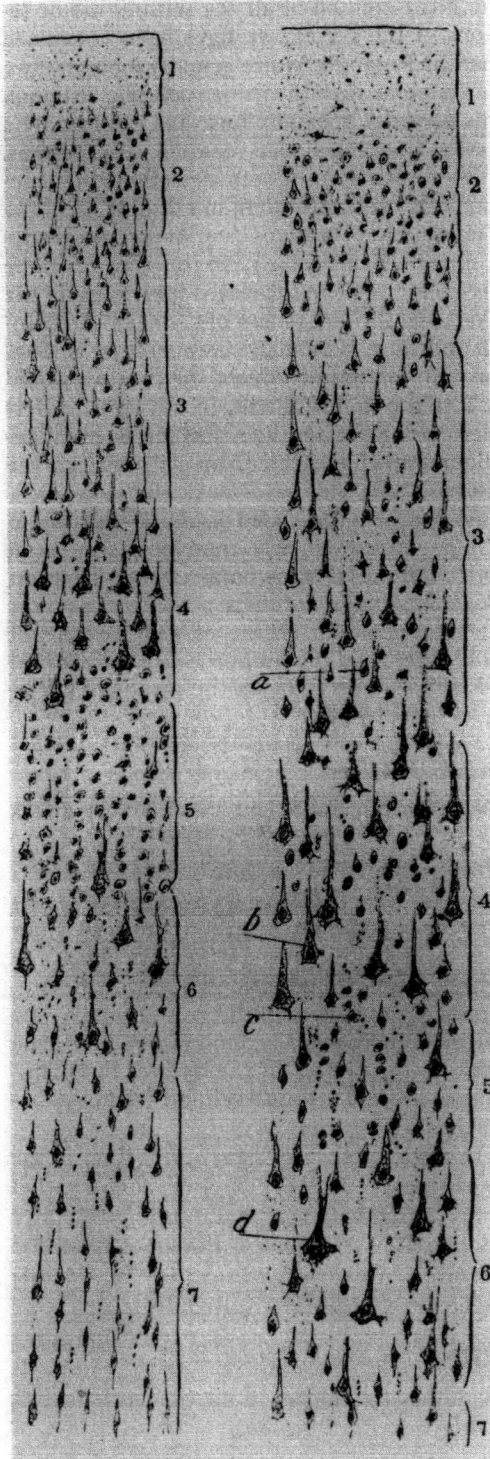

Layer of the Medium Pyramids

In this layer, the precentral gyrus differs from the postcentral in two important features: it possesses a greater thickness, which can reach nearly double, as shown in fig. 2^B [*fig. 88*], and, furthermore, its cells are more widely separated as a consequence of the great richness of the intercalated plexuses. In the deep portion of this layer, small pyramids and small stellate cells are very abundant.

Layer of the Superficial Large Pyramids

It also presents a greater thickness in the precentral gyrus in comparison with the postcentral, extending more deeply to the level of what in this area is the layer of the deep large pyramids. As a consequence of this, the number of superficial large pyramids is much larger in the precentral gyrus than in the postcentral. The unequal development, in both gyri, of the medium and large pyramids is well appreciated by measuring the thickness of the third and fourth layers together; this thickness ranges from [1.25 to 1.40 mm] in the precentral, while it only reaches from [0.70 to 0.80 mm] in the postcentral.

Layer of the Granule Cells

It is quite rudimentary in the precentral gyrus, with regions in which it cannot be distinguished. It is not surprising, therefore, that it has passed unnoticed by some, all the more so because frequently some sequences or small islands of large pyramids obliterate it by invading the terrain of the fifth layer to link the fourth with the sixth. But, in fact, although few in number, and not always associated in a continuous layer, the granule cells appear always in between the large deep pyramidal formation (fourth, fifth, and sixth layers), and

[*FIG. 88*] Fig. 2. Structure of the limiting gyri of the Rolandic [region]. (Method of Nissl.) The figure on the right corresponds to the precentral gyrus and on the left to the postcentral. *1*, plexiform layer; *2*, small pyramids; *3*, medium pyramids; *4*, superficial large pyramids; *5*, small stellate cells; *6*, deep large pyramids; *7*, layer of the fusiform and triangular cells.

they can be recognized with a good apochromatic [lens], thanks not only to their small size but also to the polygonal and spindle shapes that many of them possess. Sometimes, the granular formation, completely blurred in one place, is reestablished in another, appearing in the form of rounded or vertically elongated small islands. Such inequalities of the granular layer depend in part, in our opinion, on the irregularities of position of the superficial giant pyramids, which in the deeper part [of the fourth layer] trace a steplike or festooned line, going down at some points until they enter the domain of the sixth layer, and going up at others, permitting the reestablishment of some granular accumulations. In several regions of the precentral gyrus, it has seemed to us that the granule cells have partially emigrated over the superficial large pyramids. Anyway, there is no doubt that the deepest plane of the layer of the medium pyramids contains many small elements with short axon, with the same morphological properties as the granule cells, although they hardly ever form a well-defined stratification. Hammarberg has also seen small pyramids in it (*ganglionic cells* of this author). All of the diminutive cells, [which are] scarce in number, would thus form two irregular bands, which could be distinguished by the designations of *external granular formation* and *internal granular formation.*

With regard to the postcentral gyrus, the granule cell layer, according to what we have stated above, appears well developed, and it is constantly present at all parts of the gyrus. Its thickness does not reach, however, that possessed by the homonymous layer in the association areas. Contrary to the dictum of Hammarberg, who attributes to the superior portion of the postcentral gyrus the same properties as the precentral, we believe we have perceived a structure very similar in the whole postcentral gyrus; thus, the granule cells appear nearly up to the interhemispheric border.

Layer of the Deep Giant Pyramids

It reaches a much lesser development in the precentral gyrus than in the postcentral, as shown in fig. 2 [*fig. 88*]. In general, the pyramids here are not as voluminous as in the fourth layer; nevertheless, from time to time, there appears a type of large size that probably corresponds to the giant cells of Betz, [and which] Hammarberg also draws in this same layer (fig. 2, *d*) [*fig. 88*].

The largest pyramids found by us in the said layer inhabit the fundus and banks of the Rolandic fissure (precentral gyrus); their size ranges between 35 and 45 μm. The homologous cells of the postcentral gyrus reach only 24 to 30 μm. Otherwise, in this gyrus, the most voluminous pyramids are not those of the sixth layer but those of the fourth, in which we have found some with a size of 28 to 32 μm. It can thus be affirmed, with Betz, that the size of the pyramids increases in the regions situated anterior to the Rolandic fissure, although there exist some exceptions that we will specify when we deal with the association cortex.

Layer of the Fusiform and Triangular Cells (Polymorphic Cells)

In this layer, hardly any differences exist between the two gyri; it has seemed to us, however, that the layer is thicker in the postcentral than in the precentral gyrus. This compensates to some extent for the proportionately lesser development of the first four layers of the postcentral gyrus.

Fundus and Walls of the Rolandic Fissure

In order to observe the relative extent of each of these two types of structure, as well as the transitions that link them, we have studied, with the Nissl method, the banks and fundus of the fissure of Rolando. Our exploration reveals that both gyri keep their own structure until the very fundus of the fissure, in which there exists a region of transition where the anatomical characters of each are mixed. This region is characterized for its extraordinary richness in [blood] vessels of some caliber which dot with holes the full thickness of the sections, and for the enormous development of the plexiform layer. On crossing from the postcentral to the precentral gyrus, it is noted that the fourth layer, or layer of the superficial large pyramids, gains progressively in thickness, and that the granule cells, previously disposed in a well-marked layer, infiltrate between the said large pyramids, [so that the granule cell layer] loses its character as an independent formation. In the places where the large pyramids of the fourth layer form a gap, the granule cells reappear, constituting irregular small islands. But, in general, the small stellate cells are disseminated throughout the whole thickness of the fourth, third, and fifth layers, with some larger concentrations, however, beneath the large pyramids of the fourth layer, that is to say, constituting a rudimentary fifth layer. Near the above-mentioned region of transition are the largest pyramids of the fissure of Rolando and precentral gyrus. A special characteristic of the fundus of the fissure is the relative abundance of horizontal and especially of piriform or limiting cells in the plexiform layer.

We are now going to enter into a detailed examination of each cerebral layer, exposing the concordant revelations of the several methods we have used, particularly that of Golgi.

This description will be common to both central gyri; however, we must declare that most of the good silver chromate preparations that serve as a basis for the text and figures relate to the precentral gyrus.

First [or] Plexiform Layer

[When] examined in the adult human cortex stained by hematoxylin or with the Nissl method, [this layer] presents that well-known reticulated and pale aspect characteristic of all regions rich in axonal and dendritic arborizations. The cellular poverty of this layer was already noticed by Meynert, who believed he could recognize [in it] some small nerve cells with unknown properties; but in Meynert's time, the inadequacy of the methods did not allow one to appreciate the nature of the said elements, so that Golgi could, with the approval of many authors, take them to be neuroglial cells. Nowadays, when much more valuable analytical resources have been applied to the study of this layer, it is not permissible to ignore [the fact] that in addition to numerous cells of Deiters,[c] there exist in it, as Golgi discovered, some authentic nerve cells, the principal kinds of which have been discovered by us.

In fact, it is not necessary to resort to the methods of Golgi and Ehrlich to distinguish the nerve cells; even in Nissl or hematoxylin preparations, two classes of cell bodies are observed strewn in the thickness of the pale plexus: diminutive pale somata, bereft of clear processes, provided with a small nucleus, and corresponding to neuroglial cells; and more voluminous cell bodies, provided with obvious processes, endowed with a voluminous nucleus, which evidently represent nerve cells.

Under the 1.30 Zeiss apochromatic [lens], the nerve cells show some differences in structure, position, and form, which we reproduce in fig. 3 [fig. 89], in which three varieties of neurons can be observed: first, small cells with polygonal nucleus, scarce in protoplasm, devoid of [Nissl granules], and scattered in the whole thickness of the plexiform layer, although they are more evident in the superficial half (fig. 3, c, d) [fig. 89]. Such cells, around which two or three neuroglial nuclei sometimes lie, probably correspond to our cells with short axon (medium and small types); second, triangular or piriform marginal cells, possessing protoplasm quite rich in [Nissl] granules, and with several dendrites, one of which constantly descends (fig. 3, a, b) [fig. 89]. Such cells, which are very rare (in fig. 3 [fig. 89], have been reproduced the only two cells that were in the section studied), are, in our opinion, none other than the special marginal cells (Cajal'sche Zellen of Retzius, Retzius'sche Zellen of Kölliker), described by Retzius in the human cortex; third, finally, the deep half or the lower two-thirds of the said layer possesses certain relatively voluminous fusiform, triangular, or stellate cells (fig. 3, g, e, f) [fig. 89] which correspond, positively, to our deepest horizontal, fusiform, or triangular cells (special cells of Cajal and Retzius, situated in lower levels of the first layer). The nucleus of such cells is oval or triangular in section, and contains a loose-stained mesh and one or two clearly apparent nucleoli. Around the protoplasm, which possesses some thin

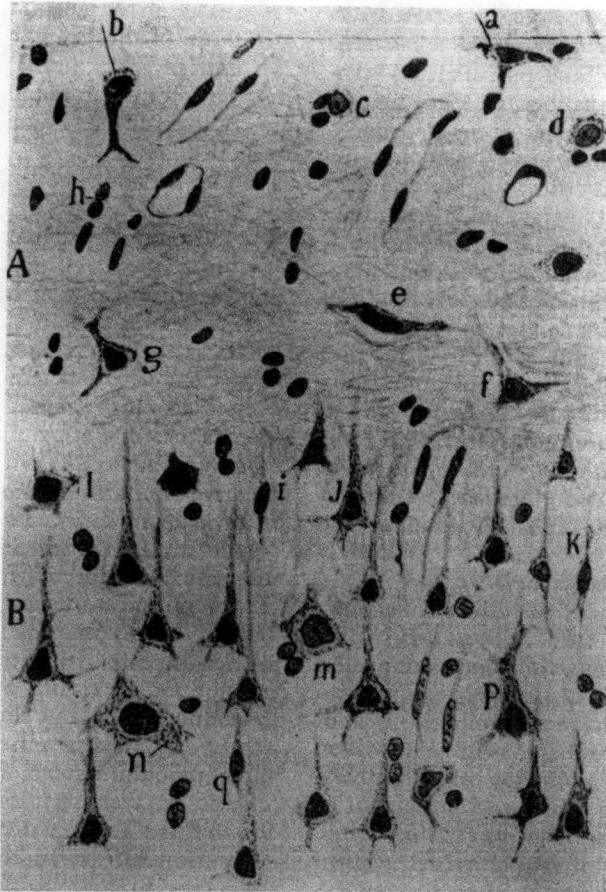

[*FIG. 89*] Fig. 3. Cells of the first and second layers of the precentral gyrus. (Method of Nissl.) 1.30 Zeiss objective. *A*, plexiform layer; *B*, layer of the small pyramids; *a*, *b*, piriform or triangular marginal cells; *c*, *d*, small cells with short axon; *e*, *f*, *g*, horizontal cells; *h*, neuroglial cells; *i*, *q*, *k*, fusiform or bitufted cells; *m*, *n*, *l*, large cells with short axon; *p*, true pyramids. (In the molecular layer, the nerve cells shown are from an area three times larger.)

[Nissl] granules, the surrounding [neuropil] is retracted.

It is not possible to confuse the minute neuroglial cells scattered in the first layer with any of these nerve cells. Besides the smallness of the nucleus, a feature quite distinctive of the cells of Deiters, this [neuroglial] cell is characterized, according to what we have pointed out in other work,[33] by the disposition of the nuclear chromatin, which, instead of forming central frames or blocks as in the neurons, constitutes a peripheral net which, on focusing through it, has the appearance of a mem-brane of nuclein. [The cell] also lacks the large nucleolus so common in neurons.

For the rest, the Nissl preparations also show that the neuroglial cells are disseminated almost equally throughout the whole thickness of the plexiform layer, and not especially concentrated beneath the pia as some authors have supposed (fig. 3) [*fig. 89*]. Not uncommonly, they are disposed in series of three or more, and some of them appear to accompany the capillaries, as pointed out by Andriezen.[34]

If, instead of the method of Nissl, we apply that of Weigert, we will observe, as was recognized some time ago by Kölliker,[35] Exner,[36] and others using the methods of potassium and osmic acid, tangential medullated fibers, some of considerable caliber. In these preparations, the plexiform layer appears divided into three planes: submeningeal rim, free of medullated fibers, according to Martinotti,[37] and rich in neuroglial fibers; a middle stratum thicker than the first, in which lie thick horizontal medullated fibers; and an inferior stratum, which in some places is almost as thick as the middle stratum, and is composed of scarce, thin, myelinated fibers that are irregularly oriented, although with a dominant horizontal direction. Where these fibers are condensed in the deeper part, a special zone or lamina, is formed—the *stria of Bechterew*, described by Kaes. In the motor region of the cortex, this stria seems to us to be lacking or to be very rudimentary.

The Weigert preparations do not illustrate sufficiently the origin of all of these fibers for us. But comparing such preparations with well-impregnated Golgi [preparations], one is easily convinced that the thick tangential fibers belong to the large horizontal cells and represent their medullated and very long axons, as we stated in our first work on the cortex and as confirmed recently by Bottazzi. It is true that there are authors like Kölliker who admit the possibility that such thick myelinated fibers come from the deep cerebral layers and even from the white matter; but this opinion vies with the fact that the caliber of the ascending fibers arriving at the first layer is constantly smaller than that of the thicker tangential fibers. Let us add that the level at which the ascending or Martinotti fibers turn horizontally is almost always lower than that corresponding to the robust horizontal fibers.

To proceed further with the structural analysis of the plexiform layer, it is necessary to resort to the method of silver chromate applied, according to what we have said earlier, to the child of a few days. This method allows us to recognize in the said layer the following elements:

1. The [dendritic] tufts of the pyramidal cells of all the underlying layers, including those formed by the radial [dendritic] shafts of the deepest cells, that is to say, those of the layer of fusiform cells (seventh layer).
2. The terminal [dendritic] tufts of some cells with short axon in the second and third layers.
3. The dendrites and axons of the intrinsic horizontal cells.
4. The dendrites and axonal ramifications of the intrinsic cells with short axon.
5. The terminal arborizations of the ascending fibers of Martinotti and of the fibers from the white matter.
6. The neuroglial elements.

Terminal Tufts of the Pyramids

Golgi and Martinotti have already observed that the [dendritic] shafts of some pyramids arrive at the plexiform layer of the cerebrum, and they even reproduce in the illustrations attached to their works some ramifications of the same; but only we[38] in mammals and Retzius in man have demonstrated the true disposition of the terminal portion of the shaft. This shaft does not end in sharp-pointed, vertical branches, linked to vessels or to neuroglia, as Golgi thought; instead, when they arrive at the plexiform layer, and sometimes before, they devolve into a tuft of dendrites that in coming away, naturally, at acute angles, do not delay in becoming more or less horizontal, sometimes running over long trajectories through the various levels of the layer. The contour of these branches, as well as the shaft from which they arise, bristles with simple or bifurcated collateral appendages, as we first demonstrated with silver chromate and later with methylene blue. Such appendages, whose free termination is as evident in the preparations of Golgi as in those of Cox and Ehrlich, have been erroneously estimated by Hill[39] to be the beginning of an incompletely stained interstitial plexus.

The extent, shape, and robustness of the dendritic tufts present large variations even on those which belong to cells of the same layer; thus, for example, there are diffuse tufts widely extended in the horizontal direction but poor in branches; others are more abundant in dendrites but occupy a less extensive field; finally, there are some formed by thick branches, whereas others present thin threads of short length.

It is very difficult to classify all of these forms into dominant types because of the transitions that [occur from one to the other], and [it is] more difficult still to determine to which cells they belong, since, as we have already said, the pyramids of the same layer can exhibit different tufts; nevertheless, it is possible to affirm that the tufts formed by thick and long branches belong to superficial and deep giant pyramids; that the ones formed by ascending thin branches [that are] varicose, relatively poor in spines, and extended up to near the pia correspond to superficial small or medium pyramids; that the dense tufts of thin thread[-like dendrites], but bearing long spines, must be attributed to the more superficial bitufted cells (fig. 4, F, J) [fig. 90]; that, finally, the thin varicose fibers poor in spines, and ending in an undivided or very moderately ramified tip (fig. 4, H, I) [fig. 90], belong to the cells of the deepest layers (pyramidal, fusiform, and triangular cells of the sixth and seventh layers and small pyramids of the fifth).

With regard to the levels of the plexiform layer to which the tufts of each layer of pyramids correspond, Bevan Lewis notes that the dendrites of the small pyramidal cells (layer of polygonal cells of this author) are given off in the lowest level of the said layer, whereas the tufts of the medium and large pyramids are distributed preferentially in the superficial part. Our studies in man have convinced us that there is so much variation in this that it is impossible to assign with any certainty special levels of the plexiform layer to each stratum of pyramids. The only thing that it is possible to affirm is that the tufts of the medium and small pyramids occupy with some frequency levels higher than those of the larger [pyramids], a disposition that is also observed in the visual cortex. But there is no lack of tufts of large pyramids that extend throughout almost the whole thickness of the first layer, as can be seen in the preparation reproduced in fig. 4, G [fig. 90].

Are all the pyramids represented in the first layer by a terminal tuft?

Previously, Golgi believed he had observed

that the shafts of the pyramids of the deep third of the cortex did not reach the first layer, and we, Retzius, and Kölliker were in favor of such an opinion. Nevertheless, the careful study of excellent preparations of the cerebrum of the cat of fifteen days to one month, and of the human cortex on the thin or concave portions of the gyri, has revealed to us that every pyramidal, fusiform, or triangular cell with long axon, irrespective of the layer it inhabits, is represented in the plexiform layer by one or several dendrites. The difference between the superficial and deep cells rests on the first sending a robust tuft to the said layer, whereas the second only sends a poorly or nonramified filament. That is to say, the deep cells (sixth and seventh layers) assign the greater part of the collector apparatus to the middle and deep layers (fourth, fifth, sixth, and seventh layers), reserving for the first layer only a thin appendage; while, by contrast, the large pyramids of the sixth layer and the medium and small pyramids of the fourth, third, and second send the major part of the cellulipetal arborization to the plexiform layer. All of these morphological peculiarities and many others that we have to refer to in relation to the cells with short axon can be summarized in these two propositions, whose generality suffers from very few exceptions: first, the neurons with long axon have a radial orientation, and send a plumed fiber or [dendritic] shaft to the plexiform layer; second, the neurons with short axon affect a nonradial direction and lack a shaft or tuft destined for the molecular layer.

Horizontal or Special Cells of the First Layer

These singular elements, discovered by us in the cortex of small mammals and confirmed by Retzius in the human cerebrum, are also found in great abundance in the whole motor cortex. Since we have dealt with them already in our study of the human visual area, here we will merely add some details obtained from our recent preparations.

Of course, we have confirmed in the said cortex the opinion already expressed in another work,[40] namely that the majority of the

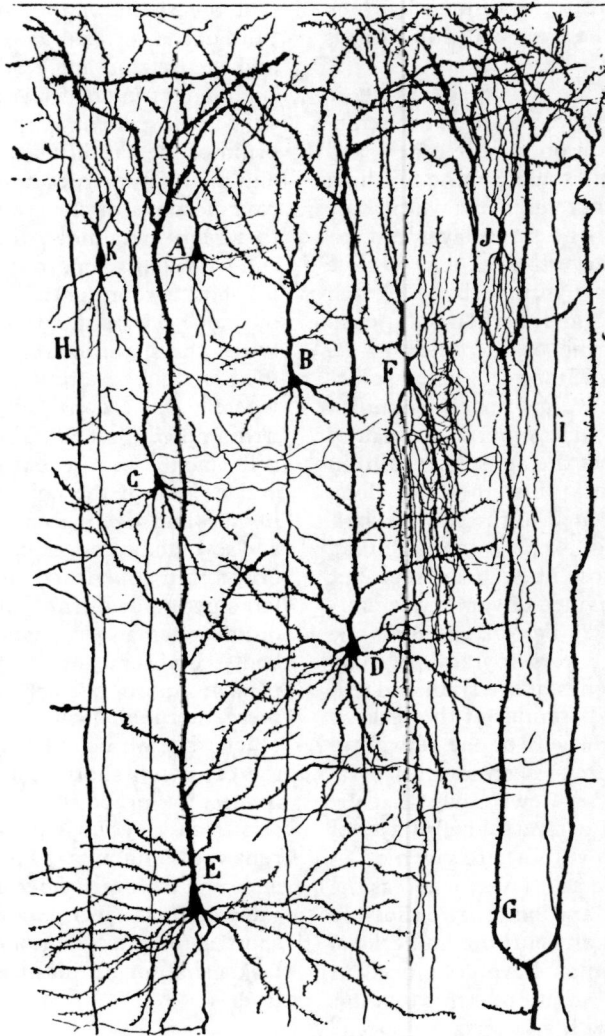

[*FIG. 90*]   Fig. 4. First, second, and third layers of the precentral gyrus of the cerebrum of a child of one month. *A, B, C,* small pyramids; *D, E,* medium pyramids; *F,* bitufted cell, whose axon formed terminal nests; *G,* dendritic shaft emanating from a large pyramid of the fourth layer; *H, I,* thin dendritic shafts of cells of the sixth and seventh layers; *J,* small bitufted cells; *K,* fusiform cell with long axon.

ascending branches arising at a right angle from the tangential fibers constitute an embryonic disposition that disappears or is transformed in the days following birth.

The special cells of the child of one month [are] devoid of almost all of these innumerable nail-shaped vertical small branches and present an aspect very different from that in the fetus, as can be noticed in fig. 5 [*fig. 91*], where we reproduce several cells of this kind taken from the precentral gyrus. Among the surviving processes, there are three categories: first, short dendrites arising from the soma or from the thick dendritic shafts, and ending freely at a short distance (fig. 5, *c*) [*fig. 91*]; second, quite long tangential fibers, arising now from the

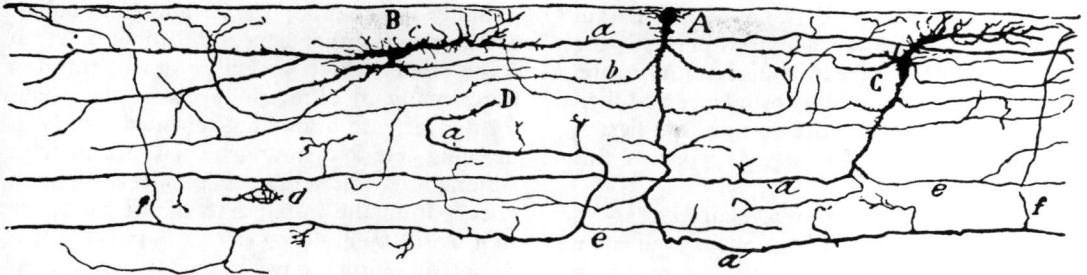

[*FIG. 91*]   Fig. 5. Some horizontal cells of the first layer of the motor cortex (precentral gyrus) of the child of more than a month. *A*, marginal or piriform cell; *B*, bipolar cell; *C*, triangular cell; *D*, axon of a nonimpregnated cell; *e*, thick initial collaterals; *d*, branches terminating in short varicose ramifications; *b*, tangential or long dendrites; *c*, short dendrites.

soma, now from some descending dendritic shaft, and which, after branching prolifically, terminate freely in the different levels of the plexiform layer, and preferentially in the most superficial part (fig. 5, *b*) [*fig. 91*]; and, finally, a robust fiber, arising from a pole of the fusiform or deep triangular cells or from a descending shaft of the piriform or marginal cells, which runs horizontally for a very long trajectory. Now then, the first two kinds of processes, which, because they are sketched out in the fetal period, were already seen and well-represented by Retzius, likely correspond to dendrites; and this is vouched for also by the fact of their being covered over a rather large part of their trajectory, with some appendages or collateral spines; but the last kind [of process], that is to say, the robust and long fiber, probably represents the axon (fig. 5, *a*) [*fig. 91*].

In the fetus and newborn child, the identification of the axon is almost impossible, because all the cellular processes exhibit an equally smooth aspect, maintain the same direction, and give off small branches at right angles terminating underneath the pia. The close packing of the cells and the prodigious number of tangential fibers are also a cause of obscurity. In addition, as the cerebrum develops, the horizontal cells suffer an important change, whose steps are as follows. Many of the short ascending dendrites that ended beneath the pia are atrophied, being transformed into short processes, freely ending in the thickness of the plexiform layer; some of the long

horizontal dendrites, without losing their original directions, seem to become greatly shortened, since it is now possible to follow them until their terminal branches, and they do not now arise at right angles, but at varied angles, and neither do they end exclusively underneath the pia, but in different levels of the first layer (fig. 5) [*fig. 91*]. Finally, in the midst of so many changes, there is a process that maintains its smoothness, original direction, and [propensity] to give off branches at right angles, acquiring progressively the exclusive features of an axon. This process, which in the adult appears enclosed in a myelin sheath, is so long that in certain cases we have been able to follow it over two to four millimeters without any indications of it being about to terminate. Thus, at present, we believe *that the true characteristic of the axon of the special cells is its enormous length and, therefore, the perfect maintenance of its individuality for a very long distance, in spite of the collaterals that it gives off.* Conversely, the tangential dendritic fibers do not maintain their individuality for long distances, suffering numerous bifurcations at acute angles and freely ending in the thickness of the layer under study.

The process which at present we estimate to be an axon has already been represented by us in mammals, and especially by Retzius in man; but the absence of a highly pronounced morphological differentiation and the almost equivalence in length shown in the fetal cerebrum by the long tangential axon and dendrites caused Retzius, no less than us, a few doubts. Anyway, there is no doubt that in many cells Retzius saw and drew perfectly the axon, which he represents descending to the deepest levels of the plexiform layer and then running in a horizontal direction (see figs. 2, 3, and 4 of plate XV in the paper of this author).[41]

The study of the axon is relatively easy in the cerebrum of the child of one or one and a half months, thanks to a change that occurs in the impregnability of the special cells. Instead of all the processes of the horizontal cells being stained, as in the fetal period, their axons and collaterals almost exclusively attract the silver chromate; [this is a] circumstance that establishes already a difference in chemical organization between the two categories of fibers. In such preparations, it is seen that the axon is generally very robust (in many cases, its diameter is more than twice that of the thicker fibers of Martinotti); moreover, it is observed that its initial trajectory is often descending, tracing not a few times a large turn (fig. 5, D) [fig. 91], from whose salient angle or curve a long collateral which runs in the opposite direction to the axon occasionally arises. Finally, it is observed that the principal branch or trunk, once it becomes horizontal, traverses a very long distance without ever descending out of the plexiform layer, in which, as a general rule, it always occupies the same level. Besides these thick axons, there is no lack of other thinner [axons], originating from horizontal cells of smaller size. All of these thick and thin axons extend through the several levels of the plexiform layer; but the most robust seems to be concentrated in the middle third, a peculiarity that fits with the well-known fact that it is this portion of the first layer that exhibits the thicker medullated fibers in Weigert-Pal preparations.

The above-mentioned axons give off collaterals; in some, they are very rare, it being possible to reveal on them only two or three small branches over a distance of a tenth of a millimeter; in others, such collaterals are more abundant, two varieties of branches being distinguishable, as can be seen in fig. 5, d [fig. 91]: very short collaterals originating at right angles and terminating by means of bifurcated, thickened, short branches, or by a small, ap-

parently pericellular basket; and long collaterals, arising either at a right angle or at an acute angle, which go up or down, running horizontally in different levels of the plexiform layer, and branching repeatedly without us being able to distinguish their termination. Among the collaterals, those already noted, arising from the initial arch of the axon, are well worth mentioning (fig. 5, e) [fig. 91], [for these] sometimes have such robustness that they seem to represent branches of bifurcation of the axon. These thick branches almost always follow a direction opposite to that of the [primary] axon. Finally, some thick axons also show long, descending collaterals that penetrate the border of the second layer and ramify among the most superficial pyramids.

In conformity with what has already been shown by Retzius, the tangential fibers or long dendrites of the fetal cerebrum run in all directions, although always inside the confines of the first layer. The same happens with the axons; however, we believe we have often detected a dominant direction perpendicular to the general orientation of the gyrus; thus, in the central gyri, most of the tangential fibers run in the anteroposterior direction, covering the whole or a large extent of the convexity of the gyrus. The enormous length of such axons shows us that the horizontal cells constitute a system of external fibers of association, [running] not only between somewhat separated zones of the same gyrus but between neighboring gyri. It is also very possible that many of the robust and very long medullated fibers that we have revealed with the aid of the Ehrlich method in the cerebral first layer of the adult cat[42] represent axons of the horizontal cells.

With regard to the dominant morphological types of special cells in the motor cortex, they are the same ones Retzius pointed out in the human fetus and which we have described in the visual cortex of the child of a few days. There exist, therefore, the piriform or marginal type; the horizontal, fusiform [type]; the triangular [type]; and the stellate [type]. Some of these have been reproduced in figs. 5 and 9 [figs. 91, 95].

The *monopolar or limiting type* is already seen, according to what we said above, in Nissl preparations of the adult cerebrum (fig. 3) [fig. 89]. In Golgi preparations, it exhibits a triangular or piriform soma, from which some short dendrites originate, the uppermost of which are extended horizontally in the external limit of the plexiform layer; a thick descending shaft covered with some short dendrites having not a few spines, and from which arise some long arciform or horizontal processes (long dendrites or tangential fibers of Retzius), terminating freely in different levels of the first layer; a very robust axon that is a prolongation of the vertical shaft and is almost always installed in the deep third of the plexiform layer (figs. 5, A; 9, A) [figs. 91, 95].

The *bipolar type* also shows a soma often covered with short dendrites, and a thick polar process, from which emanate many short and long horizontal dendrites, and a very long process arising at the opposite pole and with all the attributes of the axon (fig. 5, B) [fig. 91].

The *stellate and triangular type* is the one that shows more morphological variations. From the soma arise three or more stem processes that quite promptly resolve themselves into many short and long horizontal dendrites, some of which have an arciform course and ramify and terminate in the superficial frontier of the layer under study. The complexity of the horizontal fibers makes the axon difficult to recognize; in spite of that, in some cases we have been able to reveal it, having noticed that it arises from one of the thick descending processes, becoming horizontal and running for an enormous distance. Sometimes it cannot be readily followed, because it takes a perpendicular direction with respect to the long dendrites; thus, when the dendrites are cut lengthways in the sections, the axon is sectioned crossways.

What forms do the horizontal cells adopt in the adult cerebrum? The great metamorphosis that these elements undergo in the fetal period, and the impossibility of impregnating them by the Golgi method beyond the second postnatal month in the child, obliges us to be somewhat cautious about this subject. Considering, however, that in the child of one and a half months the pyramids and other cells of the gray matter have already their definitive shapes, and that this is usually determined by

the time the collaterals of the axon appear well differentiated, and taking also into account that Nissl preparations show in the plexiform layer of the adult cortex cell bodies whose morphology, according to what we have said above, coincides with the above-mentioned horizontal cells of Golgi preparations obtained in the child of few days, we can [then] presume that the general form of such cells will subsequently suffer few changes; these will perhaps affect only the length of the processes and the relative positions of the somata, which could change somewhat in relation to the development and [final shaping] of the [dendritic] tuft of the pyramids and of the complete appearance of the arborizations of the fibers of Martinotti.

The possibility of such changes becomes a reality when a Nissl preparation of the cortex of a child of a few days is compared with another of the adult cerebrum. It is noticed, for example, that in the adult the distances that separate the nerve and neuroglial cells of the plexiform layer are much greater than in the cerebrum of the child, and the marginal cells (limiting horizontal or piriform cells) are also more numerous in the child than in the adult. Such differences stem, in our opinion, from two causes: first, that the first layer does not increase in thickness on account of the formation of new cells, but because of the growth of the processes of its constituent nerve and neuroglial cells, which would be separated successively as a consequence of the progressive differentiation of the [dendritic] tufts of the pyramids, [and this] is not complete, perhaps, until the adult period; second, that according to our investigations[43] and those of Schaper,[44] Athias,[45] and Terrazas,[46] the submeningeal zone or rim of the cerebral cortex is the place where the most embryonic cells of the plexiform layer lie, from which level cells could descend to the various levels of the first layer as they differentiate, in a manner similar to what happens in the cerebellum. Thus, it would not be at all strange if some piriform elements should represent embryonic forms of the stellate or fusiform cells, situated at a lower level, transforming during that progressive sinking that we alluded to with a loss of the monopolar shape. However, not all of the piriform cells suffer this change, because, by dint of exploring sections of the adult cerebrum, we have been able to reveal (method of Nissl), as mentioned above, some monopolar or triangular cells very close to the peripheral rim (fig. 3) [*fig. 89*]. One is also persuaded that the submeningeal border is the place where the most embryonic elements of the molecular layer are located by the finding, frequent even in the cerebrum of the child of fifteen days, of cells of short axon, with the shape of neuroblasts or in slightly more advanced phases (fig. 7, *E, D*) [*fig. 93*].

Similarly, it is very possible that even in the first days after birth, some horizontal cells persist in the neuroblast phase, which would explain certain pear shapes provided with bent and horizontal long processes that we have sometimes observed in the visual cortex (see [Cajal 1899a] fig. 5, *I*) [*fig. 68*].)

Cells of the Plexiform Layer with Short Axon

First described by us in the cortex of the rabbit and rat,[47] confirmed later with the help of methylene blue in the adult cat,[48] they have not been a subject of special verification in recent years. Thus, Retzius did not describe them in his classical works on the special cells of the plexiform layer of man. Kölliker does not seem to have seen them either, and Schaffer[49] and Bevan Lewis, who believe that they have impregnated them with the Golgi method, refer them not to the molecular layer but to the external portion of the second layer or layer of the small pyramids, a layer these authors designate with the name of layer of *superficial polymorphic corpuscles* (Schaffer) or of *polygonal cells* (Bevan Lewis).

In fact, neither Schaffer nor Bevan Lewis has seen our polygonal cells of the plexiform layer, and we are more convinced of this judgment when the mentioned authors talk about the arborization of the short axon of such cells, [for they] suppose that the largest part of the arborization is not distributed in the first layer, as we stated, but in the second layer or the layer of the small pyramids. The cells that Schaffer and Lewis have impregnated are the relatively numerous cells with short axon, located in the underlying layer (most external level), and to which we have also dedicated some attention in previous papers concerning the cortex of the cat and the visual cortex of man.

As we can see in fig. 6 [*fig. 92*], which we have taken from one of the mentioned works, the methylene blue reveals a considerable number of cells with short axon in the plexiform layer of the cat. They will perhaps be no less abundant in the human cortex; but, unfortunately, here it is not feasible to apply the method of Ehrlich, the only analytic procedure that reveals them completely. Even so, and in spite of the inconsistency of the silver chromate impregnation, the motor cortex of the child of fifteen to twenty days exhibits numerous cells of this kind, situated inside the limits of the first layer, as proven in figs. 7 and 8 [*figs. 93, 94*]. In fig. 7 [*fig. 93*], we reproduce several of the cells that inhabit an extent of a tenth of a millimeter in the same section. Although there are preparations in which they

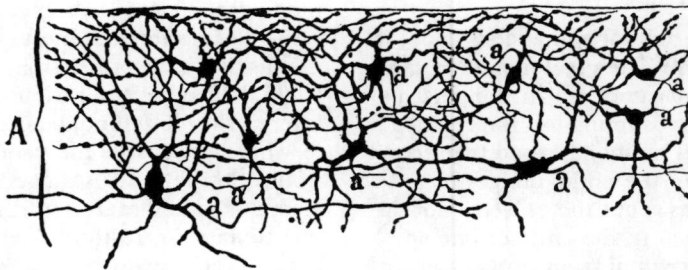

[*FIG. 92*]   Fig. 6. Cells with short axons in the plexiform layer of the cerebrum of the adult cat. Method of Ehrlich-Bethe. *a*, axons.

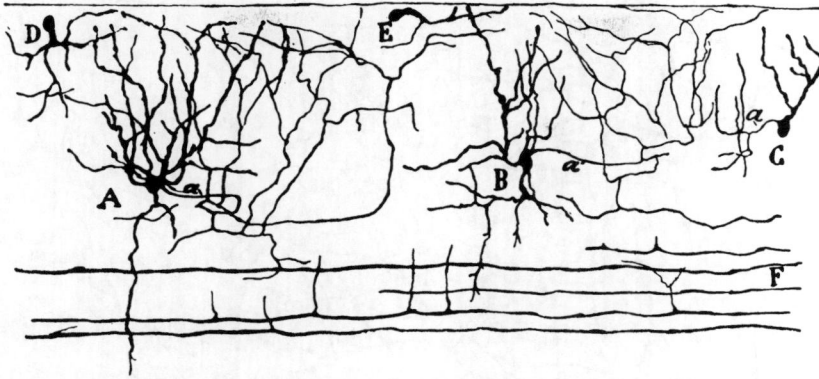

[*FIG. 93*]   Fig. 7. Several kinds of cells with short axons in the plexiform layer. Precentral gyrus of a child of one month. *A, B,* types of medium size; *C,* diminutive type; *D, E,* rudimentary cells with short axon; *F,* tangential fibers or axons of horizontal cells.

are numerous, it is necessary to confess, however, that in many cases, no doubt because of the excess induration of the superficial layers of the blocks or by virtue of other unknown conditions, the said cells fix the silver chromate less well than the underlying pyramids and even less well than the large horizontal cells.

We will not dwell thus on this point, superabundantly treated in our previous article, and here we will restrict ourselves to presenting some of the types that are observed in our preparations of the motor cortex. That their localization is in the thickness of and not beneath the first layer is proven by the fact that below them lie the long rows of tangential fibers, whose deep limit marks the true border of the plexiform layer.

The cells with short axon present a variety of forms: polygonal, triangular, stellate, and even ovoid. The latter, together with the piriform type, are typical of the smaller elements. From the angles of the soma arise divergent dendrites several times divided, provided with varicosities and spiny appendages (ordinarily they have fewer spines than the tufts of the pyramids), and extended through the whole thickness of the first layer, in whose more external part they are preferentially concentrated. With regard to the axon, it usually originates from a side of the soma or from a thick lateral dendrite, runs more or less horizontally, tracing some turns, and resolves itself into a

terminal arborization, whose branches are mainly ascending.

Although the morphological varieties of these cells are very numerous, it is possible, on the basis of their size and of the extent of the axonal arborization, to place them in four categories.

a. Medium Type or [Type] of Regular Thickness (fig. 7, A, B) [fig. 93]

This is without argument one of the most abundant cells of the first layer, in which they prefer the middle and deep levels. Their dendrites are mainly ascending, and the axon is almost always horizontal and distributed at no great distance from the parent soma.

b. Thick type

It is quite rare. In our preparations of the human motor area, only two cells of this kind are seen. Besides their exceptional size, these cells are characterized by the robustness and length of their dendrites, some of which are descending and go down through the layer of the small pyramids, ending in it or going on to the limits of the third layer (fig. 8, B) [fig. 94]. The axon is robust, runs clearly in a horizontal direction, giving off some collaterals and terminating in an unknown manner. It is probable that these elements correspond to certain large cells found by us in the plexiform layer of the adult cat (method of Ehrlich) and whose

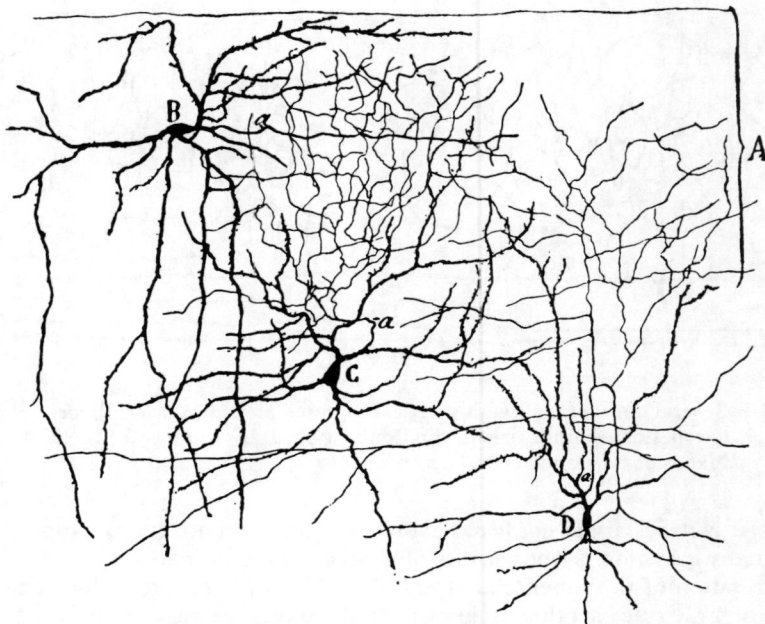

[*FIG. 94*]   Fig. 8. Voluminous cell types with short axons in the precentral gyrus (child of twenty-five days). *A*, plexiform layer; *B*, giant cells of this layer; *C*, large cell with ascending axon; *D*, cell whose axon is distributed in the first and second layers.

horizontal axon arborized inside this layer, but at a long distance from the cell body.

For the rest, the presence of spines up to the terminal portions of the dendrites and the absence of rigorously tangential processes enable one to differentiate clearly these large elements from the special or horizontal cells mentioned above.

[*c.*] *Diminutive Type*

Besides its smallness, it is characterized by its ovoid or piriform shape and by exhibiting a very thin axon, arborized in the surroundings of the cell (fig. 7, *C*) [*fig. 93*]. Some of these elements have in the child of fifteen to twenty days a very embryonic disposition, being situated close to the pia and showing a stem [process] divided in short small branches, among which it is not possible to distinguish clearly the axon (fig. 7, *D, E*) [*fig. 93*].

[*d.*] *Neurogliaform Type*

Similar to the dwarf cells described in the visual cortex, this element lies preferentially in the deeper half of the first layer, and it is clearly distinguished from the others because of the tight and very complicated, delicate, terminal arborization.

Ascending Fibers of Martinotti

They are very abundant in the human motor cortex, as proven by sections stained by the Weigert-Pal method, in which, as recognized by several authors, they are represented by thin medullated fibers which, arising from several layers of the gray matter, ascend, now vertically, now obliquely, up to the plexiform layer, where they become horizontal staying preferentially in the deep third, that is to say, beneath the thick tangential, medullated fibers (fig. 29)^D [*fig. 115*]. In silver chromate preparations, the fibers of Martinotti are quite frequent, it being noticed that they come not from pyramids, as was stated by [Martinotti], but from fusiform, triangular, or stellate cells provided with numerous ascending and descending dendrites, as we first demonstrated in animals with smooth cerebra. There exist several cellular types with axons destined for the plexiform layer. Here are those found in our preparations of the human motor cortex.

Fusiform or Voluminous Triangular Type

It corresponds to the cells properly called cells of Martinotti, and is localized through the whole cortex, as we will see below. Its processes are ascending and descending, but the ascending ones may or may not arise from a common shaft; they usually never reach the plexiform layer, nor do they give rise to a terminal tuft. The axon usually arises from an ascending dendrite (which confirms the law of conservation of matter) and, after giving off collaterals to several layers, reaches the first, where it bifurcates, giving rise to horizontal branches with opposite directions, or it bends to become horizontal and ramifies over a long

trajectory in the first layer. The collaterals of these horizontal fibers extend through the whole first layer, but it seems to us that they are especially concentrated in the lower half, a territory preferentially inhabited by the horizontal cells.

Dwarf Stellate Cell

Among the cells with ascending axon, there exists one, still not described, characterized by its small size and the form of its axonal arborization (fig. 9, G) [fig. 95]. It lies in the layer of the small pyramids and has a triangular or fusiform shape. Its very delicate axon ascends directly, and it resolves itself, when it reaches the lower frontier of the plexiform layer, into a plexus of very thin threads and narrow meshes, extending at least halfway up the first layer, but including also a portion of the second layer.

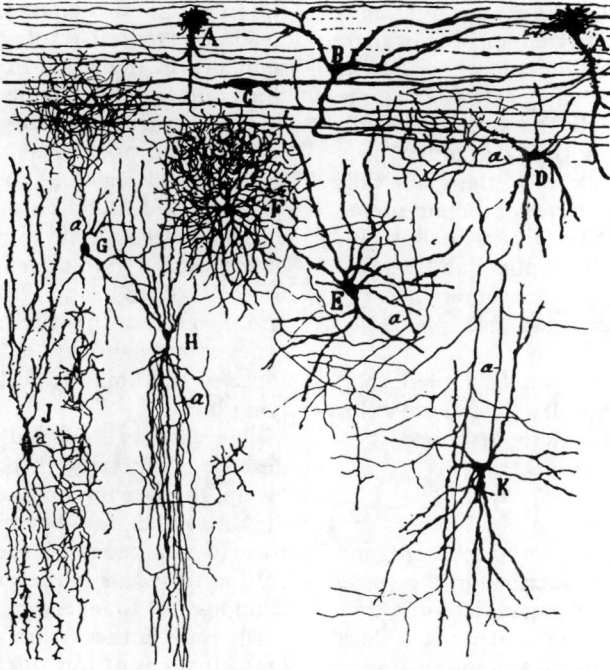

[*FIG. 95*] Fig. 9. Plexiform layer and [layers] of the small and medium pyramids of the motor cortex of the cerebrum of a child of one month. A, B, C, horizontal cells of the plexiform layer; D, E, F, cells with short axon of the second layer; G, cell with ascending axon to the first layer; H, J, bitufted cells; K, large cell with short axon of the third layer.

Cells of Medium Size and Diffuse Axonal Arborization

The just-mentioned cell is notable for the smallness of the soma and the tightness of the axonal arborization; in [the cell of medium size], the cell is larger, having much longer dendrites and a thin ascending axon, with a tortuous course, which resolves itself into an arborization with a broad extent of thin, flexuous, small branches that leave quite extensive spaces or meshes. This arborization also extends to the superficial level of the second layer (fig. 8, *C*) [*fig. 94*].

Second Layer or Layer of the Small Pyramids

This is one of the better-delimited layers of the cortex, being distinguished by the smallness and close-packed nature of the cells that inhabit it (fig. 3, *B*) [*fig. 89*]; when it is examined in good Nissl preparations with the help of the Zeiss 1.30 apochromatic [lens], in it can be recognized three kinds of cellular elements: legitimate pyramids characterized not only by their form but also by the abundance of [Nissl substance] in the soma (fig. 3, *p*)[E] [*fig. 89*]; large polygonal or stellate cells that are rich in protoplasm [but] poor in [Nissl granules] and which probably correspond to the giant cells with short axon in the silver chromate preparations (fig. 3, *m, n*) [*fig. 89*]; and finally, minute fusiform cells with elliptical and vertical nucleus, and which are none other than the bitufted cells with short axon (fig. 3, *K, I*) [*fig. 89*].

The Golgi method permits a complete analysis of the morphology of all of these cells, [each of] which will be briefly described.

Small Pyramids

They correspond entirely in shape, size, and characteristics to those described in the visual cortex. With a conical or pyramidal form, they give off at the base several thin dendrites, short in length and repeatedly dichotomized, and at the apex they form an ascending [dendritic] shaft, which is longer the deeper the location of the parent cell body. Naturally, those situated at the frontier of the plexiform layer possess a very short shaft, or they lack it, giving

off a tuft of dendrites very close to the soma; such a disposition is presented more frequently in animals (rabbit, cat, rat) than in man, where it is not rare to observe legitimate pyramidal elements, even at the very border of the first layer (fig. 3) [*fig. 89*].

When we dealt with the visual cortex, we referred to the motives by which [K.] Schaffer and Schlapp make the more superficial elements of this layer a nerve stratum which they call the layer of the *superficial polymorphic cells*. Bevan Lewis also recently accepts this subdivision, which has been based as much on the abundance in it of cells with short axon as on the irregular form of the cells improperly called pyramidal. This subdivision seems to us to be insufficiently justified, at least in man, for two reasons: first, because even when the cells with short axon are abundant in the superficial level of the layer of the small pyramids, they are present also through its whole depth, as well as in the underlying [layers]; second, because the lack of an [apical dendrite], and thus the triangular or stellate shape that is observed in some frontier pyramids, is a necessary consequence of their proximity to the first layer; third and last, because in the characterization of the layers and differentiation of the cells, the pure morphological criterion (form of the soma) must always be subordinated to the connections and direction of the axon and dendrites, criteria that in this particular case oblige us to regard the above-mentioned frontier cells of the second layer as legitimate pyramids, because the direction and other properties of the axon and dendrites coincide with those of the homonymous cells of the underlying layers.

The axon of the small pyramids is thin, it descends vertically through the underlying layers, and it is incorporated in the radial bundles in which the enormous distance of the trajectory impedes the identification of its arrival at the white matter; but if such an arrival is impossible to recognize in man, in those animals such as the mouse and rat in which the gray cortex is of less thickness, it is not a difficult task to visualize the continuation of the said axons with medullated fibers of the white matter.

During the trajectory of these axons, they give off, at the level of the second layer and even of the third, three, four, or more very delicate collaterals, which, in order to visualize in man, it is necessary to use the 1.30 Zeiss apochromatic [lens]. Such collaterals, which in animals are more robust, like the parent cells, divide several times, and the resultant branches run horizontally or obliquely in the thickness of the layer under study, traversing long trajectories. In the newborn child, these collaterals have not reached their complete development, and it seems that they may be lacking in some cells, a circumstance that explains well why Kölliker had not been able to find them. In fact, this scientist has made his observations, as is proven in fig. 726 of his book,[50] in cerebra [that are too embryonic] at a period during which the axons are still devoid of branches. We have already found collaterals in the cerebrum of the child of eight days; but only in that of one month or a month and a half is it possible to reveal the divisions and subdivisions of the collaterals, although it is not always possible to follow them to their terminations because of their extreme length.

A few collaterals arising from the axon of the frontier pyramids describe a recurrent course and send their small branches to the external limit of the second layer and even into the very interior of the first layer. K Schaffer[51] has given an exaggerated importance to this recurrent disposition which he has observed on the pyramids of the cat, since he supposes, in agreement with the opinion of Lenhossék on the cellulipetal conductor role of motor collaterals in the spinal cord, that the said cerebral recurrent fibers constitute a collector apparatus for [impulses][F] generated in the plexiform layer. The said author adds further that the dendrites and cell body would not have a role as conductors, in which he comes back, in a sense, to the opinion of Golgi and his disciples, in regard to the merely nutritive role of the dendrites and soma.

We already said when we dealt with the visual cortex that militating against the doctrine of the cellulipetal conductor role of the nervous collaterals of the pyramids is the fact that recurrence and the arrival [of the collaterals] at the plexiform layer is not the rule but the exception. In the motor cortex, this same fact is confirmed: most of the collaterals of the small pyramids are distributed in the thickness of the second and third layers, putting them apparently in contact with the somata and dendritic shafts of the congener cells. The retrograde course [of collaterals] has seemed to us to be somewhat more frequent from the deepest pyramids of each layer, which can be attributed to the fact that there are more congener cells in the superimposed planes than at the level where the parent cell lies.

It cannot be hidden that there is still much to elucidate regarding the functional significance of the initial collaterals. But if we remember the cases in which the connections of these fibers are better known, for example, [those of] the motor [axons] of the spinal cord, [those of] the axons of the Purkinje cells in the cerebellum, those originating from the thick axons of the giant pyramids of Ammon's horn, those emanating from the mitral cells of the olfactory bulb, etc., one feels inclined to consider such branches as a system of association among congener cells. The [impulse], arriving at the axon from the soma, would propagate to cells with an equivalent physiological role located in adjoining points of the gray matter, whose complementary discharge would perhaps be necessary to reinforce the initial [impulse] and increase the number of conductors of the cellulifugal nervous impulse. If such an assumption is admissible, the direction of the initial collaterals would be a merely adaptive consequence of the position of the collaborative cells in the discharge. Thus, in Ammon's horn (inferior region or [region] of giant pyramids), these branches are ascending (*ascending fibers* of Schaffer), because the collaborator pyramids lie in the superior plane of this organ; in the cerebellum, they are also ascending, because the cells of Purkinje reside in the same row and above the [level of] emergence of the above-mentioned branches, which are therefore obliged also to follow a retrograde course; finally, in the cerebrum and other centers, the vast majority of the collaterals assume a horizontal or oblique direction with respect to the plane of the gray matter, because almost all of the cells with equal physiological significance inhabit the same stratum and equal or neighboring cellular rows.

We must not, however, pass over in silence the existence of collaterals that seem to be interrelated with cells of a diverse functional nature. Such happens with the granule cells of the fascia dentata, whose initial collaterals are distributed in an underlying plexiform layer inhabited by robust cells with long axons. This leads us to think one of two things: either that these collaterals have not the same significance as the initial [collaterals] of the cells with long axon, representing rather an early portion of the terminal arborization; or that there are definitely cells that, when they become activated, request by means of their initial collaterals the collaboration not only of congener cells but of cellular elements of a different physiological category. We are more inclined in favor of the first than of the second opinion; forcing us to this preference is the consideration that the above-mentioned granule cells constitute a special type of cell with short axon (its arborization is proximal, since it is located in the neighboring portions of the gray matter, establishing connections with [apical] shafts of giant pyramids), which enters into relationships, like all the cells of this kind, with cells of other characteristics, that is to say, with cells with long axons situated at no great distance. Hence, by means of the initial collaterals, the [impulse] arriving at one cell is propagated to other congener [cells], converting the individual discharge into a collective one; it is an idea supported by the fact that cells such as the ganglion cells of the retina whose conduction must be individual, corresponding to the essentially analytical function of the visual sense, lack initial collaterals. This same fact reveals how gratuitous is the opinion of [K.] Schaffer, when he adduces an exclusive collector role to the initial collaterals, since, if that were the case, the nervous [impulse] would not be able to pass from the retina to the optic nerve.[52]

Cells with Short Axon

They are very abundant in the second layer, being scattered irregularly through the whole layer, although they are found especially in its external half. The distinguishable cell types are completely similar to those described in the visual cortex. Among them are, first, large polygonal cells with robust axon; second, bitufted fusiform cells; third, arachniform or dwarf cells.

1. Polygonal or Stellate Cells

These cells, which correspond to those large, pale, and stellate somata that appear in Nissl preparations, show the same properties as the homologous elements of the visual cortex. In figs. 8 and 9[G] [figs. 94, 95], we reproduce some cells of this type, taken from the precentral gyrus. On the basis of the direction and distribution of the axon, it is possible to distinguish the following types: (a) stellate cell with more or less horizontal axon, ramified in the thickness of the layer under study and at quite some distance from the soma (fig. 8, D) [fig. 94]; (b) stellate cell with short axon arborizing diffusely in the vicinity of the cell (fig. 9, E)[H] [fig. 95], exactly reproducing the disposition of the so-called cells of Golgi, observed in the human cortex by this author, Mondino,[53] and Martinotti[54]; (c) stellate or triangular cells with ascending arciform axon, the arborization of which embraces a large portion of the second layer and part of the third (fig. 9, K)[I] [fig. 95]; (d) very robust stellate cells, provided with long dendrites and a descending axon ramifying in the lower level of the second, in the third, and maybe in the fourth layers; (e) robust stellate cell, whose ascending axon is distributed as much in the thickness of the first layer as in the upper part of the second layer (fig. 8, C)[J] [fig. 94].

2. Bitufted Cells

They are very abundant in the second layer, as shown in the Nissl preparations, in which they appear, as we said above, in the form of thin, oblong elements provided with an elliptical and vertical nucleus (fig. 3, K, i) [fig. 89]. In our preparations of the motor cortex stained by the method of Golgi, two varieties of these cells are seen.

a. *Small Bitufted Type* Its axon resolves itself into vertical ramifications of great length. This cell corresponds entirely to the one described in the visual cortex (fig. 9, H)[K] [fig. 95].

b. *Bitufted Type of Medium Size* (figs. 10, A, B; 9, J)[L] [figs. 96, 95]. Such a cell, whose soma is almost the size of that of the small pyramids, has already been seen by Retzius, as revealed by an examination of the figures in his works;[55] but this author does not give a particular de-

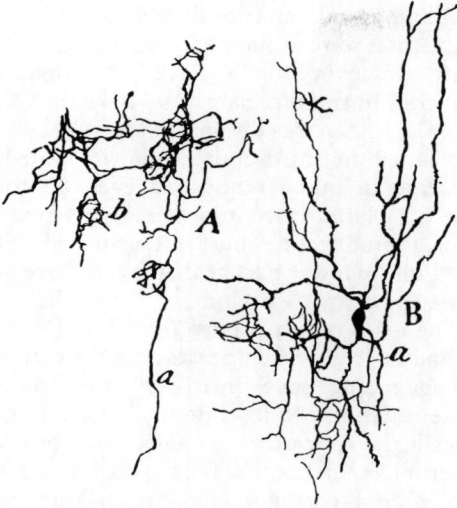

[*FIG. 96*] Fig. 10. Bitufted cells of medium size of the second layer. *A*, axon with pericellular nests impregnated in isolation; *B*, complete cell.

scription of it, simply considering it a small pyramid.

Such a cell, like the dwarf bitufted cells, shows two ascending and descending bundles of dendrites, but these are of greater thickness and are provided with long collateral spines. The ascending tuft is not limited to the second layer, but reaches the first, often extending up to the upper part of the plexiform [layer]. The axon is of medium caliber, and arises either from the upper or from the deeper part of the soma; and at a short distance, it bifurcates, and its divisions and subdivisions at a short distance from the cell engender a dense, varicose arborization, forming nests or nervous plexuses that surround the cell bodies of the small pyramids. In fig. 10 *A* [*fig. 96*], we reproduce in detail one of these axons that gave rise to six or seven nests. Fig. 4, *F* [*fig. 90*] shows another cell of the same type whose axon formed less individualized nests.

3. Dwarf Cells

They correspond to two varieties: (a) dwarf stellates, whose very delicate, varicose, and smooth dendrites can hardly be differentiated from the small branches of the dense arborization of the axon; and (b) stellate or fusiform cells, somewhat thicker, whose axon, which is

initially thin and ascending, gains in thickness on its way up and resolves itself into a very dense plexus, located in the external portion of this layer or in the very heart of the plexiform layer. When we dealt with the ascending axons or axons of Martinotti, we mentioned these singular cells, whose axonal arborizations together engender a very tight and continuous plexus, located at the point of transition between the first two layers.

Layer of the Medium Pyramids

This layer is relatively thick in the motor cortex and appears formed by the same cellular elements as the second (pyramids, small and large cells with short axon). But its pyramids are more voluminous, and among them a much more extensive plexus is observed whose composition we will examine later. In fig. 4 [*fig. 90*], we reproduce some pyramids of this layer, which are not very different, except with respect to size, from those located in the second layer.[M] In this figure, it can be noticed how the [apical] shaft, simple or bifurcated, reaches the plexiform layer, where it resolves itself into one or several tufts; and how the axon, which is descending, enters the radial bundles, after giving off numerous collaterals to the second and third layers. In some cells, we have counted up to seven collaterals.

Layer of the External Large Pyramids

As the third layer gets deeper, its pyramids gradually increase in diameter, and its basal dendrites reach a greater length and more complex ramification. At the level of the fourth layer (which it is not possible to distinguish from the third because of the transition between them), the pyramids reach their maximum thickness but keep the same shape and mode of branching. In these more robust cells, the soma shows a triangular shape with quite a wide base (compared with the pyramidal cells of the sixth layer), and from their contours arise thick and long lateral dendrites, whose direction is usually horizontal and oblique, and basal dendrites that are generally very robust and run an oblique, descending course (fig. 11, *4*) [*fig. 97*]. The [apical] shaft is usually single; there are cells, however, that

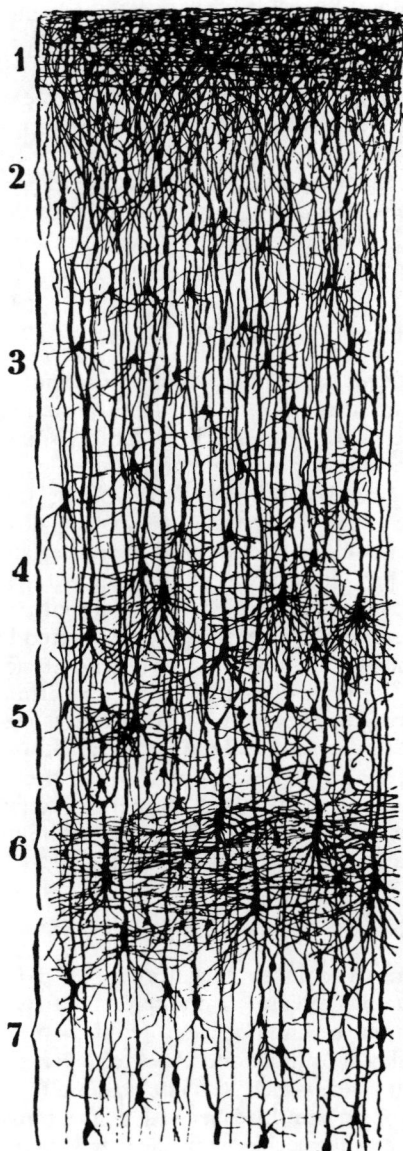

[FIG. 97] Fig. 11. Some layers of the postcentral gyrus of the child. *1*, plexiform layer; *2*, small pyramids; *3*, medium pyramids; *4*, external large pyramids; *5*, layer of the small pyramids and stellate cells; *6*, deep large pyramids; [*7*, medium pyramids and triangular cells]

have [an apical dendrite that is] double or bifurcated at some distance from its origin. This shaft, single or double, gives off numerous branches in the first part of its trajectory, that is, while it traverses the fourth layer; but when it reaches the third and second, its branches decrease in number and can even be completely lacking. Once it has arrived at the first layer, it produces a robust tuft, ordinarily confined in the lower part of that layer; there are, however, many exceptions.

The axon is very robust (fig. 12, *a*) [*fig. 98*], and at its origin often possesses a little inflexion shaped like an S; [it is] very wide and has some roughness to its contour that sometimes gives it the appearance of a dendritic process. After it has run the first four to six hundredths of a millimeter, the first collaterals arise, generally branching at an acute angle, and extending over such a wide territory that even in a child of eight days it is impossible to observe the whole arborization in one section. The number of collaterals ranges from four to eight, which are distributed preferentially in the fourth and fifth layers. Some recurrent small branches can also invade the third layer or layer of the medium pyramids.

Superficial Giant Pyramids of the Precentral Gyrus

The fourth layer is much thicker in the precentral than in the postcentral gyrus, as can be proven perfectly in the Nissl preparations. Furthermore, in the precentral gyrus, it is observed that the manner of branching of the somatic dendrites and of the [apical dendritic] shaft, possessed by the deepest cells of this layer, have a similar character to those of the giant cells of the sixth layer.

In fig. 12 [*fig. 98*], we reproduce the most common forms of these cells in the child of one month. The excessive development of the somatic dendrites that can be distinguished as basals and laterals is especially noticeable. The basals descend more or less obliquely and cover with their very long ramifications a large part of the fourth and fifth layers, and they can even enter the sixth; whereas those originating from the sides of the soma and from the initial part of the [apical] shaft run commonly trans-

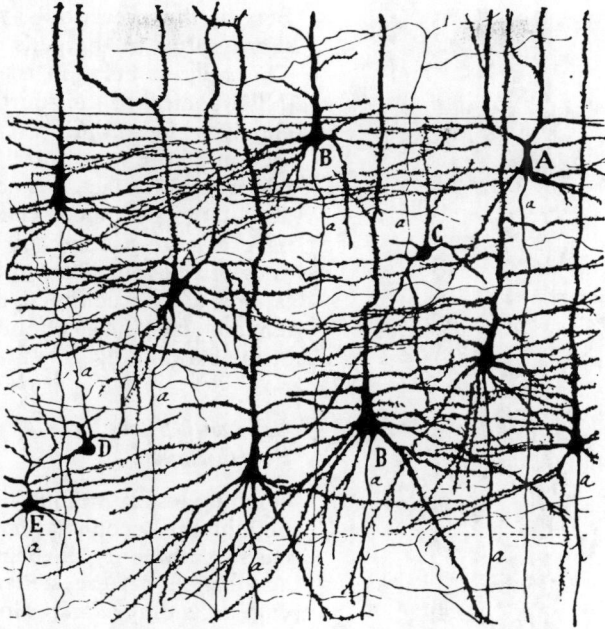

[*FIG. 98*]   Fig. 12. Layer of the external large pyramids of the precentral gyrus. *A,* pyramids with bifurcated shaft; *B,* pyramids with undivided shaft; *D,* cells with short axon destined for this same layer; *C,* cell with short axon distributed in the superimposed layer (superficial granular formation); *a,* axon.

versely, going through long horizontal trajectories and forming, by interweaving at very acute angles with those originating from neighboring cells, complicated dendritic bundles. The plexiform aspect and the relative cellular poverty of the fourth layer are mainly due to the extent of such bundles and to the enormous length of the dendrites. With regard to the [apical dendritic] shaft, it is robust and often goes undivided up to the plexiform layer, where it resolves itself into the well-known terminal bouquet. With respect to its ramification, the shaft can be divided into two segments: thick or initial part, situated in the sixth, fifth, and fourth layers, from which arise numerous horizontal dendrites; thin or superficial part, devoid of or very poor in branches, corresponding to the upper layers.

Often, the [apical] shaft is bifurcated in the thickness of the sixth or fifth layer, and the two branches are, with regard to their ramification [in the plexiform layer] like the undivided shafts. Sometimes, by means of further branching, four or more ascending shafts are formed that give rise to as many bouquets of dendrites in the plexiform layer, as shown in fig. 4, *G* [*fig. 90*]. Kölliker has also observed this disposition.

All of these morphological variations seem to us to be due to the necessity for multiplying the surfaces for reception of impulses. Hence, these surfaces of connection would not have the same extent in all the pyramids, it being very probable that those which give rise to several tufts and are represented in the first layer by means of an extensive horizontal ramification would also be the ones that receive a major flow of impulses from the terminal nerve fibers.

It is known, thanks to the investigations of Nissl, Hammarberg, and many others, that the somata of the large pyramids of the fourth layer have many very apparent [Nissl bodies]. We have revealed them already in the process of differentiation in the fetus of eight months, and they are well developed in the child of fifteen to twenty days. In general, the largest [Nissl bodies] appear first in the large cells of

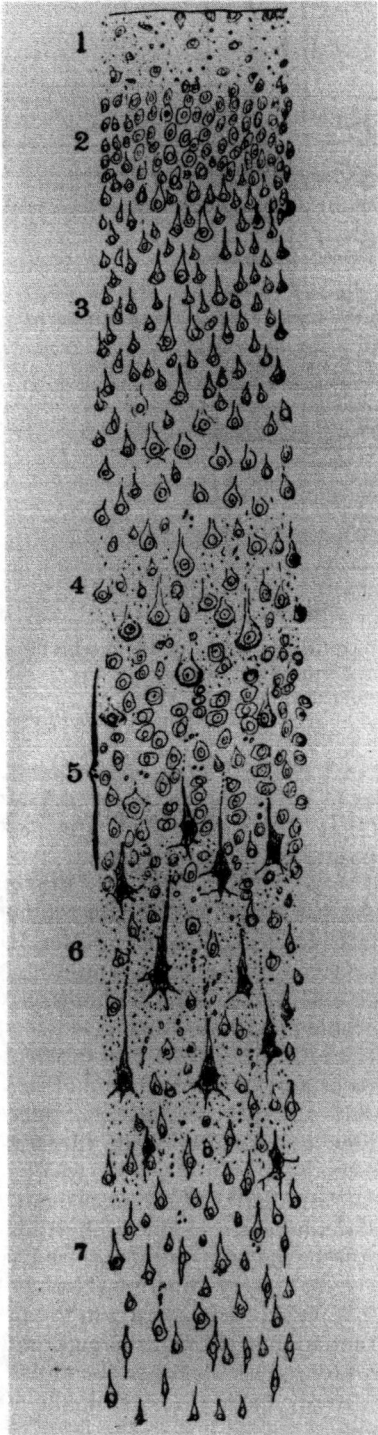

Betz of the precentral gyrus, and they arise shortly after in the cells of the fourth layer. This relative delay in the appearance of the [Nissl bodies] of the fourth layer can be seen clearly in fig. 13 [*fig. 99*], which represents a section of the postcentral gyrus of a child of fifteen days. In fact, it is noticed that while the deep large pyramidal cells of the sixth layer have a large number of [Nissl] clusters, the ones of the fourth enclose only small granulations, usually confined, by means of the violent action of the alcoholic fixation, to the base of the axon.

Cells with Short Axon of the Third and Fourth Layers

They are less numerous here than in the thickness of the second layer, but they are never lacking, three types being distinguished in abundance: (a) the stellate or fusiform type with ascending axon prolonged up to the plexiform layer; (b) the triangular or thick stellate [type] whose ascending, horizontal, or descending axon is distributed in the thickness of the fourth and third layers; (c) the bitufted type with its two varieties, small and medium. As we described these elements when we dealt with the visual cortex, and also in above paragraphs when we talked about the cells of this kind that are resident in the second layer, it excuses us from giving a new description here.

Fifth Layer or Layer of the Small Pyramids and Stellate Cells

Since the fifth layer, rudimentary in the precentral gyrus, appears well developed in the postcentral, it is there that we have preferentially focused our explorations with the Golgi method. The following description, based on the revelations of the silver chromate, will also be applicable to the precentral gyrus, to the

[*FIG. 99*] Fig. 13. Section of the postcentral gyrus of a child of fifteen days. *1*, plexiform layer; *2*, small pyramids; *3*, medium pyramids; *4*, external large pyramids; *5*, layer of the small pyramids and stellate cells; *6*, layer of the deep large pyramids; *7*, fusiform and triangular cells.

posterior portion of the first and second frontal gyri, and to the paracentral lobule, but with the following exception: the cells of the fifth layer, which in the postcentral gyrus are found in a well-delimited area intermediate between both layers of giant pyramids, are in the precentral gyrus irregularly disseminated in the whole thickness of the fourth layer, and especially concentrated above and below this, forming, in fact, two rudimentary and discontinuous granular formations.

To have an idea about the extent, number, and form of the cells of the fifth layer, it is suitable to begin with the study of Nissl preparations, in which already three classes of cells can be distinguished: voluminous and medium pyramids, few in number and completely similar to those located in the bordering layers (fig. 14) [fig. 100]; quite rare cells with triangular, stellate, ovoid, or semilunar shape, of large size and provided with abundant protoplasm and poor in [Nissl granules] (fig. 14, c, d) [fig. 100]; and finally, a multitude of close-packed minute cells, frequently arranged in vertical series (granule cells of the authors). Among these small [cellular] elements, the most abundant of the fifth layer, and responsible for giving to the layer its special physiognomy, are distinguished two varieties: (a) small pyramidal cells which Kölliker has succeeded in impregnating, although incompletely, with silver chromate, and which appear disseminated in the whole fifth layer, although being somewhat more abundant in its deepest levels (figs. 14, b; 15, A, B) [figs. 100, 101]; (b) minute stellate, ovoid, or fusiform cells, scarce in protoplasm, provided with pale, hardly perceptible dendrites, and often arranged in vertical rows or small islands. These cellular elements are distinguished from the small pyramids on account of their spindle shape and the shape of the nucleus, which is not triangular as in the pyramids, but spheric and ovoid, enclosing, instead of a nucleolus, a loose chromatic mesh. These nuclei are distinguished from neuroglial nuclei by reaching a larger size, and because their chromatin is not arranged in a peripheral mesh. Thus, according to what has already been said, the nucleus of these cells is similar to that of the smallest pyramids (second layer) and to that of the granule cells of

the cerebellum, all cells that have as a common feature the lack of centralization of the chromatin[N] (fig. 14, a) [fig. 100].

The method of Nissl reveals nothing to us about the disposition of the processes of all these cell types of the fifth layer; therefore, in order to complete our knowledge about them, it is necessary to resort to the method of Golgi, applied to the cerebrum of the child of fifteen to thirty days. In well-impregnated preparations, it is also confirmed that the fifth layer contains several kinds of cells, which can be grouped in two general categories: first, cells with long axon; second, cells with short axon.

Cells with Long Axon

a. Small Pyramids

Such cells, which have already been mentioned by several authors, correspond quite well to the type of small pyramid described by us in the sixth and seventh layers of the visual cortex. The minute soma gives rise to three, four, or more thin basal dendrites, ramifying at no great distance inside the confines of the fifth layer; from the upper part arises a thin apical shaft, which, after supplying some collateral branches to this layer, goes almost straight up to the plexiform layer, where it divides into a small number of thin dendrites, with few spines. With regard to the axon, which Kölliker does not seem to have seen, it leaves from the base of the soma, descends vertically, crossing the sixth and seventh layers, and very likely arrives at the white matter, continuing as a thin medullated fiber. Because of its length and delicacy, we have never been able to follow it further than underneath the layer of the deep giant cells.

The most interesting feature of these cells is the arrangement of their [axonal] collaterals. To the number of two, three, or four, such branches arise from the proximal part of the axon, and some acquire, after describing an arch with a concavity upward, a recurrent course, going up to the height of the fifth layer, with some of them passing beyond; perhaps they reach the first layer; however, the delicacy of their size and the great complexity of the superimposed nervous plexuses have made it impossible for us to follow them com-

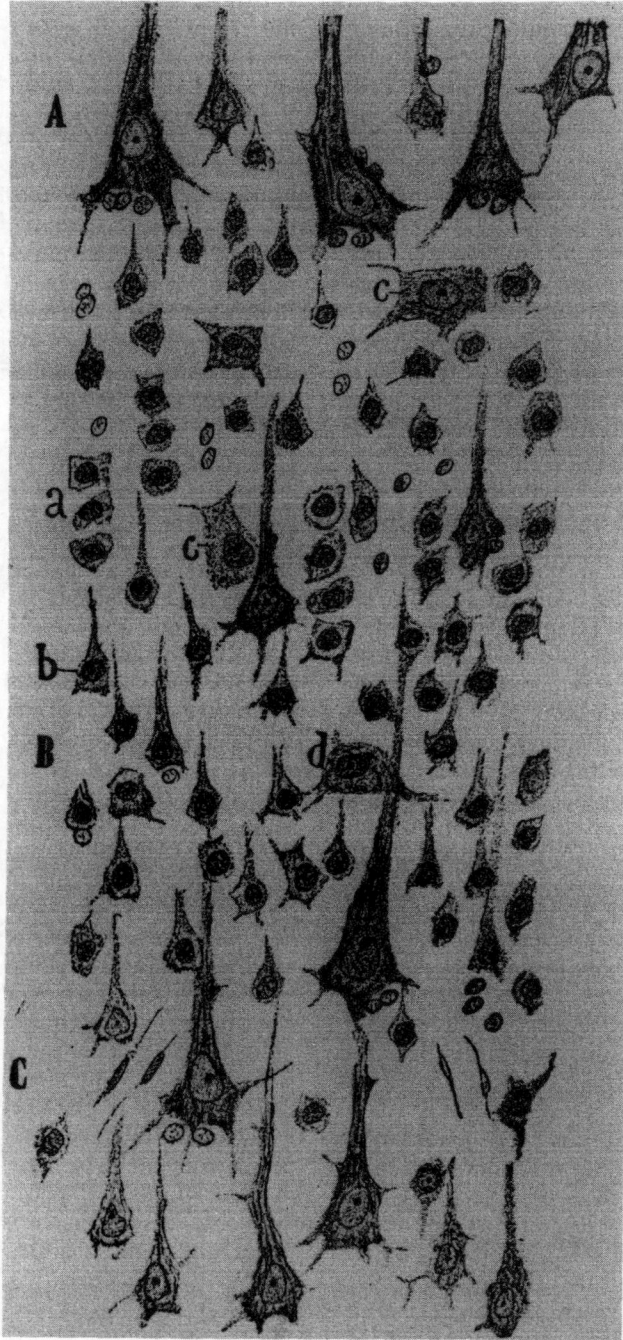

[*FIG. 100*] Fig. 14. Layer of the granule cells of the middle portion of the postcentral gyrus of an adult man. (Method of Nissl.) Zeiss 1.30 objective. *A,* deeper row of the superficial large pyramids; *B,* layer of the granule cells; *C,* sixth layer or [layer] of the deep large pyramids; *a,* polygonal small granule cells; *b,* diminutive pyramid; *c, d,* large stellate cells.

218

pletely. In some cells, as shown in fig. 15, *A, B* [*fig. 101*], the first collateral is so robust that it could be regarded as the true continuation of the axon, causing the vertical fibers descending toward the white matter to be regarded as the collaterals. Finally, there is no lack of cells that engender several axonal arcades, from which three or more recurrent collaterals arise. In such cells, the fiber destined for the white matter sometimes resembles a thin collateral arising from the convexity of an arch (fig. 15, *C*) [*fig. 101*]. All the mentioned collaterals, except the ascending branches, are distributed in the thickness of these layers, as well as in the upper portion of the next layer, complicating the nervous plexus that surrounds the deep large pyramids.

Regarding the richness in collaterals of such cells and the connections they establish with cells located in several layers, we think that it is very probable that their principal role would be to carry some particular excitation, collected by the soma, [apical dendritic] shaft, and its terminal tuft, to the giant pyramidal cells of

the bordering layers; but as there exists, in addition, a descending branch destined for the white matter, it is necessary to admit also that a part of that impulse is communicated to other distant foci of the gray matter. Besides these small pyramids with robust arciform collaterals, there is never any lack of pyramids of common type, in which the said [collateral] branches neither are more voluminous than the axon nor adopt a recurrent course. These common types seem to us to be more numerous in the precentral gyrus than in the postcentral.

b. Large Stellate Cells

These elements are much less common than the preceding cells, and so far we have impregnated them only in the postcentral gyrus of the child of fifteen to twenty days. In their form and position, they seem to correspond to those thick stellate or semilunar cells with abundant protoplasm revealed in the fifth layer of the postcentral gyrus by the method of Nissl (fig. 14, *c*) [*fig. 100*]. In Golgi preparations, they appear like the elements of the same name in the visual cortex; that is to say, they possess a stellate soma from whose angles arise several divergent processes, ramifying in the thickness of the fifth layer, and a descending robust axon, prolonged perhaps down to the white matter, and which gives off in its initial trajectory several transverse or recurrent and arciform collaterals, distributed in the thickness of the said layer (fig. 15, *D*) [*fig. 101*].

The stellate cells are impregnated with difficulty. Perhaps their distribution is very uneven in the human cortex. In the motor regions of animals (cat and dog), we have found them to be more abundant and situated above the giant pyramids.

c. Large and Medium Pyramids of Common Type

These cells usually are not absent, and on account of their morphological properties they must be regarded as homologous to the giant pyramids of the fourth layer. In fig. 15, *E* [*fig. 101*], we reproduce a pyramid of this class, whose dendritic arborization was completely similar to that of the ordinary pyramids.

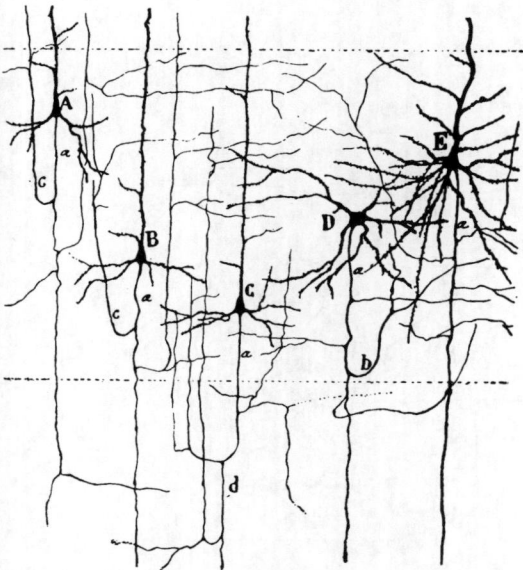

[*FIG. 101*] Fig. 15. Cells with long axon of the fifth layer taken from several locations of the human motor area. *A, B, C*, small pyramids; *D*, stellate cell with long axon; *E*, ordinary large pyramid; *a*, axon; *b, c*, recurrent thick collaterals.

Cells with Short Axon

They are still more numerous than those with long axons, and they correspond to several types, some of which have already been described when we dealt with the fourth and fifth layers of the visual cortex. Here are the most common.

a. Stellate or Fusiform Cells with Ascending Axon Divided in Long Horizontal Branches

As shown in fig. 16, *A, D* [*fig. 102*], these cells reside at different levels of the fifth layer, and they may have several sizes. The divergent dendrites, with few spines, are distributed in the thickness of the layer, and the axon resolves itself into very long horizontal collaterals and terminal branches, some of them so long that they can be followed for two or more tenths of a millimeter. From the course of such horizontal branches, several small branches usually arise at an oblique angle and are distributed in different levels of the fifth layer.

b. Cells with Ascending Axon Distributed in the Fourth Layer

In the previous type, the terminal branches and collaterals of the axon seem never to leave the fifth layer, but in this [other] type of cell, which can be considered as a variety of the previous type, the axon, without the detriment of giving off horizontal branches, reaches the fourth layer, in which it gives off some collaterals, and there it descends again to the layer of origin (fig. 16, *C*) [*fig. 102*]. In other cases, the small ascending branch is a collateral of one of the branches of the terminal bifurcation of the axon, as shown in fig. 16, *B* [*fig. 102*].

c. Cell Whose Axon Goes up to the Plexiform Layer and to the Second and Third Layers (fig. 16, F) [*fig. 102*]

Certain stellate, ovoid, or triangular cells, of larger size than the previous ones, possess a thick ascending axon, which, after supplying some branches to the fifth layer, ramifies in

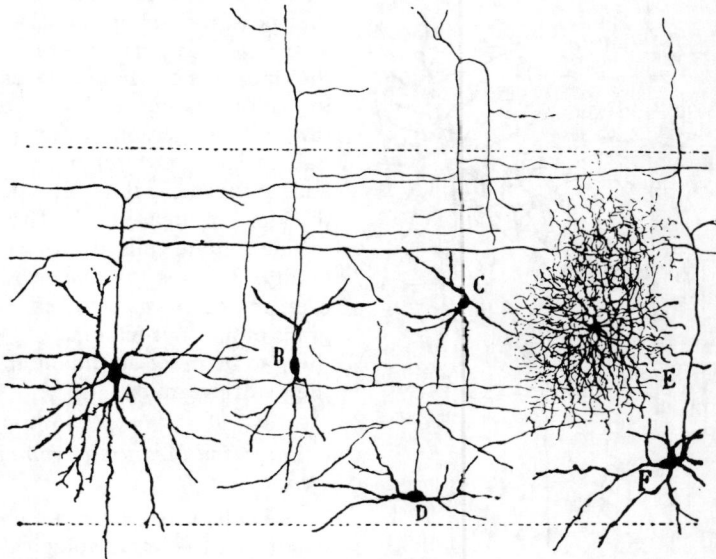

[*FIG. 102*] Fig. 16. Cells with short axon of the fifth layer taken from several locations of the motor cortex of a child of one month. *A, D,* cells with ascending axon, with horizontal branches distributed in the fifth layer; *B, C,* cells with arciform axon giving off branches to the fourth layer; *F,* cells whose axon went up to the plexiform layer.

the fourth and third layers, resolving itself into a multitude of small oblique and horizontal branches. Finally, in some cases, we have also revealed the arrival of the axon at the first layer, where it behaved like the axons of Martinotti. Similar cells likewise exist in the fourth and third layers, but, because of its very long trajectory, it is not always possible to reveal the arrival of the axon at the first layer.

In summary, although our investigations on this point are insufficient, we are inclined to admit in the fifth layer several kinds of cells with ascending axons distributed at different levels, where they could take the name of the layer in which the axon is preferentially arborized. Thus, we would have cells of Martinotti or cells destined for the first layer, cells related to the second, to the third, etc. Let us hasten to say, however, that in almost all of these cells, the axonal ramification embraces several strata.

d. Diminutive or Arachniform Cells

Although not as numerous as in the visual cortex, they are found in all the planes of the fifth layer, and are not lacking either in the neighboring layers. In fig. 16, E [fig. 102], we reproduce one of them in which the axon resolved itself into a very thin ascending nervous plexus.

e. Bitufted Cells with Axon Resolved into Small Tufts of Vertical Threads

They are completely similar to the homonymous cells of the superficial layers, so we will not make a particular description.

From all that has been said, it results that the fifth layer or layer of the granule cells is an intermediate place of the cortex in which are concentrated the cells with short axon or of intracortical association.

Granule Cells of the Precentral Gyrus

The preceding description can be applied in its broad outline to both central gyri, but to complete our knowledge about the granule cells, it will be convenient to expose the variations in the disposition of these cells in the precentral gyrus.

As we have said previously, the granule cells of this motor region are distributed in two unequal formations: one external, situated above the superficial large pyramids and intermingled with many medium pyramidal cells; and the other internal, situated underneath the fourth layer and generally better distinguishable than the external. In fig. 17, A, C [fig. 103], we reproduce these two substrata of granule cells, where one can observe, with some variations, almost all the cells reproduced in figs. 15 and 16 [figs. 101, 102].

The *external granular formation* contains the following types: first, some small and medium pyramids, as previously described (fig. 17, e) [fig. 103]; second, stellate, triangular, or fusiform cells of medium volume, provided with not very long divergent dendrites, and whose axon is arborized inside the external granular formation (fig. 17, f) [fig. 103]; third, vertical fusiform cells, whose ascending axon, after giving off branches to this formation, is ramified in the superimposed layers, in some types seeming to go up to the plexiform layer (figs. 17, c, d) [fig. 103]; fourth, bitufted cells, but with relatively thick dendrites that are very flexuous and so entangled that it is difficult to follow them, the axon resolving itself into a tight ramification, in which arciform and recurrent branches, destined for the vicinity of the cell, are abundant (fig. 17, b) [fig. 103].

In the *internal granular formation* can also be observed, first, extremely abundant fusiform, ovoid, or triangular cells with ascending axons that give off numerous collaterals both to the formation they inhabit and to the fourth layer, for which they seem especially destined (fig. 17, h) [fig. 103]; second, vertically arranged, thin fusiform or triangular cells that are often lance-shaped, provided with long ascending and descending polar dendrites, and with an axon that, after giving off some branches to the deep granular formation, seems to be distributed in the fourth layer or layer of the large pyramids, some axons going further, since they cross the layer of the medium pyramids and perhaps reach the plexiform layer (fig. 17, j, n) [fig. 103]; third, stellate or fusiform cells with short ascending or de-

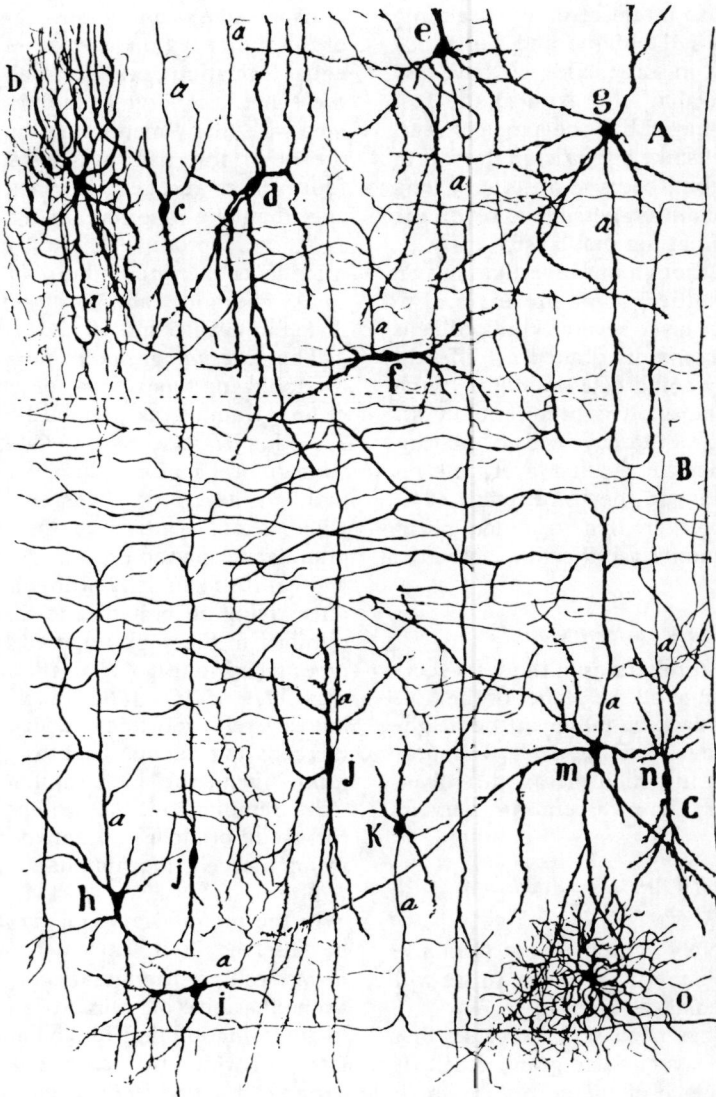

[*FIG. 103*]   Fig. 17. Layers that contain small stellate cells of the precentral gyrus of a child of one month. *A*, superficial granular formation; *B*, layer of the superficial large pyramids; *C*, fifth layer or deep granular formation; *a*, axons; *b*, large bitufted cell; *c*, *d*, cells with ascending axon of the superficial granular formation; *e*, small pyramid; *f*, cell with axon resolving into horizontal branches; *g*, cell with descending axon with arciform branches; *h*, *m*, cells whose axon ramified in the fourth layer; [*j*], *n*, thin fusiform cells with very long ascending axon.

scending axons distributed inside the granular formation under study, of which we draw in fig. 17, *I* [*fig. 103*] a type whose axon was thin and ascending and resolved itself into a delicate arborization and another thicker cell whose descending axon gave rise to long horizontal and vertical branches (fig. 17, *k*) [*fig. 103*]; fourth, arachniform cells of the type that has been described several times (fig. 17, *O*) [*fig. 103*]; fifth, a few bitufted cells.

Stellate Cells Whose Axon Is Resolved into Very Long Horizontal Branches

Besides the cited elements, the two above-mentioned granular formations, as well as the thickness of the fourth layer or layer of the superficial large pyramids, contain a special very numerous cell characterized by its stellate shape, the thinness and enormous length of its divergent dendrites, and especially the behavior of its axon (figs. 17, *m;* 18), [*figs. 103, 104*]. This process follows a variety of directions, although commonly it is ascending or descending, and at no great distance, sometimes close to its origin (fig. 18, *E*) [*fig. 104*], it bifurcates, resolving itself into a series of horizontal and oblique branches of great length. In fig. 18 [*fig. 104*], we reproduce some of these cells taken from the precentral gyrus. The limited dimensions of the drawing do not allow us to give a sufficient idea of the unusual length and complexity of the axon branches, which sometimes have the peculiarity of increasing in thickness

as they go away from the parent axon. Another peculiarity (which we think is only probable, since we do not have complete proof of it) consists of the fact that the furthest branches of the arborization resolve themselves into pericellular terminal baskets or nests, connected with the medium and giant pyramids of the sixth layer (fig. 19) [*fig. 105*].

Pericellular Nests

In certain preparations of the precentral gyrus of the child of twenty to thirty days, at the level of the layer of the giant and superficial pyramids are found delicate axonal plexuses that perfectly outline the soma and [apical] shaft of the said cells. We said something about these nests when we dealt with the giant cells of the visual cortex; here we only will add some details that we have tried to reproduce in fig. 20 [*fig. 106*]. The pericellular arborization consists of numerous small fibers, which are complicatedly interwoven, giving rise in their

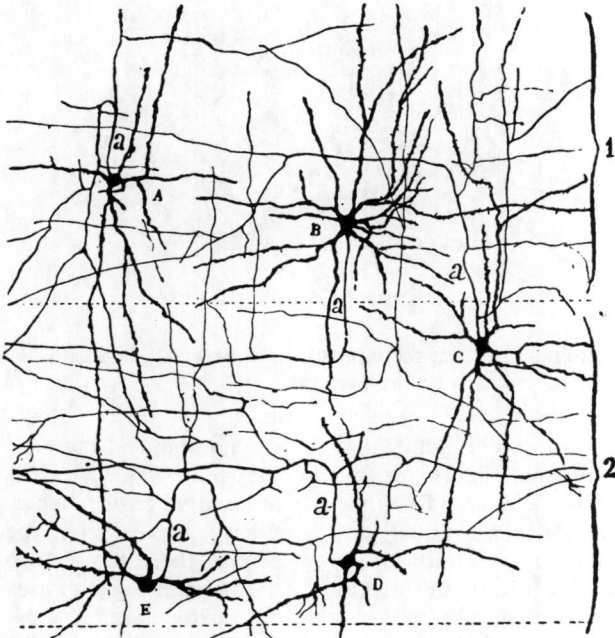

[*FIG. 104*]   Fig. 18. Stellate cells with axon divided into very long horizontal branches, probably generating terminal nests. *A, B,* cells of the superficial granular formation; *C, D, E,* cells of the fourth layer or [layer] of the external large pyramids; *a,* axon (precentral gyrus).

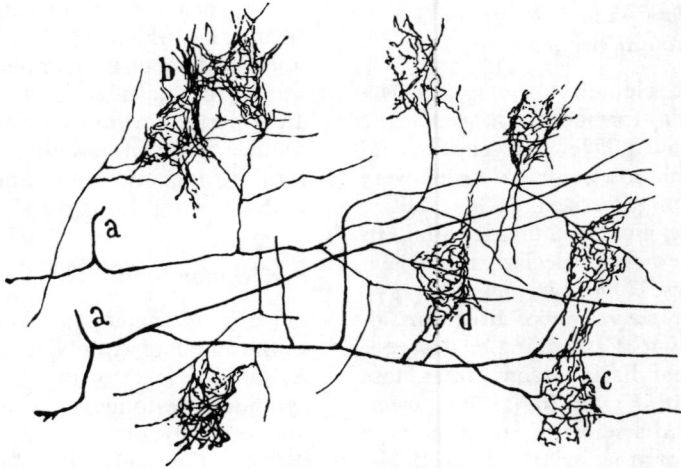

[*FIG. 105*]   Fig. 19. Pericellular arborizations of the layers of the external medium and giant pyramids of the motor cortex of a child of twenty-five days. *a*, axons dividing into long horizontal branches; *b*, *c*, *d*, pericellular baskets.

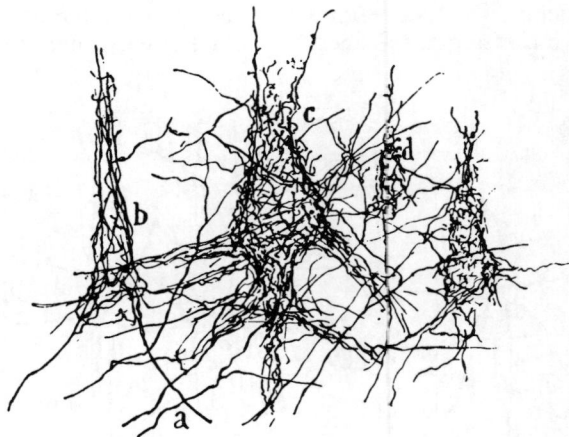

[*FIG. 106*]   Fig. 20. Pericellular nests of the layer of the superficial giant cells of the precentral gyrus. *a*, afferent fibers; *b*, external nest of a thin cell; *c*, large nest.

course to many short varicose branches that terminate freely. If the small fibers are followed outside the nest, it is observed that they do not come from a single afferent fiber, but from several, which also supply ramifications to several terminal baskets. It is not unusual to see a fiber giving some branches to a nest and even forming a part of it, to leave afterward and to be exhausted in other nearby pericellular plexuses. In certain cells, the perisomatic plexus is prolonged for a certain distance along the apical shaft and basal dendrites, as is shown in fig. 20, *c* [*fig. 106*], becoming exhausted when it reaches the first bifurcations. What is the origin of the constituent nerve fibers of these nests? In preparations in which the pericellular plexuses appear well impregnated, the staining is exclusive; thus, it is not possible to follow the fiber of origin to any parent cell. The only thing that can be observed is that such afferent fibers arise at acute angles from other, thicker branches with oblique or horizontal directions, which run for a long distance in the layer of the large pyramids. On occasions, it can be observed that two thick horizontal fibers from a short descending trunk arise by means of a bifurcation; these in their turn divide into numerous branches with several directions, some of them entering pericellular plexuses. This arrangement has been represented in fig. 19 [fig. 82] of our paper on the visual cortex. The impossibility of showing the continuity of such fibers with intrinsic nerve cells led us at first to the idea that the nests originate from sensory nerve fibers arriving from the white matter, but this opinion is contrary to certain evidence, among which we will cite the following: first, that the sensory fibers, as we will see below, have their main place of termination not in the layer of the giant pyramids but higher up in the superimposed layer of the medium pyramids; second, that in the preparations where the sensory plexus is well impregnated, as is shown in fig. 27 [fig. 112], special nests for the large or the medium pyramids are not observed, but instead [there is] a diffuse intercellular plexus, comparable to that of the visual fibers in the layer of the granule cells of the occipital cortex; third, that the features of the ramifications of the sensory fibers do not look like the arborizations of the peripyramidal nests. Moreover, the disposition of the fibers that give rise to the nests is very similar to the axons with long horizontal branches of the stellate cells of the fourth layer and adjacent granular formations; to which we must add that sometimes the axonal branches of the latter give off short branches that seem to surround the somata of the pyramids. Thus, at present, we are inclined to think that the large stellate cells, provided with long dendrites (fig. 18) [fig. 104] and an axon giving rise to horizontal or oblique ramifications of enormous length, represent the origin of the peripyramidal nests or baskets. Thus, there would come to be reproduced in the cerebrum the anatomical arrangement discovered by us in the cerebellum (basket cells of the molecular layer), in Ammon's horn[56] (cells with horizontal axon distributed around the pyramids of this organ), and in the fascia dentata (cells with ascending axon ramifying around the granule cells).

For the rest, the nests referred to have nothing to do with those that Semi Meyer[57] has claimed to observe with the methylene blue method in the cells of the guinea pig or with the superficial meshes described in the cerebral pyramids of the cat by Bethe[58] and Nissl.[59] In fact, the arrangement described by Meyer is nothing more than a pericellular precipitate of methylene blue, produced by the fixative (ammonium molybdate). Such a precipitate in the folds of the membrane, coupled with the incomplete staining of some neuroglial fibrils or small pericellular nerve fibers, can create the illusion of a genuine nervous plexus; and the meshes mentioned by Bethe and Nissl, according to our indications,[60] do not represent a pericellular nervous mesh, but the periphery of the protoplasmic reticulum, or perhaps the limiting membrane of the cell, a membrane that, as occurs with other cells, might be reticulated and in certain cases attract the methylene blue by means of the precipitating action of the fixative of Bethe.° Recently, Turner and Hunter[61] have also described in the cerebrum of the guinea pig, and in other nervous sites of the same animal, pericellular meshes that they have stained with the method of Meyer (subcutaneous injection of methylene blue during life). The figures shown by these authors resemble somewhat better the baskets described by us, as some pericellular nerve fibers can be seen in them, but also, like Meyer and Bethe, they have erroneously taken for an arborization of terminal centripetal nerve fibers the superficial protoplasmic mesh of the cell and perhaps certain folds of the membrane originating from the retraction of the protoplasm. For the rest, these experts Turner and Hunter seem to ignore all our works about the effects of the methylene blue on nervous centers,[62] a charge that we must level equally at Meyer.

Granule Cells in the Cerebrum of Mammals

When the motor region of the horse, cat, and dog is observed with the help of the method of Nissl, as in the human, a relatively simple stratification of the precentral gyrus is revealed. It corresponds to the type of four layers indicated by us[63] in the rabbit and rat (1, molecular layer; 2, layer of the small pyramids; 3, layer of the large pyramids; and 4, layer of the polymorphic cells). A layer of granule cells thus does not exist. Nevertheless, a watchful examination with the Zeiss 1.30 objective allows us to notice that above the giant pyramids (third layer), and much more abundant than in the bordering strata, there are certain small-sized stellate or fusiform cells, scattered irregularly in the deeper plane of the second layer. Often, in this place, which corresponds to the layer of the medium pyramids of the human, the pyramids proper that inhabit it have a smaller diameter than those situated in higher planes.

The Golgi preparations allow us to recognize the exceptional richness in small cells of the mentioned suprapyramidal zone. Among the cells that are found in this place, there are some very similar to those described in the human cortex. In fig. 21 [*fig. 107*], we have reproduced the most typical, namely, first, small pyramids with descending axon provided or not provided with a thick arciform collateral (fig. 21, *E*) [*fig. 107*]; second, stellate cell with long descending axon, whose initial collaterals

seem to be distributed in the border formation of the large pyramids (fig. 21, *B, C*) [*fig. 107*]; third, thick downy fusiform cells, whose ascending axon bifurcates, giving rise to very long horizontal branches (fig. 21, *F*) [*fig. 107*]; fourth, relatively thick, bitufted cell, whose axon resolves itself into some very close vertical threads that embrace this layer and the underlying layer of large pyramids (fig. 21, *G*)[P] [*fig. 107*]; fifth, stellate cells corresponding to the neurogliaform or dwarf cells of man. The latter cells, of which we reproduce in fig. 22 [*fig. 108*] the most common varieties found in the motor cortex of the cat of twenty-five days, are located preferentially above the layer of the large pyramids, but extend also into the thickness of this layer and even to the deep layer or layer of the polymorphic cells. The cell body is small or medium, and its very numerous and thin dendrites run in all directions, becoming extremely flexuous and acquiring a delicately varicose appearance. With regard to the axon, in the smallest types (fig. 22, *A, B*) [*fig. 108*], it is hardly distinguishable from the delicate dendrites and gives rise, at a

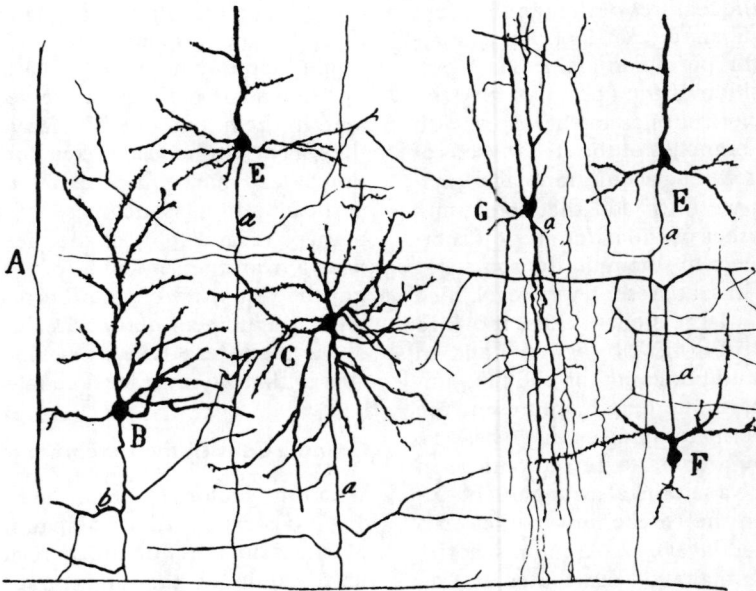

[*FIG. 107*]   Fig. 21. Small pyramids and stellate cells of the motor [cortex] of a cat of twenty-five days. *A*, layer situated above the large pyramids; *B, C*, cells with descending long axons; *E*, small pyramids; *F*, cell with ascending axon, divided into long horizontal branches.

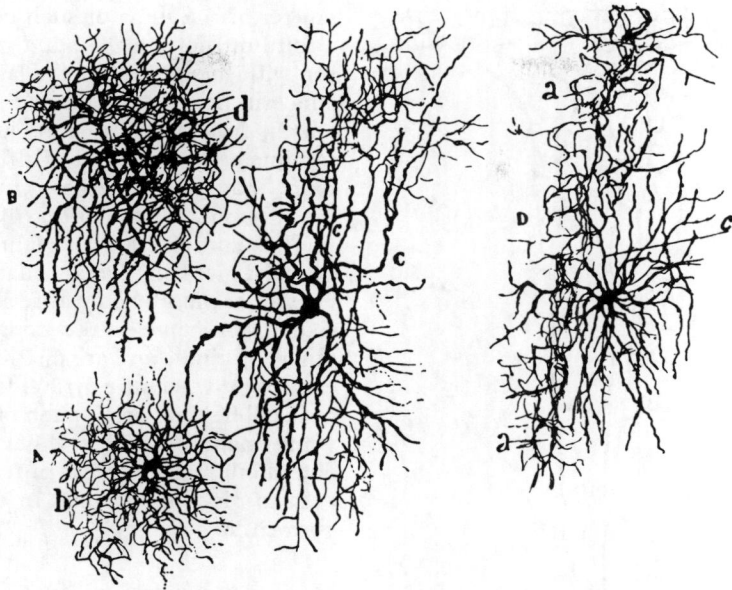

[FIG. 108]   Fig. 22. Cells with short axon from the region of the medium and large pyramids of a cat of twenty-five days. A, B, neurogliaform or small types; C, D, types of medium size; a, pericellular nerve plexuses; c, axon; d, [axonal] nests.

short distance, to a very dense arborization of extraordinary delicacy, distributed in proximal pericellular nests.

In the largest types (fig. 22, C, D) [fig. 108], the axon is more distinct, and its less complex terminal arborization forms looser plexuses than the previous variety, although it also forms, at least in some cases, pericellular nests, arranged in series (fig. 22, a) [fig. 108].

Sixth Layer or Layer of the Deep Large Pyramids

Both in the precentral and in the postcentral gyrus, there is found beneath the fifth layer a very dense axonal-dendritic plexus, sometimes arranged in horizontal bands, populated by three categories of cells [that are] quite separate from one another: pyramidal cells of large size; pyramids of regular size; and numerous cells with short axons.

Large Pyramids

They are easily recognizable in Nissl preparations by their richness in [Nissl granules], the elongated form of the soma, and the robustness of the basal dendrites. These pyramids are scarce, and they form clusters or pleiades in the precentral gyrus in which they reach their largest size (cells of Betz); [by contrast], in the postcentral gyrus, they are more abundant but commonly of smaller diameter than the superficial large pyramids.

Even more than their size, such cells are characterized by the richness and enormous length of their somatic dendrites. These, in the manner of those originating from the pyramidal cells of the fourth layer, are distinguished as *descending*, or arising from the base, as *laterals of the soma* which have a long horizontal trajectory, and as *laterals of the radial* [dendritic] *shaft* [which are] generally horizontal but of less length than the previous ones. The [apical dendritic] shaft, simple or bifurcated, goes up to the plexiform layer, where it is distributed in a tuft of horizontal and oblique branches (fig. 23) [fig. 109].

The stature of these giant types, as well as the thickness and length of their dendrites, increases with age. With regard to the soma, this

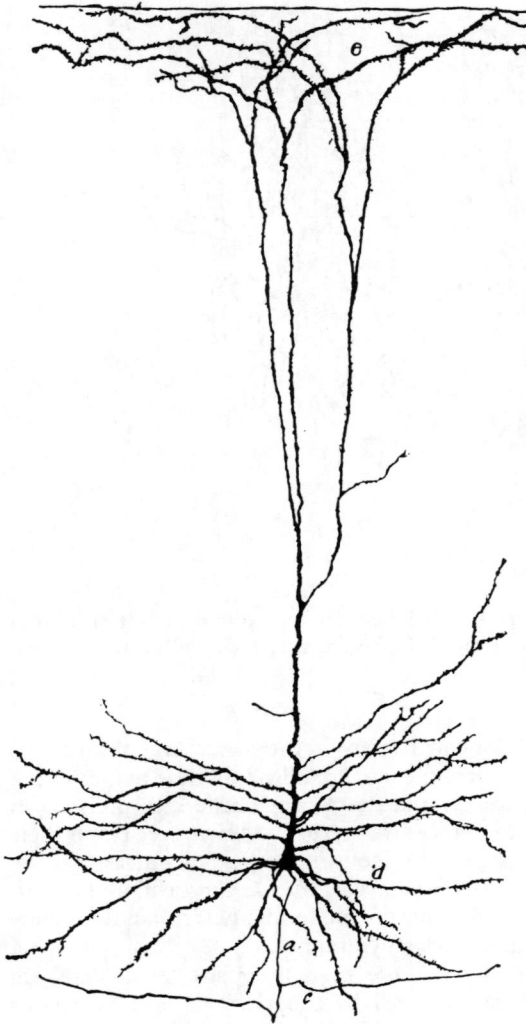

[*FIG. 109*] Fig. 23. Deep giant pyramid of the postcentral gyrus of a child of thirty days. *a*, axon; *c*, collaterals, *d*, long basal dendrites; *e*, terminal tuft.

increment can already be proved by comparing Nissl preparations of the cerebrum of the newborn child with those of the adult. But to make a comparative study of the dendrites, it is necessary to use the method of silver chromate. By means of the slow or semislow procedure, we have been able several times to impregnate the cells of Betz of the adult cerebral cortex, and we have ascertained that the di-

ameter of the soma of such cells increases by a third or more in the adult man in comparison with the child. But the largest differences concern the length of the basal dendrites which, from thirty to forty hundredths of a millimeter in the child of fifteen days, reach more than one millimeter in the adult (see figs. 23 and 24) [*figs. 109, 110*].

The axon of the deep giant pyramids is robust and gives off several collaterals (from four to eight or more). Some arise and ramify in the sixth layer between the congener pyramids; others originate and are distributed in the seventh layer, where the pyramids of medium size reside. The final destination of the axon is the white matter, which we have often seen it enter both in the cerebra of fetuses of the seventh to ninth month and in that of the newborn child.

Medium Pyramids

Except for their size, they possess the same properties as the previous ones.

Cells with Short Axons

They have a variable size and shape, for which it is necessary to distinguish a number of types:

1. Cell with ascending short axon. It is quite common, with a stellate, triangular, or fusiform shape, and it possesses divergent dendrites that ramify inside the confines of the layer. The axon is ascending and resolves itself into small terminal, more or less horizontal branches distributed both in the thickness of the sixth layer and in the deep planes of the fifth.
2. Fusiform or stellate cells with very long ascending axons extending perhaps up to the first layer.
3. Arachniform and bitufted cells.

Seventh Layer or Layer of the Medium Pyramids and Triangular Cells

This layer, which corresponds to the fourth [layer] or [layer] of the polymorphic cells of mammals and to the layer of fusiform cells of Meynert in the human cortex, appears more or less extensive, depending on the gyri under

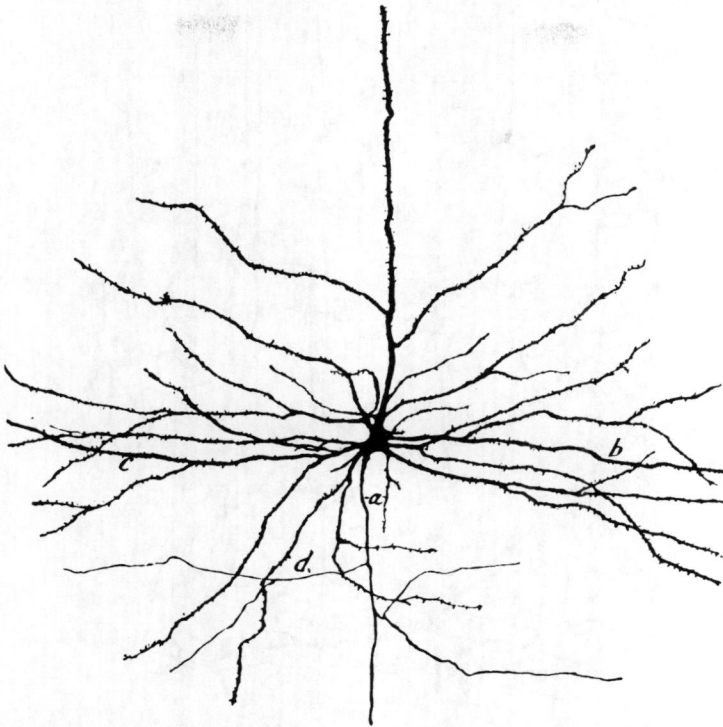

[*FIG. 110*]   Fig. 24. Deep giant pyramid of the motor region of a man of thirty years. *a*, axon; *c*, [*b*], dendrites that were followed for more than one millimeter; *d*, collaterals.

study. In the postcentral gyrus (fig. 1, 7 and 1, 8) [*fig. 87*], especially at the level of the convex parts, it almost always appears divided into two wide strata: one superficial, formed by a large number of medium pyramids, triangular cells, and fusiform cells; and the other deep, poor in cells because of the voluminous bundles of white matter that cross it radially, and composed almost exclusively of thin and fusiform cells.

These two layers are not well distinguished in the precentral gyrus, it being possible to include both together under the common designation of *layer of the polymorphic cells or layer of the fusiform and triangular cells.*

In the description that follows, we will refer to the postcentral gyrus in which, as we have exposed, it is possible to separate two sublayers, the seventh and the eighth.

The most common [cellular] elements of the seventh layer are reproduced in fig. 25 [*fig. 111*]. These are, among the cells with long axon, medium pyramids, triangular cells, and fusiform cells; and, among those of short axon, fusiform cells with ascending axons, stellate cells or cells of Golgi, and arachniform cells with very short and richly arborized axons.

Medium Pyramids

These correspond completely to the common type, showing a very long [apical dendritic] shaft that reaches up to the plexiform layer, several descending and oblique dendrites arising from the soma, and, finally, a descending axon that can be followed down to the white matter, and from whose initial course arise four, five, or more collaterals, distributed in the thickness of the seventh and eighth layers (fig. 25 A) [*fig. 111*].

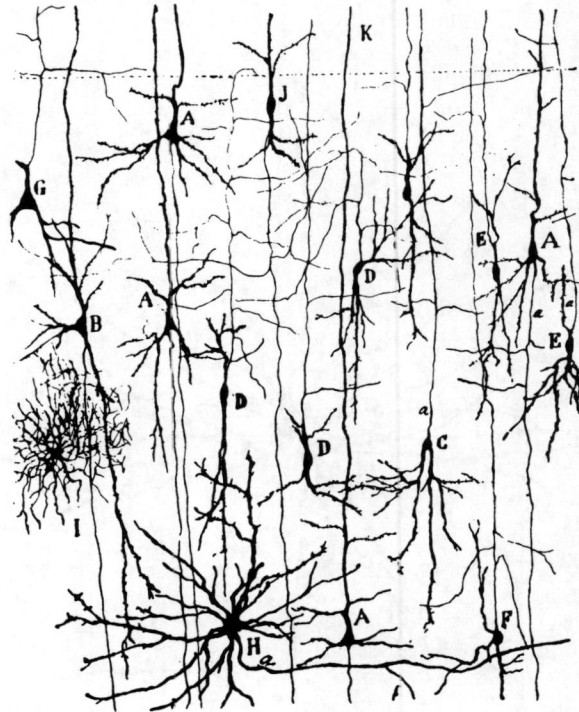

[*FIG. 111*]   Fig. 25. Cells of the seventh layer of the highest part of the postcentral gyrus. Child of one month. *A*, pyramid of medium size; *B*, triangular cells; *C*, *D*, [*E*], *F*, *G*, cells with ascending axons; *H*, large stellate cell with horizontal axon; *I*, arachniform cell; *a*, axon.

Triangular Cells

As with the preceding cells, they have a radial shaft prolonged up to the first layer, but they [are distinguished] from the genuine pyramids by two important features: they have, instead of a deep tuft of dendrites, a long descending [dendritic] shaft that ramifies very deeply in the thickness of the seventh and eighth layers; and they exhibit a lateral short [dendritic] shaft, quickly ramifying as a group of dendritic branches (fig. 25, *B*) [*fig. 111*]. The axon is descending and, as with that of the pyramids, enters the white matter.

Fusiform Cells (fig. 25, *J*) [*fig. 111*]

Instead of the pyramidal and triangular types, this cell with long axon sometimes adopts the shape of a spindle, with two long radial dendrites, the ascending destined for the first layer, and the descending, not very long, forming a tuft of dendrites. Also, the axon enters the white matter after giving off two or three collaterals.

Cells with Short Axon

They correspond to three main varieties, namely (a) cells with ascending axon, destined for the superimposed layers; (b) cells with short axon, arborized in the thickness of the seventh layer (fig. 25, *D*) [*fig. 111*]; (c) arachniform cells or cells with very short axon (fig. 25, *I*) [*fig. 111*].

Among all of these varieties of cells with short axon, the one that seems to dominate is the first. As seen in fig. 25, *E*, *C*, *F*, *G* [*fig. 111*], these cells lie in several planes of the layer, although they usually prefer the upper part of it; their form is often that of a spindle, with two [dendritic] shafts, ascending and descending, promptly resolved into terminal branches; the triangular (fig. 25, *G*) [*fig. 111*], spherical, and semilunar (fig. 25, *C, F*) [*fig. 111*] forms are not rare either. In some cases, the ascending processes are short and the descending dendrites very long, which gives them the appearance of inverted pyramids already recognized by Golgi. The axon is thin, coming frequently, in harmony with the law of conservation of matter, from an ascending dendrite, and, giving off some collaterals to the seventh layer, it finally gets lost in the superimposed layers.

Let us add still, for completeness, that in some cases we have achieved the impregnation of a thick stellate cell, whose axon ran horizontally, giving off (fig. 25, *H*) [*fig. 111*] robust ascending, descending, and oblique collaterals. Although we have not seen the destination of the axon, we think it probable that these are cells with horizontal short axons, destined to establish associations at large distances.

Eighth Layer

Beneath the accumulation of cells represented by the preceding elements starts a layer [that is] very thick in the axial region of the gyri, much [thinner] in the lateral portions of these, and very thin or completely indistinguishable from the seventh in the concave portions. The cells of this stratum have mainly a spindle shape, and they are arranged in radial series, separated by thick bundles of white matter; but others are also found, such as triangular and even pyramidal cells, provided with very long polar dendrites. In Nissl preparations, it is not rare to see around the soma of these elements two or more neuroglial nuclei.

In fig. 26 [*fig. 112*], we have reproduced the most abundant cells of the eighth layer of the postcentral gyrus of the child of one month. There can be seen (a) fusiform cells provided with a long radial process, likely to be prolonged up to the first layer, with a descending [dendritic] shaft sometimes very long and divided at acute angles and, finally, with a descending axon from which arise some initial, often recurrent collaterals (fig. 26, *A*) [*fig. 112*]; (b) genuine pyramidal cells completely equal

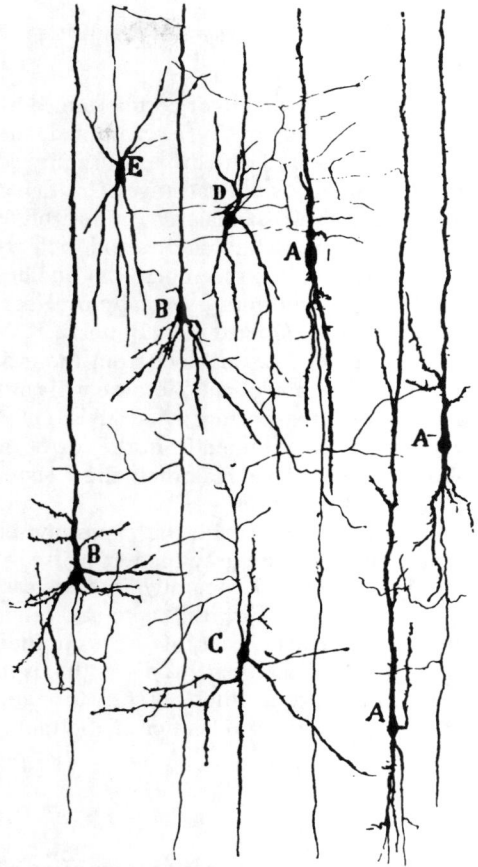

[*FIG. 112*]   Fig. 26. Cells of the deep portion of the seventh or eighth layer. *A*, fusiform cells; *B*, true pyramids; *C, D*, cells with short axons; *E*, cells with ascending axons to the upper layers of the cortex.

to those of the preceding layer (fig. 26, *B*) [*fig. 112*]; (c) stellate, fusiform, or triangular cells with ascending short axon which sometimes ramifies in the surroundings of the parent cell (fig. 26, *D*) [*fig. 112*], at others at a higher plane (fig. 26, *C*) [*fig. 112*], at others, finally, at much higher levels that we have not been able to determine (fig. 26, *E*) [*fig. 112*].

It is probable that some of these ascending long axons correspond to fibers of Martinotti, because in the rabbit and mouse, where it is easier to follow the course of the nerve fibers, the deepest layer or the layer of polymorphic cells always contains fusiform or stellate cells, whose axon goes up to the first layer.

Fibers and Nervous Plexuses of the Motor Cortex

When a section of the motor cortex stained by the method of Weigert-Pal is examined, the gray matter appears crossed by an infinity of medullated fibers, some arranged in radial bundles and others, the majority, in horizontal plexuses. Both the radial bundles and the parallel plexuses have been seen perfectly and described by many authors, especially by Kaes, Vulpius, Edinger, Obersteiner, Bottazzi, Kölliker, etc. This excuses us, too, from the task of describing them in detail. Here we will concentrate only on exposing what silver chromate preparations obtained from the cortex of the human and higher mammals show about such fibers and plexuses.

To proceed in order with the exposition of the nerve fibers of the gray matter, it is convenient to divide them, naturally, into two categories: *endogenous fibers*, that is to say, originating from intrinsic cells of the examined cortical region; and *exogeneous fibers*, that is to say, originating from other nervous foci and ending freely in the gray matter of the motor cortex.

Exogeneous Fibers

In our work on the cerebral cortex of small mammals,[64] we pointed out the existence of some robust myelinated fibers coming from the white matter, which, after entering the gray matter with a variety of directions and tracing large turns in their ascending course, terminated in a free arborization of enormous extent and located preferentially in the superficial half of the cortex.

With respect to the origin of such singular fibers, we did not make, at that time, a definite pronouncement; but Kölliker,[65] who confirmed the existence of these fibers in the rat, rabbit, cat, and dog (*fibers of S. Ramón* of this author), and who saw them to descend to the corpus striatum, supposes that they have a sensory nature and are continuous with the ascending fibers of the ribbon of Reil or medial lemniscus; their cells of origin resided thus in the bulbar nuclei of the bundles of Goll and of Burdach;[Q] unless it should be proved, as some authors want, that the ribbon of Reil has at the level of the optic thalamus an intermediary station, because in such a case the cited centripetal fibers of the motor cortex would arise from this.

Examining again the preparations that we used for our first papers on the cortex of the mouse, rat, and rabbit, we have ascertained that, in agreement with Kölliker, the cited centripetal fibers in fact come from the corona radiata, and thus, they may very well represent second-order sensory conductors. This opinion acquires great credibility if we have in mind, first, that all the sensory areas have terminal arborizations originating from thick fibers coming from the corona radiata; second, that the sensory pathways are developed before those of intracerebral association, from which it is deduced that in the period in which such arborizations of the motor area are developed (newborn mouse and rabbit, human fetus after the seventh month), other exogeneous ramifications with which they could be mingled still have not reached the gray matter; third, that the mentioned thick fibers of the motor area cannot be mistaken either for those of the other sensory territories, as they are distributed and terminate in a different manner from the visual, olfactory, and acoustic fibers.

The last argument represents an anatomical criterion of some value, which when properly applied will allow us to recognize, on account of the presence of the cited sensory arborizations, the location and extent of the motor area in the [cerebral cortex] of diverse mammals. In fact, apart from the features of cellular morphology and of stratification studied above, the motor cortex is recognized in all mammals, *because it exhibits a dense plexus of very thick exogeneous fibers, situated at the level of the medium pyramids, that is to say, above the external large pyramids.* In man, we have found this plexus only in the precentral gyrus and posterior portions of the first two frontal gyri; but, although the inconsistency of the silver chromate reaction does not allow us to formulate categorical judgments, especially if these are negative ones, we consider it to be extremely probable that the mentioned plexiform disposition extends to the whole, genuinely sensory-motor cortex.

This plexus is easily recognizable, as we have also said, because of the precocity of its appearance; thus, it is necessary to study it in human fetuses of the seventh and later months. In the newborn child, its impregnation is very uneven, showing only some of its horizontal fibers with occasional ramifications; in the child of one month, it is very rare to stain exogeneous terminal ramifications, because the myelin already covers, in part, the course of the sensory fibers.

In fig. 27 [fig. 113], we have tried to reproduce the several portions that constitute the sensory plexus. On the right are shown some fibers in isolation, whose terminal arborizations can easily be followed, whereas on the

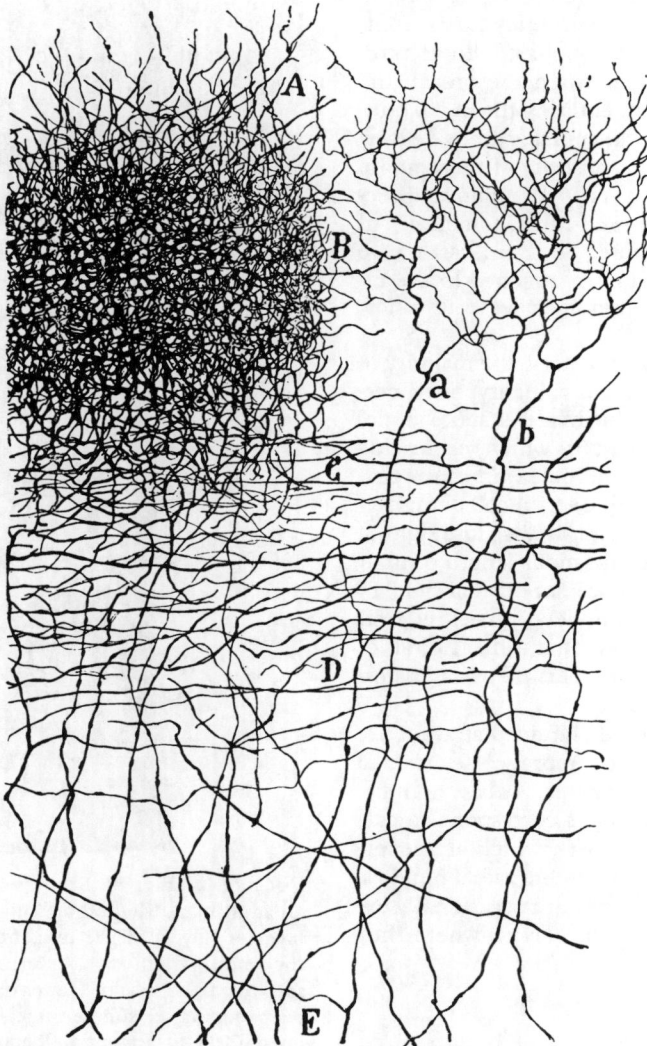

[FIG. 113]   Fig. 27. Sensory plexus of the cortex of the precentral gyrus. Human fetus of seven to eight months. A, terminal branches to the upper limit of the third layer; B, very dense terminal plexus of the layer of the medium pyramids; D, middle plexus of horizontal fibers; E, deep plexus of thick oblique fibers; a, b, terminal arborizations.

left we show a place where all the sensory ramifications were impregnated.

The sensory plexus can be divided into three principal zones: *deep zone* or zone of oblique fibers; *middle zone* or zone of the horizontal fibers; *superficial zone* or zone of the terminal arborizations.

Deep Zone

At its deeper limit, and even in the very white matter, are observed certain thick fibers, commonly thicker than the axons of the voluminous pyramids, which, when they reach the gray matter, instead of entering the radial bundles to follow a vertical course, run in a diversity of directions. The majority of them go up to the underlying layers in an oblique direction and trace angles and turns, sometimes of enormous extent; some, however, can go up almost vertically and even attached to the radial bundles, which they later leave to follow other courses.

During this initial trajectory, the majority of the fibers retain their individuality, but a certain number of them bifurcate at acute angles or give off thick collaterals, which, on leaving the stem, go up to the middle layers of the cortex (fig. 27, *E*) [*fig. 113*]. Certain collaterals follow horizontal trajectories, and we lose sight of them because of the enormous length of their course. What we think for sure is that none of the sensory fibers of the deep plane gives off ramifications to the cells that inhabit it; all of them seem to us to be fibers of passage, destined for other layers.

The sensory fibers of the deep stratum are also visible in the adult cerebral cortex stained by the Weigert-Pal procedure. As is seen in fig. 28, *f* [*fig. 114*], these fibers correspond to certain thick myelinated fibers, which are generally oblique with respect to the radial bundles, which they cross, and they are occasionally extended up to the middle plexus, where they become horizontal.

Middle Plexus

This plexus, which in the precentral gyrus corresponds to the layer of the external giant [pyramids], is characterized by containing a large number of thick myelinated fibers arranged horizontally or interwoven at acute an-

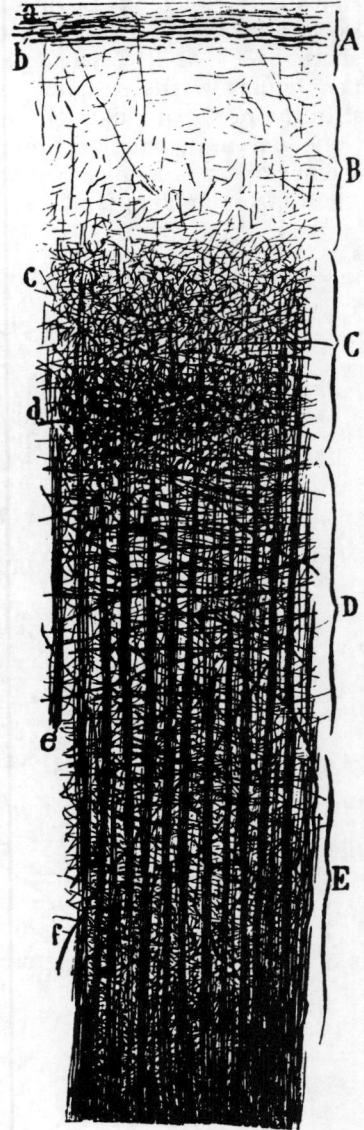

[*FIG. 114*] Fig. 28. Section of the motor gyrus of an adult man. Method of Weigert-Pal. *A*, plexiform layer or [layer] of the tangential fibers; *B*, layer of the small pyramids; *C*, external portion of the sensory plexus or stria of Gennari; *D*, middle plexus; *E*, deep plexus; *a*, submeningeal rim free of medullated fibers; *b*, tangential fibers; *c*, thin plexus for the medium pyramids; *d*, horizontal fibers; *e*, radial bundles; *f*, oblique sensory fibers.

gles. Such an arrangement results because the branches of the sensory fibers do not usually run straight to their place of arborization, but before and once they arrive at the layer of the superficial large pyramids, they become horizontal, undergo several branchings, and keep the same direction over distances so long that it is impossible in most cases to observe in a single section the whole course. So, in fig. 27 [fig. 113], the terminal fibers *a* and *b*, whose detailed arborizations are shown, do not come directly from the deep plexus but from the horizontal fibers of the middle [plexus].

The middle plexus also appears to lack terminal arborizations; only in its superficial third which corresponds to the first rows of thick pyramids are there found some small, thin ramifications and intercellular arborizations. From this it follows that (at least in the term human fetus) the somata of the superficial and deep large pyramids probably lack direct contacts with sensory ramifications. This circumstance also argues in favor of the endogenous character of the baskets of peripyramidal nests described above, because, commonly, the large cells of the encephalon (pyramids of Ammon's horn, Purkinje's cells of the cerebellum) always keep the cell body for the reception of nervous arborizations arising from cellular elements with short axon, whereas they dedicate the principal dendritic shaft and the terminal dendritic shaft to the reception of exogeneous ramifications.

Superficial Plexus

Its richness in fibers and the density of its meshes are so great, when the impregnation is complete, that from this aspect the sensory plexus can only be compared to the visual plexus of the calcarine fissure.

To appreciate it fully, it is necessary to examine those places where only some arborizations have been stained (fig. 27, *a, b*) [fig. 113]. In these places, it is observed that the sensory fiber reaches the terminal plexus from below, bifurcating quickly in the deeper aspect of the plexus, and the resulting branches, which are repeatedly subdivided, ascend sinuously and more or less obliquely to form an extensive and extremely complicated arborization, in which the cell bodies of the medium pyramids

and of the cells with short axon show up in the clear. The higher small branches of this tight plexus are varicose and extend up to the deep half of the layer of the small pyramids; however, the vast majority of these ramifications is limited to the third layer or layer of the medium pyramids, having their maximum concentration above the external large pyramids, in a place notable for its richness in small stellate cells (superficial granular formation). We have not seen any sensory fiber arrive at the plexiform layer.

The arrangement we have just described harmonizes well with what the Weigert-Pal preparations show us. Although the vast majority of the fibers of the terminal plexus lack myelin, the main branches must have a medullated sheath, as in such preparations a dense plexus of thin threads, not as rich as that impregnated with the silver chromate, is observed located above the layer of the external large pyramids and in the thickness of the third layer (fig. 28, *c*) [fig. 114]. This myelinated plexus is none other than that called by the authors *stria of Gennari, external medullary lamina* (Kölliker, etc.).

To what cells are the sensory arborizations related? The preparations in which these ramifications are well stained reveal only the hollows occupied by the [cellular] elements of the third layer, but not the cells themselves; attending, however, to the considerable number of these spaces and to the density of the intercalated sensory plexus, it is permissible to think that a contact relationship is established with all the cells situated in the layer of the medium pyramids, and perhaps especially with the numerous cells with short axon located in the same layer, cells whose mission would be to propagate the impulse arriving in the said layer to pyramids situated at several layers.

The very abundant bitufted cells located in the thickness of the third layer and deep part of the second could also be regarded as intermediary links between the sensory fibers and the pyramids. We have already said that the large pyramids and polymorphic cells do not appear to have a direct relationship with the sensory arborizations; nevertheless, and although the connection [to these pyramids and polymorphic cells] may perhaps occur via the cells with short axon, we must not forget that the [apical dendritic] shafts of those cells destined for the first layer pass through the sensory plexus, and they are in a position thus to enter into intimate contact relationships [with the plexus]. Let us add, still, that the sensory excitation can also be transferred to the plexiform layer by means of the cells with ascending axon of Martinotti, which, by connecting with new series of neurons (cells with short axon, horizontal cells of the plexiform layer), would propagate it to [apical dendritic] tufts of pyramids located in other radii of the gyrus or perhaps in other gyri.

Because of all that has been said, we find unacceptable the view of Bevan Lewis, who attributes an exclusive sensory function to the layer of the small pyramids. If the layer of the cortex that directly receives the influence of the sensory fibers might be considered sensory, only the layer of the medium pyramids and particularly its deep levels strewn with stellate cells would deserve by rights such an attribution. But if any element that receives directly or indirectly the tactile, painful, or thermal impulse is sensory, then it is necessary to confess that the totality of the motor cortex deserves such a designation, given that all its cells are capable of entering into activity under the influence of the stimulation carried by the centripetal fibers.

For our part, we believe that any attempt at intimate localization, by layers or by neurons, of the different physiological activities involved in sensory-motor function (motor or reflex automatism of the cerebrum, tactile or painful sensation, voluntary movement, etc.) is still very premature. So far, it is only possible to conjecture that, as in the assumption for the visual cortex, the layer where the sensory fibers terminate is the place of tactile, thermal, and painful sensation; that the large cells of the fourth and sixth layers constitute the place where the motor impulse starts; and, finally, that the innumerable cells with short axon of the diverse cortical layers, and especially of the first, represent the intermediary pathways of association between the sensory fibers and the motor pyramids. And now [on the wings of fancy], we can also imagine that, from the

third layer, the supposed place of sensation, the remains of the tactile, painful, etc., image drift by a special route to other regions of the cerebrum, where they would be transformed into memories. But let us hasten to confess that all of these are only suppositions, more or less acceptable, but without any basis in physiological experimentation or pathological anatomy.

Sensory Plexus of the Cortex of Small Mammals

The sensory plexus under study also presents quite analogous features in the motor region of the cat, dog, rabbit, and mouse.

In fig. 29 [*fig. 115*], we reproduce the sensory arborizations of the cerebrum in a cat of four days. It is also observed that the originating fibers arriving in the gray matter are exceptionally thick (fig. 29, *F*) [*fig. 115*]. In their ascending course through the layer of the polymorphic cells, they follow a variety of directions; the oblique dominate and give off occasional collaterals, which appear to be distributed in quite separate radii of the gyrus (fig. 29, *b*) [*fig. 115*]. When they reach the layer of the giant pyramids, they become oblique or horizontal, but the course followed in this direction is much shorter than in man, the entire course of each fiber being easily followed, in a single section, as seen in fig. 29, *E* [*fig. 115*]. The middle plexus or plexus of horizontal fibers is not, therefore, as distinct in the cat as in man. Finally, when such fibers reach the upper limit of the third layer or layer of the giant pyramids, they give rise to the terminal arborization, [which is] much less dense and complicated than the homologous plexus in man and composed of varicose branches, arising commonly at acute angles, and extending through the whole layer of the medium pyramids (fig. 29, *D*) [*fig. 115*]. The upper small branches reach the deep levels of the layer of the small pyramids, but without reaching the upper part of it or invading the plexiform layer (fig. 29, *c*) [*fig. 115*].

In the rabbit, rat, and mouse, the disposition of the sensory fibers that we have just exposed is also repeated, confirming likewise that the terminal arborizations have a maximum den-

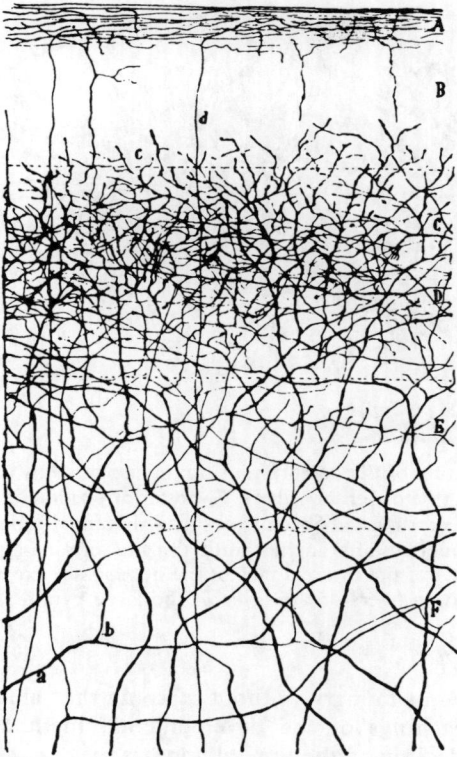

[FIG. 115]   Fig. 29. Sensory plexus of the motor [cortex] of a cat of a few days. A, plexiform layer; B, layer of the small pyramids; C, D, layers of the medium pyramids; E, layer of the giant pyramidal cells; F, layer of the polymorphic cells; a, trunk of a sensory fiber; b, bifurcation; c, small terminal branches; d, fiber of Martinotti.

sity above the layer of the most voluminous pyramids.

We will not describe here in detail, therefore, the course and ramifications of the above-mentioned fibers, all the more because we already have made a quite complete description of them in our monograph in *La Cellule*.[R] We will concentrate for the moment on adding some data, obtained in recent investigations.

In the first place, we must say that the ascending ramifications to the first layer, of which we showed some examples in our figures of the above-mentioned monograph, are not as frequent as we imagined at that time but truly exceptional, so much so that they are

lacking completely in some good impregnations of the newborn and eight-days-old mouse, as well as in the rabbit of one week and in preparations in which the arborizations of the layer of the medium pyramids were perfectly stained (fig. 30, A) [*fig. 116*].

The second point deals with the origin of the fibers. In the mouse, they definitely come from the corona radiata; [then] they ascend in the plane of the cortical white matter, running in a horizontal direction for long distances and giving off at this level some branches; finally, as we have said, they take an ascending course to bifurcate and terminate. The area occupied by the whole arborization reaches in the mouse an enormous extent in relation to the volume of the cerebrum, as can be observed, although with difficulty, in fig. 30 [*fig. 116*].

The third point is about the total area occupied by the motor cortex in the cerebrum of the mouse and rat. This task seems feasible if, as everything seems to prove, the doctrine of Munk and Flechsig about the sensory-motor character of the cerebral foci of projection is true. With this settled clearly, and considering, as we have said above, that the sensory arborizations possess special, almost specific features, the method that we must follow to provide such a determination will be to observe *what is the extent of cortex in which the sensory arborizations are found.*

This method, properly brought to the other sensory regions of the cortex, will allow us also to establish a rational parcelation with an anatomical basis of the various cortical territories (since the mode of ramification and the place of connection of the centripetal fibers is different in each nervous center) and gather together some data to pronounce in due course and opportunely on an interesting dispute arising since the appearance of the important doctrine of Flechsig about the centers of association and projection, namely whether in the smooth-brained mammals there also exist these two kinds of cortical foci, or whether, as that author requires, these animals possess only the phylogenetically older centers, i.e., those designed as the *substratum* of sensations and motor impulses. The investigation and adoption of other principles of the individuality of the cortical areas are all the more nec-

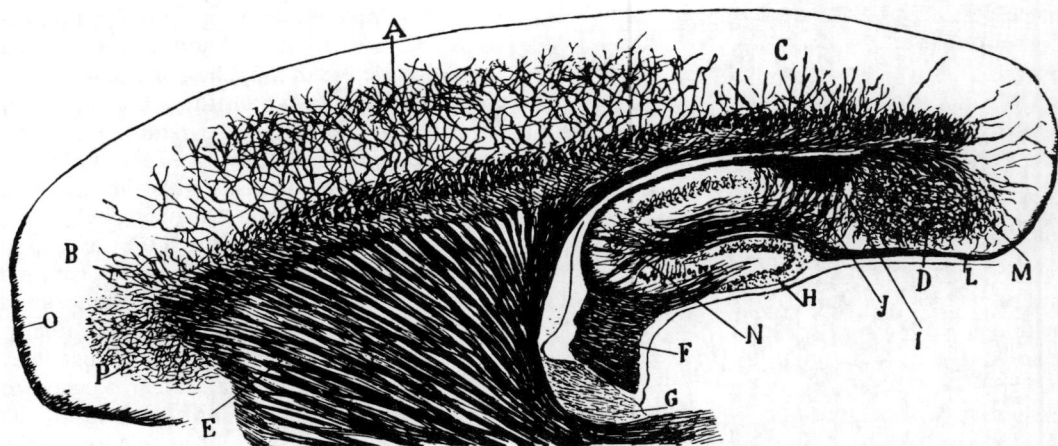

[*FIG. 116*]   Fig. 30. Somewhat lateral, anteroposterior section of the cerebrum of the mouse of a few days. *A*, sensory arborizations of the motor area; *B*, frontal pole free of sensory fibers; *C*, posterior portion of the cortex in which centripetal fibers are later [to arrive]; *D*, plexus of visual fibers; *E*, corpus striatum; *F*, fimbria; *H*, fascia dentata; *I*, thick bundle of fibers that originated bunches of branches ramifying and terminating in the plexiform layer of Ammon's horn (*J*); *L*, plexiform layer of the internal face of the hemisphere covered with horizontal nerve fibers; *M*, visual bundles; *N*, ascending fibers of the layer of the large pyramids of Ammon's horn.

essary because that adopted preferentially by Flechsig (existence or absence of centrifugal or projection fibers) has been the object of some justified criticism. It is known, in fact, that several authors, among whom can be cited Dejerine,[66] Mahaim,[67] and Siemerling,[68] have shown the existence of fibers of projection in cortical regions that Flechsig considered to lack them and hence [he thought] concerned only with functions of association. For our part, we will add that in the mammals of small size (rabbit, rat, and mouse), the Golgi method has always revealed to us fibers of projection in all the cortical regions, although the motor region is the richest in conductors of this kind. This inquiry is all the more straightforward because in the mouse and rat a few days old or newborn, it is very common to obtain preparations where all the nerve fibers (sensory and projection) have been exclusively impregnated, in the absence of cells and dendritic processes. The preparations of this kind, arranged in serial sections, are excellent for the study of the cerebral pathways, as they allow one to follow each fascicle through almost the whole brain and to determine with certainty its origin, course, and termination.

In summary, without scorning the valuable teachings of the developmental method of Flechsig on the time of appearance of myelin, we believe that, in order to determine the extents of the sensory and association areas, preferably the principle of the existence or absence of sensory nervous arborizations coming through the corpus striatum must be applied. Thereby, the sensory areas incorrectly called centers of projection by Flechsig will be characterized because certain parts of the gray matter contain specific plexuses of centripetal fibers, whereas the foci of association will have as a common negative attribute the lack of such plexuses. We do not mean by this that the association areas lack terminal plexuses, but they possess a different character, being formed by thinner fibers, of late appearance, and probably related to association fibers coming from the sensory or sensory-motor areas. The association areas could also have centrifugal fibers.

As Flechsig has pointed out, the later appearance of their fibers is a distinctive characteristic of the association areas. This feature can be appreciated not only with the method of Weigert but with that of Golgi, as we have had the occasion to observe repeatedly in the cerebrum of the human and of mammals. Therefore, in the newborn child, as in some small mammals (mouse, cat, and rabbit), the association areas are distinguished in Golgi preparations because of the almost total absence of the terminal exogenous fibers and for the excessively embryonic appearance of the pyramidal cells and cells of the plexiform layer. In this respect, the silver chromate method resembles the method of Weigert-Pal, as it only stains well the nerve fibers that have reached a certain maturity, that is to say, in a period very distant from that in which the myelin sheath appears.

Extent of the Motor Area in the Mouse, Rat, and Rabbit

We have already said that in these animals the centripetal fibers of the sensory areas can be completely impregnated with relative ease. In no mammals, however, are results obtained as secure as in the mouse of a few days old. As we show in fig. 30 [*fig. 116*], which reproduces a rather lateral, anteroposterior section of the cortex of this rodent, the very robust and precocious sensory arborizations embrace a large part of the cerebrum, almost two-thirds of the vault (fig. 30, A) [*fig. 116*]. Nevertheless, two regions devoid of sensory arborizations are observed: one situated above Ammon's horn (fig. 30, C) [*fig. 116*] and the other corresponding to the frontal pole (fig. 30, B) [*fig. 116*]. In these territories are seen small terminal fibers, few in number, generally thinner, but very poorly arborized or totally undivided, with features, in short, different from those characteristic of the sensory arborizations. There is no doubt that such fibers are in a very early developmental phase.

Finally, below the frontal pole (fig. 30, P) [*fig. 116*] and behind Ammon's horn, very dense, thin plexuses are perceived that it is not possible to mistake for the sensory plexuses. The last of these (fig. 30, D) [*fig. 116*] seems to us to correspond to the visual region, being therefore homologous to the one we have described in the calcarine fissure.

If, instead of longitudinal sections, frontal or transverse sections behind the corpus callosum are studied (fig. 31) [*fig. 117*], the appearance of the cortex that results is very instructive, as it is recognized that the area of the sensory arborizations ceases medially at some distance from the interhemispheric fissure (fig. 31, *a*) [*fig. 117*], and that laterally the plexus of robust fibers is interrupted (fig. 31, *b*) [*fig. 117*] or greatly attenuated, before somewhat further laterally another plexus, with a character somewhat different and very dense in its superficial plane, commences (fig. 31, B) [*fig. 117*]. This new lateral plexus, situated in the descending and lateral portion of the cortex, probably represents the acoustic area, which in the mouse appears well developed, although not as much as the sensory. It follows, therefore, that the motor area occupies an anteroposterior elongated area that expands over a large part of the cortical vault but is not extended either to the occipital or frontal pole or to the sphenoidal lobule or to the internal region of the hemispheres. Anteriorly, the motor areas approach one another, but neither in the rat nor the mouse do they reach to the interhemispheric fissure; they approach closest somewhat to the superior edge of the fissure without reaching it.

A similar position is occupied by the sensory areas of the rabbit, an animal in which the centripetal arborizations are extended more or less over the whole area considered to be motor by the physiologists.

Do Association Areas Exist in Smooth Cerebra?

If the anatomical rule of Flechsig (absence of fibers of projection) is used to pass judgment about this point, only one region of the cortex would be considered an association area. This is the gray matter on the internal face of the hemispheres, from which we have never seen fibers destined for the corpus striatum to arise. The majority of the long axons of this region are reunited above and to the sides of the corpus callosum to form a very robust anteroposterior bundle (fig. 31, *c*) [*fig. 117*] which we have followed easily in serial sections down to Ammon's horn, in whose plexiform layer it arborizes and terminates, often having constituted a large part of the formation that the authors call *longitudinal fibers of the gyrus fornicatus and fornix longus of Forel.*

But if we prefer the above-mentioned cri-

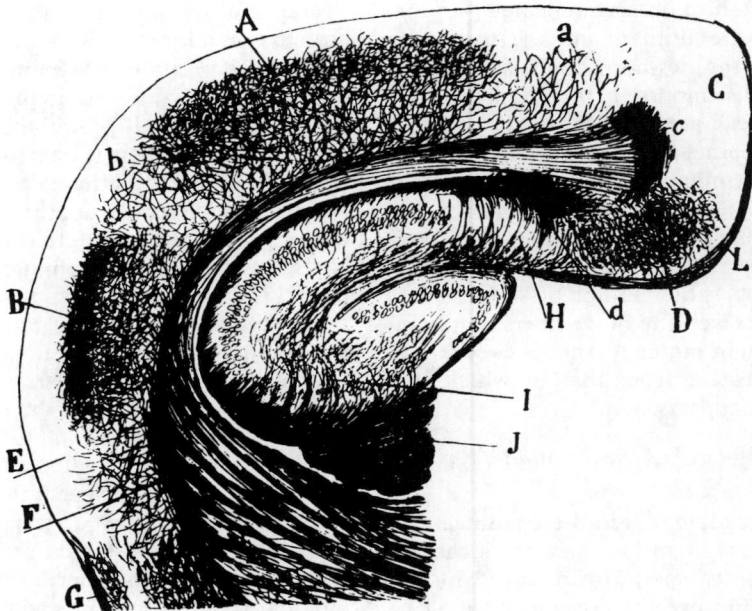

[*FIG. 117*]   Fig. 31. Transverse section of the cerebrum of a mouse a few days old. The section passes behind the corpus callosum. *A*, sensory plexus of the motor region; *B*, acoustic nerve plexus; *C*, internal portion of the hemisphere free of sensory plexuses; *D*, probably visual plexus; *E*, zone without sensory plexuses; *F*, corpus striatum; *G*, olfactory region.

terion (absence of specific arborizations coming from the corona radiata), it must be recognized that the cerebrum of the small mammals also contains some areas of association or ideation, although of small extent and rudimentary. These areas, characterized by their poverty in small terminal fibers at a period in which the centers of sensation have robust fibers and very dense plexuses and because of the impossibility of following their exogenous fibers down the corpus striatum, have not yet been completely studied by us. But, nevertheless, we are inclined to think, with the hope that subsequent investigations will confirm our assertion, that all the cortical areas that in fig. 31 [*fig. 117*] (corresponding to the mouse of a few days) possess associative and memory function lack well-formed centripetal plexuses, namely the gray matter of the whole internal face of the hemisphere (fig. 31, *C*) [*fig. 117*]; the pole and inferior face of the frontal lobule; the superior area of the occipital pole (fig. 31, a^S) [*fig. 117*]; a small space situated between the sensory, motor, and acoustic areas (fig. 31, *b*) [*fig. 117*]; another sit-

uated between this and the olfactory cortex (fig. 31, *E*) [*fig. 117*]; and some more which the deficiency of our observations do not allow us to determine exactly.

The doctrine that we have just exposed harmonizes essentially with that of Flechsig on the anatomicophysiological duality of the cerebral cortex. This cortical duality seems to us, even a priori, eminently rational. The principle of the division of labor that must prevail in the cerebrum more than in any other organ requires that the organs that elaborate the sensation are other than those that have the task of registering memories. In addition, there are other reasons and arguments belonging to physiology and human pathological anatomy which this is not the occasion to specify in detail. We only disagree with Flechsig about the adoption of his anatomical criterion to distinguish the foci of sensation and of ideation (the presence or absence of special centripetal arborizations) and in our acceptance, not only for man but for all mammals, of the two categories of cerebral areas. In our opinion, between the cerebrum of man and that of the mouse, there are only differences of degree, not of quality; consequently, all the differentiated cortical regions endowed with a particular structure and function in the human cerebrum must be represented also, with the necessary reductions and simplifications, in the mammals, and perhaps in other lower vertebrates.

To establish, as Flechsig does, such a contrast in organization between the gyrencephalic and lissencephalic mammals would be legitimate if comparative psychology would reveal to us a similar contrast in relation to psychic acts. But who will be able to consider the cerebrum of the small mammals, whose structural plan, from what we know well, fits perfectly with that of man, as a mere mechanism of reflex acts, an exclusive theater of sensations and motor impulses? Who will deny that in their congruent reactions the said mammals are driven sometimes not only by the sensation but by the residues of those already passed, that is to say, by visual, olfactory, tactile, and acoustic memories? And if for these reminiscences man possesses appropriate registering areas, why are they not possessed also by the lower mammals? An organ that performs in an animal several functions presents an adequate structural complexity for this functional plurality. Therefore, if we admit that the centers of projection of the small mammals have the job both of sensation and of ideation and volition, their intimate organization might be more complex in them than in man, just as happens with the optic lobe of the fishes, batrachians, and reptiles, whose fine structure is much more complicated than the superior colliculus of mammals. In the latter example, the double mission as the organ of motor reflexes and of visual sensations permits such complexity; but in the present case, the contrary occurs as the areas of sensation of the small mammals possess a structure organized certainly according to the design in man, but much more simple.[T]

Plexuses of Centripetal Fibers in the Postcentral Gyrus

The postcentral gyrus also possesses certain terminal nervous plexuses, formed by robust exogenous fibers, but their impregnation is only possible in the child of eight to fifteen days, that is to say, at a much later period than that in which the sensory plexus of the precentral gyrus is stained.

The afferent axons to the postcentral plexus have seemed to us, in general, less dense than those of the precentral sensory plexus; they come from the white matter in a variety of directions; they cross, commonly obliquely, the seventh and eighth layers, having some bifurcations beneath the granule cells, that is to say, the thickness of the seventh and sixth layers, without constituting a well-defined plane of horizontal fibers as in the precentral gyrus; and, finally, they resolve themselves into a very dense arborization of delicate small branches that form by their reciprocal interweaving a horizontal plexus or band located in the middle regions of the cortex, with no lack of small branches distributed outside the frontiers of this band. The true situation of such a plexus is difficult to determine exactly, because, as often happens in the Golgi preparations, when well-impregnated terminal centripetal arborizations are obtained, the cells are not stained, or they are stained in very small numbers, and it is not possible, therefore, to establish the cellular stratum to which the plexus corresponds. Nevertheless, on comparing the plane of the arborization in a preparation of Golgi with one of Nissl of the same region under study, we are inclined to fix the position of the densest and most intricate region of the said plexus in the layer of the granule cells (fifth layer), that is to say, beneath the superficial large pyramids. The highest branches would not go beyond the level of the medium pyramids.

We do not know the significance of this plexus, which we have also found, although less completely stained, in the association areas; its somewhat specific position and aspect, by comparison with the precentral gyrus, has prevented us from accepting without reticence its sensory character.[69]

Callosal Fibers

Omitting the already old opinion of Hamilton, refuted by several authors and in which it was guessed that the corpus callosum is formed by interweaving projection fibers, it is now generally thought that this commissure represents a system of horizontal conductors destined to join together homotopical points of the cortex.

It is reasonable to presume, therefore, that the motor areas of the cerebrum possess a special system of callosal fibers, thanks to which the functional synergy of both hemispheres would be achieved, and perhaps also the storing in the association areas of the opposite side of a large part of the memories of tactile, thermal, and sensory impressions of contralateral origin.[70]

But from the moment that it is sought to determine by anatomical means to what extent such presumptions are legitimate, the difficulties are so grave that they make the solution of the problem almost impossible, especially in the human cerebral cortex, where it is never possible to follow sufficiently the callosal fiber or to distinguish its aspect or its particular manner of distribution in the gray matter from those of the association fiber. At this point, we are wrapped in a darkness that we will perhaps only be able to dispel in the future by anatomicopathological methods allied with procedures for the staining of fibers.

In the small mammals, in which we have particularly studied this question, the difficulties are less exhausting, thanks to the shortness of the distances and to the not unusual fortunate chance that in Golgi preparations the fibers of the corpus callosum are stained almost exclusively. Even so, we have only managed to clarify very incompletely the origin and termination of these fibers. Here are, anyway, some observations that are confirmations and extensions of those published in 1891.[71]

In the transverse sections of the cerebrum of the mouse and rat of four to eight days, the corpus callosum appears perfectly developed; in it are distinguished two planes of fibers that differ in their origins, although they are joined intimately in their trajectory: the *superficial* and the *deep* planes. The superficial, often exclusively impregnated (which reveals perhaps a certain priority of development), originates in the motor area, particularly from the most superior region close to its midline; it goes down to the plane of the corpus callosum, contributing some of its more internal fibers to the most lateral bundles of the large anteroposterior arciform fasciculus of the white matter

(longitudinal fibers of the gyrus fornicatus and fornix longus); then, after lying horizontally beneath this formation, it arrives at the opposite side, again curving inward to enter, at different radii, the motor cortex of the other hemisphere. The callosal fibers appear more abundant in the point of transition between the internal or interhemispheric and the external cortex, which perhaps is merely a consequence of the great thickness of the gray matter in that region. A singular fact is that the cortex of the interhemispheric fissure and the gray matter of the striae of Lancisi lack callosal fibers, or at least, if they exist, they must be notably scarce.

The deep callosal plane, situated beneath the preceding, consists of fibers coming from much more lateral regions of the cortex, perhaps of the acoustic area and areas of transition to the motor [area].

Carefully examining the fibers of the superficial plane or *intermotor fibers,* during their course in the gray matter of both sides, it is observed that their caliber is very thin, in comparison with the axons of the large and medium pyramids, and they are often arranged in small vertical bundles whose filaments end progressively in several cortical layers, but especially above the layer of the large pyramids. At this point, the impregnation is almost always interrupted; only in a few cases is it possible to follow some callosal fibers up to the layer of the small pyramids. It has never been possible for us to see them enter the molecular layer. The vast majority of these fibers maintain perfectly their individuality over their whole course, without exhibiting branches either in the gray matter or in the white matter.

Nevertheless, as we pointed out in other work,[72] a few callosal fibers are bifurcated or give off collaterals before arriving in the contralateral motor region, leading, therefore, [to the belief] that the said fibers must have connections with two or more different parts of the opposite motor area, or perhaps with the motor area and with other sensory or association areas. Such a disposition is, however, less frequent than what we had thought at first.

Thus, a first point can be considered as resolved: the participation of the corpus callosum in the construction of the motor area. This participation can be elevated to the category of a general anatomical role, since, according to our observations, the callosal fibers also enter in part the acoustic areas; and everybody knows that the anterior commissure principally represents a link between the two olfactory cortices (bulbar and sphenoidal), as well as the fornix, which is generally considered as a commissure laid down between the two Ammon's horns.[73] We can admit, then, fearless of being wrong, that between the sensory areas of one hemisphere and those of the contralateral side, there exist transverse pathways of union, although at present it is not possible to determine if this union is established between isodynamic or between heterodynamic groups of pyramids in the homonymous regions.

Are the callosal fibers collaterals of [other] axons, or [are they] direct axons? In our opinion, the corpus callosum, as we pointed out in the work mentioned so many times, consists of both categories of fibers. One is inclined to think that collaterals of axons, either of projection or of association, enter the corpus callosum, because it can be seen that collaterals of some of these axons, once they arrive in the plane of the corpus callosum, are incorporated into the fibers of this structure and are comparable to them in thickness, course, and direction. In spite of this, it is not feasible to be quite sure that such collaterals reach the midline and result in true commissural fibers, because the long trajectory unfortunately prevents them from being followed completely. Thus, the participation of this flow of collaterals in the construction of the corpus callosum has to be expressed as a probable opinion and not as a demonstrated fact.

Much more important, it appears to us, is the contingent of direct axons. As we had recognized and Kölliker has confirmed,[74] the large majority of the callosal fibers comes from the small cells of the cortex, and particularly from small and medium pyramids.

In fact, on following many of these [terminal] fibers backward, sometimes they are observed to increase in thickness and end in a thick extremity that has the appearance of the starting point of an axon. Finally, in some cases, we have revealed a link between these axon origins and true pyramids. For the rest, the absence of collaterals in the initial trajectory of these fibers, a circumstance which is doubtful, can be easily explained by remembering that in the period that such axons are easily impregnated with silver chromate (mouse of four to ten days), the axons of the medium and small pyramids and of the polymorphic cells have still not given off such small branches.

A more arduous undertaking is to determine in these preparations of the cortex which is the terminal callosal fiber, distinguishing it from the fiber of origin. In the mouse of four days and the rabbit of eight days, it is sometimes possible to recognize the terminal fibers because of their greater thinness than the parent fibers, their notably varicose aspect, and the presence of some bifurcations. However, the majority of such terminal callosal fibers are not branched, ending in varicose free tips, either ascending or oblique. For the rest, it would be very risky to affirm that the terminal callosal fibers behave the same in the adult mouse; on the contrary, it might very well happen that later in development they would give rise to some more or less complicated terminal arborizations.

There exists, however, an anatomical fact that lends much verisimilitude to the opinion that the terminal callosal fibers do not reach, even in the adult phase, a great richness of branches; this fact is that any thin axon or collateral, as much in the spinal cord as in the cerebrum, either does not branch or does so very moderately (examples: granule cells of the cerebellum, granule cells of the fascia dentata, small cells of the habenular ganglion, etc.). Let us confess, at any rate, that this point requires further new and more penetrating explorations.

Up to this point, [we have described] the corpus callosum of small mammals. It is natural to presume that the motor area of man also contains fibers and in obviously greater numbers than the mouse. But which among the fibers that the Golgi method allows us to discover in the human cerebral cortex are the callosal fibers? We have already said that we can only conjecture about the origins of the exogenous fibers terminating in the said cortex. Thus, the following assertion of ours must be taken as a possibility only, namely that the terminal callosal fibers correspond to certain little branched, thin threads that are found both in the white matter and in the second and third cellular layers of the motor cortex.

When the nerve fibers of the axis of the precentral gyrus are studied, it is observed, of course, that among the thick and medium fibers, either endogenous or sensory, there exist a few that are particularly delicate and from time to time bifurcated, especially in the vicinity of the gray matter. The resultant branches can undergo further bifurcations, and the daughter branches reach the superimposed gray matter in very different parts of the same gyrus. The further destination of these thin, small branches has constantly escaped our examination.

This fact must be linked with another about which we have not yet spoken in the course of this work.

This is the existence, in certain preparations of the motor cortex of the child of fifteen days to one month, at the level of the layer of the small and medium pyramids, of a plexus of fibers of extraordinary richness and whose more interesting features are the dominant vertical orientation of its fibers, the penury of ramifications of the fibers, and the extreme delicacy of their caliber, which does not exceed, in general, $0.2~\mu m$. Such extreme delicacy obliges the use of the 1.30 Zeiss objective to observe them properly.

Some fibers form vertical small bundles, others run in a dispersed manner, and there is no lack of some that cross the shafts of the pyramids obliquely and with a variety of inclinations. The higher small fibers reach the plexiform layer, where, not unusually, they are bifurcated, but these are scarce; the vast majority end in different planes of the second layer or [layer] of the small pyramids. When the fibers are followed downward, it is observed that they submerge in the vicinity of the layer of the giant cells, in which they lose their vertical course, acquiring a flexuous trajectory, and escape observation.

It has been impossible for us to follow them down to the white matter, to observe their link with the innumerable short axons ramifying among the second, third, and fourth layers. The fibers that resemble them most are the fibers that form the vertical small bundles of arborizations of the bitufted cells, but the absence or the extreme poverty of their ramifications distinguishes them at first sight from the latter.

In summary, could not these threads, whose origin appears to us to be very enigmatic, represent the terminations of the callosal fibers? This is a question whose answer must be reserved for the future. For the present, it is enough for us to point out that in the upper layers of the motor cortex, there are located a multitude of thin fibers of an axonal nature that apparently are not continuous, either with the collaterals of the pyramids or with the arborizations of the cells of short axon, or with the sensory ramifications, and which, by exclusion, could very well be terminal branches of callosal fibers. It is clear that there is no strong reason to exclude other origins, for example, to reject the possibility of their being association fibers, among which, as we have said elsewhere, there are also collateral branches of a thickness comparable to the callosal fibers.

Association Fibers

In the human motor region, all our efforts to identify exogenous association fibers by special characteristics or particular connections have been in vain. We must, however, presume that they exist and that perhaps they are very numerous, coming from the several association areas and perhaps from other sensory areas.

In the mouse, the presence of these fibers does not present any doubts, although they are rather more scarce than would be expected. In fact, the immense majority of the fibers entering the motor area of this animal are callosal or sensory fibers. It is possible, however, to observe, especially in longitudinal sections of the cerebrum of the mouse of four to fifteen days, some very long anteroposterior association fibers which become more abundant as in sagittal sections we come closer to the territory of the arcuate fasciculus.[U] These fibers appear scattered in the deep two-thirds of the motor cortex, showing some ascending or oblique collaterals, and they are distributed in several parts of the area. Their origin is still doubtful; some of them can be followed forward to an accumulation of large cells situated in the frontal region ahead of the corpus callosum.

The arcuate fasciculus is, without doubt, the more important route of association in the cerebrum of rodents. But the majority of its fibers lack relations with the motor cortex, representing a system of communication between Ammon's horn and the gray matter of the interhemispheric fissure. If it has some relationship with the motor area, this could only be established in the most extensive portion of the fasciculus. But we will deal with the probable connections of the large anteroposterior association route of the small mammals in other work, when we study the olfactory cortex.

Collaterals of the White Matter

By analogy with what happens in the white matter of the spinal cord, medulla, and pons, it appears likely that the white matter of the cerebrum also has collateral [axon] branches, whose distribution would occur in the superimposed gray matter. This definitely happens in the cerebrum of small mammals, where all the association bundles exhibit small collateral fibers, although [they are] few in number. These are particularly visible in the white matter of the arcuate fasciculus, striae of Lancisi, white cortex of Ammon's horn, etc. Those of the arcuate fasciculus can be followed up to the molecular layer.

In the human cerebrum and particularly in the white matter of the gyri, the collaterals are few in number, and of those that exist it is impossible to decide if they belong to association fibers, to exogenous fibers, to terminal sensory fibers, or to the axons of the pyramids located in the superimposed cortex.

However, our personal impression, based especially on the study of the cortex of rodents, is that the majority of the collaterals arising from the white matter come from association fibers; the projecting axons, the callosal, and sensory fibers very rarely give off collaterals; when they branch in the white matter, the common mode of division is a bifurcation.

Endogenous Fibers

Long Axons

These are the axons of the small, medium, and large pyramids of the granule, fusiform, and polymorphic cells. As is well known, such axons form small vertical bundles; begin at the level of the medium pyramids with a few, barely approximated fibers; and are progressively thickened by the incorporation of new axons until they reach the white matter, where they get lost.

We have already spoken about the collaterals arising from such axons as they traverse the gray matter, as well as about the plexuses that they engender throughout almost the whole depth of the cortex. Here we will add only that in man such collaterals can reach an enormous length, and they constitute a system of association over both short and long distances between pyramids of the same layer or of immediately adjoining layers. The majority of the fibers of the interradiate plexuses are none other than the collaterals of pyramidal axons. Needless to say, all of these collaterals have a myelin sheath on their main axons and thick branches but lack it on the small, varicose terminal branches.

When they reach the white matter, the majority of the axons continue as a single nerve fiber. The bifurcations, which are observed with relative frequency in the cerebrum of small mammals, are scarce in the human motor cortex. Up till now, we have only been able to confirm them in the case of a few axons arising from pyramidal or fusiform cells of the seventh and eighth layers. The divisions often have the form of a Y or a T. It is not rare to see that one of the branches is thinner than the other. Sometimes, the thin branch, after running in the opposite direction, changes plane to become deeper than its fellow. Such thin branches likely go to other parts of the gyrus, so they must be regarded as association fibers, although, needless to say, nothing certain can be stated about their destinations.

The relative rarity with which the endogenous axons in the white matter of man divide perhaps arises simply from technical difficulties, for example, the impossibility of exploring their whole very long trajectory through the white matter. In the mouse and rat, as a consequence of the narrowness of the band of white matter that separates the gray cortex from the corpus striatum or from the lateral ventricle, the bifurcations and collaterals of association are obliged to be concentrated in a narrow region, amenable to analysis; but in man, such divisions might occur anywhere in the white matter and according to the law of economy [of matter] at points favorable to and different for each fiber from the same area. It would, therefore, be very desirable to make a complete exploration of the white matter of the human cerebrum with the methods of Golgi and Ehrlich from this point of view.

With regard to the cerebrum of the cat, we have made a partial study with the aid of the Ehrlich procedure[75] and have been persuaded that the divisions and collaterals exist only near the gray matter and not in the axes of the gyri or at a distance from these. We must not forget, however, a potential cause of error that we have not always been able to discount: the possibility of taking the dichotomizing of a sensory afferent fiber for the division of an endogenous or projection fiber.

Arborizations of the Cells with Short Axon

They have already been exposed when dealing with the corresponding layers of the motor cortex. The plexuses they give rise to are of an extraordinary density and richness, not only in the motor cortex but also in the whole human cortex, forming without doubts one of the anatomical features more characteristic of this and proving the superior organization of the cerebrum of man. Unfortunately, the delicacy, intricacy, and spread of such arborizations; the absence of corresponding limits to the layers; and the impossibility, with a few exceptions, of labeling the cells with which they form connections make a systematic study of them almost impossible.

Here it is appropriate to say only that all the layers of the cortex are rich in nerve plexuses engendered by cells with short axon and, particularly, those in the layers of the small and medium pyramids; and that, usually, the dense and thin arborizations originating from the

small or medium cell types are in relationship with the somata and initial portions of the [apical dendritic] shafts of the pyramids, whereas the loose arborizations, of long branches, coming from cells of large size, appear to enter into transverse, oblique, or parallel contact with the [apical] shafts and other dendrites of the pyramids. There are, however, exceptions to this rule, which does not seem to us to be applicable entirely to the cells with short axon of the first or plexiform layer.

Another fact that we believe to be unquestionable is the lack of myelin on the terminal arborizations of the short axons. About that, one can be easily persuaded in comparing the Golgi and Weigert preparations. In the latter, the vast majority of the thin medullated fibers with an oblique or horizontal direction among the [radial bundles] of the axons of projection, and in the second and third layers, correspond sometimes to sensory or callosal branches and sometimes to collaterals of the pyramidal axons. The axons of Martinotti and the horizontal cells of the first layer must be regarded from this point of view as long axons, because they are provided with a myelin sheath.

Conclusions

From all of this long and fatiguing study of the motor cortex, a study that is far from being terminated, some general conclusions can be made, among which the most important appear to us to be the following.

1. The precentral gyrus and the posterior portions of the first and second frontal [gyri] have a different structure from that displayed by other cortical regions.

The peculiarity of this structure consists of the lack of a well-differentiated layer of granule cells (the granule cells are scattered above and below the fourth layer), the enormous thickness of the layers of the medium and superficial large pyramids, and the presence of a specific nerve plexus, composed of robust exogenous fibers and situated at the level of the medium pyramids.

2. The postcentral gyrus resembles, at least in a large part of its extent, the association cortex, because, like the latter, it has a well-defined layer of granule cells, a thin layer of me-

dium and superficial large pyramids, and a special exogenous nerve plexus, located in a position different from that in the frontal cortex. Consequently, it is permissible to suspect one of two things: either that the postcentral gyrus represents a special motor region that has demanded, because of the peculiar nature of its activities, a structure somewhat different from that of the companion gyrus, or that the motor significance attributed to it is incorrect, and it has, at least in a large part of its extent, the physiological characteristics of association cortex. In the latter case, it could be suggested that it represents a focus of ideomotor association, whose excitation because of its proximity to the sensory-motor areas would produce, like the direct stimulus of the pre-Rolandic structures, movements in particular muscular groups.

3. The motor cortex gives off and receives callosal fibers; perhaps it receives also fibers originating in other brain territories and gives off in its turn nervous fibers probably terminating in special centers of association so far undetermined.

4. In the manner of the visual cortex, the motor presents also the common structural features [of all cortex] (plexiform layer, layers of the medium and small pyramids, etc.), and [also] the singular features by which it is recognized, [i.e.], the sensory plexus of the third layer and the size and considerable number of the giant pyramids.

5. Since the layer of medium pyramids is the special place where the sensory fibers are distributed, it can be conjectured that these cells constitute the substratum of tactile, painful, and thermal sensations and the starting point of the fibers destined to bring residues or memories of such perceptions to other points of the cerebrum.

6. Although it is impossible to specify the real roles of the several kinds of pyramids, the results of our overall investigations make it quite permissible to advance the hypothesis that the pyramidal tract arises from the giant pyramids and to no small extent from the medium pyramids, while the callosal pathway has its principal but not exclusive origin in the small pyramids and perhaps also in the polymorphic cells.

Cajal's Notes

1. We must express here our gratitude to the director and physicians of the Foundling Hospital of this city, and particularly to our valued friend Dr. Figueroa, for the facilities they have placed at our disposal and for the material necessary for our investigation.

2. An abstract of the present work was the subject of one of three lectures given at Clark University (Worcester, Mass.) on the 8th, 10th, and 12th of last July. The English text of these lectures is now in the course of publication [Cajal, 1899c].

3. T. Meynert, Manual of Stricker. *Vom Gehirne der Säugethiere*, p. 704 [1872].

4. Betz, Ueber die feinere Struktur der menschlichen Gehirnrinde, *Centralblatt f. die med. Wissensch.*, nos. 11, 12, 13, 1881.

5. Bevan Lewis, Researches on the Comparative Structure of the Cortex Cerebri. *Phil. Trans.*, 1880.
Bevan Lewis and Clarke, The Cortical Lamination of the Motor Area of the Brain, *Proceedings of the Royal Society*, Vol. 28 [1878].

6. Golgi, Sulla fina anatomia degli organi centrali del sistema nervoso, Milano, 1886.

7. S. Ramón y Cajal, Textura de las circunvoluciones cerebrales en los mamíferos inferiores, Barcelona, December 1890.
——, Sobre la existencia de colaterales y bifurcaciones en las fibras de la substancia blanca del cerebro, December 1890.
——, Sur la structure de l'écorce cérébrale de quelques mammifères, *La Cellule*, Vol. VII, 1891.

8. Retzius, *Biol. Unters.* N.F., Vol. V, 1893; and Vol. VI, 1894.

9. Karl Schaffer, Zur feineren Struktur der Hirnrinde und über die funktionelle Bedeutung der Nervenzellenfortsätze, *Arch. f. Mikros. Anat.*, Bd. 48, [Pt.] IV, 1897.

10. Bevan Lewis, The Structure of the First or Outermost Layer of the Cerebral Cortex, *Medical Journ.*, Edinburg, June 1897.

11. E. Veratti, Ueber einige Struktureigenthumlichkeiten der Hirnrinde bei den Säugethieren. *Anat. Anzeiger*, no. 14, 1897.

12. [E.] A. Schäfer, The Spinal Cord and Brain, Vol. III, part 1. *Quain's Elements of Anatomy*, 10th ed., 1893.

13. Hammarberg, *Studien über Klinik und Pathologie der Idiotie*, etc., published by Dr. S. E. Henschen, Upsala, 1895.

14. A. Kölliker, *Handbuch der Gewebelehre.*, 6th edition, Vol. II, 1896.

15. Edinger, *Vorlesungen ueber den Bau der nervösen Centralorgane*, 6th edition, Leipzig, 1899.

16. Schlapp, Der Zellenbau der Grosshirnrinde des Affen, etc. *Arch f. Psychiatrie.* Vol. 30, 189[8].

17. Tuczek, Ueber die Anordnung der markhaltigen Nervenfasern in des Grosshirnrinde, *Neurolog. Centralbl.*, 1882.

18. Zacher, Ueber das Verhalten der markhaltigen Nervenfasern in der Hirnrinde bei der Progressiven Paralyse, etc. *Arch. f. Psych. u. Nervenkunden*, 1887.

19. Bechterew, Zur Frage über die äusseren Associationfasern der Hirnrinde. *Neurol. Centralbl.*, 1891.

20. Vulpius, Ueber die Entwicklung und Ausbreitung des Tangentialfasern in der menschlichen Grosshirnrinde während verschiedener Alterperioden. *Arch. f. Psych. u. Nervenk.*, 1892.

21. Kaes, Beiträge zur Kenntnis der Reichtums der Grosshirnrinde des Menschen zur markhaltigen Nervenfasern, *Arch. f. Psychiatr. u. Nervenk.* H. 3, 1893.

22. Bottazzi, Intorno alla corteccia cerebrale, e spezialmente intorno alle fibre nervose intracorticali dei vertebrati, 1893.

23. Nissl, *Allgem. Zeitschr. f. Psych.*, Bd. 50, [1894–95].

——, *Neurolog. Centralbl.*, nos. 2, 3, 1895.

24. Azoulay. See Dejerine, *Anatomie des centres nerveux*, Vol. I, 1895. (Figure 338, drawn by Azoulay.)

25. Van Gehuchten, *Anatomie du système nerveux de l'homme.*, etc., 3rd edition, Vol. 1, [1900].

26. Flechsig, *Gehirn und Seele*, 1896, Leipzig. *Die Localisation des geistigen Vorgänge insbesondere der Sinnesempfindungen des Menschen*, Leipzig, 1896.

27. Siemerling, Ueber Markscheidenentwickelung des Gehirns und ihre Bedeutung für die Localisation (*Versammlung d. Vereins d. Deutsch. Irrenärzte zu Bonn.*, 17 Sept. 1898).

28. Ballet and Faure, Atrophie des grandes cellules pyramidales dans la zone motrice de l'écorce cérébrale, *Société Méd. des Hôpitaux*, 30 March 1899.

29. Dotto and Pusatteri, *Rivista di Patol. Nervosa e Mentale*, no. 1, 1897.

30. Marinesco, Sur les altérations des grandes cellules pyramidales consécutives aux lésions de la capsule interne, *Revue Neurologique*, 1899.

31. E. Lugaro, Genesi delle circunvoluzioni cerebrali e cerebellari, *Rivista di Pat. Ner. e Ment.*, Vol. II, 1897.

32. See Conference at Clark University, July 1899.

33. S. Ramón y Cajal, Estructura del protoplasma nervioso, *Rev. Trim. Microgr.*, Vol. I, 1896.

34. Andriezen, *British Medical Journal*, July 1893.

35. Kölliker, *Handbuch der Gewebelehre*, 1st edition, 1852.

36. Exner, Zur Kenntnis vom feineren Bau der Grosshirnrinde, *Sitzungsber. d. Kais. Akad. der Wissensch. in Wien*, 1881.

37. Martinotti, Beitrag zum Studium der Hirnrinde, etc., *Intern. Monatsch. f. Anat. u. Physiol.*, Vol. VIII, 1890.

38. Kölliker and some authors attribute this discovery to Retzius. In fact, it is only right to admit that we are indebted to the illustrious Swedish scientist for the first detailed description and exact representation of the terminal tuft of the pyramids in man (Ueber den Bau der Oberflachenschicht der Grosshirnrinde beim Menschen und bei den Säugethieren, *Biologiska Foreingens Förhandlingar*, Vol. III, January–March 1891, nos. 4–6); but, before Retzius, they were already observed by us in small mammals, as is proven by the attached figure of our first work and by several passages of the text, in which the *peripheral arborization of the shaft of the pyramids* is explicitly mentioned (Textura de las circunvoluciones cerebrales de los mamíferos inferiores. Preliminary note with two plates, 30 November 1890). Let us add, also, that in another note (Sobre la existencia de células nerviosas especiales en la primera capa de los circunvoluciones cerebrales, *Gaceta Médica Catalana*, 15 December 1890), alluding to the connections occurring in the first layer, we said: "to this purpose (to be related to terminal nerve fibers), all the pyramidal cells send to the first layer a dendritic shaft that *is* richly *arborized* among the above-mentioned nerve fibers, ending by small free branches bristling with spines and impressed gulfs." [*sic.* We believe that this may refer to elongated spines with bifurcated necks or to gaps between spines. See chapter 1 in this volume]. There is even a passage in another work, in which the terminal *cup* of the pyramids is spoken of; but we will not insist more on this point, limiting ourselves to remembering that Retzius himself, giving proof of an impartiality rarely imitated, confesses in his above-mentioned work that the form of the terminal ramification of the shaft "has been considered by me in the same way as he himself considers it, according to the details of a small figure in our cited paper of the 30th November of 1890."

39. Hill, The Chrome Silver Method, Presidential Address to the Neurological Society., *Brain*, London, 1896. Bevan Lewis, The Structure of the First or Outermost Layer of the Cerebral Cortex, *Edinburgh Medical Journal*, June 1897.

40. S. R. Cajal, Las células de axón corto de la capa molecular del cerebro, *Rev. Trim. Microgr.*, Vol. II, 1897.

41. Retzius, Die Cajal'schen Zellen der Grosshirnrinde des Menschen, *Biol. Unter. Neue Folge.*, Vol. VI, 1894.

42. Cajal, *Rev. Trim. Microgr.*, Vol. II, 1897.

43. S. R. Cajal, Sur les fibres nerveuses de la couche granuleuse du cervelet, etc., *Intern. Monatsch. f. Anat. u. Physiol.*, Bd. VII, 1890.

44. Schaper, Einige kritische Bemerkungen zu Lugaros Aufsatz ueber die Histogenese der Körner, etc., *Anat. Anzeiger*, no. 13, 1895.

45. Athias, Structure histologique de la moelle du têtard de la grenouille, *Bibliogr. Anatom.*, Vol. V, 1897.

46. R. Terrazas, Notas sobre la neuroglia del cerebelo y el crecimiento de los elementos nerviosos, *Rev. Trim. Microgr.*, Vol. II, 1897.

47. S. R. Cajal, Sobre la existencia de células nerviosas especiales en la primera capa de las circunvoluciones cerebrales, *Gaz. Med. Catalana*, 15 December 1890.

——, Textura de las circunvoluciones cerebrales de los mamíferos inferiores. Preliminary note, Barcelona, 30 Nov. 1890.

48. S. R. Cajal, Las células de cilindro-eje corto de la capa molecular del cerebro, *Rev. Trim. Microgr.*, Vol. II, 1897.

49. K. Schaffer, Zur feineren Struktur des Hirnrinde über die funktionelle Bedeutung der Nervenzellenfortsätze, *Arch. f. Mik. Anat.*, Vol. 48, 1897.

50. A. Kölliker, *Handbuch*, 6th edition, Vol. II, [1896] p. 644 and following.

51. [K.] Schaffer, *loc. cit.* [page 420].

52. The doctrine of Schaffer, in that it denies the conductor role of the dendrites, is so gratuitous and arbitrary and contrary to all the facts of the peridendritic and perisomatic relationships discovered over the last twelve years that we regard it as completely idle to refute it. If Schaffer would limit himself, like Lenhossék, to regarding the initial collaterals as a particular system of dendrites, a remnant of the collector apparatus of the neurons of invertebrates, such an opinion would still offer large difficulties, but it would fight the facts to a much lesser extent. Furthermore, his conjecture, limited in this way and stripped of its arbitrary denial of the receptive capacity of the soma and dendrites, would fit perfectly with our theory of axipetal polarization. The [impulses] could go from the collaterals to the axon in a cellulifugal direction, without the necessity of passing retrogradely through the soma. For the rest, the theory of axipetal polarization seems each day more probable, especially since Bethe has demonstrated that in the invertebrates the nervous excitation does not need to be propagated to the soma, passing from the dendrites or initial collaterals to the axon and its terminal arborization. With regard to the objections that Van Gehuchten raises against this new formulation of the theory of dynamic polarization (*Anatomie du système nerveux de l'homme*, 3rd edition, [1900]), [these objections] have very little force, as we will probe in another work.

53. Mondino, Richerche macro-microscopiche sul centri nervosi, Torino, 1887.

54. Martinotti, Su alcuni migloramenti della tecnica della reazione al nitrato d'argento nei centri nervosi, etc., *Annali di Freniatria e Scienze Affini.*, Vol. I, 188[7].

55. Retzius, Die Cajal'schen Zellen der Grosshirnrinde beim Menschen und bei Säugetieren, *Biol. Unter.*, N.F., Bd. V, 1893. See in plate 4, fig. 6, the cells labeled k.p.

56. S. Ramón y Cajal, Estructura del asta de Ammon y fascia dentata, *Anal. de la Sociedad Española de Historia Natural*, Vol. 22, 1893.

57. Semi Meyer, Ueber die Funktion der Protoplasm. Fortsätze de Nervenzellen, *Abhand. d. Sachs ges. d. Wiss*, 189[7].

58. Bethe, Ueber die Primitivfibrillen in den Ganglienzellen von Menschen und anderen Wirbelthieren, *Morphol. Arbeit. v. Schwalbe*, Vol. 8, Part I, 1898.

59. F. Nissl, Nervenzellen und graue Substanz, *Münchener Medizinischen Wochenschrift.*, nos. 31, 32, 33, 1898.

60. S. Ramón y Cajal, La red superficial de las células nerviosas centrales, *Rev. Trim. Micr.*, Vol. III, 1898.

61. W. Aldren Turner and W. Hunter, On a Form of Nerve Termination in the Central Nervous System, etc., *Brain*, Spring 1899.

62. These are: El azul de metileno en los centros nerviosos, *Rev. Trim. Microgr.*, Vol. I, 1896; Las espinas colaterales demostradas por el azul de metileno, *Rev. Trim. Microgr.*, Vol. I, 1896; Las células de cilindro eje corto de la capa molecular del cerebro, *Rev. Trim. Mi-*crogr., Vol. III, 1897; La red superficial de las células nerviosas centrales, *Rev. Trim. Microgr.*, Vol. III, 1898.

63. S. Ramón y Cajal, Sur la structure de l'écorce cérébrale de quelques mammifères, *La Cellule*, 1891.

64. S. Ramón y Cajal, Sur la structure de l'écorce cérébrale de quelques mammifères, *La Cellule*, June 1891.

65. Kölliker, *Lehrbuch der Gewebelehre des Menschen*, 6 Aufl., Bd. II, 1896, p. 666.

66. Dejerine, Sur les fibres de projection et d'association des hemisphères cérébraux, *Compt. Rend. des Séances de la Société de Biol.*, 20 February 1897.

67. Mahaim, Centres de projection et centres d'association du cerveau, *Annal. de la Société Médico-chirurgicale de Liège*, 1897.

68. E. Siemerling, Ueber Markscheidenentwickelung des Gehirns, etc., *Versam. des Vereins der Deutsch. Irrenärzte zu Bonn am 17 Sept. 1898 gehal. Vortrage.*

69. At the time that we wrote the study on the visual cortex, our observations on the motor cortex had focused, preferentially, on the postcentral gyrus. It was precisely in this gyrus that we observed for the first time a nervous plexus of exogenous fibers which, imbued as we were with a preconception about the structural unity of the motor cortex, we generalized prematurely to the precentral gyrus. Later, when we discovered the sensory plexuses of this new territory, and we ascertained that their main place of distribution was the layer of the medium pyramids, we had to restrict the said generalization, being convinced that in regard to the disposition and localization of these plexuses, the two mentioned gyri are not equal. The indications, thus, that we made about this point in our first report (Visual Cortex, *Rev. Trim. Micr.*, 1899 p. 62) and in our lectures at Clark University (Comparative Study of the Sensory Areas of the Human Cortex, *Clark University Decennial Celebration*, Worcester, 1899, p. 370 and following) must be taken as alluding to the postcentral gyrus and not to the whole motor area.

70. See Cajal, Estructura del kiasma óptico, etc., *Rev. Trim. Micr.*, 1898, p. 59 and following.

71. Cajal, Sur la structure de l'écorce cérébrale de quelques mammifères, *La Cellule*, Vol. VII, part I, 1891.

72. *Loc. cit.*, p. 37 and following.

73. Cajal, Ueber die feinere Struktur des Ammonshorns, *Zeitschr. f. wiss. Zool.*, Bd. 56, 1893.

74. Kölliker, *Lehrbuch der Gewebelehre*, 6th edition [1896].

75. Cajal, El azul de metileno en los centros nerviosos, *Rev. Trim. Microg.*, Vol. I, 1896, p. 193.

Editors' Notes

A. Cajal's words.

B. The original incorrectly says 3.

C. Neuroglial cells.

D. The original incorrectly says fig. 27.

E. The original incorrectly says fig. 30.

F. Cajal uses the word *currents* here and in many other places.

G. The original incorrectly says *7* and *8*.

H. The original incorrectly says 8, *E*.

I. the original incorrectly says 8, *K*.

J. The original has fig. 7, *D*, which appears to be incorrect.

K. The original has fig. 8, *H*.

L. The original has fig. 8, *I*.

M. The original incorrectly says *third* layer.

N. i.e., its failure to be condensed into a nucleolus.

O. See [*fig. 42*] in chapter 9 in this volume.

P. Reference to fig. 21, *G* added by us.

Q. The gracile and cuneate nuclei and fasciculi.

R. See chapter 5 in this volume.

S. The original, apparently incorrectly, says 30, *a*.

T. Here ends the first, longer portion of this paper, which appeared in the *Revista Trimestral Micrográfica* 4:117–200, 1899. What follows is the conclusion, which appeared in the same *Revista* 5:1–11, 1900.

U. Presumably the cingulum.

17

Studies on the Human Cerebral Cortex III: Structure of the Acoustic Cortex

[*Revista Trimestral Micrográfica* 5:129–183, 1900]

The analytical study that follows deals with the human sphenoidal cortex,[A] specifically with the first temporal and insular gyri, regions that the pathologists think are the principal cortical site of auditory function. This functional localization has also been confirmed, in broad outline and allowing for species differences, in gyrencephalic animals, such as the dog and monkey (Munk, Luciani, Seppilini, Ferrier, Monakow, etc.). Thus, Munk has proven, using the ablation method, that the acoustic area in the dog is located in the center of the second and third sphenoidal gyri. With this cortical area bilaterally removed, the animal ceases reacting to acoustic stimulation. Such a region must be considered a pure sensory center, on the whole comparable to the visual area of the occipital pole of the cerebrum. It would not be thus a center of ideation or of sensory memories, but the cortical region where auditory perception takes place. The area for the memories of sounds, that is to say, the cortical place from whose activity the understanding of words results, would be located lower down, not far from the sphenoidal pole. The ablation of this region of cortex in the dog causes verbal deafness, which is the total incomprehension of commands and of the significance of all kinds of noises and sounds.

The results of the anatomicopathological methods agree with the teachings of physiological experimentation. When the secondary acoustic routes arising from the inferior colliculus are interrupted, ascending degeneration is observed which terminates in the sphenoidal lobule of the cerebrum; and vice versa, if this lobule is removed, it leads to degeneration and atrophy that descends to the inferior colliculus and medial geniculate body (Monakow).

In man, the acoustic region of the cerebrum has a more extensive area than in animals and shows a greater complexity, without doubt dependent on the anatomical adaptation to the faculty of spoken language and to musical intelligence. According to Dejerine, the region of language in man includes the whole surroundings of the sylvian fissure and the gyri of the insula, extending from behind those to the supramarginal gyrus and to a portion of the base of the occipital lobule. Inferiorly, its limits are marked by the inferior margin of the first sphenoidal gyrus. Similar localizations have been established by other pathologists, particularly Monakow, Wernicke, etc.

Unfortunately, an accurate determination of the acoustic localizations in man is still needed. It will be necessary, on the one hand, to determine exactly the cortical area of the sonorous, musical, and verbal sensations, separating it from the place in which are located the acoustic memories and the ideomotor coordinations involved in speech; on the other hand, it will have to distinguish correctly the areas corresponding to the several kinds of acoustic memories. Such localizations not having been established in exact detail, we must be content, in order to be useful for us as a guide in our anatomical explorations, with a total or global physiological localization of both acoustic sensations and memories. The exact place of acoustic sensation is unknown, but it is known that it is located in the upper part of the sphenoidal gyrus, as proven by the cases reported by Wernicke, Friedlander, Pick, and others, in which a more or less complete softening of the sphenoidal lobules led to complete deafness.

In the absence, therefore, of a physiological localization that allows us to separate topographically the acoustic areas of association from those of projection, we have no other recourse than to explore methodically the whole sphenoidal cortex, excluding the piriform lobule and Ammon's horn, whose olfactory significance cannot be doubted.

In the present work, our main purpose has been to find out if, as happens in the visual cortex, the auditory cortex is also distinguished from other areas by some anatomical peculiarity which, coinciding topographically with the auditory physiological localizations, would be useful to us as a guide to trace better its limits. And, as all the pathologists give as the preferred place of mental audition the anterior half of the first sphenoidal gyrus, we will begin our anatomical examination of the human sphenoidal cortex by the exploration of that convolution.

Faithful to our method, we have used as material for study the child of a few days (newborn and of fifteen, twenty, and thirty days), in which the method of Golgi gives quite good results. To complete our reports, we have re-sorted also to the adult human cortex, stained by the methods of Nissl and Weigert-Pal.

I. Cortex of the First Sphenoidal Gyrus

The data that are available about the structure of the sphenoidal cortex in general, and about the first gyrus in particular, are little abundant and imprecise.

According to Betz,[1] the cortex of the three temporal gyri is characterized by the existence of a thick fifth layer (layer of the fusiform cells) and by the presence in the third layer, or layer of the large pyramids, of small [cellular] elements.

C. Hammarberg,[2] who for the first time has submitted all the gyri of the human cortex to a systematic study with the Nissl method, observes in the *superior temporal gyrus* the following layers:

First or molecular layer, composed of some isolated cells without a characteristic disposition. Its thickness is 0.20 mm.

Second layer or [layer] of the small pyramids. The size of these cells is 9 by 15 μm, increasing in size with depth until the layer becomes merged with the third.

Third layer or [layer] of the large pyramids. The deepest cells of this layer have a size 20 by 30 μm, but the superficial ones do not exceed 12 by 22 μm.

Fourth layer or [layer] of the granule cells. It is constituted of small pyramids and of irregular cells.

Fifth layer or [layer] of the ganglionic cells. In it, large pyramids of 20 by 30 μm are mixed with medium or small pyramids 10 by 18 μm.

Sixth layer or [layer] of the fusiform cells. It is extremely thick, measuring 1.20 mm in thickness. It is composed of elongated and fusiform cells that measure 9 by 30 μm.

The medial, inferior, and internal temporal gyri are distinguished from the [superior temporal] gyrus in that the cells of the third layer and of the fifth (ganglionic cells) are larger, but without reaching giant size.

According to Schlapp,[3] the sphenoidal cortex corresponds to the so-called *second cortical type* of this author, that is to say, that in which the layers of the *pygnomorphic giant* cells appear divided in two strata by the insertion of a layer of granule cells. Altogether the layers are:

First layer or [layer] of the tangential fibers. It is thinner than in the first or motor type.

Second layer or [layer] of the external polymorphic cells. (Small pyramids of other authors.)

Third layer or [layer] of the parapygnomorphic cells. (Medium pyramids.)

Fourth layer or [layer] of the pygnomorphic pyramids. (Superficial giant pyramids.)

Fifth layer or [layer] of the granule cells. Corresponding to the fourth layer of Hammarberg; contains small multipolar cells of 6 by 6 μm or 6 by 7 μm.

Sixth layer or [layer] of pygnomorphic pyramids. Corresponds to the deep half of the layer of the large pyramids of the motor cortical type. These cellular elements do not reach the size of the cells of the latter type of cortex.

Seventh layer or [layer] of the internal polymorphic cells. (Fusiform cells of Meynert.)

When dealing with the significance of the layer of the granule cells, Schlapp affirms that such minute cellular elements cannot be regarded as association neurons, since they are particularly abundant in genuinely sensory regions; probably, they intervene and are necessary in the act of proper sensation, even when it is impossible at the present to determine the nature of this collaboration.

Such are the few anatomical data that we have been able to collect about the auditory region of the sphenoidal lobule. It is obvious that our knowledge about the morphology and relationships of the cells of this part of the gray matter leaves a lot to be desired and requires new and more careful explorations. In the following pages, we will expose the results of our explorations.

Enumeration of the Layers and Examination with the Methods of Nissl, Weigert, and Golgi

Perpendicular sections of the first temporal gyrus of the adult human reveal in the Nissl sections the following layers:

First layer, plexiform or molecular [layer] of the authors; second layer or [layer] of the small pyramids; third layer or [layer] of the medium pyramids; fourth layer or [layer] of the giant pyramids; fifth layer or [layer] of the granule cells or small nerve cells; sixth layer or [layer] of the deep medium pyramidal cells; seventh layer or [layer] of the fusiform and triangular cells.

These layers have very unequal thickness and development. Thus, the plexiform layer is thinner, as Schlapp says, than the corresponding layer in the motor cortex, ranging in thickness between twenty and twenty-two hundredths [of a millimeter]; the layer of the small pyramids, very rich in cells, measures twenty-six to twenty-eight hundredths [of a millimeter]; the [layer] of the medium pyramids contains a lesser number of cells and measures about forty hundredths [of a millimeter]; the [layer] of the large pyramids has a thickness similar to that of the plexiform layer; that is to say, about twenty hundredths [of a millimeter], an exiguous height compared with the notable development of this same layer in the motor cortex; the [layer] of the granule cells ranges between twenty-four and twenty-eight hundredths [of a millimeter]; the [layer] of the deep medium pyramids, which is not well delimited from the lower part of the last layer, is extremely robust, adding up to seventy to seventy-five hundredths [of a millimeter]; there still remains for the last or seventh layer a space of fifty to fifty-five hundredths [of a millimeter]. The thickness of the deep layers together, that is to say, the fifth, sixth, and seventh, is somewhat larger than that of all the other layers, so that if the gray matter were divided at the layer of the granule cells, it would result in two horizontal portions of almost equal thickness.

The above measurements have been made on the convex or apical parts of the gyrus; but, as usually happens, the flat or lateral sides of these, corresponding to the sulci, as well as the concavities, show a rather small thickness. Only the first or plexiform layer does not appear to decrease but rather increases in thickness; the other layers are thinner, the second decreasing in thickness to eighteen or twenty hundredths [of a millimeter]; the third to thirty-five and the fourth to eighteen; the fifth layer or [layer] of the granule cells decreases a

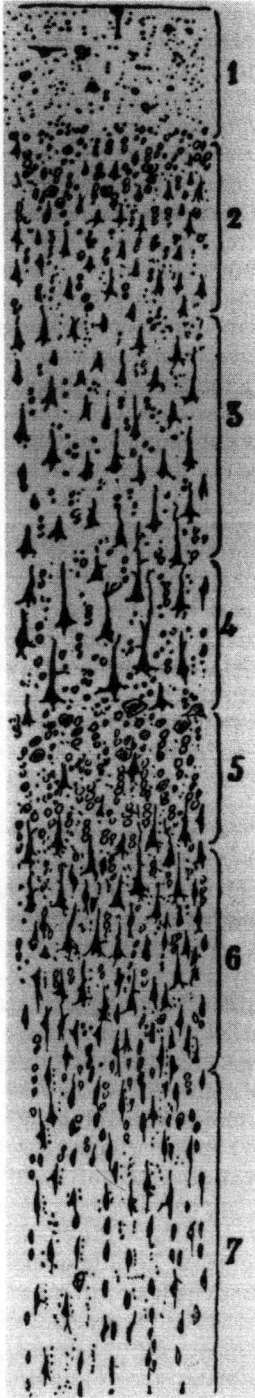

little; but, however, the last two layers have lost robustness since, instead of totaling one hundred twenty or one hundred thirty hundredths [of a millimeter], they only total seventy-five or eighty hundredths [of a millimeter]. This decrease in thickness is compensated, but only partially, by a denser packing of the cells that inhabit the layers.

Plexiform Layer

Its appearance in Nissl preparations coincides with that of the motor region.

Besides the neuroglial nuclei, which are often accumulated in small islands, there are observed some cells with a voluminous nucleus that correspond to the large horizontal cells and to the medium and small cellular elements with short axon.

The large horizontal cells are scarce, only an occasional one of the piriform and marginal type being found (fig. 1) [fig. 118]. There is no lack, however, of fusiform elements, horizontally oriented in the thickness of this layer, but the perferred localization for this cellular type seems to us to be the deep third of the layer, where they many times adopt an oblique and even vertical orientation. In the good Nissl preparations, it is also observed that the small and medium cells with short axon are frequently accompanied by a circle of neuroglial cells, so as to avoid untoward contacts with [apical dendritic] tufts of pyramids.

The Weigert-Pal method shows in the superficial half of the first layer the known tangential fibers, some of them reaching an unusual thickness (fig. 2) [fig. 119]. The deep half of the plexiform layer lodges thinner medullated fibers with several orientations and arranged in a loose plexus.

The thick tangential fibers run in several directions and often transversely with respect to the gyrus, and they can be followed for enormous distances, without any tendency to sink

[FIG. 118] Fig. 1. Transverse section of the first temporal gyrus of an adult man. Nissl method. 1, plexiform layer; 2, small pyramids; 3, medium pyramids; 4, superficial large pyramids; 5, granule or small stellate cells; 6, deep medium pyramids; 7, fusiform cells.

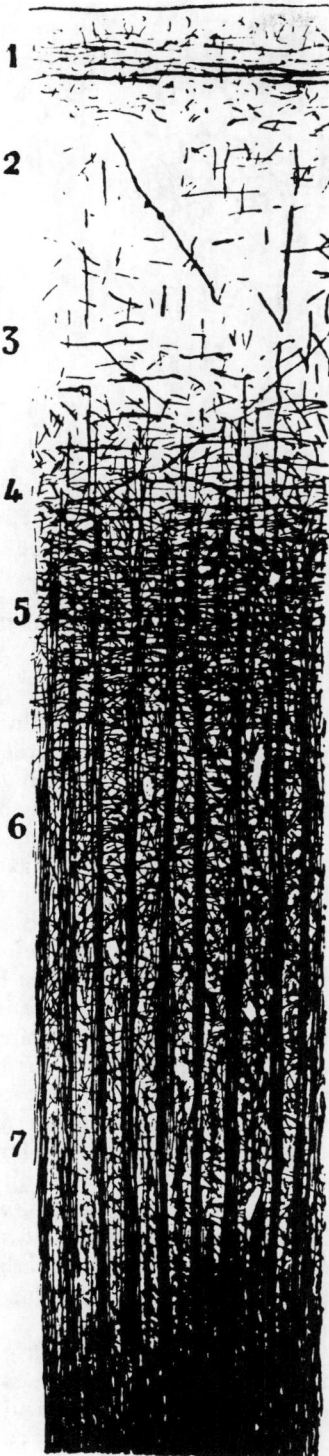

deeper into the cortex. Their unusual thickness and the fact of not being in continuity with radial myelinated fibers allow us to suspect, following what we previously said in our study of the motor cortex, that such fibers represent the axons of the horizontal cells. With regard to the thinner medullated fibers, located outside and below the tangential fibers, these belong, as we will see later, to the preterminal arborizations of the ascending myelinated fibers of Martinotti.

The Golgi method impregnates very well the cells and fibers of the plexiform layer, but because they show no special features in the sphenoidal region, we will refrain from repeating here the description that we have made in previous works. In fig. 3 [fig. 120], which corresponds to the sphenoidal cortex of a child of one month, we show several types of special cells (piriform, triangular, fusiform types, etc.). In it appear also a small cell with short horizontal axon and two more [cellular] elements of this kind, whose axon was descending and gave rise to a dense arborization located in the deepest plane of this layer and in the upper limits of the second (fig. 3, *f*) [fig. 120].

In the silver chromate preparations, in which the fibers and nerve plexuses are well impregnated, the plexiform layer exhibits a large number of nerve fibers with a different significance and origin. These fibers can be divided by their orientations into horizontals and verticals.

The *horizontal fibers* (fig. 4) [fig. 121] form three planes: the central, superior, and inferior. The central or intermediate plane includes, preferentially but not exclusively, the axons of the special or horizontal cells, axons that are recognized easily by their great thickness, varicose aspect, excessive length, and the presence of collaterals arising at right angles, and ending in modest and short arborizations. Overall, some collaterals of these axons reach a considerable length, descending down to the layer of the small pyramids (fig. 4, *G*) [fig. 121].

[*FIG. 119*] Fig. 2. Section of the first sphenoidal gyrus of man. Weigert-Pal method. The numbers correspond to those of the layers.

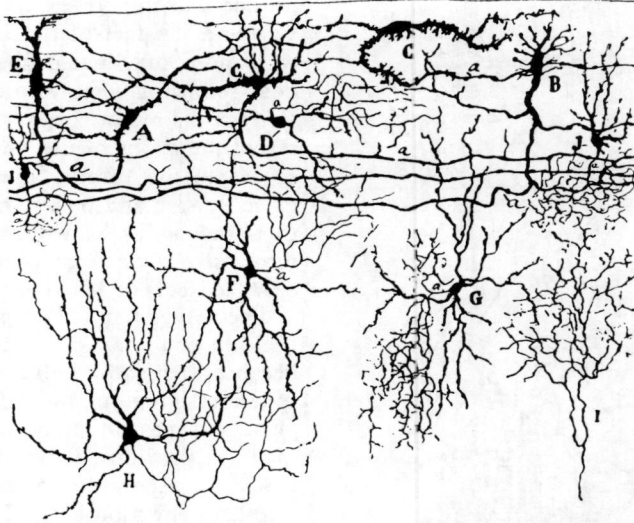

[*FIG. 120*]   Fig. 3. Cells of the first and second layers of the cortex of the child of one month. *A*, triangular cell; *B*, piriform cell; *C*, horizontal fusiform cells; *E*, vertical bipolar cell; *D*, cell with loose short axon; *J*, cells with thin axon and giving rise to a tight arborization at the frontier of the second layer; *F*, *G*, *H*, cells with short axon of the second layer; *I*, ascending thin axon terminating in the superficial plane of the second layer.

The more external or submeningeal plane is the preferred point of arborization of the ascending fibers of Martinotti, which, often bifurcating, become resolved into varicose collaterals often arranged in pericellular plexuses. Such nests or plexuses, which we reproduce in fig. 4, *H* [*fig. 121*], enter into contact with the cell bodies of the horizontal or special cells of the first layer. Finally, the inferior plane or limit of this layer is also a point of convergence of terminal arborizations of ascending axons, although the plexus here originated is looser and weaker than at the external or submeningeal frontier. As is shown in fig. 4, *E* and *K* [*fig. 121*], some fibers of Martinotti send terminal branches not only to the external plane but also to the interior of the plexus of the plexiform layer.

With regard to the *vertical fibers*, the majority represent ascending fibers of Martinotti, arising from fusiform or stellate cells scattered through the whole cortex. In fig. 4 [*fig. 121*], we reproduce the ascending fibers that appear in good preparations of the auditory cortex of the child of one month. For greater clarity, we have not reproduced the cells of origin. Notice

that such fibers belong to three main varieties: first, ascending robust axon, little or not branched in its trajectory through the pyramids, and ending by a bifurcation situated in the external plane of the first layer (fig. 4, *D*) [*fig. 121*]; second, ascending robust axon which gives off numerous branches when it crosses the third and second layers and ends in a large number of horizontal branches, often bifurcated, in the deep plane of the first layer (fig. 4, *F*) [*fig. 121*]; third, ascending axons that are characterized by frequently describing at their origin an arciform bend (fig. 4, *E*) [*fig. 121*], and especially by providing in their initial portion several thin collaterals with a vertical course, either ascending (fig. 4, *E*) [*fig. 121*] or descending (fig. 4, *K*) [*fig. 121*]; and fourth, finally, thin flexuous threads which, when followed downward, are observed to represent the upper branches of the axonal arborization of a bitufted cell of medium size (fig. 4, *L*) [*fig. 121*].

From the preceding brief description, the ascending nerve fibers constitute in man a complicated system of intracortical association, by means of which a double connection is carried out with the pyramidal cells: a direct connection originating and formed by the initial collaterals of the said fibers, with the [dendritic] shafts of the immediately adjacent pyramids; and an indirect and distant connection, established by means of the special cells of the first layer, which with their cell bodies enter into contact with the mentioned arborizations, and they are related probably by means of their axon to groups of pyramids located at a great distance. It is necessary, however, to confess that the latter relationship is very conjectural, because the position of the terminal arborization of the axons of the special cells of the first layer has not yet been discovered.

Finally, let us mention still, to be complete, the existence of certain oblique ascending fibers, commonly thin, and whose origin we have not been able to determine. Perhaps they represent recurrent collaterals of axons of pyramids (fig. 4, I) [fig. 121].

Layer of the Small Pyramids

In Nissl preparations, it consists of numerous tightly packed cells of medium or small size, separated by a scanty amount of intercellular plexus. Among them, in the most superficial planes of this layer, there also show up some pyramidal elements (of 10 by 15 μm), which are recognizable as much by their shape as for exhibiting a relatively large volume; they are recognized also for having a protoplasm with a particular affinity for the basic aniline dyes. But, in fact, the dominant cells are not the pyramids but those of short axon, characterized in such preparations by having a triangular, fusiform, or polygonal shape and weak staining with thionin. It is not rare to observe the soma of such minute cells seemingly retracted from the inside of the membrane. Occasionally, if the second layer is examined with a good apochromatic [lens], here and there one stumbles across relatively large triangular or polygonal cells that correspond, as observed in Golgi preparations, to voluminous cells with short axons.

For the rest, the Golgi method does not reveal in the second layer any special cell that we do not already know from the study of other cortical regions. In fig. 6, a, b [fig. 123], we re-

produce some medium and small pyramidal cells, whose axon was followed over a large distance; from its initial course arose four, five, and more collateral branches of which some ran upward and arrived with branches up to the very frontier of the plexiform layer. However, other pyramids (fig. 6) [fig. 123] were very modest in [the number of] axon collaterals.

The cells with short axon are, as we have said, more numerous than the pyramids, and they belong to all the types described in the visual and motor cortex. To save useless repetitions, we will limit ourselves to reproducing in figs. 3 and 5 [figs. 120, 122] the most frequent types observed in our preparations. Notice the following.

(1) Large stellate type, provided with an axon [that is] highly branched over a short distance (fig. 3, H) [fig. 120]. (2) Small stellate type, whose axon is arborized in the limits of the first and second layer with some small branches penetrating the plexiform layer (fig. 3, F) [fig. 120]. (3) Also a minute type, situated near the latter layer and whose thin axon formed two arborizations, one ascending and the other descending (fig. 3, G) [fig. 120]. Of this same kind, we reproduce in figs. 5, A and B [fig. 122] two cells of larger size and more deeply situated, in which the ascending arborizations arrived at the plexiform layer, and the descending went down to the center of the layer of the medium pyramids. (4) Large or medium stellate type with descending axon arborized to a large extent in the third layer and deep portion of the second (fig. 5, C, B) [fig. 122]. (5) Finally, cells of medium or small size, situated in several planes of the second layer and even in the upper part of the third, and whose thin axon with an ascending course gives rise in the external third of the second layer and boundary of the plexiform to a very complicated and dense arborization, inside the meshes of which are lodged a group of small pyramids. These cells are abundant also in the motor and visual cortex, perhaps even more so than in the acoustic cortex (fig. 3, I) [fig. 120].

Third Layer or Layer of the Medium Pyramids

Quite well demarcated from the second layer, it is smoothly continuous with the fourth,

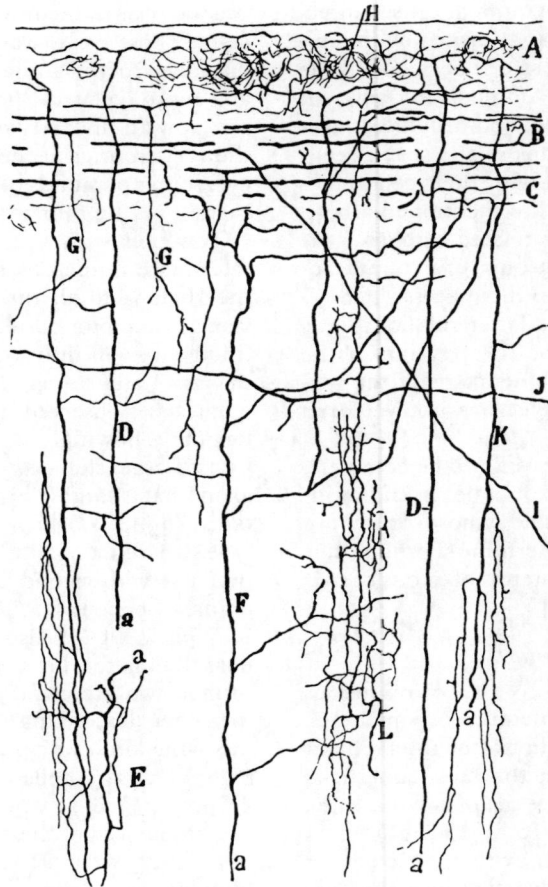

[FIG. 121]   Fig. 4. Plexiform layer and fibers of Martinotti of the cortex of the child of one month. *A*, external plane of the first layer; *B*, middle plane; *C*, internal plane; *D*, thick and little branched fibers of Martinotti; *E*, fibers that at their origin formed bundles of vertical collaterals; *F*, fiber with a wide arborization; *G*, collaterals of tangential fibers; *L*, upper branches of an axon of a bitufted cell; *a*, origin of the axon.

from which it is only possible to separate it artificially. The Nissl method shows in it pyramids of a size of 13 by 20 μm, whose protoplasm appears splashed with thin [Nissl granules] and meshes. Between the cells exist wide spaces, occupied, without doubt, by dendritic arborizations and axonal plexuses.

The main cells stained by the silver chromate in the third layer appear in figs. 5 and 6 [figs. 122, 123]. They are distinguished as pyramids or cells with long axon, and as cells with short axon.

The *pyramids* do not offer any morphological novelty. The axon was followed to near

the white matter, it being presumed that it is continued as a medium [myelinated] fiber of this; the majority of the collaterals arising from the axon run in oblique or horizontal directions, and they are related to the [apical dendritic] shafts of the underlying medium pyramids and perhaps also to the [apical] shafts of the large pyramids that cross the third layer (fig. 6, *f*) [fig. 123].

With respect to the *cells with short axon*, they are very numerous and adopt a large variety of shapes. Having been almost all described in our works on the visual and motor cortex, we will here only mention the main types: first, large fusiform type, whose ascending axon terminates in the plexiform layer after giving off several collaterals in the thickness of the second and third layers; second, voluminous stellate type (fig. 6, c) [fig. 123], provided with ascending dendrites extending up to the first layer, and with an axon that first descends for a certain distance, tracing an arch from which arise descending collaterals, then goes up vertically and is distributed in the plexiform layer, behaving as the fibers of Martinotti; third, large and medium stellate types with descending or ascending horizontal axon, but arborized at short distance from the cell; fourth, tufted cells. These elements are very numerous in the acoustic cortex, extending through all the layers, particularly the second, third, and fourth, and adopting a large variety

of forms and sizes. However, three varieties can be separated.

a. Large bitufted cell, provided with quite robust ascending and descending dendrites, and with an ascending or descending axon, whose branches form a weak and loose arborization, disseminated over an extensive radial perimeter (fig. 5, D) [fig. 122].

b. Medium and dwarf bitufted cells, whose two tufts are composed of very thin and varicose dendrites extended in paintbrush form and hardly distinguishable from the axonal arborizations. The axon, of extreme delicacy, runs in an axial direction and forms very complicated small radial bundles of varicose threads applied to the apical dendritic shafts and cell bodies of the pyramids (fig. 5, F) [fig. 122]. A variant of this cellular type has a more

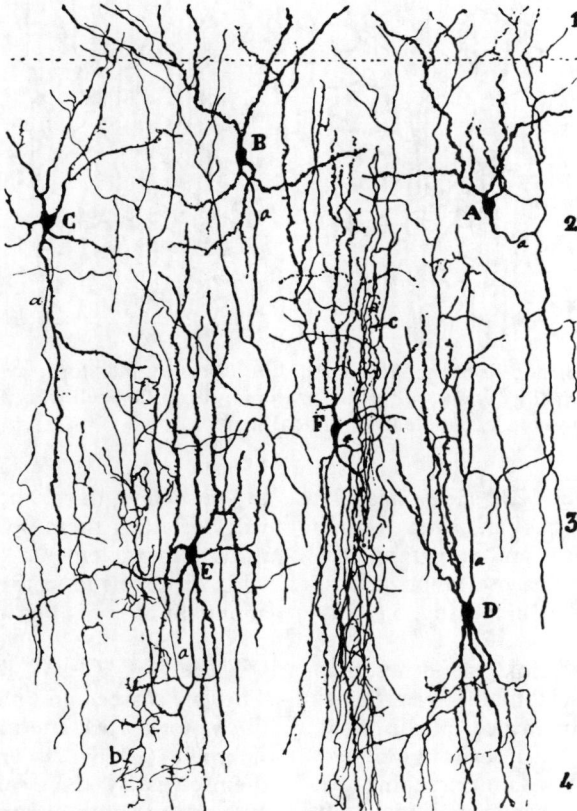

[FIG. 122]   Fig. 5. Cells with short axon observed in the second and third layers. 1, plexiform layer; 2, small pyramids; 3, medium pyramids; A, B, C, large cells with axon forming vertical small branches; D, E, F, several types of bitufted cells; a, axon.

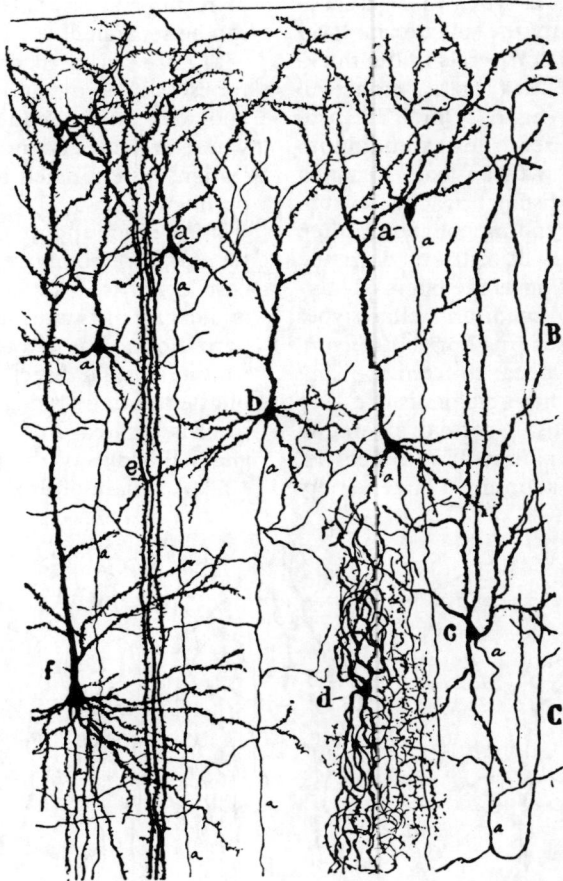

[*FIG. 123*]   Fig. 6. Pyramidal cells of the second and third layers. *A,* plexiform layer; *B,* small pyramids; *C,* medium pyramids; *a, b,* small pyramids; *f,* medium pyramid; *d,* bitufted cell with flexuous dendrites; *c,* cell with arched and ascending axon; *e,* bundle of pyramidal shafts.

robust size (fig. 5, *E*) [*fig. 122*], shows strongly spiny dendrites, and has an axon whose branches, often arciform and recurrent, terminate in pericellular varicose arborizations, probably related to the pyramids (fig. 5,*b*) [*fig. 122*].

c. Bitufted cells with crinkly dendrites, that is to say, undulating and folded over themselves to form a complicated plexus, and whose axon gives rise to a vertically dilated dense arborization, but without reaching the extreme length of the previous types (fig. 6, *d*) [*fig. 123*]. Still, we would have to add, to be complete, the giant horizontal cells specific to the acoustic cortex, cells that are not lacking

in the second, third, and fourth layers; but we will deal with them below when we describe the cellular elements of the sixth layer, in which it seems to us they are somewhat more abundant.

Fourth Layer or Layer of the Giant Pyramids

They are scarce in number in comparison with the motor cortex, and in size are not very considerable (20 by 28 μm). Some distinguish themselves by their volume in comparison with the medium pyramids. As can be seen in fig. 7, *a* [*fig. 124*], they have a triangular soma from whose deep portion arise long and numerous basal dendrites and an apex which is elongated as a [dendritic] shaft prolonged up to the plexiform layer. An arrangement that is perhaps not exclusive to this cortical region is shown in fig. 6, e [fig. 123]: the [apical dendritic] shafts of the large pyramids ascend together in tight fascicles to the upper part of the second layer, where they diverge in order to reach separately the plexiform layer. It is probable that on these bundles of [dendritic] shafts are ramified the small bundles of axonal arborizations formed by the axons of the small and medium types of bitufted cells. The fourth layer also includes some cells with short axon belonging mainly to the bitufted types and to the large [types] with ascending axon of Martinotti, or of the [type with an] axon branched and terminating at a short distance.

Fifth Layer or Layer of the Diminutive Cells (Layer of the Granule Cells)

The examination of this layer, even in Nissl preparations, reveals a large variety of cellular forms and shapes. The large forms (of 20 by 20 μm or more) are scarce, and they correspond to spheroidal, polygonal, or stellate cells, rich in protoplasm and provided with several divergent dendrites; these cellular elements are scattered through the whole fifth layer, but they seem to us to be somewhat more abundant in the external third of the same, below the giant pyramids. It is not unusual, either, to observe them forming groups of two or three. The protoplasm commonly has a great paleness in the Nissl preparations, showing an extremely pale [Nissl] meshwork, but sometimes the protoplasmic material is more abundant, staining the cell body a dark shade, almost as dark as the cell bodies of the large pyramids.

With respect to the small cellular elements, whose size usually does not exceed 7 to 9 μm, they are much more numerous and are arranged in vertical pleiades in which the cell bodies are often in intimate contact. Such cells show a pale and scanty protoplasm, almost bereft of [Nissl] granules, and two or more clear, hardly perceptible processes that immediately get lost in the confusion of the intercellular plexus. Among the forms adopted by these minute cells in Nissl preparations are included the pyramidal, which corresponds, without

doubt, to small pyramidal cells of the common type; the fusiform, provided with two polar processes; and the polygonal or globose, from whose contours arise thin dendrites. The latter types probably represent cells with short axon.

So much for the revelations of the method of Nissl, which cannot show us in detail the real morphology of the granule cells. Fortunately, the silver chromate stains these cellular elements quite well, as we show in figs. 7 and 8 [figs. 124, 125], together with the polygonal and fusiform cells of a more considerable size. Let us notice the great analogy existing between all of these cells and those already mentioned by us in the homonymous layer of the motor cortex.

As in [the motor cortex], such cellular elements must be distinguished as cells with long axon and as cells with short axon.

a. Small Pyramids. They are indistinctly located in the whole fifth layer; nevertheless, they are somewhat more abundant in the deep half of the same, although there are many exceptions to this. They have the morphology of common pyramids; that is to say, they have a radial, undivided [apical dendritic] shaft that runs up to the plexiform layer, a medium or small soma (of 10 by 12 or 14 μm), with a triangular appearance, but more often ovoid and even spheroidal, from which arise some delicate and not very long lateral and descending dendrites, and, finally, a thin axon that has the peculiarity of resolving itself into a system of small nervous arcades, continued as ascending collaterals. From the point of view of the arrangement of the axonal arborization, two types of small pyramids can be distinguished: first, cells whose axon, although very slender and of smaller diameter than the collaterals, is not completely exhausted in forming these and descends more or less obliquely down to the white matter (fig. 7, f) [fig. 124], after giving off in its deep trajectory, that is to say, below the nervous arcades, some horizontal or oblique collaterals, and which has seemed to us to be the most common type; second, less abundant cells in which the axon is exhausted completely when it gives off the arciform collaterals, in such a way that no axonal thread down to the white matter can be seen, and if

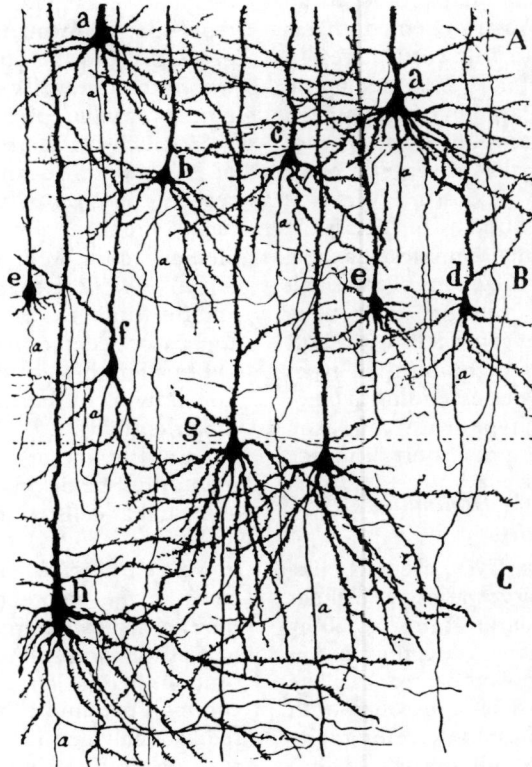

[*FIG. 124*]   Fig. 7. Cells of the fourth (*A*), fifth (*B*), and sixth (*C*) layers of the first sphenoidal gyrus of the child of twenty-five days. *a*, superficial large pyramids; *b*, *c*, small pyramids of the fifth layer; *e*, *d*, *f*, pyramids with axon forming in part arciform collaterals; *g*, *h*, large pyramids of the sixth layer.

some descending fiber is observed, it is not the continuation of the axon but represents some thin collateral arising from the convexity of an arch and ramifying in the fifth or sixth layer (fig. 7, *e*) [*fig. 124*]. In both types of cells, the ascending collaterals are very robust, and, going up parallel to the [apical dendritic] shaft, numbering two, three, four, and more, reach the fourth layer and even the third, in which they are prolixly branched; near their origin, and sometimes when they trace the initial arcades, the said ascending collaterals also give off oblique and horizontal branches, perhaps destined to enter into contact with the [apical dendritic] shafts of the nearby pyramids.

b.   Large   and   Displaced   Medium   Pyramids. They are rare, but usually there is no lack of medium or large pyramids in the fifth

layer, completely equal to the giant and medium pyramids of the bordering layers (fig. 7, *c*, *g*) [*fig. 124*].

c. Cells with Short Axon. Such [cellular] elements, which constitute the essential formation of the fifth layer, include several types. The most frequently observed in our preparations are:

1. Fusiform cell of medium size and provided with ascending and descending long dendrites, arising commonly from polar shafts (fig. 8, *A*) [*fig. 125*]. The axon arises from the upper shaft, goes up giving off collaterals to the fourth and third layers, and perhaps reaches the first layer. This cell represents probably some category of the cells of Martinotti.

2. Cell of medium and sometimes large size,

of triangular or stellate shape, with long and divergent dendrites, and provided with an ascending axon that gives rise, at the level of the upper limit of the fifth layer or in the broad thickness of the fourth, to very long horizontal or oblique collaterals, without lacking also some with a descending course (fig. 8, *B, C*) [*fig. 125*]. It will be remembered that this type is also frequent in the motor and visual cortex.

3. Fusiform or triangular cell of medium or small size, whose ascending axon is ramified in the external third of the fifth layer and thickness of the fourth (fig. 8, *F*) [*fig. 125*]. In relation to the spread and amount of branching of the axon, there exist many variants of this cellular category.

4. Fusiform or stellate, medium-sized cell with flexuous and intertwined dendrites, whose axon is extended vertically over the area of the fifth layer, resolving itself into a very tight and radially elongated plexus with thin axonal ramifications in which the cell bodies

of the granule cells show up as clear spaces (figs. 8, *E*; 9, *A, B*) [*figs. 125, 126*].

These cells have seemed to me rather abundant, and between them and the neurogliaform [cells] we observe numerous phases of transition. When many of them are impregnated at the same time, their axonal arborizations, of extreme delicacy and notably varicose and granular, are very close together and intermingled, giving rise in the layer of the granule cells to a continuous and very dense plexus. This plexus forms numerous pericellular nests, and it is so vast and widely extended that it surpasses the limits of the fifth layer, spreading to the fourth, although in the fourth it appears much looser and with large gaps.

5. Dwarf or neurogliaform cells, provided with thin and short dendrites, and bearing a delicate axon resolving itself into tight branches of short extent (fig. 8, *D*) [*fig. 125*].

6. Cell of medium size and spindle- or tri-

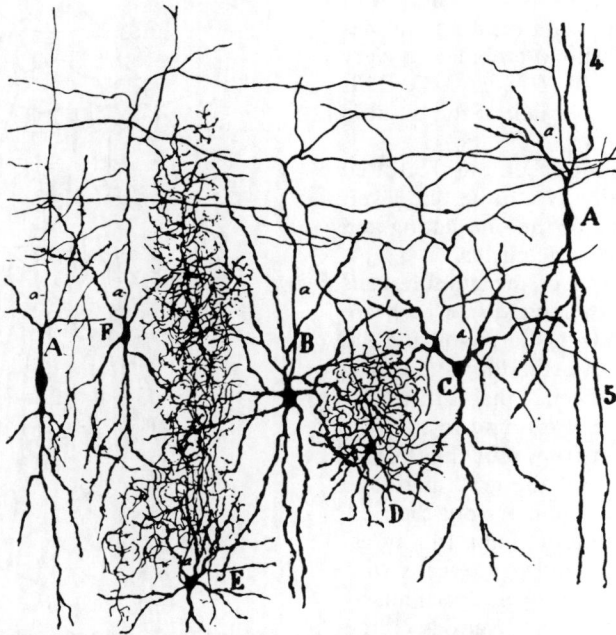

[*FIG. 125*]   Fig. 8. Several types of cells with short axon of the fifth layer. Child of one month. *A,* fusiform cells with ascending axon; *B,* cell with axon resolving itself into very long horizontal branches; *C, F,* cells with less extensive axonal arborizations; *E,* neurogliaform cell with axon resolving itself into a very complicated plexus interspersed with nests; *D,* neurogliaform cell with a dense axonal arborization; *4,* layer of the superficial large pyramids; *5,* granule cells.

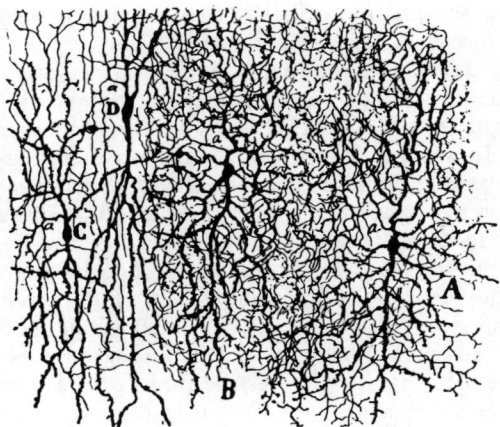

[*FIG. 126*] Fig. 9. Axonal plexus originating in the fifth layer from the ramifications of the axons of the elongated neurogliaform cells and from some of the bitufted cells.

angular-shaped, provided with thin, vertical, almost smooth, very long, separated, undulating dendrites extended over a considerable area of the gray matter; its axon, arising from a dendrite, is divided into ascending and descending branches, which embrace a very widespread field (fig. 10, *D*) [*fig. 127*]. This type seems to us to be a variant of the bitufted cell.

7. Small and medium, common bitufted cells of the type described in the second layer. They are characterized by the undulating and curly arrangement of the dendrites.

In summary, the layer of the granule cells represents the cortical territory, in which are concentrated the cells with short axon and the [cellular] elements with ascending axon. It is not that the mentioned cells inhabit this layer exclusively, as they are also found in the others, at least their main types, but they prefer this intermediate place of the gray matter as the best strategical point to carry out their assignment, which is, without doubt, that of establishing connections with all the cells with long axon of the cortical layers, particularly with the large and medium pyramids of the fourth and sixth layers. The associative character of the cells of the fifth layer is demonstrable even in its small pyramids, whose collateral axonal arborization, formed by branches thicker than the continuation of the [parent] axon, resembles in its disposition more that of the cells with short axon than that of those with long axon. On account of this, we are led to presume that the layer of the granule cells, as in the visual cortex, is a place of preferred termination of exogenous fibers, perhaps of second-order acoustic fibers.

Sixth Layer or Layer of the Deep Medium Pyramids

This layer contains [cellular] elements of very diverse forms and sizes, but among them seems to predominate, especially in the most superficial planes of the layer, the pyramidal type, with a size a little bit superior to that of the medium pyramids (16 by 28 μm).

There are, however, cells whose structure approaches very much that of the pyramids of the fourth layer, from which they are differ-

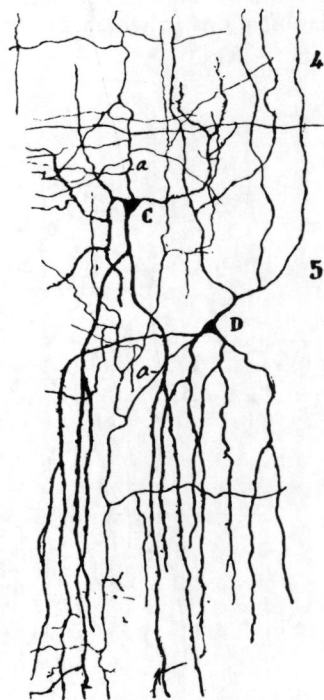

[*FIG. 127*] Fig. 10. Cellular types with short axon of the fifth layer. *C*, cell with descending long [dendritic] tuft and ascending axon; *D*, cell provided with a double and very long tuft of dendrites; *a*, axon; [*4*, layer of superficial giant pyramids; *5*, granule cell layer]

entiated only in presenting a somewhat narrower basal portion.

By means of the Golgi method, the following cellular types are revealed in this layer.

1. Medium and Large Pyramids. Provided with one or more [apical dendritic] shafts prolonged up to the first layer, a descending tuft of basal dendrites, and an axon capable of being followed down to the white matter and from which arise four or six collaterals, ramifying in the thickness of the sixth layer (fig. 7, *g, h*) [*fig. 124*].

2. Triangular Cells with Descending Axon. Analogous to the ones described in the motor cortex, they have two radial [dendritic] shafts, descending and ascending, the latter

prolonged up to the first layer, and a thick lateral process from which arises a short shaft dividing into dendrites. The axon descends down to the white matter (fig. 11, *J*) [*fig. 128*].

3. Fusiform Cells with Ascending Axon. This type is very abundant, both in the sixth layer and in the seventh, surpassing perhaps the pyramidal cell. It has a diversity of shapes, although the bipolar type with ascending and descending dendrite, both dividing into a tuft of branches, predominates. The axon arises from the upper [dendritic] shaft; it crosses the layer of the granule cells, and perhaps reaches the plexiform layer, up to whose vicinity we have sometimes followed it. In its initial portion, it gives off several collaterals to the sixth layer (fig. 11, *E, G*) [*fig. 128*].

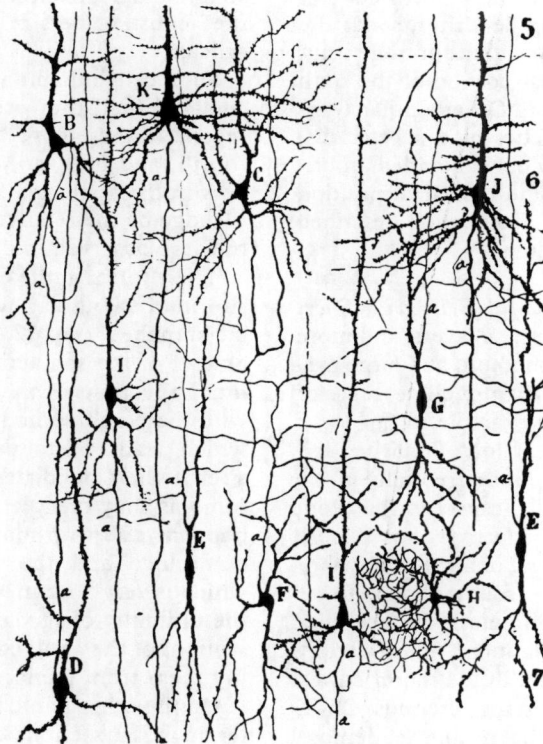

[*FIG. 128*]   Fig. 11. Several cellular types of the sixth layer and beginning of the seventh. Child of one month. *5,* layer of the granule cells; *6,* layer of the deep medium pyramids; *D,* large cell with ascending long axon; *J, K,* large pyramids with long axon; *C,* large polygonal cell with long axon, whose axon gave off three robust ascending collaterals; *E, G,* tiny cells with long, ascending axon; *F,* cell with short axon forming horizontal branches; *H,* neurogliaform type; *I,* small fusiform or pyramidal cells.

4. Pyramidal or Triangular Cells. Either of medium or large volume, provided with a radial [dendritic] shaft that reaches up to the plexiform layer, and with an axon that, after first descending for a certain distance, traces an arch with its convexity down and then goes up, getting lost in the superimposed layers, in which it ends in an unknown manner (fig. 11, *B, C*) *[fig. 128]*. From the descending portion as well as from the arch arise some transverse and descending collaterals. We do not know if some of them reach the white matter. These elements are very similar to the small pyramids with arciform collaterals of the fifth layer; they differ from them, however, in being in general more robust and because they do not have more than a single axonal arcade.

5. Triangular or Stellate Cell of Medium Size and with Ascending Short Axon. This cellular type, with not very long dendrites, sends the axon to ramify in the layer of the granule cells, as well as in the external portion of the sixth layer (fig. 11, *F*) *[fig. 128]*. Other similar types exist whose axon branches at a shorter distance, giving rise to a widely extended arborization that reproduces the typical disposition of the so-called cells of Golgi, well described by Mondino and Martinotti.

6. Cells of Golgi or Colossal Cells with Short Axon. The sixth and seventh layers, and more rarely the layers of the medium and large pyramids, contain certain giant stellate cells, of which we reproduce an example in fig. 14, *E* *[fig. 131]*. They have very long dendrites oriented in all directions but preferentially in the radial direction, and with respect to the axon, which is quite thick, it shortly forms a loose arborization with very long oblique or horizontal branches that can be followed sometimes about a tenth of a millimeter. This cellular type is, in our opinion, a more robust variety of the cellular type found in the motor cortex at the level of the deep giant pyramids. On it, however, we have not been able to demonstrate any pericellular arborizations. Overall, these nests are not lacking here, particularly around the large pyramids, but they are neither as noticeable as in the motor cortex, nor

have we been able to determine the origin of their fibers.

7. Minute Neurogliaform Cells See (fig. 11, *H*) *[fig. 128]*.

Specific Cells of the Auditory Cortex

The cells so far described, with some variations in form, inhabit the other cortical areas, but the ones we are now going to describe we have found only in the auditory cortex. This absolute constancy with which they are represented in the first sphenoidal gyrus (they have never been absent in twenty or twenty-one impregnations with the method of Golgi) obliges us to consider them as the principal anatomical characteristic of the cortical center of audition, although, so far, we have not been able to elucidate either their connections with the acoustic fibers or their physiological significance.

Such cells inhabit all the cortical layers except the first; they are little abundant in the second layer, more frequent in the third, fourth, and fifth, and present in larger numbers in the sixth and seventh layers, if we are to judge by the relative abundance with which they are observed in our preparations.

Their form, in the Golgi preparations, is fusiform or triangular, with very robust horizontal branches[B] (fig. 12, *A, D*) *[fig. 129]*, the diameter of the somata reaching 30 by 40 to 60 μm. In sections of the adult cerebrum stained with the Nissl method, they appear quite thin, which leads us to presume that such cells stretch their dendrites at the expense of the soma as they complete their development, as happens also with many other cells. This circumstance and the paleness of the soma, which is very poor in [Nissl granules], explains the difficulty of recognizing them in the thin sections of the adult cortex, and in distinguishing them from the large cells with short axon.

On the other hand, they show up much better in Nissl sections of the cerebrum of the child of fifteen days to a month and a half, in which they have a larger size than the large pyramids and exhibit a protoplasm rich in [Nissl material]. It is noticed also in these

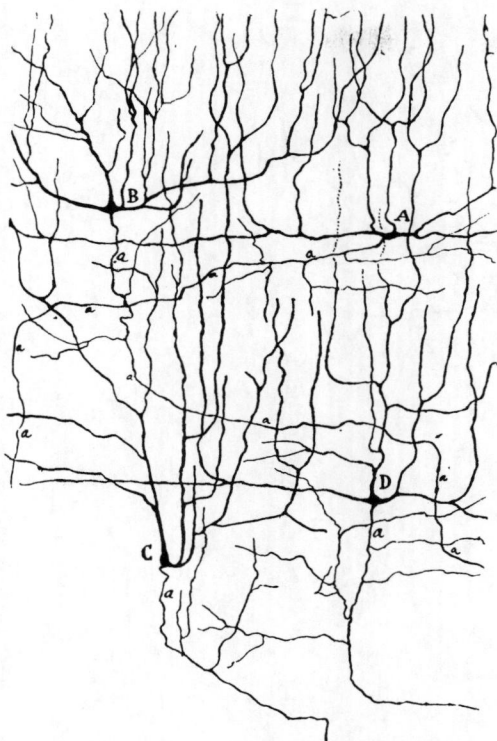

[FIG. 129] Fig. 12. Four giant specific cells of the first sphenoidal gyrus of the child of one month. *A, B,* cells found in the fourth layer; *C, D,* cells found in the sixth; *a,* axon. In this figure, only a part of the dendritic arborization appears. Zeiss A objective.

preparations of the child that the cited cells are more abundant in the sixth and seventh layers than in the others; however, their number is always scarce, as more than three of them rarely appear in a single field examined with the C objective of the microscope.

In the silver preparations, the shape of the specific cells varies according to the orientation of the section. If this is horizontal, the soma is triangular or stellate, with two or more divergent and horizontal branches of enormous extent; there are branches that can be followed about one tenth of a millimeter. Such processes have a rough contour; they give off at intervals ascending branches, sometimes in parallel, which go up more or less vertically, some of them managing to cross two and three

superimposed layers. With the exception of the few cells of this type located in the third layer, whose dendrites can go up to the boundaries of the first layer (fig. 13) [*fig. 130*], the ascending branches of the rest rarely reach the second layer. In their course toward the surface, these branches divide several times, tracing at their points of division little arches with a concavity upward (fig. 12, *A, D*) [*fig. 129*] and covering with little branches a considerable cortical region. For the rest, such dendrites are distinguished well from those belonging to the pyramids by lacking [dendritic] spines or by having them only rarely. Some cells also exhibit long descending dendrites, as can be appreciated in fig. 13 [*fig. 130*].

Altogether, the ascending, descending, and horizontal processes embrace a considerable volume, perhaps reaching, in some cells, more than a cubic millimeter. However, the processes of the cells located in the seventh layer are extended over a more exiguous field, they often lack descending branches, and the ascending ones are shorter, which appears to result from the narrowness of the radial spaces left free by the bundles of medullated axons.

The axon is very robust and generally arises from the deep or lateral portion of the soma; if first descends a certain distance, then it frequently bends obliquely or horizontally, running through several layers of the cortex for long distances, sometimes without showing a clear tendency to descend to the white matter (fig. 12, *B*) [*fig. 129*]. In other cases, after an oblique and horizontal course, the said axon becomes progressively vertical and descending, approaching, although rarely in a straight line, the deep cortical layers. This disposition, the great length of the axon, and the fact of our never having been able to observe on it a terminal arborization incline us to consider the cells under study as cells with long axon. And, although in the vast majority of these cells we have not been able to observe the arrival of the axon down at the white matter, since this is impeded by the turns and the staircaselike trajectory that the axon describes, in two or three cases we have been more fortunate. One of these cells, in which the axon was followed more deeply, is shown in fig. 13 [*fig.*

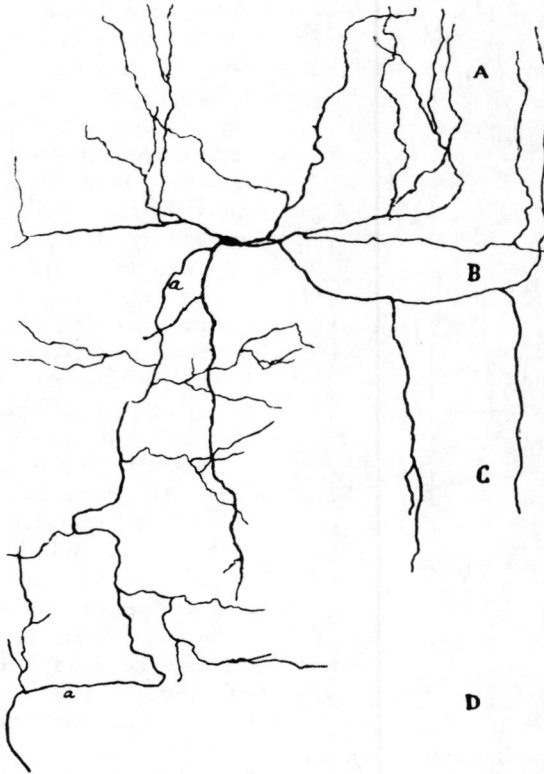

[*FIG. 130*]   Fig. 13. Specific giant cell of the sphenoidal cortex of the child of one month. In order to save space, the axon has only been drawn over a portion of its trajectory. *A*, layer of the small pyramids; *B*, medium pyramids; *C*, superficial large pyramids; *D*, granule cells; *a*, axon. Examination at low magnification.

130], in which we do not present, however, more than half of the observed trajectory. This cell was located in the layer of the medium pyramids, and its axon, oblique at the beginning, after tracing wide curves, became descending, being followed down further to the sixth layer, where it still maintained almost its original diameter, and it appeared to be incorporated into a bundle of fibers arriving from the white matter. We have also observed the arrival at the white matter [of the axon of] some cells of this kind located in the sixth and seventh layers.

Already from their initial trajectory, these axons give off collaterals, in number three, four, or more, which are prolixly branched over an extensive area of the gray matter (fig. 13) [*fig. 130*]. Some of these collaterals, as seen

in fig. 12 [*fig. 129*], have a recurrent course. In the cell represented in fig. 13 [*fig. 130*], more than ten collaterals were counted whose secondary ramifications were notably thin and ran preferentially in the horizontal direction.

It is impossible to formulate a reasonably solid hypothesis about the functional significance of such singular [cellular] elements of the auditory cortex, which are comparable in many ways to the large stellate cells of the visual cortex. This obscurity would have been dispelled in part if we had had the good fortune to reveal the terminal axonal branches arising from such cells; but all the efforts made to find perisomatic arborizations, as well as a special relationship of the dendrites to the plexus of the fifth layer, have so far been unsuccessful.

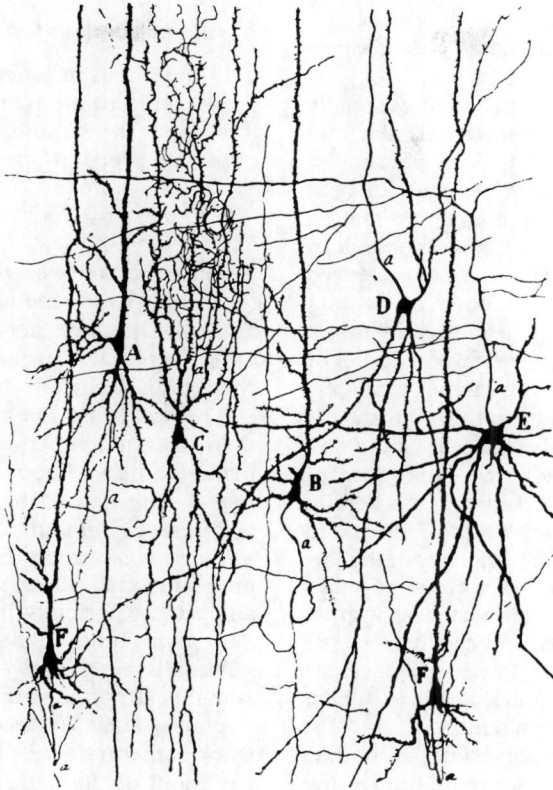

[*FIG. 131*] Fig. 14. Several cellular types of the seventh layer. Child of one month. *A*, triangular cell with long axon; *F*, somewhat ovoid pyramids with short basal dendrites and recurrent axon collaterals; *B*, pyramid provided with collaterals more robust than the descending portion of the axon; *C*, large bitufted cell; *E*, giant cell with short axon forming long horizontal collaterals.

Seventh Layer or Layer of the Fusiform Cells

It includes the same cellular types as in the motor cortex, that is to say, a multitude of fusiform cells with ascending axon, many cells with short axon, and some fusiform triangular cells and even pyramids with descending axons destined for the white matter.

In fig. 14 [*fig. 131*], we reproduce the cells more frequently found in our preparations. In *A*, we represent a triangular cell quite abundant in this layer, although not so much as in the preceding layer. It has a [dendritic] shaft that goes up to the first layer and a long axon continued as a myelinated fiber of the white matter. The lateral and inferior [dendritic] shafts resolve themselves into tufts of den-

drites. The cell that we show in *B* is a genuine pyramid, but on it are still observed ascending or transverse robust axon collaterals as in certain cells of the superimposed layers.

As has been seen, such cells characterized by the presence of arciform collaterals and by the thinness of descending [parent] axon are not lacking in the fifth, sixth, and seventh layers, although it has seemed to us that their main localization is the fifth.

In the seventh layer, there are also robust cells with ascending axons, perhaps prolonged up to the first layer. One of them of giant size is reproduced in fig. 14, *D* [*fig. 131*]; another smaller one appears in fig. 11, *D* [*fig. 128*]. Sometimes, the ascending axon of these voluminous types runs first in a descending direction, gives off some collaterals in the region situated below the cell, and then goes up, perhaps as far as the plexiform layer.

Another very common type, and especially abundant near the white matter, is the medium pyramid (fig. 14, *F*) [*fig. 131*], poor in descending dendrites and provided with an axon that is incorporated into the white matter. Such a kind of cell, which is also abundant in the visual and motor cortex, is characterized especially by the recurrent course of its axon collaterals, which go up to ramify in upper planes sometimes of the seventh, sometimes of the sixth layers. This peculiarity is very interesting, as it demonstrates two things: first, that whatever the plane of distribution of the collaterals, these cannot advance their place of origin, which is invariably situated at a certain distance from the starting point of the axon; second, that because of the exigency of the law of economy of space or on account of other conditions, many cells are located at a great distance from the territory where their axonal collaterals are distributed, forcing these collaterals to follow a retrograde course to reach their natural place of termination.

The bitufted cells are not lacking in the seventh layer. The one that we reproduce in fig. 14, *C* [*fig. 131*] had a medium size and spiny, varicose, ascending and descending dendrites, in part extended into the white matter, and it had an ascending axon that resolved itself not into bushes of threads but rather into loose pericellular arborizations. As can be seen, the bitufted cells represent a constant anatomical feature of all the cerebral layers (except the first), and their axonal arborization is adjusted to the form and orientation of the cellular elements with long axon, to which they must be related.

In general (there are exceptions), the tufted cells are more voluminous the deeper they are located, and their axonal arborizations increase in complexity and density as the cell body becomes smaller.

To finish with the elements of the seventh layer, we will just mention the fusiform cells with long descending axon, the neurogliaform cells, and the giant and medium-sized stellate cells provided with short axon, soon forming long horizontal branches, of which we show an example in fig. 14, *E* [*fig. 131*].

Nervous Plexuses of the Auditory Cortex

To study them in order, we will expound first those demonstrated in the Weigert preparations and then those revealed in the silver chromate preparations.

Medullated Fibers and Plexuses in Weigert Preparations

When a transverse section of the auditory cortex stained by the method of Weigert-Pal is examined, the same nervous plexuses found in other cerebral territories are observed, but with some slight variations (fig. 2) [*fig. 119*].

The first layer is poorer in medullated fibers than the motor cortex, and reveals three planes of nerve fibers: *a*) *external* or submeningeal *plane*, thin and made up of thin and very scarce fibers, that run in all directions; (b) *middle plane*, much thicker, composed of robust tangential fibers, some of them very long and almost perfectly parallel to the gyrus; (c) *deep plane*, quite thick, in which fibers of exiguous diameter show up, also oriented horizontally, although with less regularity than the previous ones. We have already said that the thick tangential fibers belong very probably to the axons of the large special cells of the first layer, whereas the less voluminous fibers of the three planes, and particularly those of the first and third, represent the terminal branches of the fibers of Martinotti, and perhaps also of fibers coming from the white matter.

Comparing these preparations of the adult cortex with those obtained in the child of a few days, and stained with silver chromate, some differences attract attention. It is noticeable that the whole plexiform layer has decreased in thickness in the adult, and that the plane containing the tangential fibers is more flattened and contains a notably smaller number of them than in the silver preparations of the child of one month. Such differences result, in our opinion, from the fact that many of the tangential fibers that appear in the cerebrum of the child are not axons but horizontal dendrites, destined perhaps to atrophy or to change their original orientation. Another cause of the narrowing of the plane of the tangential fibers, which suffers a superficial dilation during the development of the plexiform layer, could be the progressive insertion of the [apical dendritic] tufts of pyramids between the special cells which would perhaps oblige the [latter] cells and their axons to slide tangentially, proportionately shortening their trajectories. Anyway, we must not forget that the Golgi method only reveals more or less embryonic dispositions that will undergo transformation in adulthood, as functional differentiations require new anatomical adaptations.

The layers of the small and medium pyramids are very poor in medullated fibers. Almost all that cross these layers vertically belong to the so-called fibers of Martinotti, and they are thinner than the already mentioned robust tangential fibers. Occasionally, however, a thicker ascending fiber is observed with a very deep origin and which may represent either a centripetal fiber arriving from the white matter or the axon of the giant stellate or fusiform cells with ascending axons of the sixth and seventh layers. With regard to the horizontal and oblique fibers, they are scarce and commonly thin, and they do not form a plexus in the strict sense. Almost all correspond to the collaterals of the medium pyramids and to branches of the fibers of Martinotti. This poverty of thin fibers in the Weigert preparations and the position and orientation of the few such fibers revealed in them prove that all the innumerable axons and axonal arborizations of the bitufted and stellate short axon cells (small, medium, and giant types) lack a myelin sheath.

Sometimes, some robust medullated fiber is observed crossing the third layer more or less horizontally; such fibers, which coincide in position with certain voluminous fibers of the Golgi preparations, probably represent, as we shall see later, centripetal fibers.

The fourth layer or layer of the large pyramids (fig. 2, 4) [fig. 119] is much richer in medullated fibers, which are distinguished as verticals and transversals. The verticals, initially dispersed, do not delay in joining together in small radial bundles, which appear completely constituted at the deep level of this layer. As is known, such bundles are composed of axons of small, medium, and large pyramids, and perhaps of a centripetal fiber and some fiber of Martinotti. The interradial plexus or [plexus] of the horizontal and oblique myelinated fibers is moderately rich, increasing progressively

downward, until it becomes merged with the more complicated and dense plexus located in the layer of the granule cells.

The majority of the fibers of the interradial plexus of the layer of the superficial large pyramids represents probably collaterals of axons of large and medium pyramids; but to it also contribute, as we shall see later, a number of horizontal and oblique branches arising from centripetal fibers, and also thick axons of the special acoustic cells.

At the level of the fifth layer or [layer] of the granule cells, the interradial plexus reaches its maximum in complexity and richness (fig. 2, 5) [fig. 119], it being possible to compare it, both in position and in physiological significance, to the dense plexus or the stria of Gennari of the visual cortex and to that characteristic of the third layer of the motor cortex. However, this plexus in the cerebral region under study has no fibers as voluminous, or so complicated, as in these other cortical territories. To it contribute, besides the radial bundles, an infinity of thin or medium myelinated fibers that run horizontally, or obliquely, and not a few robust fibers that cross almost at a right angle the mentioned bundles and are prolonged over considerable distances.

In the middle of the meshes, the minute cell bodies of the granule cells show up. The plexus in question extends somewhat less densely into the sixth, seventh, and eighth [white matter] layers, showing, the deeper it is situated, a greater richness in robust fibers parallel to the [surface of the] gyrus, the majority of which must be regarded as exogenous or centripetal fibers. Anyway, it has seemed to us that the thinner fibers and the narrower spaces of the plexus correspond to the cited layer of the granule cells.

It is easy to understand that, given such a complexity of fibers, the complete pursuit of each fiber to the white matter and the determination of its origin and termination will be impossible. In the motor area, it is relatively easy to reveal the arrival of sensory fibers at the intermediate stria or nervous plexus of the third layer, thanks to [their] notable thickness and to [their] almost always oblique or staircaselike course, but not so in the auditory cortex, because the centripetal fibers have a diameter that does not usually surpass that of the axons of the large pyramids and also because they are much less numerous and follow a great variety of courses in the deep cortical regions.

Plexuses in Golgi Preparations

As can be presumed, the good preparations of the Golgi method in the child of fifteen days to one and a half months reveal clearly not only the fibers [that can be] impregnated by the hematoxylin, but an enormous amount of unmyelinated small fibers, arranged in very complicated and inextricable plexuses. We will not enter now into a meticulous description of these plexuses, because we have dealt with them already in previous works. Here we will limit the description to some observations about the properties and distributions of the exogenous fibers that form them.

Thick Exogenous Fibers Terminating in the Plexus of the Layer of the Granule Cells

At first, when the Golgi preparations of the auditory cortex in which fibers are well impregnated are examined, these exogenous conductors do not attract attention. In fact, the number of such fibers is scarce, and their thickness is not so great as to catch at once the eye of the observer. By dint of examining [many] preparations, however, we will finish up by discovering in some sections moderately thick fibers that reach the plexus of the fifth and bordering layers from the white matter. In some fortuitous sections, these fibers will appear almost exclusively stained. These fibers cross, either radially or obliquely, the seventh and sixth layers, and once arrived in the thickness of the latter layer or at the level of the fifth, they become progressively horizontal, bifurcating on their way and giving rise to very long branches that trace flexuosities to accommodate to the granule cells and pyramids, over very long distances. As is seen in fig. 15, *a* [*fig. 132*], the majority of these fibers are arranged parallel to the cerebral surface and give off at intervals some thin collaterals that are lost in the fifth layer, forming a rich plexus but less dense than the one produced in the visual and motor areas.

In general, these few collaterals also have a horizontal course, but it is difficult to follow their route. In addition to the fibers that are seen to arrive from the white matter in a perpendicular section of the first sphenoidal gyrus, there exist others that it is not possible to follow backward to the white matter, because they come perhaps in a crosswise direction, that is to say, parallel to the gyrus. Many such fibers, whose branches reinforce the plexus of the fifth layer, could very well be exogenous fibers with the same origin [as the exogenous fibers mentioned above] but with a different and extremely oblique initial course.

Not all the fibers with an exogenous appearance are arborized in the layer of the granule cells; many also run horizontally over long trajectories in the fourth layer, and there is no lack, either, of analogous fibers dispersed in the sixth and seventh layers. There are places in which it is impossible to distinguish the plexus located in these layers from that located in the thickness of the granule cell [layer], so perfect is the continuity of the plexuses and so great the similarity in the course, direction, and branching pattern of their constituent fibers. Such a widely distributed spread of the exogenous fibers constitutes one of the most serious difficulties that impede good structural study of this cortical region. There are fibers that reach up to the third layer, in which they trace long horizontal trajectories, and they are distinguished by their thickness from the collaterals of the pyramids and from the branches of the cells with short axon that pass through this layer (fig. 15, *c*) [*fig. 132*].

From whence come the exogenous fibers ramifying in the fifth and bordering layers? It is impossible to answer this question with any semblance of certainty. The difficulty is all the greater because the vast majority of the horizontal thick fibers of the sixth, fifth, and fourth layers reach such great length that they are never seen to [ascend from] the white matter, and it is not possible thus to resolve definitely the question of their exogenous nature. But, nevertheless, considering that a few fibers of this kind positively [can be traced] down to the white matter, it does not appear reckless to suppose that many of them, at least, definitely represent the continuations of centripetal conductors. Accepting this, if we think of an analogy and we remember that in other cortical re-

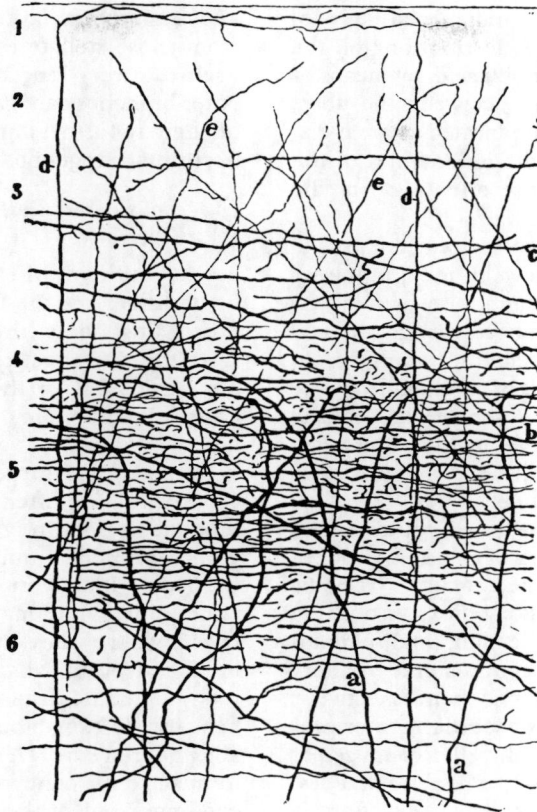

[*FIG. 132*]   Fig. 15. Nervous plexuses of the sphenoidal cortex of the child of twenty-five days. Method of Golgi. *1,* plexiform layer; *2,* small pyramids; *3,* medium pyramids; *4,* external large pyramids; *5,* layer of the granule cells; *6,* layer of the deep medium pyramids; *a,* centripetal fiber; *b,* robust horizontal centripetal fibers; *c,* thick horizontal fibers of the third layer; *e,* thin oblique threads; *d,* long ascending fibers to the first layer.

gions, in the visual, for example, where the centripetal fibers ramifying in the layer of the granule cells represent very probably second-order visual fibers, it would be possible to suppose here that the said exogenous plexuses of the sphenoidal cortex also include terminal, second-order acoustic fibers, perhaps coming from the medial geniculate body.

With such an assumption, guesses can be made about the manner of connection of the said fibers and about the mechanism of propagation of [nerve impulses] in the auditory cortex. The exogenous fibers would enter into contact relationships, first, with the cell bodies and [apical dendritic] shafts of many pyramids of the sixth, fifth, and fourth layers; second,

with the [dendritic] shafts and somata of the special acoustic cells located precisely in the layers in which the said exogenous fibers are preferentially distributed; and third, with the somata and dendrites of the innumerable cells with short axon located in the layer of the granule cells. But the last connection is equivalent to a contact relationship with the pyramids, since the axons of the granule cells and of all kinds of bitufted cells of the fifth layer definitely engage in contact relationships with the somata of the cells with long axon. We would have, therefore, both direct and indirect or remote connections between the terminal acoustic fibers and the cells of projection or pyramids: the first occur between the acoustic fibers and the pyramids and special cells located in the sphere of distribution [of the fibers]; the second are established, by means of the cells with short axon, between the fibers and the pyramids that are located at great distances, either in the radial orientation of the gyrus or in the transverse orientation of the gyrus.

To identify these probable connections is to trace the customary flow of the [impulses]. Therefore, the acoustic impulse arriving by the centripetal fibers, and absorbed by the several listed cells, will be able to emerge from the cortex via three kinds of conductors: by the robust axons arising from the special acoustic cells, by thin axons of the medium and small pyramids, and by the thick axons of the large pyramids and triangular cells.

Let us add that these three routes correspond to the three types of physiological coordination required theoretically (acoustic memories, motor-acoustic reflex, association with areas of visual ideation, and perhaps [integration] with the contralateral auditory area). [These pathways] may be, respectively: that which must convey acoustic memories is via the special cells; the impeller of muscular reflexes is via the large pyramids; and that destined for the interhemispheric associations is via the small and medium pyramids. [To allocate these functions to the path mentioned] is to formulate a conjecture [that is] certainly plausible but completely devoid of anatomicophysiological support and without more significance than to indicate to the future [investigator] one of several possibilities that it is convenient to bear in mind for orienting ideas and interpreting data.

The exogenous plexuses of the fourth, fifth, and sixth layers are additionally complicated by an infinity of branches of endogenous axons, the meticulous analysis of which we will not enter into here. It will be enough to remember that in the plexus of the fifth layer participate (a) axon collaterals of the medium and small pyramidal cells of the layer of the granule cells; (b) collaterals of numerous ascending fibers arising from the cells of Martinotti, located in the sixth and seventh layers; and (c) terminal arborizations of many cells with ascending short axon, located in the fifth

and underlying layers and very particularly from those stellate cells whose axon resolves itself into very long horizontal branches. The latter branches can often be mistaken, because of their robustness and enormous length, for horizontal exogenous fibers.

Exogenous Fibers Destined for the Plexiform or First Layer

Several authors, when dealing with the medullated fibers of the typical cortex, have supposed that some myelinated fibers coming from the white matter would have their point of termination in the plexiform layer, after crossing perpendicularly all the interposed layers.

In our recent impregnations of the auditory cortex, we have often been able to reveal very long fibers relatively thick and bereft of or with very modest numbers of collateral ramifications, which were followed, from sites very close to the white matter, up to the plexiform layer, where they turned horizontally and branched prolifically after traveling for very long tangential distances. Will these radial fibers also be exogenous conductors? It is probable, but not sure. Here it is possible to err and to mistake for centripetal fibers the robust ascending axons of the colossal cells of Martinotti, which are located in the seventh layer and sometimes very close to the white matter (fig. 15, *d*) [*fig. 132*].

Thin Fibers Distributed to the Second, Third, and Fourth Layers (fig. 15, *e*)[*fig. 132*].

Already in our study on the motor cortex, we called attention to the frequency with which in certain impregnations there are found in these layers, and especially in the second and third, a prodigious number of very delicate, varicose threads, sometimes with a vertical course, but more often oblique and even transverse. Almost all of these threads, some of which are shown in fig. 15, *e* [*fig. 132*], end by a varicosity or by a bifurcation either in the thickness of the plexiform layer or in the several planes of the second layer; they run undivided downward for long distances, and generally cease to be visible, either for lack of impregnation or for other reasons, before the sixth layer; often, as they become deeper, they thicken slightly, converging with others, and form small vertical or oblique bundles, whose origin we have still not been able to establish.

Such fibers give rise to a very rich plexus (not as dense in the auditory region as in the motor, although this difference can result from better or worse impregnation) in the second and third layers, and they appear to be attached to the [apical dendritic] shafts of the pyramids; will they be perhaps the terminal branches of the callosal or association fibers? We do not know; we can only assure [the reader] that they do not represent recurrent collaterals of pyramids, or ascending fibers of Martinotti, or axon collaterals of the special acoustic cells, or, finally, ascending branches of the bitufted cells. But since these fibers have not been followed to the white matter, it is clear that it is not possible to exclude at all an endogenous origin. It is reasonable, for example, to imagine that they represent thin ascending axon collaterals coming from those small pyramids or granule cells whose axons form a little arch from which vertical threads arise. They could be, lastly, collaterals from the white matter or perhaps also the uppermost branches arising from the axons of the cells with short axon located in the fifth, sixth, and seventh layers. So this is a question that requires subsequent and more careful investigations.

Auditory Cortex in Other Gyrencephalic Mammals

In order to complete our studies on the subject, we have explored also the temporal gyri of the dog and cat, also using the methods of Nissl and of Golgi. The most beautiful preparations have been obtained in the cat of twenty to twenty-four days, a period in which all the cells, excluding the first rows of small pyramids, have reached almost completely their morphological perfection.

As is known, the [temporal] lobe of the dog and cat shows three parallel descending gyri[C] that become fused at the [ventral] pole of the lobe. According to Munk, the acoustic area will be located in the dog in the inferior portion of the two posterior gyri, which are the thickest.

One presumes that the cat has the same localization. Anyway, we must point out that our observations have been focused on the central regions of both posterior gyri,[D] in which we have found, with slight differences, an identical structure.

We will not consider if the structural data that we have gathered in the said region are general [for the whole cortex or unique to the acoustic region], because our comparative studies between the sphenoidal cortex and the other cerebral areas of the cat and dog are still very incomplete. Anyway, in spite of the deficiencies of the analysis, we believe that we can affirm that the cortical areas of the mammals show much less structural contrast [from area to area] than in man, which explains well why several authors have only been able to recognize in the mouse, rabbit, and cat a single structural plan, the so-called *typical cortex.*

The Nissl method reveals in the [temporal] gyri of the dog and cat the following layers: first or *plexiform;* second or [layer] *of the small pyramids;* third or [layer] *of the medium pyramids;* fourth [layer] *of the granule cells* or *small pyramids and stellate cells;* fifth [layer] or [layer] *of the giant pyramids;* sixth or [layer] *of the tight-packed fusiform and triangular cells* (layer of the *polymorphic cells* of the rabbit and mouse); seventh *fibrocellular layer* or [layer] *of the scarce triangular and large fusiform cells.*

As can be seen, the cat and dog lack the layer of the superficial large pyramids, which is replaced by medium pyramids. The granule cells do not constitute, either, a layer as well defined as in the human cortex; in fact, this layer is nothing but a deep portion of the layer of medium pyramids in which the cells with short axon are more abundant than in other layers. The fifth layer is well marked by the appearance of large intercellular spaces, as well as by the presence of robust pyramids; these spaces, indicative of interstitial plexuses, get narrower again at the level of the sixth layer, whose cellular elements are situated very close together. Finally, the seventh layer is well recognized by the wide bundles of white matter that separate the cells, which are scarce, have a bipolar, triangular, or stellate shape, reach a voluminous size comparable and sometimes superior to that of the giant pyramids, and often show crowns of neuroglial nuclei. The thickness of the sixth and seventh layers together on occasions is equal to the sum of all the other layers, except in the concavity of the gyri, in which the latter predominate.

We will not give here a detailed description of all the cells that the Golgi method reveals in the cerebrum of the cat and dog. Many of them are identical to the ones located in the motor and visual cortex, and they have been well described by the authors who have studied the typical cortex.

We will limit ourselves at present to drawing attention to some [cellular] elements that appear to correspond in their more substantial characteristics to those already described in the human temporal cortex.

Plexiform Layer

In the cat and dog, it is nothing special. In it are observed the tangential fibers, that is to say, the horizontal axons of the special cells (rarely impregnated), the terminal arborizations of the fibers of Martinotti, and the axonal ramifications of cells with short axon, which are similar on the whole to those already described by us in other work.[4]

Second and Third Layers or Layers of the Small and Medium Pyramids

Besides the well-known pyramidal types, some of them reproduced in fig. 16, A [*fig. 133*], this layer is inhabited by several categories of cells with short axon.

Among them we must mention:

a. A type of relatively large bitufted cell, whose axon forms an arborization of ascending and descending little branches, less complicated and shorter than those belonging to the homonymous type of the human cortex (fig. 16, I) [*fig. 133*].

b. Robust or medium-sized stellate or triangular cells, provided with divergent long dendrites and an axon that forms an extensive and loose arborization extending over a large portion of the second and third layers.

In some preparations, we have found also certain very robust axonal arborizations, whose very long branches embrace the second, third, and fourth layers; some of them went up to the

thickness of the plexiform [layer]. We have not yet impregnated the parent cells, but they must be of giant size [because of the very extensive arborization].

c. Cells with ascending axon ramifying either in the first, second, and third layers or in just the plexiform layer.

Layer of the Granule Cells

It contains also, as in the human cortex, cells with long and short axon.

a. The cells with long axon have a pyramidal shape and similar properties to the corresponding cells of man. As can be seen in fig. 16, C, D, E [*fig. 133*], the axon collaterals of these cells describe little arches and run mainly in a recurrent [course], to terminate in the thickness of the third and second layers. With regard to the deeper portion of the axon, it has a smaller diameter than the collaterals, and it is prolonged down to the white matter. There are, besides, in this layer many medium pyramids, identical to the common pyramids, as is shown in fig. 16,[E] B [*fig. 133*].

b. Large or medium bitufted cells with axon moderately branched in a radial direction (fig. 16,[F] *f*) [*fig. 133*].

c. Large or medium stellate or globular cells, whose axon gives rise to a dense vertical arborization extending through the whole thickness of the granule cell layer. It is not rare to see that this ramification forms parallel and radial series of pericellular nests. As examples of such cellular elements, which correspond without doubt to the cells with a prolixly arborized axon that we already described in the layer of the granule cells of the sphenoidal region of man, we show two cases in figs. 16, H, and 17, A [*figs. 133, 134*].

d. Neurogliaform type (fig. 17, C) [*fig. 134*]. It is larger generally than the corresponding cell in the human cortex, and it is distinguished not only by the delicacy and density of the arborization of the axon but also by the considerable number and strongly varicose aspect of the dendrites.

e. Large stellate cell with an axon loosely arborizing in this and bordering layers (fig. 17, B) [*fig. 134*].

f. Fusiform cell with ascending axon forming long horizontal branches (fig. 17, D) [*fig.*

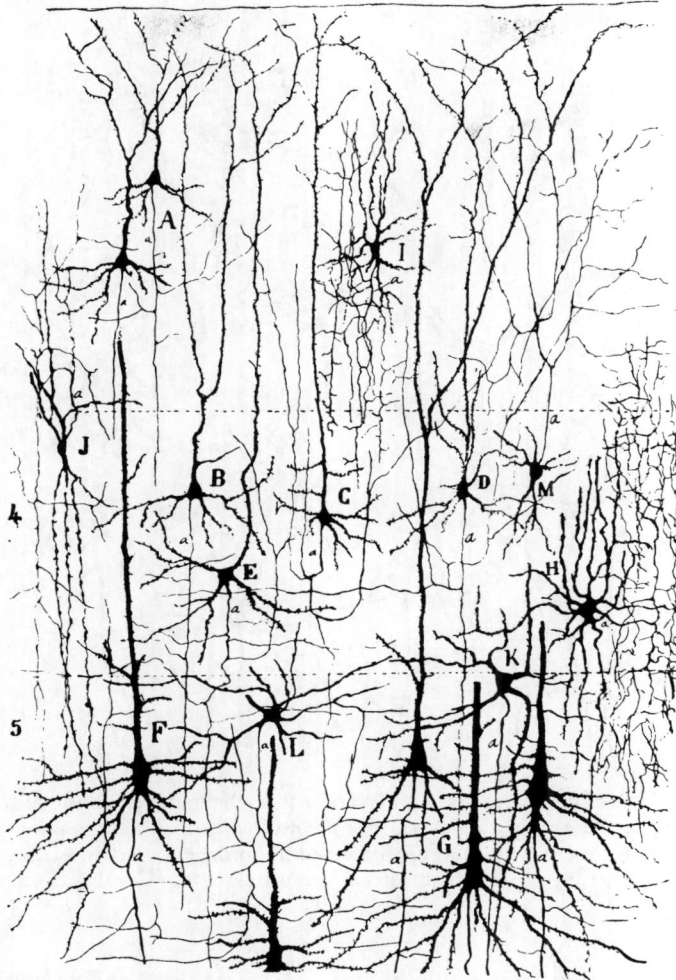

[*FIG. 133*]   Fig. 16. Several cellular types of the sphenoidal cortex of the cat of twenty-four days. *4,* layer of the granule cells; *5,* layer of the giant pyramids; *A,* small and medium pyramids; *B,* medium common pyramid of the fourth layer; *C, D,* granule cells with ascending axon collaterals terminating in the second and third layers; *E,* stellate cell with radial [dendritic] shaft; *F, G,* giant pyramids; *H,* giant bitufted type with very dense axonal arborization; *J, I,* bitufted cell of medium size and with poorly branched axon; *K,* cell with descending long axon; *L,* large stellate cell with short axon dividing in long horizontal branches; *M,* cell with ascending axon ramifying in the second and third layers.

134]. It will be remembered that this type exists also in the human cortex.

g. Triangular stellate or fusiform cell, whose axon is ramified prolixly in the upper layers, that is to say, in the second and third (fig. [16], *M*) [*fig. 133*].

h. Fusiform, triangular, or globular cell that lacks a radial [dendritic] shaft but gives off a descending long axon (figs. 16, *K;* 17, *E*) [*figs. 133, 134*]. Less abundant here than in the underlying layers, having, instead of an ascending [dendritic] shaft, a short tuft of varicose branches that do not pass the upper border of the fourth layer, and one or two robust descending [dendritic] shafts.

The axon can be followed down to the white

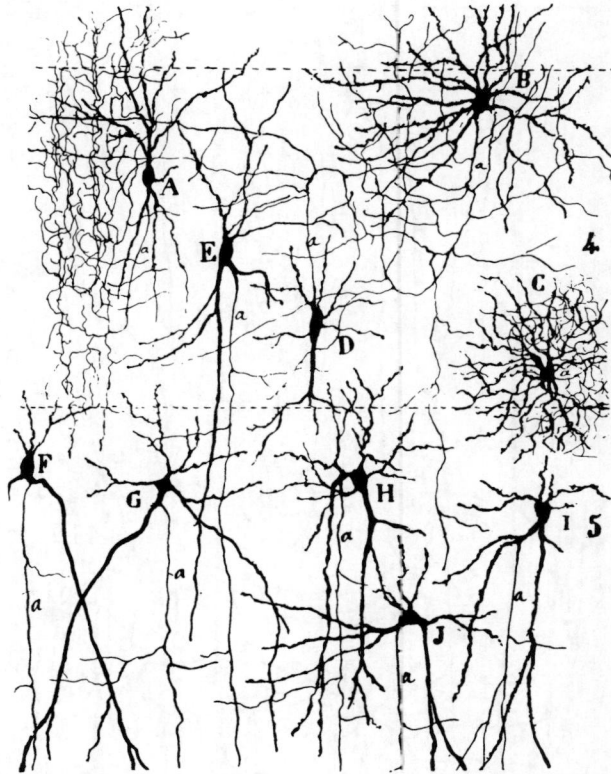

[*FIG. 134*]   Fig. 17. Cells of the fourth and fifth layers of the sphenoidal cerebrum of the cat. *4,* layer of the granule cells; *5,* layer of the giant pyramids; *A,* type of bitufted cell; *C,* neurogliaform cell; *B,* stellate cell with short axon; *D,* fusiform cell with short axon divided in horizontal branches; *E, F, G, H, I, J,* morphological varieties of a cellular type devoid of an [apical dendritic] shaft and with a descending long axon.

matter, where often it divides into a thin and a thick branch. Do these cells correspond to the special acoustic cells? We do not know. To resolve this point, it would be necessary to explore the whole cortex and to see if the mentioned cells exist exclusively in the [temporal] region; we have not yet had time to make such an exploration. Anyway, the referred elements do not coincide with the special cells except in the absence of a radial [dendritic] shaft; they lack the giant size, the horizontal direction, and the long ascending dendrites.

Layer of the Large Pyramids

It lodges robust and elongated giant and medium pyramids, from whose somata arise long and horizontal dendrites (fig. 16, *G, F*) [*fig.*

133]. The thick and descending axon can easily be followed down to the white matter.

Besides this pyramidal type, bitufted cells, stellate cells with short axon ramifying in the thickness of the layer (fig. 16, *L*) [*fig. 133*], and especially the already mentioned cell devoid of an [apical dendritic] shaft and provided with a descending long axon are also observed.

The latter type is very frequent in the fifth layer (fig. 17) [*fig 134*], and it exhibits a great variety of forms: mitral (*J*), stellate (*G*), triangular (*H, I*), ovoid (*F*), etc. The collaterals of the axon are ramified, especially in the fifth and sixth layers.

Another cell with a somewhat special form is shown in fig. 16, *K* [*fig. 133*]. Its general form is stellate, like the previous type, but it is distinguished from it in that one of the ascending dendrites, instead of terminating at a short distance [from the parent cell], goes up, after tracing a turn, to the plexiform layer.

Sixth Layer or Layer of the Triangular and Fusiform Cells

It contains triangular, stellate, pyramidal, and fusiform cells, provided with a radial dendrite that reaches the first layer and an axon incorporated into the white matter. There is no lack here (perhaps they are even more abundant than in the preceding layer) of cells with short axon of all kinds and of the stellate cells devoid of a radial shaft, but with an axon prolonged down into the white matter.

Seventh or Fibrocellular Layer

It exhibits a series of isolated cells or cells separated by septa of white matter. In it are found, in addition to the types of the preceding layer which here commonly reach a larger size, these two other types:

a. Upside-down pyramidal cell, that is to say, with a descending dendritic shaft and with an ascending axon prolonged up to the first layer (fig. 18, F) [fig. 135].

b. Giant stellate cell from whose soma arise long and divergent dendrites, and whose axon, very thick and varicose, is incorporated into the white matter after giving off long recurrent collaterals. This cellular type, which appears very abundant in the seventh layer, although it is not lacking in the sixth, approaches more than any others the special cellular element of the human auditory cortex; but we do not dare identify it with this, because it lacks the most characteristic features, namely the preferential horizontal orientation of the dendritic shafts and the numerous ascending secondary branches.

In summary, in the [temporal] cortex of the dog and cat, there are cellular types similar to those in the human cortex, but the morphological variants they present make the comparison difficult. Nevertheless, both cortices coincide in some characteristics: presence of a layer of granule cells containing similar cel-

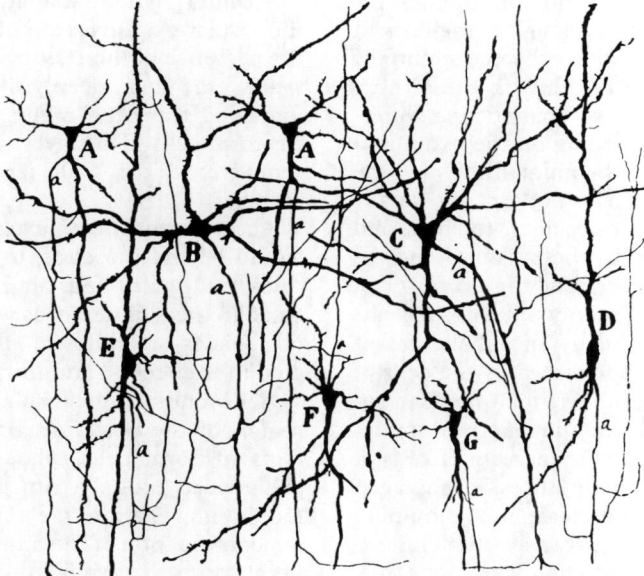

[FIG. 135]   Fig. 18. Some cellular types of the seventh layer of the sphenoidal cortex of the cat of twenty-four days. A, G, cells devoid of radial [dendritic] shafts and with long descending axons; B, C, giant stellate types with axon incorporated into the white matter; D, E, fusiform types with long axon and provided with a radial [dendritic] shaft; F, upside-down pyramidal cell or cell of Martinotti.

lular elements with short axon; excessive development of the deep layers; existence of cells with long axon but devoid of an [apical dendritic] shaft; etc. It is also curious to find in the cat cellular forms that seemed characteristic of the human cortex, such as the neurogliaform and the bitufted types, [though] somewhat modified.

If, after the preceding succinct analysis, and having in mind the data relating to other sensory cortical regions, [anyone] would ask us what is the cardinal difference that distinguishes the cerebrum of man from that of the higher mammals, we would answer unhesitatingly that it is none other than the extraordinary abundance of the cells with short axon, and especially of the tufted cells.[G] To such superabundance of cells of association at short distance is due the notable development of the layer of the granule cells (the place where the said cells are concentrated) and the cellular richness of the layer of the small pyramids in man.

Thus, for us, there is no doubt that the cells with short axon, and especially the most abundant [types], that is to say, the bitufted, perform an important function in the performance of psychic acts, although at the present time it is impossible to specify the nature of that function. There are thus in the sensory cerebrum two factors of construction differently associated, depending on the evolutionary stage reached by the animal: the *old phylogenetic factor,* which is not lacking in any cerebrum, from the batrachian to man, and which is represented by the pyramids and the centripetal sensory fibers; and the *relatively recent phylogenetic factor,* since it only appears well developed in the gyrencephalic mammals, and which is represented by the cells of short axon with their diversity of morphological types. Certainly, the human cerebrum has not progressed only by the increase of cells of association over short distances; it has been also advanced by the increase in the number of small and medium pyramids, perhaps extending fibers of association over long distances, and in addition by the more complete differentiation of the cells located in the plexiform layer.

II. Cortex of the Insula

Considering the insula as a territory subordinate to the auditory cortex, it is of interest to find out if its gyri have the same structure as the first sphenoidal [gyrus] or if they show individual characteristics revealing some special physiological task.

With this aim, we have studied recently, both with the method of Nissl and with that of Golgi, the insular gyri, and the results obtained, as yet rather incomplete because we have only achieved a small number of good impregnations, prove that the insular gray matter has unique structural characteristics, thanks to which it can be easily differentiated from the cortex of the other cerebral regions. These features concern the singular morphology of the pyramids and the thickness and distribution of the layers common to all the gyri.

The data obtained so far about the subject are scarce and incomplete. Our bibliographic investigation on the theme only allows us to record here incomplete observations, mainly in relation to the number of layers and their extent.

Meynert,[5] who first analyzed in some detail the insular gyri, gives as characteristic of these the presence of the *claustrum,* that is to say, of a new gray layer, deeply situated and well demarcated from the others, and composed of fusiform cells. This layer would be the representative of the fifth layer of the general cortex.

According to Betz,[6] exclusive to the insula would be the presence, in the fifth layer, of thick multipolar cells similar to the ones located in the claustrum, as well as the existence of pleiades or groups of small pyramids situated in the second and third layers.

For Mondino,[7] the insular and especially the region of the posterior marginal sulcus contains fusiform cells, whose dendrites, which are divided prolixly, run parallel to the surface. With regard to the claustrum, he sees in it a continuation of the anterior lip of the temporal cortex that would [thus] invade the white matter of the insula.

If we are to believe Obersteiner,[8] the insular cortex differs little if at all from the common type of cortex, presenting the classical five layers of Meynert.

Hammarberg,[9] who has studied very meticulously all the cortical regions, devoted little attention to the insular region. Here is the stratification that this author describes in the *short* [insular] *gyri:*

First layer or molecular [layer].
Second and third layers. They are composed of small and large pyramids.
Fourth layer. Little pronounced and thin; it is composed of small pyramids, as is shown in fig. 1, plate 3, of the work of the said author.
Fifth layer or ganglionic [layer]. It is composed of cells of 10 by 15 μm.
Sixth layer or layer of fusiform cells. It is very thick, measuring 1.20 mm; it contains cells of 4 by 8 μm.

Simple inspection at low power of a Nissl section of the insular gyri shows very clearly that the insular cortex has unique features, mainly in the slight thickness and resolution of the layer of the granule cells, in the scarcity of giant pyramids, and in the enormous thickness of the sixth layer or layer of the fusiform cells, which is seen divided in two by a septum of white matter.

Between the several layers of gray matter, in the insula there is much less contrast and demarcation of the layers is decidely more difficult than in other cortical regions. Nevertheless, by studying comparatively Nissl preparations obtained in several cerebra, we have been able to recognize the following stratification.

First or Plexiform Layer

It is thin, since it does not usually exceed eighteen hundredths [of a millimeter], and it contains, as is shown with the Nissl method, scarce horizontal or special cells. The special cells appear well stained with the Golgi method and do not differ from those above mentioned. In this layer also reside [cellular] elements with short axon, and in it there exists

a plexus rich in threads [that are continuations of the fibers] of Martinotti.

Second Layer or Layer of the Small Pyramids

Comparing it with that of the same name in the sphenoidal cortex, it appears narrower and poor in pyramidal cells. Almost all its [cellular] elements appear to be cells with short axon. The pleiades of pyramids about which Betz talks are not demonstrated with clarity. The Golgi method reveals the same composition as in the sphenoidal cortex.

Third Layer or Layer of the Medium Pyramids

It embraces a great thickness of the cortex, no less than one hundred to one hundred twenty hundredths [of a millimeter]. In the Nissl preparations, it is noticed that it is composed of medium pyramids with a size of 12 to 15 by 18 to 20 [μm] [and] separated by rather extensive spaces. In the deep part of this layer, the cellular stature increases very little; thus, it is not possible to recognize a layer of superficial large pyramids or fourth layer of other cortical regions.

The silver chromate reveals only known [neural] elements in this layer. Besides the pyramids and the cells with ascending or descending short axon, here there are a large number of bitufted cells primarily of a medium and large size.

Fourth Layer or Layer of the Granule Cells

It is little pronounced, and, rather than a separate layer, it appears to be a region of the third layer, in which are concentrated somewhat more the cells with short axon scattered through other territories. In the cortex of the child of one month (Nissl method), this layer is more pronounced than in the adult. In this the thickness does not surpass eighteen to twenty hundredths [of a millimeter].

The method of Golgi reveals here the same [cell] types as in the sphenoidal cortex. Dominating are the stellate or fusiform cells with short or long ascending axon and the bitufted and neurogliaform cells. There is no lack also of small or medium pyramids with robust and arciform axon collaterals.

Fifth Layer or Layer of the Pyramidal and Large Fusiform Cells

This layer reaches a thickness of thirty to sixty hundredths [of a millimeter], and in it appear somewhat bigger pyramidal cells, though they do not surpass, however, 10 or 12 μm of thickness per 30 or 40 μm length. In general, the pyramids of this layer observed in the Nissl preparations present a certain transverse narrowness of the soma that distinguishes them at first glance from the giant cells of other cortical regions.

Besides the frankly pyramidal types, there are observed especially in the adult cortex long fusiform cells provided with two robust radial polar processes and with an oblong nucleus, sometimes elongated like a little rod, as in fibroblasts. At the level of the starting point of the ascending or descending processes, there is often observed a swelling formed by the accumulation of a brown pigment. This layer contains also bifurcated cells, that is to say, cells supplied with two thick ascending dendrites and one descending, and likewise some irregularly disseminated, small, or polyhedral fusiform cells lodge there.

The method of Golgi allows us to determine better the morphology of the cellular elements of this layer. Because they show some interesting peculiarities, they deserve that we pay some attention to their study.

As is observed in fig. 19 [fig. 136], taken from the insula of the child of one month, the cellular types with long axon that inhabit the fifth layer are of three kinds: first, true pyramidal cell analogous to the one present in the acoustic cortex, from which it differs in being somewhat thinner and in having the basal dendrites larger, descending and not very long (fig. 19, A, B) [fig. 136]; second, triangular, bifid, or trifid cell (fig. 19, E, F) [fig. 136], characterized by showing two, three, or more ascending dendritic branches capable of being followed up to the plexiform layer, and a basal dendrite forming at a certain distance a tuft of descending

and diverging thin dendrites, from the inferior pole of which dendritic pedicle there arises the axon that does not differ from that of the pyramids, either in its direction or with respect to its collaterals; third, fusiform type with descending tuft (fig. 19, C, D) [fig. 136], the cell more abundant and characteristic of the fifth layer, being also present, although fewer in number, in the adjoining layers. It has an oblong and thin soma, which sometimes resembles a simple thickening of the radial dendrite; from the inferior pole arises a descending [dendritic] shaft, generally devoid of branches, and which, at a certain distance, somewhat variable for each cell, forms an elegant tuft of thin descending dendrites; the radial or [apical shaft] goes up across the fourth and third layers and reaches the plexiform layer, where it gives rise to a tuft [of dendrites]. Usually, this radial [dendritic] shaft is bifurcated in the thickness of the fourth layer, thus giving rise to two terminal tufts. Lastly, from the sides of the soma as well as from the initial portions of the polar [dendritic] shafts arise some delicate horizontal dendrites. With regard to the axon, as in the previous type, it arises from the inferior portion of the descending process and goes down to the white matter after giving off, in its initial trajectory, some collaterals with a horizontal or oblique and even recurrent course.

At first sight, the singular morphology of the cells of the fifth layer, surely homologous to pyramids in functional significance, raises the idea of a radial stretching suffered by the cells due to lateral compression. But these cellular forms are only to be observed in certain cortical regions (insula and olfactory cortex, as we will see in other work): they are lacking in the protuberant portions of the ordinary gyri, and there is the easily demonstrable fact that by the side of the fusiform cells there are true pyramids, so we are obliged to renounce this supposition [of lateral compression].

This morphological phenomenon probably represents an adaptation to the position and disposition of the terminal arborizations of the centripetal fibers, and it must be governed by the laws of the conservation of mass or protoplasm, about which we have insisted in other works.[13]

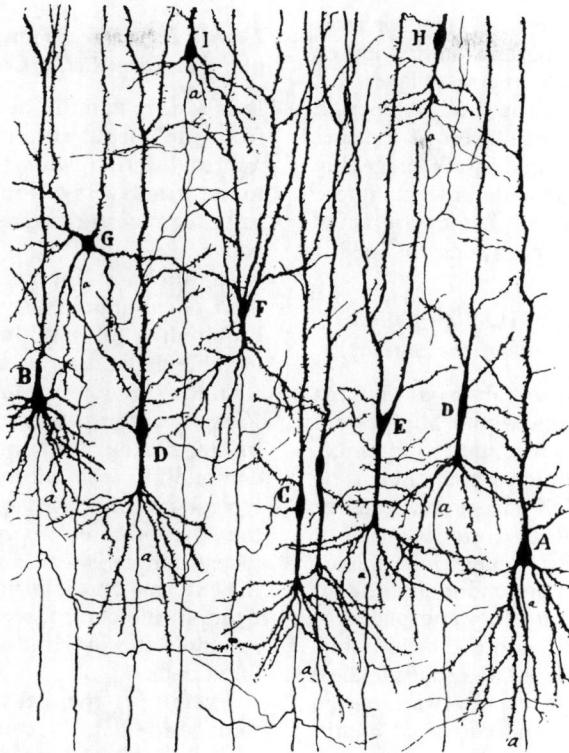

[*FIG. 136*] Fig. 19. Vertical section of the cortex of the insula of the child of one month. Fifth layer or [layer] of the pyramids and large fusiform cells. *A, B,* ordinary large pyramids; *D, C,* fusiform cells with descending [dendritic] tuft; *E, F,* cells provided with two or more ascending [dendritic] shafts prolonged up to the first layer; *G,* stellate cell with two radial dendritic shafts; *H, I,* small cells with long axon of the fourth layer; *a,* axon.

Sixth Layer or Layer of the Small Fusiform and Triangular Cells

The transitions existing between this layer and the previous one make it impossible to identify a well-pronounced border. In the Nissl preparations, it is only seen that the relatively large pyramids of the fifth layer, as well as the robust fusiform cells, are progressively disappearing, ceding their positions to smaller stellate fusiform, triangular, or pyramidal cells. In the most superficial portions of this layer, the cells mentioned still keep their radial orientation, but in the deepest planes, this is lost almost completely, the dendrites being oriented in all directions. Also attracting attention in the deep plane is the great frequency with which most of the triangular, stellate, or fusiform cells are bordered with neuroglial crowns. There are some cells that appear surrounded by fifteen or sixteen neuroglial nuclei.

The sixth layer embraces a great extent of the insular cortex; in the adult man, its thickness is not less than three hundred fifty hundredths [of a millimeter] (convex parts).

Examining this layer in the Golgi preparations of the child of one month or a month and a half, it shows a similar structure to that reported in our previous work. In it are found true pyramids with long axon; fusiform and triangular cells with axon prolonged down to the white matter; globular, triangular, or fusiform cells with ascending axon, either long and extending to the superficial layers or short and forming terminal arborizations distributed at the level of the seventh and sixth layers.

An interesting fact also is the existence in the fifth, sixth, and seventh layers of the specific acoustic cells described in the preceding study on the first sphenoidal gyrus. Those found are few in number, but they are never lacking in the good impregnations obtained.

Seventh Layer or Layer of the Fibrocellular Substance (Extreme Capsule of the Authors)

Below the preceding layer is observed a lamina of white matter, between whose bundles are disseminated nerve cells separated by distances more or less great. Although scarce, there is no lack of these cells, which have a triangular or stellate shape and show an average stature of 12 by 20 μm. The dendrites have no preferred orientation, going in all directions, and the somata have no orientation. In some places of this layer, the cells are more concentrated, forming islets or pleiades. The total thickness of the fibrocellular layer reaches two hundred to two hundred fifty hundredths [of a millimeter].

The neuroglia of this region are abundant, and although they are less frequent than in the preceding layer, pericellular crowns are also observed.

In the light of the Golgi method, the fibrocellular layer appears made up of a plexus of nerve fibers oriented in all directions, among which are found irregularly disseminated, voluminous, and medium stellate and triangular cells, whose axon we have not been able to follow adequately because of the turns of its course. However, attending to their features and to their direction, it has seemed to us that the majority of these axons belong to the long class, and we believe that they are continuous with myelinated fibers of the medullary plexus in the middle of which they lie.

For the rest, such [cellular] elements, whose dendrites are varicose and with an intertwined course, lack a radial shaft, and thus they are not represented in the plexiform layer by a terminal tuft; some, however, whose shape is triangular, show a long dendrite oriented upward, but this can never be followed sufficiently to determine its destination.

Eighth Layer or Layer of the Deep Stellate and Fusiform Cells (Claustrum of Meynert)

It is a deep lamina of gray matter separated from the corpus striatum by a layer of white matter (external capsule) and outwardly joined to the true layers of the insula by the fibrocellular formation or transitional zone described above.

Its thickness in the adult man is not less than one hundred fifty to one hundred sixty hundredths [of a millimeter], and it is quite variable depending on the region.

In the opinion of Meynert, the claustrum or Vormaier, constitutes an integral part of the insular cortex, containing fusiform cells that do not differ from those of the fifth layer of the typical cortex (layer of fusiform cells), and they are oriented mainly parallel to the surface. Such cells would reside preferentially in the external and internal portions of the claustrum; in the central areas, cells that somewhat resemble the pyramids would be the predominant cells.

Examining the claustrum in Nissl preparations of the adult, it reveals to us a large number of multipolar nerve cells, irregularly arranged, and separated by a quite wide interstitial plexus. In general, the size of its cells is quite larger than that of the cells of the sixth and seventh layers, and notably superior to that of those inhabiting the underlying corpus striatum. True pyramidal cells do not exist; if some of [the cells] imitate this form, they always lack the radial [dendritic] shaft oriented toward the surface. Anyway, although the cellular elements of this region lack a determined orientation, it has seemed to us, however, that the majority of the dendritic branches run in the horizontal orientation or parallel to the cortex. Many cells have likewise their somata stretched in the same direction, a peculiarity already mentioned by Meynert.

In fig. 20 [fig. 137], we reproduce some of the most abundant cells of the claustrum of a child of one month stained with silver chromate. Notice that these cells are of two kinds: large, with a triangular or stellate shape (fig. 20, A) [fig. 137]; and of medium or small size, among which are observed globular (C), fusiform (B), and starlike (D) shapes.

The large cells give off four, five, or more

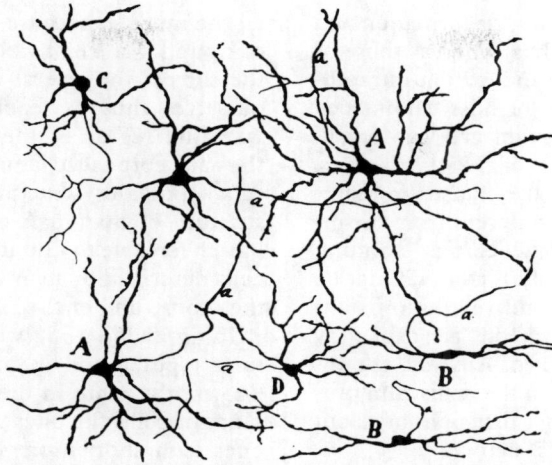

[*FIG. 137*]   Fig. 20. Cells of the claustrum of the child of twenty-five days. *A,* giant stellate type; *B,* small fusiform type; *C,* sphenoidal type, perhaps with short axon.

robust dendrites several times branched which are divergent, extending for long distances and running in all directions, terminating, however, in the bosom of the same layer. The axon is robust, follows a variety of directions, and is continuous with a medullated fiber. In some cells, the axon was definitely observed ascending, going up to the proximity of the fibrocellular layer, but, not having been able to determine the destination of the axon, we do not know the significance of the mentioned cells. Anyway, it is undoubted that they represent stellate cells with long axon.

With regard to the *medium and small cells* (fig. 20, *B, C, D*) [*fig. 137*], they give off thinner and shorter processes, often extended in the plane of orientation of the claustrum, and they have a thin axon from which some collaterals arise. In the globular cell (fig. 20, *C*) [*fig. 137*], the axon seems to resolve itself into a loose terminal arborization, thus identifying the said cell with the cells with short axon or sensory type of Golgi; but in other cells, the said axon does not show branches, and because of this we are inclined to consider such cellular elements as cells with long axon continuous with a myelinated fiber of the white matter (although about it we have no decisive proof, as the cells that we have found well impregnated are still few).

The absence in the claustrum of vertical fu-

siform cells with an [apical dendritic] process crossing the external layers of the cortex and terminating at the level of the plexiform [layer] makes us presume that this gray formation has a certain independence from the insular cortex, and it cannot be considered, as desired by Meynert, as an annex or dependency of the last layer or layer of the fusiform cells. We must not forget that in the common regions of the [cortex], the last layer or layer of the fusiform or polymorphic cells appears constantly coordinated with the superimposed layers, from whose axons it receives collaterals and across which it always sends the radial [dendritic] shafts of its cells, prolonged up to the first layer. Furthermore, the relatively considerable size of the cells of the claustrum and their predominantly stellate form also indicate a difference or contrast between these cells and those that inhabit the last two layers of the insular cortex.

Neither is it possible to identify the [claustrum] with the corpus striatum. This is characterized, leaving aside the fibrous factor, by showing a very tight network of small stellate cells that are rich in divergent dendrites, and the vast majority of them are provided with a short axon loosely arborized in the surroundings of the cell body, features that we do not meet in the cells of the claustrum. Even in Nissl preparations, notable differences are observed between the cells of this formation and of the corpus striatum; thus, whereas those of [the claustrum] are large and exhibit intraprotoplasmic clots and nets [of Nissl substance], those of the corpus striatum are very small, pale, and almost bereft of Nissl granules, whereby we deduce that the claustrum represents a special formation different from the insular cortex and from the corpus striatum, whose physiological significance it will not be possible to determine definitively until its anatomical connections with the adjacent gray territories are better known. Anyway, the inadequacy of our studies on the claustrum prohibit us from formulating a firm opinion about its anatomicophysiological nature.

The insular cortex also contains very complicated nervous plexuses. Many thick horizontal fibers that run and are ramified in the layers of the granule cells and of the large fusiform cells have seemed to us to represent exogenous conductors; but the rarity of good impregnations has impeded us from making a complete study of these fibers and from determining with any certainty their origin and final disposition.

In summary, the structure of the insular cortex can resemble in broad outline that of the auditory cortex (first sphenoidal gyrus), some of whose singular features it reproduces, because it has special giant cells with long axon (our special acoustic cells); but it also has some unique characteristics, among which we include the absence of a layer of large superficial pyramids, the exiguousness and indeterminate character of the layer of the granule cells, the presence of a fibrocellular seventh layer, the appearance of the claustrum, and especially the singular form of the pyramids of the fifth layer.

Corpus Striatum

Our numerous attempts at impregnation of the gyri of the insula of Reil with the method of Golgi have led us sometimes to achieve excellent preparations of the adjacent regions of the external capsule and corpus striatum.

It is not our intention, neither would it be appropriate in this place, to make a meticulous study of the structure of the corpus striatum, all the more so because it is a task entrusted to our pupil, La Villa, who has been working on the subject for several months. We will limit ourselves thus to report here that in many ways the region of the lenticular nucleus of the said corpus [striatum], adjacent to the insula, coincides structurally with the corpus striatum of mammals of small size, since we have been able to find in it the several kinds of cells described by us in the corpus striatum of the mouse and of the rabbit.[11]

In fig 21 [fig. 138], we show the several cellular types found in our preparations. As is known, there are in the [corpus striatum] two kinds of cells: the ones with long axon and the ones with short axon. Between them are observed two classes of terminal fibers: thick fibers arriving probably from [lower centers], and collateral fibers arising from the bundles of the corona radiata.

Of the cells with long axon, the more common type is shown in fig. 21, B [fig. 138]. It is a cell of medium size and with robust and long dendrites; its axon, after a wide turn and after giving off several collaterals, enters a bundle of medullated fibers, running in a descending direction.

But, in addition to this type, there exists another of a gigantic size, much more infrequent than the preceding and characterized by showing very long and robust divergent dendrites (fig. 21, C) [fig. 138] and a long axon, apparently descending and incorporated into the medullated bundles. For the rest, this giant cell can already by observed in the Nissl preparations, confirming that it is rare, stellate, and has a soma rich in [Nissl granules], comparable to that of a motor cell.

The cells with short axon belong to three types. (a) Common cells of medium size and stellate form, provided with numerous, spiny, divergent dendrites that are not very long, and with a short axon that has been already described by the authors, mainly by Marchi,[12] us, Calleja, and Cl. Sala (birds) (fig. 21, A) [fig. 138]. (b) Dwarf or neurogliaform cell with a spherical soma and poor in dendrites which are thin and varicose, and provided with a thin axon resolving itself quickly into a very dense and delicate terminal arborization, in which the unstained somata of nerve cells show up as

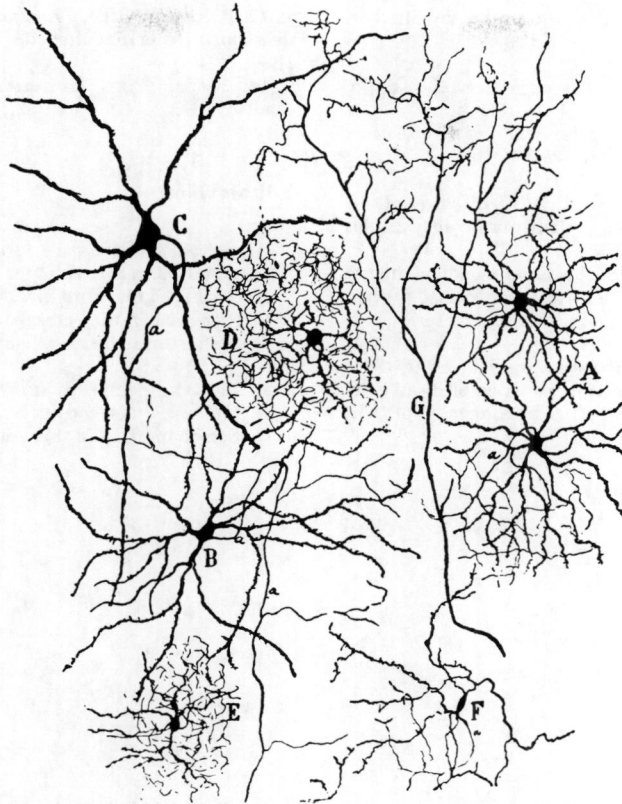

[*FIG. 138*] Fig. 21. Some cellular types of the caudate nucleus, taken from the region adjacent to the claustrum. *A*, cells with short axon and of small size; *B*, cell with descending long axon; *C*, giant cell with long axon.

clear spaces (fig. 21, *D, E*) [*fig. 138*]. This type has been mentioned by my brother[13] and Cl. Sala[14] in the basal ganglia of lower vertebrates. (c) Fusiform or triangular cell, provided with long and intertwined varicose dendrites (fig. 21, *F*) [*fig. 138*].

As an example of the terminal centripetal fibers, we reproduce in fig. 21, *G* [*fig. 138*] one of the most completely impregnated. Notice the frequent preterminal dichotomies, and notice the delicate, short arborizations by which the secondary and tertiary branches terminate; these arborizations are arranged sometimes in loose nets and are probably related to the cells with long axon of medium size. In the rabbit and mouse, we have observed several times that these arborizations form dense plexuses shaped like small islands quite well demar-

cated, in which are lodged a pleiad of nerve cells. It is very possible that all these cells correspond to the category of cells with long axon; however, about them we do not yet have precise observations.

Cajal's Notes

1. Betz, *Centralblatt. f.d. Mediz. Wissensch.*, nos. 11–13, 1881.
2. C. Hammarberg, *Studien über Klinik und Pathologie der Idiotie, nebst Untersuchungen über die normale Anatomie der Hirnrinde*, Upsala, 1895.
3. M. Schlapp, Der Zellenbau der Grosshirnrinde der Affen *Macacus Cynomolgus.*, Arch f. Psychiatrie., Vol. 30, [583–607, 1898].
4. S. R. Cajal, Las celulas de cilindro-eje corto de la capa molecular del cerebro, *Rev. Trim. Micrográfica*, Vol. II, 1897.

5. Meynert, *Handbuch der Gewebelehre,* by Stricker, 187[2].

6. *Loc. cit.*

7. Mondino, Ricerche sui centri nervosi, Torino, 1887.

8. Obersteiner, *Anleitung bei Studium der nervösen Centralorgane,* 3rd ed., Wien, 1897.

9. *Loc. cit.*

10. See *Revista Trimestral Micrográfica,* [Vol. II, 1897], Leyes de la morfología y dinamismo de la células nerviosas.

11. Cajal, Algunas contribuciones al conocimiento de los ganglios del encéfalo. V. Cuerpo estriado, *Anal. de la Socied, Españ. de Historia Natural,* 2nd series, Vol. III, Session of 1 August 1894.

See also *Corps strié: Bibliographie anat.,* no. 2, 1895.

12. Marchi, Sulla fina struttura dei corpi striati e dei talami ottici, *Rev. Speriment. di Freniatria.,* Vol. XII, 1887.

13. P. Ramón Cajal, *Trabajos de la sección de técnica anatómica* de la Facultad de Medicina de Zaragoza, 1889.

14. Cl. Sala Pons, La corteza cerebral de las aves, Madrid, 1893.

Editors' Notes

A. *Sphenoidal* is Cajal's term for temporal cortex. See chapter 18 in this volume.

B. Cajal uses the word *arms.*

C. Presumably, the ectosylvian (and sylvian?) gyri.

D. We assume, the middle and posterior ectosylvian gyri.

E. The text incorrectly says fig. 14.

F. The text incorrectly says fig. 14.

G. See chapter 15 in this volume.

18

From: Studies on the Human Cerebral Cortex[1] IV: Structure of the Olfactory Cerebral Cortex of Man and Mammals

[*Trabajos del Laboratorio de Investigaciones Biológicas de la Universidad de Madrid* 1:1–140, 1901–1902]

By general agreement among the neurologists, the central olfactory system comprises two nervous stations or points of [synaptic connections]: first, the *primary center* represented by the *olfactory bulb;* second, the *secondary centers* consisting mainly of the *piriform lobule* and, additionally, the gray matter subjacent to the upper parts of the internal and external olfactory roots (*gray matter of the bulbar pedicle,* of the *frontal lobe,* of the *olfactory tubercle,* etc.); finally, almost all the authors would claim that further *tertiary or terminal stations* exist among which the principal would be Ammon's horn. But, as we will see later, the acceptance of direct communicating pathways between the primary and secondary olfactory foci on the one hand and Ammon's horn, fascia dentata, septum lucidum, gyrus cinguli, supracallosal striae, etc., on the other hand meets with great difficulties when subjected to anatomical investigation.

A careful comparison of the structure, position, and connections of the said centers with those of the corresponding visual, tactile, and acoustic systems allows us to recognize that the first or *olfactory bulb* is homologous to the ret-

ina (not to the whole retina but to the inner plexiform layer, ganglion cell layer, and [optic nerve fiber layer]), to the ventral and lateral [cochlear nuclei] in the medulla, and to the [dorsal column nuclei] of this same center. The second station or *sphenoidal cortex*[A] represents probably a cortical center of projection or of sensation (in the sense of the theory of Flechsig). If this homology is admissible, there would be lacking in the central olfactory system (at least in the sequence and position in which the other systems have it) the *intermediary* or thalamic *station,* consisting in the visual pathways of the *lateral geniculate body* and *pulvinar,* in the tactile of the *lateral thalamic* [nucleus],[2] and in the auditory of the *medial geniculate body.*[3] The connections that certain authors have supposed between the second olfactory foci and the *stria* [*medullaris thalami*], or between the *column of the fornix* and the thalamus, cannot be considered, because they would exist (which is very debatable) not as intermediary centripetal thalamic stations but rather as reflex foci in which centrifugal pathways arise.

The present paper, which is a continuation

of the previous ones,[4] will deal in particular with the structure of the secondary olfactory focus or sphenoidal cortex. However, with the aim of making this work complete and in order to present to the reader a picture of the whole of the central organs of the olfactory system, we will deal also, although superficially and in summary form, with the olfactory bulb, the anterior commissure, the interhemispheric cortex, Ammon's horn, and other foci and secondary pathways that are supposed to be connected with these centers.[B]

II. Secondary Olfactory Relays

As we have just seen, the first link or olfactory relay resides in the glomeruli, the starting point of the pathways represented by the mitral cells.

The axons of these central neurons run backward, forming several pathways that assail the pedicle of the olfactory bulb, in the superficial or molecular layer of which they are concentrated. The principal pathway that gathers together the vast majority of the mitral axons is that situated on the external and inferior side of the olfactory pedicle, that is to say, the *external root* of the authors. The horizontal

sections show clearly that mitral fibers enter this root from all the bulbar regions, the ones from the external face of the bulb directly, those from the superior, inferior, and internal faces horizontally or transversely.

There exist, however, other accessory pathways.

One of them, which we will designate the *superior root*, is formed on the superior face of the pedicle of the olfactory lobe, ending in the vicinity of the frontal pole of the cerebrum.

Another less apparent pathway is observed on the internal inferior face of the pedicle, ending, apparently, in the olfactory tubercle. Such is the *medial root* of the authors. All of these pathways do not always appear clearly demarcated. In fact, they are none other than segments of the superficial fibrillar capsule that surrounds the bulbar pedicle, and which has a region of great density and concentration: the external root.

But besides these superficial pathways formed by the aggregation of the axons of the mitral cells, there is another central pathway to which we have already alluded. This system of thin fibers resident in the axis of the bulb results from the grouping of the delicate axons of the tufted cells (not mitrals), of small, medium, and large [size].

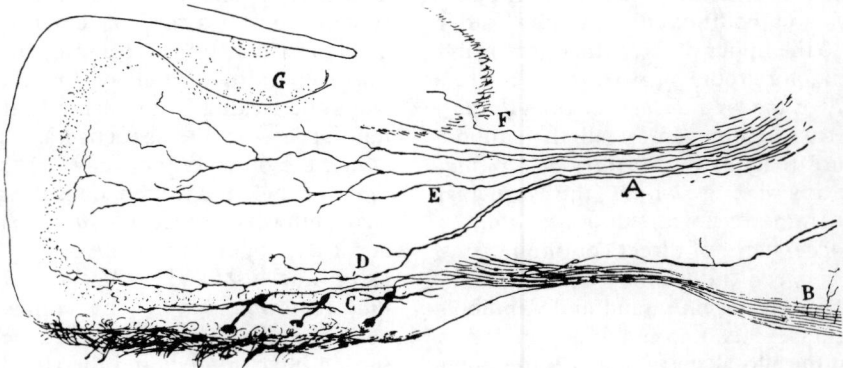

[*FIG. 139*]   Fig. 7. Olfactory bulb of a mouse of eight days. Axial section. The fibers of the anterior commissure can be seen arriving and ramifying among the granule cells. *A*, anterior commissure; *B*, external root of the olfactory bulb; *C*, layer of mitral cells; *D*, fibers arborizing in the internal plexiform layer; *E*, branching commissural fiber; *F*, commissural fiber apparently coming from the cortex of the bulbar peduncle; *G*, accessory olfactory bulb.

Principal Pathway or External Root of the Olfactory Bulb

This root is a robust white bundle, triangular in section, which first goes along the external and inferior side of the pedicle of the olfactory bulb, then crosses in an anteroposterior, somewhat oblique direction toward the exterior of the inferior face of the frontal lobe, and finally is submerged in the plexiform or superficial layer of the piriform lobe of animals or in the hippocampal gyrus of man, which it traverses from forward to backward. Over such a long trajectory, the fibers of the said root, thick at its origin, successively become thinner, and they are placed, at the level of the sphenoidal cortex, in the external half of the piriform lobe, and especially near the external fissure or delimiting frontier of this lobe with the rest of the cerebral cortex (*limbic or rhinal fissure* of the authors).

The continuity of the fibers of the external root with the nerve cells of the bulb, suspected some time ago by Gudden, Ganser, Golgi, and other authors, was completely demonstrated by us in the bulb of the small mammals, as well as by van Gehuchten, Retzius, Calleja, and Kölliker. In fig. 7,[C] B [*fig. 139*], taken from the newborn mouse, this continuity is shown clearly. Löwenthal, using the method of Marchi,[5] has also ascertained this fact, today covered with controversy.

In its very long anteroposterior trajectory, the external olfactory root gives off a prodigious number of collaterals originating at a right or acute angle and arborizing in the plexiform layer of the bulbar or underlying cerebral cortices. The last branches or terminal fibers, notably thinner, are exhausted in the sphenoidal cortex, give off equal collaterals, and terminate in the same manner, that is to say, by means of varicose and extensive branches, extending through the thickness of the plexiform layer. In certain cases, we have seen some displaced root fibers, that is to say, detached from the superficial stratum, which run in the second layer of the sphenoidal cortex, tracing large turns and flexuosities. In their trajectory, they give off collaterals to the deep layers. The existence of these displaced root fibers, [which are] relatively easy to impregnate in the cat, explains the fact stated by Löwenthal that secondary degeneration can be observed in the second or deeper layers of the cortex covered by the external root when the olfactory bulb is removed.

The collaterals of the external root, which form one of the most intricate plexuses observed in the nervous centers, were discovered by us[6] in the brain of the mouse; later, Calleja[7] made a meticulous description that was confirmed by Kölliker and others.

An interesting fact is that such collaterals are arborized almost exclusively in the thickness of the molecular or plexiform layer of the frontal and sphenoidal cortex, and since it is in this layer that the [dendritic] tufts of the pyramids terminate, it follows that the olfactory excitation carried by the external root [makes contact with] the cortical cells by the dendrites of the [apical] shaft, to be propagated to the soma, and finally to the axon of the pyramids.

In spite of our first presumptions, such an arrangement of the sensory terminations does not represent a general anatomical law for all the sensory areas of the cerebrum, since our recent investigations[8] persuade us that in other cortical regions, such as the motor and visual, the centrifugal sensory conductors have their final arborization in deep layers of the gray matter (*layer of the granule* cells in the visual cortex, *layer of the medium pyramids* in the motor).

Let us point out that, even in the olfactory cortex, as recognized by Kölliker, it is not rare to observe also some of the above-mentioned collaterals, descending beyond the plexiform layer; these long collaterals are very rare in the mouse and rabbit, [but] less scarce in the cat and dog, and are arborized at the level of the somata of the small pyramids or superficial polymorphic cells.

The gray cortex receiving the fibers of the external root includes three regions: the *pedicle of the olfactory lobe*, the *frontal lobe*, and the *external territory of the sphenoidal cortex*. The three cerebral territories possess essentially the same structure, as Calleja pointed out in his excellent work on the subject. But in regard to the sphenoidal cortex, there exist sufficient structural differences to justify a separate study of this cerebral region, which can be regarded as the principal secondary relay of the olfactory excitations.

Structure of the Bulbar and Frontal Cortex Underlying the External Root

The cortex of the *olfactory tract*, and the frontal lobe covered by the external root, has been well studied by Calleja, who distinguishes the following layers: first, *fibrillar or [layer] of the external root;* second, *molecular or plexiform;* third, of the *small and large pyramids;* fourth, of the *polymorphic cells;* and fifth, of the *white matter* [*fig. 140*].

1. Fibrillar Layer. [This] is none other than the mass of anteroposterior fibers of the external root. In this layer, one has to consider the innumerable descending collaterals of the olfactory fibers already mentioned, and some terminal fibers that, as recognized by Golgi and confirmed by Calleja, descend obliquely through the molecular or plexiform layer to ramify, and to form, not a mesh, as was

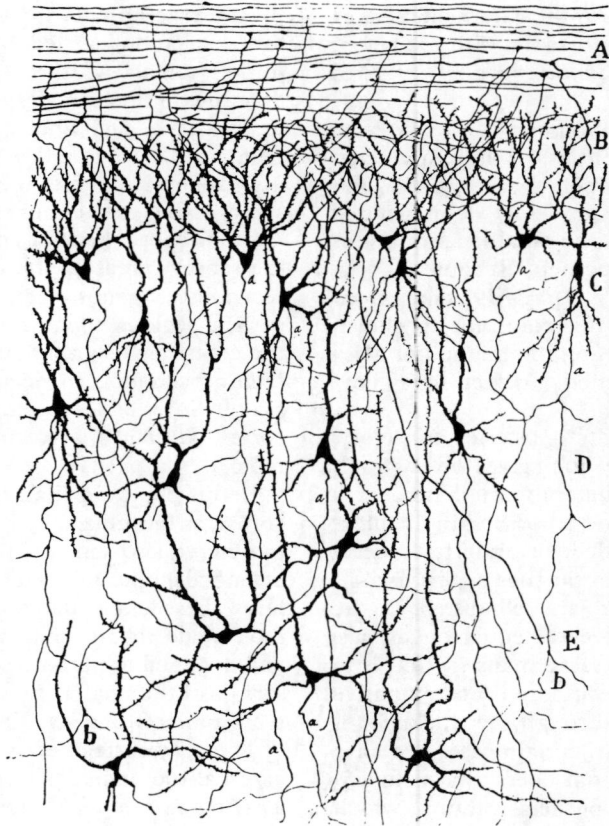

[*FIG. 140*]   Fig. 10. Cortex of the frontal region covered by the external root. *A*, layer of the olfactory fibers; *B*, plexiform layer; *C*, layer of the superficial polymorphic cells; *D*, layer of the pyramids; *E*, deep polymorphic cells; *b*, bifurcations of the axons. Rabbit of twenty-five days. [The legends appended to the figures from the chapter on the olfactory cortex in the *Histologie du système nerveux* are often more complete than in the original Spanish work. We have therefore used the more extensive versions in making our translations.]

thought by the Italian histologist [Golgi], but a varicose, perfectly free ramification limited to the second layer, in conformity with the observations of the latter author.

2. Molecular Layer. It has an unusual thickness and reveals the same structure as the other cortical regions, that is to say, it is composed of a dense plexus, to which contribute the tufts of the pyramids; the dendrites of the intrinsic horizontal cells, either with long axon or with short axon; the nervous arborizations of ascending fibers of Martinotti; and finally, as we already said, the collaterals and terminals of the fibers of the external root.

3. Layer of the Small and Medium Pyramids. This layer, which perhaps would be better designated *layer of the superficial polymorphic cells,* as, in fact, it contains extremely variegated shapes, forms a flexuous and undulating band quite clearly demarcated from the bordering layers.

As is observed in fig. 10, C [*fig. 140*], the most superficial cells of which it is composed have a semilunar, mitral, and triangular shape, and they usually lack descending dendrites, possessing four or more ascending processes extending through the molecular layer. But, as they occupy a deeper plane, such cells are, with regard to their shape, more similar to the pyramids, being provided with an [apical dendritic] shaft promptly resolved into a terminal tuft, and with a group of descending dendrites, sometimes gathering together in a bundle or like a paintbrush.

In all these cells, the axon is descending, and it gets lost in the white matter after giving off some collaterals, frequently ramified in the deepest plane of this layer, in which reside the most voluminous pyramids. For the rest, the configuration of the neurons of the layer is very variable, it being possible to observe, even in deep planes, numerous cells whose shape is triangular, stellate, or fusiform, although they do not lack a radial dendrite destined for the second layer.

4. Layer of the Polymorphic Cells. It consists of voluminous cells, sometimes larger than the large pyramids of the preceding layer, which have a great variety of forms: stellate, triangular, fusiform, mitral, etc. Also, such cells lack that radial orientation typical of the pyramids, as the dendrites go in all the directions; one of their processes, however, after describing a varied course, usually runs toward the surface and assails the molecular layer. The axon is descending, gives off some collaterals, and is incorporated into the white matter. In some cells, generally of medium volume and with a spindle shape, the axon is ascending and is arborized in the second and third layers.

5. Layer of the White Matter. With a plexiform aspect and not lacking in some polymorphic cells, this stratum constitutes the point of convergence of the axons of the cells resident in the superimposed layers. Such fibers are not arranged, as in the typical cortex, in radial bundles, but engender an irregular and labyrinthine plexus. But, in spite of the confused and complicated nature of their trajectories, it is possible to appreciate that the majority of these axons, after a flexuous course through the layer under study, gain the corpus striatum and are continuous with a fiber of the corona radiata. Considering that almost all these fibers supply one, two, or even more long collaterals at the level of the deep portion of their trajectory, it does not appear risky to conjecture that, of both branches, the thinner is destined for the anterior commissure. In fig. 11, *a* [*fig. 141*], we also show cells of the layer of the polymorphic cells, whose axons are bifurcated, and one of their branches, sometimes the thicker and posterior, gets lost among the fibers of the commissure or at least in the fibrillar plane from which it comes, whereas the other is directed forward, perhaps to be arborized in the cortex of the bulbar pedicle.

In summary, the fibers or conductors of second order, originating in the bulbar and frontal cortex underlying the external root, follow two pathways: most go deeply backward, to gain the head of the corpus striatum and to be incorporated into the corona radiata; others run medially and backward and enter the anterior commissure. We do not know if some of them reach Ammon's horn, as we have not been able to follow such fibers sufficiently.

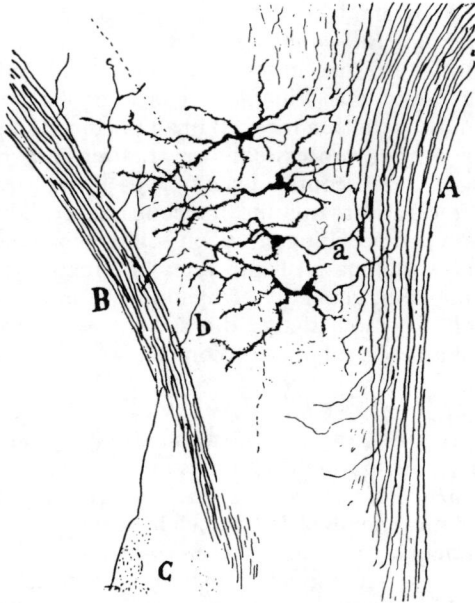

[*FIG. 141*]   Fig. 11. Horizontal section of the cerebrum of the mouse of ten days. *A*, plane of the fibers of the anterior commissure; *B*, external root; *C*, end of the olfactory bulb; *a*, bifurcated axons; *b*, plexiform layer.

III. Structure of the Hippocampal Gyrus[D] and of the Piriform Lobule

We are particularly interested in the organization of this cortical region, because it is the principal point of termination of the lateral [olfactory] stria and because it shows a highly characteristic structure. Olfactory collaterals terminate preferentially in the bulbar and frontal cortices underlying the said stria, whereas the parent fibers have the sphenoidal cortex as their ultimate destination.

In man, these terminal branches do not form a bundle visible to the naked eye, because when they reach the hippocampal gyrus they are dispersed over a considerable area of the plexiform layer without forming tight, small bundles. However, in animals (rabbit, mouse, guinea pig, etc.), the arrival of the fibers can be seen standing out by virtue of their white color against the gray background of the piriform lobule, in which they diverge like a fan before finally vanishing.

The structure of the hippocampal gyrus in man and that of the piriform lobule in animals have been little studied. In general, the authors have distinguished in the hippocampal gyrus two regions or segments: the *subiculum*, or portion adjacent to Ammon's horn, recognizable by showing a plexiform layer furrowed by thick bundles of white matter; and the principal portion, distant from [Ammon's] horn, in which an organization almost identical to that of the other [cerebral] gyri has been supposed.

However, some authors, among whom we must cite Betz, Obersteiner, Dejerine, Hammarberg, and especially Calleja and Kölliker, have recognized some structural peculiarities exclusive to the piriform lobule and hippocampal gyrus.

One of the most typical features of the cortex of the subiculum is the presence, at the level of the layer of the small pyramids, of pleiades of cells separated by ascending bundles of white matter which were already recognized by Betz,[9] who named them *cortical glomeruli*.

For his part, Obersteiner,[10] who studied also the structure of the subiculum, found in this a very thick molecular layer formed by the accumulation of many nerve fascicles (*substantia reticularis*). At the level of the second layer, he also observed the cellular accumulations of Betz, as well as the bundles of white matter that separate them; and, finally, in the third layer he thought he could see only large pyramids. He did not give details about the rest of the hippocampal gyrus.

In a study of Ammon's horn and the fascia dentata,[11] we reported some data about the subiculum and the zone of transition between this and [Ammon's] horn. In the subiculum, we recognized the typical four layers of the cortex of small mammals: the molecular [layer], [the layer] of the small pyramids, [the layer] of the large pyramids, and [the layer] of the polymorphic cells. We have pointed out that the superficial bundles of the molecular layer were continuous with the *lamina medullaris circonvoluta* and with the *stratum lacunosum* of Ammon's horn, and included two kinds of fibers: some arising probably from [Ammon's horn] and terminating in the subiculum, and others arising in the subiculum and bordering regions of the sphenoidal cortex (piriform lobule), which, concentrating first in the subventricular white matter, would ascend arranged in bundles through the subicular cortex and would terminate in Ammon's horn. The axons of Martinotti, originating from deep cells of the subiculum, would also participate in the formation of these ascending pathways. But at that time, our studies did not allow us to recognize that the contingent of exogenous fibers of this ascending pathway greatly exceed the endogenous fibers and those of Ammonic origin, to such an extent that they can be considered, as we will see below, as an afferent system whose parent cells are located in the adjoining gyri.

Dejerine,[12] using the method of Weigert, has examined the structure of the subiculum, in which he observed a molecular layer rich in tangential fibers, which form a festooned plexus in its deep limit, and whose teeth penetrate between the small pyramids. From the vertex of the festoons arise radial bundles that are incorporated into the white matter of the gyrus. The second layer or [layer] of the small pyramids is interrupted by the festoons of white matter. The third layer or [layer] of the large pyramidal cells contains large pyramids of 40 μm in length, which are located, especially, in the deep parts of this layer; their long radial [dendritic] shafts are arborized in the molecular layer and give to the third layer a radial aspect which has led to its being named the *stratum radiatum*. The fourth layer or layer of the polymorphic cells seems identical to that in the other central [cortical] areas. The white matter shows two planes of nerve fibers: the thin or deep represent the collaterals of the axons of the subiculum and form part of the *psalterium* or interammonic commissure; the external, which are thicker, represent the axons of the pyramids of the subiculum and Ammon's horn, and probably establishes relations with the posterior fascicle of the *cingulum,* whose fibers bring Ammon's horn into relationship with the hippocampal gyrus and distant gyri of the cerebral cortex.

One neurologist who had dedicated more attention to the theme we are dealing with, exploring equally all the regions of the hippocampal gyrus with the method of Nissl, was Hammarberg.[13] According to this author, the *gyrus hippocampi* shows on its more external half or part more distal with respect to Ammon's horn a similar texture to the temporal gyri, except that the first layer is particularly thick, increasing further in thickness as it nears the Ammon's horn. In agreement with Betz and Obersteiner, he observed the small islands of the second layer and the ascending white bundles. In his opinion, the recognizable layers are, first, molecular [layer]; second, layer of the small and large pyramids (layers 2 and 3 of other cerebral regions); third, layer poor in cells with some small pyramids and occasional irregular cells; fourth, layer of the ganglionic cells; and [fifth], layer of the fusiform cells. The latter two are very reduced in thickness.

In the medial regions of the gyrus, where the islands are well defined, the following two planes are observed: superficial or of small pyramids, and deep or of voluminous pyramids; but at the level of the subiculum, the positions of these two planes of pyramids are altered, the large pyramids being pushed outward to invade the spaces that separate the pleiades of minute cells and giving rise in this way to a row of islands composed alternately of small and voluminous cells, which is a characteristic arrangement of this cortical region. In this same internal portion of the hippocampal gyrus, the deep plane, not interrupted by the second layer, cannot be separated from the underlying ganglionic layer; both together form a wide cellular band of about 0.60 mm.

Finally, Hammarberg illustrates his description by reproducing two sections, one of the subiculum and the other of the central portion of the *hippocampal gyrus.* In the latter figure the second layer appears divided in two superimposed pleiades, one of small and the other of large pyramids.

But the works of Hammarberg show us little about the morphology of the cells and their connections. This hiatus has begun to be filled with the investigations made, with the help of the Golgi method, by Calleja[14] and Kölliker.[15] We will talk about them in the course of this work. Also we ourselves gave some information, although incomplete, about the histology of the subiculum of small mammals.[16]

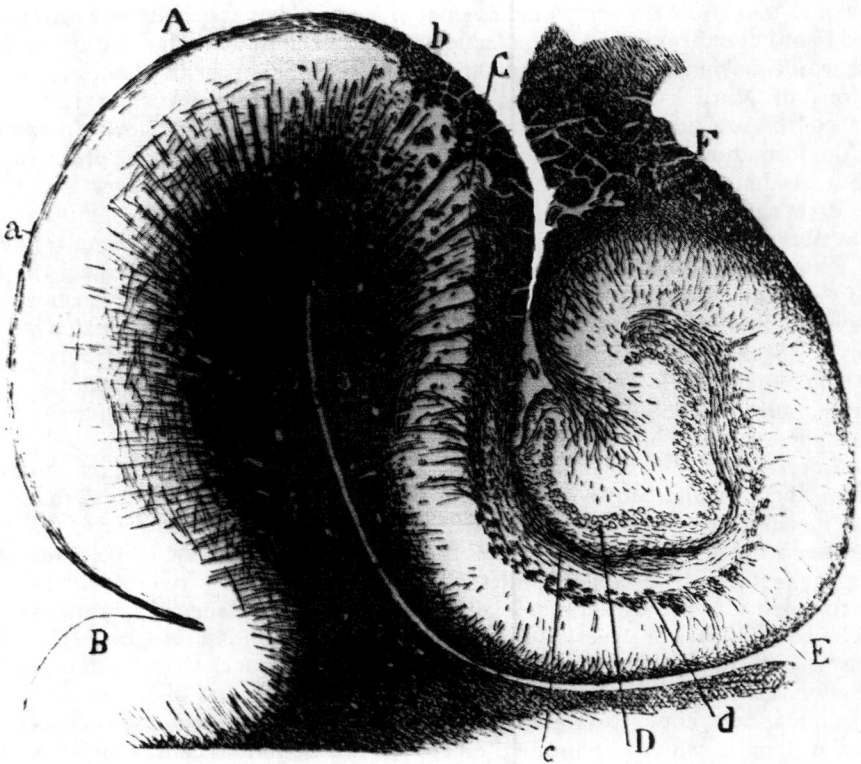

[*FIG. 142*]   Fig. 12. Section of Ammon's horn and the hippocampal gyrus of an adult man. Method of Weigert-Carmine. *A,* hippocampal gyrus; *B,* inferior sphenoidal [gyrus]; *C,* subiculum; *D,* granule cells of the fascia dentata; *E,* cortex of Ammon's horn; *F,* fimbria; *a,* plexiform layer; *b,* plexus of superficial fibers of the subiculum; *c,* pathway of Ammon's horn continuous with the latter; *d,* deep pathway continuous with the collaterals of the giant pyramids.

Our present observations have fallen on the hippocampus of man, which has been studied with the methods of Nissl, Golgi, and Weigert. The Golgi method, in particular, was used in the child of fifteen days to two months, and it has allowed us to collect many details about the structure. To complete our reports, we have had recourse also to the piriform lobule of the cat, dog, rabbit, and mouse, in which, at ages ranging between eight days and one month, splendid and very expressive silver chromate preparations were obtained.

A transverse section of the human hippocampal gyrus, stained with the Nissl method, reveals the following layers: first, *plexiform or molecular layer;* second, *layer of the large polymorphic cells;* third, *layer of the medium tasseled cells;* fourth, *layer of the large tasseled cells;* fifth, *layer of the fusiform and triangular cells or of the deep polymorphic cells;* and sixth, *layer of the white matter.*

As follows from this enumeration, the sphenoidal cortex lacks two important layers: that of the granule cells and that of the giant pyramids. This peculiarity and, as we will see later, the absence of many types of cells with short axon that are abundant in other regions of the human cortex give us already to understand that the gray matter of the hippocampal gyrus has not reached in man the level of development of other sensory areas. It is not correct, however, to affirm that this cerebral region is in the process of atrophy in comparison with animals, for in spite of the *microsomatic* nature of man, the histology of the gyrus, as well as of Ammon's horn, has a positive advantage over the corresponding centers of the macrosomatic mammals.

Not all regions of the hippocampal gyrus exhibit the same appearance in Nissl preparations. From the point of view of the distribution of the cells and number of layers, three regions or sectors must be distinguished, namely the *subiculum,* the central portion or crown of the hippocampal gyrus, and the *external lateral portion* bordering the limbic or rhinal sulcus.

1. Ammonic Portion or Subiculum

[This] is easily recognizable (fig. 13) [*fig. 143*], for the enormous thickness reached by the plexiform layer, the relative thinness of the layer of pyramids, and the presence of accumulations or islets of very small cells disseminated in the thickness of the first layer.

These islets consist of packed pyramidal cells whose size is so tiny that they do not exceed 7 μm; exceptionally, some are observed with [diameters of] 12 to 16 μm. Underneath the cellular accumulations are sometimes found traces of cells that almost join the islands with the underlying layer. The number of islets is scarce: in a transverse section of the subiculum, rarely more than three or four are found; usually, there is one of colossal size, completely embedded in the nervous plexus of the first layer (fig. 13, A) [*fig. 143*].

The extraordinary occurrence of small nerve fiber bundles in the first layer of the subiculum has almost entirely squeezed the special cells out of the first layer. However, exploring carefully with the Zeiss 1.30 apochromatic [lens], it is observed that, although scarce, there is no lack of a few cells scattered between the bundles and particularly accu-

mulated in the most superficial plane of the first layer. It is common to see them surrounded with a crown of neuroglial nuclei. Apparently, among them the medium or small polygonal cells with short axon predominate.

The second layer of the subiculum shows several irregular rows of medium pyramids and polymorphic cells, which in certain places approach each other so much that they constitute true islands (fig. 13, *b*) [*fig. 143*]. Frequently, this layer shows interruptions situated in front of the islets of the first layer, which interruptions are occupied by ascending bundles of white matter, as can be observed by comparing the Nissl preparations with those of Weigert-Pal (fig. 13, *a*) [*fig. 143*]. [See also fig. 12, *C,* our *fig. 142.*]

Well-differentiated third, fourth, and fifth layers are not observed in the subiculum. In place of them is observed a cellular band of rather voluminous pyramids, extending from the layer of the polymorphic cells to the white matter. Often, this pyramidal formation is arranged in parallel vertical series, and in other cases in very irregular forms of grouping as a consequence of the presence of radial or perforating bundles of white matter.

Finally, the latter exhibits an extraordinary thickness, invading and surrounding the deep fusiform cells which lie between the nervous fascicles.

2. Central Ammonic Portion

[This] must be divided into two regions: one bordering the subiculum, devoid of islets, crossed by ascending fiber bundles, and which, to talk directly, we will name the *presubicular region;* and the other external and extensive, characterized by the presence in the second layer of alternating islets of giant and medium polymorphic cells. We will call the latter territory, which is the most important of the hippocampal gyrus, the *external sphenoidal or olfactory region.*

a. Presubicular Region. This part of the cortex, adjacent to the subiculum, has particular characteristics that allow us to differentiate it clearly from the adjacent territories (fig. 14) [*fig. 144*].

It differs from the olfactory portion by lack-

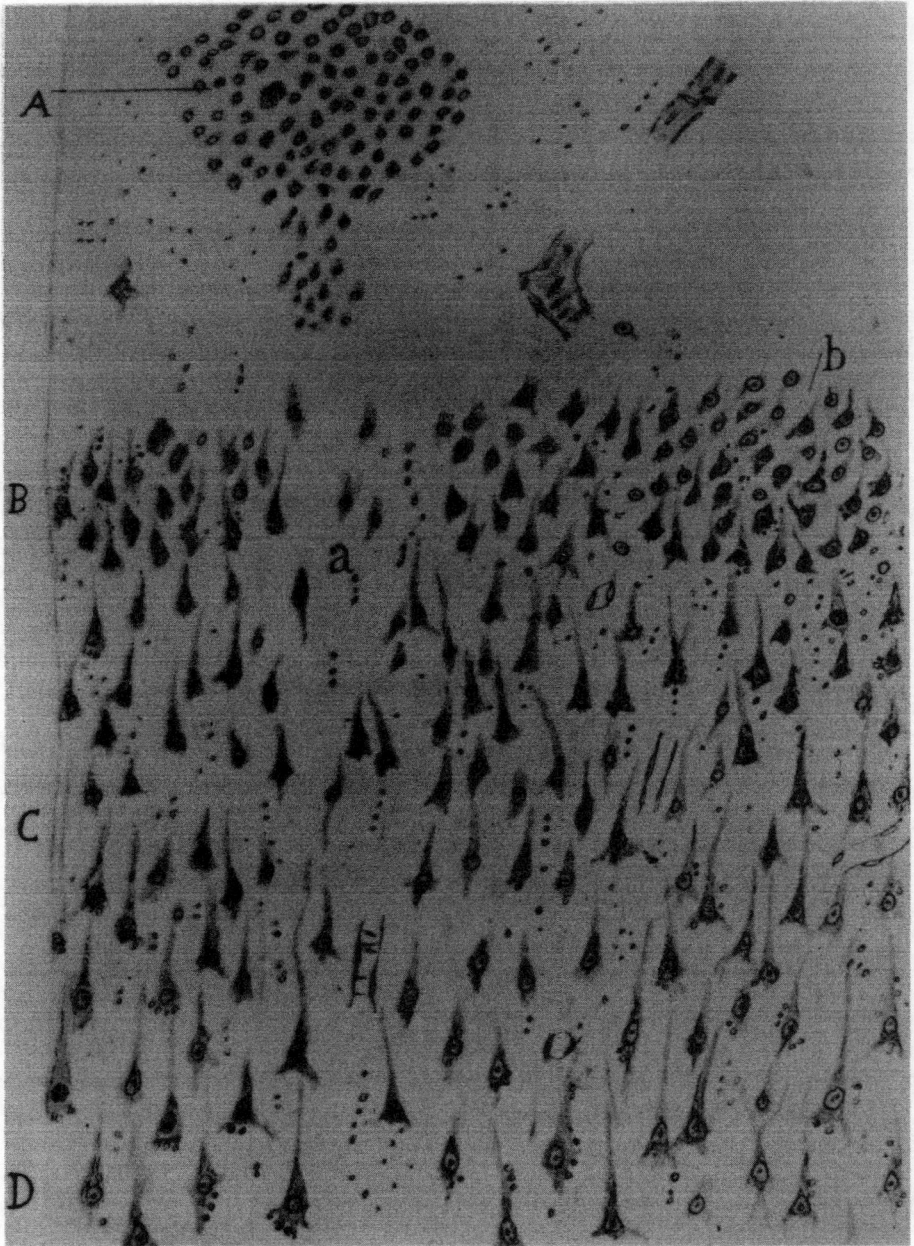

[*FIG. 143*]   Fig. 13. Transverse section of a piece of the human subiculum. Method of Nissl. *A*, plexiform layer with an islet of small cells; *B*, layer of the medium and small pyramids; *C, D,* deep layers of pyramids; *a*, territory through which perforating bundles pass; *b*, a point where the pyramids are concentrated in a pleiad.

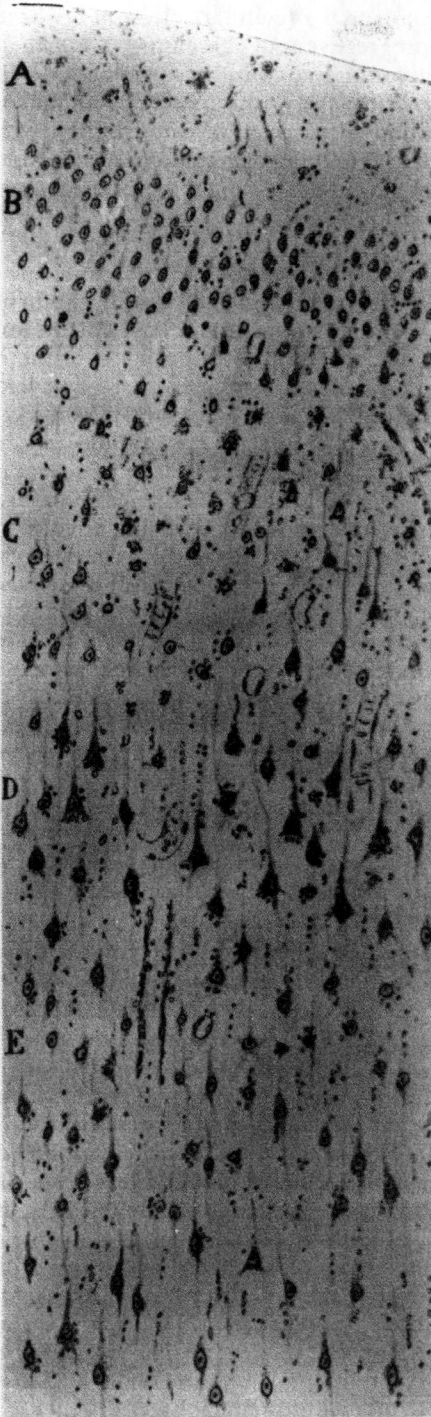

ing the layer of the giant polymorphic cells and from the subiculum by showing a more complicated [arrangement] of layers and especially a plexiform third layer filled with small cells. Its layers are: (1) *Plexiform,* in which lie piriform horizontal cells and cells with short axon. (2) *Layer of the small pyramids and fusiform cells,* made up of a band (not arranged in islands but uneven) of small fusiform, triangular, and pyramidal cells, and occasionally somewhat voluminous polygonal cells, probably with short axon. (3) *Deep plexiform layer.* It is an extensive band poor in cells, among which appear small and medium pyramids and some stellate and triangular cells of variable size. This layer is the principal point of ramification of an important pathway coming from the white matter. (4) *Layer of the medium and large pyramids,* among which some fusiform and triangular cells show up. In certain places, these cells appear in series because of the presence of ascending fiber bundles. (5) Finally is the layer of the *fusiform and triangular cells,* similar to that in the other cortical regions, but little different from the previous layer because of the similarity of the cellular sizes and the existence of transitions between them. The latter two layers, especially the fifth, appear in the Weigert-Pal preparations to be invaded by numerous fiber bundles that in the frontal sections are shown cut across. Also in the third and second layers are observed some isolated small bundles continuous with the deep white matter and with the tangential fibers of the first layer.

b. External or Olfactory Portion of the Central Ammonic Region. It is extemely distinct and the best studied by the neurologists, particularly by Hammarberg. As this author affirms, beneath the first layer, which here has already a normal thickness, appear some islets of cells,

---

[*FIG. 144*] Fig. 14. Section of the middle and external layers of the cortex of the presubiculum in man. Method of Nissl. *A,* plexiform layer; *B,* small pyramids and fusiform cells; *C,* deep plexiform layer; *D,* layer of medium and large pyramids; *E,* layer of fusiform and triangular cells.

in which voluminous cells are mixed with dwarf cells. As is seen in fig. 15, B [fig. 145], the accumulations of giant cells are more or less globular and of variable size, ranging between [400 and 600 microns]. These pleiades are separated from the rest of the layer of polymorphic cells by means of a semicircular ring almost bereft of neurons. The cells that inhabit the said accumulations are gigantic, having a greater size than that of the large pyramids of the fourth layer (of 24 to 30 μm) and showing a polygonal shape, provided with several processes, among which the ascending predominate. With regard to the pleiades of small cells, they consist of minute elements of 7 to 12 μm in diameter, with a pyramidal shape and endowed with several processes, one of which runs upward to ramify in the plexiform layer. In general, such islands of minute pyramids are usually less extensive than the previous [pleiades of large cells], and they occupy a somewhat more superficial plane inside the layer of the polymorphic cells.

Beneath the layer of the islets, a broad *plexiform layer* shows up; [it is] poor in small and medium pyramids, which in many places seem to be disoriented. Their size increases slightly in the deep plane of this layer, forming a transition to the next or *fourth layer,* which is inhabited by large and medium pyramids concentrated in irregular lines and in part also disoriented.

Finally, there comes a *fifth layer,* composed of polymorphic cells, the majority of which are fusiform and triangular and with their inferior part prolonged down into the thickness of the white matter. In the transition between the fifth and fourth layers, there are recognized some granule cells or small pyramidal and stellate cells, irregularly disseminated and without, therefore, constituting an individualized stratum. In summary, the cited region consists of the following layers: first, *plexiform;* second, *of the polymorphic cells or of the islands;* third, *deep plexiform or of the medium pyramids;* fourth, *of the large pyramids;* and fifth, *of the fusiform and triangular cells.*

3. External or Fissural Portion of the Hippocampus

As we move toward the external side of the hippocampal gyrus, the islets of gigantic cells

disappear, and its [cellular] elements, whose size is progressively decreasing, are arranged in a regular and continuous formation. They form, in this way, [though] not without some transition of disposition (interruption of the stratum, irregular aggregations of cells), the second layer of small pyramids of the common cortex. Quite before reaching the bottom of the limbic fissure, the gray matter acquires the features of the association areas, showing up successively and with total clarity the first or plexiform layer, the second layer of the small pyramids, the third layer or [layer] of the medium pyramids, the fourth layer or [layer] of the superficial large and giant pyramids, the fifth layer or [layer] of the granule cells, the sixth layer or [layer] of the deep large and medium pyramids, and the seventh layer or [layer] of the fusiform or triangular cells.

In the small mammals, the structure of the piriform lobule, observed with the method of Nissl, coincides in its fundamental features with that of the human gyrus hippocampi. The layers, however, appear very simplified. In the rabbit, guinea pig, and mouse, it is possible to recognize a *subicular* region, another *presubicular* [region], and finally, the *principal* or *olfactory* [region].

In the *subiculum,* there is observed a thick first layer, rich in nerve fibers, which do not form thick bundles as in man but thin and plexiform bundles. This layer lacks the islets of small pyramids. Beneath the plexiform layer begins the layer of the medium pyramids, which is extended down to the white matter without showing well-defined subdivisions. A similar arrangement is observed in the cat and other gyrencephalic animals.

The *presubicular region* is very distinctive, being recognizable by the presence (fig. 16) [fig. 146] of a thick *second layer,* composed of very small pyramids more or less grouped in certain places. Beneath this, there exists, as in man, a *plexiform band* inhabited by scarce and minute pyramidal, stellate, or fusiform cells. It comes after the *layer of the large,* not very voluminous *pyramids,* and, finally, the layer of the *polymorphic cells,* which are cells commonly of a small size and with a globular, ovoid, or fusiform [shape] and oriented preferentially in the horizontal direction.

In the cat, the presubicular region is very

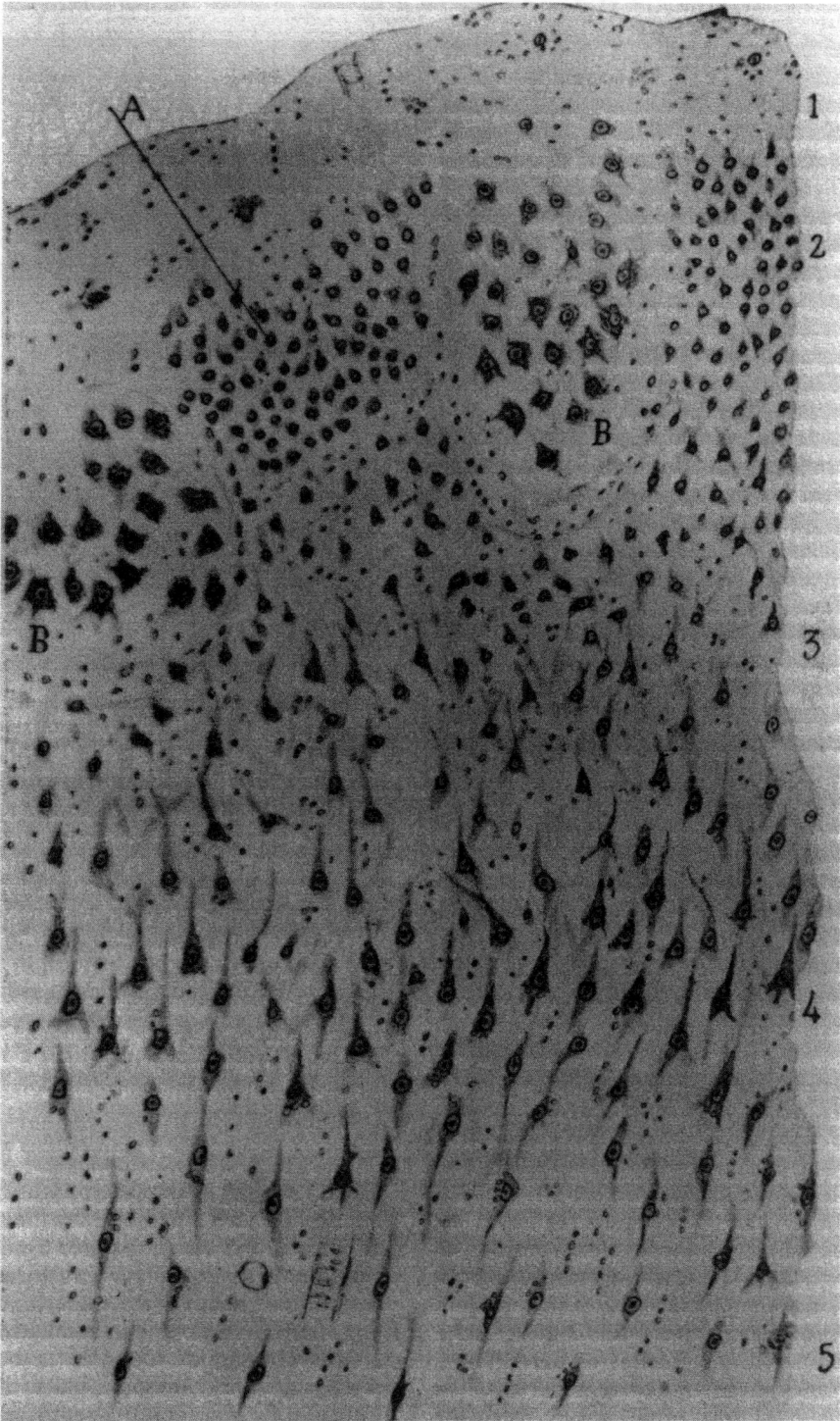

[*FIG. 145*]   Fig. 15. Section of the olfactory region of the human hippocampus. Method of Nissl. The numbers label the layers. *A,* islet of small pyramids; *B,* islet of giant polymorphic cells.

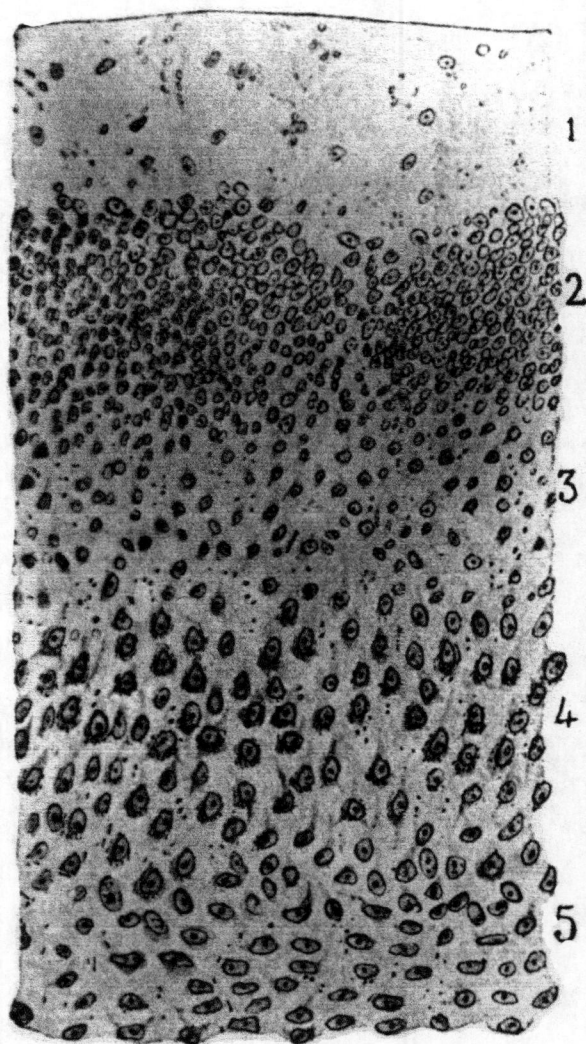

[*FIG. 146*]   Fig. 16. Section of the presubicular region of the piriform lobule. Method of Nissl. Guinea pig.

extensive and much richer in cells. It is differentiated from the homologous region of the rabbit and guinea pig especially by showing an extensive second layer, whose most superficial cells are, in some places, congregated in islets, and by showing a third layer, almost exclusively composed of a plexus of nerve fibers, that becomes more and more superficial the closer it is to the subiculum, until it meets the plexiform layer of [the subiculum].

With regard to the *olfactory area,* it is recognized (guinea pig, rabbit) by the presence of a robust *second layer* inhabited by giant stellate cells, not arranged in islets as in man but in a continuous band with slight condensations and alternating rarefactions. Neither are islets of dwarf pyramids found in it, but it is observed, however, in some places [to contain] little groups of minuscule cells irregularly disseminated in the thickness of the second layer, and whose examination requires the use of a good objective. The other layers differ little from the corresponding layers in man.

In the cat, the second layer or [layer] of the polymorphic cells contains large cells that form a continuous series in the anterior portions of the sphenoidal lobe, but in the posterior portions, bordering the visual area, they are fragmented in flattened pleiades. Beneath the gaps appear plexiform strips poor in cells. The third layer is plexiform and consists of fusiform and triangular cells and large pyramids, and, finally, the fourth layer, still poorer in cells, shows smaller cells that have a variety of shapes, although the fusiform shape predominates.

All the mentioned regions do not seem to be connected with the olfactory fibers. As we will see below, the olfactory stria only penetrates the medial and lateral portion of the piriform lobule of mammals. And comparing these clearly olfactory regions with the corresponding regions of the human hippocampal gyrus, it is possible to affirm that this lacks direct olfactory connections, like the subiculum and presubicular region (internal part of the center of the gyrus), and the walls and fundus of the limbic fissure.

Up to this point, we have studied in man the layers and aspect of the gyrus hippocampi as revealed with the method of Nissl. In the next pages and in order of layering, we will expose the data on the structure that the silver chromate has allowed us to collect both in man and in the mammals.

Olfactory Area

1. Plexiform Layer

Its appearance differs depending on the area of the gyrus under study. In the subiculum, as is well known and as already appreciable in the Nissl and Weigert preparations, the thickness of this layer is very great, and it also appears disrupted by the invasion of the deep white matter; but at the commencement of the medial sphenoidal portion, the normal constitution of the layer reappears, and the layer becomes maximally differentiated in the external portion of the center of the hippocampal gyrus.

At the level of this territory, which represents, as we have already said, the true olfactory area, the plexiform layer exhibits a new factor, that is to say, tangential fibers continuous with the lateral stria of the olfactory bulb. Thanks to this addition, the first layer becomes organized into two sublayers or planes: *external plane or sublayer of the root fibers; internal plane or plexiform sublayer in the strict sense.*

The first plane contains mainly neuroglial cells with long processes and the mentioned root fibers. The latter, which are medullated, as appreciated in the Weigert preparations, run in the sagittal direction, showing a diameter clearly less than that of the fibers of the lateral stria from which they come. This peculiarity is easily understandable remembering the large number of collaterals given off from the parent fibers during their presphenoidal trajectory, that is to say, in the frontal and olfactory lobes.

Occasionally, we recognize here also, as in the frontal cortex, oblique or descending collaterals scattered and ramifying in the plexiform layer and in the layer of the giant polymorphic cells.

The *plexiform sublayer* exhibits the typical composition of the cerebral molecular layer. In it stand out, first, fusiform or triangular cells provided with long dendrites and a horizontal axon (*cells of Cajal,* according to Retzius), of which we reproduce in fig. 17, A [*fig. 147*] some examples taken from the child of eight days; second, the dendritic tufts of the innumerable small, medium, and large pyramids situated in the underlying layers; third, small cells with short axon ramifying in the thickness of this sublayer; and fourth, terminal axonal ramifications originating either from the ascending axons of Martinotti, from recurrent collaterals of pyramids, or, finally, from cells with short axon located in the second layer. It is not our purpose to describe meticulously all of these elements, since they are not exclusive to the sphenoidal cortex and they have been repeatedly studied in our previous works on the cerebral visual and motor areas.

For the present, we will limit [ourselves] to mentioning the cells with short axon found in the plexiform layer of the hippocampal gyrus of man and mammals. These cellular elements are shown in the drawings of figs. 20 and 21 [figs. 150, 151]. Among them, attention is drawn to an ovoid or triangular type located in the broad plexiform layer or at its border with the underlying layer; from its cell body arise ascending and descending dendrites and a short axon which runs horizontally over a long distance, ending by means of collaterals that are mainly ascending, in the thickness of the layer under study (fig. 21, A) [fig. 151]. Another interesting type is represented by minute cells whose axon is thin and descending and quickly arborized, forming a dense and thin ramification extending into the underlying layer (fig. 20, C) [fig. 150]. Finally, in the

human cortex, as reproduced in fig. 24,[E] A, B, and E [fig. 154], we show several ascending axonal branches distributed in the plexiform layer and originating from the large and medium cells with short axon.

2. Second Layer or [Layer] of the Giant Polymorphic Cells

Named by Calleja, who has carefully explored this layer in the rabbit and mouse, the *layer of the semilunar and horizontal triangular cells*, it consists of several rows of densely packed cells, whose morphology and arrangement are somewhat variable depending on the portion of the olfactory area under study.

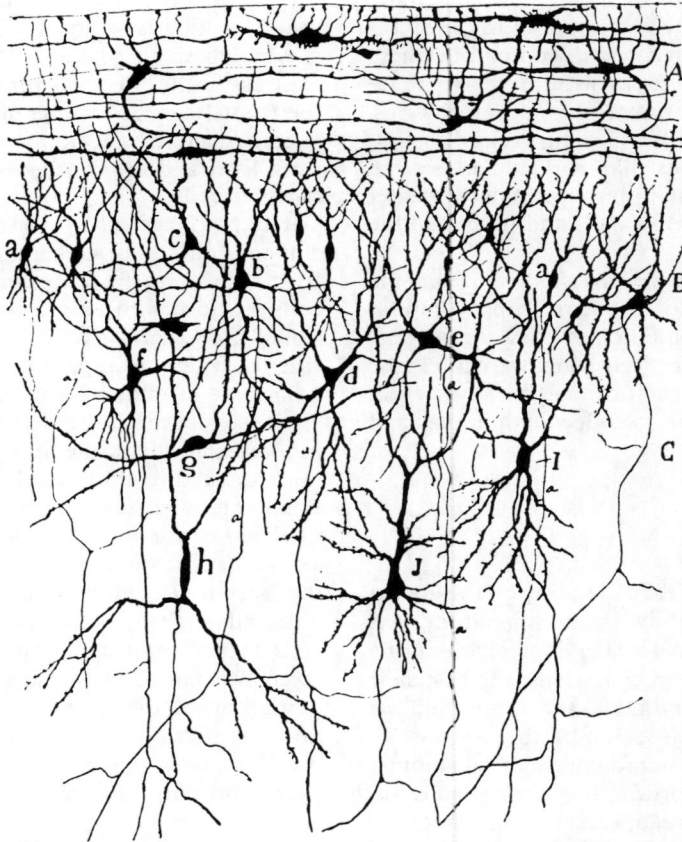

[FIG. 147] Fig. 17. Section of the first and second layers of the olfactory region of the hippocampal gyrus of the child of twenty days. A, plexiform layer with its horizontal cells; B, layer of the large polymorphic cells; C, beginning of the layer of the small tasseled cells. ([From a] region [situated] a short distance from the presubiculum.)

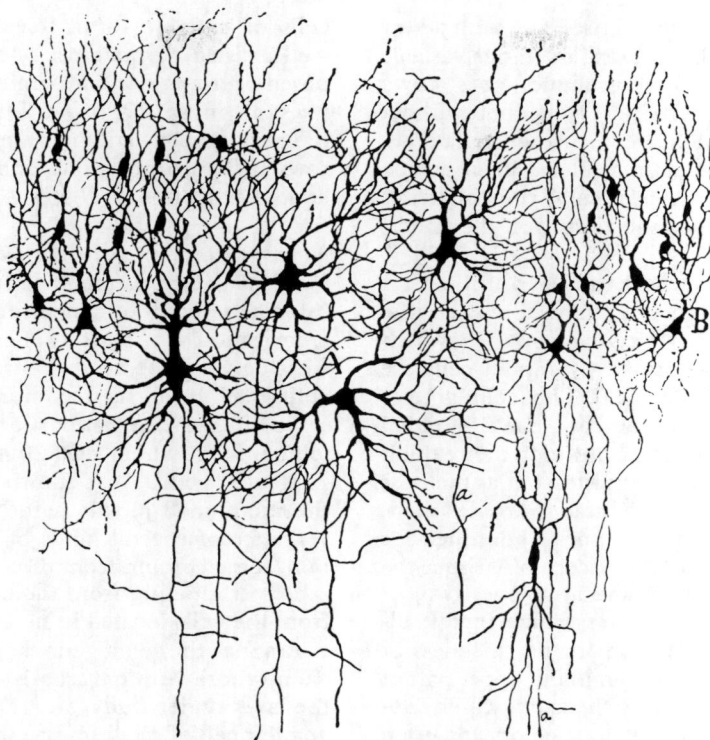

[FIG. 148]   Fig. 18. Cells of the layer of the giant polymorphic cells of the olfactory region of the hippocampal [gyrus] of the child of one month. A, islets of large cells; B, islets of small pyramids.

In the region adjacent to the presubicular territory, this layer constitutes a continuous band of large cells intermingled with medium and even small cells, as is shown in fig. 17, B [fig. 147]. But in the parts in which the Nissl preparations show the alternating islets of large and small cells, the appearance is very characteristic and notable (fig. 18) [fig. 148].

The cells of the large-celled islets are gigantic and have an extremely variable shape, but with the stellate type with numerous, thick, divergent, and quickly branching processes predominating. Some cells lack the radial [dendritic] shaft, which appears replaced by two or three dendrites arborizing in the first layer; in others, generally the deepest of each pleiad (fig. 18, A) [fig. 148], a radial dendrite does appear, although [it is] short and quickly arborized into its terminal branches. Also, these cells are characterized by the profusion of the secondary and tertiary branches of the lateral and descending dendrites that often give rise to dendritic plexuses similar to those of the cells of the inferior olive. With respect to the axon, it is very robust and descends to the white matter, not without having given rise to several collaterals; some of them are recurrent and arborized among the cells of the same pleiad [from which they arise]. It is not rare to observe on the said axon premature bifurcations, as is shown in fig. 18, A [fig. 148]; both branches seem to descend and to be continuous with myelinated fibers of the white matter.

The islets of small cells are narrower and are located in a plane somewhat more superficial (fig. 18, B) [fig. 148]. They contain ovoid, fusiform, or pyramidal cells of minute size that increase somewhat with depth. The majority of these cells are provided with a radial [dendritic] shaft quickly bifurcating and arborizing in varicose ascending branches; with thin and granular descending dendrites, whose distribution is usually limited to the interior of the [islet in which they arise]; and with a very delicate axon which, after an initial variable course [that is] often oblique, goes down through the underlying layers, not without first giving off delicate recurrent collaterals, distributed in the cellular pleiad [from which it arises]. In the deepest cells, the collaterals can also establish connections with the underlying cells.

In those places where the layer of the giant polymorphic cells is not arranged in islets, the cells form several irregular rows, in which some medium and small pyramidal cells are scattered (fig. 17) [fig. 147]. The [cellular] elements of the external rows lack a radial [dendritic] shaft, in place of which they exhibit [multiple] ascending dendrites; but as the cells come to occupy a deeper plane, a robust shaft, from which arise the [dendrites] destined for the first layer, becomes discernible. From the inferior part of the soma arise one, two, or more descending dendrites, which rapidly dichotomize and terminate in the thickness of the second layer, and even in the upper part of the third. With regard to the axon, which usually has an irregular initial trajectory and often arises from a descending [dendrite], it goes down to the deeper regions, not before giving off near its origin some collaterals ramifying in the thickness of the second layer and even in the first.

With respect to the small pyramidal or fusiform cells intercalated among the polymorphic giant cells of the regions devoid of islands, their shape and other features [make them] correspond to the classical type of pyramidal cell. They have an [apical dendritic] shaft, basal dendrites often originating from a [single] descending shaft, and a thin and descending axon that gives rise to some collaterals (fig. 17, a, b) [fig. 147]. In the cat, in which we have been able to study better than in man the axon of some small cells of the second layer, it is observed frequently that these collaterals have a recurrent course and are arborized in a complicated manner among the somata of their companion cells (fig. 20, A, B) [fig. 150].

In the mouse, rabbit, and cat, as Calleja demonstrated, the layer under study is simpler than in man, and, instead of a solid crowd of cells of variable form, it exhibits two quite well-defined formations: one external, composed of triangular and semilunar cells which we show in fig. 19, A [fig. 149]; and the other internal, thicker, and made up of two or more rows of fusiform, ovoid, and even true pyramidal cells (fig. 19, B) [fig. 149].

Nervous Plexuses and Cells with Short Axon of the Second Layer. The layer under study represents the point of concurrence and terminal arborization of an infinity of endogenous fibers which give rise to a very dense plexus not well delimited above. Its maximum richness is observed in the external portion of the piriform lobule, from which figs. 20 and 21 [figs. 150, 151] [are taken]. As is shown in these figures, the mentioned plexus is formed by the convergence of several kinds of axonal arborization, some coming from the endogenous cells, others originating from the bordering cells or from the cells located in neighboring layers.

Among the endogenous cells with short axon, whose terminal arborizations extend into the layer under study, are: (1) An ovoid or triangular cell of medium size whose descending axon forms a loose arborization, rich in secondary and tertiary branches and exclusively located in the second layer (fig. 21, C) [fig. 151]. Some cells of this kind inhabit the superficial frontier of the second layer and even the very plexiform layer (fig. 20, C) [fig. 150]. (2) Minute globular cells provided with thin and varicose dendrites and an axon forming a delicate and dense terminal ramification that surrounds the somata of the polymorphic cells and forms at some points true nests. Some such cells are located deeply or at the inferior frontier of the second layer (fig. 21, J) [fig. 151].

The said two cellular types belong to the cortex of the cat. In man, perhaps because of the poorer condition of the material that we have used, we have not been able to impregnate them. However, we have stained in the second layer certain relatively large cells with a short axon which is to a large extent ascending, and whose branches, [although we do not know if they] reach the first layer, have as their principal place of distribution, the second layer (fig. 24, A, B, C) [fig. 154].

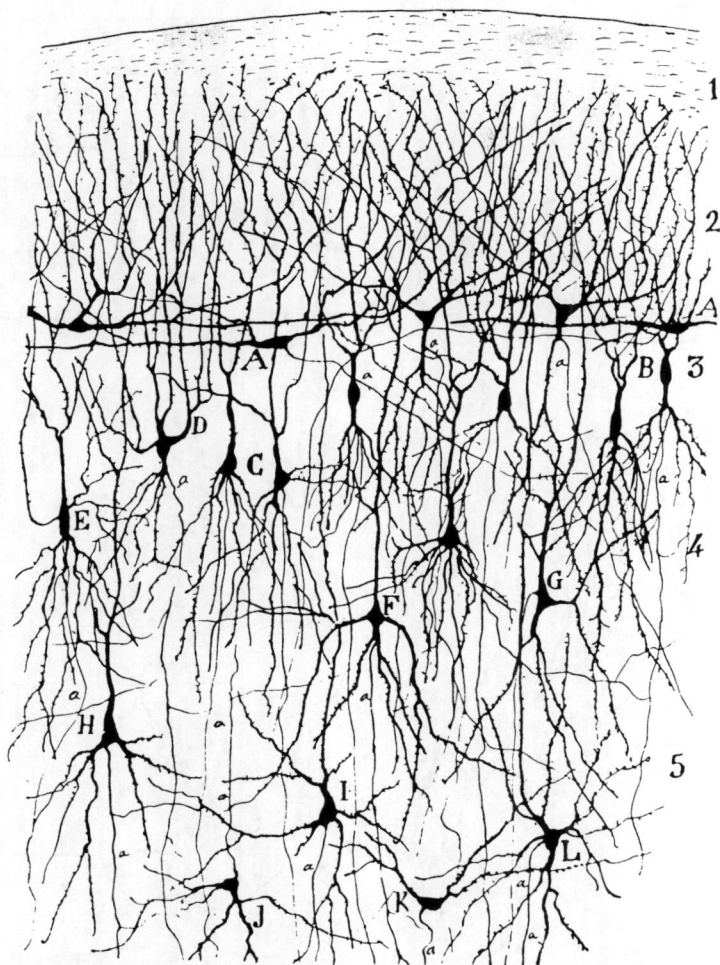

[FIG. 149] Fig. 19. Transverse section of the sphenoidal lobule of the cat. 1, olfactory fibers; 2, plexiform layer in the strict sense; 3, layer of the large polymorphic cells; 4, layer of the medium and small pyramids; 5, layer of the triangular and fusiform cells; A, triangular and semilunar cells of the second layer; B, fusiform cells of the second layer; C, D, E, different types of tasseled cells.

The nerve fibers coming from cells more or less distant from the second layer belong to the following varieties: (1) Recurrent collaterals, arising from the axons of the superficial polymorphic cells and distributed almost exclusively in the thickness of the second layer (fig. 20, A, B) [fig. 150]. (2) Upper collaterals originating in large cells with short axon, located in the third layer. In fig. 21 [fig. 151], from the cortex of the cat, we reproduce one of these cells (D), and in fig. 24 [fig. 154], which repro-

duces the cells with short axon found in the human limbic cortex, we show another (E), whose ascending axon provides branches to the second, third, and fourth layers. (3) Terminal arborizations of ascending axons arising from cells situated in the third layer or perhaps deeper. A cell of this kind, but of small size and with a pyramidal shape, is shown in fig. 20, H [fig. 150]. Certain large cells found in the human cortex (fig. 24,[F] F, G) [fig. 154], whose appearance corresponds to that of the

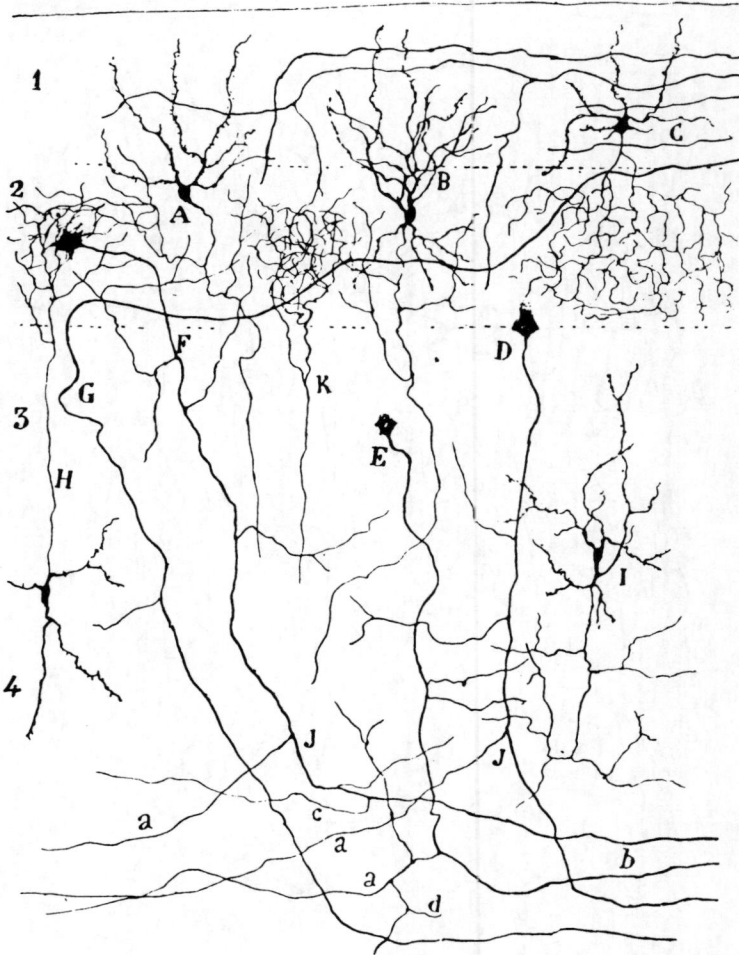

[*FIG. 150*] Fig. 20. Transverse section of the olfactory sphenoidal region of the cat of twenty days. *A, B,* cells with long axon of the second layer; *C,* cell whose axon is arborized in the second layer; *D, E, F, G,* axons of large cells located in the second and third layers; *H, K,* ascending fibers terminating in axonal nests in the second layer; *H,* cell with [one of these] ascending axons.

large-sized cells of Golgi, equally collaborate in the formation of said plexus, to which they send a long ascending, moderately branched fiber among the giant polymorphic cells. (4) Dense arborizations forming complex pericellular nests, continuous with an ascending fiber coming from very low down and which also may give off a small collateral branch to the third layer. Such interesting fibers that, so far, we have only observed in the cortex of the cat seem to come from cells with ascending axon

located in deeper layers; however, we must record that we have not been able to demonstrate the continuity of these fibers with the ascending axons of the cells of the fifth and sixth layer (fig. 21, *E*) [*fig. 151*].

Layer of the Tasseled Pyramids

Kölliker and Calleja, independent of each other, discovered that the medium and large pyramids of the sphenoidal cortex, as well as those of the subradicular region of the frontal

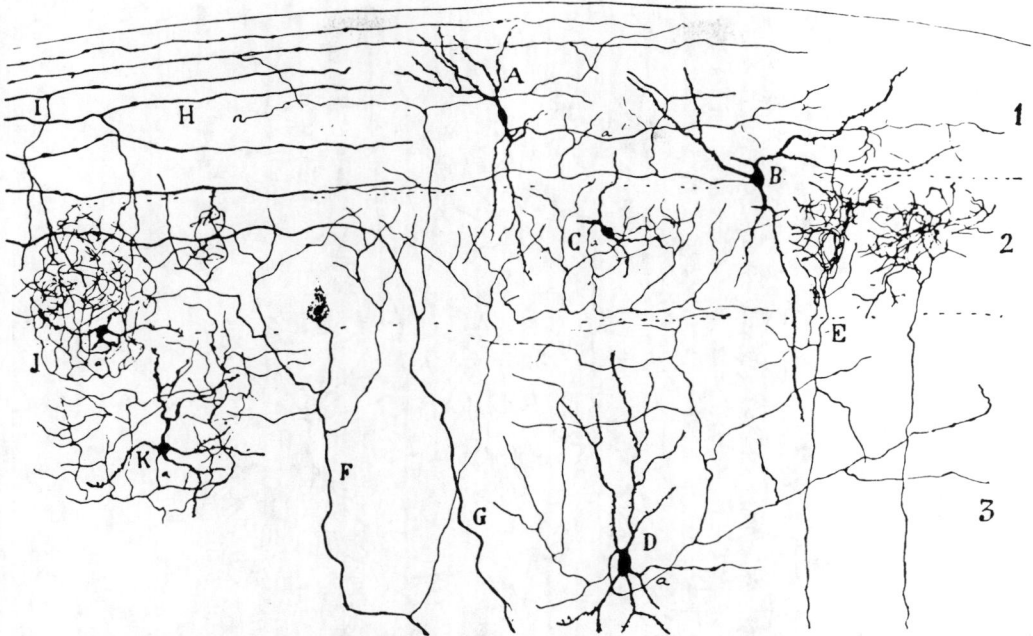

[*FIG. 151*]   Fig. 21. Cells with short axon in the olfactory sphenoidal cortex of the cat. *1*, plexiform layer; *2*, layer of the large polymorphic cells; *3*, layer of the medium and large tasseled cells.

lobe, appear with their basal dendrites gathered together into a descending paintbrushlike arrangement, giving them an unusual physiognomy; but they did not indicate well the part of the cortex in which this peculiarity is observed, nor did they verify that they occur in man, since Calleja observed them only in the mouse and Kölliker in the young cat. We have been able to impregnate the mentioned cells in the mouse, cat, and dog and in the child of one to two months, having noticed that they do not extend throughout the whole piriform lobule but are confined to the olfactory region, that is to say, to the central and external portion of [the piriform lobule]. This interesting morphological peculiarity is lacking, as we will see later, both from the subiculum and from the presubicular region; it begins on the ammonic side of the territory under study, and becomes more noticeable as we move closer to the limbic fissure. Near this [fissure], the descending tufts are less dense, and disappear completely in the fundus of the sulcus.

In man, the arrangement is much more ac-

centuated and more elegant than in the mammals, as we show in fig. 22 [*fig. 152*]. The basal dendrites of the medium and large pyramids, instead of paintbrushes, seem to form cottony tassels composed of an infinity of varicose, curly, spiny, and extremely intricate threads. In the small and medium pyramids, the fibrillar tuft is of singular delicacy and complication, whereas in the large pyramids, situated in the deepest plane, the threads, which are thicker, can be more easily followed. The tassels are so typical that because of them it is possible to recognize the sphenoidal olfactory cortex at first glance. Often, the [apical dendritic] shaft, at a certain distance from the soma, exhibits several horizontal thin dendrites, and it is not rare to see, when the cell body instead of being pyramidal has a spindle shape (fig. 22, *C*) [*fig. 152*], that the descending tuft arises from a descending radial dendritic process. Only two more details [are required] to finish with [the description] of such singular arrangements: dendrites never arise from the sides of the soma [of a tasseled cell], which is a rare circumstance, since, commonly, no pyr-

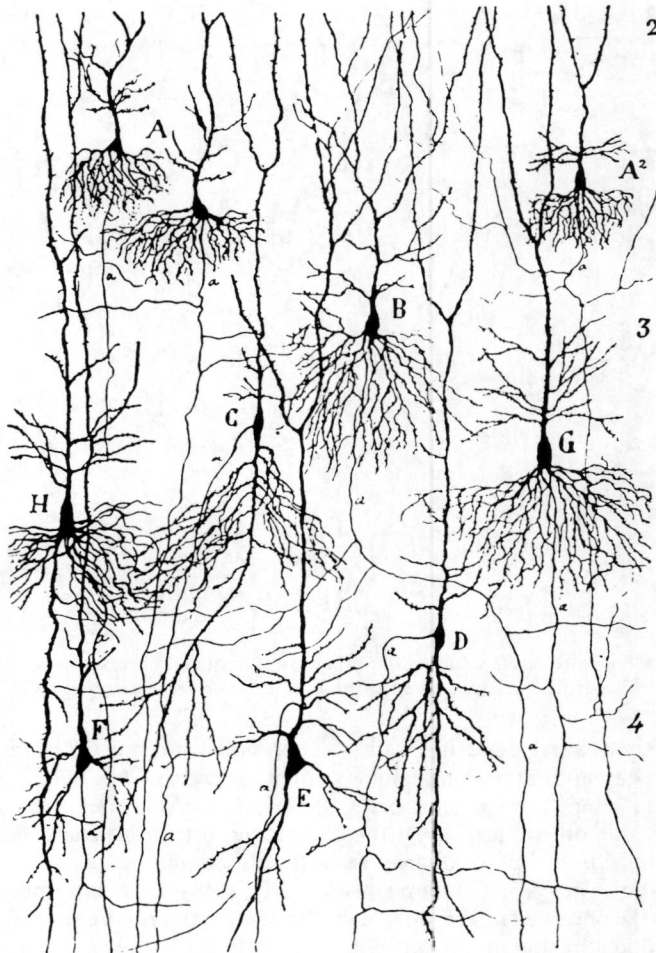

[*FIG. 152*] Fig. 22. Section of the olfactory sphenoidal cortex of the child of one month. In this figure appear the layers of the medium and large tasseled pyramids and the beginning of the fourth layer or [layer] of the polymorphic cells. *A*, small tasseled cells; *B, G, H,* large tasseled cells; *D*, fusiform cell with a lateral axon; *E*, triangular cell with arciform axon; *F*, common pyramid.

amid lacks lateral processes; however, at the sides of the soma, between the basal cottony tassel and the lower dendrites of the [apical dendritic] shaft, there constantly remains a space completely free of dendrites (fig. 22, A^2, *G*) [*fig. 152*].

The axon originates from the basal portion of the soma, except in the fusiform cells in which it can also arise from one side; it descends more or less radially, giving off some collaterals, and, either at the level of the infe-

rior polymorphic cells or farther away, it usually divides into a thick branch directed deeply and a thin branch oriented toward the surface. Sometimes, as is observed in fig. 22, *B* [*fig. 152*], the said axon is bent resolutely toward the depths, giving rise at the point of inflexion to two or more small branches. In the cases of bifurcation, each resultant branch can, in turn, give off collaterals.

In the cortex of the cat and dog, the paintbrushlike cells or *double pyramids,* as Kölliker calls them, exhibit an axon arranged in the same way; that is to say, it often changes its descending course, tracing turns and ending, either far from or close to the white matter, by dividing into a thick internal branch and a thin external branch frequently cut in cross-section. The first fiber has seemed to us to run forward in the subventricular plane of the white matter to enter finally the lenticular nucleus of the corpus striatum; it represents, therefore, a fiber of projection. The other branch could constitute a fiber of intracortical association or perhaps also a fiber of the anterior commissure.

Layer of the Deep Polymorphic Cells or Layer of the Fusiform and Triangular Cells

As is observed in fig. 23, A, B, C [*fig. 153*], where we show the most common cells of this layer in man, the morphology is extremely varied. There can be recognized frankly fusiform cells, provided with two robust ascending

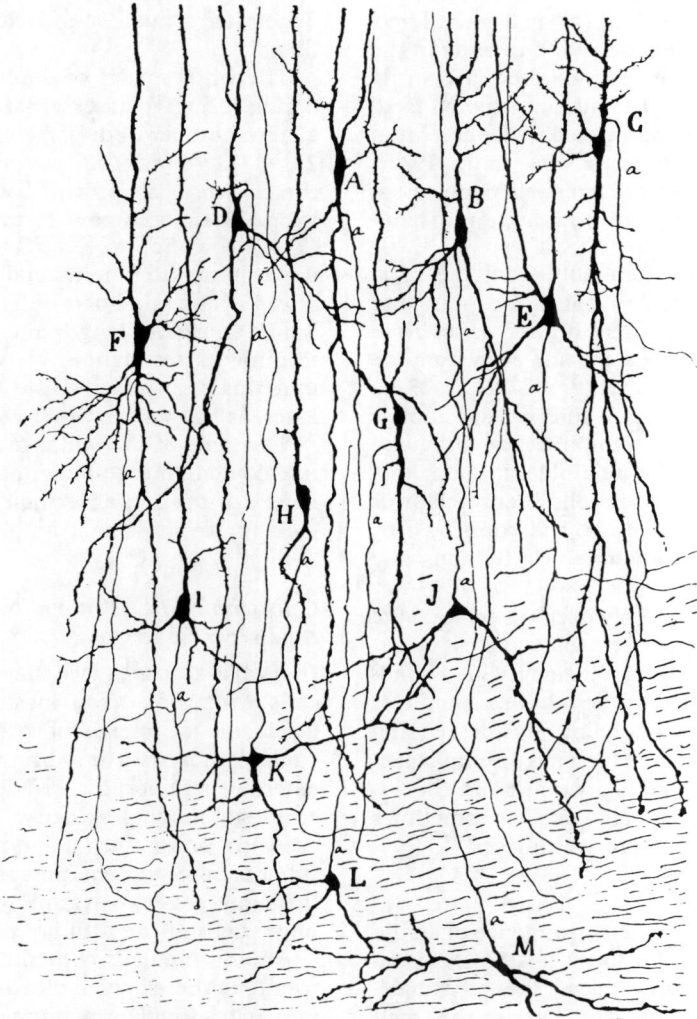

[*FIG. 153*]   Fig. 23. Section of the deep layers of the olfactory sphenoidal cortex of the child of one month. *A, B, C, D, E, F, G, H,* several types of fusiform and triangular cells; *K, L, M,* cells of the white matter provided with ascending axons.

and descending [dendritic] shafts (fig. 23, *A*, *C*, *H*) [*fig. 153*], the latter often prolonged into the white matter and the other up to the plexiform layer; others have a more or less pyramidal shape (fig. 23, *B*, *E*) [*fig. 153*]; finally, there are also triangular cells with a short lateral [dendritic] shaft quickly forming dendritic branches additional to the long ascending and descending processes.

In the majority of these cells and even in the true pyramidal cells, there is usually no lack of a robust and elongated descending dendrite (fig. 23, *A*, *B*, *D*) [*fig. 153*], [of such a kind] similar to that likewise observed frequently in the cells situated in the superimposed layers (fig. 22, *D*, *H*) [*fig. 152*]. This anarchy of [cell] forms can also be appreciated in the cerebrum of the cat, in which, as we show in fig. 19, *H*, *I*, *L* [*fig. 149*], there are irregularly mixed triangular, pyramidal, fusiform, and even semilunar cells.

The axon arises generally from the basal portion of the soma, except in the triangular and fusiform cells, where it often arises from the lateral side of the soma and even from the ascending radial dendrite (figs. 22, *E*, *D*; 23, *C*, *D*) [*figs. 152, 153*]. When such a disposition is accentuated, the said axon traces an arch with inferior concavity that resembles in shape that of the [shepherd's] crook cells discovered by us in the optic lobe of birds, and confirmed by Van Gehuchten, Kölliker, P. Ramón, and Riss.

The layer of the polymorphic cells in the subiculum of the mouse, rabbit, and cat is particularly rich in cellular elements with ascending axon. Almost all of them have a spindle or ovoid shape with ascending and descending dendrites; their axon, which has a complicated and flexuous course, is distributed in the superimposed layers, it being possible sometimes to follow it up to the plexiform layer.

White Matter

It is the general point of convergence of all the long axons of the fusiform, tasseled, and superficial polymorphic cells. This zone, extremely thick in man, constitutes in the small mammals a thin subventricular layer, in which it is noticed that the dominant direction of the fibers is toward the interior and forward, as though in search of the lenticular nucleus of the corpus striatum. A careful examination of the bundles of the white matter reveals that their exist two categories of fibers: thin and perhaps continuous with the collaterals or [the parent] axons of medium and small pyramids; and thick, continuous with large tasseled pyramids and with voluminous fusiform and polymorphic cells. We have not been able to find centrifugal fibers coming from the white matter, except in the subiculum and presubicular region, which, as we will show below, are penetrated by two large systems of exogenous fibers.

The white matter of the human sphenoidal cortex (central and external regions) contains a large number of dispersed nerve cells. In fig. 23, *K*, *L*, *M* [*fig. 153*], we reproduce some of them, almost all provided with an ascending axon. Their dominant form is the triangular (*J*) or ovoid. Some cells (*K*) are like an upside-down pyramid. The ascending axon was followed over a large part of its vertical itinerary, but its enormous length did not allow us to determine its destination. We suppose, however, that this axon reaches the first or plexiform layer, as happens in other cortical areas.

The cells of the white matter with ascending axon are more uncommon in the olfactory cortex of the cat; nevertheless, they are never lacking; we show an example in fig. 19, *J* [*fig. 149*].

Cells with Short Axon and Nervous Plexuses of the Deeper Layers

In previous pages, we have mentioned the cells with short axon located in the second layer and the plexus of endogenous and exogenous fibers surrounding the somata of the external polymorphic cells. Similar plexuses, although much less dense and complicated, are also present in the other layers of the sphenoidal cortex, particularly in the layer of the large tasseled pyramids and [among] the upper cells of the fifth layer.

Among the cells with short axon that contribute to these axonal plexuses are the following: first, a small or medium cell with descending axon, arborized in the thickness of the fourth and fifth layers (fig. 20, *I*) [*fig. 150*]; second, robust ovoid or triangular cell, whose horizontal or ascending axon gives rise to a large number of horizontal or oblique branches (fig. 21, *D*) [*fig. 151*]. [Cell] types analogous to these, although more abundant, are also observed in the human cortex, as we show in fig. 24, *D, F, G* [*fig. 154*]. Often, the axon whose course is descending traces an arc with a superior concavity, and later goes up to fill with horizontal and oblique branches a considerable cortical area (fig. 24, *F*) [*fig. 154*].

The plexuses just mentioned are widely extended and consist of fibers that run in all directions; but in some territories of the human olfactory area, especially in its external portion, the layer of the large tasseled pyramids exhibits a plexus arranged as a horizontal band, in which small nerve fibers parallel to the cortex predominate. To this plexus of parallel branches, long horizontal collaterals originating in medium and small pyramids preferentially contribute; [these cells are] located either in the said layer or in the preceding [layer]. Also contributing to it are the oblique and horizontal collaterals of ascending axons with an initial arciform course and numerous small branches arising from cells with short axons.

In summary and to conclude, we will say

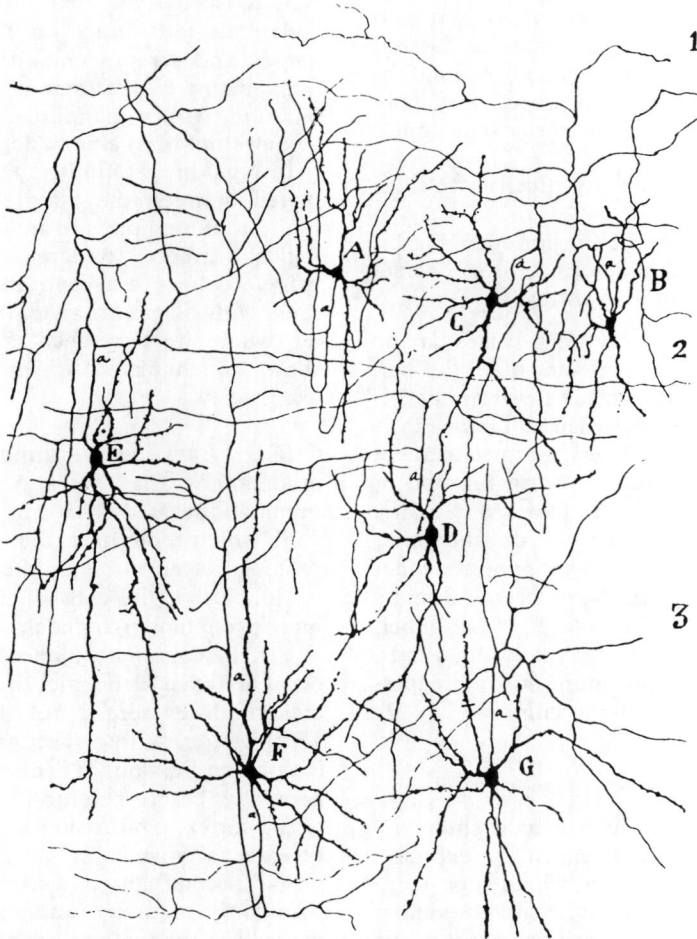

[*FIG. 154*] Fig. 24. Cells with short axon found in the cortex of the hippocampal gyrus of the child of one month. *1*, plexiform layer; *2*, layer of the external polymorphic cells; *3*, layer of the tasseled pyramids.

that the olfactory cortex of the hippocampal gyrus has a highly characteristic structure that is distinguished easily from the other cortical areas by the following positive and negative features:

1. For presenting, instead of a layer of small pyramids, a layer of giant polymorphic cells that in some places are arranged in islands alternating with groups of small cells.
2. For the presence, at the bases of the medium and large pyramids, of tassels of thin dendrites.
3. For the absence of a layer of granule cells and [of a layer] of giant pyramids.
4. For the superficial distribution, that is to say, in a broad plexiform layer, of the sensory or exogenous nerve fiber ramifications which, as is known, are distributed in the deep layers in the visual and motor areas.
5. For the relative poverty of cells with short axon.
6. For the absence of the innumerable bitufted and neurogliaform cells so characteristic of the human cortex.

Thus, the human olfactory cortex is the least human or [least] perfected of all the sensory areas. The stamp of the lower animals is revealed even in the superficial situation of the plexus of exogenous fibers, an arrangement that reproduces a feature of organization of the cerebral cortex of the lower vertebrates. Such structural stagnancy is, on the other hand, easy to understand if we remember that the sense of smell is in the process of atrophy in man, or at least in a quiescent state, which is quite different from the rest of the senses, which tend to become more and more perfected in man and higher mammals.

Region of the Subiculum

As we said above, the subiculum is characterized by these three features: first, the excessive robustness of the first layer, which appears invaded by numerous ascending nerve bundles arriving from the white matter; second, the presence in the said first layer of islets of small and medium pyramids; and, third, the structural simplicity of the underlying layers that together are reduced to a continuous formation of pyramids of medium and regular dimension.

First or Plexiform Layer

Examined in man with the method of Golgi, this layer presents an infinity of robust nerve bundles with a parallel orientation which pass successively from the subiculum to the molecular layers of Ammon's horn and the fascia dentata. In the transverse sections of the gyrus hippocampi, the majority of these fibers appear obliquely or cross-sectioned. When following them individually over long trajectories, it is observed that they give off many collaterals, distributed in the *stratum lacunosum* and *stratum radiatum* of Ammon's horn, with a few of them dedicated to the subiculum, with a manner of termination that we have not been able to determine.

In Nissl preparations, there appear disseminated between the bundles of fibers some neurons of medium size about whose morphological attributes we cannot say anything because we have not been able to impregnate them with silver chromate. In the cat and rabbit, where we have seen them stained, they show the characteristics of cells with short axon.

Cellular Islets. Seen distinctly in the Nissl preparations, they are also stained in Golgi preparations, as is shown in fig. 25, *A, F* [*fig. 155*], which reproduces the islands of the first subicular layer of the child of fifteen days.

Notice that the cells of these pleiades are more ovoid than pyramidal, and have a smaller size in the superficial planes than in the deepest. The radial [dendritic] shaft ends with several dendrites spread out in the superficial white matter. With respect to the axon, which is thin and flexuous, it is directed deeply, and, generally, before reaching the deepest layers of the cortex, it bifurcates into an internal and an external branch (fig. 25, *b*) [*fig. 155*]. In its initial trajectory, it gives off several collaterals, commonly recurrent and distributed among the cells of the same cellular pleiad (fig. 25, *A*) [*fig. 155*]. A notable peculiarity is that the cells of the underlying layers usually avoid the

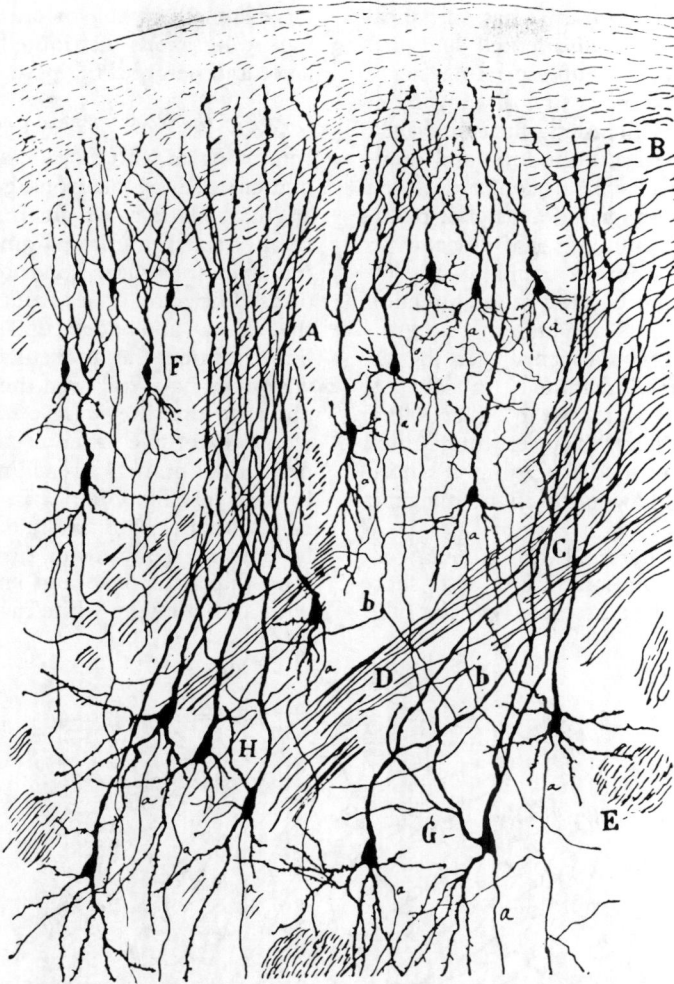

[*FIG. 155*] Fig. 25. Section of the hippocampal gyrus of the child of fifteen days. Subicular region. *A*, islets of small pyramids; *B*, mass of superficial white matter; *C, D*, bundles of fibers that descend to the deep white matter; *F*, another islet; *H*, medium and large pyramids whose dendrites go up in the septa of white matter; *b*, terminal bifurcation of the axon.

pleiades or islets of pyramids, since, instead of passing through them with their long radial [dendritic] shafts, they simply gather together between the said territories, that is, in the thickness of the septa of white matter that separate them; thus, thick bundles of interpyramidal dendrites are engendered, whose [terminal] tufts are extended up to the most superficial part of the cortex.

Layer of the Medium and Large Pyramids

Beneath the plexiform layer, there begins, at an irregular toothlike frontier, a thick formation of quite voluminous pyramids, which extends to near the white matter. The most superficial of these cells sometimes have an ovoid and fusiform shape, but their size differs little from that of the deep pyramids (fig. 25,

G, H) [*fig. 155*]. Each pyramid has an [apical dendritic] shaft, often disoriented and displaced by the presence of ascending nerve bundles and by the necessity, already mentioned, of respecting the islets of the first layer, in which they arborize; quite long and ramified lateral dendrites; basal dendrites, even longer but never arranged in a tassel or paintbrush; and, finally, an axon that descends to the white matter, where it seems to pass toward the interior, more or less in the direction of Ammon's horn. Its penetration into Ammon's horn is observed, especially, in the subiculum of the small mammals, in which it can also be verified, as shown in fig. 26, *b* [*fig. 156*], that the said fiber bifurcates into a thick internal branch destined for Ammon's horn and a thin branch that gets lost in the subicular white matter.

Among the said pyramids, the human cortex shows constantly some cells with short axon, either of the small stellate type or of the large stellate type. Nor does it lack cells with ascending axons distributed in the molecular layer and neighboring planes of pyramids.

Layer of the Polymorphic Cells

Intermingled with horizontal bundles of white matter lie several neurons, generally with a triangular, stellate, or fusiform shape and of smaller size than the pyramids of the preceding layer and whose dendrites run in all directions. The axon arises from the upper part of the soma and goes up, giving off small branches near the molecular layer. In rodents, where we have followed these axons best, it is observed that they give off branches over the whole extensive layer of the pyramids, the final small branches reaching up to the plexiform layer (fig. 27, *g*) [*fig. 157*]. Besides the cells with ascending axon, there are also in this layer some pyramids or fusiform cells with a long radial dendrite and an axon continuous with a fiber of the white matter.

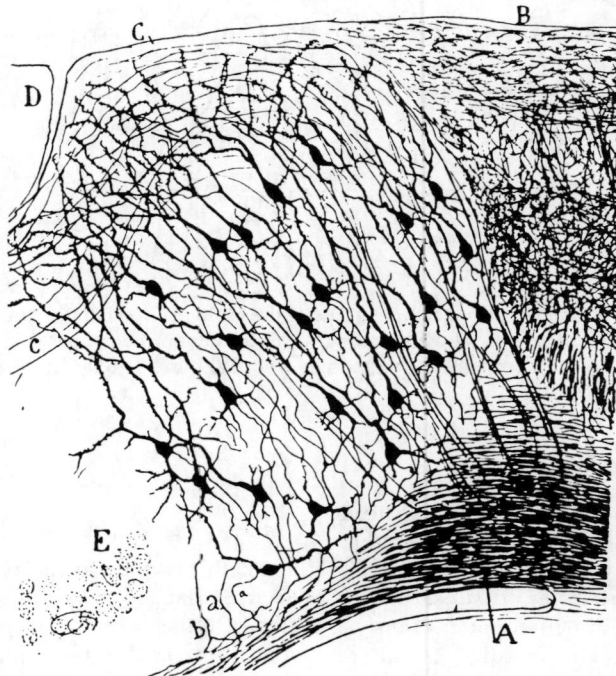

[*FIG. 156*] Fig. 26. Sagittal section of the subiculum of the mouse of fifteen days. *A*, commissural bundle; *B*, presubiculum with its terminal plexuses; *C*, subiculum; *D*, fascia dentata; *E*, beginning of the pyramids of Ammon's horn; *a, b*, subicular axons penetrating Ammon's horn.

White Matter

It represents a huge formation in man [but is] less voluminous in the rodents, and it extends from the thickness of the preceding layer to the proximity of the ventricle. Externally, this massive fibrous structure is continuous with the no less robust one lying underneath the presubicular region, and internally it successively becomes thinner on passing to form the white matter of the alveus. The Weigert-Pal preparations, especially in the rodents, reveal the existence, at the subicular angle of the ventricle, of two planes of nerve fibers: the deep or subventricular plane composed of thin medullated fibers (fig. 27, D) [fig. 157], and the superficial plane formed by thick medullated fibers.

The subventricular plane or [plane] of *thin myelinated fibers* (fig. 27, D) [fig. 157] has few connections with the subiculum. A careful examination in serial sections stained either with the method of Golgi or with that of Weigert (small mammals) shows that the said fibers are commissural axons arising in a special region at the occipital lip and which form a longitudinal pathway that increases in thickness from bottom to top, at least in its inferior half, by the addition of new contingents; this pathway, on reaching the midline, passes under the corpus callosum, to form the *psalterium dorsale.*

With regard to the thick myelinated fibers, they constitute, as we will see, another important exogenous pathway that in all the vertebrates studied by us lies constantly at the level of the subicular angle of the ventricle. By contrast with the aforementioned pathway, this one decreases from bottom to top, disappearing almost completely in proximity to the psalterium dorsale and in being progressively displaced toward the interior, that is to say, toward Ammon's horn. As is well known, from this pathway there are detached small bundles that cross the subicular cortex (along different radial lines) and invade the plexiform layer to enter finally Ammon's horn, by inclining both medially and laterally. We will deal later with the origin and termination of this powerful exogenous pathway.

The subiculum also receives branching nerve fibers. As is seen in figs. 27, *a,* and 30, *h*

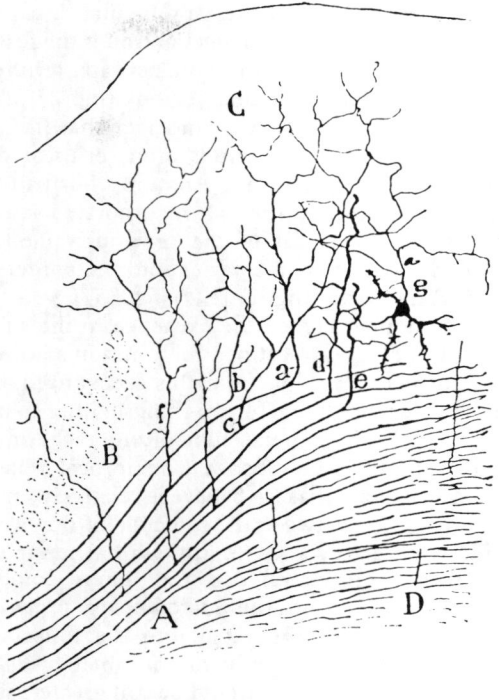

[*FIG. 157*] Fig. 27. Piece of the subicular region close to [Ammon's] horn of the mouse. *A,* penetrating bundle in the alveus; *D,* commissural optic pathway; *C,* axonal arborizations terminating in the subiculum; *a, b,* terminal fibers; *d, e,* centrifugal axons birfucating in the white matter.

[*figs. 157, 160*], from the white matter between the great exogenous pathway and the first pyramids of Ammon's horn arise numerous collaterals originating at right or obtuse angles, which arborize among the subicular cells, generating a complicated plexus that does not seem to extend up to the plexiform layer. In addition, it is also observed that the arrival and branching of the terminal fibers lead to the formation of a loose and rich arborization. Such fibers evidently come from Ammon's horn, since they are seen extending [backward] over a long trajectory into the territory of the alveus. In their preterminal portions, they behave in two ways: some, which are in the minority, simply bend to enter and ramify in the subiculum (fig. 27, *b*) [*fig. 157*]; others, [which are] the most numerous, are divided into a thick terminal branch with a subicular distribution and a thin branch that continues the former course of the axon and perhaps terminates in distant subicular regions (fig. 27, *a*) [*fig. 157*]. Finally, let us remember that from the subiculum come axons often bifurcated into a branch penetrating Ammon's horn and a generally thinner branch incorporated into the solid fiber mass of the previously mentioned exogenous pathway or into the bordering white matter (fig. 27, *e, d*) [*fig. 157*].

The double fact of the existence in the subiculum of fibers destined for Ammon's horn and of fibers coming from this seems to give us to understand one of two things: either that between both centers, subiculum and Ammon's horn, is established a reciprocal relationship, a fact that we believe is relatively unlikely, or that between the subicula [of the two sides] there exists, as occurs with Ammon's horn, a commissural pathway. There could equally arise from the subiculum a projection pathway incorporated into the fimbria, whereby the assumption of the analogy between the two centers would be still greater, as it is well known that the fimbria carries the principal pathway of projection of Ammon's horn.

Presubicular Region of the Sphenoidal Cortex

The application of the Golgi method to the analysis of this cerebral territory has not given in man such good results as in animals. In general, its cells are developed later than those of the olfactory cortex, as a consequence of which it has often happened to us that we have not found, [even] in the same sections in which the olfactory region was well impregnated, any completely stained cell [in the presubiculum]. Anyway, the results obtained, although very defective, are sufficient to justify the affirmation that this territory of the hippocampal gyrus has unique features in no way similar to those of the adjacent territories.

Plexiform Layer

It lacks olfactory fibers, both in man and in animals. However, in it lie a multitude of medullated fibers arriving from the white matter underlying the ventricular angle, as is well seen in the Weigert-Pal preparations. In man, we have also found all the usual features of construction of this layer, especially the large horizontal cells and the cellular elements with short axon.

Layer of the Small Fusiform and Pyramidal Cells

In fig. 28, 2 [*fig. 158*], we reproduce some of these cellular elements, whose form is extremely variable, although ovoid and fusiform shapes predominate. From their upper part arises a thin radial [dendritic] shaft that arborizes in the first layer, whereas from the deeper part there arises either a group of delicate basal dendrites or a [single dendritic] shaft quickly resolving into some small descending branches. The thin axon, sometimes somewhat oblique near its origin, descends to get lost in the deep layers, after supplying two or three recurrent collaterals of great delicacy to the second and first layers.

In the mouse and rabbit, as is shown in fig. 29, 2 [*fig. 159*], the fusiform type is predominant in the second layer, alternating with occasional pyramids and globular cells. The shortness of the distances has allowed us to follow the axon down to the white matter, where it seems to be continuous with a thin nerve fiber of the superficial exogenous pathway.

[Internal] Plexiform Layer

This cell-poor layer, underlying the second, lodges small and medium cells, the majority, belonging perhaps to the fusiform type with ascending or descending axon, quickly ramifying in the thickness of the layer or prolonged up to the second and first layers. Such fusiform cells, of which we show three examples in fig. 28, *a, c* [*fig. 158*], seem to us to represent somewhat modified varieties of the bitufted cells of other cortical regions. The layer contains, besides, stellate cells with short axon of the common type (fig. 28, *b*) [*fig. 158*] and medium and small pyramids.

In the mouse, besides the medium and small pyramids and occasional cells with ascending axon destined for the first layer (fig. 31, *C*) [*fig. 161*], we have found in the superficial plane of layer, and particularly concentrated in the deep plane of the first layer.

But the principal feature of construction of the third layer is a very dense plexus, formed by the terminal ramifications of innumerable exogenous fibers, coming from the white matter underlying the ventricular angle. The presence of this exceptionally rich plexus distinguishes, at first glance, in good Golgi preparations, the presubicular region from the subiculum and from the olfactory portion of the piriform lobule. The extent and richness of this plexus in man make it impossible to analyze it with profit; but in the mouse of twelve to twenty days, it can be studied perfectly (fig.

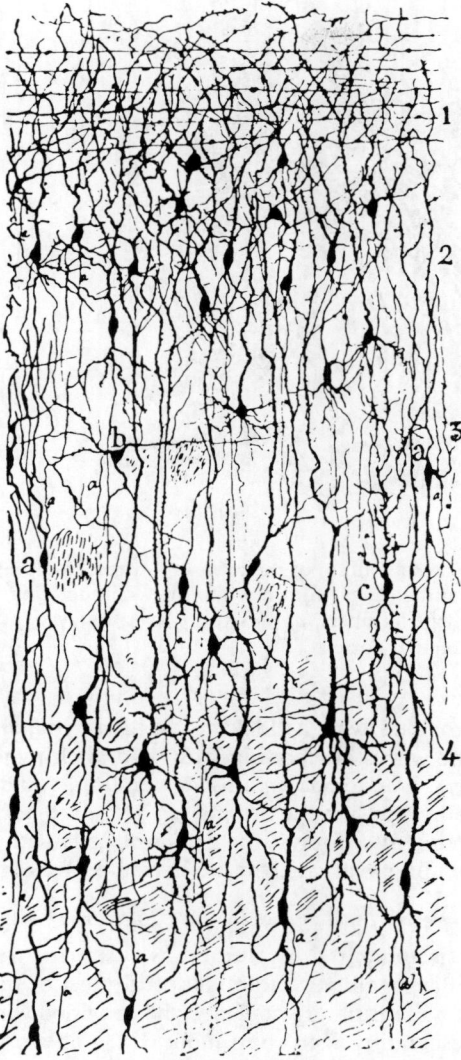

[FIG. 158]   Fig. 28. Section of the presubicular region of the human gyrus hippocampi. 1, plexiform layer; 2, layer of the small fusiform and triangular cells; 3, plexiform layer; 4, layer of the medium pyramids; a, fusiform cells with short axon; b, stellate cell with short axon; c, fusiform cell with ascending axon and spiny dendrites.

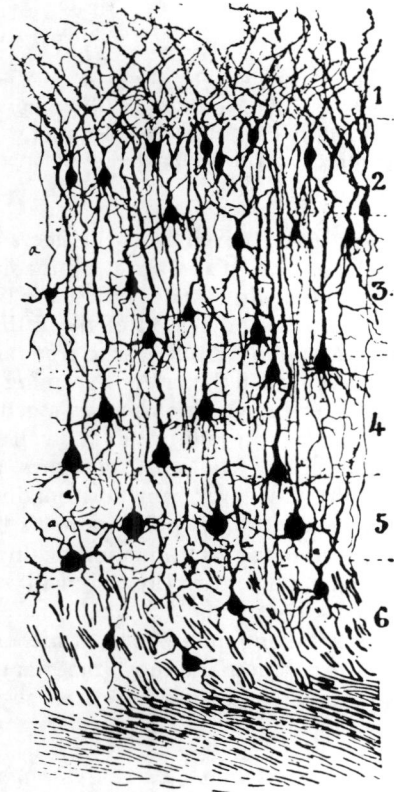

[FIG. 159]   Fig. 29. Section of the presubicular cortex of the mouse. 1, plexiform layer; 2, layer of the fusiform cells; 3, plexiform layer; 4, layer of the medium and large pyramids; 5, layer of the spheroidal cells with ascending axon; 6, layer of the polymorphic cells and the plexiform white matter.

this layer certain relatively large globular cells, with radiated and varicose dendrites, and whose axon, commonly horizontal or ascending, is resolved quickly into a dense arborization distributed around the cells of the second

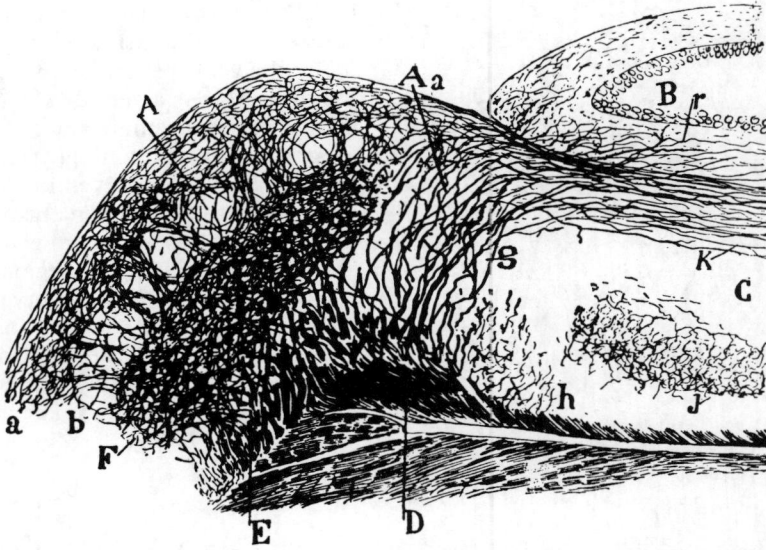

[*FIG. 160*]   Fig. 30. Sagittal section of the subiculum and presubiculum of the mouse. *A*, presubiculum; *B*, fascia dentata; *C*, Ammon's horn; *D*, commissural optic bundle; *E*, plexiform white matter underlying the presubiculum; *F*, dense terminal plexus of exogenous centripetal fibers; *a*, plexiform layer; *b*, layer of the fusiform cells; *g*, perforant bundles; *h*, collaterals to the subicular cortex.

30, *F*) [*fig. 160*], observing that its fibers arise mainly from the plane most immediately [adjacent] to the white matter; these are bifurcated repeatedly at the level of the fifth and sixth layers, and are resolved into free ramifications that cover all the layers, excepting only the second, across which pass many ascending small branches, forming irregular small bundles. Many of the said small branches, after reaching the first layer, run horizontally beyond the subiculum to enter Ammon's horn. About the origin and termination of this important exogenous pathway, we will speak later.

The above-mentioned plexus, which must be one of the richest and most important that exists in the nervous centers, we have also impregnated in the cat and rabbit.

Layer of the Medium and Large Pyramids

This sphenoidal region lacks the voluminous giant pyramids, and the ones that do appear in this layer do not surpass the size of medium pyramids. As is seen in fig. 28, *4* [*fig. 158*], even the pyramidal shape is rare; triangular and fusiform shapes are more abundant, and they are provided with a thick apical [dendritic] shaft and with a descending, quickly branching process. The axons, mainly descending, could be followed to the white matter. Here are not infrequently [found] the fusiform cells with ascending axon and the stellate cells of Golgi.

Layer of the Triangular and Fusiform Cells

It is inhabited by numerous fusiform, triangular, ovoid, or pyramidal cells, most of them of a medium or small size and provided with a descending axon continuous with a fiber of the white matter. The bifurcations are abundant. Some [cellular] elements with a fusiform or triangular shape, devoid of a long radial [dendritic] shaft, send their axons to the superficial layers.

In the rabbit and mouse, this deep layer, [which is] easy to analyze because of its short extent, exhibits two sublayers: the *external* (fig. 29, 5) [*fig. 159*], narrow and almost exclusively inhabited by voluminous spheroidal or piriform cells, with ascending axons prolonged up to the first layer; and the *internal*, wider, invaded by bundles of the white matter, and in which reside piriform, triangular, or ovoid

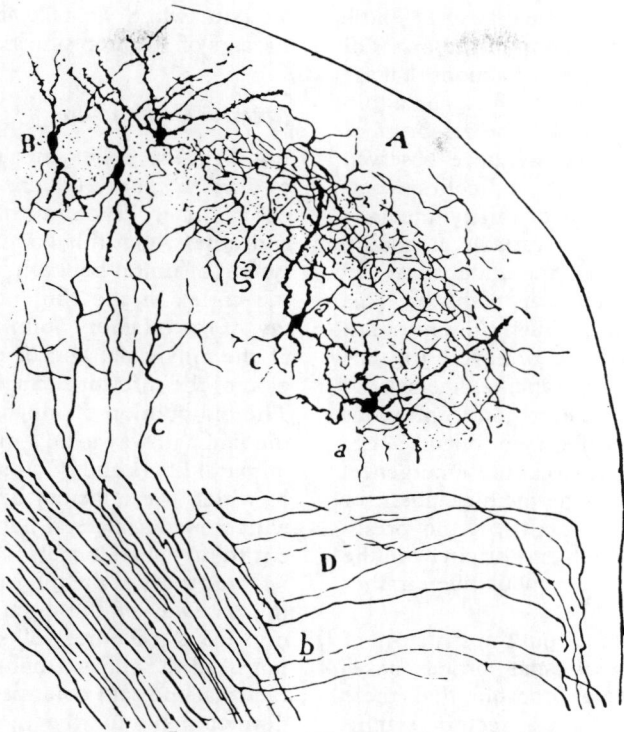

[*FIG. 161*]   Fig. 31. Cells with short axon of the presubicular cortex (*A*) of the mouse. *A*, plexiform layer; *B*, fusiform cells; *D*, perforant optic fibers arising from the white matter of the subiculum; *a*, axons of the cells with short axon; *c*, axons arising from the presubiculum and incorporated into the commissural optic pathway.

cells of a much smaller size and provided either with a long axon continuous with a fiber of the white matter or with an ascending axon (fig. 29, *6*) [*fig. 159*]. The external sublayer appears at some points interrupted and without a well-marked differentiation, in certain presubicular regions.

White Matter

In man, this formation acquires an enormous thickness, extending from the proximity of the ventricle to the fifth layer and further on. In Golgi preparations from the child of fifteen days, a period in which the myelin has still not appeared in the presubicular white matter, the bundles of fibers go up to the third layer and invade the whole fourth and fifth layers.

Such a richness in fibers, producing large topographic variants in the form and disposition of the layers, makes it impossible to try to

find out the origin, trajectory, and termination of the exogenous fibers, and presents no little difficulty in following the endogenous axons.

On account of these difficulties, we had recourse to those small mammals, such as the mouse, guinea pig, and rabbit, in which the white matter is reduced to the minimum. In these animals, it is easily recognizable that the presubicular white matter, like that of the subiculum, has two formations of fibers: a *deep* or subventricular, composed of thin fibers (fig, 41, *G*) [*fig. 167*], which, as shown in serial sagittal and frontal sections, are continuous with the dorsal psalterium; and another *superficial*, underlying the presubicular cortex, formed by thick myelinated fibers arranged in small bundles that sagittal sections reveal obliquely or cross-sectioned (figs. 30, *E*; 41, *e*) [*figs. 160, 167*].

The fibers forming this superficial plane of

the white matter are of three kinds: (1) Those representing the continuation of the axons of the presubicular cortex, continuations that are often fibers that bifurcate in a thick and a thin branch. In sagittal sections of the cerebrum of the mouse of four days, we have observed sometimes that one of the branches, commonly the thicker, runs definitely medially and then forward (after a variable ascending trajectory in the fibrous plane under study), to enter the commissural optic pathway. This continuity is especially visible in the most lateral sagittal sections of the cerebrum (fig. 31) [*fig. 161*]. (2) Numerous branched fibers arriving from the white matter and continuous with the dense plexus aforementioned. (3) Let us also add for completeness the emergence, from the mentioned plane of thick fibers, of collaterals destined to ramify in the presubicular cortex, and which may originate in the same manner from endogenous fibers rather than from exogenous fibers.

The preceding notes about the structure of the subicular and presubicular cortices makes the opinion extremely probable that these sphenoidal territories lack olfactory significance. And our thinking on this matter is based not only on the special texture of such regions but also on the fact of these areas being interposed in the course of important association pathways that do not come either directly or indirectly, as we will point out, from primary and secondary olfactory foci.

IV. Pathways Originating from the Sphenoidal Cortex[G]

The inferior sphenoidal or olfactory cortex possesses, like all the sensory areas, three centrifugal pathways: first, *a commissural pathway,* by means of which it enters into communication with the homonymous cortex of the contralateral side; second, *a projection pathway* which, after traversing the corpus striatum and descending with the pyramidal system, terminates in the motor foci of the [medulla oblongata] and spinal cord; third, *an internal pathway of association,* which links mainly the anterior parts with the posterior parts of the sphenoidal cortex. We will deal with the pathways originating in the presu-

biculum when we talk about the exogenous streams of Ammon's horn.

Anterior Commissure

It is a general belief since the important works of Ganser[17] and Gudden, confirmed by Edinger, Kölliker, Elliot Smith, Löwenthal, Probst, and others, that this commissure represents a system of union between symmetrical parts of the cortex of the rhinencephalon, that is to say, of the olfactory bulb, of the piriform lobe, of the amygdala, and of the subradicular region of the inferior surface of the frontal lobe. The old opinion of Meynert, who considered the said pathway to be a mixed system of commissural fibers and of crossed fibers, by means of which the olfactory bulb would be linked with the contralateral hemisphere, is at present rightly abandoned.

The proofs of the interolfactory character of the pathway of the anterior commissure are numerous and quite well known, so that we do not need to indicate them here. Omitting the fact that the said commissure reaches a great development in the macrosmatic animals (mole, dog, rabbit, mouse, etc.) and a weak development in the microsmatic, there are two [other] completely decisive facts of observation. (1) One of them is the symmetrical degeneration of the cited commissure when the nervous foci from which [its fibers] come are removed. We, like Löwenthal and Probst, have cut the olfactory bulb in the rabbit and guinea pig, and have consistently observed degeneration in the anterior half of the commissure, that is to say, in the bulbar portion of the same, which is prolonged on the normal side up to the layer of the granule cells of the olfactory bulb. When the piriform lobe is lesioned, the degeneration is limited to the posterior or sphenoidal portion of the commissure. (2) But the decisive proof of the olfactory commissural character of the pathway under study is given by the direct anatomical observation of vertical and horizontal sections of the cerebrum of small mammals, previously stained with the procedure of Weigert and even better, as we have made, with that of Golgi. These serial sections show without any doubt that the anterior commissure, as demonstrated by Ganser and as confirmed by Edinger, Obersteiner, Kölliker, and others, consists of two bundles: one anterior with a horseshoe shape, whose arms run forward, entering the olfactory bulbs; and another posterior, whose horns, directed backward, get lost in the thickness of the piriform lobe and in the vicinity of the sphenoidal cortex.

Anterior or Bulbar Portion of the Commissure

As is seen in fig. 32, A [fig. 162], the fibers of the *anterior or interbulbar portion* are thin, although not as thin as those of the posterior portion; they run in a compact transverse bundle at the level of the midline, without

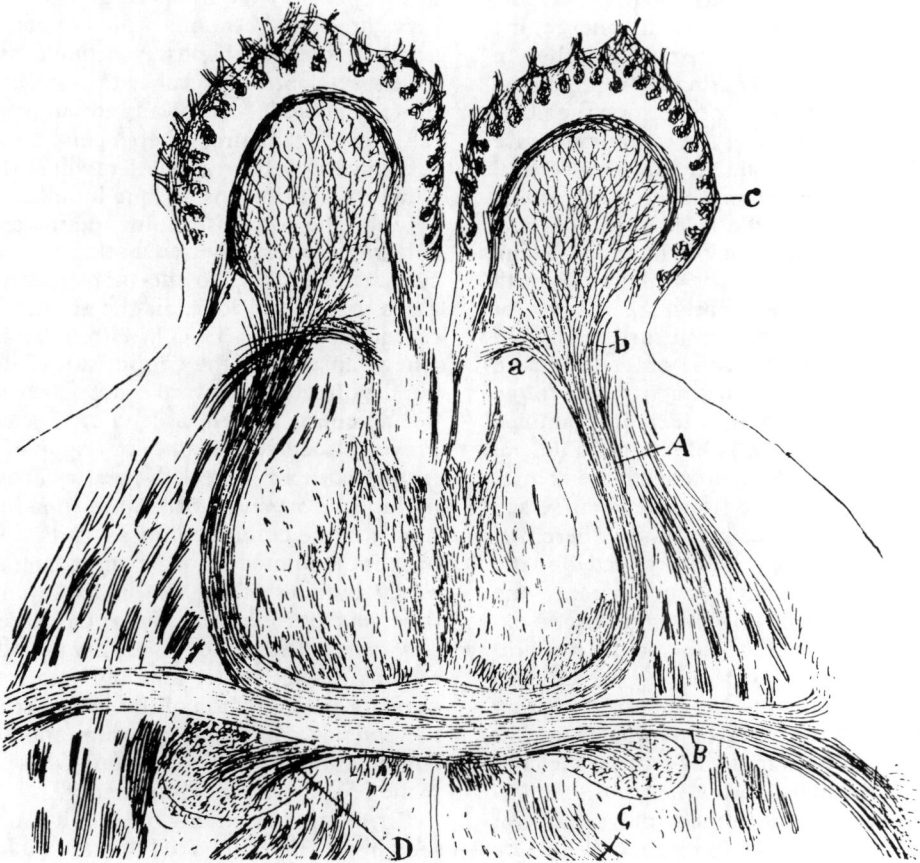

[FIG. 162] Fig. 32. Horizontal section of the brain of the newborn mouse. Anterior commissure and olfactory bulbs. A, anterior portion of the commissure; B, posterior or sphenoidal portion; C, columns of the fornix; D, bundle incorporated into the pathway of projection of the sphenoidal cortex; a, superior terminal bundle of the commissure; b, principal or external bundle; c, plexus of commissural fibers in the internal plexiform layer.

branches or deviations, and once they arrive in proximity to the corpus striatum, not far from the *great olfactory projection pathway,* they curve to become dorsoventral and reach the frontal lobe. At the level of the head of the corpus striatum, the bundle diverges in a fan-shaped manner, being concentrated in three principal radiations: the *external* or thick, destined for the lateral and inferior half of the bulb and its pedicle; the *intermediate,* distributed in the internal bulbar sector; and the *internal,* which runs directly medially, tracing an arc with a posterior concavity and getting lost in the superior bulbar region, as well as in the cortical gray matter lying above the olfactory pedicle. In their long trajectory, the fibers of the anterior bundle of the commissure give off only very rare collaterals all with a vertical course and with an unknown destination. Only when they arrive at the layer of the granule cells do ramifications and dichotomies begin. In summary, therefore, and in harmony with the data revealed [previously] the anterior or bulbar portion of the commissure consists of olfactory neurons of second order, that is to say, of direct axons originating from the tufted cells of one side, and which are ramified among the granule cells of the contralateral side; and as these [cells] propagate the contralateral impulse received from the said fibers to the mitral and tufted cells, it results, therefore, that each olfactory excitation collected by the bulb of one side is split into two streams: one *direct,* which will flow to the homolateral external root, draining into the homolateral limbic cortex; and the other *indirect,* which runs in the anterior commissure and, propagating to the contralateral mitral and tufted cells, will also be transmitted along this route to the contralateral sphenoidal cortex. Thus, the unilateral stimulus is transformed into a bilateral one, and the [sensory] impression collected by one group of olfactory bipolar cells will provoke the uniform activity of almost the whole central olfactory system.

According to Ganser, the anterior portion of the commissure would also supply some bundles to the internal capsule, which would propagate them to the piriform lobe. Kölliker has confirmed [the presence of] this bundle in the rabbit but not in the mouse. We have not been able, either, to observe it clearly in this animal, from which figs. 32 and 33 [*figs. 162, 163*] have been taken.

Sphenoidal Portion

This bundle of the commissure is also perceptible in fig. 32, B [*fig. 162*], where it is seen near the midline plane, closely attached to the bulbar portion, being situated between this and the [columns of the fornix] that appear transversely sectioned. But a fruitful examination of this pathway requires comparison of transverse or frontal sections with horizontal sections. In these, it is observed that when [the sphenoidal portion] reaches the cortex of the piriform lobe, it is resolved into an infinity of fan-shaped radiating fibers, penetrating the deep layers of the gray matter, where they engender a tight plexus. A long bundle, situated between the corpus striatum and the sphenoidal gray matter, directed backward, provides commissural fibers to the more posterior regions of the said lobe. In the frontal section reproduced in fig. 33, G [*fig. 163*] can be seen a new radiation of the commissure. The thick bundle directed backward is not observed here, but a robust, arched, ascending fascicle that provides fibers to the superior region of the olfactory cortex is revealed; this, on arriving in the upper part and quite diminished in thickness, has the contingent of axons that remain in it incorporated into the most lateral horizontal bundles of the corpus callosum. It is thus very possible that the anterior commissure receives fibers not only from the olfactory regions of the frontal lobe but also from the upper or lateral region of this lobe; in this way, the ends of the corpus callosum and anterior commissure form a continuous whole in the plane of the cortical white matter.

Besides this ascending bundle, it can also be seen in fig. 33, F [*fig. 163*] that the bulk of the fibers of the sphenoidal portion of the commissure radiate out into the cortex situated anteriorly, and are there distributed in the third, fourth, and fifth layers.

How do the frontosphenoidal fibers of the anterior commissure begin and terminate? Here is a subject about which no author has been able to formulate a relatively precise opinion. Kölliker confesses to ignorance on

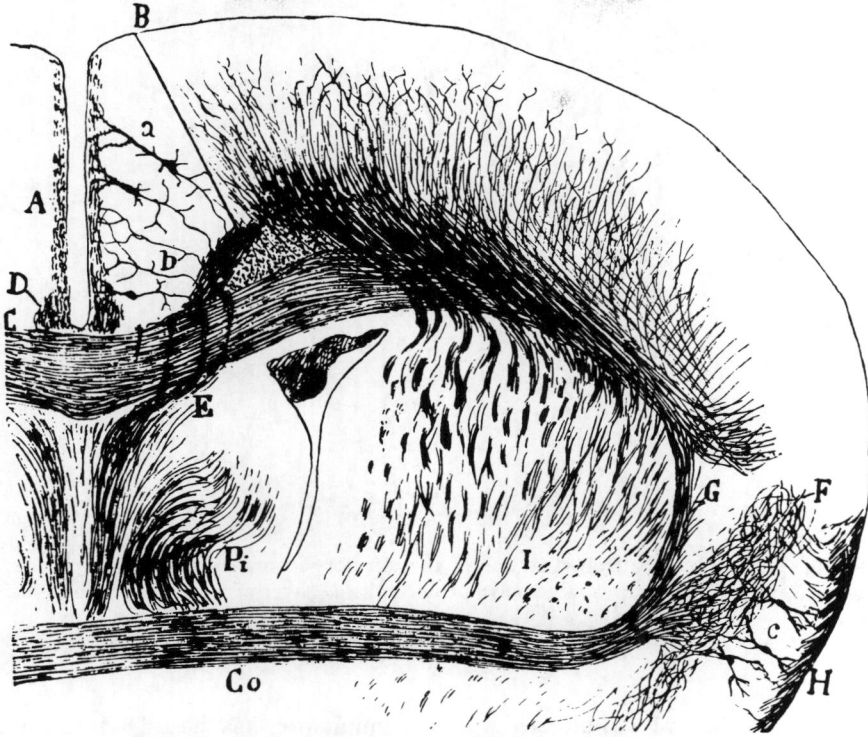

[*FIG. 163*]   Fig. 33. Frontal section of the cerebrum of a mouse of four days. *A*, interhemispheric cortex; *B*, cingulum; *C*, corpus callosum; *D*, internal stria; *E*, fornix longus; *F*, plexus of collaterals of the interhemispheric cortex; *G*, ascending prolongation of the anterior commissure; *H*, fibers of the external olfactory root; *Co*, anterior commissure; *Pi*, anterior pillar of the fornix.

the kinds of relations that are established between the said fibers and the cells of the piriform lobe, and we, after persistent attempts to resolve this problem in small mammals (mouse and rat), have hardly achieved any advance beyond the histologist of Würzburg.

As is seen in fig. 33, *c* [*fig. 163*], the posterior commissural fibers are centripetal and centrifugal; that is to say, some begin and others terminate in the piriform lobe of each side. The terminal fibers tracing a curving course gain the layer of white matter, and on arriving among the polymorphic cells and the pyramidal cells (third layer) which in the newborn mouse are not well developed, the fibers ramify prolixly and engender a very dense termi-

nal plexus. It is precisely this plexus, which we reproduce in somewhat simplified [form] in fig. 33, *F* [*fig. 163*], that is the largest obstacle to the determination of the origins of the axons, because when these appear stained, the plexus is almost always completely impregnated, and, by the abundance of its fibers and their very complicated trajectory, prevent the axons originating in this region from being followed successfully. However, in a few cases, we believe that we have seen that the commissural fibers are none other than the long, deeper nervous collaterals originating from the axon of cells of the piriform lobe. In fig. 34, *d*, *e*, *f* [*fig. 164*], we reproduce several cells whose axon ran backward, entering the corona

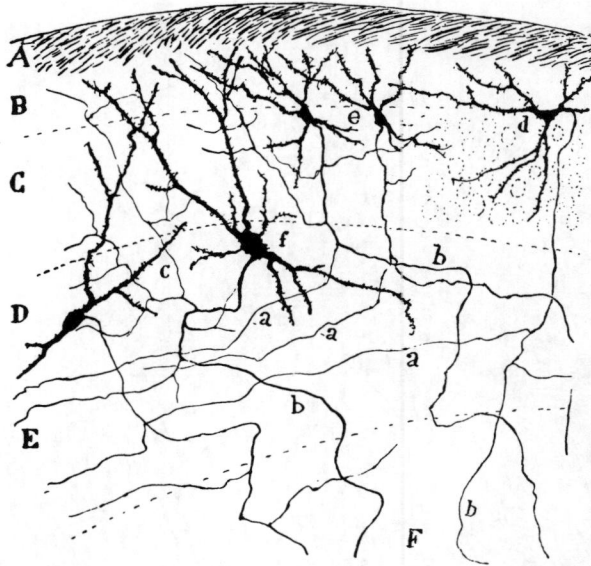

[*FIG. 164*]   Fig. 34. Portion of a frontal section of the olfactory frontal cortex (mouse of a few days). *A,* olfactory fibers; *B,* plexiform layer; *C,* large polymorphic cells; *D,* layer of the pyramidal and fusiform cells; *E,* white matter.

radiata, whereas a collateral was directed upward to the plane of entrance of the anterior commissure. When we studied the sphenoidal cortex of man and of the cat, we pointed out also that many of the axons originating in this region gave off at the level of the white matter one or two thin, long collaterals that could very well enter the anterior commissure; a similar disposition is also very common in the mouse, where it is observed in almost all the cells, including the superficial polymorphics. Because of all this, we are inclined to think that the commissural fibers of the sphenoidal portion represent in their vast majority long collaterals of the cells of the piriform lobe, and very particularly of the frontal region of the same. By this we do not pretend to exclude the involvement of direct axons from cells of medium volume; their participation is observed in the olfactory lobe and in certain regions of the bulbar pedicle (see fig. 11, *a*) [*fig. 141*], and it would not be strange if they should exist also in the region of the piriform lobe. For the rest, the existence of afferent fibers ramifying in the piriform lobe and probably linked with the

commissure has already been indicated by Kölliker.

Besides the connections described, the posterior arm of the commissure receives an important bundle of the projection or centrifugal pathway of the sphenoidal lobe, a pathway extraordinarily robust in the rodents, and which the authors know by the name of *stria cornea, taenia semicircularis,* etc.

As shown in figs. 32, *D,* and 35, *B* [*figs. 162, 165*], at the moment that this robust pathway of projection gets close to the external side of the septum lucidum and passes behind the anterior commissure, a group of its fibers, the most dorsal and superior, to be precise, separates from the large centrifugal stream and enters the commissural system. It is very possible that these fibers are of two kinds, centripetal and centrifugal, and that by means of them an association is established between the deepest and posterior portions of the sphenoidal lobe of both sides. The fascicle alluded to, which has been very well described by Kölliker, could be called the *posterior arm of the commissure.* Its position in relation to the other two appears clearly in fig. 32, D [fig. 162]. We will talk later about the origin of the *taenia,* and we will review the ideas of Kölliker on the significance of the same.

In man, the anterior commissure is less well known than in animals. It is thought, nevertheless, and apparently proved by the investigations of Meynert, Henle, Dejerine, Brissaud, Edinger, and others, that its structural plan coincides substantially with that of the macrosmatic vertebrates. In it can be recognized also the two bundles, *anterior* and *posterior;* but it has not been possible to establish their terminal connections with security because of the difficulty of applying direct anatomical methods to the subject and especially on account of the excessive distance which makes the efficient pursuit of the fibers impossible. There is no doubt, however, that from examinations of transverse sections of the human cerebrum the said commissure, as in animals, establishes relationships not only with the hippocampal gyrus and with the frontal and bulbar olfactory regions but also with the sphenoidal gyri.

Motor or Projection Pathway of the Sphenoidal Cortex

As is well known, from the entire sphenoidal cortex come nerve fibers destined for the corona radiata, which, at first concentrated near the ventricle and then running forward, gain the lenticular nucleus and enter the cerebral peduncle. Following completely this important pathway in gyrencephalic mammals is extremely difficult because of the length and curvature of its trajectory; however, in the guinea pig and especially in the mouse, it is an easy task to follow the whole of its complicated curve and to reveal its entrance into the peduncle.

In fig. 35, B [fig. 165], we reproduce a frontal section of the cerebrum of the mouse of a few days, in which the entire course of the cited

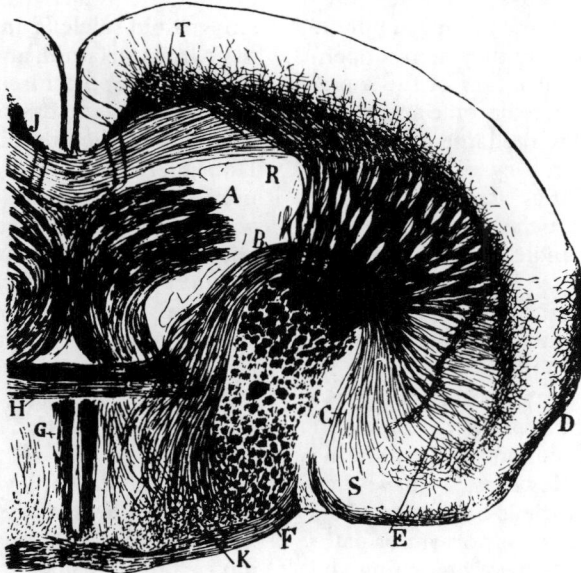

[FIG. 165]   Fig. 35. Frontal section of the cerebrum of a mouse of four days. (The section is so thick that it is equivalent to three ordinary sections.) A, columns of the fornix; B, olfactory projection pathway; C, origin of this pathway in the sphenoidal cortex; D, olfactory sphenoidal cortex; E, lenticular nucleus of the corpus striatum; F, optic tract; G, middle radiation of the septum; H, anterior commissure; J, cingulum; K, olfactory pathway of projection; R, caudal nucleus of the corpus striatum; T, arcuate or superior longitudinal bundle of the cerebrum.

pathway appears. In fact, it is impossible to see the totality of the olfactory projection bundle in only one thin section, but it is feasible in a very thick and transparent frontal section, [which is] somewhat oblique from forward to backward. Notice that this bundle comes equally from the external and medial sphenoidal cortex, that is to say, from that underlying the expansion of the external olfactory root, and from the internal region or amygdaloid nucleus. From all of these places, the fibers go upward and forward, arranged in thin bundles, crossing the gray nuclei of the lenticular nucleus of the corpus striatum, to converge finally in a compact and robust bundle that is situated above the thick bundles of the motor pathway (fig. 35, *B*) [*fig. 165*]. Once at this point, they go medially, describing an arc with an inferior concavity and situated underneath the epithelium of the ventricle; then they pass inside the bundles of the cerebral peduncle, and outside the septum lucidum, occupied at this level by the columns of the fornix; they then cross behind the sphenoidal portion of the commissure, to which they send, as we have already mentioned, a bundle of thin threads; and finally they arrive, opening their small bundles like fans, at the suprachiasmatic white matter, to become anteroposterior and to be added to the large peduncular formation, inside which they will occupy the most internal and inferior area. Some of the descending bundles are more internal, separate from the main bundle, mix with the descending pathway of the septum (fig. 35) [*fig. 165*], and end precisely in the same area of the cerebral peduncle in which the olfactory bundle of projection ends.

In this very long trajectory, the cited olfactory pathway does not give off collaterals; if these exist, it still does not possess them in the mouse of eight days. However, we have seen inside the lenticular nucleus bifurcated fibers arriving from the inferior portion of this pathway, which give indications of branching and terminating in the olfactory cortex. Their branches, however, could not be followed to their terminations because of the labyrinthine trajectory that they have when they arrive in the deep layer of the said cortices. In their terminal or descending portion, that is to say,

during their trajectory toward the suprachiasmatic region, the small bundles of this system of projection are separated by numerous fusiform, triangular, or ovoid nerve cells, provided with divergent dendrites and whose axon has seemed to us to descend, incorporating the peduncle and becoming anteroposterior. These cells correspond perhaps to the basal nucleus of Ganser.[H]

The pathway we have just described is none other than the *stria cornea* or *taenia semicircularis* of the human cerebrum, a bundle of white matter that runs superficially between the corpus striatum and the optic thalamus in the floor of the lateral ventricle. About the origin and termination of this pathway there is much uncertainty, due to the impossibility of revealing, by means of the method of Weigert and in the higher mammals, the effective connections of the fibers. Thus, Kölliker,[18] who has dedicated much attention to this point and has studied the said pathway in Weigert preparations of the rabbit, is inclined to admit that the stria has its main origin in the cortex at the pole of the ventricular inferior horn, in the amygdaloid nucleus and lenticular nucleus of the corpus striatum, and has its termination in front of the optic chiasm in a gray nucleus that is identical to the basal ganglion of Ganser.

A similar dictum has been pronounced by Honegger,[19] who also supposed that connections existed between the said pathway and the claustrum, the anterior column of the fornix and the optic thalamus. To Dejerine,[20] the taenia represents an olfactory pathway of third order, which contains fibers arising from the amygdala and terminating in the olfactory area, and fibers that arise in the anterior perforated substance and septum lucidum, and whose terminal arborizations would be in the amygdala.

In fig. 36 [*fig. 166*], we reproduce the trajectory of the fibers of the mentioned pathway in the lenticular and amygdaloid nuclei of the mouse of fifteen days. Notice that the vast majority of the fibers do not run subventricularly, as Kölliker thinks, but pass through the lenticular nucleus, to be directed toward the exterior and to assail the very complicated deep plexus of the olfactory sphenoidal cortex, a plexus in which the axons of the cells of this

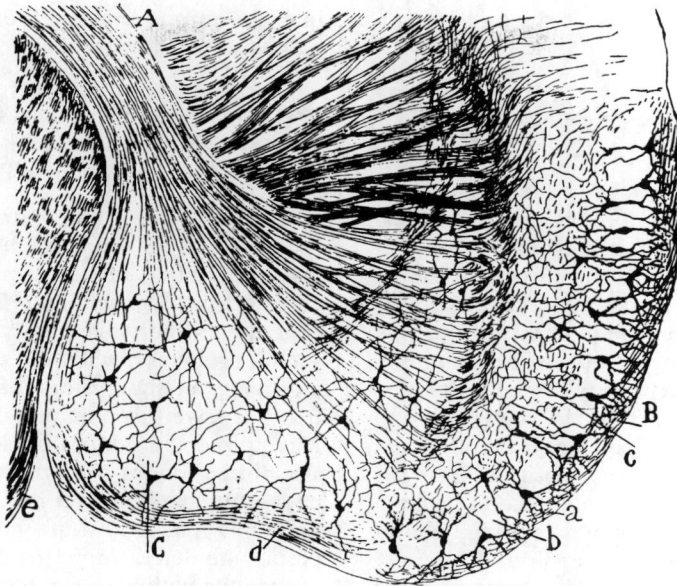

[*FIG. 166*]   Fig. 36. Frontal section of the sphenoidal cortex of the mouse of fifteen days. *A,* pathway of projection of the sphenoidal cortex; *B,* olfactory cortex; *C,* amygdaloid nucleus; *a,* layer of olfactory fibers; *b,* layer of large polymorphic cells; *c,* plexus of the deep layers; *d,* tangential bundle of the amygdala; *e,* optic tract.

cortical region are going to end, after tracing many flexuosities. The amygdaloid nucleus definitely receives fibers, but so far it has not been possible for us to reveal the continuity of any axons with the axons of the cells in this nucleus. Even more, we believe that the majority of the amygdaloid cells, like those in the lenticular nucleus, are cells with short axon that resolves into extensive free arborizations. Even in the largest cells of the said nuclei, the axon usually bifurcates at no great distance, and the trajectory of the branches is so extensive and complicated that it is not possible to ascertain their continuity with the fibers of the projection pathway. It is very possible, furthermore, that the fibers destined for the amygdaloid nucleus are fibers of termination and not fibers of origin, and that they are arborized in the cortex of [the amygdala], from which originates an arciform border pathway (fig. 36, *d*) [*fig. 166*], which skims underneath and inside the said nucleus and ends, as we have observed in more anterior sections of the sphenoidal cortex, in the large pathway of the inferior and internal portion of the cerebral peduncle.

In summary, and without granting that the problem is definitively resolved in all its points, we believe that we can affirm that the *stria semicircularis* represents a mixed commissural and projection pathway of the sphenoidal olfactory cortex. The vast majority of its fibers would arise from the cells of this cortex, and a small portion of the same would possibly originate (or perhaps terminate) in the cortical portion of the amygdaloid nucleus.

With regard to their terminations, the bulk of the fibers would enter the cerebral peduncle, whereas some contingents would terminate, after being incorporated in the anterior commissure, in the contralateral sphenoidal olfactory cortex.

For the rest, the amygdaloid nucleus seems to us, as Kölliker affirms, an annex of the corpus striatum and not an olfactory center. Direct olfactory fibers do not penetrate it, since those of the external root stop, as is observed in fig. 36, *B* [*fig. 166*], in the inferior apex of the sphenoidal cortex. Neither in Marchi preparations is it possible to reveal the entrance of degenerated fibers into the said nucleus (preliminary section of the bulb and olfactory lobe).

Dorsoventral Association Pathway of the Sphenoidal Cortex

When horizontal sections of the cerebrum of the mouse that pass through the sphenoidal region are examined, it is observed that, besides the white matter concentrated in the vicinity of the corpus striatum and lateral ventricle, there exists in the thickness of the gray cortex a multitude of robust fibers running dorsoventrally, which are in all the gray layers of the said cortex except the molecular and that of the superficial polymorphic cells. Such fibers are so long that the majority go from the dorsal pole of the sphenoidal lobe to its anterior end and the frontal olfactory region; others are somewhat shorter, ending in intermediate regions. In their course, some of them often change direction, getting close to the white matter or also to the molecular layer, but without apparently leaving the olfactory cortex, in which they arborize and terminate.

The cited fibers have seemed to us to represent, in their majority, branches of bifurcation of axons of projection of cells in the layer of the superficial polymorphic cells and of underlying cells. Some, however, resemble direct axons of intrinsic cells because of their notable thickness.

For the rest, the existence of intragriseal association fibers arising by the bifurcation of axons of projection (either inside the gray matter or in the white matter) does not constitute a unique feature of the olfactory cortex; we have found it also as a general structural feature in other cortical regions in the brains of the mouse, rabbit, and guinea pig. Even more, we believe, as the result of our recent investigations (which we will publish opportunely), that the majority of the fibers of projection give off long-distance association fibers, and that a good part of the association systems described in the human cerebrum by the authors are not direct or exclusive pathways established between two cerebral nervous territories, but bundles of collaterals or branches of bifurcation arising from the course of projection of fibers whose main branch, incorporated

into the corpus striatum, constitutes a motor pathway.[1]

VIII. Systems of Exogenous Fibers That Penetrate Ammon's Horn and the Fascia Dentata; Spheno-Ammonic Pathway

One of the more transcendental points about the anatomy of Ammon's horn is the origin and termination of its exogenous fibers. Nobody will be surprised, therefore, given the exceptional importance that the resolution of such a problem has for the elucidation of the physiological significance of Ammon's horn, that we have given it very special attention. Having recognized, of course, that the excessive dimensions of the structures and the richness of the white matter in the gyri of the cat, dog, and man constitute an insurmountable obstacle to determining the origin of the cited exogenous pathways, we have worked preferentially (with both the method of Weigert and that of Golgi) in the rabbit, guinea pig, and mouse. In the last especially, the more demonstrative preparations have been obtained, as proven in the following figures.

But before entering into the exposition of our observations, let us survey the state of the question. In general, the authors suppose that the exogenous fibers of Ammon's horn and the fascia dentata come from the olfactory ganglia, entering them in the column of the fornix. They add, furthermore, that relationships exist between the gyrus uncinatus and the cingulum, on the one hand, and Ammon's horn on the other; but they tell us nothing about the origin and termination of the fibers or the precise positions of the [contact] relationships.

But let us cite particularly some authoritative opinions.

Kölliker, who has studied the fornix and the septum lucidum of several mammals with the help of the Weigert method, is inclined to accept that the secondary olfactory centers (piriform lobe, pedicle of the bulb, olfactory tubercule, etc.) send axons to Ammon's horn, but along the following route: first, they would arrive at the olfactory radiation of the *septum lucidum* (*radiation* of Zuckerkandl), from which they would reach (some passing through the corpus callosum, others attaching to the genu

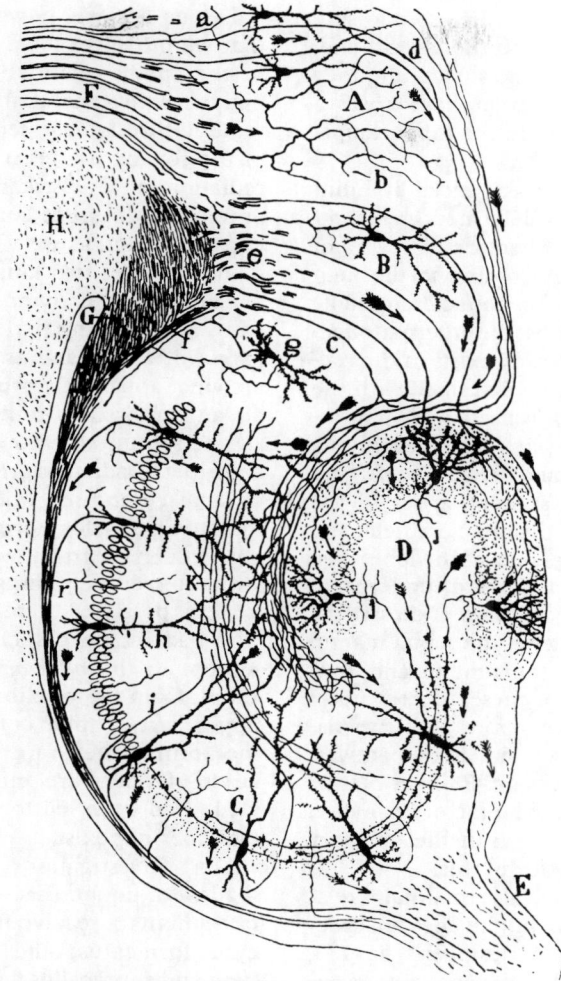

[*FIG. 167*]   Fig. 41. Scheme of the structure and connections of Ammon's horn. *A*, ganglion of the occipital pole; *B*, subiculum; *C*, Ammon's horn; *D*, fascia dentata; *E*, fimbria; *F*, cingulum; *G*, crossed angular bundle; *H*, corpus callosum; *a*, axons penetrating the cingulum; *b*, cingular fibers terminating in the focus of the occipital pole; *c*, perforant spheno-ammonic fibers; *d*, perforant cingular fibers; *e*, plane of the superior spheno-ammonic fibers; *g*, cell of the subiculum; *h*, pyramidal cells of the superior region of Ammon's horn; *i*, ascending collaterals of the large pyramidal cells; *j*, axon of a granule cell; *r*, collaterals of the fibers of the alveus. [Items *h–r* are not indicated in the caption appearing in the original paper, nor in the *Textura*. We have taken these from the caption for the same figure as reproduced in chapter 31 of the *Histologie*.]

of this) the white matter of the cingulate gyrus; from there, they would then go to Ammon's horn, where they would perhaps be continuous with those branched centripetal fibers that we had seen to leave the alveus,[21] and terminate in the strata *radiatum, lacunosum* and *moleculare* of [Ammon's] horn. Kölliker[22] does

not give details about the point of arrival at this center. We do not know, thus, if the door of entrance for the said olfactory pathway is the subiculum or the column of the fornix. Perhaps it is the latter, for, in the opinion of [Kölliker], between the subiculum and Ammon's horn, the relationship is not centripetal but centrifugal; that is to say, the axons arising from Ammon's horn pass to the alveus, and, going up in the cortex of the subiculum, they arborize in it, and from it perhaps arises a new pathway terminating in the hippocampal gyrus.

A similar dictum was pronounced by Edinger, the author who has dedicated special attention to the study of olfactory pathways of the lower vertebrates. According to the neurologist of Frankfurt,[23] the olfacto-ammonic pathway is represented by the internal olfactory radiation, which already exists in the reptilian brain, and which he described with the name of *tractus cortico-olfactorius septi.* The ascending olfactory pathway, described in the mammals by Zuckerkandl (*Riechbündel der Ammonshornes* of this author), arises in the medullary substance of the olfactory field, and especially in the internal face of the lobe, then running medially and backward, underneath the genu of the corpus callosum, it crosses the septum and, finally, reaches the septal margin of the fornix to enter the fimbria and Ammon's horn. One part of these afferent fibers would be crossed in the septum, but the majority would constitute a homolateral pathway. In other passages of his book, Edinger betrays the suspicion that the cited olfactory radiation of the septum has its origin in the olfactory bulb, perhaps in the cortex of this.

Ammon's horn would also maintain relations with the cingulum, but he does not specify how this takes place. In [Edinger's] fig. 183, the cingulum, as reproduced, appears as an extended pathway from the olfactory lobe to near the subiculum, whereas in [his] fig. 379, where the fascicles of long-distance association fibers are shown, the said bundle appears prolonged posteriorly to the sphenoidal pole of the cerebrum. It is seen from this that the thoughts of Edinger fluctuate between several opinions. With regard to the *gyrus fornicatus,*[1] he doubts greatly that it maintains connections with Ammon's horn.

The ideas of Kölliker and Edinger, which reproduce in part the already old opinions of Broca, Honegger, Ganser, and Zuckerkandl, are shared by the majority of modern neurologists, such as Turner, van Gehuchten, Elliot Smith, Löwenthal, etc.

Let us declare, however, that all the work that we ourselves have devoted to confirming in the small, essentially macrosmatic, mammals the existence of an olfactory pathway extending through the septum into the columns of the fornix, has been in vain. Naturally the radiation of Zuckerkandl exists, but in our opinion it does not come from the olfactory cortex; in fact, as we will see in other work,[24] it incorporates two kinds of fiber: descending or centrifugal, arriving from the gyrus fornicatus and forming part of the so called *fornix longus* cf Forel, and ascending or centripetal, arriving, apparently, from the cerebral peduncle and arborizing in the septum.

The septum definitely receives, therefore, a centripetal radiation arriving from lower levels of the cerebrum; but these fibers, whose [putative] olfactory origin we have not been able to demonstrate, terminate in the septum without ever trespassing beyond its borders. It is very possible, therefore, that the authors who had included such afferent fibers to the septum in the *olfactory radiation* of Zuckerkandl, from the proximity of the same, in the upper part of their course, to the column of the fornix (there are places in which both kinds of fibers are mixed up and intermingled), had been led to believe in a continuity that does not exist.

Our investigations prove, without any shadow of doubt, that Ammon's horn and the fascia dentata receive fibers originating in the gyrus fornicatus, others come from the *indusium* and supracallosal striae, and especially in a very robust system, truly colossal in the small mammals, originated from a singular ganglion located at the posterior border of the spheno-occipital cortex, a ganglion whose nature we have not been able to determine[25] in spite of many investigations. Let us add still, for completeness, the group of fibers coming from the subiculum and penetrating the alveus of Ammon's horn. In summary, this organ and the fascia dentata, are penetrated by and are the destination of the cited spheno-ammonic pathway, of the *cingulum,* of the *nerves* of Lancisi, and of the pathway originating in the cells of the subiculum, or *subiculo-ammonic pathway.* Notice that all these pathways have their door of entrance in the white matter of the subiculum and presubiculum, centers that can be considered as the atrium for the afferent fibers to Ammon's horn and the fascia dentata.

With regard to the centrifugal system of Ammon's horn, it is none other than the fimbria and its continuation as the column of the fornix and radiation of the *tuber cinereum*. The so-called *fornix longus* of Forel does not appear to have relations with Ammon's horn; according to the general opinion, confirmed by us, it comes from the gyrus fornicatus and perhaps also from the indusium, representing the projection or peduncular pathway of the cells in these centers.

Spheno-ammonic Pathway

At the posterior border of the spheno-occipital cortex of the mouse, rabbit, and guinea pig, immediately underneath that concavity in which the upper surface of the superior colliculus lodges, lies a nervous nucleus perfectly demarcated from the rest of the cerebral cortex, from which it is distinguished, especially in Golgi preparations (fig. 43, A) [*fig. 169*], by exhibiting a very tight nerve plexus in the middle and superficial layers. To avoid prejudgments, and alluding to its position at the angle formed by the posterior border of the occipital lobe, where it is continuous with the sphenoidal [lobe], we will call this ganglion the *angular or spheno-occipital center*. The Nissl method reveals in this cortical subdivision a more complicated texture than that of the other cerebral regions, for, besides the four classic layers, it presents a new deep layer, formed by granule cells, and another superficial or second [layer], made up of stellate cells. The details of the structure of this singular focus and the possible conjectures about its nature will be found in other work in this same journal.[K]

For the moment, we wish to state that from the giant and medium pyramidal cells and the stellate cells of this focus comes a very robust association pathway, directed toward Ammon's horn. This pathway is none other than the bundle situated in the white matter of the subiculum, from whose superficial portion, as many authors have seen, come ascending radiated bundles that, after crossing the portion of the subiculum closest to Ammon's horn, reach the molecular layer of this (*stratum lacunosum et moleculare*) to ramify and terminate in its thickness (fig. 42, A), [*fig. 168*]. But the subicular and presubicular white matter contains besides, as we explained previously, another pathway situated above and behind the preceding one (fig. 42, C) [*fig. 168*]; this is the pathway of the cingulum with which we will deal later.

The large spheno-ammonic pathway consists of three formations or bundles: the *angular or crossed bundle* (we call it *angular* because it is located in the fundus of the subicular fold), the *perforant bundles* or direct spheno-ammonic [pathway], and the *spheno-alvear pathway*.

Angular Bundle or Commissural Spheno-ammonic pathway

When sagittal sections of the cerebrum of a small mammal, previously stained with the method of Weigert or of Golgi, are examined, there appears in the white matter of the subiculum, underneath the lateral prolongation of the splenium of the corpus callosum and above Ammon's horn, a very robust and well-demarcated bundle, triangular in section, and whose fibers show up from the callosal [fibers] by being thicker, and from the cingular and perforant spheno-ammonic [fibers] by being somewhat thinner (fig. 42, B) [*fig. 168*].

This bundle runs transversely and somewhat obliquely from down to up, from the cerebral cortex of the spheno-occipital border up to the midline, where it is installed beneath the splenium of the corpus callosum, above the terminal portion of Ammon's horn, constituting, finally, a large portion, if not the totality, of what Ganser and Kölliker have called the *dorsal psalterium*. The determination of the origin and course of so important a pathway is very easy in sagittal sections of the cerebrum of the mouse of a few days. As we show in figs. 43 and 44 [*figs. 169, 170*], which reproduce very lateral sagittal sections, the fibers of the said bundle represent the continuation of the axons of the superior extremity of the angular or sphenoidal focus (*B*). This part of the ganglion possesses a thinner and tighter tex-

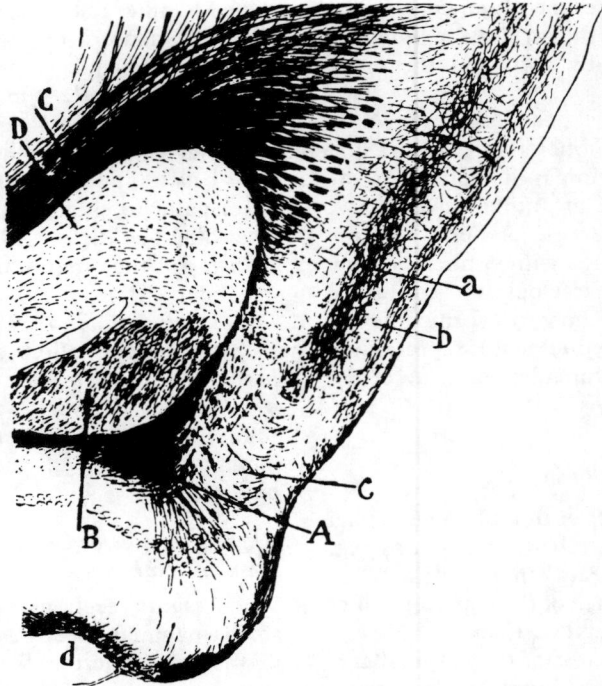

[FIG. 168] Fig. 42. Sagittal section of the cerebrum of the guinea pig. A, section of the ascending perforant ammonic pathway; B, crossed spheno-ammonic angular bundle; C, cingulum; D, corpus callosum; a, intermediary terminal plexus of the nucleus of the occipital pole; b, layer of the small pyramids; c, subiculum; d, fascia dentata. (Method of Weigert-Pal.)

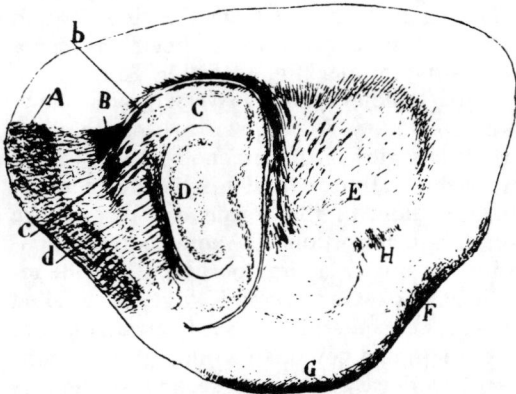

[FIG. 169] Fig. 43. Very lateral sagittal section of the brain of the mouse of a few days. A, angular or spheno-occipital focus; B, angular or crossed bundle; C, superior portion of Ammon's horn; D, fascia dentata; E, corpus striatum; F, external olfactory root; G, sphenoidal olfactory cortex; H, anterior commissure; c, superior perforant bundles of Ammon's horn; d, inferior perforant bundles; b, spheno-alvear pathway. (Method of Golgi.)

ture than that of the rest of the cortex, and arising from it are very numerous axons which first run in a straight line forward, but near the ventricular angle they bend to be directed medially and upward. Thanks to this change of direction, the sagittal sections show such fibers sectioned transversely or obliquely. The continuation of the cited axons with the fibers of the spheno-commissural or angular bundle is verified, commonly at a simple inflection; it is not rare, however, [to see] their division into two branches: one thick, which forms the mentioned bundle, and the other directed laterally, and perhaps destined to gain the corpus striatum and be continuous with the corona radiata. Such bifurcations appear better in horizontal than in sagittal sections, in which naturally both branches are shown endways and cannot be easily followed.

When the sagittal sections are more medial (fig. 45, B) [fig. 171], the angular ganglion has already disappeared, and the crossed spheno-

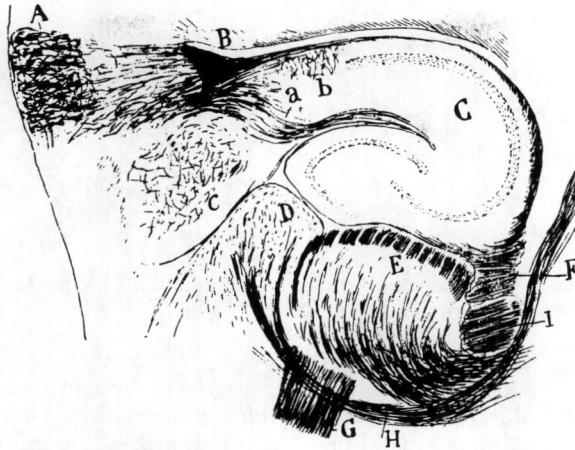

[FIG. 170]   Fig. 44. Very lateral sagittal section of the cerebrum and Ammon's horn of the mouse of eight days. A, lateral border and superior end of the angular or spheno-ammonic focus; B, crossed ammonic bundle; C, Ammon's horn; D, medial geniculate body; E, lateral geniculate body; a, ascending perforant spheno-ammonic pathway. (Method of Golgi.)

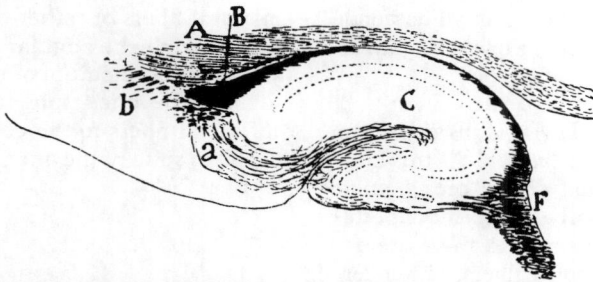

[FIG. 171]   Fig. 45. Another, more internal sagittal section of Ammon's horn and angular or crossed spheno-ammonic bundle. A, corpus callosum; B, crossed spheno-ammonic bundle; C, Ammon's horn; F, fimbria; a, superior perforant spheno-ammonic fibers. Mouse of eight days. (Method of Golgi.)

amonic pathway constitutes a bundle [that is] triangular in section and remains located at the ventricular angle, beneath which it has been displaced a little forward, having abandoned completely the external ependymal wall and covering the deep frontier of the subiculum and a small part of the alveus. The closer we are to the midline, the more is the triangle formed by the perimeter of the said bundle elongated, and its fibers gain more space above the alveus (fig. 46, B) [fig. 172].

Finally, in the sections that pass through the midline or near it, the angular bundle is presented flattened from downward to upward, attached to the corpus callosum, from which it

is separated by fibers of the fornix longus of Forel, and inferiorly extending over a large part of the alveus or superior frontier of Ammon's horn [which is] rudimentary in this place [fig. 175].[L] Often, the angular fibers are shown arranged in separate bundles (fig. 48, B) [fig. 174], which are extended in an oblique thin layer from behind forward and from upward to downward, thanks to which the splenium of the corpus callosum is linked with the more superior commissural bundles originating from the base of the fimbria.

This medial trajectory of the crossed spheno-ammonic pathway is also clearly and expressively observed in frontal sections of the

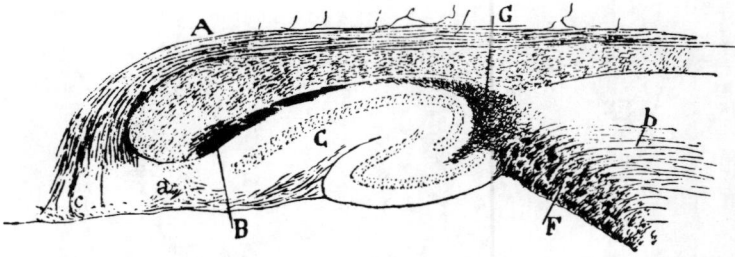

[*FIG. 172*]   Fig. 46. Sagittal section that passed through the cingulum. *A*, cingulum; *B*, angular or crossed bundle; *C*, Ammon's horn. Mouse of eight days. (Method of Golgi.)

cerebrum, which pass through the splenium of the corpus callosum. In these sections, the said pathway is presented as a transverse band of white matter, separated from the corpus callosum by the fornix longus, and lying down between the two subicula over the crowns of both horns of Ammon. In their transverse and central course, the fibers do not appear to change plane or give off collaterals; only uncommonly have we observed a small descending branch that could belong to extraneous fibers of the spheno-ammonic type.

Lateral Termination of the Angular Pathway or Crossed Spheno-ammonic Bundle. As this bundle arrives at the region of the presubicular ganglion, and particularly at the most posterior and inferior regions of this, there are detached from it some robust fibers, either terminal or collateral, which penetrate the cortex of the said focus and engender among the cells a very dense and complicated arborization, with which we have already dealt (fig. 47, *C*) [*fig. 173*]. Such terminal fibers, which represent a portion of the angular pathway, appear to come in the majority or exclusively from the midline. And since the plane of the mentioned pathway also receives axons originating from the pyramidal cells of the presubiculum, which in large part run medially, as we show in fig. 51, *a* [*fig. 177*], it would not be surprising if the mentioned fibers arborizing in the presubicular cortex would represent axons originating from the homonymous, contralateral focus. However, it is not at all possible to exclude a participation in the plexus of the presubicular cortex of fibers originating in the spheno-occipital focus.

Anyway, the fact that fibers detached from the angular pathway terminated in the presubiculum proves that this system is at least double, containing crossed conductors arriving both from the angular nucleus and from the presubiculum. Only the application of anatomicopathological methods, perhaps that of Marchi, might definitively resolve whether both contingents represent exclusively commissural fibers or rather crossed association fibers, linking the angular ganglion of one side and the presubiculum of the contralateral side.

Does the cited spheno-ammonic commissure send fibers to the contralateral Ammon's horn? In spite of the attention we have devoted

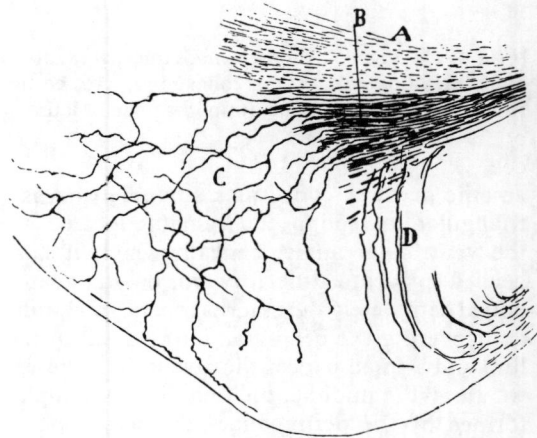

[*FIG. 173*]   Fig. 47. Sagittal section of the subiculum and presubiculum of the mouse of four days. *A*, corpus callosum; *B*, angular bundle; *C*, precommissural focus; *D*, perforant spheno-ammonic bundles. (Method of Golgi.)

to observing the course of the fibers of this bundle, we can say nothing sure about this particular. In several preparations, we have noticed that once the said pathway has passed the midline and arrived at the subiculum of the contralateral side, collaterals and terminal [fibers] with a perforant course were detached and assailed the plexiform layer to enter Ammon's horn; but such fibers had their origin in deep and plexiform levels of the bundle, levels in which the superior perforant spheno-ammonic fibers are mixed up and intermingled with fibers arriving from the cingulum. So it would be impossible to say if the totality of such conductors comes from the cingulum or if a good part of them originates also from the contralateral angular bundle. Anyway, we do not conceal that the latter opinion seems to us the more natural and acceptable. If such an opinion were to be definitely ascertained by experimentation, a good contingent of the angular bundle could be considered as a crossed pathway established between the spheno-occipital ganglion of one side and Ammon's horn of the opposite side, in contradistinction to the direct spheno-ammonic pathways, about which we will talk later.

Let us add, finally, to end this study of the crossed bundle, that at its starting point, in the spheno-occipital focus there are always observed, as we will describe below, centripetal fibers, that is to say, [fibers] arborized in the intermediate nervous plexus of this central focus. Such fibers are not very numerous; if we have to judge by our preparations, they have a point of termination in the superior cellular conglomerate of the angular ganglion, a place

[to which] also come the majority of the centrifugal fibers making up the crossed spheno-ammonic pathway.

In summary, from our observations as a whole about the destination of the fibers of the angular or crossed pathway, it appears very probable that this important transverse bundle consists of at least three categories of conductors: commissural fibers of the presubiculum, commissural fibers of the spheno-occipital focus, and crossed spheno-ammonic fibers. It is clear that at the present state of investigation it is impossible to determine the proportions of each of these fibers or the precise positions that they occupy in sections of the large angular bundle.

The crossed spheno-ammonic pathway that we have described is none other than the *dorsal psalterium* of Ganser and of Kölliker, a transverse pathway [that is] extremely developed in the rodents, and which almost all the authors regard as an interammonic commissure. In fact, Ammon's horn and probably also the subiculum send their commissural fibers to the fimbria and to the *suprafimbrial* bundle of the midline (see below), a general destination also of the projection fibers of those structures. For the rest, that the dorsal psalterium (our *crossed angular or spheno-ammonic pathway*) is extraneous to the fimbria and to the extraventricular alveus, and has few or weak connections with Ammon's horn, is a dictum professed by some authors, among whom we must cite Honegger,[26] who supported the existence of a connection between the said infracallosal commissural bundle and the superficial white lamina of the subiculum. Dejerine[27]

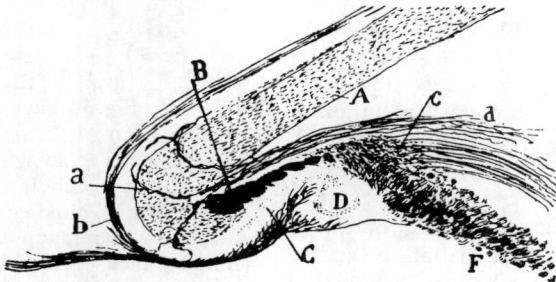

[*FIG. 174*] Fig. 48. Sagittal section close to the midline. *A*, corpus callosum; *B*, dorsal psalterium; *b*, nerves of Lancisi; *C*, Ammon's horn; *D*, fascia dentata. Mouse of eight days. (Method of Golgi.)

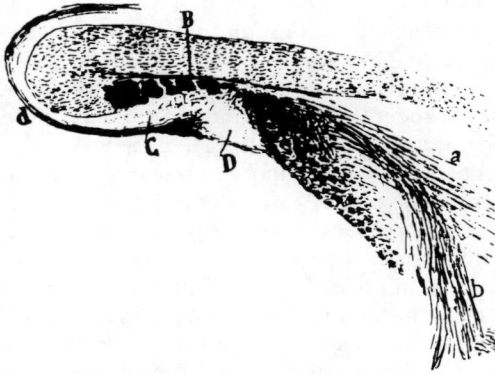

[*FIG. 175*] Fig. 49. Medial sagittal section. *B*, crossed spheno-ammonic pathway; *C*, rudimentary Ammon's horn; *D*, rudiment of fascia dentata; *d*, internal supracallosal stria and fasciola cinerea. Mouse of ten days. (Method of Golgi.)

also admits this link, but affirms (which, at least in the small mammals, we believe doubtful) that the said pathway likewise receives fibers from the cingulum and from the intraventricular alveus. For this author the dorsal psalterium would represent not only an interammonic commissure but also a means of crossed association between the gyrus fornicatus and the contralateral Ammon's horn.

Systems of Perforant Spheno-ammonic Fibers

When dealing with the subiculum, we mentioned the existence of small bundles of fibers that, originating in the white matter, perforate the gray cortex, and are prolonged up to the plexiform layer of the said center and of Ammon's horn. Now we are going to add some details about the origin and termination of such fibers.

Sagittal sections are less appropriate for the study of the origin of the perforant fibers. In them, however, especially when they are very lateral and pass through the angular ganglion or its vicinity, two facts of some importance can be ascertained, namely; first, that the said fibers do not come from the crossed or angular bundle, but directly from the cortex of the homolateral spheno-occipital ganglion and from the medial or inferior portions of this; second, that the perforant bundles are distinguished by their position and directions as *su-*

perior or *ascending* [bundles], which innervate the superior segment of Ammon's horn (superior arched portion of this), and *inferior* oblique or transverse [bundles], which innervate the inferior portions of the said center.

Superior Perforant Bundles. As appears in fig. 54, *F* [*fig. 180*], the superior part of the spheno-occipital focus sends to Ammon's horn, besides the commissural or angular pathway, a group of robust, loose, and plexiform bundles, which are situated in the white matter of the subiculum, behind the cited pathway and in a plane more superficial to it (fig. 51, *D*) [*fig. 177*], and which are converted, finally, into perforant bundles. The sagittal sections show these bundles transversely sectioned (fig. 50, *b*) [*fig. 176*], whereas those parallel to Ammon's horn (fig. 52, *C*) [*fig. 178*] show them lengthways. The closer the sagittal sections are to the midline, the poorer they appear in perforant fibers, which are lacking completely or reduced to weak vestiges in the midline or commissural region. In fig. 50, *b* [*fig. 176*], we show these fibers as they appear in sections of the

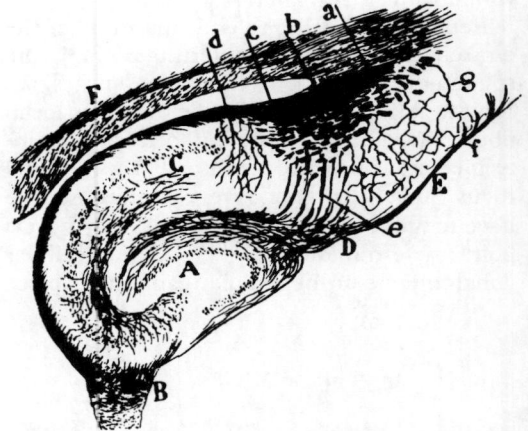

[*FIG. 176*] Fig. 50. Sagittal section of the height of Ammon's horn. *A*, fascia dentata; [*B*], fimbria; *C*, Ammon's horn; *D*, subiculum; *E*, presubiculum; *a*, ascending loose bundles situated underneath the presubiculum; *b*, bundles of the same kind situated beneath the subiculum; *e*, perforant spheno-ammonic bundles of the subiculum; *c*, angular or crossed bundle; *d*, collaterals of the spheno-alvear pathway; *g*, terminal fibers in the presubiculum. Mouse of ten days. (Method of Golgi.)

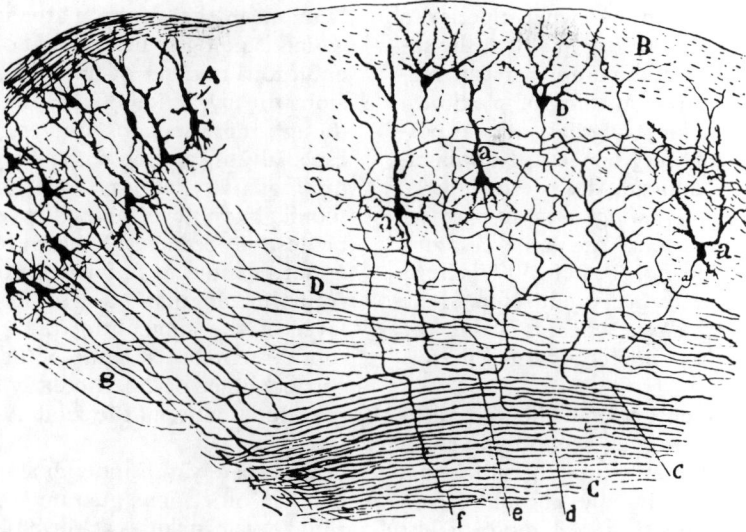

[*FIG. 177*]   Fig. 51. Horizontal and oblique section from inside to outside of the posterior region of the spheno-occipital cortex of the mouse of twelve days. *A*, superior end of the angular focus; *B*, presubicular ganglion; *C*, angular or crossed bundle; *D*, bundles destined to form the ascending perforant spheno-ammonic pathway.

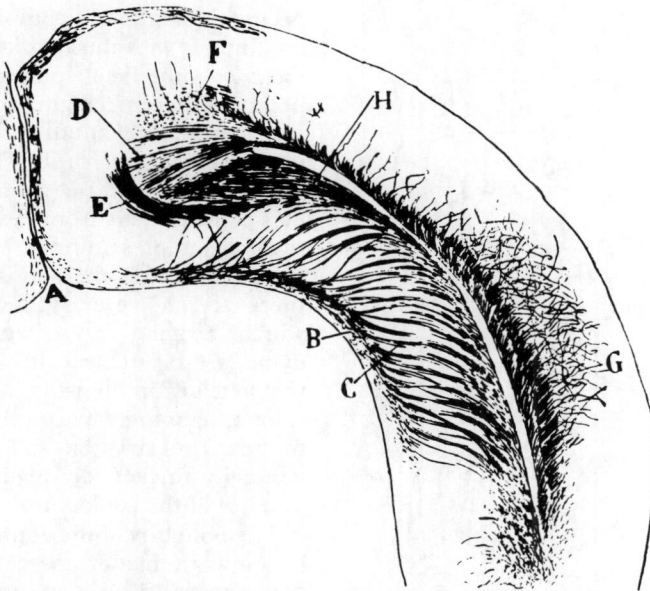

[*FIG. 178*]   Fig. 52. Longitudinal section of the superior portion of the subiculum. *A*, interhemispheric fissure; *B*, subiculum; *C*, superior perforant spheno-ammonic bundles; *D*, corpus callosum; *E*, cingulum; *H*, angular or crossed bundle.

intermediate region and somewhat superior to Ammon's horn, in a territory in which the superior end of the presubiculum persists. Notice that the plane of the thick or plexiform fibers that flank the large angular pathway posteriorly possesses a wing beneath the subiculum and another beneath the presubiculum. From the presubicular wing come in part terminal fibers (others leave the large commissural bundle) which fig. 50, g [fig. 176] shows to be relatively simple, because it refers to the mouse of a few days, whereas from the [subicular] wing arise numerous small perforant bundles (e).

The origin of such perforant fibers is difficult to establish in sagittal sections. Even in the most lateral, the only ones useful for that purpose, the perforant bundles appear beneath the ventricular angle sectioned more or less obliquely, and their penetration into the spheno-occipital focus can be recognized by the general bulk of the bundle, though not by individual fibers. In perfectly horizontal sections, the difficulties are less, and they reveal very clearly that the perforant fascicles come from a mass of oblique or longitudinal fibers

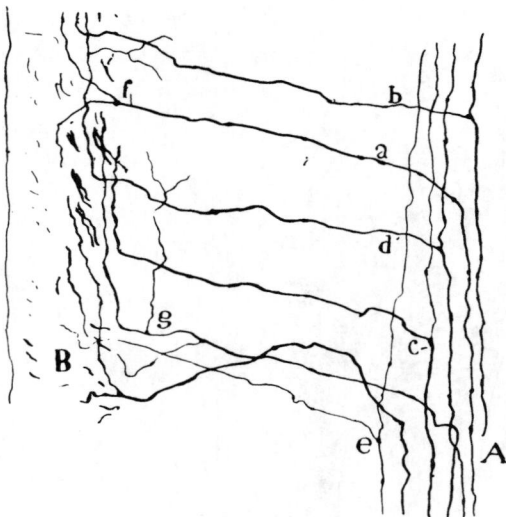

[FIG. 179]   Fig. 53. Details of the superior perforant spheno-ammonic bundle represented in fig. 52 [fig. 178]. A, ascending fibers of the subicular white matter; B, molecular layer of the subiculum; a, b, c, e, perforant collateral and terminal fibers.

lying near the ventricular angle, a mass in which is going to lie, for that cerebral side, an enormous number of horizontal axons arising from the pyramids of the angular focus. Although these sections are very demonstrative, especially if, as frequently happens, the only impregnated pathways are the spheno-ammonic, they nevertheless leave something to be desired; because of their great obliquity, it is not possible to follow the individual axons from the angular nucleus to the molecular layer of the subiculum; they will always be found sectioned at some point of their extracortical trajectory, particularly at the levels of the white matter of the subiculum and its deep layers.

Fortunately, this individual tracing of the fibers, an efficacious guarantee against all possibility of mistake, is achieved in sections [that are] not precisely horizontal but somewhat oblique in the lateral direction, in such a way that in one hemisphere they pass above the corpus callosum and in the other through the superior end of the angular focus, the commissural pathway, and the presubiculum. As seen in fig. 51, A [fig. 177], two planes of fibers originate from the superior end of the spheno-occipital ganglion: a compact or deep [plane] continuous with the angular bundle (C), and a loose or superficial [plane] whose fibers are bent at different heights to pass to the deep layers of the subiculum and to be transformed into perforant fibers (D). This same figure reveals, besides, that the majority of the cited fibers come directly from the medium and large pyramids, representing terminal fibers, that is, continuous with the axons of the said cells; there are, however, spheno-ammonic fibers which, arriving in the vicinity of the ependyma, are bifurcated into an anterior branch that gets lost in the white matter of the hemisphere, seemingly by running in the direction of the corpus striatum, and an internal branch, generally thicker, destined for the perforant bundles of the subiculum.

The obliquity of the course of these bundles in the white matter and cortex of the subiculum appears clearly in fig. 52, C [fig. 178], which reproduces a frontal section parallel to the axis of Ammon's horn. In this figure can be appreciated the extraordinary fibrillary

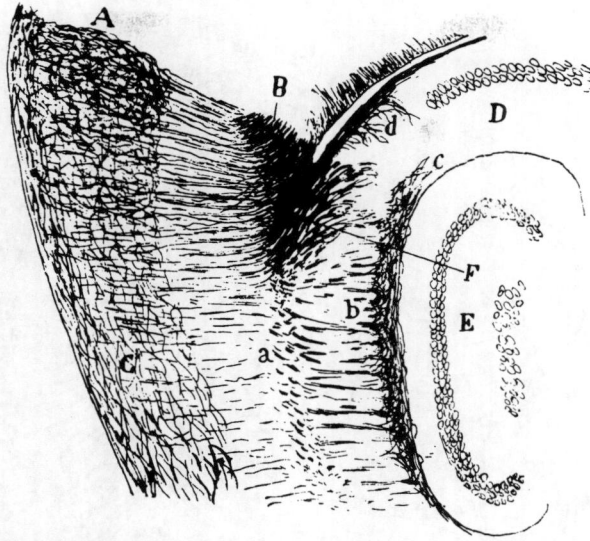

[FIG. 180] Fig. 54. Very lateral sagittal section of the spheno-ammonic focus and Ammon's horn, similar to that of fig. 43 [fig. 169], but at higher magnification. A, superior portion of the focus; F, perforant spheno-ammonic bundles located inside the subiculum; a, b, inferior perforant bundles; E, fascia dentata; B, angular bundle; C, inferior portion of the superior spheno-ammonic focus; D, Ammon's horn; c, molecular layer of Ammon's horn; d, fibers of the spheno-ammonic pathway of the alveus. Mouse of ten to twelve days. (Method of Golgi.)

richness of the perforant system, whose bundles are aggregated in the molecular layer of the subiculum, coming up to the superior terminal portion of this.

In their longitudinal course in the white matter of the subiculum, the perforant fibers give off from time to time collaterals that run as terminal [fibers] through the subicular cortex and gain the plexiform layer. In fig. 53, A [fig. 179], we show the details of this disposition and the usual form of the ramifications, among which attention is called to the frequency with which certain thick fibers divide into a terminal thick branch, promptly converted into a perforant fiber, and a thin branch that still continues a certain distance in the horizontal direction to end also in the same manner (c).

Inferior Perforant Fibers. From the medial and inferior regions of the spheno-occipital ganglion comes a large number of small bundles less robust than the superior perforant [bundles], arranged in vertical series and des- tined for the inferior segment of Ammon's horn. These bundles are revealed easily in the very lateral sagittal sections (Fig. 54, a) [fig. 180], verifying that they run first to the ventricular angle, at which they are bent, taking a transverse direction (on account of which they appear sectioned transversely in the cited sections), to penetrate, finally, in a horizontal or oblique direction the subicular cortex and Ammon's horn.

The detailed following of these perforant axons can be achieved perfectly in horizontal sections that include, besides the inferior segment of Ammon's horn, the ventral regions of the spheno-occipital ganglion.

As can be noticed in fig. 55, B [fig. 181], the said axons, the majority originating from the medium and large pyramids of the spheno-occipital cortex, are concentrated before assailing the subiculum in a white subventricular lamina that runs transversely until it reaches the apex of the subicular angle, here, after concentrating, such a fibrillar stream is fragmented into a group of divergent small bun-

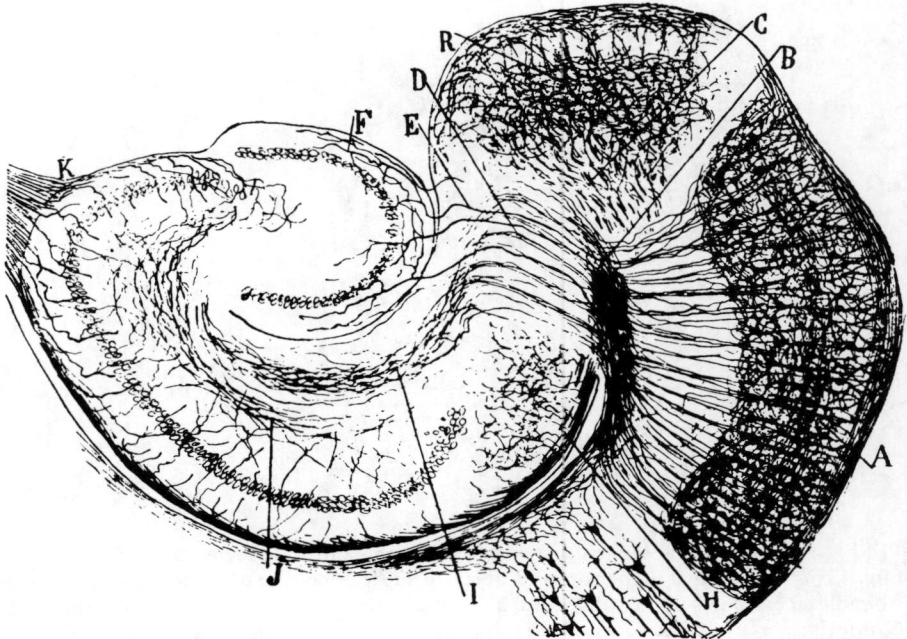

[*FIG. 181*] Fig. 55. Horizontal section of the spheno-occipital focus and of Ammon's horn immediately underneath the plane of the angular bundle. *A*, spheno-occipital focus; *B*, point where the inferior perforant spheno-ammonic bundles meet; *D*, perforant fibers; *E*, fibers destined for the fascia dentata; *H*, alvear spheno-ammonic pathway and plexus that it engenders in the subiculum; *I*, distribution of the perforant fibers in the stratum lacunosum of Ammon's horn; *J*, plexus of collaterals of Ammon's horn; *F*, fibers terminating in the fascia dentata; *K*, fimbria; *R*, deep plexus of the subiculum. Mouse of fifteen days. (Method of Golgi.)

dles, which are disseminated over a quite extensive area of the subiculum, and, crossing the cortex of this almost horizontally, they go up to the plexiform layer and Ammon's horn.

The details of the origin and initial trajectory of these fibers are shown in fig. 56., *a, b, d* [*fig. 182*]. Among them, the thicker fibers have the less complicated trajectory, passing almost directly from the spheno-ammonic ganglion to the cortex of the subiculum and without ramifying on their way (*d*). Others are bifurcated in the plane of the white matter and engender a direct perforant fiber and another that continues for a certain distance in the tangential direction (*a*). Finally, there are also some, one of the branches of which passes to the spheno-ammonic pathway of the alveus (fig. 56, *b*) [*fig. 182*], whereas the other, after a variable tangential course, becomes perforant. The bifurcation can appear prematurely, as is shown in fig. 56, *f* [*fig. 182*].

Termination of the Perforant Fibers. Whatever origin they may have, whether they represent either collaterals or terminal [fibers], ascending or inferior perforant [fibers], their manner of termination is the same. Once arrived at the first layer, they suddenly change direction, all running toward the terminal portion of Ammon's horn, and consequently in a transverse direction with respect to this and to the subiculum. By virtue of this turn, in frontal section, the cited subicular and ammonic plexiform layer shows the fibers sectioned transversely or obliquely, whereas in sagittal sections of the cerebrum (which are essentially transverse with respect to Ammon's horn), they appear obliquely and even transversely sectioned.

In figs. 57, *E*, and 58, *a* [*figs. 183, 184*], which reproduce, at different magnifications, sagittal sections of the brain of the mouse, the terminal trajectory of the perforant fibers can be well studied. In these same figures, it is noticed that the spheno-ammonic ramifications invade the whole extents of the molecular and lacunosum layers of Ammon's horn, as well as the whole plexiform layer of the fascia dentata.

Here is what we have observed about the manner of terminal ramification of the perforant fibers. From this aspect, they can all be classified as three kinds: direct fibers to the fascia dentata, fibers destined for Ammon's horn, and mixed fibers, that is to say, ramifying in these two centers.

a. The *direct fibers to the fascia dentata* are perhaps the most robust of all, although there is no lack of some of a medium thickness; first they run for a certain distance through the plexiform layer of the subiculum without branching, and on arriving at the fascia den-

tata, they divide into two streans: the posterior, formed ordinarily by fibers of medium thickness, which are incorporated into the posterior or superficial portion of the fascia dentata; and the anterior, in which the thick fibers that penetrate the anterior portion predominate. Arriving in this way at the plexiform layer of the fascia dentata, the fibers of both streams are bifurcated, or they ramify in a more complicated fashion, extending their small branches over long trajectories in a direction parallel to the cited layer and engendering a dense plexus coming into intimate contact with the dendritic shafts of the granule cells. Some thick fibers pass, without stopping or giving off small branches, through the whole thickness of the plexiform layer of the fascia dentata, and when they are close to the layer of the granule

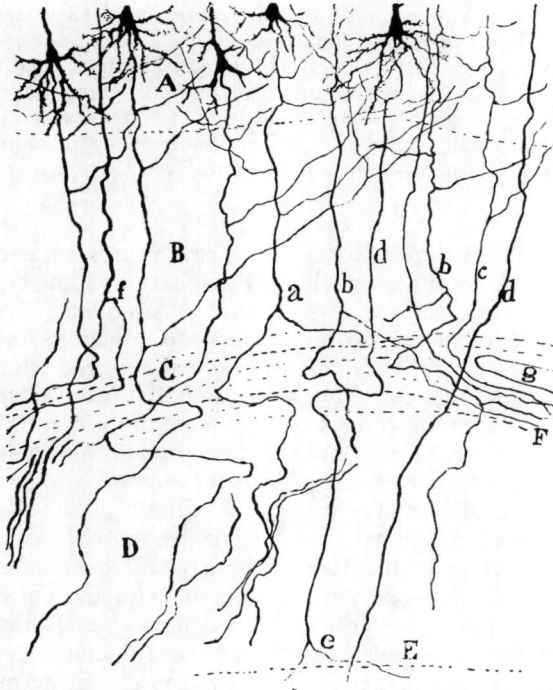

[*FIG. 182*]   Fig. 56. Details of the origin and penetration of the fibers of the spheno-occipital focus in the subiculum. *A,* layer of the large pyramids of the same; *B,* layer of the granule cells; *C,* plane of subicular white matter; *D,* subiculum; *g,* angle or external border of the lateral ventricle; *a, b,* bifurcated fibers; *d,* thick fibers now bifurcated; *E,* external plexiform layer of Ammon's horn; *F,* place where the spheno-ammonic perforant fibers meet; *c,* nonbifurcated thin fiber; *e,* bifurcation of a fiber in the external plexiform layer of the Ammon's horn; *f,* premature bifurcation of a perforant spheno-ammonic fiber. Mouse of fifteen days. (Method of Golgi.)

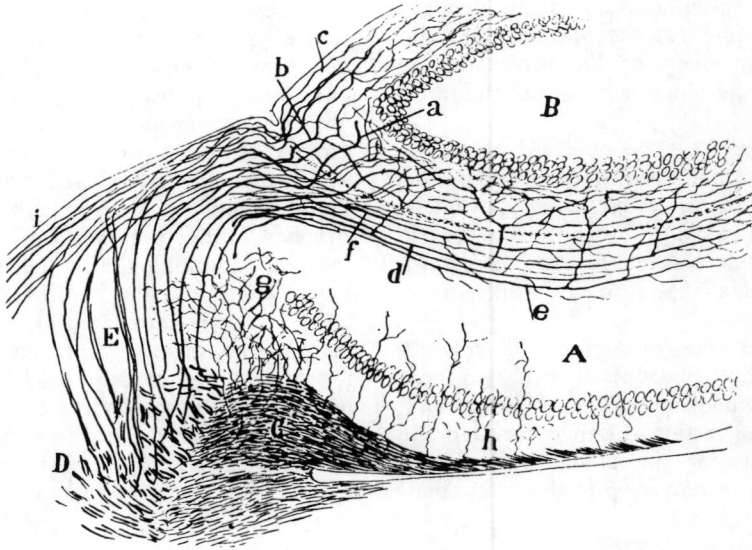

[*FIG. 183*] Fig. 57. Course and termination of the superior perforant fibers (sagittal section of the cerebrum). *A*, Ammon's horn; *B*, fascia dentata; *C*, angular or crossed bundle; *D*, ascending pathway from which the perforant spheno-ammonic fibers leave; *E*, perforant bundles; *a*, thick fiber penetrating the molecular layer of the fascia dentata; *b*, bifurcated afferent fiber; *c*, afferent fiber going to the free portion of the fascia dentata; *d*, plane of the afferent fibers of the molecular layer of Ammon's horn; *e*, fiber that gives rise to perforant fibers to the fascia dentata; *f*, nonbifurcated fibers destined only for Ammon's horn; *h*, collateral of the angular fascicle. Mouse of fifteen days. (Method of Golgi.)

cells, they change direction, becoming longitudinal or parallel to this center and escaping from observation.

The fascia dentata can be reached by its own spheno-ammonic fibers or by the collaterals of the mixed fibers at any point of its curve; but there is a preferred place where the vast majority of the cited fibers penetrate. This door of entrance in some preparations appears occupied by a very robust bundle (section of a vertical, more or less condensed lamina) that corresponds to the proximity of the angle of the fascia dentata (figs. 58, *b;* 57, *b*) [*figs. 184, 183*].

b. The *fibers destined for Ammon's horn* are the most numerous, it being possible to follow them easily in the sagittal sections from the perforant bundles to the border of the ammonic formation (fib. 58, *a, c*) [*fig. 184*]. When they reach the plexiform layer of the subiculum, they behave in one of several ways: the majority of them curve inward without branching, entering some of the longitudinal small bundles of the stratum lacunosum; oth-

ers are bifurcated at the point of inflection, giving an ascending branch, that is to say, parallel to Ammon's horn, and another with the opposite direction; finally, some are resolved into two or three branches with a similar direction that run inside Ammon's horn and are installed in different planes of the stratum lacunosum and molecular layer (*lamina medullaris circonvoluta*).

c. Finally, the *mixed fibers* correspond in their general characteristics to the preceding, from which they differ in being, in general, more robust, and especially because they give off one or several thick branches penetrating the fascia dentata, in whose molecular layer they arborize and terminate (fig. 57, *d, e*) [*fig. 183*]. In some cases, the branch destined for the fascia dentata represents the continuation of the axon, it being possible to estimate the other, which is prolonged toward the molecular layer of Ammon's horn, as a collateral (*d*).

Since in man there exists, as is well known (see. fig. 12) [*fig. 142*], a very robust bundle of

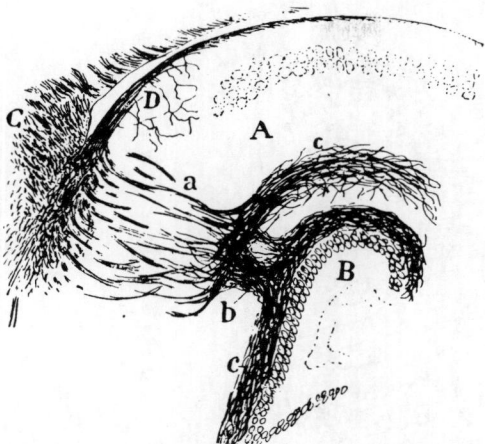

[*FIG. 184*]   Fig. 58. Sagittal and somewhat oblique section of Ammon's horn and fascia dentata of the mouse of twelve days. *A*, Ammon's horn; *B*, fascia dentata; *C*, crossed angular bundle; *D*, alvear spheno-ammonic bundle; *a*, superior perforant bundle; *c*, prolongation of this in the molecular layer of Ammon's horn; *b*, pathway destined for the fascia dentata. (Method of Golgi.)

white matter in the ammonicosubicular angle and numerous thick perforant bundles that go up to the *stratum lacunosum et moleculare* of Ammon's horn and to the *lamina medullaris circonvoluta* and fascia dentata, it can be presumed that he possesses also a sphenoperforant ammonic pathway, as well as an angular or crossed spheno-ammonic bundle.

Such a supposition is highly probable, since recent observations have persuaded us that the cited pathways, as well as the spheno-occipital nucleus from which they arise, exist in the cerebrum of the dog and cat, where they reach an extraordinary robustness. The angular focus occupies in these animals the most elevated and transversely thinner posterosuperior portion of the piriform lobe (see below).

Optic Alvear Pathway[M] (fig. 55, *H*) [*fig. 181*]

When lateral sagittal sections are examined, that is to say, those including the angular focus and sectors of Ammon's horn, it is constantly noticed that in the medial region of the said ganglion, beneath the territory from which the commissural bundle arises, there originates a group of axons that, after being situated

beneath [the commissural] bundle, turns abruptly at the ventricular angle, assailing the alveus, and runs a certain distance on the surface of this, running forward and upward, until finally it gets lost among the endogenous fibers of Ammon's horn.

As we said above, such alvear fibers, whose spheno-occipital origin we consider unquestionable, supply an infinity of collaterals ramifying through the whole cortex of the subiculum, and particularly in a triangular area bounded above by the commissural bundle, behind by the small perforant bundles, and below and anteriorly by the first aggregations of the ammonic pyramids (figs. 59, *D;* 58, *D*) [*figs. 185, 184*].

Fig. 27, *a, d,* [*fig. 157*], in which we show in detail these fibers as they appear in sagittal sections, reveals that not all the collaterals or terminal fibers of the alvear bundle come from the homolateral angular focus; they also originate from the ammonic or posterior portion of the alveus and either terminate, after a prior inflection, ramifying in a large area of the subicular cortex, or they bifurcate into a thick terminal branch, distributed in this cortex, and a thin branch, which follows its course laterally, getting lost among the fibers of the angular or commissural bundle and its vicinity.

About the origin of such fibers, we can say nothing positive. To formulate a somewhat precise opinion, it would be necessary to follow the alvear spheno-ammonic fibers over their whole extent, as well as the cited fibers arriving from the posterior alveus, a task that, even in the newborn mouse and in the most favorable sections, is completely impossible. The fact that the alvear spheno-ammonic fibers do not appear to be totally consumed in the subiculum, but are prolonged toward Ammon's horn over a long trajectory, suggests the conjecture that the referred afferent fibers of the interior could represent alvear spheno-ammonic fibers from the contralateral side.

The plane of the alvear white matter contains also, as we said when we dealt with the subiculum, axons originating in cells of [the subiculum] and prolonged toward Ammon's horn. Some are divided into a posterior branch to the alveus and an anterior branch that gets lost among the fibers of the angular or crossed

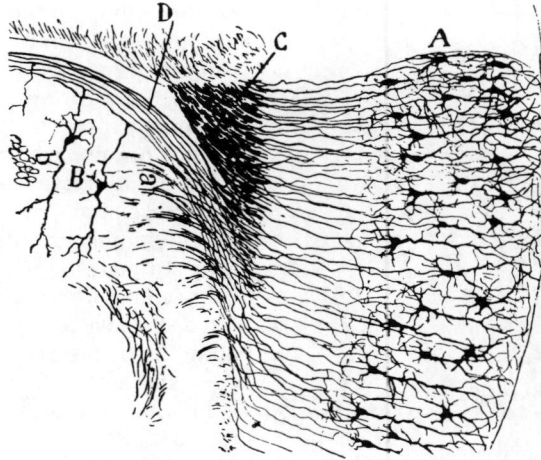

[*FIG. 185*]   Fig. 59. Details of the origin of the angular or crossed bundle and superior perforant bundles. (Very lateral sagittal section.) *A*, spheno-occipital focus; *C*, angular bundle; *B*, subiculum; *D*, alvear spheno-ammonic pathway; *a*, superior perforant bundles; *b*, cell of the subiculum with a bifurcated axon. Mouse of fifteen days.

bundle or in the deep planes of the perforant fibers. We do not know the course and ultimate destination of the said fibers.

The cortico-ammonic connections that we have just studied raise interesting anatomico-physiological problems. We do not dare, however, to draw any physiological conclusion from the revealed facts before we know with security the functional significance of this very singular occipital-sphenoidal center, which seems to us to exist in all mammals.

We hope that the physio-anatomico-pathological experiments on the said focus that we are soon going to undertake in the rabbit and guinea pig will allow us to resolve definitively this interesting problem, getting rid of the legitimate scruples that at present hinder us from formulating some secure opinion about the physiological significance of Ammon's horn, a significance that must be linked probably with that of the angular center from which it receives the vast majority of its afferent fibers.

As we will see later, there is no lack of indications that allow us to consider the angular focus as a special area of the apparatus of olfaction. Perhaps it receives from the inferior sphenoidal cortex some pathway so far unknown. In such a supposition, the large

spheno-ammonic pathways that we have described could very well represent the legitimate and perhaps unique perforant olfactory pathway to Ammon's horn, a center that, in its turn, would come to be an olfactory area of the third or fourth order. As we will point out later, this conjecture has the advantage of harmonizing well with the general opinion of the neurologists which regards the whole piriform lobe of mammals as an olfactory center, and with the negative data resulting from our observations, that is, with the absence of olfactory pathways coming from Ammon's horn through the septum lucidum and columns of the fornix.

IX. Interhemispheric Cortex and Gyrus Fornicatus; Cingulum

Before commencing study of the cingulum or supracallosal cortico-ammonic pathway, it will be convenient to analyze succinctly the structure of the gray matter from which it arises, which is none other than the cortex of the gyrus fornicatus in man and of the interhemispheric region in rodents.

The only author who has made a reasonably careful examination of the fine structure of the said gyrus (first and second limbic [gyri]) in man is Hammarberg.[28] According to this researcher, the cingulate gyrus consists of, first, molecular layer; second, layer of the small pyramidal cells; third, layer of the large pyramids; and fourth, layer of the fusiform cells. It lacks the fourth layer or layer of the granule cells. The second consists, in fact, not of pyramidal forms, but of globular forms, which were considered fusiform by Betz. As we approach the corpus callosum, the layers become thinner, the cells decreasing in thickness. In the zone of transition to the corpus callosum, there persists no more than the molecular layer, a set of the pyramids, and some cells of the fourth layer which lie horizontally.

Our observations in man, made in Nissl preparations, confirm in essence the assertions of Hammarberg, but add some details. As revealed in fig. 60 [*fig. 186*], the said layers are first, molecular or plexiform layer characterized by its notable thickness; second, layer of the small fusiform and pyramidal cells; third, plexiform layer poor in cells; fourth, layer of the large pyramids and giant fusiform cells; fifth, layer of the deep medium pyramids; and sixth, layer of the white matter and polymorphic cells.

In the fourth layer, true giant cells do not exist, but [there are] voluminous pyramids, which in the inferior plane of the layer appear mixed irregularly with some long and robust fusiform cells that resemble the specific cells of the insular cortex. This layer, as well as that of the medium pyramids, is not as thick in the cingulate gyrus by comparison with the corresponding layers in other gyri, from which the said gyrus is differentiated especially by the plexus of nerve fibers of the third layer and by the predominant fusiform character of the cells of the second.

This somewhat special structure does not appear to correspond only to the inferior two-thirds of the cingulate gyrus; in the superior part of this, the layers thicken, the plexus of the third layer becomes less apparent, and the large fusiform cells of the fifth layer vanish. Taking into account this fact and considering, besides, that the cingulum comes very principally, as the Weigert preparations show, from the inferior portion of the said gyrus, we believe it probable that only this part of the cin-

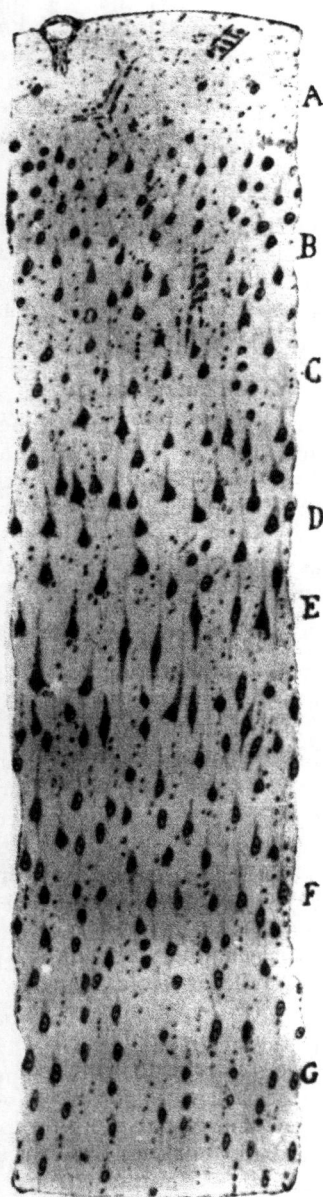

[*FIG. 186*] Fig. 60. Section of the inferior region of the cingulate gyrus of man. *A*, plexiform layer; *B*, layer of the small fusiform and pyramidal cells; *C*, deep plexiform layer; *D*, layer of the large pyramids; *E*, large fusiform cells; *F*, layer of the polymorphic cells; *G*, layer of the polymorphic cells and of the white matter.

gulate gyrus must be considered homologous to the interhemispheric cortex of the rodents.

The whole supracallosal gyrus in neither the cat nor the dog appears to correspond to the mentioned interhemispheric region. Thus, in the cat, the Nissl preparations only reveal a texture analogous to the cingulate cortex of the rodents in the inferior half or three-fourths of the supracallosal gyrus. The superior portion contributes the majority of its fibers of projection to the corona radiata, this being directed laterally above the corpus callosum.

In rodents, the cingulum comes from the whole internal face of the hemisphere, and, consequently, it may be presumed that the totality of the interhemispheric cortex has the special features that we just noticed in the cingulate gyrus of the gyrencephalic animals. In fact, those features that it presents are much more accentuated than in man, cat, and dog.

Thus, as is seen in fig. 61 [fig. 187], in the guinea pig, rabbit, and mouse, a transverse section of the interhemisphere cortex, when stained with the Nissl method, shows the following layers: (1) naturally, attention is called to the great thickness of the plexiform layer (more than twice that in the superior region of the hemisphere) that lodges some cells with short axon and a large number of medullated fibers. (2) Underneath this layer appears a granular formation that resembles the granule cell [layer] of the fascia dentata. Such cells are very close to each other, forming several rows, and have spindle or ovoid, sometimes triangular forms. (3) Then appears a plexiform layer dotted with pyramidal cells of small or medium size, underneath which appear, successively, the layers of the large pyramids (fourth layer) and of polymorphic cells (fifth layer). The latter encloses ovoid or fusiform cells of medium and even small size, resident between the little radial nerve bundles.

In summary, the interhemispheric cortical region shows up from the rest of the hemisphere of the rodents on account of the enormous development of the plexiform or first layer; the substitution of the layer of the small pyramids by a layer of fusiform and ovoid cells; the poverty of giant and medium pyramidal cells, which are arranged in relatively narrow strata; and the presence, as we will detail later, of a dense nerve plexus at the level of the third layer. This particular aspect of the interhemispheric cortex ceases near the superior border of the hemispheres, the plexus of the third layer gradually disappearing, the granule or fusiform cells of the second layer being converted into genuine pyramids, and all the layers increasing in thickness.

But the fine structure of the interhemispheric region can only be revealed by the Golgi method. So far, we have only applied it successfully in small mammals, particularly in the mouse of eight to fifteen days, to which fig. 62 [fig. 188] refers. In this animal, the robustness and proximity of the cingulum to the midline and the thinness of the layers are favorable circumstances for the structural analysis, as we pointed out already in our old work on the cerebral cortex.[29]

Plexiform Layer

It is characterized by the extraordinary abundance of its nerve fibers which engender an extremely dense plexus. It contains, besides, small and medium cells with short axon terminating inside the layer, and the terminal [dendritic] tufts of all the cells of the underlying layers.

The nervous plexus consists of the following elements:

1. Collaterals of the White Matter of the Cingulum

These collaterals, discovered by us many years ago,[30] are very numerous; they arise at right angles from the fibers of the cingulum, ascending, branching through the inferior layers; and they terminate in the plexiform layer by means of a wide and loose arborization (fig. 62, b) [fig. 188].

2. Terminal Fibers Arriving from the White Matter

In horizontal sections are found, although infrequently, ascending fibers detached from the white matter, and which form in the entire gray matter of the region under study an extensive arborization, particularly concentrated in the first layer (c). The axons of origin can-

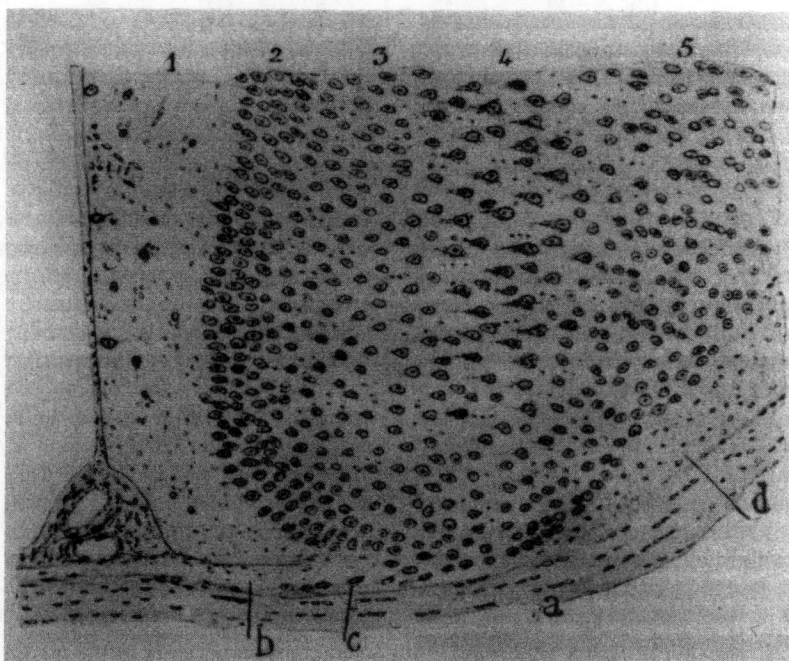

[*FIG. 187*]   Fig. 61. Section of the inferior portion of the interhemispheric cortex of the guinea pig. Method of Nissl. *1*, plexiform layer; *2*, layer of the fusiform cells; *3*, deep plexiform layer; *4*, layer of the large pyramids; *5*, layer of the polymorphic cells; *a*, corpus callosum; *b*, cortex of the supracallosal striae; *d*, cingulum; *c*, nerve cells of the longitudinal striae.

not be followed except over a short trajectory through the cingulum; thus, we do not know if they include ascending fibers arriving through the corpus callosum [together] with the bundles of the fornix longus of Forel, or the terminal portions of association branches of bifurcation arising from axons originating in the gyrus fornicatus.

3. Ascending Fascicles of the Cingulum

In frontal sections of the anterior half of the interhemispheric cortex, we have sometimes seen certain, perfectly stained robust fascicles that, detaching from the most internal portion of the cingulum (fig. 63, *B*) [*fig. 189*], crossed obliquely the gray matter and gained the plexiform layer, where they turned to become tangential, notably strengthening the terminal nervous plexus of this layer. As is observed in fig. 63, *A* [*fig. 189*], the majority of these fibers in the first layer follow an oblique course forward and upward, invading a part of the su-

perior cortex and perhaps establishing connections with other cerebral regions. A good number of such ascending cingulate fibers seem to end in the interhemispheric cortex, and on them collaterals are observed, some destined for the first layer, others distributed in the underlying layers (fig. 63, *a*) [*fig. 189*].

4. Ascending Axons of Martinotti

They come from the fusiform, ovoid, or stellate cells, distributed through the whole thickness of the cortex, but particularly located in the fourth and fifth layers (fig. 62, *a, f*) [*fig. 188*].

Layer of the Ovoid and Triangular Cells

In small mammals, it consists of several rows of very tight cells that, in Nissl preparations, exhibit the appearance of the granule cells of the fascia dentata or of the retina. In Golgi preparations, they possess an ovoid, triangular,

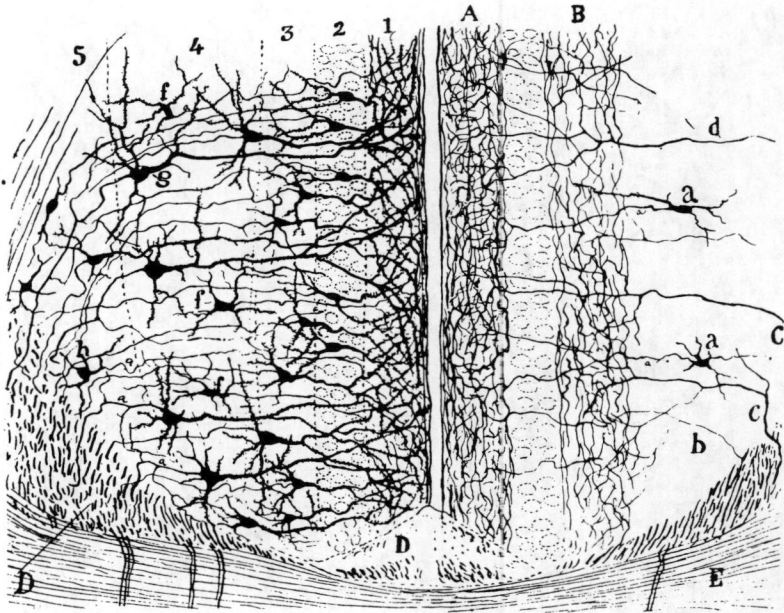

[*FIG. 188*]   Fig. 62. Vertical transverse section of the interhemispheric cortex of the mouse of eight days. *A*, superficial plexiform layer; *B*, deep plexiform layer; *D*, cingulum; *E*, corpus callosum; *a*, cells with ascending axon; *b*, collaterals of the cingulum; *c, d*, terminal fibers of this; *g*, large pyramidal cell; *f, h*, cells with ascending axon. (Method of Golgi.)

or fusiform shape [fig. 62, 2]^N [*fig. 188*]. Their cell bodies are smooth and only give rise to [dendritic] processes at their poles. These processes are usually one or two ascending and terminating by means of tufts in the plexiform layer; one or two descending and resolving into several small branches at the level of the third or deep plexiform layer; and a thin axon that arises, either from the soma or from the descending [dendritic] shaft, crosses to the [third] layer, giving off collaterals, and gains, finally, the cingulate white matter, where it is continuous with a thin medullated fiber.

Deep Plexiform Layer

So called because at its level there exists a very dense nervous plexus, almost as rich as that of the first layer, and formed by the accumulation of collateral or terminal arborizations of the following fibers: (a) collateral branches of fibers detached from the white matter; (b) terminal branches of collaterals arising from the

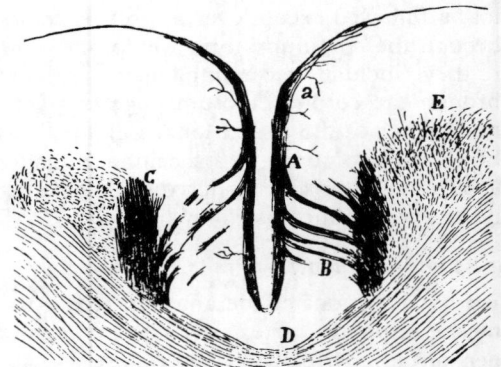

[*FIG. 189*]   Fig. 63. Frontal section of the cerebrum of the mouse. Anterior portion of the interhemispheric [white] matter. *A*, plexiform layer of the interhemispheric cortex; *D*, corpus callosum; *C*, cingulum; *B*, perforant bundles terminating in the plexiform layer; *E*, transverse section of the arcuate fasciculus; *a*, collaterals originating from ascending fibers of the cingulum and terminating in the plexiform layer and underlying layers. (Method of Golgi.)

cingulum; (c) thin collaterals originating from the axons of the cells of the second layer; (d) terminal ramifications and collaterals originating from underlying cells with ascending axons (fig. 62, *B*) [*fig. 188*].

But, in addition, this layer contains some small and medium pyramids (fig. 62, *3*) [*fig. 188*] and some occasional cells with short and ascending axon.

Layer of the Medium and Large Pyramids

As is seen in fig. 62, *4* [*fig. 188*], such cells are the true pyramidal type, having a radial [dendritic] shaft ramifying in the first layer, basal dendrites distributed inside the fourth or in the underlying layer, and a robust axon that runs laterally and downward, to be continuous with a fiber of the cingulum. From this axon several collaterals arise, some of which are recurrent and can gain the third layer and even the first. Ordinarily, the cells lying in the deepest plane are the most voluminous, and they almost merit the name of giant cells (fig. 62, *g*) [*fig. 188*]. In the cited layer, cells with ascending axon are never lacking.

Layer of the Polymorphic Cells

In this layer [fig. 62, *5*]° [*fig. 188*], which is narrow and with a triangular form, lie some pyramidal cells of medium size, cells of similar volume but with a triangular shape, and occasional ovoid or fusiform cells with ascending axon, prolonged up to the first layer, where they ramify (fig. 62, *h*) [*fig. 188*].

The special structure of the interhemispheric cortex is extended, as we have already said, in the mouse, rabbit, and guinea pig, over the whole internal face of the hemispheres, extending, besides, forward to the frontal pole and downward around the hemispheres to the middle part of or somewhat beyond the posterior border of the occipital lobe, that is to say, until the point at which the presubicular area begins.

In all this enormous area of gray matter, the same layers appear, and essentially the same connections are established; however, there are two regions in which some variations of disposition are presented. They are the *precal-*

losal ganglion, which is the portion of the interhemispheric gray cortex situated immediately above the olfactory bulbs; and the *arcuate ganglion or ganglion of the occipital pole,* an extensive gray band extending from the superior part of the occipital pole to the presubiculum [*fig. 190*].[P]

Precallosal Ganglion

Not far from the pedicle of the bulb and underneath and in front of the callosal genu, the interhemispheric cortex is characterized by the great development of the first layer, into which numerous perforant bundles of the cingulum penetrate; by the thinness of the cingulum, which is reduced to an arched lamina that flanks the genu of the corpus callosum; and, finally, by the reduction in thickness of the focus, at the expense of which the gray matter of the frontal pole increases.

The *arcuate focus or [focus] of the occipital pole* was already analyzed at another time by us.[31] It is characterized, especially, by the great development of the plexus of the third layer, which is, in large part, medullated, as is shown by Weigert-Pal preparations (fig. 42, *a*) [*fig. 168*]; [also] by the great richness in medium

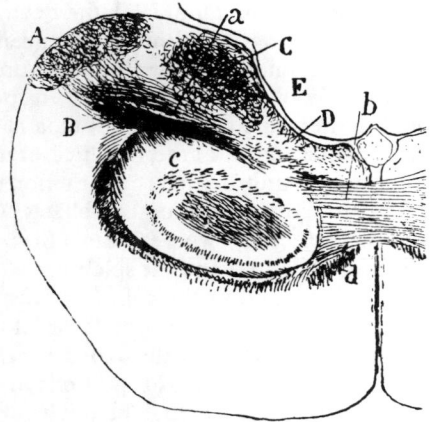

[FIG. 190] Fig. 64. Somewhat oblique horizontal section of one cerebral hemisphere of the mouse of a few days. *A,* angular focus; *C,* presubicular focus; *B,* crossed angular bundle; *D,* focus of the occipital pole; *E,* superior colliculus; *a,* initial stream of perforant bundles; *b,* corpus callosum; *c,* Ammon's horn; *d,* cingulum. (Method of Golgi.) [Ventral is up.]

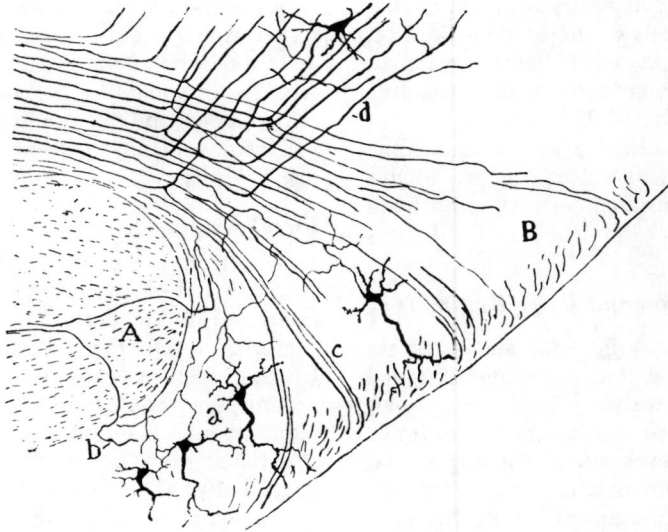

[FIG. 191]   Fig. 65. Sagittal section of the posterior or occipital end of the cerebrum (mouse of ten days). A, splenium of the corpus callosum; B, focus of the occipital pole; a, cells of the inferior portion of this focus, whose axons went toward the cingulum; b, fibers destined for the fornix longus; d, bifurcated axons; c, perforant fibers to the plexiform layer of the focus of the occipital pole.

and large pyramidal cells (third and fourth layers); and especially by being the origin of a large number of postero-anterior fibers of the cingulum. In fig. 65, d [fig. 191], the behavior of the axons originating in this territory can be observed. The ones coming from the upper part, that is to say, from the true occipital pole, descend to the plane of the cingulum, and the majority divide into an anterior thick branch and a posterior thin branch; the anterior one runs forward, being continuous probably with a fiber of projection; whereas the other descends more or less behind the splenium of the corpus callosum and finally gains, by crossing the gray matter, the plexiform layer of the ganglion under study. But the axons originating in the medial and inferior portions of the focus are usually ascending, being incorporated in part into the cingulum and in part into the fornix longus of Forel, which, in order to reach, they perforate the splenium of the corpus callosum. In their trajectory in the gray matter, they give off recurrent collaterals (fig. 65, a) [fig. 191] and some long branches, ascending or descending, that run into the underlying white matter and whose destination is

difficult to establish. The terminal fibers, the majority of which come from the cingulum, are very abundant in the focus of the occipital pole, engendering a plexus extending through all the layers, although particularly concentrated in the third. In fig. 68, J [fig. 194], we reproduce some of these terminal fibers, detached from the cingulum; frequently, at the point of inflection of the fiber, where it becomes ascending, there arises a collateral that runs for a certain distance in the white matter.

The special situation of the focus under study on the internal face of the occipital pole, and the presence in it of an intermediate stria of white matter, comparable to the stria of Gennari in the cortex of the human calcarine fissure, made us incline in our first work on the subject to the view that the said focus is the visual area of rodents. But at present, after a careful analysis of the whole interhemispheric cortex, which has revealed to us the great analogy existing between the focus at the [occipital] pole and the supracallosal gray matter, plus the fact that the said focus of the occipital pole receives exclusively fibers from the cingulum, it not being possible to demonstrate in it the entry of fascicles coming from the corona radiata and consequently from the secondary optic foci, we have completely abandoned our old opinion.[Q]

White Matter of the Gyrus Fornicatus

When a complete series of frontal sections of the mouse, guinea pig, and rabbit stained by the method of Weigert or of Golgi, is studied, there is observed, above the corpus callosum and immediately underneath and outside the interhemispheric gray matter, a robust bundle of white matter, which was already studied and delineated by Ganser.[32] According to [Ganser], this bundle, perfectly demarcated in the rodents, would be independent of the internal capsule and would correspond probably to the superior longitudinal fascicle of man. Its probable mission, says Ganser, is to link the several territories of the gyrus fornicatus. In our work of 1890,[33] we also reproduced the cited bundle, although without distinguishing its regions, proving for the first time that its axons originate in the interhemispheric gray matter, and that they follow an anteroposterior course. But, it not having been at that time our aim to analyze the connections of the cingulum, we said nothing about its manner of termination in [Ammon's] horn.

Kölliker[34] appears not to have subjected this interesting point to a detailed analysis with the method of Golgi. In his descriptions and figures, he represents the cingulum as a very long sagittal, supracallosal bundle, from which perforant fibers destined to form the fornix longus of Forel are detached. But about its posterior and anterior termination, nothing is specifically shown to us. The cingulum of man, on which several authors have worked, particularly Beevor, has received more attention.

In the opinion of Beevor,[35] the cingulum of man would be a complex formation, consisting of fibers with several origins, as suggested by the fact that when it is sectioned and [the ensuing] secondary degeneration in it examined, its fibers never degenerate completely, either forward or backward. Three groups or successive segments of fibers would form it: the *anterior,* the *horizontal,* and the *posterior.*

The *anterior bundle or portion,* resides underneath the genu of the corpus callosum and connects the anterior perforated substance and the internal olfactory root with the frontal lobe. The *horizontal fascicle* constitutes the main portion of the cingulum, that is to say, the supracallosal [part], and would establish connections between the frontal extremity of the hemisphere and limbic gyri on the one hand and the superior gyri of the internal cerebral face on the other. Finally, the *posterior segment* lies in the thickness of the hippocampal gyrus and, posteriorly, interrelates the fusiform [gyrus], the lingual lobe, and the temporal pole. Neither Ammon's horn nor the amygdaloid nucleus would receive [fibers] derived from this cingulate pathway.

For Edinger,[36] the gyrus fornicatus is only apparently continuous with Ammon's horn, and he much doubts its olfactory character; he admits, however, that the cingulum is connected, although he does not say how, with that nervous center. In one figure, [he shows] the posterior distribution of the fibers of this sagittal system as far as the sphenoidal gyri.

Dejerine[37] considers the cingulum as the bundle of association of the rhinencephalon. Its fibers do not extend the entire length of the bundle, but represent short pathways renewed several times and terminating in the adjacent gyri. In its posterior extremity, the cingulum would constitute a layer of sagittal fibers, heavily stainable by hematoxylin, and located in the internal extremity of the diverticulum of the subiculum.

Elliot Smith,[38] who has dedicated a good study to Ammon's horn and the fornix of lower mammals, does not appear to have seen the supposed connections that link the gyrus fornicatus with the white matter of the piriform lobe; however, he tells us that one part of the fibers of the gyrus fornicatus perforates the corpus callosum and forms part of the precommissural fascicle or olfactory radiation of Zuckerkandl, and could be followed until near the [optic] chiasm. Ganser also gave a similar opinion some time ago.

As is seen, the generality of the authors are inclined to consider the cingulum as a pathway of multiple association, composed of short fibers and extending from the hippocampal gyrus to the anterior perforated space. The existence in it of long fibers as extensive as the bundle thus appears doubtful, and it is not known where and how its fibers terminate at the two anterior ends.

My observations made on small mammals prove peremptorily these four fundamental facts: first, the cingulum contains, besides short pathways equivalent to those mentioned by Beevor in the human cortex, a very long pathway that occupies the whole or almost the whole length [of the cingulum]; second, the cingulum terminates posteriorly, at least in large part, by means of free aborizations in the thickness of the subiculum and Ammon's horn; third, the anterior extremity of the cingulum descends not to the olfactory region but to the corona radiata, representing thus a pathway of projection; fourth, finally, the fibers of the cingulum arise in cells of the interhemispheric cortex, equivalent to the cingulate gyrus of the human cortex.

Let us detail now the composition, trajectory, origins, and terminations of the cingulum or principal white matter of the gyrus fornicatus, such as they appear in the preparations of Golgi in small mammals.

Let us begin by establishing that we do not regard all the supracallosal white bundle, situated underneath the fissural gray matter of the rodents, as homologous to the cingulate pathway of man. In fact, this robust sagittal bundle, whose section is semilunar in the rabbit and mouse, consists of two very different bundles. (1) The *internal bundle or bundle of thick fibers,* situated immediately underneath the specific gray matter, afore-described, and originating from the cells of the same. This fascicle seems to us to correspond completely to the cingulum of man, so that from now on we will designate it the *cingulum* or *sagittal bundle of the gyrus fornicatus.* (2) The *external bundle* or bundle of thin fibers, which we will call *arcuate or superior longitudinal fascicle of the hemispheres.* This important bundle, situated on the outside of the preceding [bundle], is much wider and forms a superior and lateral eminence. The analysis of its fibers has proven to us that it represents a pathway of association between the anterior and posterior regions of

the superior cortex of the hemispheres. Its fibers do not intervene, consequently, in the formation of the cingulum, nor do they maintain relations with Ammon's horn. We consider it probable that the cited arcuate fascicle corresponds to the *arcuate or longitudinal bundle* of Burdach in man, as we already noted in other work. It could likewise represent in part the *occipitofrontal* bundle of Forel and Onufrowicz. Both pathways, well developed and differentiated in man, would perhaps be merged in small mammals into a single sagittal bundle (figs. 33; 63, *C, E*) [*figs. 163, 189*].

The two mentioned portions of the supracallosal white matter, namely the cingulum and the arcuate bundle, appear little separated in Weigert-Pal preparations, but they are perfectly differentiated in those of Golgi. Already, on another occasion, we have remarked on the singular property possessed by the silver chromate of staining exclusively, in the embryonic animals or in those a few days old, certain nervous pathways to the exclusion of others, a fortunate circumstance that permits the easy following of the axons from their origins to their terminations. This preference (which depends probably on a certain peculiar chemical state of all the nerve fibers that are close to the time of apperance of a myelin sheath) is verified especially in the cingulum, which is shown, as seen in fig. 63, *C* [*fig. 189*], to be stained completely over its whole extent, showing up, besides, from the rest of the white matter on account of the exceptional robustness of its fibers. In the said frontal sections, it is observed also that the cingulum forms a mass increasing in thickness from the front to the back, reaching to a maximum in the proximity of the occipital pole.

To appreciate clearly the origin and termination of the cingulate fibers, the more demonstrative sections are the sagittals and horizontals. In the hotizontals, of which we reproduce one somewhat schematized in fig. 66, *A* [*fig. 192*], three kinds of fibers appear with complete evidence in the cingulum.

1. Direct axons originating from the interhemispheric pyramids, which run backward, gaining the splenium of the corpus callosum and focus of the occipital pole.

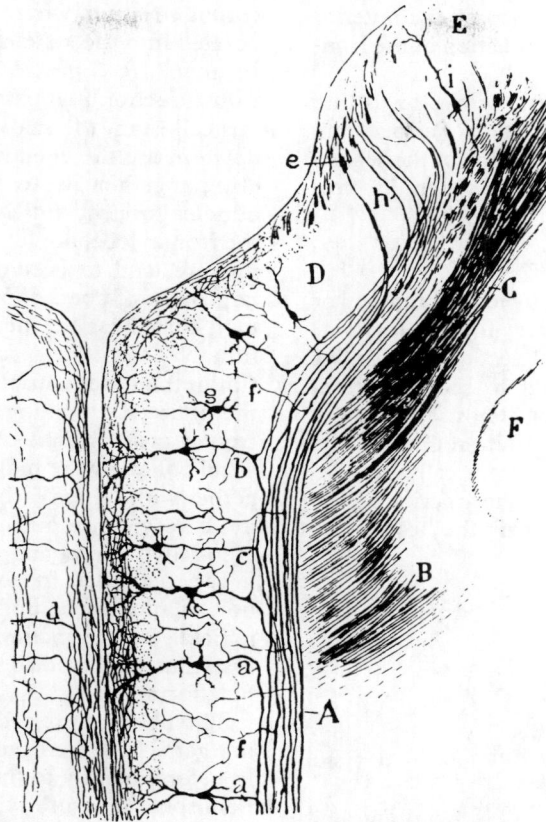

[*FIG. 192*]   Fig. 66. Horizontal section of the cerebrum of the mouse of eight days. *A*, cingulum; *B*, corpus callosum; *C*, crossed angular or spheno-ammonic bundle; *D*, focus of the occipital pole; *E*, subiculum; *F*, Ammon's horn tangentially sectioned; *a*, axon directed forward; *b*, axon bifurcated into anterior and posterior branches; *f*, collaterals terminating in the interhemispheric cortex; *g*, cells with ascending axons; *c*, posterior branch originating from the bifurcation of an axon; *d*, collaterals of the white matter of the cingulum, terminating in the molecular layer; *e*, perforant fascicles sectioned more or less transversely; *h*, perforant fascicles destined for the subiculum; *i*, pyramidal cells of the subiculum. (Method of Golgi.)

2. Direct axons of the same origin, which run forward, rounding the genu of the corpus callosum, and assail the anterior end of the septum lucidum. Such axons are much more numerous than the preceding ones, and especially abundant in the supracallosal region of the interhemispheric cortex (fig. 66, *a*) [*fig. 192*].

3. Axons bifurcating into a thin frontal and a thick dorsal branch or, conversely, into robust frontal and thin dorsal branches or, finally, divided into two equal branches. The posterior or caudal branch is directed in the majority of cases backward, toward the focus of the occipital pole; the anterior or frontal, after going through the superior face of the callosal commissure, gets lost in the corpus striatum (figs. 65, *d;* 66 *b*, *c*) [*figs. 191, 192*].

These bifurcated fibers constitute the large majority of the cingulate fibers, a good many of which correspond to the variety in which the caudal branch is thinner than the frontal (fig. 66, *b*) [*fig. 192*]. It is thus permissible to affirm that the fibers of the posterior portion of the cingulum are mainly dorsal branches originating from axons of the interhemispheric cortex, whereas the fibers of the anterior portion represent the continuation of the frontal branches.

The behavior of the first proves to us that they constitute, in fact, a system of association, while the course and destination of the second tell us that they represent a system of projection.

Termination of the Anterior Branches

What happens subsequently to the branches or to undivided fibers [that are] directed forward? The very anterior frontal sections, as well as the sagittals [cut] parallel to the cingulum, show us very clearly that almost all of these postero-anterior fibers, after rounding the genu and rostrum of the corpus callosum, descend, forming bundles, to the anterior part of the septum lucidum, and gain the head of the

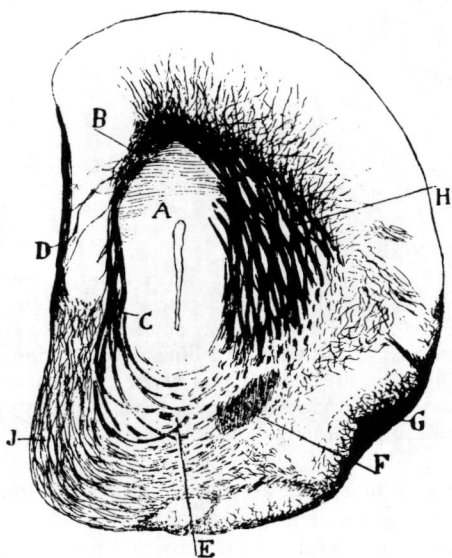

[*FIG. 193*] Fig. 67. Transverse section of the frontal lobe of the mouse of four days. *A*, frontal radiation of the corpus callosum; *B*, anterior portion of the cingulum; *C*, anterior descending bundles of the cingulum; *D*, plexiform layer of the anterior end of the interhemispheric cortex with perforant fibers arriving from the cingulum; *E*, region where the bundles of the cingulum become sagittal; *F*, anterior commissure; *G*, external olfactory root; *H*, corpus striatum; *J*, fibers of projection of the anterior extremity of the interhemispheric cortex. (Method of Golgi.)

corpus striatum, where they are finally incorporated into the system of fibers of projection. In fig. 67, *B*, *C* [*fig. 193*], which reproduces a frontal section that passed in front of the corpus callosum, the said fibers were seen going down inside the ependymal epithelium, gathering together in arciform and loose small bundles to assail finally the inferior plane of the frontal lobe, not far from the anterior commissure, and to become incorporated in the large mass of fibers of projection, mainly olfactory, that cross the head of the corpus striatum. Not all of the descending cingulate fibers run to the corpus striatum; some, as shown in the figure (*D*), coming from the inside of the frontal prolongation of the corpus callosum, assail obliquely the molecular layer, where, together with others earlier arrived, they engender a very dense plexus of nerve fibers, preferentially parallel and vertical. Since we have never succeeded in observing the incorporation of such ascending fibers into the corona radiata, we are inclined to consider them as branches of association terminating in the plexiform layer.

The fibers of projection that pass in front of the genu of the corpus callosum seem to me to belong mainly to the neurons of the interhemispheric fissure lying in the anterior half of this. The ones arising from the more posterior cells, particularly those in the focus of the occipital pole, with the aim of avoiding the long, roundabout course that would result if they had to associate with the anterior ones, [in order] to gain the corpus striatum, perforate the corpus callosum at different points, and, after penetrating the space that lies between this commissure and the dorsal psalterium, they descend through the septum into the inferior levels of the corpus striatum.

Such perforant fibers are none other than the descending small bundles of the fornix longus of Forel, well described by Ganser, Honegger, Edinger, and, especially Kölliker, who has demonstrated them recently in the human cortex. In the opinion of this scholar, the perforant fibers would probably contain ascending and descending [types], the ascending emerging perhaps from the medial mamillary body and terminating in Ammon's horn; the descending come probably from the gyrus for-

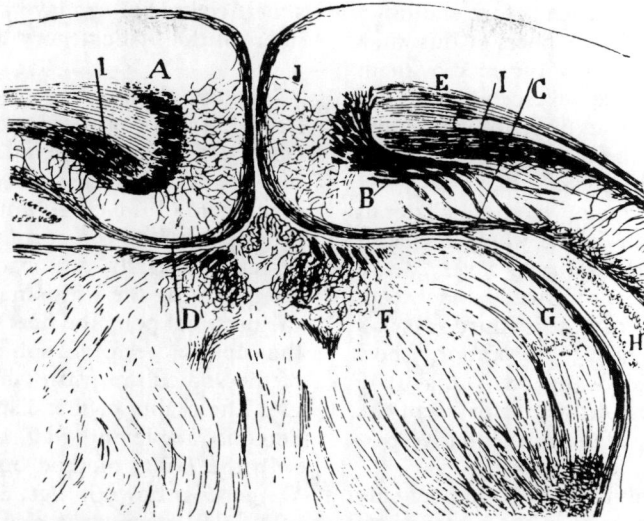

[*FIG. 194*]   Fig. 68. Frontal section of the cerebral hemispheres behind the corpus callosum (mouse of ten days). On one side, the section passes through a more anterior plane than on the other. *A,* cingulum of one side transversely sectioned; *B,* cingulum that arched to be placed underneath the angular or crossed bundle; *C,* perforant bundles directed to the subiculum; *D,* fibers of the interhemispheric plexiform layer continuous with the superficial ones of Ammon's horn; *E,* corpus callosum; *F,* focus of the habenula; *G,* lateral geniculate body; *I,* crossed spheno-ammonic bundle; *J,* plexus of collateral and terminal fibers originating in the cingulum. (Method of Golgi.)

nicatus, penetrate the corpus callosum more frontally than the others, descend to the septum, participate in the *septal olfactory radiation* of Zuckerkandl, and terminate, finally, in the basal ganglion[R] of Ganser.

Our studies have not allowed us to confirm the existence in the fornix longus of ascending fibers, which, if they exist, could very well run not only to Ammon's horn but to the same cortex of the gyrus fornicatus.

As revealed by figs. 33, *E,* and 48, *a* [*figs. 163, 174*], in which the descending portion of the fornix longus appears, the cited perforant fibers are gathered, after having crossed the corpus callosum, near the midline, in the very septum lucidum, from whence they go down flexuously to inferior levels of the cerebrum, merging in their trajectory with the olfactory radiation of Zuckerkandl and with the fibers of the inferior fornix. As the [olfactory] radiation is incorporated, as we will see later,[39] into the corona radiata, without touching the olfactory foci, with which, apparently, the inferior fornix does not establish relations either, we be-

lieve that the fornix longus represents the pathway of projection of the posterior and medial portions of the gyrus fornicatus, a pathway that, for reasons of economy of trajectory and of protoplasm, is made through the corpus callosum, instead of by following the ordinary route.

Posterior Terminations of the Fibers of the Cingulum

The posterior branches of bifurcation of the axons originating in the interhemispheric cortex can be classified, from the point of view of their manner of termination, in three categories: first, fibers terminating in the cortex of the focus of the occipital pole; second, perforant fibers destined for the plexiform layer of this ganglion; and third, fibers destined for the subiculum and Ammon's horn.

1. Fibers Destined for the Focus of the Occipital Pole. [These] are numerous. The majority of them represent collaterals or terminal branches of fibers that still continue their

course for a certain distance before ending in the same manner. In some fibers of this kind, it is observed that at the bend formed by them when they turn [to become] ascending, a thin collateral (terminal for its direction) arises and is incorporated into the plane of the cingulate fibers destined for the subiculum.

These fibers as a whole, whether collaterals or terminals, generate in the whole cortex of the focus of the occipital pole a very dense plexus, especially concentrated underneath the layer of the fusiform cells (third layer), a place where the Weigert preparations show also a very dense plexus (fig. 68, *f*) [fig. 194]. The upper branches of this plexus assail the first layer, in which they from extensive parallel arborizations.

The cited terminal fibers are found not only in the cited focus but also in the posterior regions of the supracallosal interhemispheric territory. They correspond to the thick perforant fibers, drawn in figs. 62, *d, c* [fig. 188]. The plexus that such fibers generate in the third and first layers is notably reinforced by the arborizations of the axons of Martinotti, axons that are very abundant in the whole interhemispheric cortex (figs. 66, *g;* 62, *a*) [figs. 192, 188], and which, on arrival at the superficial plexiform layer, often become postero-anterior, running long trajectories before terminating.

2. Perforant Fibers Destined for the Plexiform Layer of the Focus of the Occipital Pole. They are also very numerous, being observed especially in the middle and inferior regions of the cited ganglion. As revealed by fig. 65, *c* [fig. 191], these fibers, which are usually thin, form isolated bundles that cross the cortical layers without branching, assailing the plexiform layer where they bend, traverse long trajectories, and give off collaterals. Since in the sagittal sections the majority of these fibers appear transversely sectioned, we must suppose that they run in the same direction as the occipital focus, going down in the direction of the subiculum, which perhaps they enter. The large distance that such tangential fibers must traverse until they reach the latter focus prevents us from ascertaining if they positively penetrate it, or if they are exhausted earlier in the

superficial plexiform layer, like the branching fibers of the first category.

3. Bundles Destined for the Subiculum. Serial frontal sections of the posterior portion of the cerebrum of the mouse, guinea pig, and rabbit reveal with complete clarity that the principal contingent of the cingulum goes down around the splenium of the corpus callosum, then is directed laterally and backward, and later, after forming the white matter of the focus of the occipital pole, the fibers enter the plane of the superior perforant spheno-ammonic fibers of the subiculum, with which they intermingle. The reality of this disposition, very easily demonstratable in small mammals, not only with the Golgi method but also with that of Weigert, is shown in figs. 66, *e*, and 68, *C* [figs 192, 194], where it is also seen that the cingulate fibers are situated underneath the angular or commissural bundle, and penetrate successively and in a very oblique direction the cortex of the subiculum, to gain the plexiform layer of this, and assail Ammon's horn. The details of the origin of this new kind of subicular perforant fiber correspond to the same dispositions described when we dealt with the spheno-ammonic perforant fibers; that is to say, the ascending fibers sometimes are simple collaterals of fibers that descend to zones closer to Ammon's horn, other represent terminal fibers, and others, finally, thick branches originating from axons that still continue their initial course for a certain distance, reduced to a thin collateral.

At first sight, it seems that the spheno-ammonic perforant fibers must be easily confused with the cingulate fibers, and, in fact, their separation is difficult in sagittal sections, but in frontal sections, and especially in those parallel to the subiculum (fig. 52, *E*) [fig. 178], they are distinguished by their different directions: the superior perforant spheno-ammonic fibers run from below upward and from lateral to medial, whereas the cingulate fibers run from above downward and from medial to lateral. In some places, both kinds of perforant fibers are observed at the same time, and their crossed direction can be easily noticed.

From all that we have exposed about the white matter of the interhemispheric cortex, it follows that this cerebral focus gives origin to three classes of exogenous fibers: fibers of projection destined for lower levels still unknown; fibers of association at short distance, destined to link somewhat separated areas of the same interhemispheric ganglion; and fibers of association at long distance, terminating in the subiculum and Ammon's horn. Do commissural or callosal fibers also exist in the interhemispheric cortex? In man, such fibers appear to exist (see, for example, Dejerine); but in the small mammals, as we have indicated in another work,[40] we have not been able to reveal them, a negative fact that would be of great theoretical importance if it could be generalized to other association areas of the cerebrum. Perhaps the callosal fibers originating in the human cingulate gyrus come exclusively from the superior portion, not the cingulate [area], and [are] not specific for this area.

A great lacuna still remains to be filled in this brief study about the structure and connections of the interhemispheric cortex: the origin and termination of its centripetal fibers. [This is] lamentable ignorance, since so long as we do not know the origin and functional nature of the afferent fibers, it will be impossible to extract from the indicated facts any reasonably secure physiological deduction.

General opinion, since the memorable works of Broca, requires that the limbic gyri are the place of distribution of primary or secondary olfactory fibers. However, all our efforts to find such afferent sensory fibers have failed completely. The analysis to which we have submitted the cerebral bundles of fibers that in small mammals appear to link the limbic cortex with the septum lucidum, olfactory tubercle, bulbar pedicle, and head of the corpus striatum, etc., has persuaded us that these fibers represent centrifugal or descending pathways that pass near the olfactory foci, with which they have no more than relations of vicinity.[s]

[X] Inferomedial Cortex of the Frontal Lobe

It is not our purpose to deal in detail here with the question of the structure of the limbic gyri and of their relationships to the olfactory radiations. Our purpose is limited to the state-

ment that in the fissural cortex or [cortex] on the medial surface of the frontal lobule (infracallosal cortex) of small mammals, we have not been able to observe the entrance of any primary or secondary olfactory pathway.

This cortex possesses, as we have mentioned above, very special characteristics. Absence of stratification, disorientation of the dendrites, existence of voluminous cells of variable shape, mixed with cells of smaller size, and the presence among the cells of a great number of small bundles and tangential fibers, mostly with a descending course—such are the characteristics that allow [us] to recognize, at first glance, this cortical territory in Nissl, Weigert, and Golgi preparations.

We show two figures of this territory, both taken from the mouse of eight days. One (fig. 67, $\mathcal{J}^T$) [fig. 193] shows a frontal section examined at low magnification. Even in this, it can be seen that the cortex here is striped tangentially with a multitude of almost parallel fibers, which, on arriving at the inferior plane of the frontal lobule, incline laterally to become finally sagittal, and enter the great olfactory projection pathway. In fig. 72^U, A [fig. 195], which represents, at higher magnification, a portion of the same interhemispheric region, it is clearly seen that the parallel axons come from certain triangular, stellate, or fusiform cells of voluminous or medium size, devoid of radial orientation, and lying at all the cortical levels. The axons of the most superficial [cells] usually also run superficially in the cortex without emitting collaterals (at least in mammals a few days old), while those originating from the deepest [cells] run through the deep zones and can even be associated with the projection pathway of the cingulum, which lies very close (fig. 72, C) [fig. 195]. But not all the fibers which cross this cortex in a parallel orientation emanate from intrinsic cells; some, the most superficial and especially thick [fibers], come from the septum lucidum, being continuous, as we will see later, with the *radiation* of Zuckerkandl.

We have observed few free exogenous arborizations in this cortical territory; the ones represented in our preparations seemed to come from below, [from] the region of the corona radiata. It was not possible to determine

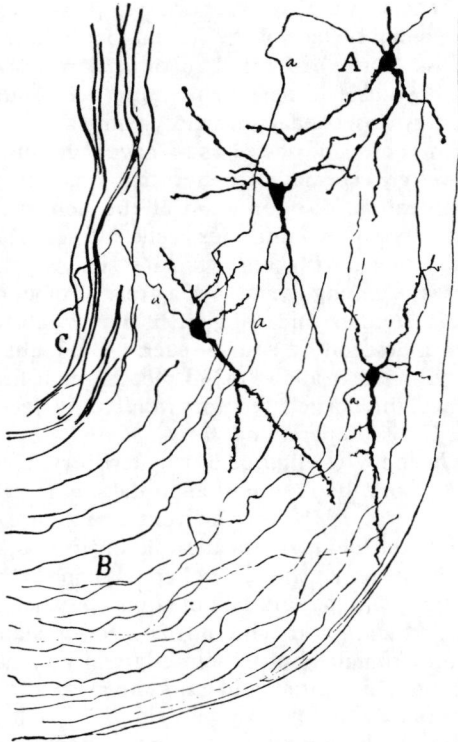

[FIG. 195]   Fig. 72. Cells of the infero-internal region of the frontal lobule. *A, B,* large cells; *C,* anterior descending bundles of the cingulum. Mouse of twelve to fifteen days. (Method of Golgi.)

their origin. In any case, none of them seemed to run in the direction of the olfactory bulb, nor were they continuous with olfactory fibers of second order. Nor does the method of Marchi reveal degeneration in this cerebral region, after sectioning of the olfactory bulb.

In short, the cortex of the internal surface and most posterior portion of the frontal lobule has a great similarity to the gray matter of the septum lucidum, with which it is continuous in part, and in whose connections it perhaps participates.

General Conclusions

The following propositions can be considered as the general conclusions of the preceding work on the sphenoidal cortex and on the other systems and pathways generally considered as olfactory:

1. We must consider as secondary olfactory centers all those which undoubtedly receive fibers from the lateral, medial, or superior [olfactory] roots. Such centers, all of which possess a similar structure, are the cotrex of the olfactory lobule (bulbar pedicle), the frontal cortex underlying the lateral [olfactory] root, and the external region of the sphenoidal cortex.

2. The subiculum, the presubicular area, and Ammon's horn do not seem to possess direct olfactory fibers.

3. The amygdala, the septum lucidum, the limbic gyri and interhemispheric cortex, the supracallosal striae, the prechiasmatic fissural cortex, etc., apparently lack direct olfactory relationships. The supposed connections between the olfactory bulb and the [olfactory] tubercle are probable, but not perfectly demonstrated.

4. The afferent pathways of Ammon's horn are the posterior prolongation of the cingulum, the occipital ends of the supracallosal striae, the superficial white matter of the interhemispheric cortex, and a very important pathway originating in a special ganglion, situated at the posterior lip of the hemispheres, over the olfactory sphenoidal cortex and beneath the presubiculum.

5. This special ganglion furnishes both a direct and a crossed ammonic pathway, both terminating in the plexiform layers of Ammon's horn and the fascia dentata.

6. We do not know the physiological significance of the spheno-occipital or angular ganglion from which these systems arise. So far, we have not been able to observe in it the arrival of fibers coming from the lateral olfactory root or those of the tertiary olfactory pathways. Besides, this cortical region is perfectly distinguished by its very special structure from the secondary olfactory centers, and particularly from the olfactory sphenoidal cortex. If in the future it would be possible to observe the entry and termination in this focus of some olfactory collateral, direct or indirect, there would be ipso facto demonstrated the existence and point of arrival in Ammon's horn of olfactory fibers, fibers that nowadays are gratuitously supposed to arrive via the septum lucidum.

7. The sphenoidal lobule contains, besides, an important focus adjacent to the subiculum, the presubiculum, also with a special texture, and whose fibers mainly enter the angular or crossed bundle and the dorsal psalterium.

Cajal's Notes

1. This work forms a part of an extensive mémoíre, which, under the title *Orígenes y terminaciones de los nervios olfativo, óptico y acústico en los vertebrados,* was presented to the Real Academia de Medicina de Madrid as an application for the Martínez y Molina Prize. The excessive delay in printing this extensive monograph (the manuscript and the drawings were submitted in June of 1901) has obliged us to anticipate publication (with the permission of the Academy) of some of the more original chapters of the same.

2. Cajal, Contribución al estudio de la vía sensitiva central y estructura del tálamo óptico, *Rev. Trim. Microgr.,* Vol. V, 1900.

3. Cajal, Die Endigung des äusseren Lemniscus oder die sekundäre akustische Nervenbahn, *Deutsche Mediz. Wochenschrift,* 17 April 1902.

4. See *Revista Trimestral,* Vols. IV and V.

5. Löwenthal, *Ueber das Riechhirn der Säugethiere,* Braunschweig, 1897.

6. Cajal, Sobre la existencia de bifurcaciones y colaterales de los nervios sensitivos y sustancia blanca del cerebro, *Gaceta Sanitaria de Barcelona,* April 1891.

7. Calleja, La región olfatoria del cerebro, Madrid, 1893.

8. See our works on the structure of the motor, visual, and acoustic areas of the cerebrum, *Rev. Trim. Microgr.,* Vols. IV and V.

9. Betz, *Centralblatt. f. d. medicin. Wissensch.,* nos. 11–13, 1881.

10. H. Obersteiner, *Anleitung beim Studium des Baues der nervösen Centralorgane,* Leipzig, 1892.

11. S. Ramón y Cajal, Estructura del asta de Ammon, *Anales de la Socied. Españ. de Historia Natural,* Vol. XXII, 1893.

12. Dejerine, *Anatomie des centres nerveux,* Paris, Vol. I., 1895.

13. Hammarberg, *Studien über Klinik und Pathologie der Idiotie,* etc., Upsala, 1895.

14. Calleja, La región olfatoria del cerebro, Madrid, 1893.

15. Kölliker, *Lehrbuch der Gewebelehre,* Vol. II, p. 723 [1896].

16. S. R. y Cajal, Estructura del asta de Ammon y fascia dentata, etc., *Anal. de la Socied. Españ. de Historia Natural,* Vol. XXII, 1893.

17. Ganser, Vergleichend-anatomische Studien über das Gehirn des Maulwurfs, *Morphologisches Jahrbuch,* Bd. 7, 1882. See also from the same author: Ueber die vordere Hirnkommissur der Säugethiere, *Arch. für Psych.,* Vol. IX [1878].

18. Kölliker, *Lehrbuch der Gewebelehre,* Vol. II, p. 715 [1896].

19. Honegger, Vergleichend-anat. Unter. über den Fornix, etc, Geneva, 1886.

20. Dejerine, *Anat. des centres nerveux,* Vol. II, 1901. See also: *Compt. Rend. Société de Biol.,* 1897.

21. S. R. Cajal, Estructura del asta de Ammon., *Anal. de la Socied. Españ. de Historia Natural,* Madrid, 1893.

22. Kölliker, *Lehrbuch der Gewebelehre,* Vol. II, pp. 789, 790 [1896].

23. Edinger, *Vorlesungen über den Bau der nervösen Centralorgane des Menschen und der Thiere,* etc., 6th edition, Liepzig, [1899].

24. S. R. Cajal, Estructura del septum lucidum, *Rev. Trim.,* Vol. VI, [1902].

25. See Cajal, Sobre un ganglio especial de la corteza esfeno-occipital de los roedores. See in this same volume.

26. Honegger, Vergleichend-anatomischen Untersuchungen über den Fornix, etc., *Rec. de Zool. Suisse.,* Vol. V, 1890.

27. Dejerine, *Anatomie des centres nerveux,* Vol. II, 1901, p. 296.

28. Hammarberg, *Studien über Klinik und Pathologie der Idiotie,* etc., Upsala, 1895.

29. S. Ramón Cajal, Structure de l'écorce cérébrale de quelques mammifères, *La Cellule,* 189[1].

30. S. R. Cajal, Pequeñas comunicaciones anatómicas II: Sobre la existencia de colaterales y bifurcaciones en las fibras de la sustancia blanca del cerebro, December 1890.

31. S. R. Cajal, Estructura de la corteza occipital de los pequeños mamíferos. *Anales de la Sociedad Española de Historia Natural,* Vol. XXII, 1893.

32. Ganser, *Loc. cit.*

33. Cajal, *La Cellule,* Vol. VII.

34. Kölliker, *Lehrbuch der Gewebelehre,* Vol. 2, p. 780, fig. 803, [1896]. See also: Ueber Fornix longus von Forel und die Riechstrahlungen im Gehirn des Kaninchen, *Verhandl. des Anat. Gesellsch.,* 1894.

35. Beevor, On the Course of the Fibres of the Cingulum and the Posterior Parts of the Corpus Callosum and Fornix in the Marmoset Monkey, *Phil. Transactions,* 1891.

36. Edinger, *Vorlesungen ueber den Bau der nervösen Centralorgane,* etc., 6th edition, [1899].

37. Dejerine, *Loc. cit.,* p. 749 and following.

38. E. Smith, *Journ. of Anat. and Physiol.,* Vol. 32, 1898.

39. S. R. Cajal, Textura del *septum lucidum.* See this volume.

40. S. R. Cajal, Estructura de la corteza motriz., *Rev. Trim.,* Vol. V, [1899].

Editors' Notes

A. The sphenoidal cortex of animals is now usually termed *temporal cortex* and was so translated by Azoulay in the *Histologie du système nerveux.* See his footnote on page 686 of the second volume of that work.

B. [Here follows Chapter I (pages 2–20), devoted to the olfactory bulb. We recommence our translation with Chapter II on page 20.]

C. The text incorrectly says 6.

D. By *hippocampal gyrus,* Cajal means the modern parahippocampal gyrus, not the hippocampus proper. The latter he names by its separate parts: Ammon's horn, fascia dentata, and subiculum.

E. The original text incorrectly says 22.

F. The original text incorrectly says 22.

G. See note A in introduction.

H. The olfactory tubercle.

I. [Here (at page 77) follows Chapter V on the superior olfactory tract, Chapter VI on the olfactory tubercle, and Chapter VII on Ammon's horn. We recommence our translation on page 90 but reproduce fig. 41 [*fig. 167*] from Chapter VII, since it is alluded to later in the text.]

J. The cingulate gyrus.

K. See chapter 19 in this volume. The angular focus is probably the medial entorhinal area.

L. Inserted by the editors. This figure appears here as well as in the *Textura* and the *Histologie,* but it is not mentioned in any of these works.

M. We cannot determine the reason for Cajal's use of the adjective *optic* here. In the German translation of 1903 and in the *Textura,* he calls the comparable section "Spheno-Ammonic Alvear Pathway," and in the *Histologie,* he calls it "Temporo-Ammonic Alvear Pathway."

N. Inserted by the editors.

O. Inserted by the editors.

P. Inserted by the editors. This figure appears here as well as in the *Textura* and the *Histologie,* but it is not mentioned.

Q. See chapters 6 and 28 in this volume.

R. The olfactory tubercle.

S. [Here (at page 132) follows Chapter X on the supracallosal striae and the inferomedial cortex of the frontal lobe. We translate only pages 138–140, dealing with the last mentioned area of the brain and with Cajal's general conclusions on the olfactory cortex.]

T. The text, apparently incorrectly, says *A.*

U. The text incorrectly says 74.

19

On a Special Ganglion of the Spheno-Occipital Cortex

[*Trabajos del Laboratorio de Investigaciones Biológicas de la Universidad de Madrid* 1:189–206, 1901–1902]

At several points in our study of the olfactory cortex and Ammon's horn,[1] we have alluded to a special focus at the posterior border of the cerebral hemispheres from which arise three robust pathways terminating in Ammon's horn and the fascia dentata. To complete the study of this center, whose afferent pathways have already been described in detail, we are going to give here some new data on its structure and possible physiological significance.

Topography of the Angular or Spheno-occipital Focus[2]

When horizontal sections of the cerebrum that pass through the union of the occipital and temporal lobes are examined in the mouse, guinea pig, or rabbit, there appears, at the point at which the cortex of the external face of the hemispheres is curved to become internal and continuous with the presubiculum, a special cortex very different in appearance and manner of stratification from that seen in the adjacent regions, and from which it can be separated very accurately. This is the *angular focus*, which we can study equally well in very lateral sagittal sections, that is to say, in those

that pass through the center of the superoposterior extremity of the temporal lobe.

The sagittal sections reveal clearly the superior and inferior limits of the focus under study. In fig. 1, *B* [*fig. 196*], taken from a cat, and at very low magnification, we reproduce one such section that is very appropriate for appreciating the real position of the occipito-temporal nucleus. Notice that it begins at the height of the sphenoidal olfactory cortex, in front of the superior limit of the lenticular nucleus, superiorly ending at the inferior edge of a short transverse gyrus, which in the [cat], crosses the caudal border of the occipital lobe. The deep frontier of the focus is adherent to the white matter of the subiculum, which, in fig. 1, *B* [*fig. 196*], is shown sectioned lengthways. In the rabbit and mouse, the macroscopical superior limit is not observed as clearly as in the cat, because of the absence of the mentioned transverse gyrus; it can, however, be determined, as we show in fig. 4 [fig. 199], at the angle or very sharp point at which the piriform lobe is terminated superiorly.

The internal and external lateral limits are shown with complete clarity in the transverse sections, these being represented respectively

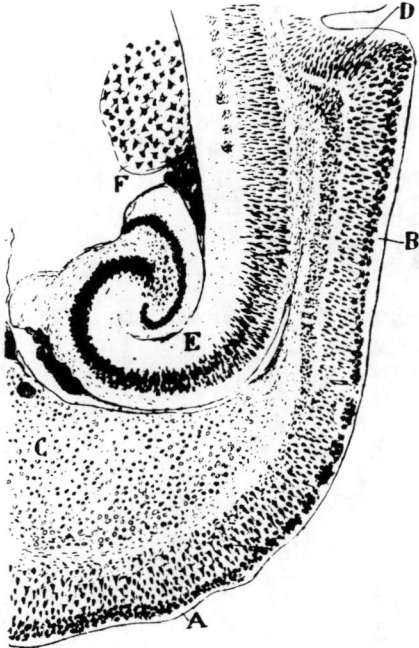

[FIG. 196] Fig. 1. Central sagittal section of the piriform lobe of the cat of one month and a half. Nissl method. A, sphenoidal cortex, clearly olfactory; B, spheno-occipital focus; D, superior termination of this focus at the level of the transverse gyrus; C, lenticular nucleus; E, Ammon's horn.

by the presubiculum and the superior prolongation of the *rhinal fissure.*

Such sections, stained with the Nissl method, reveal the following stratification: first, *plexiform layer;* second, *layer of the large stellate cells;* third, *layer of the medium and large pyramids;* fourth, *deep plexiform layer;* fifth, *layer of the horizontal cells;* sixth, *layer of the granule cells or small pyramids;* seventh, *layer of the polymorphic cells;* eighth, *layer of the white matter.* The third is the thickest of all these strata, forming more than a third of the whole cortex, and that of the horizontal cells is thinnest, at many points being seen to be represented by one or two discontinuous rows of cells.

The referred stratifications are presented almost in the same manner in the mouse, rat, rabbit, guinea pig, dog, and cat. Fig. 3 [fig. 198] corresponds to the last animal and represents

a portion of the sagittal section drawn in fig. 1, B [fig. 196], at higher magnification.

1. Plexiform Layer

It shows the classic histological construction of this layer [as seen throughout] the whole cortex, namely (a) fusiform, globular, or stellate cells with short axon of which we show some examples in fig. 5 a^A[fig. 200]; (b) horizontal cells (figs. 7^B and 5) [figs. 202, 200], apparently less frequent than the previous ones; (c) dendritic tufts originating from the underlying pyramids and ascending dendrites of the neighboring stellate cells; (d) ascending fibers of Martinotti; (e) recurrent axon collaterals of cells resident in deep layers.

Of all the cited elements, there is one that is dominant and brings character to the plexiform layer, explaining the great thickness of the layer in this cerebral region. This element is represented by fibers and ascending collaterals, which reach the plexiform layer in very great abundance and at all levels of the layer, but, especially at deep levels adjacent to the stellate cells, they become parallel, engendering a very dense and extremely widespread plexus. Among the elements of this intricate plexus, certain robust ascending axons show up on account of their thickness; these, once transformed into tangential [fibers], run preferentially from down to up, traversing at different levels of the first layer almost the whole extent of the focus, and resolving into numerous collaterals, arborized not only in the said layer but also and very particularly in the layer of the large stellate cells. None of these thick fibers trespasses over the frontier of the angular nucleus to invade the supero-internal occipital cortex. Nor in the inferior part have we seen them leave the cited ganglion. Commonly, when they are followed to their origin, it is verified that, after a variable ascending trajectory, they sink into the middle or deep gray layers, and their impregnation suddenly ceases, as if the silver chromate would [avoid] the parent cell. Such descents of the main [axonal] trunk are observed preferentially in the inferior fourth of the focus. Furthermore, as we will see later, it is very frequent to see axons originating from cells with ascending

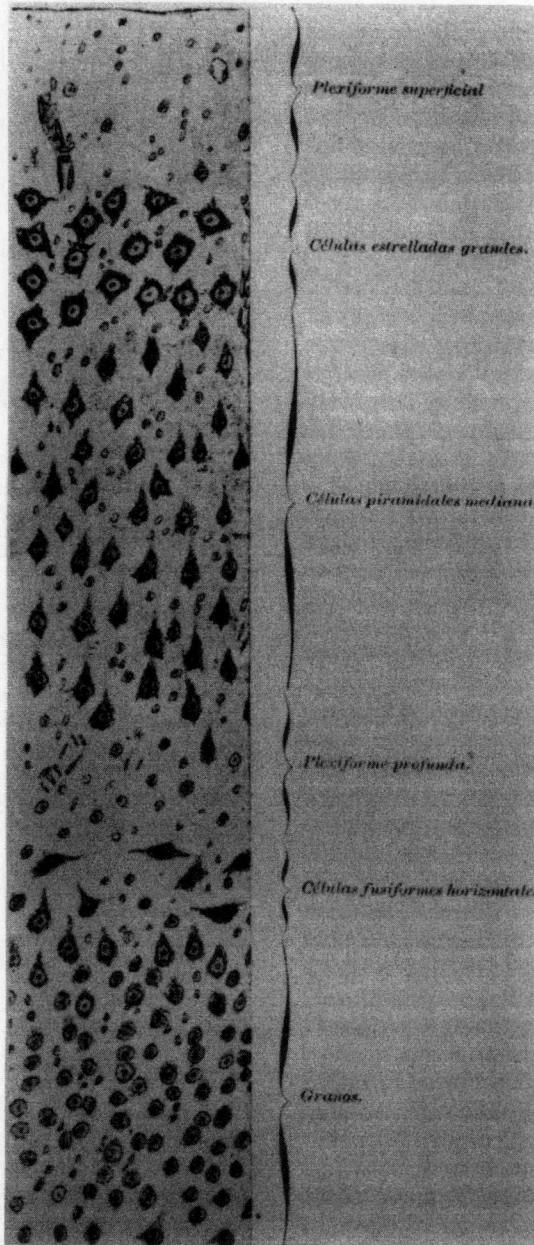

Plexiforme superficial

Células estrelladas grandes.

Células piramidales medianas

Plexiforme profunda.

Células fusiformes horizontales

Granos.

[FIG. 197]   Fig. 2. Transverse section of the spheno-occipital cortex of the adult rabbit. Superficial plexiform layer; layer of the large stellate cells; layer of the medium pyramidal cells; deep plexiform layer; horizontal fusiform cells; layer of the granule cells. (Nissl method.)

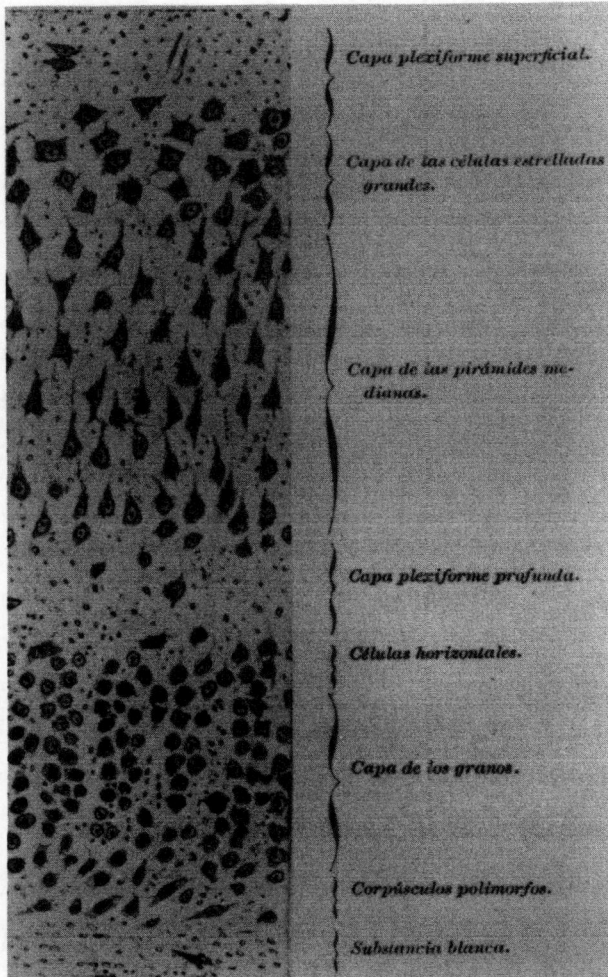

[*FIG. 198*] Fig. 3. Longitudinal section of the spheno-occipital cortex of the cat of one month and a half. Nissl method. (Lower magnification than in the previous figure.) Superficial plexiform layer; layer of the large stellate cells; layer of the medium pyramidal cells; deep plexiform layer; horizontal cells; layer of granule cells; polymorphic cells; white matter.

axons going up to the first layer and to be continued as thick, medium, or thin tangential fibers. Altogether, this leads us to believe that the mentioned thick tangential fibers represent the peripheral trajectory of endogenous conductors; however, we do not consider this point sufficiently elucidated.

2. Layer of the Large Stellate Cells

The Nissl preparations show us such cells to be of regular size (24 to 30 μm), of a polygonal or stellate form with abundant protoplasm filled with [Nissl] granules and a voluminous nucleus. Generally, they are arranged in two or three irregular rows of cells, somewhat separated by an interstitial plexus. In some places, there is observed a tendency to assemble in poorly delimited accumulations or pleiades.

The Golgi preparations confirm the indicated morphology and add some data relative to the behavior of the processes. The dendrites, as can be appreciated in fig. 5, *A* [*fig. 200*], are abundant, flexuous, and spiny; they

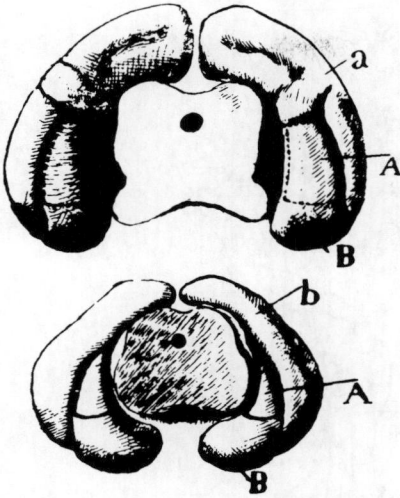

[FIG. 199] Fig. 4. Posterior edge of the cerebral hemispheres of the cat and rabbit. A, angular focus; B, sphenoidal olfactory focus; b, ganglion of the occipital pole.

emerge from all sides of the soma, run in several orientations, [and are] repeatedly divided. The ascending ones among them, of variable number, are distributed in the first layer, but they do not arise from an [apical dendritic] shaft and are no thicker or longer than the descending and lateral [dendrites], a peculiarity that distinguishes these cells, at a glance, both from the cerebral pyramids and from the cells of the second layer of the subiculum, presubiculum, and olfactory sphenoidal cortex.

The axon is robust and descending; it originates either from the soma or from an inferior dendrite, traverses all the underlying gray layers, and is continuous with a fiber of the white matter. During its initial trajectory, and during its passage through the extensive third layer, it gives off four, five, or more collaterals, some horizontal or oblique and others recurrent; some of [the recurrent collaterals], like the initial collaterals of the giant stellate cells of the human visual cortex, are as thick or thicker than the descending continuation of the [parent] trunk. The recurrent collaterals are distributed both in the second layer and in the thickness of the first, whose nervous plexus they make more complicated; the deeper collaterals are distributed almost exclusively in

the different levels of the third layer (figs. 7, B; 5, A), [figs. 202, 200].

Besides the cited cells, the second layer contains some pyramidal cells, cells with short axon, and certain triangular neurons with a very oblique ascending [dendritic] shaft, and whose axon appears to run horizontally. In fig. 7, e [fig. 202], we show one of the latter cells, whose morphological properties we have not been able to analyze completely.

Between the cells of the second layer, there exists an extremely complicated nervous plexus in whose formation participate, besides the intrinsic cells with short axon, collaterals and terminals of tangential fibers of the first layer and the terminal arborizations of cells with ascending axons resident in the third layer (fig. 6, B, b) [fig. 201].

3. Layer of the Medium Pyramids

The sections stained with basic aniline [dyes] show that this wide layer contains several planes of pyramids of medium size, similar to those of the common cerebral cortex (fig. 2 and 3) [figs. 197, 198]. The cells placed near the second layer are usually somewhat smaller than those resident in the vicinity of the fourth, but often this difference in size is little accentuated. Although the majority of such cells have a pyramidal shape, there is no lack of fusiform, globular, or even triangular cells. In any case, from the soma there always arise one or two radial [dendritic] tufts destined for the first layer, some lateral dendrites branching at quite a long distance, and several basal dendrites, more or less descending, but without constituting the tassel or typical tuft of the olfactory sphenoidal pyramids. The descending dendrites, coming from the deepest rows of pyramids, are concentrated in the fourth or [deep] plexiform layer, engendering a very dense feltwork, beyond which few dendrites pass.

In addition, the following cells inhabit the third layer:

a. Small, fusiform, or triangular cells provided with an ascending axon, arborized in the cited layer, as well as in the second and first [layers] (fig. 6, a, b) [fig. 201].

b. Voluminous and downy fusiform cell, analogous to that resident in the human visual

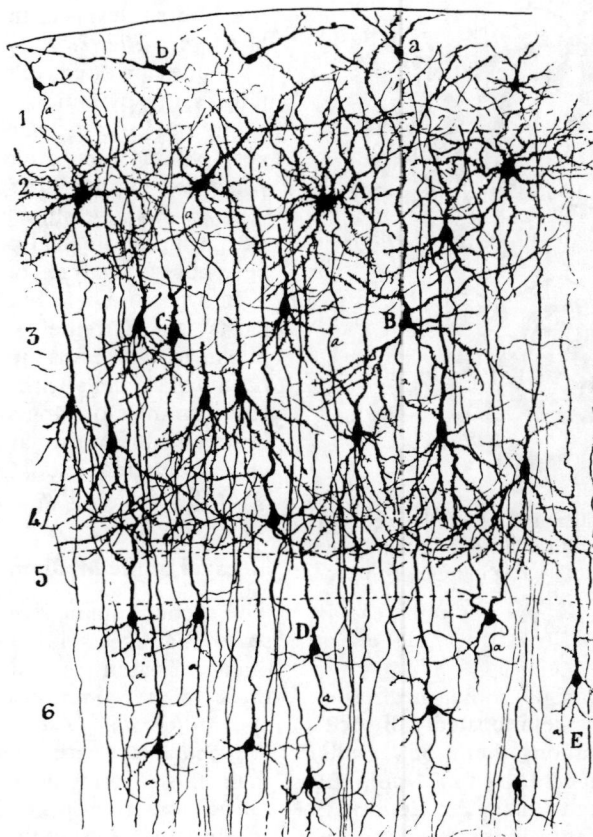

[*FIG. 200*] Fig. 5. Horizontal section of the angular focus of the mouse of eight days. *1*, plexiform layer; *2*, layer of the large stellate cells; *3*, layer of the medium pyramids; *4*, plexiform layer; *5*, layer of the horizontal cells; *6*, layer of the granule cells; *A*, stellate cell; *B*, pyramid; *C*, fusiform cell with short ascending axon; *D*, *E*, granule cells.

cortex (fourth layer), provided with external and internal [dendritic] tufts and with an ascending axon, divided in long horizontal fibers, ramified mainly in the second layer (fig. 5, *C*) [*fig. 200*].

c. Stellate cells with short axon ramifying at a short distance (classic type [II cell] of Golgi).

The third layer, like the second and the fourth, shows in well-impregnated Golgi preparations an axonal plexus of extraordinary richness which offers the peculiarity of being suddenly cut off toward the deep third of the gray cortex, that is to say, at the frontier of the fifth layer. The unusual and exceptional richness of this plexus, one of the thinnest, most intricate, and richest that can be seen in the

central nervous system; its restriction to the fourth layer; and its sudden cessation at the superior, inferior, internal, and external frontiers of the focus under study constitute one of the characteristic features of this [area] and an infallible means of preventing its confusion with bordering cortical regions, all of which either do not reveal any stained plexus (as happens almost constantly in the cerebrum of the mouse of four or six days), or they possess a much less rich [plexus] of very diverse localization and appearance. The sections presented in figs. 54 and 55 [*figs. 180, 181*, in chapter 18 of this volume] give an idea, although not an exact one, of the appearance, richness, and situation of this singular plexus.

d. Free arborizations of terminal or collateral nerve fibers coming from the white matter.

Third and Fourth Layers at the Superior End of the Focus

The form, dimensions, and abundance of the [cellular] elements of these layers vary little in most parts of the angular ganglion; there is, however, a territory corresponding to the upper end of the same that exhibits mutations worthy of notice. To begin with, this region possesses a larger number of neurons than the others, which is due not only to the greater thickness of the third and fourth layers but

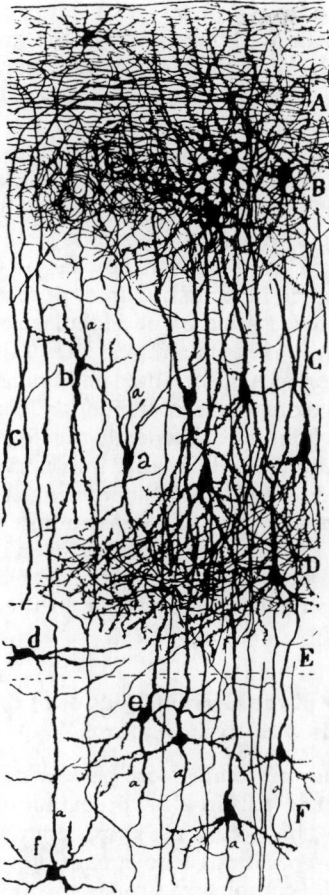

[FIG. 201] Fig. 6. Transverse section of the angular focus of the rabbit of six days. A, plexiform layer; B, layer of the stellate cells; C, medium pyramids; D, plexiform layer; E, layer of the horizontal fusiform cells; F, granule cells.

The following elements combine in order to form the cited nervous plexus:

a. Innumerable collaterals originating from the axons of the already described stellate cells (second layer), as well as from the medium pyramids (third layer).

b. Terminal axonal arborizations, coming from the cells with short axon of the third layer and from cells of Martinotti.

c. A prodigious number of recurrent or retrograde arciform collaterals of the granule cells (see below).

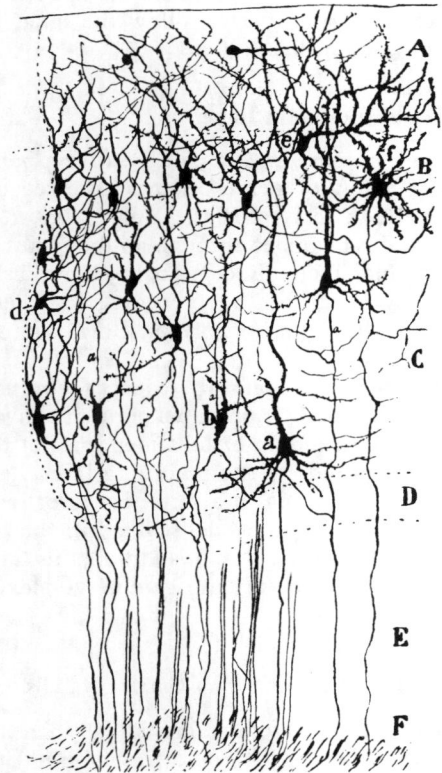

[FIG. 202] Fig. 7. Lateral sagittal section of the cerebrum of the mouse of eight days. A, plexiform layer; B, stellate cells; C, layer of the pyramids; D, layer of the horizontal cells; E, layer of the granule cells; a, medium pyramid; b, cell with ascending axon; c, d, cells of the superior limit of the focus.

also to the decrease in the volume and increased packing [density] of these [layers]. Notice, besides, that the pyramidal cells here frequently have an ovoid, triangular, or fusiform shape; that the [apical dendritic] tuft of the same appears flexuous and resolves itself into secondary branches; that, finally, the volume of the stellate cells (second layer) appears diminished, and the diameter of the dendrites is thinner (fig. 7, *B*) [*fig. 202*].

The cells lying at the very frontier of the cited territory are the most reduced in volume and the most metamorphosed; their form is almost completely stellate, without indications of an [apical dendritic] shaft, and their dendrites are thin, flexuous, and varicose, and in large part directed in a vertical direction, forming a plexus so entangled that it is hardly possible to identify and follow the long descending axon (fig. 7, *d*) [*fig. 202*].

4. [Deep] Plexiform Layer

In Nissl preparations, a pale plexiform band, almost bereft of nerve cells, is observed beneath the third layer (figs. 2 and 3) [*figs. 197, 198*], and is extended through all the cortex of the angular focus. Exceptionally, some dislocated pyramids of the preceding layer and some small, ovoid, or polygonal cells are observed in it.

The silver chromate allows [us] to recognize that this layer is the principal point of convergence of descending or basal dendrites of the deeper pyramids of the preceding layer, dendrites that, running in a variety of directions, engender an extremely dense dendritic plexus (fig. 6, *D*) [*fig. 201*]. But, in addition, this layer forms part of the very intricate nerve plexus, described above.

5. Layer of the Horizontal Fusiform Cells

Nissl preparations reveal, immediately beneath the preceding plexiform layer, a thin rim, whose rather large cells, [which are] scarce and separated, exhibit a cell body with ovoid or fusiform shape, provided with dendrites oriented preferentially in a horizontal direction (fig. 2) [*fig. 197*]. From time to time, there also appear,

as seen in fig. 2 [*fig. 197*], some large pyramidal cells similar to the residents of the third layer.

The elements of this layer are characterized by being extraordinarily refractory to the silver chromate. In all the preparations that we have, no cells appear, but their hollows [are seen] arranged in one or two irregular rows and separated by small bundles of axons that come down from the superimposed layers.

We have seen only three cells of this kind impregnated in some hundreds of sections. All three showed a large and globular soma, provided with one or two robust lateral thick dendrites, horizontally oriented and branched; and a thick axon that ran flexuously and with a parallel orientation beneath the fourth layer and resolved itself, finally, into nerve ramifications destined for the bordering layers and preferentially for the superimposed [layer]. For the rest, this layer is very poor in axonal arborizations; almost the totality of the fibers that traverse it are in passage to the superior layers (fig. 8, *a*) [*fig. 203*].

6. Layer of the Granule Cells or of the Small Pyramids with Arciform Axon

The mass of small, close-packed nuclei that this layer reveals in Nissl preparations (figures 2 and 3), [*figs. 197, 198*], appears resolved in Golgi preparations into an infinity of small pyramids, completely similar to the ones described by us in the 6th and 8th layers of the human visual cortex[3] or in the 5th layer (layer of the granule cells) of the motor cortex.

As is seen in fig. 5c, *D, E* [*fig. 200*], such cells possess a thin and long [apical dendritic] shaft terminating in the first layer, several delicate basal dendrites, and a thin axon that, first descending for a certain distance, traces an arch with an external concavity and then goes up to arborize and end in the upper layers. From the convexity of the initial arch arise one or several branches ramifying in the deeper levels of the layer under study. Sometimes, it has seemed to us that one of these descending branches is prolonged to the white matter, representing, consequently, in regard to its direction, the continuation of the axon, but in regard to its thickness, a long collateral (fig. 8, *e*) [*fig. 203*]. Neither is it rare to notice, as happens in the human visual cortex, that the axon generates not only one arch but two or three because [of the way] it resolves itself into other recurrent branches (fig. 5, *E*) [*fig. 200*].

The layer of the granule cells also presents some pyramidal cells with long axon and, especially, certain ovoid or fusiform cells with short axon, of which we draw an example in fig. 8, *b*^D [*fig. 203*].

A peculiarity of the layer of the granule cells is the poverty of the interstitial nerve plexus, which contrasts notably with the exceptional richness of the plexus located in the first, second, third, and fourth layers. Almost all the fibers that traverse the said stratum represent fibers in passage.

7. Layer of the Polymorphic and Fusiform Cells

Some polygonal, fusiform, and triangular large cells, few in number and not constituting a continuous well-demarcated stratum, are seen beneath the granule cells among the radial bundles of axons, and even in the very

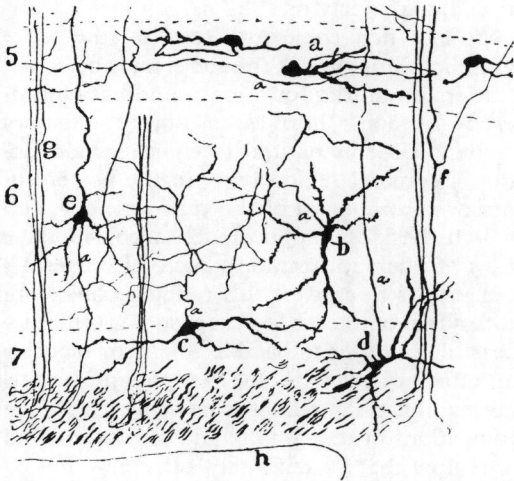

[*FIG. 203*] Fig. 8. Inferior layers of the angular cortex of the mouse. *5*, horizontal cells; *6*, layer of the granule cells; *7*, layer of the polymorphic cells; *a*, horizontal cells; *b*, cells with short axon; *c, d*, bundles of axons that cross the layer of the granule cells; *h*, ventricle.

white matter; most of them, as is seen in fig. 8, *c, d* [*fig. 203*], belong to the category of cells provided with ascending axon ramifying in the thickness of the preceding layers.

White Matter

a. Centrifugal fibers. We have dealt already, in our study of the afferent pathways of Ammon's horn, with some details about the composition of the white matter of the spheno-occipital focus, and of the course of the centrifugal fibers.

Here we will limit ourselves to remembering that all the fibers originating from the pyramids, from the large stellate cells, and from some of the granule cells descend through the inferior layers gathered together in small bundles, and, on arriving at the white matter, they bend to form the following pathways: first, the *crossed spheno-ammonic bundle* or dorsal psalterium; second, the *superior perforant spheno-ammonic pathway* of Ammon's horn; third, the *spheno-alvear bundles or pathway;* and fourth, the *inferior perforant spheno-ammonic pathway.*

But, although the immense majority of the fibers of the angular temporo-occipital focus are incorporated in the said pathways, there are also fibers, either direct or collaterals or branches of bifurcation, which are concentrated near the ventricle in a thin white lamina and then go forward and upward and perhaps enter the corpus striatum and corona radiata. In fig. 9, *a* [*fig. 204*], we show a section on which is traced, somewhat schematically, the possible direction followed by this centrifugal pathway. Naturally, the enormous length of the trajectory of this pathway and the change of direction of its fibers during their forward course have impeded us from following them completely; we cannot thus affirm at all their penetration into the corpus striatum and corona radiata.

b. Centripetal Fibers. When we dealt with the nerve plexus of the third and fourth layers, we identified the centripetal fibers coming from the white matter as being involved in the same.

In fig. 10, *a, b* [*fig. 205*], we reproduce such

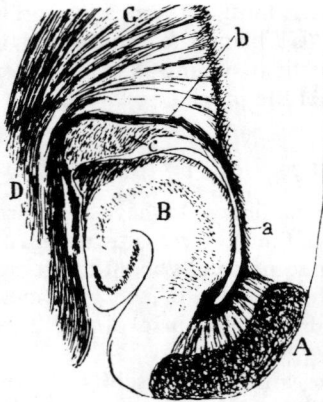

[FIG. 204] Fig. 9. Horizontal section of Ammon's horn, corpus striatum, and angular focus (mouse of eight days). A, angular focus; B, Ammon's horn; C, corpus striatum; D, internal capsule; a, b, nerve bundles that appear to leave from the angular focus.

fibers as they are observed in sagittal sections of the cerebrum of the mouse of eight days. Notice that they are commonly thick axons which gain the fourth layer obliquely, in which, or before reaching it, they bifurcate, and by means of successive dichotomies engender in the full thickness of the fourth, third, and second layers a plexus of flexuous and varicose branches and with an extremely intricate and labyrinthine course. Some fibers, before reaching the fourth layer, run horizontally for a certain distance, giving off ascending collaterals. The granule cells do not appear to receive any branches from such fibers.

In general, the full extent of the spheno-occipital focus receives centripetal fibers, but there is a place found in the most superior portion of the said ganglion to which arrive a larger number of the same. It is not, therefore, strange that in this cellular territory the nerve plexus is more dense than in the rest of the ganglion, or that in complete impregnations it appears covered by an almost black blot of silver chromate. The majority of the afferent fibers to this territory come from the commissural bundle or dorsal psalterium of the authors. However, it is not rare to see also arriving and arborizing in the said place or superior end of the focus under study some thick centripetal fiber, coming perhaps from the un-

derlying white matter or from the medial portions of the ganglion (fig. 10, c) [fig. 205]. We have also sometimes observed ascending collaterals coming from the white matter, arriving and ramifying in the fourth and third layers.

Conjectures about the Physiological Significance of the Angular Cortex

The importance of the ganglion under study comes from its very robust links with Ammon's horn and the fascia dentata. Such connections are so notable that they necessarily imply a functional unity of the two centers, in such a way that it can be said without fear of error that if the angular ganglion is olfactory then Ammon's horn must be olfactory, if optic then [Ammon's horn is] optic, etc.

Unfortunately, when one reaches this point, only conjectures can be made. Three suppositions, of course, occur: (a) the focus in question is a secondary or tertiary olfactory center; (b) the said ganglion represents the visual area or a part of the visual area of rodents and carnivores hitherto unknown; (c) it is finally, a special region of unknown character and peripheral connections.

a. The first conjecture rests on the topographical situation of the focus and the scientific tradition that for a long time has considered Ammon's horn as a higher olfactory center. It seems natural to consider as olfactory a cerebral region lying in the posterosuperior continuation of the piriform lobe, and which, besides, supplies such a considerable flow of fibers to Ammon's horn. However, all our efforts to convert this rational conjecture into a real opinion have been, so far, little successful. In order to be able to affirm securely an olfactory character for the spheno-occipital cortex, it is essential not to be content with the indications of topography and of proximity to a region that is definitely olfactory, but to prove, without room for doubt, that the said gray focus is penetrated either by fibers of the external olfactory root or by fibers originating in the medial and anterior portions of the piriform lobe. Here are some of the observations [that are] little favorable toward this conjecture: (1) Marchi preparations (cutting of the

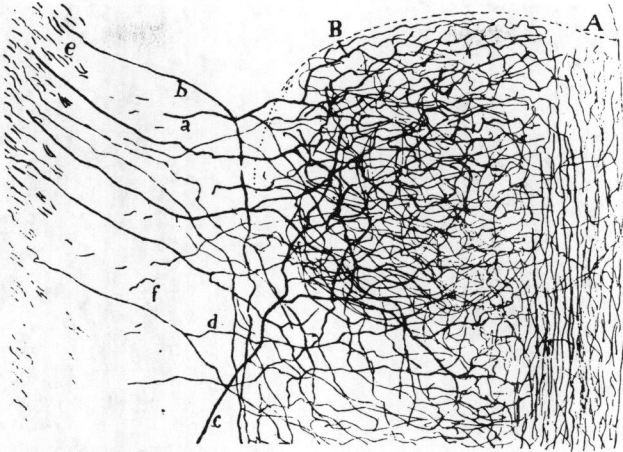

[*FIG. 205*]   Fig. 10. Section of the superior extremity of the angular or spheno-occipital focus. *A*, plexiform layer; *B*, plexus of centripetal nerve fibers.

olfactory bulb and its pedicle) never allow [one] to follow, in the rabbit and guinea pig, a trace of oily droplets into the angular focus. The degenerated fibers appear only in the foci underlying the external root,[E] and they do not extend beyond the inferior sphenoidal cortex. (2) In Golgi preparations of the mouse and rabbit (sagittal sections of the piriform lobe), the layer of the olfactory fibers lying on the surface of the sphenoidal cortex progressively becomes thinner from forward to backward, and it cannot be followed into the spheno-occipital focus. (3) When sagittal sections of the piriform lobe that include the inferior sphenoidal portion and the angular focus stained by the method of Weigert-Pal are examined in the adult dog and cat, these sections allow us to follow easily the medullated fibers of the external root, successively diminishing in diameter and number, up to the vicinity of the latter focus. The submeningeal rim of the angular cortex, which is the place where the inferior sphenoidal region exhibits the [fiber] contingents of the external root, is free of medullated fibers, or, if it presents some, they do not seem to be continuous with the olfactory fibers. The tangential fibers of the spheno-occipital regions lie in the deepest levels, and they seem to come, as we have already said, from cells with ascending axons. (4) These same tangential fibers, instead of in-

creasing from upward to downward and from backward to forward, as would occur if they were olfactory [fibers], increase from downward to upward, reaching their maximum, as revealed in Weigert-Pal sections of the cat and dog, in the vicinity of the transverse or limiting gyrus. (5) The structure of the sphenoidal olfactory cortex is extremely different from that of the spheno-occipital focus, as seen in the preceding descriptions. The contrast is clear even in the Nissl preparations, as can be noticed by comparing figs. 12 and 11 [*figs. 207, 206*], which represent, respectively, sections of the olfactory sphenoidal cortex and of the temporo-occipital focus of the cat of one month and a half. (6) Finally, both foci are not similar in their connections, since while the principal pathway of the piriform lobe goes to the corona radiata, that from the angular focus terminates in Ammon's horn.

b. As indications of the visual significance of the center under study, there can be counted, first, the existence in it of a special layer of stellate cells, very similar in morphology to those of the calcarine fissure or human visual area; second, the presence of a layer of deep granule cells provided with arciform axons and analogous to the corresponding [cells] of the visual cortex of a man; third, the existence of a very dense intermediate plexus in which converge, as in the [visual] cortex, numerous

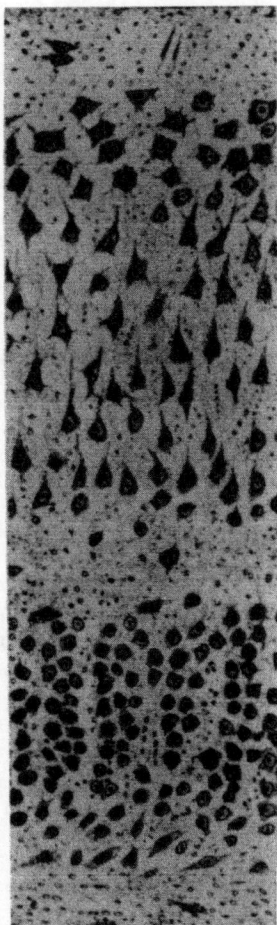

[FIG. 206]   Fig. 11. Spheno-occipital cortex of the cat. (Nissl method.)

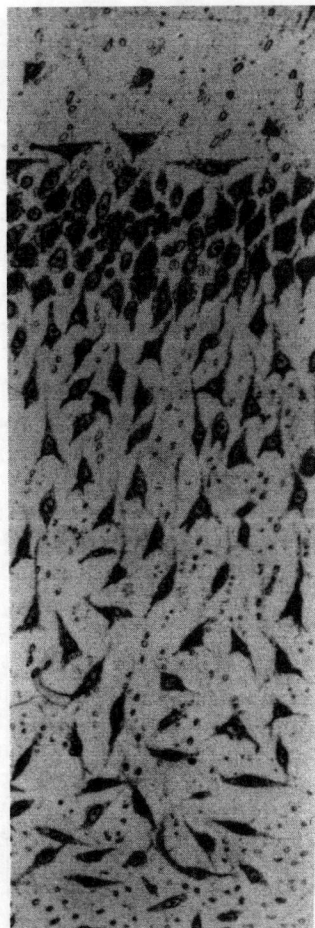

[FIG. 207]   Fig. 12. Olfactory sphenoidal cortex of the cat. (Nissl method.)

exogenous fibers; fourth, finally, the consideration that the ganglion of the occipital pole in rodents that we had considered optic in nature appears little different in structure and connections from that of the interhemispheric gray matter (from both come the cingulum and the fornix longus of Forel), forcing us, therefore, to localize the visual areas in the said animals in other territories. But very important reasons militate against these indications.

Experiments involving excitation of the region generating conjugate movements of the eyeballs, made by Munk[4] and Obregia[5] in the dog and by Steiner[6] in the cat, rabbit, and other mammals, have allowed [us] to localize the visual area of the said animals, not on the internal face of the occipital lobe or in the occipitotemporal intermediate region (posterior border), the localization of the focus under study, but on the external surface of the occipital lobe and on a part of the parietal. The schemes of Munk and Obregia on the visual center of the dog and cat are definitive and even mark the region of the posterior segments of the three superior sagittal gyri (A, A₁,

A), on which the quadrants of the retina are projected. On the other hand, the negative anatomical argument, that is to say, the absence in rodents and carnivores of an external occipital region that exhibits the texture of the human calcarine fissure, would only have strength had the external face of the occipital lobe of the said animals been the target of precise and careful applications of the methods of Golgi, Weigert, and Nissl. But we have not noticed that this meticulous examination, very interesting from several points of view, has yet been made.[7]

c. The third conjecture can only prosper from the inadmissibility of the others. In order for it to be possible to consider the said focus as a special sensory area, or as an association area in the sense of the doctrine of Flechsig, it would be necessary to eliminate totally, and by virtue of rigorous anatomical and physiological experiments, the two previous possibilities, and also to determine positively the centers or sensory pathways with which the spheno-occipital ganglion makes connections.

Which of the three conjectures must be preferred? In fact, in the absence of anatomico-pathological experiments that indicate the origin of the afferent pathways to the angular focus, or of physiology to illustrate its functions, there is no secure base on which to rest any hypothesis. However, we must not conceal that we feel a particular predilection for the first conjecture, that is to say, for the one which supposes that the spheno-occipital cortex in question represents a tertiary olfactory area, which would be linked by means of pathways at present unknown with the infero-anterior sphenoidal cortex. The said center could thus be a special olfactory territory, in which would develop activities little different from those that are developed in the rest of the piriform lobe. In this supposition, any difficulty rests on revealing the tertiary pathways that must associate the superior sphenoidal cortex with the inferior; at least, it should be possible to demonstrate, which we think probable, [that there is a] continuation of the fibers of the external [olfactory] root up to the height of the angular focus.

This hypothesis has, among other advantages, the following. First, it fits well with the general opinion that considers the entire piriform lobe as an olfactory region, and that also considers Ammon's horn as a tertiary olfactory center, something like the area of olfactory memory. Second, it fits very well with the negative results of all our efforts to confirm the existence of the olfactory pathway of the septum, as well as other supposed associations between Ammon's horn and anterior olfactory foci.

After all that has been exposed, it is natural and logical to suppose that the route or pathway of union between the olfactory area and Ammon's horn and the fascia dentata is none other than the spheno-ammonic pathways as a whole originating in the angular cortex. The authors would not, therefore, have been mistaken when they predicted the physiological nature of Ammon's horn but when they indicated the origin and course of the afferent olfactory pathways of this center, pathways that would not pass anteriorly but posteriorly, taking advantage of the proximity (now well comprehensible) that exists in all mammals between the inferior region of Ammon's horn and the posterosuperior pole of the piriform lobe.

Cajal's Notes

1. See, in this same volume: Afferent pathways of Ammon's horn [see chapter 18].
2. With the aim of not prejudging the physiological significance of this center, which, as we will see later, is in doubt, and to avoid periphrasis, we will call it the *angular or spheno-occipital nucleus*, alluding to its intermediate position between the occipital lobe and the temporal or sphenoidal [lobe], that is to say, in the obtuse angle that both lobules form when they meet. [The area is undoubtedly what we would now call the medial entorhinal area.]
3. S. R. Cajal, Estructura de la corteza visual humana, *Rev. Trim. Micrográfica*, vol. IV, 1899.
4. Munk, *Ueber die Funktionen der Grosshirnrinde (Gesammelte Mittheilungen)*, 2nd edition, Berlin, 18[89].
5. Obregia, Ueber Augenbewegungen und Sehsphärenreizung, *Arch. f. Anat. u. Physiol.*, Phys. Abtheil., 1890.
6. Steiner, Die Funktionen des Centralnervensystems und ihre Phylogenese, 1888 [and 1890]. See also Sinnessphären und Bewegungen, Pflüger's Arch, 1891.
7. Some tentative analyses of the regions of the ver-

tebrate that Munk, Obregia, and Steiner estimate as visual, recently made by us, prove positively that in the cat, dog, and rabbit, the external occipital cortex contains a region with a special structure, a region that, as we had recognized in other work, extends to the edge, tip, and posterior border of the occipital lobe, but has its area of maximum differentiation on the external face of the cerebrum.

Editors' Notes

A. The original text says 4*a*.
B: The original text says 4.
C. The original text says fig. 15.
D. In the original, 8, *B*.
E. The lateral olfactory tract.

PART IV

The Years of Consolidation (1904–1911)

The *Textura* and the *Histologie*

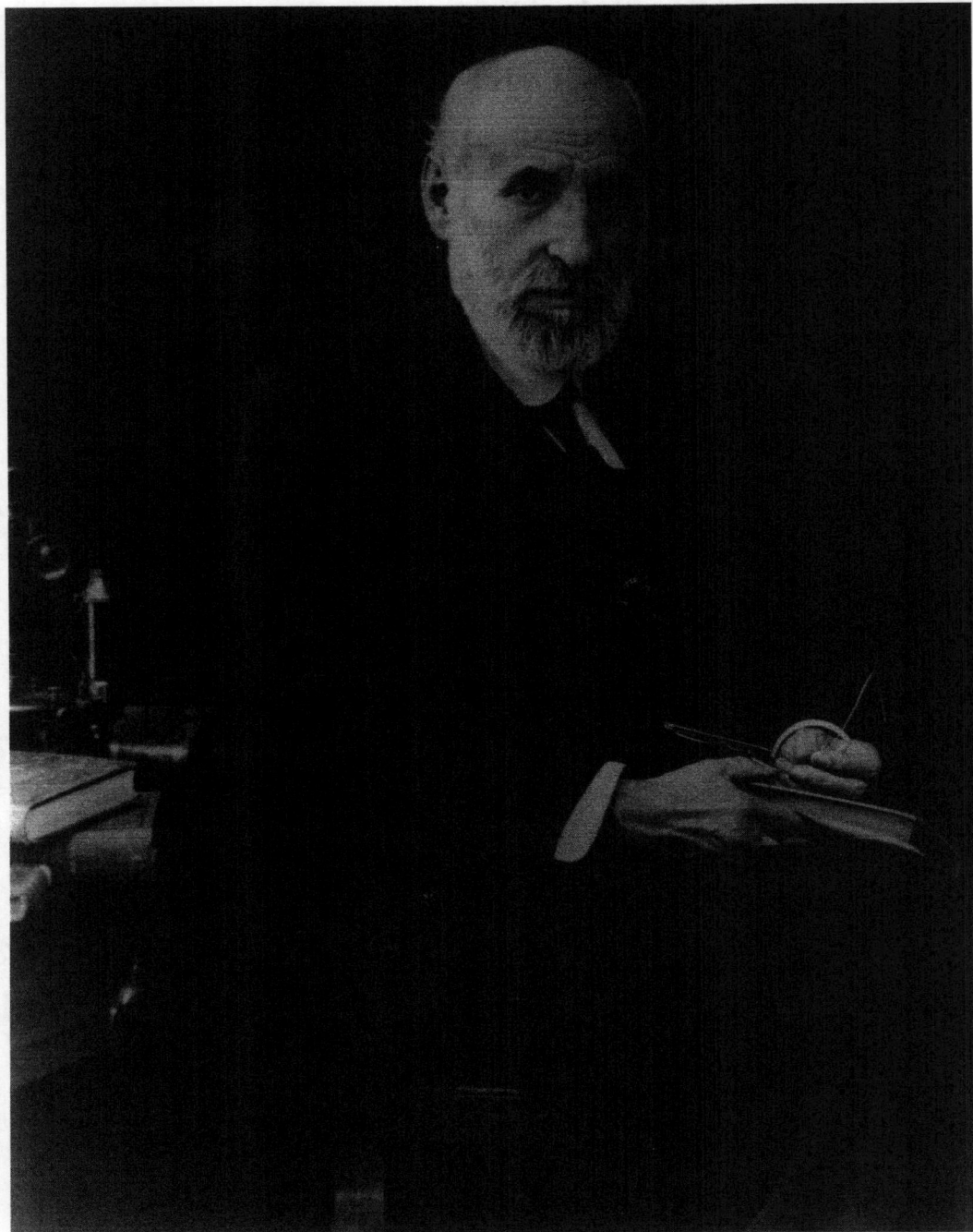

Santiago Ramón y Cajal. This photograph, probably taken in 1922, when Cajal was aged seventy, is in the collection of one of the editors of this volume.

20

Introduction

Most of the details from Cajal's works of 1899–1902 on the human cerebral cortex were incorporated into thirteen chapters[A] on the cerebral cortex in the second part of the second volume of the *Textura del sistema nervioso del hombre y de los vertebrados,* which was published in 1904.

By this time, Cajal's thoughts on the cerebral cortex had been consolidated, and he was able to write a lengthy general account of the organization of the human cortex at the cellular level (his chapter 37, which is chapter 21 in this volume), to precede the chapters on the major areas (his chapters 38–45, which is chapter 22 in this volume). In the general account, Cajal draws primarily on material taken from his papers of 1899–1900 on the human cortex. We can already detect some of the general ideas he had brought forward in his Croonian lecture and in his lectures before the Academy of Medical Sciences in Barcelona (chapters 7 and 8 in this volume). Among items of note is his final conclusion that the special cells of layer I do not possess multiple axons, as he had previously supposed. There is also a description of neuroglial cells (which

fails to identify oligodendrocytes), an account of the neurofibrillar structure of pyramidal cells, and a description of the Golgi complex and certain intranuclear inclusions, most of which are taken from short, previously published communications.

Chapters 46, 47, and 48 of the *Textura,* corresponding to chapters 23, 24, and 25 in this volume, are also interesting in that the first two chapters bring together data from many of Cajal's earlier studies (particularly from that published in *La Cellule* in 1891) in order to make general statements about the comparative anatomy and histogenesis of the cerebral cortex. These studies (especially that on comparative structure) can also be seen as developing out of the earlier lectures. The third chapter is unique in that it surveys the then current theories on functional localization and sensory-motor interactions in the cerebral cortex, reflecting the level of understanding of brain function then extant. It is noteworthy that Cajal largely confines himself to anatomical considerations either in support of or against the more functionally oriented theories of others.

The thirteen chapters of the cerebral cortex were translated by Azoulay for the second volume of the *Histologie du système nerveux de l'homme et des vertébrés* (1911), and Cajal made few textual additions to them other than an occasional paragraph. Azoulay made no effort to "improve" on Cajal and limited himself to clarifying a few phrases, eliminating an occasional pejorative phrase, and inserting references to more recently published work. In both the Spanish and French versions of the book, the chapters on visual, sensory-motor, olfactory, and auditory cortex are considerably abbreviated in comparison with the original publications translated in Part III of this volume. However, in the general account of the human cerebral cortex, appearing as chapter 37 in the *Textura* and as chapter 24 in the *Histologie* (chapter 21 in this volume), Cajal was able to incorporate a large proportion of the original figures, which were excluded from the chapters on the individual areas, as well as a number of new figures.

The added figures are relatively few in number; most of them, as well as any additions to the accompanying text, relate to the neurofibrillar structure of the cortical cells. These additions were made possible by his use of the reduced silver nitrate method, introduced into his laboratory at about the time of publication of the *Textura*.

Cajal began experimenting with reduced silver nitrate in 1903, and he is adamant in his autobiography (Cajal, 1917) that he arrived at his version of the method independent of Bielschowsky, who introduced the early versions of his method in 1902 and 1903.

In his autobiography, Cajal implies that he first became acquainted with some version of the reduced silver nitrate method at the International Medical Congress held in Madrid in 1903, when the Italian Donaggio displayed some neurofibrillar preparations but refused to divulge the secret of his method. Cajal says that thereafter he made many attempts to develop a silver-based neurofibrillar stain, but these attempts initially failed. Finally, he hit on the idea of a block staining process in which the silver nitrate is reduced by pyrogallol. This was later modified several times, notably by the addition of a step involving fixation in ammoniacal alcohol prior to immersing the tissue in silver nitrate.

Cajal's version of the reduced silver nitrate method was published in Spanish and in German translation in 1903 (Cajal 1903b–e); other versions were described in several papers in 1904.

Accompanying this part of the translation are only those new figures that Cajal prepared either for the books themselves or for minor papers that we have not translated. All the other figures he used in the book chapters are from works translated in the preceding chapters of this volume. We have indicated where these can be found in our text and, where necessary, have indicated any changes made in the captions between the original publication and the textbook. The added figures of reduced silver preparations are in chapter 21 of this volume. The figures in the chapters on comparative anatomy and on the development of the cortex (chapters 23 and 24 in this volume) are mainly of Golgi preparations, many of them taken from the *La Cellule* paper of 1891 (chapter 5 in this volume). A few come from other sources, some not Cajal's. The final, theoretical chapter (chapter 25 in this volume) contains a small number of schematic diagrams of some interest.

We have translated only four of the thirteen chapters on the cerebral cortex from the Spanish *Textura*: chapter 37 on the general plan of the structure of the cortex; chapter 46 on the comparative structure; chapter 47 on the histogenesis; and chapter 48 on "anatomico-physiological considerations." In the few places where additions were made to the text of the French *Histologie,* we have added translations of them from the latter work. The chapters on the visual, sensory-motor, auditory, and olfactory cortex (chapters 38–46 in the original) contain little of significance that is not described at greater length in the original research papers, so we have translated only those of their introductions that contain updated references, as well as an occasional passage dealing with regions of cortex, such as the association areas that were not the subjects of other publications by Cajal. These passages, translated from the French *Histologie,* appear in chapter 22 of this volume.

To the best of our knowledge, the general account of the human cortex (chapter 21 in this volume) was not published elsewhere or translated other than for the *Histologie*. A German translation by Bressler of the last three chapters, taken from the *Textura*, appeared in 1906 as the fifth part of the series that included translations of the 1899–1901 papers on the human cortex (Cajal, 1906b). Much of the chapter on development also appeared in *Studies in Neurogenesis* (Cajal, 1929).

Editors' Note

A. The chapters are numbered 37 through 48, but there are two chapters numbered 44, no chapter 45, and two chapters numbered 46. This was corrected in the *Histologie*, where the chapters are numbered 25 through 36.

21

General Plan of the Structure of the Cerebral Cortex

[From: *Textura del sistema nervioso del hombre y de los vertebrados*, Vol. 2, Pt. 2, (Madrid: N. Moya, 1904), chap. 37, pp. 792–864; also published in French as chap. 24 of *Histologie du système nerveux de l'homme et des vertébrés*, Vol. 2, pp. 519–598 (Paris: Maloine, 1911)]

Layers of the gray matter of the gyri. Plexiform, of the small pyramids, of the medium and large pyramids, of the granule cells, of the deep large pyramids, of the deep medium pyramids and of the fusiform cells. White matter and its relations with the gray. Connections of the cerebral cells. Historical notes about cortical structure.

As is well known, the *anterior vesicle of the cerebrum* of vertebrates, excepting fishes, possesses a vault or cortical region, separated from the corpus striatum or primordial ganglion by a cavity (lateral ventricle), and in which are housed the higher functions of the nervous system. It is to be presumed that the extent and the structural complexity of this gray layer are intimately related to the psychological advancement of each vertebrate. Thus, in the batrachians and reptilians, where it makes its appearance for the first time, the cortex is limited almost completely to the central projection of the olfactory sensory surfaces; in birds, as shown by the experiments of Munk, a visual sphere is already elaborated beside the olfactory [region], and finally, in the mammals, the cortex represents an ensemble of centers, each one of them linked to a periph-

eral sense. There are, thus, visual, acoustic, sensory, gustatory, and olfactory cerebral territories, respectively responsible for receiving and transforming into sensations the impulses carried by the centripetal pathways originating in the corresponding sense [organs]. Besides these sensory regions, there should also exist, according to Flechsig, in man and gyrencephalic mammals, intercalated cortical territories (centers of association), without direct connections with the lower motor centers or with the sensory apparatuses, and whose role would be to associate and combine in a thousand ways the sensory impressions furnished by the sensory areas, elaborating very complex psychic processes. From this it is seen that, if the theory of Flechsig is correct, the cerebral cortex comes to have a double projection of the sense [organs]: *direct or of first order,* made up of the cited central sensory areas; *indirect or of second order,* made up of cerebral areas at which arrive the centripetal pathways originating in the preceding [areas]. In other words, the sensory cerebrum represents a synthesis of all the sensory surfaces of the organism; the cerebrum of association represents only the sensory cerebrum. This [latter] becomes, therefore, a synthesis of a synthesis and a projection of a projection.

As is well known, the cerebral cortex consists of two superimposed formations: the *gray matter,* a soft layer of gray pink color, notably vascular, situated at the surface immediately underneath the pia; and the *white matter,* a much harder formation, which occupies all the space existing between the gray layer on the one hand and the ventricles and corpus striatum on the other. It is also a common fact of observation that the gray cortex appears smooth in the lower vertebrates and even in the small mammals (mouse, guinea pig, rabbit, etc.), whereas in the mammals of large size, and especially in the monkey and man, it is found to be folded *(gyrencephalic animals),* offering eminences or gyri and sulci or anfractuosities. We will see later that, smooth or folded, the cerebral cortex obeys in its essentials the same structural formula.

Our study of the cortex will include five parts: in the first, we will deal, in general, with the construction of the human cerebral cortex and that of the gyrencephalic animals, that is to say, without reference to a particular territory; in the second, we will expose the regional cortex, that is to say, the cerebral territories that possess particular structural features; in the third, we will analyze the [cortex] in the small mammals and lower vertebrates; in the fourth, we will give some information on cortical histogenesis; and in the last, there will appear those physiopsychological inductions that are more naturally detached from the whole of the dynamic, anatomicopathological, ontogenic, and phylogenetic structural data, in relation to the cerebrum. The last chapter will form, to the extent permitted by the scarcity of objective data, an essay on the theory of the cerebrum.

Structural Plan of the Cerebral Cortex: Layers of the Cortex

The gray matter of the gyri is not homogenous. Even to the naked eye, it shows indications of stratification, especially in the occipital regions, where an intermediary white line *(stria of Gennari or of Vicq d'Azyr)* shows up;

but the number and composition of such strata can only be determined with a microscope and in preparations stained with carmine, hematoxylin, and basic aniline [dyes].

Omitting the regional differences that will be revealed later, there can be differentiated in the human cerebrum and in that of gyrencephalic animals (monkey, dog, cat, etc.) seven concentric layers, namely:

1. *Plexiform layer (layer poor in cells* of Meynert, *molecular* of many authors, etc.).
2. *Layer of the small pyramids.*
3. *Layer of the external medium and large pyramids.*
4. *Layer of the dwarf pyramids and stellate cells (granule cells* of the authors).
5. *Layer of the deep large pyramids.*
6. *Layer of the deep medium pyramids.*
7. *Layer of the triangular and fusiform cells.*

1. Plexiform Layer

This layer, [which has] a finely granular appearance in carmine preparations and is clearly plexiform in Ehrlich or Golgi sections, is not very rich in intrinsic neurons. It represents mainly the territory of connection and contact of two orders of exogenous elements: the terminal dendritic tufts of the pyramidal cells and the ascending arborizations of numerous cells with short axon lying at several cortical levels. As a place of interneuronal connection, it resembles completely the plexiform layers of the retina and the molecular [layer] of the cerebellum (fig. 658, *1) [fig. 87].*

In fig. 659, *A [fig. 89],* we show the appearance of this layer and that of the following [layer] in a Nissl preparation. Its poverty in nerve cells is noted, as mentioned some time ago by Meynert, plus the relative abundance of nuclei of neuroglia. This predominance of the supporting framework led Golgi to suppose erroneously that the first layer is inhabited exclusively by radiated neuroglial cells intimately linked with the blood vessels. But as we demonstrated some time ago,[1] the neurons are absolutely constant, belonging to several varieties of the class with short axon.

The analysis of this cerebral layer with the methods of Ehrlich, Golgi, and Weigert allows us to distinguish in it the following structural features: first, *small and medium cells with short axon;* second, *large horizontal cells,* provided with semilong tangential axons; third, *terminal dendritic shafts* of pyramids and other cells of the underlying layer; fourth, *ascending axonal arborizations* of cells with semilong axon, also resident in deeper strata; fifth, *cells of Deiters or neuroglia.*

Cells with Short Axon of the Plexiform Layer

First described by us in the cortex of the rabbit and rat,[2] then confirmed with the aid of the methylene blue [method] in the adult cat, these cells have not been the subject of special verification in the last years. Thus, Retzius does not illustrate them in his classic works on the special cells of the plexiform layer of man, Kölliker does not appear to have seen them either, and Schaffer[3] and Bevan Lewis, who believe they have impregnated them with the method of Golgi, place them not in the molecular layer but in the external portion of the second [layer] or that of the small pyramids, a layer that these authors designated by the name *layer of the superficial polymorphic cells* (Schaffer) or *layer of the polygonal cells* (Bevan Lewis). In fact, neither Schaffer nor Bevan [Lewis] has seen our polygonal cells of the plexiform layer, and we convince ourselves all the more of this opinion, since when the said authors talk about the arborizations of the short axon of such cells, they suppose that the majority of the branches of the same do not extend through the first layer, as we showed, but in the second layer or [layer] of the small pyramids.

As can be seen in fig. 660 [*fig. 92*], which we take from one of the above-mentioned works, the methylene blue reveals in the plexiform layer of the cat a considerable number of cells with short axon. These cells, becoming larger with depth, inhabit the whole thickness of the said layer; have a polygonal, triangular, or ovoid shape; and are provided with numerous radial dendrites, mainly ascending. As occurs in all the preparations of Ehrlich, the final branches of such processes appear heavily varicose, being concentrated especially in the superficial half of the layer.

The study of the axon must be done in Golgi preparations. As we show in fig. 661 [*fig. 52*], taken from the cat of a few days, this process, whose direction varies although the tangential dominates, after a variable course and tracing some turns, resolves into a free arborization that does not go beyond the confines of the first layer. With respect to the length of the axon and robustness of the cell, it is possible to distinguish in the cat, dog, and rabbit two cellular varieties: small, globular and stellate cells with short axon, promptly ramified (fig. 661, A, B) [*fig. 52*]; larger, fusiform or triangular cells, usually lying in the deep third of the layer, and whose robust and horizontal axon engenders an extensive arborization.

In man, not only do the referred cells exist, but they present, as would be presumed, a large variety of morphological types. Attending to the volume of the soma and extent of the terminal axonal arborization, the following categories can be distinguished.

a. Medium Type or Type of Regular Size (fig. 663, A, B) [*fig. 93*]. This is without doubt one of the most abundant cells of the first layer, in which it prefers the middle and deep levels. Its dendrites are mainly ascending, and the axon, almost always horizontal, is distributed at no great distance from the location of the soma.

b. Large Type. In addition to their exceptional size, these cells are characterized by the robustness and length of their dendrites, some of which are descending and go down through the layer of the small pyramids, ending in it or at the border with the third (fig. 662, B) [*fig. 94*]. The axon is robust, runs resolutely horizontally, giving off some collaterals and ending in an unknown manner. It is probable that these cells correspond to the large cells with horizontal axon described earlier in the cerebrum of the cat and dog.

c. Diminutive Type. It is characterized, in addition to its smallness, by its ovoid or piriform shape and because it exhibits a very fine axon, arborized in the vicinity of the cell (fig. 663, C) [*fig. 93*]. Some of these [cellular] elements have, in the child of fifteen to twenty days, a very embryonic disposition, lying near the pia and showing a shaft dividing into short small branches, among which it is not possible to distinguish clearly an axon (fig. 663^A D, E) [fig. 93].

d. Neurogliaform Type. Similar to the dwarf cells lying in deeper layers, and on which we will dwell later, this cell preferentially inhabits the deeper half of the first layer, and it is easily distinguished from the others by the tightness and great complication of the delicate terminal arborization.

Horizontal Cells

Our already old studies on the cerebral cortex of the small mammals[4] allowed us to observe a singular kind of voluminous nerve cell, with a spindle or triangular shape, and characterized by the smoothness, horizontality, and enormous length of its polar processes, as well as by the circumstance that several of the thin branches arising from the shafts have the appearance of axons (fig. 665) [fig. 65]. In the rabbit especially, there are cells to which, taking morphological criteria (length, smoothness, thinness of the axon, ramification at right angles, etc.) exclusively into account, two or three axons could be attributed. But the studies made with methylene blue in the cerebrum of the cat,[5] the observations of Retzius[6] in the human fetus and of Veratti[7] in the rabbit, and the new works undertaken by us on the cerebral anatomy of the newborn child[8] have persuaded us that among the polar or collateral processes of the shafts only one deserves to be regarded as an axon. This is a relatively thick fiber, rather more robust than some dendritic branches, with a very long horizontal course (such that it is not possible to see its end in a single section, no matter how thick), and from which arise at a right angle or at obtuse angles collaterals [that are] mainly ascending and which terminate exclusively in the first layer. The cells that concern us are less numerous in the mammals (rabbit, cat) and occupy several planes of the plexiform layer, preferentially the deep border close to the layer of the small pyramids.

For the rest, the dendritic character of the

long polar processes becomes clear with the method of Ehrlich, in the cerebrum of the cat. As is seen in fig. 664, A [fig. 50], such processes, smooth and without spines during their initial trajectory and prior to the main dichotomies, become heavily varicose in their last branches; varicosities are never seen on the [parent] axon. Let us add also that Weigert-Pal preparations reveal in the first layer the existence of thick tangential nerve fibers [that are] not continuous with fibers of Martinotti, and which correspond probably, as we demonstrated in our first work on the cortex, to the thick axons of the horizontal cells.[9]

The horizontal cells of man are much more abundant and robust than in animals, deserving a particular description. Among them, we must distinguish two stages: the fetal and the adult or definitive forms.

Fetal Form. The strange morphology of these cells in the human fetus, first observed by Retzius,[10] is shown in fig. 665, A, B, C [fig. 65]. Notice that several morphological types exist (fusiform, triangular, stellate, and piriform), on all of which are recognized one or several thick radial dendrites, terminating underneath the pia, two or more robust and very long polar branches that run horizontally, tracing short small arches corresponding to the branching intervals, and an infinity of ascending collaterals, each originating at a right angle at the level of a varicosity of the preceding processes and ending constantly underneath the pia in the form of a terminal sphere.

As each cell commonly supplies a large number of horizontal branches (*tangential fibers* of Retzius), the abundance of these in good impregnations is considerable, engendering in the several levels of the plexiform layer an important system of parallel fibers so extremely long that, commonly, it is not possible to observe their termination (fig. 665) [fig. 65]. Among them are mixed up the axons of the horizontal cells whose similarity to the polar dendrites is such that it is impossible to distinguish the two. The peculiarities appear also in newborn small mammals, especially the long varicose horizontal and parallel dendrites; but the rarity of cells capable of being impregnated makes their observation very difficult and fortuitous.

Adult Horizontal Cells. Retzius, who confirmed in human fetuses the cited horizontal cells and first detailed their singular ontogenic features, has not been able to impregnate them after birth. It has therefore been impossible for him to determine their definitive form, although he considers it probable that they do not suffer great changes in their further development. But the observations that we have been able to make in the twenty-five to thirty days after birth allows us to affirm, first, that the majority of the ascending collaterals of the tangential branches described by Retzius are embryonic dispositions destined to atrophy in the days following birth, disappearing one month or two months later, except for a small branch that later will change direction and arborize in the first layer; second, that the very long horizontal polar processes remain indefinitely, constituting through the full thickness of the plexiform layer a system of horizontal fibers provided with scarce and thin small branches disseminated at all levels of the layers; third, that one of these horizontal branches, usually thick and representing the axon, being characterized by acquiring a myelin sheath, runs horizontally over an enormous course and gives off at intervals collaterals aborizing around the cells with short axon of the first cerebral layer.

The details pertaining to the morphology of these cells, such as is presented in the child of one month or one month and a half (in the adult, we have not been able to stain them so far), are reproduced in figs. 665 and 666 [*figs. 65, 91*], in which are recognized several morphological types already mentioned by Retzius.

The *monopolar type* or limiting type is already observed in Nissl preparations of the adult cerebrum (fig. 659, *a, b*) [*fig. 89*]. In Golgi preparations, it exhibits a triangular or piriform soma, from which arise some short dendrites, the upper ones being extended horizontally at the external border of the plexiform layer; a thick descending shaft, covered with some short dendrites and not a few spines, and from which arise some long arci-form processes (long dendrites or tangential fibers of Retzius) or horizontal processes freely terminating at different levels of the first layer; and a very robust axon, [which is] the continuation of the vertical [dendritic] shaft, and almost always situated in the deep third of the plexiform layer (figs. 665, *B, G;* 666, *A*) [*figs. 65, 91*].

The *bipolar type* also displays a soma often covered with short dendrites, a thick polar process from which emerge many short and long horizontal dendrites, and a very long process originating from the opposite pole and with all the characteristics of the axon (fig. 666, *B*) [*fig. 91*].

The *stellate and triangular type* is the one that has the most morphological variations. From the soma arise three or more shafts, which quite soon give rise to many short and long horizontal dendrites, some of which possess an arciform course and ramify and terminate at the external frontier of the layer under study. The complicated [nature] of the horizontal fibers makes it difficult to recognize the axon; even so, in some cases, we have been able to detect it, having noticed that it arises from one of the thick descending processes, becoming horizontal and running for enormous distances (figs. 666, *C;* 665, *E*) [*figs. 91, 65*].

In fig. 666, *d, e* [*fig. 91*], we also show some details of the collaterals of the axons. It is noticed, of course, that in some axons these branches are very rare, arising at intervals of one-tenth of a millimeter or more. In others, they are more abundant, as is seen in fig. 666, *d* [*fig. 91*], which shows two kinds of branches: short, little branches, terminating by means of a bifurcation in small, short, thickened branches or by a small, apparently pericellular basket; and long collaterals, originating either at a right angle or at an acute angle, which go up or down, running horizontally at different levels of the plexiform layer and repeatedly ramifying, without our having been able to determine their terminations. Among the collaterals, there are very worthy of mention those originating from the initial bend of the axon (fig. 666, *e*) [*fig. 91*], which sometimes have such a robustness that they seem to represent branches of bifurcation of [the parent axon].

These thick branches almost always follow a course opposite to that of the axon. Finally, some thick axons also show long descending collaterals (fig. 674, G) [fig. 121], which penetrate the frontier of the second layer and ramify among the most superficial pyramids.

The axons of the horizontal cells never descend to the underlying layers, leading us to suppose that they terminate in the first layer, although so far we have not been able to reveal their termination. These fibers occupy the several levels of the plexiform layer, but the most robust appear to be concentrated in the middle third, a peculiarity that fits with the well-known fact that this part of the first layer is the one that exhibits the thickest medullated fibers in Weigert-Pal preparations.

Terminal Tufts of the Pyramids

Golgi and Martinotti have already observed that the [dendritic] tufts of some pyramids arrive at the plexiform layer of the cerebrum, and they even reproduced in the plates attached to their works some ramifications of the same; but only ourselves[11] in the mammals and Retzius[12] in man demonstrated the true disposition of the terminal portion of the [dendritic] shaft. This shaft does not end by sharp-pointed vertical branches, linked with blood vessels or with neuroglia, as Golgi thought, but, when it assails the plexiform layer and sometimes before, it resolves itself into a tuft of dendrites that, diverging at acute angles, do not delay in becoming more or less horizontal, running sometimes over long trajectories in several levels of the referred layer. The contours of these branches, as well as of the shaft from which they arise, bristle with simple or bifurcated collateral appendages, as we demonstrated first with silver chromate and later with methylene blue. Later, when we deal with the pyramids, we will describe the variations in the disposition of these tufts.

Ascending Nerve Fibers Ramifying in the First Layer

In all the layers underlying the first, there are neurons whose axon, instead of being directed toward the white matter, runs toward the plexiform layer, where, bifurcating or bending, it forms long and branched horizontal fibers.

With these fibers, which we have designated fibers of Martinotti, we will deal later when we describe the parent cells.

Neuroglial Cells

We will deal with these when we conclude the study of the cortex.

2. Second Layer or [Layer] of the Small Pyramids

This layer, also called the *layer of the superficial polymorphic cells* by Schaffer and Schlapp, is one of the best delimited of the cortex, being distinguished by the smallness and close-packed nature of the cells that inhabit it. It contains four categories of cells: the small pyramids, the large cells with short axon, the diminutive cells with short axon, and the cells of Martinotti or cells with an axon terminating in the plexiform layer.

Small Pyramids or Cells with Long Axon

They are cells with a triangular longitudinal section, already observed and described a long time ago by Meynert, who gave them their name. In fact, the Golgi preparations show that they are not pyramids but rather cones, with a deep base from which the axon arises and a superficial apex continuous with a long radial process. These cells, when studied in Nissl sections (fig. 659, *p*) [*fig. 89*], reveal a soma stained by the presence of fine [Nissl bodies] and an ovoid or triangular nucleus provided with one or several nucleoli. Between the [Nissl bodies], the filamentous framework (method of [reduced] silver nitrate) is faintly seen, [though it is] somewhat more appreciable at the beginning of the radial process (man, cat, and dog) (fig. 342, B, G)[B] [*fig. 208*].

In figs. 667 and 668 [*figs. 66, 209*], which reproduce pyramids of the human [and mouse] cerebrum, can be seen the morphology and connections of these cells, on which there appear three kinds of processes: the basal dendrites, the radial [dendritic] shaft, and the collaterals of this and the axon.

The *basal processes*, in number three or more, are robust, obliquely descend, dichotomizing repeatedly, and terminate by thin ends inside the stratum under study. The *ra-*

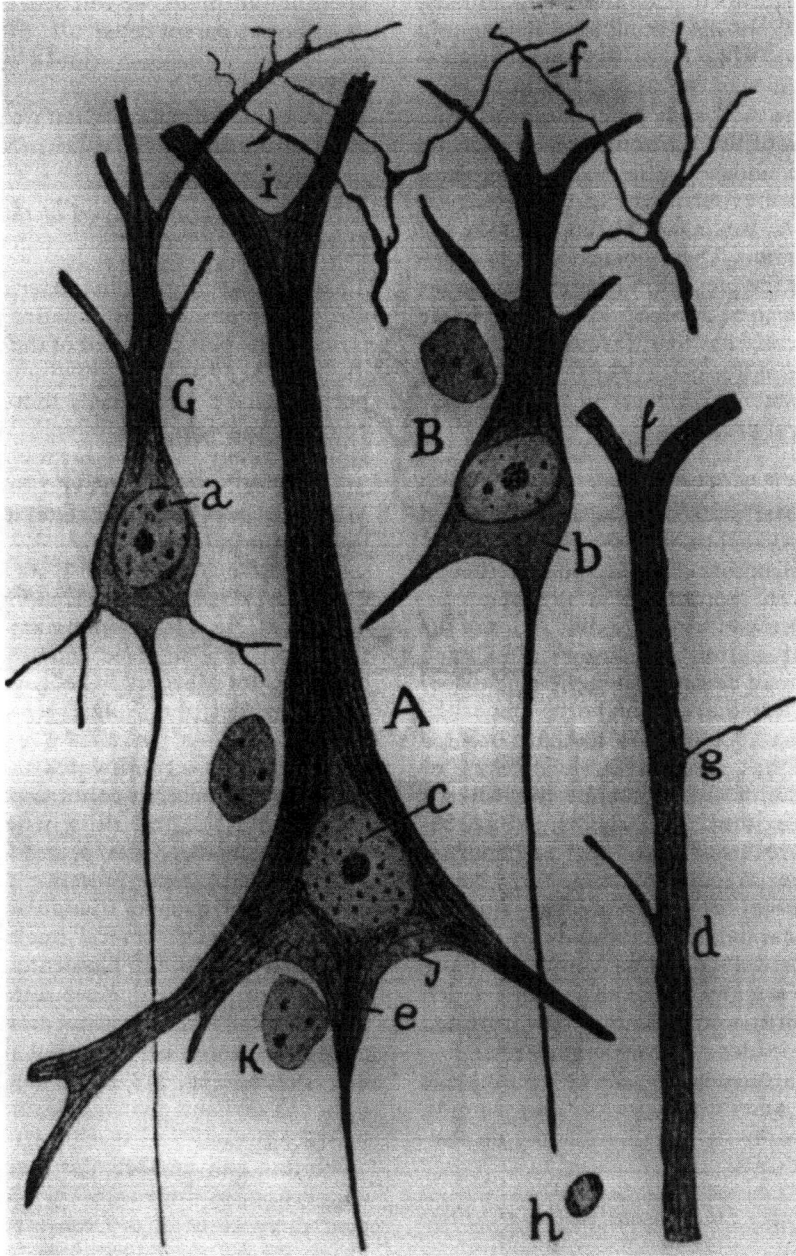

[*FIG. 208*]   Fig. 342. Nerve cells of the layer of the small pyramids; human cerebrum. Method of reduced silver nitrate (formula 1, without previous fixation). *A,* medium pyramidal cell; *B, G,* small pyramidal cells; *C,* nucleus; *a,* nucleolus; *b,* cellular region in which the neurofibrils are impregnated with difficulty. [This figure is only in the French version of the book.]

dial [*dendritic*] *shaft,* long and robust, originates at the apex of the soma and, after traversing the whole second layer, reaches the plexiform layer, in whose thickness it generates a tuft of three, four, or more repeatedly divided horizontal branches. It is not rare to see it dichotomize prematurely, that is to say, near its starting point. Naturally, the frontier cells of the plexiform layer possess a very short shaft or lack it, the tuft of dendrites arising from the superficial angle of the soma, an arrangement that appears more frequently in animals (cat, rabbit, mouse) than in man. From the course of the radial [dendritic] shaft, as well as from the surface of the soma, some dendrites commonly arise at acute angles and, ascending obliquely, get lost by ramifying at several levels of the second layer. Finally, to be complete, let us indicate that all the dendrites (except the soma and the origin of the radial shaft) are covered, as we recognized some time ago, with an infinity of delicate spiny appendages, demonstrable in both Golgi and Ehrlich preparations (fig. 668) [*fig. 209*].

The axon of the small pyramids, already seen by Golgi, is fine [and] arises from the soma or from the origin of a thick dendrite by means of an initial very prolonged cone; then it descends through the intermediate layers and enters the radial bundles, in which the enormous distance of the course in man prevents us from revealing its arrival at the white matter; however, in those animals, such as the mouse and rat, in which the gray cortex reaches little thickness, it is not a difficult task to reveal the continuation of the said axons with medullated fibers of the white matter (fig. 668 *b*) [*fig. 209*].

From the course of these axons arise, at the level of the second layer and even of the third, three, four, or more very delicate collaterals, which, in order to be well seen in man, require the use of the 1.30 Zeiss apochromatic [objective]. Such collaterals, which, in animals, like the parent cells, are more robust, are divided several times, and the resultant branches run horizontally or obliquely through the thickness of the layer under study, traversing long trajectories. In the newborn child, these collaterals have still not achieved their complete development, and even seem to be lack-

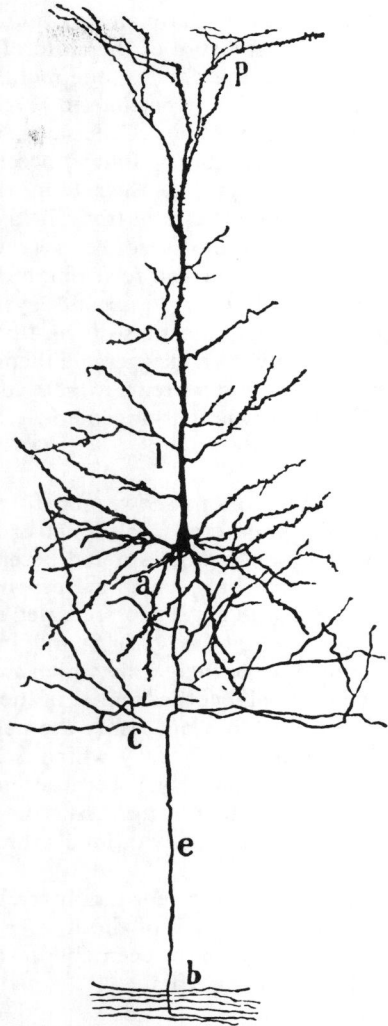

[*FIG. 209*]   Fig. 668. Ensemble of the arborizations of a pyramidal cell of the cerebrum of the mouse. *a,* basal dendritic processes; *b,* white matter where the axon [enters]; *c,* collaterals of the axon; *e,* portion of the axon bereft of collaterals; *l,* [apical] dendritic shaft; *p,* terminal dendritic tuft. (Method of Golgi.)

ing in some cells, a circumstance that well explains why Kölliker had not been able to find them. In fact, this authority has made his observations, as proven by fig. 726 of his book,[13] in cerebra that are too embryonic, at a period during which the axons are shown to be still bare of branches. We have already found collaterals in the cerebrum of the child of eight days, but only in the child of one month or a month and a half is it possible to reveal the divisions and subdivisions of the same, which are not always possible to follow, because of their extreme length, to their terminations. Some few collaterals arising from the axon of the frontier pyramids describe a recurrent course, and send the small recurrent branches to the external limit of the second layer, and even into the very thickness of the first. [K.] Schaffer[14] has given an exaggerated theoretical importance to this recurrence which, furthermore, is not a constant arrangement.

Cells with Short Axon

The Nissl preparations show, mixed up with the pyramids, numerous polygonal or ovoid cells, with a pale protoplasm and bereft of a radial [dendritic] shaft, which correspond evidently to cells with short axon revealed by the silver chromate (fig. 659, c, d) [fig. 89]. In spite of the abundance of these cells, which are concentrated especially at the frontier of the plexiform layer, this does not justify the name of *layer of polymorphic cells* by which Schaffer designates the second layer, because, in fact, both in man and in the mammals the pyramidal type, or cell type with long axon, constantly dominates.

The analysis of these cells is only feasible in good Golgi preparations of the human cerebrum, in which we have been able to differentiate the following types.

a. Voluminous Stellate Cell. Corresponding to the cell with short axon indicated in the cerebral cortex by Golgi,[15] Mondino,[16] and Martinotti,[17] this type exhibits a polygonal outline and varicose divergent dendrites that dichotomize several times. The axon, which often traces an arch above or below the cell, resolves itself into a loose terminal arborization, with long thin branches [that are] in large part vertical and horizontal. According to the extent and direction of the terminal ramification, some varieties of this cellular category, which we reproduce in figs. 669 and 662, D [figs. 95, 94], can be distinguished: (a) cell with a relatively long axon, [which is] ascending, descending, or horizontal and which gives rise to a terminal plexus at a distance from the cell; (b) cell with an axon promptly resolving itself into a terminal ramification (fig. 669, E) [fig. 95]; (c) cell whose descending axon gives rise to a vast arborization extending through the deep level of the second, the third, and sometimes the fourth layer, etc. (fig. 669, K) [fig. 95].

Although with less richness in morphological varieties, the cortex of mammals (dog, cat, rabbit) also exhibits this cellular category, as can be seen in fig. 671, a [fig. 79]. In the rabbit, the most superficial cells often have a pear shape, the deep ones being larger and with a stellate shape, the majority of which exhibit a more or less descending axon. For the rest, there are also found here numerous variants with respect to the length of the axon and extent of the field of arborization.

b. Dwarf or Neurogliaform Type. Our studies on the human cerebral cortex[18] have allowed us to recognize the existence of a very diminutive, short axon cell that, because of the size of the soma and the richness and fineness of the radiating dendrites, has deserved the name of *dwarf or neurogliaform cell*. It inhabits not only the second layer but the whole cortex, although it has seemed to us to be more abundant in the deep layers. As seen in fig. 669, F [fig. 95], it has a polygonal shape, from whose edges arise an infinity of fine, varicose, radiated processes, hardly branched, and terminating at a short distance. At first glance, these cells would be taken as small neuroglial cells with short radiations, but the lack of collateral appendages on the divergent [dendritic] processes and the undoubted presence of an axon promptly announce their nervous character. The axon is very delicate, so much so that the silver chromate stains it yellow, and at a short distance from its origin it resolves itself into a very tight arborization, whose delicate and moniliform branches require for their proper analysis a good apochromatic [lens]. On occasions, such tight arborizations are stained in isolation, that is to say, without the parent cell, which notably facilitates their examination.

This cell type also exists, although with rarity, in the cerebral cortex of the dog and cat (fig. 671, b) [fig. 79], where it reaches a somewhat larger size and displays a much more evident axonal arborization.

c. Small Cells with Ascending Axon Resolving Themselves into Very Dense Arborizations. In several regions of the human cerebral cortex, we have found[19] within the second layer, and mainly in its deeper half, some small, ovoid, or stellate cells, furnished with not very long, thin dendrites [that are] often ascending or descending (fig. 669, *G*) [*fig. 95*]. But what gives to these neurons an original physiognomy is the behavior of the axon, which is thin and ascending, and which, on arriving at the external third of the second layer, is resolved into a rich and dense terminal arborization preferentially concentrated at the border separating the first and second layers. It is common to find this elegant arborization impregnated in isolation, but from time to time the parent cell is stained simultaneously. The concentration of the cited axonal arborizations engenders between the first two layers a very dense and continuous nerve plexus, on whose bosom are observed numerous nests for the somata of pyramids (fig. 670, *A, B, c*) [*fig. 70*].

d. Bitufted Fusiform Cells. Among the cells discovered by us in the human cerebral cortex,[20] there deserve to be mentioned some small fusiform cells, oriented in the radial direction, and from whose external and internal poles arises a bundle or paintbrush of thin varicose dendrites, almost parallel and extending, especially the descending ones, over very long trajectories. Seen for the first time in the acoustic cortex, these were later confirmed in all [cerebral cortical] regions and in all cortical layers except the first. They are never lacking in the second cerebral layer, although they have seemed to us to be somewhat more abundant in the third and fourth [layers] (layer of the medium and large pyramids and layer of the granule cells).[c]

The more interesting peculiarity of this cellular type is the form of its axonal arborization. As we can see in fig. 672 *a* [*fig. 71*], this process is very delicate, and, arising from the soma or a dendrite, it follows an ascending or descending radial course and resolves itself, generally at a large distance from the parent cell, into a

paintbrush of very thin longitudinal threads. Over its long course, the axon gives off at right angles numerous collaterals that very quickly resolve themselves also into parallel and flexuous bundles of yellowish, ascending and descending varicose threads, so lengthy that they can extend through almost the whole thickness of the cortex, and so fine that for their proper analysis the 1.30 Zeiss objective is absolutely essential. In the brain of the newborn or few-days-old child, these arborizations are still somewhat thick and not very extensive; to reveal them at their complete development and to find out the extreme delicacy of their threads, it is necessary to study them in the cortex of the child of twenty to thirty days. Figs. 672 and 669, *H* [*figs. 71, 95*] give an incomplete idea of this delicacy, since the photozincographic procedure has significantly thickened the lines of the drawing.

Examining carefully each of the little [axonal] bundles, there is observed in its thickness a vertical cavity that, judging by its size, seems to correspond to the [dendritic] shaft of a large or medium pyramid. And as each cell engenders or can engender several bundles, it may be said that it could be connected with several pyramids.

The cells mentioned are extraordinarily abundant in the human cerebrum, so much so that we do not hesitate to consider them as one of its more important characteristics. In good impregnations of the motor, acoustic, and visual cortices, they are so close that the axonal arborizations or paintbrushes of one cell almost touch those formed by the adjacent [cells], giving rise to a series of very long vertical bands, embracing one, two, or three layers, and whose threads show a yellowish color due to their unprecedented thinness. Although with rarity, we have also confirmed [the presence of] such cells in the dog and cat (fig. 671, *d*) [*fig. 79*]; there they are deficient in little nerve branches, and they do not offer the extreme delicacy and length of the similar ones of man.

As a variety of the previous type, there can be considered a larger fusiform cell of less specific morphology (fig. 669, *J*; 673, *b*) [*figs. 95, 96*]. This cell has been already observed by Retzius[21] as follows from the examination of the figures of one of his publications; but this author does not give a particular description of it, considering it, without doubt, a small pyramid. Like the dwarf bitufted [cells], it exhibits two ascending and descending bundles of dendrites, but these show a greater thickness and are furnished with long collateral spines. The ascending [dendritic] tuft is not confined to the second layer, but assails the first, commonly extending to the upper part of the plexiform layer. The axon is of medium caliber; arising either from the upper or the lower part of the soma, at a short distance it bifurcates, and its divisions and subdivisions engender at a short distance from the cell [body] a dense and varicose arborization, resolving into baskets or axonal plexuses that surround the cell bodies of the small pyramids (fig. 673, A) [fig. 96].

e. Cells with Axons Ascending to the First Layer or [Cells] of Martinotti. This author was the first who mentioned the existence, in the second layer, of some pyramids whose axon, contrary to that of the common pyramids, goes up to the plexiform layer, where it ends by means of horizontal branches of variable length. [Although we believe we are fully justified in giving to these neurons the name of this scientist, we must note that][D] our observations, made both in animals[22] and in man,[23] showed two facts: first, that the cited cells are not pyramids, but globular, ovoid, or fusiform cells, devoid of radial [dendritic] shafts, although with ascending and descending varicose dendrites; second, that such elements are very abundant in all the cerebral layers, but especially in the deep third of the cortex, where they can present a large size and many morphological varieties. Later, these cells were confirmed by Retzius, Kölliker, and Schaffer.

The cells of this type, resident in the second [layer] and in part of the third layer (layer of medium pyramids) of the human cortex, belong to two categories: (a) fusiform or stellate cell, whose ascending axon supplies near its origin several vertically oriented ramifications distributed at deeper levels, while the main trunk reaches the most external portion of the first layer, to ramify in it in a complicated manner, generating a continuous plexus (fig. 674, E, K) [fig. 121]; (b) triangular or stellate

cells, usually more voluminous than the preceding, and whose axon lacks initial branches, going up to the plexiform layer, where it divides, giving rise to two or more very long horizontal branches, not without emitting before reaching the cited layer oblique and ascending branches to the second [layer] (fig. 674, D) [fig. 121]. Let us add for completeness that, on occasions, the highest branches of the axonal arborizations of bitufted cells (fig. 674, L) [fig. 121] and not a few axonal ramifications of large cells with short axon also arrive at the plexiform layer (fig. 662, C, D) [fig. 94].

3. Layer of the Medium and Large Pyramids

In Nissl preparations, there begins underneath the preceding layer, without a precise demarcation line, a very important formation of pyramids, whose sizes increase progressively from superficial to deep, until they reach the layer of the granule cells, at whose frontier the most voluminous somata are situated. This size is, on the average, in man 12 to 16 μm. The largest cells reach a diameter of 22 μm and a length of 26 or 28 μm (fig. 658, 3, 4)[E] [fig. 87].

Large and Medium Pyramidal Cells

The importance of the referred pyramidal cells, from which probably arise the long pathways originating in the cerebrum, obliges us to a somewhat meticulous structural and morphological analysis of them.

Already in the preparations of Nissl, they are easily recognized because they possess a large ovoid or triangular nucleus, in whose interior there is a voluminous nucleolus, as well as an abundant protoplasm strewn with quite thick [Nissl bodies], which are prolonged somewhat into the starting point of the radial [dendritic] process and origins of the basal dendrites. Above the nucleus and [opposite the axonal process], there is usually a thick triangular hillock.

Neurofibrils

Between the Nissl [bodies], there are observed clear passages that run from one dendrite to another, and especially from the [apical dendritic] shaft toward the region of origin of the axon. When such passages are stained by

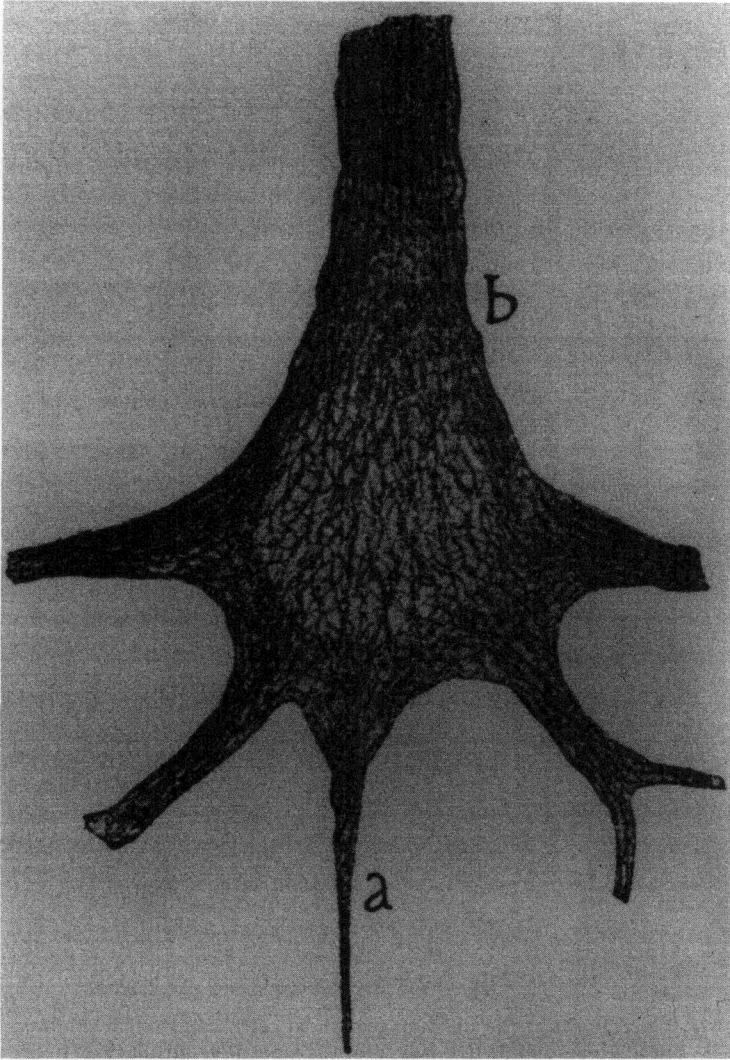

[*FIG. 210*]   Fig. 676. Neurofibrils of the soma of a large pyramidal cell; adult cat. Method of reduced silver nitrate.

the method of Bethe, and even better with our silver nitrate method, there are revealed quite clearly, as discovered by the said author, some bundles of very fine plexiform and varicose threads, which descend from the radial dendrite, separating the [Nissl bodies] and penetrating into the axon and basal dendrites (figs. 676, 677, 678) [*figs. 210, 211, 212*]. It is impossible to know (so thin are such threads) whether they anastomose or not during their course through the soma; what seems probable, from the examination of good preparations of the human, cat, and dog cerebrum, is that they maintain their independence in the interior of the dendrites, into whose branches they separate like the filaments of a small bundle.[24] A meticulous examination with the Zeiss 1.30 apochromatic objective reveals that in the radial [dendritic] shaft and thick dendrites, the *neurofibrils,* so called by Bethe, run exclusively

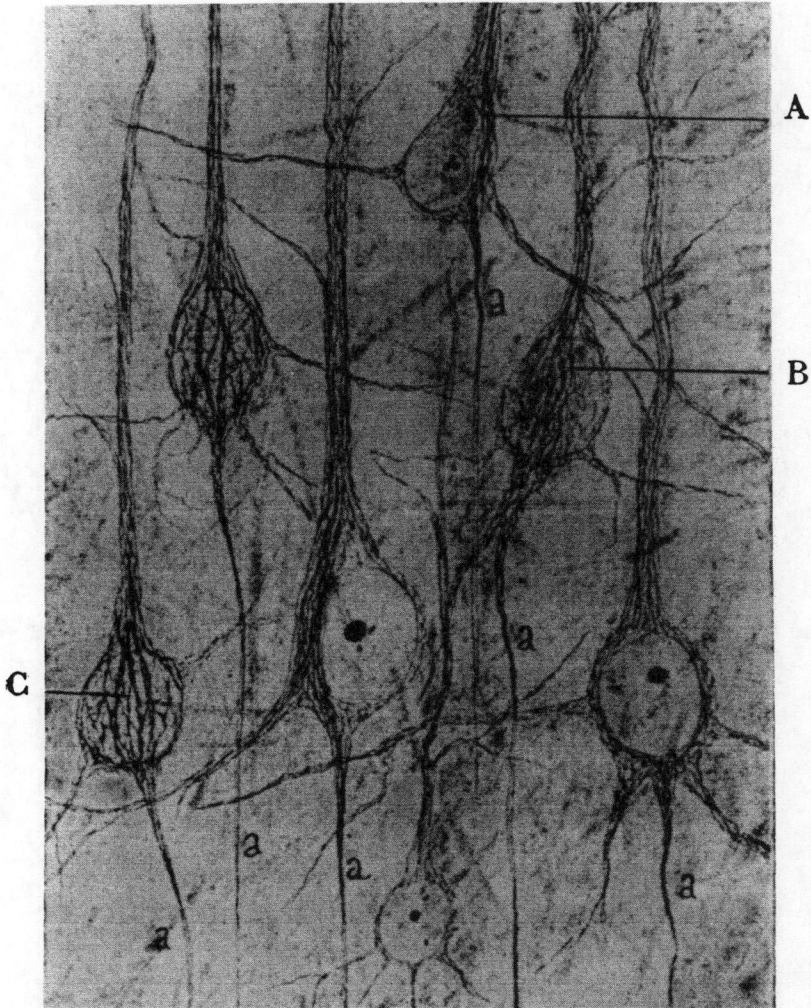

[*FIG. 211*] Fig. 677. Neurofibrils of the medium pyramidal cells; adult rabbit. Method of reduced silver nitrate. *A, B,* bundle of thick neurofibrils that run from the [apical] dendritic shaft to the axon; *C,* primary filaments seen at the surface [of the cells]; *a,* axon.

at the periphery, leaving a central space full of colorless plasma. Finally, the last small dendritic [processes], which seem to terminate freely in the broad gray matter, have only one neurofibril, although the paleness of the impregnation does not allow us, except occasionally, to reveal the final termination. From the above, it follows that the small internal fibrils of the protoplasm never leave the soma or the dendrites, forming an intracellular framework,

totally independent of the pericellular nerve arborizations, in spite of the dictum of Bethe, [Nissl,][F] and Meyer, which they have defended without having made any precise observations, that there is a substantial continuity between both formations.[25] It is worthy to note the lack of the said [neurofibrils] in the spines of the dendritic processes, as well as the existence, in the fine dendritic processes, of a relatively thick protoplasm, in the heart of which is

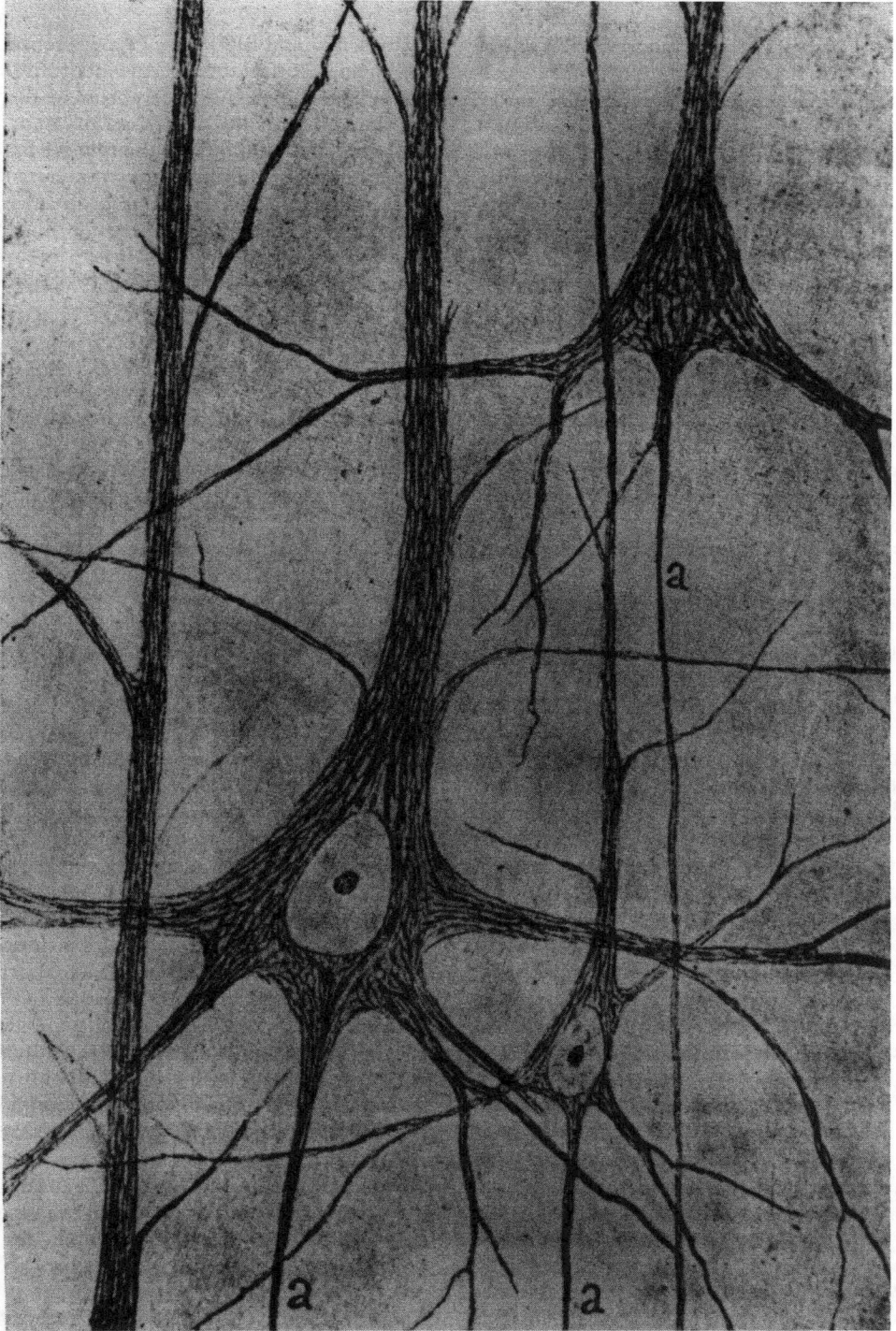

[*FIG. 212*]   Fig. 678. Neurofibrils of large and medium pyramidal cells in the human visual cortex. Method of reduced silver nitrate. *a*, axon.

found a very delicate axial neurofibril. For the rest, the absence of a relationship between the neurofibrils and the pericellular nerve plexuses is a fact recognized by Held[26] and Donaggio.[27]

With respect to the axon, it is formed by the gathering of a group of neurofibrils coming from all regions of the cell, and primarily from the radial dendrite. The passage of the neurofibrils into the axon from the apical shaft is best observed in the rabbit (fig. 677) [*fig. 211*], in which the perinuclear protoplasm is thinner than in man; neurofibrils that run from superficial to deep are arranged in flexuous and varicose bundles, inside which are seen, although without being discerned clearly, fine oblique threads or trabeculae of union (our *secondary filaments*). In the place where the axon hillock becomes thin, the fibrillar bundle is condensed into a cylinder of homogenous aspect, which descends for a certain distance into the region at which the myelin commences. At this point, the narrowing reaches a maximum, and the impregnation ceases or becomes pale, to reappear further on, that is to say, after passing the first ring of cement (fig. 678, *a*) [*fig. 212*]. Often, as is seen in the large cell of fig. 678 [*fig. 212*], there are observed in the cone of origin of the axon two layers: central, notably dense, formed by filaments that appear to come from a complicated perinuclear plexus, continous with the [apical dendritic] shaft; and cortical, looser, in which are gathered together the neurofibrils coming from the [other] dendrites. Anyway, in man, the number of neurofibrils of the protoplasmic framework is so large and their arrangement so intricate that it becomes impossible to determine their reciprocal relations; [thus,] the descriptions and figures given by Bethe and copied by several authors must be considered as strongly schematic and in large part conjectural.

[On the other hand, the drawings published by Bielschowsky,[28] Brodmann, and Schaffer,[29] taken from preparations obtained with the method of the first of these authors, are infinitely more exact. Marinesco[30] has given equally good figures of neurofibrils; he has himself indicated some new details on this subject, in particular the reticulum of large polygonal meshes that they form in the region where the cellular pigment is found.

[Figs. 677 and 678 [*figs. 211, 212*] reproduce the special appearance of the neurofibrils of the pyramids, one in the cerebrum of the rabbit, the other in the cerebrum of man. One will observe, undoubtedly, the relative scarcity of the neurofibrillar elements in the former of these mammals and their extraordinary abundance in the second. The neurofibrillar layer that surrounds the nucleus in the rabbit appears so tenuous that it forms only one bundle that continues into the axon.][G]

Intraprotoplasmic Vacuoles of Golgi and Holmgren. As we exposed elsewhere,[31] the investigations of Golgi, Veratti, Retzius, Holmgren, and others have shown inside the protoplasm of the ganglionic [spinal] neurons, as well as some few medullary nuclei, a system of tubes or vacuoles that form a mesh generally limited to the vicinity of the nucleus. Such small canals appear also in the cerebral pyramids, as Soukhanoff[32] has shown.

We have also impregnated them by applying to the cerebrum of the rabbit our special method of reduced silver nitrate,[33] as we show in fig. 679, *A, B,* [*fig. 213*]. Such small tubes are all the more thick and abundant as the pyramid becomes larger, being concentrated particularly above the nucleus, where they seem to converge on a central stem situated in the axis of the radial [dendritic] process. Toward the basilar region, the meshes are narrower, but without giving prolongations into the basal dendrites. In no case is there a communication of this lacunar system with the exterior, as Retzius[34] and Holmgren[35] claim to have observed in the [spinal] ganglion cells.

[Later investigations, made with the aid of a special formula of our method of reduced silver nitrate,[36] have allowed us to confirm the existence of the tubular apparatus in almost all the cells of the cerebrum. In figure 356 [*fig. 214*], this apparatus can be seen as it is presented in the giant pyramidal cells of the adult dog; one cannot fail to remark on the vesicular appearance of the large diverticula that are found at the origins of the dendrites.][H]

Small Intranuclear Rods. Several authors have indicated, as a sporadic fact of uncertain significance, a small, thin, intranuclear rod, especially colorable with Heidenhain's hematox-

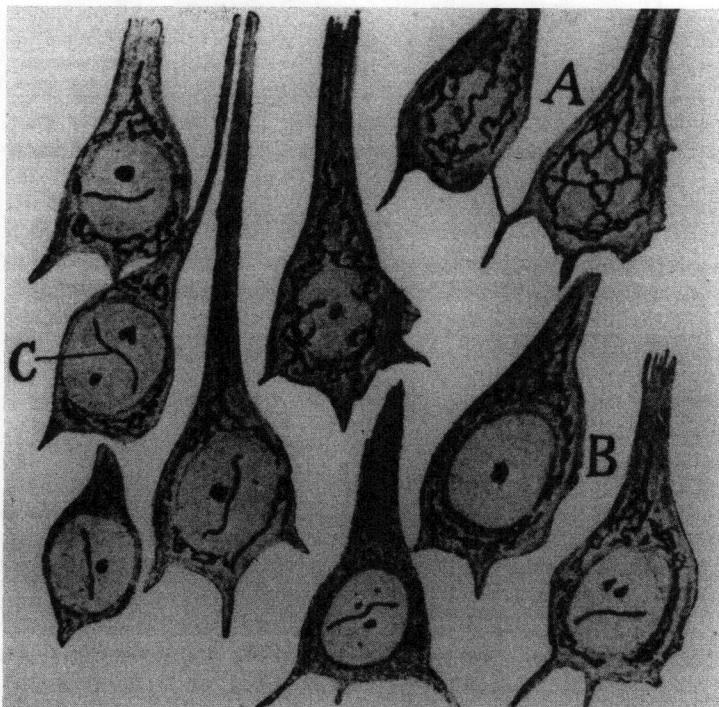

[*FIG. 213*]   Fig. 679. Deep pyramidal cells of the cerebrum of the rabbit. Method of reduced silver nitrate. *A,* intraprotoplasmic canaliculae of Golgi-Holmgren, [seen] in superficial optic plane; *B,* the same [seen] in equatorial optic plane; *C,* cells furnished with an intranuclear rodlet.

ylin (Mann, Lenhossék, Prenant, Holmgren, etc.). Our already cited silver nitrate method stained them an intense black, and they appeared constantly single, rectilinear or slightly curved, and completely independent of the nucleolus. This singular filament, whose significance is not known, resides exclusively in the medium and small cells of the deep layers (*layer of the polymorphic cells* of the rabbit) and, exceptionally, in small pyramids. So far, we have not been able to impregnate it in the cerebrum of man and gyrencephalic animals.

Pericellular Network of Golgi. When we dealt with the cerebellum, we already spoke about the existence, around the Purkinje cells and other cells, of a granular mass that, as Golgi and Bethe have demonstrated, very often presents a reticulated appearance. We have successfully applied the modified method of Ehrlich[37] to the staining of this pericellular

network, having impregnated it with great intensity in the cells with short axon of the cerebrum of the cat. As is seen in fig. 680, *A, B* [*fig. 215*], this network is flat, lies immediately outside the membrane, and exhibits narrow and rounded meshes of great regularity. It often ceases toward the thick polar [dendrites], presenting an intensely stained thickening or flange; but at other times it continues along the dendrites, progressively turning pale and elongating its meshes.

This net, confirmed also in the cerebrum by S. Meyer (method of Ehrlich), who erroneously considers it to be continuous with nerve fibers, and by Donaggio, Held, and Simarro, who have stained it by means of special methods in the spinal cord and medulla, is totally extraneous to the pericellular nerve arborizations. The observations we have recently made with a method of Bethe[38] prove that this network represents an artifact, probably a pro-

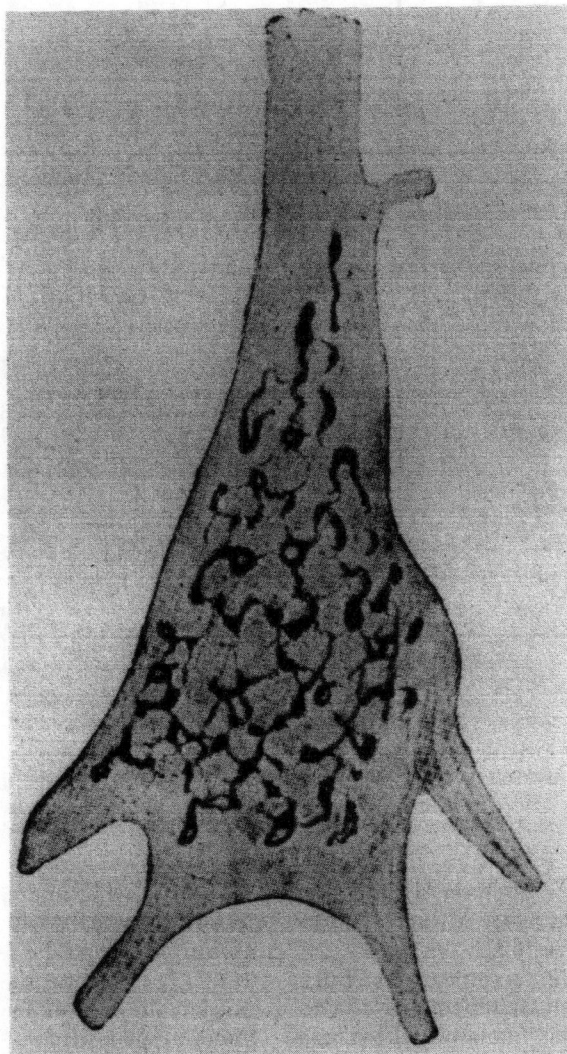

[*FIG. 214*]   Fig. 356. Tubular apparatus of Golgi-Holmgren of a giant pyramidal cell; adult dog. Method of reduced silver nitrate (special formula). [This figure is only in the French version of the book.]

tein clot, produced in the plasma of the peri-cellular spaces.[1]

[The reduced silver nitrate procedure, used by a special formula, also allows us to impregnate the pericellular mesh in the cerebrum; in this way, we have been able to reveal it around certain neurons of the cerebral cortex of the cat and dog.[39]

We show, in figs. 357 and 358 [*figs. 215,* 216], the appearance presented by the cells with short axon invested with this mesh in the cerebrum of the cat. It is seen that it invests the [cell] bodies, dendrites, and axons; in the axon, it descends to the origin of the myelin sheath, where it suddenly ceases. It is really strange that the method of Ehrlich and our special silver formula, throughout the whole cortex, impregnate the superficial mesh only

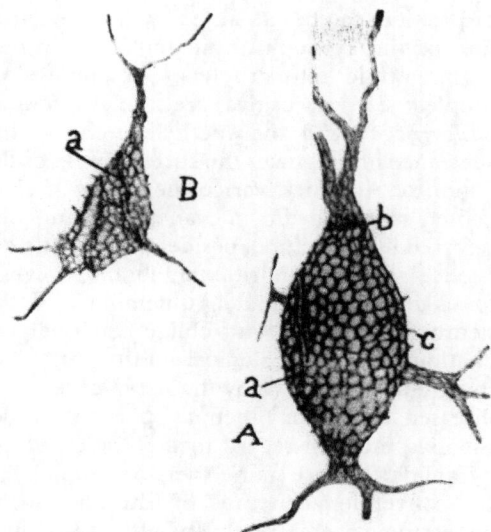

[FIG. 215] Fig. 357. Cells with short axon; cerebrum of the cat. Method of Ehrlich, slightly modified. *A*, large cell; *B*, small cell; *a*, folds of the pericellular network that could be taken erroneously for nerve fibers; *b*, polar rings strongly stained; *c*, spines arising at right angles from the cell body. [The original is in blue.]

on the cells with short axon and more particularly on the neurons whose large axons ascend to the plexiform layer.]ʲ

If, after taking a quick look at the texture of the large and medium pyramids, we want to pass to the detailed study of their morphology and the trajectory and termination of their processes, it will be necessary to resort to the method of Golgi or to that of Ehrlich.

Like the small pyramids, the giant and medium pyramids possess a conical cell body from which also emerges, upward, the radial [dendritic] shaft; downward, the basal or descending dendrites; from the sides, the oblique and horizontal processes; finally, from the deep aspect of the soma, the robust and descending axon. All of these processes reproduce the appearances already described for the small pyramids, except that they are larger and more [spine covered], traverse longer trajectories, and ramify in a much more complicated fashion than those of the small pyramids. The [apical] shaft is especially thick and very long,

and ends in the plexiform layer, where, as seen in fig. 675, *E* [*fig. 90*], it engenders an arborization of horizontal branches [that are] thicker and longer than those coming from the small pyramids. Often we have observed that this dendritic arborization extends through a deeper level of the cited layer than the [dendritic] tufts of the upper small and medium pyramids. With regard to the axon, it descends vertically and, after entering the radial nerve bundles, reaches the white matter, where, as we discovered,[40] it can divide into two branches with opposite orientations. In accordance with what Golgi observed, and as confirmed by Martinotti, us, Retzius, and Kölliker, from the initial trajectory of the axon arise four, five, or more collateral branches,

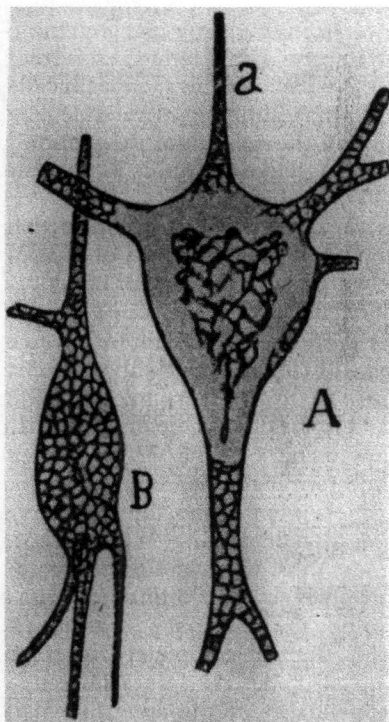

[FIG. 216] Fig. 358. Two cells with short axon of the cerebrum; adult cat. Method of reduced silver nitrate with previous fixation in formol-acetone. *A*, cell with ascending axon seen in equatorial [focal] plane; *B*, cell with descending axon seen in superficial [focal] plane; *a*, axon. [This figure is only in the French version of the book.]

which run more or less horizontally, covering with their small secondary branches a large area of the gray matter. In the cat and rabbit, the collaterals are less numerous, less long, and less branched than in man, it being possible to observe easily their termination, which is made by means of a free varicosity. It is common to see that the first collaterals run obliquely upward, entering into connection with the somata and [dendritic] shafts of the more superficial cells, whereas the deeper collaterals take a more or less horizontal direction, being connected with deeper large pyramids. The main point of origin of the cited branches is the upper third of the axon, that is to say, the portion of its course [in the third layer]; during its course in the underlying layers, collaterals are rare or completely lacking, and when they occur, they usually trace a recurrent trajectory. In any case (and this is a law that no neuron with a long axon is free from), the initial portion of the axon lacks collaterals, a portion that, although of variable length depending on the volume of the neuron, in the medium and large pyramids can be estimated to be 40 or 50 [μm].

It is very instructive to compare the Golgi preparations with the results of vital impregnation with methylene blue or method of Ehrlich. We have used this procedure successfully in the cat and rabbit,[41] being fortunate in confirming fully the findings with silver chromate with respect to the morphology of the pyramids and to the disposition of the dendrites. As we show in fig. 681 [*fig. 217*], the [dendritic] shaft and terminal tuft are very well stained a more or less intense blue, the appearance varying somewhat depending on the time of action of the air; thus, when the pieces are exposed for half an hour after infiltration with methylene blue, the terminal [dendritic] tuft will maintain almost completely its regularity, showing all collateral spines in the form of pale appendages, terminating in a dark blue sphere; in those that have remained one or two hours [exposed] to the air, the impregnation is more intense, but on the other hand, all the fine dendrites appear notably varicose and devoid of collateral appendages. The postmortem alteration that some authors, such as Renaut [of Lyon,][K] have considered a normal

disposition, can be explained by the concentration of the cyanophilic matter of the protoplasmic fluid into droplets. Sometimes, the droplets or varicosities are broken (*cyanophilorrhage*), and the methylene-blue-loving substance impregnates the surroundings of the dendrite. All thick varicosities show a clear center, surrounded by a cyanophilic rim. The referred phenomenon, besides proving the existence of a peridendritic membrane,[42] reveals to us the extraordinary vulnerability of the neuronal processes, and oblige us to be very cautious with physiological interpretations of the alterations shown by the nerve cells of the diseased cerebrum (anemias, poisonings, dementias, etc.). In regard to the somata of the pyramids, they are stained very occasionally by the conventional method of Ehrlich, usually appearing extremely pale and almost invisible. However, using other methods of impregnation (our *anaereal* reaction),[43] both the soma and the basal dendrites are impregnated, showing exactly the same morphology as with the method of Golgi.

The axon is stained better with methylene blue, but it cannot be as easily followed as in the Golgi preparations, because the impregnation usually ceases not much further than the apex of the axonal cone. By contrast, the origins of the collaterals and the points of bifurcation are very well seen, thanks to the intense blue color acquired by the nerve fibers at the level of the strangulations [nodes of Ranvier].

Cells with Short Axon

The layers of the medium and large pyramids are somewhat less rich in cells with short axon than the second layer; however, such cells are not lacking in them, the following types being recognized: (a) stellate or fusiform cell, provided with an ascending axon prolonged up to the plexiform layer, after giving off branches to the third and second layers; (b) voluminous stellate cell with a short, ascending, horizontal, or descending axon, often arciform in its initial trajectory, which engenders a diffuse arborization with long, more or less horizontal filaments, distributed in the thickness of the third layer; (c) the bitufted type, very abundant at the level of the medium pyramids, with its

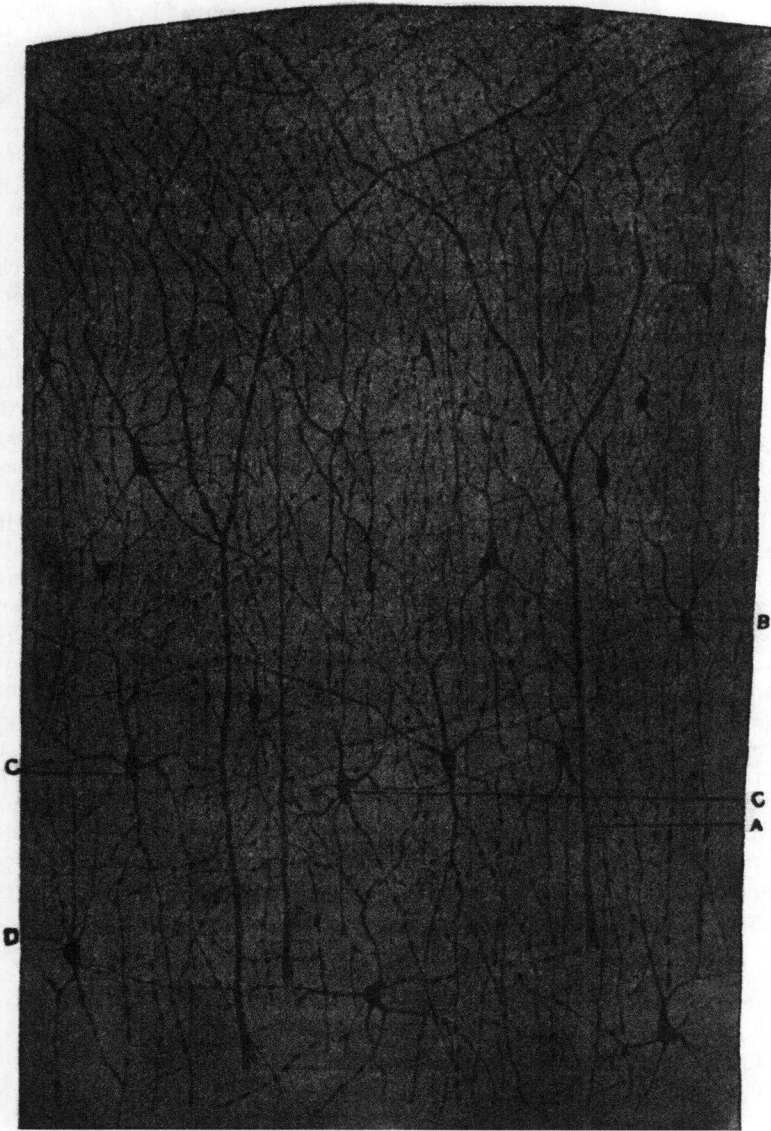

[*FIG. 217*]   Fig. 681. Section of a cerebral gyrus of the adult cat. Method of Ehrlich. All the visible cells have short axons. *A*, [apical dendritic] shaft of a large pyramidal cell; *B*, large bitufted cell; *C*, large cell with arched short axon resolving itself into long branches; *D*, cells with ascending axon. [The original is in blue.]

two varieties (small and medium size) and its characteristic nerve arborizations; (d) finally, robust cells whose axonal branches resolve themselves into pericellular nests. But about the latter cells, comparable in more than one

respect to the basket cells of the cerebellum, we must set down some details.

Discovered by us, first in the visual cortex and later in the motor [cortex], such cells probably reside in the majority of the cerebral areas of man, both in the third layer, where they seem to us to be especially abundant, and in the underlying formation of the granule cells or fourth layer. They are characterized by their stellate shape, the thinness and enormous length of their divergent dendrites, and above all the behavior of the axon (figs. 682, *a*; 683, *a*) [*figs. 104, 105*]. This process follows a variety of directions, although commonly it is ascending or descending, and at a short distance, sometimes near its starting point (fig. 682, *E*) [*fig. 104*], it bifurcates, resolving itself into a number of horizontal and oblique branches of great length.

One sees that such branches, after a very long and complicated course, resolve into pericellular arborizations which wrap around and tightly encircle the outline of the soma and the origin of the thick dendrites. The nests, in the strict sense, consist of many branches that are intertwined in a complicated manner, being composed of little branches [that are] short, varicose, and terminate by a nodule contacting the protoplasmic surface. When the branches that make up the nest are followed to the parent fibers, it is observed that they do not come from a single afferent fiber but from several, each of them furnishing filaments to several terminal baskets. It is not rare to observe that a fiber gives some little branches to a nest and may even make up the main part of it; then it leave and exhausts itself in other pericellular plexuses (fig. 683, *c, b*) [*fig. 105*].

It is not always easy to determine the origin of the constituent fibers of a nest. Sometimes, the impregnation of these occurs in isolation, as appears in fig. 684, *c, b* [*fig. 106*], in which the afferent fibers are notably thick and the nests dense and extended along the [apical dendritic] shaft and basilar dendrites. Here arises the question of whether all the pericellular plexuses that the silver chromate reveals in the human cerebrum have the same [origin.].

It is indubitable that the fine perineuronal plexuses that we reproduce in fig. 683, *a* [*fig. 105*], originate from cells with short axon; but it could happen that the robust nests would have another origin, coming, for example, from exogenous fibers ramifying in the cortex. New investigations on this point are necessary.

Recently, we have applied in adult man the method of reduced silver nitrate,[44] which stains the nerve baskets in the cerebellum and spinal cord, and we have obtained in the motor [cortex] preparations in which the large pyramids are shown surrounded by nerve arborizations of a dark brown color. These pericellular nerve branches are relatively thick, possess from time to time thick varicosities, and terminate on the somatic and dendritic protoplasm in notably thickened terminals (our *terminal clubs*). [These clubs, which are frequently very tiny, show in their interior a neurofibrillar ring that contacts the surface of the enveloped neuron. The [pericellular plexuses] are, for the most part, much less numerous than upon the nerve cells of the spinal cord and medulla oblongata, as shown in fig. 363, [*fig. 218*], in which we have reproduced the nerve plexus on a large pyramid of the cerebrum of the adult dog. This figure, which is taken from a preparation obtained by a special formula of impregnation,[45] is interesting from another point of view. It is seen that the surfaces of the neuron that are in the immediate vicinity of the capillaries and neuroglial cells are completely devoid of pericellular fibrils; these surfaces enter also into intimate contact with the capillaries or the astrocytes. The regions of the pyramidal cell that are contiguous either to the basal neuroglial cells or to the capillary vessels could thus be called *neuroglial areas and nutrient areas or poles*. It is also seen in this figure that a large number of fibrils pass from one plexus to another, entering in this way into connection successively with many pyramids.][L]

For the rest, the referred nests do not resemble at all those which Semi Meyer[46] has believed he observed with the aid of methylene blue on the cells of the guinea pig, nor [do they resemble] the superficial meshes described in the cerebral pyramidal cells of the cat by Bethe[47] and Nissl.[48] In fact, the dispositions drawn by Meyer and Bethe, as well as by Turner and Hunter,[49] have nothing to do with nerve fibers, since they correspond to the homogenous pericellular net of Golgi described

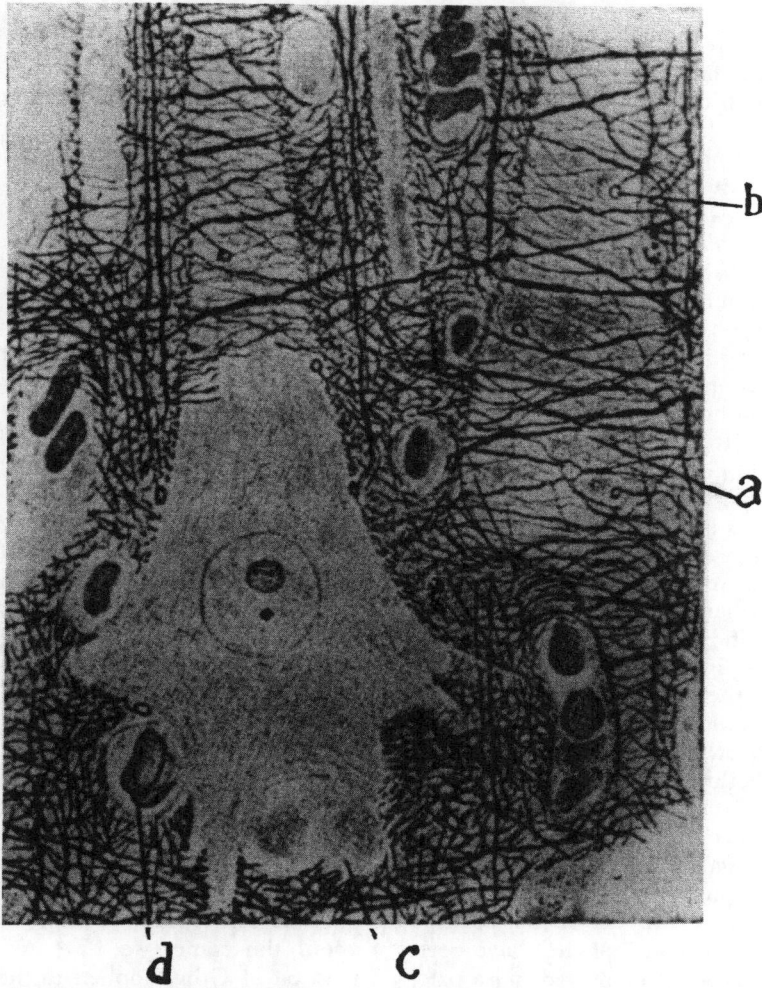

[*FIG. 218*] Fig. 363. Terminal nerve plexuses forming nests around the pyramidal cells of the cerebral cortex; adult dog. Method of reduced silver nitrate, fifth formula. *a*, nerve plexus; *b*, neurofibrillar ring of the terminal clubs; *c*, basilar neuroglial cell, and *d*, blood capillary, with their respective areas devoid of pericellular fibers. [This figure is only in the French version of the book.]

above, which, according to Donaggio,[50] Held,[51] and Simarro[52] does not have an axonal nature.

Cells with Short Axon in the Mammals. The layer of the small, medium, and large pyramids exhibits also in the cat and dog a considerable number of cells with short axon, among which are discovered the same types, although somewhat larger and morphologically more simplified than in the human cortex. Let us note that the method of Ehrlich is very useful for determining the relative abundance of such cells, because usually (common method) it impregnates simultaneously and exclusively all the cells with short axon lying in the stained region. In such preparations, it is confirmed that the above-mentioned cells are as numerous as the pyramids, being distributed with a certain regularity in the several cortical layers, except the second [layer], in which they are usually somewhat more numerous. Among the cells that particularly abound are the voluminous stellate [cells], provided with arciform axon, dividing into very long horizontal branches (fig. 681, *C*) [*fig. 217*]; the medium fusiform [cells], with fine ascending or descending axon, giving rise to less extensive arborizations (fig. 681, *D*) [*fig. 217*]; the bitufted [cells] whose axon is not sufficiently stained to be studied (*B*); and the globular, ovoid, or triangular [cells] with ascending axon, distributed in the plexiform, second, and third layers.

The preparations of Ehrlich reveal to us, besides, two details that are lacking in the [preparations] of Golgi. One is that when the dendrites are completely [stained], the methylene blue allows us to follow them over very long trajectories, revealing that the ascending [dendrites] reach very often, perhaps always, to the first layer, where they add to the complexity of the dendritic plexus therein, concentrating near the pia (fig. 681, *B*) [*fig. 217*]. The second relates to the revelation of the myelin sheath of the axon, so far never demonstrated in the cells with short axon. As we show in fig. 685, *a* [*fig. 219*], this process, whose initial trajectory hardly attracts the methylene blue, shows at the level of its dichotomies an intense impregnation (exceptionally an extreme paleness), indicating the presence of strangulations and thus the lack of a myelin sheath at these points. [Once] the main branches have been given off, they become more and more pale, the hyperchromatic portions disappearing after a short distance, which indicates that the last branches of the nerve arborization lack myelin.

4. Layer of the Small Stellate and Pyramidal Cells

Distinguished by Meynert and commonly named *layer of the granule cells,* this layer is revealed in most parts of the human cortex, where it acquires an enormous development compared with the corresponding layer in the gyrencephalic animals.

In order to gain an idea about the variety, number, and form of the cells of this layer, it is [appropriate] to begin with the study of Nissl preparations, in which there already can be distinguished three classes: voluminous and medium pyramids, few in number and completely equal to the ones lying in the bordering layers (fig. 686) [*fig. 100*]; cells also rather rare, with triangular, stellate, ovoid, or semilunar shapes, of large size and provided with abundant protoplasm and poor in [Nissl bodies] (fig. 686, *c, d*) [*fig. 100*]; and, finally, a multitude of tight, tiny cells, frequently arranged in vertical rows (*grains* of the authors), some of which have a pyramidal shape (fig. 686, *b*) [*fig. 100*], whereas others exhibit a polygonal contour and very pale protoplasm (fig. 686, *a*) [*fig. 100*].

[Among these cells are the granules in the strict sense, which are more difficult to stain by the neurofibrillar methods. When one is able to impregnate them, for example, by the reduced silver nitrate, it is confirmed that the filamentous framework forms a delicate network usually located in the vicinity of the nucleus. In certain cells, the network is more extensive (fig. 366, *A*) [*fig. 220*] and surrounds the whole nucleus; in others, it covers only a minimum part of this organelle and occupies only a very restricted area of the cell body. Be that as it may, the neurofibrils anastomose and gather together in thin bundles that penetrate into the processes of the cell.][M]

The method of Nissl shows us nothing about the arrangement of the processes of all of these cell types; to complete our knowledge about the same, we have to resort to the method of Golgi applied to the cerebrum of the child of fifteen to thirty days. In the preparations with good impregnations, it is confirmed that the fourth[N] layer lodges, in fact, several cellular varieties, which we can group in two general categories: first, cells with long axon; second, cells with short axon.

Cells with Long Axon

[These are all pyramidal cells. They are of two kinds: one sort is small, the other large and medium.][O]

a. Small Pyramids. Such cells, which were already mentioned by several authors, especially by Kölliker, possess a diminutive soma that emits three, four, or more fine basal dendrites,

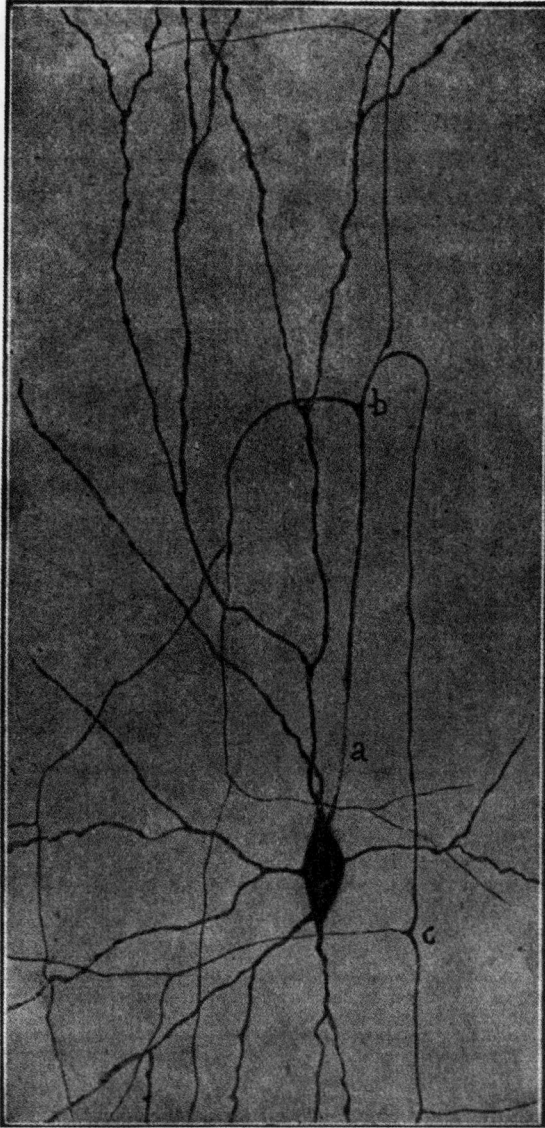

[*FIG. 219*]   Fig. 685. Large cell with short axon of the layer of the medium pyramids; adult cat. Method of Ehrlich. *a*, pale portion of the axon; *b*, portion strongly blue-stained, corresponding to an interannular strangulation; *c*, another strangulation. [The original is in blue.]

branching at no great distance inside the limits of the fourth[P] layer: from the upper part arises a thin [dendritic] shaft, which, after supplying some collateral branches to this layer, goes up almost straight to the plexiform layer, where it divides in a small number of fine, sparsely spiny dendrites. With regard to the axon, which Kölliker apparently has not seen, it emerges from the base of the soma, descends vertically, crossing the [underlying] layers, and very probably reaches the white matter, continuing as a fine myelinated fiber. We have

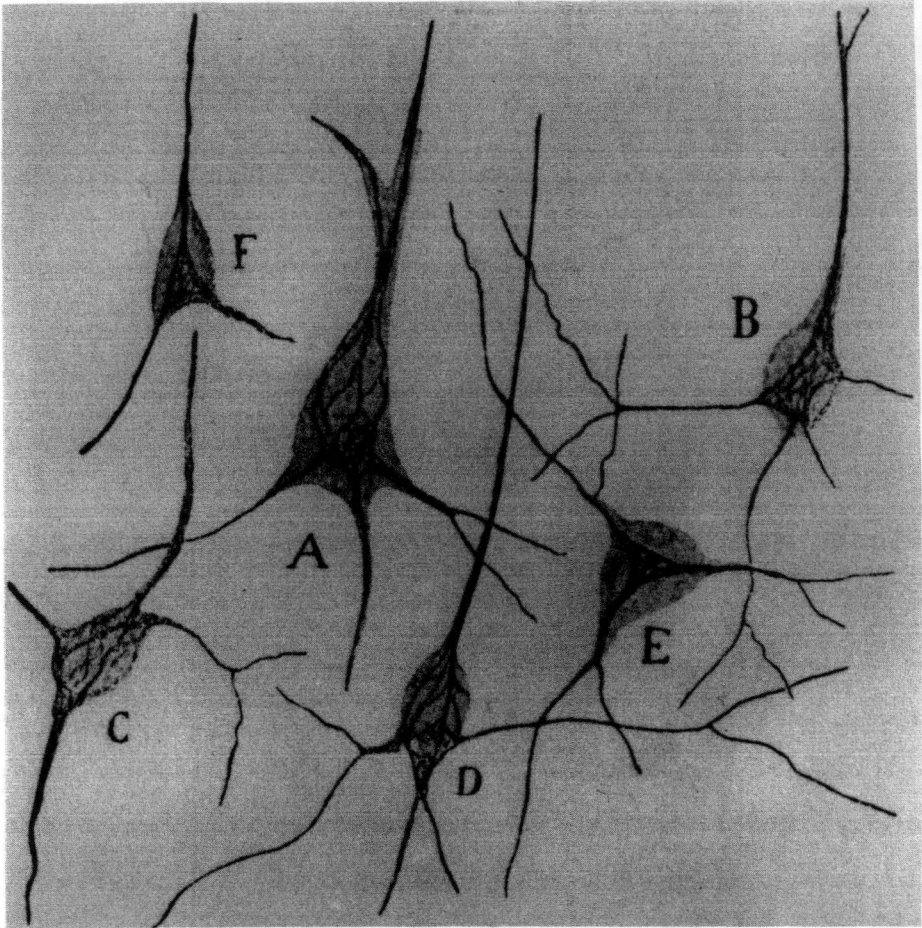

[*FIG. 220*]   Fig. 366. Small pyramidal cells or granule [cells] of the visual cortex; adult man. Method of reduced silver nitrate. *A, C, D*, cells with neurofibrillar framework arranged around the nucleus; *B, E, F*, cells whose neurofibrillar framework is situated on one side of the nucleus. [This figure is only in the French version of the book.]

never been able to follow it, because of its length and delicacy, to a point deeper than beneath the layer of the deep giant cells.

The most interesting feature of these cells is the disposition of their axonal collaterals. In number two, three, or four, such branches originate in the upper trajectory of the axon, and some of them, after describing an arc with a superior concavity, go up to the upper part of the fourth^Q layer and perhaps even beyond; perhaps they reach the first layer; anyway, their fine diameter and the great complication

of the superimposed nerve plexuses have prevented us from following them completely. In some cells, as seen at *A, B*, fig. 687 [*fig. 101*], the first collateral is so robust that it might be regarded as the true continuation of the axon, as a consequence of which the vertical descending fiber destined for the white matter would be a true collateral. Finally, there is no lack of cells which engender several axonal arcades, from which arise three or more recurrent collaterals. In such cells, the fiber destined for the white matter sometimes resembles a fine collateral arising from the convexity of an arch (fig. 687, C) [fig. 101]. All the above-mentioned collaterals, except the ascending branches, are distributed in the thickness of this layer, as well as in the upper portion of the [underlying layer], adding to the complexity of the nerve plexus that surrounds the deep large pyramids.

b. Large and Medium Pyramids of Common Type. Such cells, whose number is very variable, depending on the cerebral territories explored, are never absent from the fourth layer, coinciding completely in morphological properties with the large pyramids of the preceding layer. We reproduce them in fig. 687, E [fig. 101].

Cells with Short Axon

They are much more numerous than the cells with long axon, making up in many cortical territories a formation so thick and important that it would not be inappropriate to give their name to the cerebral layer in which they reside. They correspond to several types; some of them have already been described in the second layer.

Here are the most common.

a. Stellate or Fusiform Cells with Ascending Axon Divided in Long Horizontal Branches. As is seen in fig. 688, A, D [fig. 102], these neurons inhabit several planes of the fourth layer and have different sizes. Their dendrites, divergent and a little spiny, are distributed in the thickness of the cited layer, and the axon divides into very long horizontal, collateral, and terminal branches, some of them so lengthy that they can be followed for two or more tenths of a millimeter. From the course of such horizontal branches, further small branches that commonly arise at oblique angles are distributed to different levels of the fourth[R] layer.

b. Cells with Ascending Axon Distributed to the Fourth layer. In the previous type, the terminal and collateral branches of the axon do not appear ever to leave the fourth layer, but in this kind of cell, which may be considered as a variant of the previous type, the axon, not without deigning to emit horizontal branches, goes up through the third layer, in which it abandons some collaterals, to descend again to the layer of origin (fig. 688, C) [fig. 102]. In other cases, the little ascending branch occurs as a collateral of one of the branches of the terminal bifurcation of the axon as seen at B (fig. 688) [fig. 102].

c. Cells Whose Axon Goes Up to the Plexiform Layer and Second Layer (fig. 688, F) [fig. 102]. Certain stellate, ovoid, or triangular cells, of larger size than the previous ones, possess a thick ascending axon which, after supplying some branches to the fourth layer ramifies in the third layer, resolving into a multitude of tiny oblique and horizontal branches. Finally, in some cases, we have also observed the arrival of the axon at the first layer, where it behaves like the axons of Martinotti. Similar cells exist also in the second and third layers, but it is not always possible to observe the arrival of the axon at the first layer because of the very long trajectory.

In short, although our investigations on this point are insufficient, we are inclined to admit in the fourth layer several kinds of cells with ascending axon distributed at different levels, which [cells] could take the name of the layer in which the axon is preferentially arborized. Thus, there would be cells with ascending axon destined for the first layer, others with this process distributed in the second [layer], others in the third [layer], etc. Let us hasten, however, to set down that in almost all of these cells the nerve ramification includes several layers.

d. Diminutive or Arachniform Cells. They are found at all levels of the fourth layer and are not lacking, either, in the bordering [zones]. In fig. 688, E [fig. 102], we reproduce one of them, in which the axon resolved itself into a very fine ascending nerve plexus.

e. Bitufted Cells with Axon Resolved into Vertical Tiny Bundles or Threads.[S] They are, on the whole, similar to the homonymous cells of the upper layers, so that we will not make a particular description of them.

From what has been said above, it results

that the fourth layer or [layer] of the granule cells is an intermediate station of the cortex in which are concentrated the cells with short axon or [cells] of intracortical association. Even the small pyramids of this layer show, because of the amount and robustness of the recurrent nerve collaterals, the very significant stamp of the cells of association at short and medium distances.

5. Fifth Layer or [Layer] of the Deep Large Pyramids

In several cerebral regions, peculiarly in the so-called *gyri of association,* in the visual, acoustic, and motor [gyri] (postcentral [and precentral] gyri), there are observed one or several discontinuous rows of robust pyramids that seem to be displaced from the third layer, emigrating through the granules to the frontiers of the layer of the deep medium pyramids. Three neuronal categories inhabit the region, where they gather together and which is of very unequal extent in the same gyrus: colossal pyramids or cells of Betz, pyramids of medium size, and numerous cells with short axon.

a. Large Pyramids [or Betz's Cells].[T] They are easily recognized in Nissl preparations, because of their richness in [Nissl granules], the vertically elongated form of the soma (by contrast with the pyramids of the third layer, which are broader), and the robustness of the basilar dendrites.

Even more than by their size, they are characterized in Golgi preparations by the abundance and enormous length of the basilar dendrites, whose branchings cover a large area of the fifth and sixth layers. The [apical dendritic] shaft, often bifurcated not far from its origin, spreads a broad and loose [dendritic] tuft, the most extensive of all the pyramids, in the plexiform layer.

The size of the soma as well as the length of the basilar dendrites vary with age, as can be seen by comparing the figures that show, respectively, the cells of Betz in the cerebrum of a child (fig. 689) [*fig. 109*] and in that of an [adult] man. In the latter, some such dendrites traverse a distance of more than one millimeter (fig. 690) [*fig. 110*].

With respect to the axon, it is robust and gives off several collaterals (from four to eight or more), some originating and branching in the fifth layer among the pyramids of the same kind, others originating in and distributed to the sixth layer, in which the pyramids of medium volume reside. The final destination of the axon is the white matter, where we have seen it arrive both in the cerebrum of fetuses of the seventh to ninth month and in the newborn child.

[The neurofibrils are extremely abundant and form a very complicated framework in the giant pyramids, as can be seen in figs. 371 and 372 [*figs. 221, 222*], in which we have illustrated some specimens of these cells from man and rabbit. The disposition of the [neurofibrils] is of the fascicular type with the intervening cavities lodging the Nissl [bodies]. In man, there is observed in the basilar region and sometimes in the lateral regions of the cell body a voluminous accumulation of pigment, divided into several sections by the neurofibrils (fig. 371, c^U) [*fig. 221*]. Another interesting detail revealed by the reduced silver nitrate: the nucleolus appears made up of a considerable conglomeration of tiny spherules.][V]

b. Medium Pyramids. Except for their size, they possess the same characteristics as the [Betz's pyramids].

Cells with Short Axon

They have a variable size and shape, on account of which it is necessary to distinguish certain types.

a. Cell with Short Ascending Axon. It is quite common, with a stellate, triangular, or fusiform shape, and it possesses divergent dendrites that ramify inside the confines of this layer. The axon is ascending and resolves itself into little, more or less horizontal, terminal branches, distributed either in the thickness of the fifth[W] layer or in the lower levels of the fourth.[X]

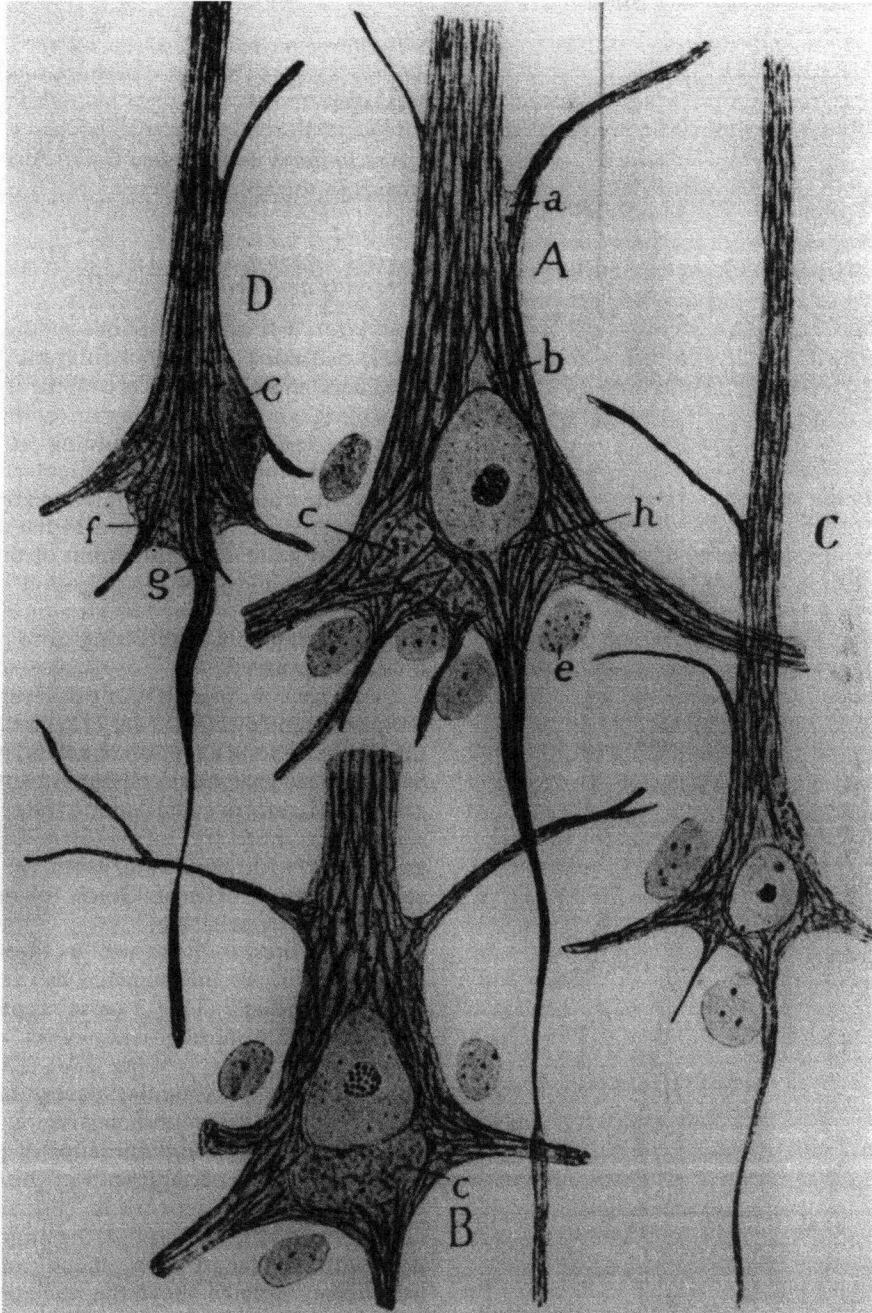

[*FIG. 221*]   Fig. 371. Giant pyramidal cells or cells of Betz of the cerebrum of man. Method of reduced silver nitrate. *a, b,* cavities corresponding to the chromatic bodies of Nissl; *c,* mass of pigment; *e,* nuclei of neuroglial cells; *f, h,* neurofibrils penetrating into the axon. [This figure is only in the French version of the book.]

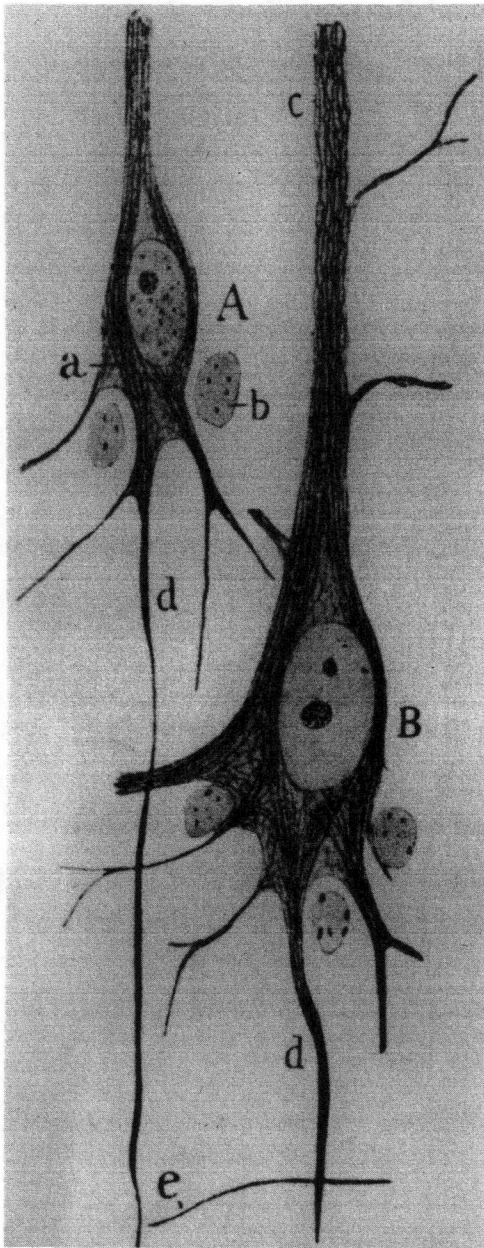

[FIG. 222] Fig. 372. Giant pyramidal cells; adult rabbit. Method of reduced silver nitrate. A, cell of medium size; B, cell of very large size; a, neurofibrillar bundles running into the axon; b, nucleus of a neuroglial cell; c, neurofibrils of the [apical] dendritic shaft; d, axon; e, collateral. [This figure is only in the French version of the book.]

b. Fusiform or Stellate Cells with Very Long Ascending Axon. [The axon] perhaps reaches the first layer.

c. Arachniform and Bitufted Cells. Already described in the second layer.

6. Sixth Layer or [Layer] of the Medium Pyramids and Triangular Cells

This layer, which corresponds to the fourth [layer] or [layer] of the polymorphic cells of mammals and to the [layer] of the fusiform cells of Meynert in the human cortex, is of greater or lesser extent, depending on the gyri under study. In some gyri, particularly at the level of the convex parts, it almost always appears divided into two sublayers [that are] recognizable by the different extent of the intercalated nerve plexuses. On the other hand, in other gyri, it is presented as an almost homogeneous formation, authorizing us to consider it as a single layer.

The most common cells of this layer appear in figs. 691 and 692 [figs. 111, 112], and, among the cells with long axon, there are: (a) medium pyramids; (b) triangular cells and inverted pyramids; (c) fusiform cells. Among the cells with short axon, there are: (a) fusiform and triangular cells with ascending axon; (b) stellate cells or sensory cells of Golgi; (c) neurogliaform or dwarf cells, etc.

[Most of these cells, as well as those of the seventh layer, are impregnated by the neurofibrillar methods. The diverse appearances that their neurofibrillar framework presents are illustrated in fig. 374 [fig. 223]. There will be noticed at c the reticular disposition of the neurofibrils in the superficial regions of the cell body; at f, the conglomeration of pigment whose position is variable and at the level of which the fibrillar network is loose and difficult to see; finally, at b and d, the empty space destined to lodge the block of Nissl [substance], situated above the nucleus.][Y]

Cells with Long Axon

a. Medium Pyramids. They resemble completely the type already described in other cerebral layers, showing a very long [apical dendritic] shaft which assails the plexiform

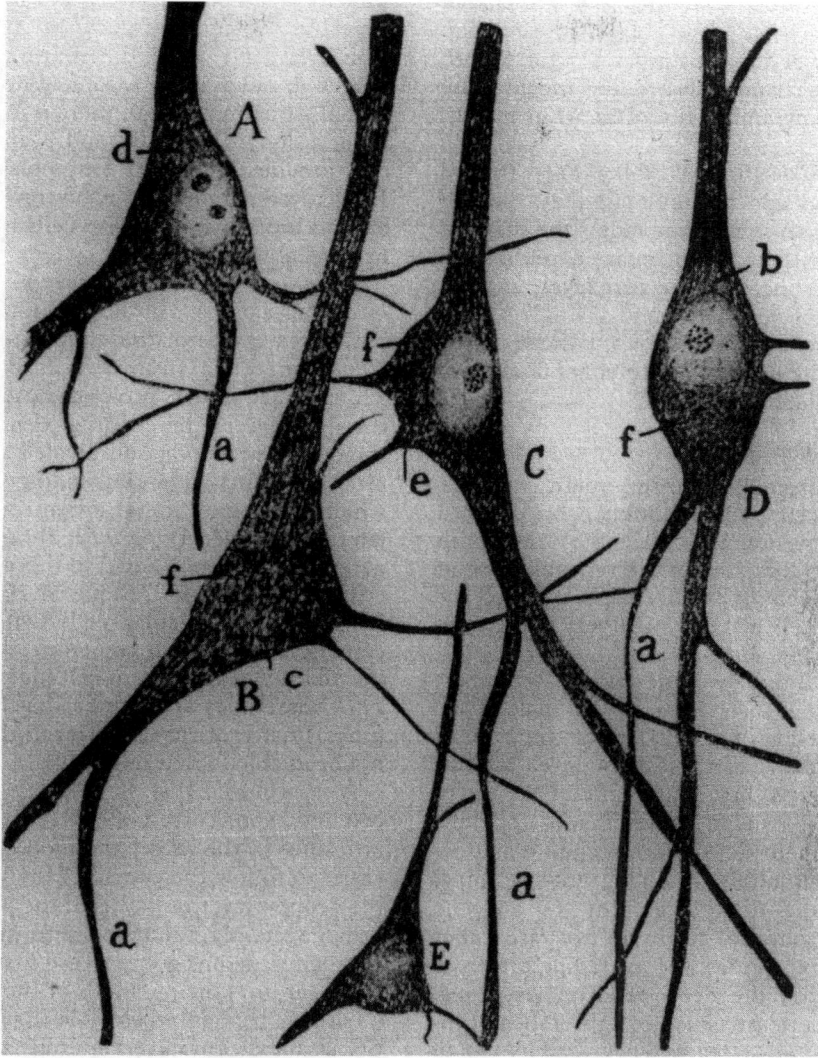

[*FIG. 223*]   Fig. 374. Cells of the layer of the fusiform neurons of the motor cortex of man. Method of reduced silver nitrate. *A, E,* small and medium pyramidal cells; *B, C,* triangular cells; *D,* fusiform cells; *a,* axon; *b, d,* site of the triangular block of Nissl [substance] above the nucleus; *c,* reticular disposition of the superficial neurofibrils; *f,* pigment accumulation. [This figure is only in the French version of the book.]

layer, several descending and oblique dendrites originating from the soma, and, finally, an axon that can be followed very easily to the white matter and from whose initial course four, five, or more collaterals, distributed in the thickness of the sixth and seventh layers, arise (fig. 691, *A*) [*fig. 111*].

b. Triangular Cells. Like the preceding cells, they possess a radial [dendritic] shaft prolonged up to the first layer, but they differ from the true pyramids in two important features: they possess, instead of a basal dendritic tuft, a very long descending [dendritic] shaft, which branches deep down, in the thickness of the seventh layer, and they show a lateral, short, and thick [dendrite], rapidly breaking up into a group of dendritic processes (fig. 691, *B*) [*fig. 111*]. The axon is descending and, like [the axon] of the pyramids, enters the white matter.

c. *Fusiform Cells* (fig. 691, *J*) [*fig. 111*]. Instead of pyramidal and triangular shapes, the cell with long axon sometimes adopts the shape of a spindle, with two long radial dendrites: ascending, destined for the first layer; and descending, not very long, and giving rise to a tuft of dendrites. The axon is also incorporated into the white matter, after giving off one, two or three collaterals.

Cells with Short Axon

They correspond to three main varieties, namely (a) cells with ascending axon, destined for the superimposed layers; (b) cells with short axon, arborizing in the very thickness of the sixth layer (fig. 691, *D*) [*fig. 111*]; (c) arachniform cell or cells with very short axon (fig. 691, *I*) [*fig. 111*].

Among all these varieties of cells with short axon, the one that seems to dominate is the first. As is seen in fig. 691, *E, C, F, G* [*fig. 111*], these neurons lie at different levels of this layer, although they usually prefer the upper part of it; their shape is often that of a spindle, with two [dendritic] shafts, ascending and descending, promptly resolving into terminal branches; the triangular form (*G*) and the semilunar spherical form are not rare either (*C, F*). In some cases, the ascending processes are short and the deep dendrite very long, which gives to the cells the appearance of inverted pyramids already recognized by Golgi. The axon is fine and frequently arises, in harmony with the law of conservation of matter, from the ascending dendrite; it emits some collaterals to the sixth^Z layer, and finally gets lost in the superimposed [layers].

7. Seventh Layer or [Layer] of the Fusiform Cells

Underneath the cellular accumulation represented by the preceding cells begins a layer [that is] very thick in the axial regions of the gyri, much thinner in the lateral portions of these, or completely merged with the sixth [layer] in the concave portions. Most cells of this layer have a spindle shape and are arranged in radial rows, separated by thick bundles of white matter, but there is also observed an occasional triangular and even pyramidal cell, provided with very long polar dendrites. In Nissl preparations, it is not rare to observe around the somata of these cells two or more neuroglial nuclei.

In fig. 692 [*fig. 112*], we have illustrated the most abundant cells of the seventh layer of the postcentral gyrus of the child of one month. There are seen (a) fusiform cells provided with a long radial process prolonged probably up to the first layer, a descending [dendritic] shaft sometimes very long and divided at acute angles, and, finally, a descending axon from which arise some initial, often recurrent collaterals (fig. 692, *A*) [*fig. 112*]; (b) true pyramidal cells completely equal to those of the preceding layer (fig. 692, *B*) [*fig. 112*]; (c) stellate, fusiform, or triangular cells, with short ascending axon, which sometimes branches in the vicinity of the parent cell (fig. 692, *D*) [*fig. 112*], sometimes at an upper level (*C*), sometimes, finally, at very high levels that we have not been able to determine (*E*).

It is probable that some of these long ascending axons correspond to fibers of Martinotti, since in the rabbit and mouse, where it is easier to follow the course of the nerve fibers, the deepest layer or [layer] of the polymorphic cells constantly contains fusiform or stellate cells whose axons go up to the first layer.

[Regarding] the pyramids of the deep layers (fusiform, triangular, etc.), do they send to the first or plexiform [layer] a terminal [dendritic] tuft? Golgi believed he could see that the [apical dendritic] shaft of the pyramids of the deep third of the cortex never reached the first layer, ending at regions quite deep to it, and we, Retzius, and Kölliker had inclined to this view. However, the careful study of excellent preparations of the cerebrum of the cat of fifteen days and of the visual cortex of the child, corresponding to the thin or concave parts of the gyri,^{53} has persuaded us that any pyramid or cell with long axon (fusiform, triangular, deep small pyramids, etc.) is represented in the first layer by one or several branched dendrites. The only difference among the pyramidal cells of the second, third, fourth, and fifth layers and those of the sixth and seventh layers rests in the extent of the peripheral [dendritic] tuft; that is to say, whereas the former engender a spray of robust and spiny dendrites, the latter limit themselves to a few thin and varicose dendrites, and even to a single fine appendage that crosses the plexiform layer more or less obliquely.

Fearless of being wrong, we can thus formulate these two principles, confirmed in both man and animals: first, any pyramid or cell with long axon furnished with a radial [dendritic] shaft, wherever it resides, sends to the first layer a tuft of dendrites or a dendritic branch; second, the vast majority of the cells with short axon, even though they are furnished with radial dendritic processes, do not have a dendritic representation in the plexiform layer.

Fibers and Nerve Plexuses of the Cerebral Cortex

When a section of a human gyrus stained by the method of Weigert-Pal is examined, the gray matter appears crossed by an infinity of medullated fibers, some arranged in vertical bundles and most in horizontal plexuses. Both the radial bundles and the parallel plexuses have been perfectly seen and described by many authors, particularly by Kaes, Vulpius, Edinger, Obersteiner, Bottazzi, Kölliker, etc.

To proceed in order with the exposition of the nerve fibers of the gray matter, it is convenient to divide them, of course, into two categories: *endogenous* fibers, that is to say, originating in intrinsic neurons of the cortical region under study; and *exogenous* fibers, that is to say, those originating in other nerve foci and freely ending in the gray matter of the cerebral[AA] cortex.

Exogeneous Fibers

a. Sensory [Fibers][BB]

In our work on the cerebral cortex of the small mammals,[54] we indicated the existence of robust fibers coming from the white matter, which, penetrating the gray [matter] at varying

orientations and tracing in their ascending course large bends, terminate by means of a free arborization of enormous extent, located preferentially in the superficial half of the cortex.

At that time, we did not pronounce resolutely on the origin of such singular fibers; but Kölliker,[55] who confirmed the existence of the same in the rat, rabbit, cat, and dog (*fibers of S. Ramón* of this author), and which he followed back to the corpus striatum, thinks that they are of a sensory nature. Having reexamined the preparations that served for our first works on the cortex of the mouse, rat, and rabbit, we have ascertained that, in effect, in conformity with Kölliker, the cited centripetal fibers come from the corona radiata, and, therefore, it is very probable that they represent sensory fibers whose cells of origin reside in the sensory centers of the optic thalamus. Naturally, each sensory area of the cortex shows, with respect to the origin and manner of termination of the said thalamocortical fibers, specific distinctions with which we will deal later. Here we will limit ourselves to setting down that the referred fibers are thicker than the efferent [fibers] of the gray matter; that they usually bifurcate in the deep cortical layers; and that the resultant branches, whose course is more or less oblique toward the surface, engender, by means of successive branching, a very dense terminal plexus horizontally extended at the level of the middle cortical layers, and preferentially through the so-called *layer of the granule cells or of the deep small pyramids* (fig. 694, C, D) [*fig. 115*].

b. Fibers of Homolateral Association

Since dynamic associations exist among the several cortical areas, we must suppose that each gyrus receives fibers originating from pyramids resident in distant regions of the same hemisphere. But this assumption, which represents a postulate from pathological human physiology and anatomy, has not received confirmation in man by means of direct anatomical methods (method of Golgi, etc.).

However, in the rabbit and above all in the mouse, we have observed many times that from the fascicles of intercortical association, for example, the *arcuate fasciculus* and *cin-*

gulum (anteroposterior pathways of the cortex near the interhemispheric fissure), there frequently arise terminal branches, which ascend to the gray matter and terminate, by means of free arborizations, in the whole cortex and preferentially in the plexiform layer.

c. Collaterals of the White Matter

By analogy with what occurs in the white matter of the spinal cord, medulla, and pons, it seems likely that the white matter of the cerebrum also presents collateral branches whose distribution would be to the superimposed gray matter. This occurs, definitely, in the cerebrum of small mammals, where all the association bundles exhibit, although in small numbers, thin collateral fibers. These are especially obvious in the white matter of the *arcuate fasciculus, cingulum, nerves of Lancisi, the white cortex of Ammon's horn and origin of the fornix, projection pathways of the olfactory, frontal and sphenoidal cortex,* etc. All of these branches go up through the gray matter, branching during their course, and reach the plexiform layer, where they engender, like the terminal association fibers, extensive tangential nerve plexuses [that are] in contact with the [dendritic] tufts of the pyramids (fig. 695, *a, c, d*) [fig. 6].

In the human cerebrum, and especially in the white matter of the gyri, the collaterals are little numerous, and of those that exist it is impossible to decide if they belong to fibers of association, to exogenous fibers, or to terminal sensory fibers, or whether they are the axons of the pyramids situated in the superimposed cortex. However, our personal impression, suggested primarily by the study of the cortex of rodents, is that the majority of the collaterals coming from the white matter have their origins in fibers of association.

d. Callosal Fibers

The cerebrum of man and of the mammals possesses a rich system of commissural fibers that can be compared with the system of the same name in the spinal cord. Three formations are concerned with this important formation: the *corpus callosum* in the strict sense, which links transversely the cortex of the superior region of both hemispheres (frontal, parietal, and occipital lobes); the *anterior commissure,* which joins the olfactory sensory cerebral cortex (cortex of sensation); and the *commissure of the fornix or interammonic commissure,* which joins the areas of olfactory association (Ammon's horn and subordinate territories).

Our already old studies on the corpus callosum of small mammals, as well as those made in recent years on the commissures of the olfactory sensory and association cortex, have led us to accept two classes of commissural fibers: *direct axons,* coming commonly from the medium and small pyramids of the opposite side; and *collateral fibers,* originating along the course of axons of association or projection, continuous, in turn, with contralateral, voluminous pyramids. All of these fibers, characterized by their great thinness, first descend to the white matter, interweaving with fibers of diverse significance; then they come near the ventricular cavity and enter the corpus callosum, inside which they run until they cross the midline and get lost in the gray matter of the contralateral hemisphere.

It is a difficult problem to determine how and where the callosal fibers are arborized. In man and gyrencephalic mammals, the enterprise is impossible because of the enormous length of their trajectory. In the mouse and rabbit of a few days, it is possible, however, to observe that the callosal fibers penetrating the gray matter of the motor area have a great thinness, possess a varicose appearance, and, after some divisions at an acute angle, they terminate by means of fine ascending threads that are prolonged at least to the layer of the medium and small pyramids. It seems probable that in the adult this arborization, so moderate in young animals, becomes much more complicated.

Although rarely, the callosal fibers emit during their course some transverse collateral, a peculiarity observed by us in the portion of the corpus callosum situated underneath the arcuate fasciculus of the mouse and rabbit. Such an arrangement leads to the assumption that the callosal fibers do not represent simple commissures destined to link homotopic and homodynamic territories of both hemispheres, but that they are fibers of combined association, thanks to which an excitation originating in a sensory area of one side is capable of interacting with several areas of the opposite [side] (fig. 695, *h*) [*fig. 6*].

Which in man are the callosal arborizations? We do not know. In certain preparations of the motor cortex of the child of fifteen days to one month, there appears at the level of the layer of the small and medium pyramids a fibrillar plexus of an extraordinary richness, whose more interesting features are the dominant vertical orientation of its fibers, the poverty of their branching, and the extreme delicacy of their caliber, which generally does not exceed 0.2 μm. Such extreme thinness obliges us, in order to appreciate them fully, to use the 1.30 Zeiss objective. Some threads form small vertical bundles, others run diffusely, and there is no lack of some that cross the [dendritic] shaft of the pyramids obliquely and at a variety of inclinations. The uppermost fibrils reach the plexiform layer, where, not infrequently, they bifurcate; but these are rare; the vast majority end at several levels of the second layer or [layer] of the small pyramids. When these fibers are followed downward, one sees them submerge in the vicinity of the layer of the giant cells, where they lose their vertical course, becoming flexuous and escaping observation. It has been impossible for us to follow them to the white matter or to observe their junction with the innumerable short axons, distributed through the second, third, and fourth layers. The most similar fibers are those that make up the small vertical bundles of [axonal] arborizations of the bitufted cells; but the absence or extreme poverty of their branches distinguishes them at first glance from the latter.

In short, might not the said threads, whose origin appears to us very enigmatic, represent the terminations of the callosal fibers? This is a question whose solution must be saved for the future.

Endogenous fibers

The long fibers originating in the gyri are, first, *projection or decending fibers;* second, *fibers of homolateral association;* third, *callosal fibers or [fibers] of contralateral association.* The short or intragriseal fibers can be distinguished in three categories: first, *semilong radial axons,* which link the deep layers with the upper layers (fibers of Martinotti and other types whose arborization does not reach the first layer); second, *semilong axons which connect distant areas of the plexiform layer;* third, *short axons* destined to connect, at short distance and in several directions, cells lying in the same [layer] or in two adjacent layers. We have already spoken about all these fibers when we dealt with the cortical layers or with the termination of the exogenous fibers. Here we will limit ourselves to describing the fibers of projection.

Fibers of Projection

This is the title of the long axons that, arising from the pyramids of the cerebral cortex (above all, large and medium [pyramids]), go down to the white matter, cross the callosal and association systems, and penetrate the corpus striatum to terminate in deep gray centers. Flechsig had thought that such descending fibers arose exclusively from the sensory areas (acoustic, olfactory, visual, motor, etc.); [this is a mistake[56]].[CC] The anatomicopathological investigations in man of Dejerine, Monakow, Siemerling, [Brodmann, Oskar Vogt, and Madame Vogt][DD] and our histological observations in small mammals prove, without any kind of doubt, that the above-mentioned fibers come from all the cortical areas, whatever their topography and functional significance. In this way, in the rodents, in which we have made a detailed analysis of the cited fibers in the majority of the cortical areas, we have found fibers of projection, directed toward the corpus striatum, even in those areas that do not receive direct sensory fibers, for example, the *interhemispheric cortex* and *Ammon's horn* (see below under olfactory cortex) which it is appropriate to consider as centers of olfactory association of ideation. The so-called *fornix longus* of Forel and the *anterior column of the fornix* represent, respectively, the projection pathways of the said gray systems.

The intragriseal course of the axons of the pyramids has already been described. We will add only, as clearly shown in the Ehrlich and Weigert preparations, that such fibers run almost in a straight line toward the white matter gathered in small bundles (fig. 693, *e*) [*fig. 114*], and, once they arrive at the white matter, they get lost among the callosal and association fibers. Sometimes, just as they reach the white matter or somewhat further on, the said axons bifurcate, engendering a thick branch with the characteristics of a main axon which submerges in the corpus striatum, and another [branch], frequently thinner, that gets lost in the plane of the callosal [fibers]. A still more common situation, about which we have to insist later, is shown in the case of the axons of projection of the mouse and rabbit. At the moment at which such fibers come near to or reach the corpus striatum, they divide into two branches: the *main* or descending, which follows the original course [of the axon], reaching the deep centers; and the accessory or association [branch], which runs parallel to the white matter and, after a variable course, ascends to the superimposed gray cortex, where it terminates by means of free arborizations.

We have also seen bifurcations in the white matter of man but much more rarely than in the small mammals. This scarcity of divisions is perhaps only apparent and engendered by purely technical difficulties, for example, the impossibility of exploring the whole very long trajectory of the axons through the white matter. Because of the thinness of the white matter in the mouse and rabbit, the bifurcations and collaterals of association are concentrated in a narrow, readily explored place; but in man, the said divisions might occupy the whole region of the oval center,[EE] making [divisions], according to the laws of economy, at points [that are] favorable and different for each fiber of the same area. A complete exploration, from this point of view, of the white matter of the human cerebrum with the Golgi, Ehrlich, [and reduced silver nitrate][FF] methods would thus be desirable.

In the cat, in which we have applied the procedure of Ehrlich,[57] the divisions and collaterals only reside near the gray matter, being absent from the axis of the gyri and at a distance [from the gray matter]. Let us not forget, however, a source of error that we have not always been able to rule out: the possibility of taking a dichotomy of an afferent sensory fiber for a division of an endogenous or projection fiber.

Medullated Plexuses of the Gray Matter

The above notions mainly refer to Golgi preparations, in which [in young or still fetal animals,][GG] both unmyelinated and [those that will later be][HH] myelinated fibers are equally impregnated. To complete this study, it is convenient now to determine which nerve fibers in the adult are covered with a myelin sheath and how these are arranged in the several layers of the gray matter.

From this point of view, examination of sections stained by the procedure of Weigert-Pal will be very instructive (fig. 696) [*fig. 114*]. Immediately observed in all the cortical layers is the existence of three classes of myelinated fibers: *vertical or radial, horizontal, and oblique.* But the numbers of these three categories of fibers vary in each layer.

First Layer

It shows preferentially horizontal or tangential fibers of two kinds: *fine fibers,* somewhat flexuous, especially located in the deeper half of the first layer and evidently continuous with the ascending axons of Martinotti; and *thick tangential fibers,* already seen some time ago by Kölliker,[58] Exner,[59] and well described by Martinotti,[60] Bottazzi, Kaes, etc., and in our opinion belonging to the robust axons of the horizontal or special cells of the first layer.

Such thick fibers, which preferentially inhabit the middle third of the first layer, can also be observed in Ehrlich preparations (tangential sections) of the cerebrum of the adult cat and dog (fig. 664, *b*) [*fig. 50*], appearing very long, provided with strangulations and bifurcations, and without any tendency to descend, this latter circumstance of which, together with their exceptional thickness, distinguishes them perfectly from the horizontal branches of the axons of Martinotti. Naturally, the terminal arborizations of both kinds of tangential fibers do not appear in the preparations of Ehrlich and Weigert because they lack a myelin sheath.

Immediately underneath the pia, there is a

thin rim completely devoid of medullated fibers, as Martinotti has observed; but in this place final nerve arborizations, as well as dendritic tufts of pyramids, are not lacking, since they are observed in the good Golgi sections of the human cortex. Such submeningeal fine plexuses (see fig. 696) [*fig. 114*] belong to ascending fibers of Martinotti.

Finally, near the second layer, the preparations of Weigert-Pal sometimes show a horizontal condensation of fine fibers that Kaes calls the *stria of Bechterew*. This line is lacking in animals and is not constant in man.

Layer of the Small Pyramids

It shows up by the poverty of its medullated fibers, which can be distinguished as three kinds: first, long vertical or oblique [fibers] which go up to the plexiform layer and represent fibers of Martinotti (fig. 696, *b*) [*fig. 114*]; second, thinner vertical [fibers] which descend to the white matter, being incorporated in the deep layers into the radial medullated bundles, and which are nothing other than axons of the small pyramids, whose initial course lacks a myelin sheath; third, fine oblique fibers, little abundant, corresponding perhaps to recurrent nerve collaterals of deep pyramids or maybe to terminal branches of exogenous fibers.

Layer of the Medium and Large Pyramids

From the beginning of the medium pyramids, the medullated plexus, loose and poor in the preceding layer, gets richer, becoming more and more dense, and showing three classes of fibers: radial fascicles, very thick horizontal and oblique fibers, and a very delicate interstitial medullated plexus.

a. The radial fascicles, poor in fibers in the upper level of the medium pyramids, are already well pronounced in the deeper level of this layer, and gain notably in thickness during their course through the following [layers], until they get lost and separated in the white matter (fig. 696, *e*) [*fig. 114*]. They are made up of axons of small and medium pyramids, to which are added more deeply robust axons of giant pyramids and other less thick [axons] of fusiform and triangular cells of the sixth and seventh layers. The preparations of Ehrlich (cat and dog) reveal on these fibers numerous strangulations [nodes of Ranvier] from which arise occasional collaterals.

b. The thick horizontal and oblique fibers are scarce and, after a variable course, become descending and continuous with thick fibers arriving from the white matter. Such fibers, which are clearly distinguished from the axons of the pyramids, thanks to their unusual diameter and to their oblique course, represent the main trunks and branches of exogenous fibers probably coming from the sensory thalamic nuclei. Their main branches and dichotomies are very well stained in the Ehrlich preparations (fig. 696, *f*) [*fig. 114*].

c. With respect to the delicate interstitial plexus, in which the somata of the pyramids show up as clear spaces (fig. 696, *c*) [*fig. 114*], our studies prove that it is nothing other than the ensemble of the fine preterminal branches of the cited sensory fibers. Comparison of the said medullated plexus [in sections stained with the Weigert-Pal method][II] with that appearing at the same position in Golgi preparations of the child of a few months (motor and visual areas) is in this respect very demonstrative.

Deep Layers

From the layer of the external large pyramidal cells to the white matter, the warp of medullated fibers shows an almost even appearance. This wide gray band is made up of a dense interstitial plexus formed by horizontal and oblique medullated fibers, which stand out, at intervals [because of their considerable diameter][JJ] an occasional voluminous exogenous sensory fiber; and the already described radial bundles or fascicles of pyramidal axons. The vast majority of the horizontal or oblique fibers correspond probably to the collaterals of the pyramidal axons.

To conclude the study of the plexuses of the gray matter, let us note that the Weigert-Pal preparations only reveal an insignificant part of the axonal arborizations. Comparing the said sections with complete silver chromate impregnations, it is easily deduced that many [cells with] short axons lack myelin (dwarf cells, bitufted cells, small cells of Golgi) as well as the final small branches of the arborizations of the [cells with] long [axons]. By contrast, the [cells with] semilong endogenous axons (cells of Martinotti, large horizontal cells of the first layer, cells with ascending axon ramifying in the second and third layers, etc.), possess, at least at the level of the trunk and initial branches, a medullated sheath.

[Terminal Plexuses]

[The preparations obtained by means of the neurofibrillary methods reveal the existence of terminal plexuses of an unimaginable richness in the gray matter of the cortex, because, with the exception of the finest little axonal branches of the cells with short axon, both the myelinated and unmyelinated fibers are found impregnated simultaneously. This simultaneity of staining, coupled with the necessity of using thin sections, unfortunately becomes an insuperable obstacle to the individual study of single fibers in the plexus. The complexity of these inter- and pericellular plexuses can be seen in fig. 363 [fig. 218], in which we have illustrated a section of the cerebral cortex of the adult dog. But this complexity is nothing compared with that observed in the cerebrum of man; in man, the cortical gray matter, including the plexiform layer, appears in well-impregnated preparations to be made up or a continuous nerve plexus dotted with cells and against which stand out by their greater thickness the radial fascicles of the efferent myelinated fibers and the axons of the sensory or afferent fibers with their main branches.]^KK

Neuroglia of the Cerebral Cortex

In the gray matter of the gyri, there are found the two kinds of neuroglia already described in the general part of this book: the kind with short and downy processes or cell of the gray matter, and the kind with very long and smooth processes or cell of the white matter.

Cells with Long Processes

They are found scattered through the white matter, corresponding completely to the type described in the general part of this book.

However, some of these cells penetrate a little into the gray matter, [where they]^LL reach to the third layer.

In the first layer, there is also found a variety of these cells indicated by Martinotti and well studied by Retzius and Andriezen. As is seen in fig. 697, A [fig. 224], it is a large cell resident beneath or at short distance from the pia, and from which arise ascending or oblique short branches, terminating at the cerebral surface, and a tuft of descending branches, rough and downy in their initial course but later fine and straight, which go down undivided through the first layer, apparently ending at several levels in the interior of the second [layer].

Cells with Short Processes

They are very numerous and reside in the whole gray matter, including the first layer, where they are particularly abundant, as has been proven by Retzius, Andriezen, and Cajal.

In fig. 697, B, D [fig. 224], which illustrates the neuroglia of a child of two months, the cells resident in the first layer still exhibit a radial orientation and peripheral branches terminating underneath the pia, [which are] embryonic features destined later to disappear. Among the [cells] resident in the plexiform layer, the kite-shaped cells and the downy fusiform [cells], comparable to a lady's boa and about which Retzius has given excellent drawings, are very interesting (fig. 697, D) [fig. 224; see also fig. 226].

The [neuroglial cells] resident in deeper layers can be free, but the majority, as was demonstrated by Golgi, Cajal, Andriezen, Retzius, Kölliker, etc., send feet to be inserted into the capillaries and small arterioles and venules. (See the first volume of this book.)

The characteristic of the cell type with short processes is, above all, the infinity of ramified appendages, as spongy as cotton waste, that cover the whole extent of each radial process. Thanks to such processes, a large part of the gray matter appears traversed by a dense neuroglial plexus, in whose tubular interstices reside the dendrites and nerve fibers. [These two types of neuronal processes are only free at the points where junctions occur between them.]^MM

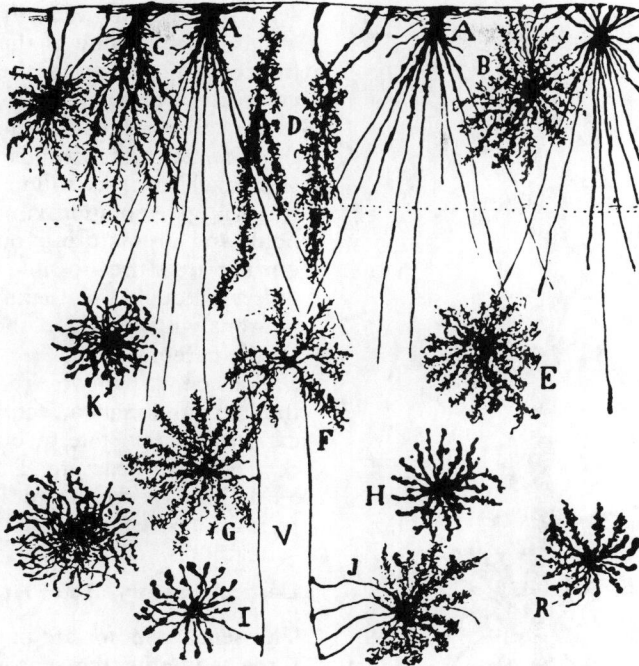

[*FIG. 224*] Fig. 697. Neuroglia of the superficial layers of the cerebrum; child of two months. Method of Golgi. *A, B, C, D,* neuroglial cells of the plexiform layer; *E, F, G, H,* neuroglial cells of the second and third layers; *I, J,* neuroglial cells with vascular pedicles; *V,* blood vessel.

According to the length and complexity of the downy or collateral appendages, several kinds of neuroglial cells can be distinguished: cells covered with fine, long, and highly branched appendages; cells with less developed and retracted appendages reduced to simple excrescences or irregular clumps (fig. 697, *K, R*) [*fig. 224*]; finally, cells whose downiness has completely disappeared, showing bare but thick and notably varicose processes (fig. 697, *I*) [*fig. 224*]. There are cells in which certain processes show a mossy arborescent downiness, while others that are shorter and retracted appear bare and beaded (fig. 697, *R*) [*fig. 224*]. Do all of these forms of neuroglial arborizations represent [different] physiological stages of the same cells or diverse degrees of postmortem alteration? We do not know; the only thing we can say is that the said morphological varieties, which recall the ameboid phases of leukocytes and the alternating stages of contraction and extension of the chromato-

phores of many animals, constantly coexist in the same gyrus and even in very restricted cortical regions.

Finally, among the more interesting neuroglial cells are the pericellular [type] already mentioned in the first part of this book (fig. 53) [*fig. 225*]. The majority of the pyramids and not a few cells with short axon possess neuroglial satellite cells, whose processes surround a part of the soma and the cone of origin of the axon. The preferred place is the base of the cell body, in the gulf existing between the [origin of the] axon and the basilar dendrites. But they are not lacking from the sides of the radial [dendritic] shaft.

Would not so curious a disposition, on which we have commented in other work,[61] have the object, given the insulating role of the neuroglia, to prevent fortuitous contacts being made on the soma and origin of the axon by adjacent dendrites and axonal arborizations with which [the cell] must not make contacts?

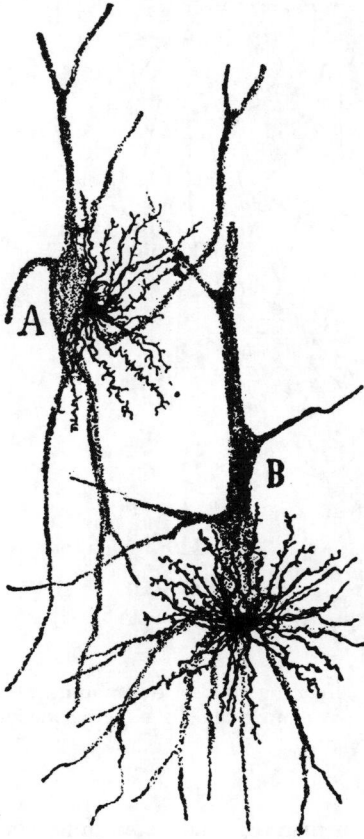

[*FIG. 225*]　Fig. 53. Pericellular neuroglial cells of the cerebral cortex of man. Golgi method. [This is fig. 82 of the first volume of the French version of the book.]

Connections of the [Neural] Elements of the Gray Cortex

This is a difficult theme, about which it is only possible at present to make a very superficial and fragmented study, because of the extraordinary complexity of the plexuses of the cortical layers and the multiplicty of connections made by each pyramid with its partners in the [same cortical] area and with homonymous cells in other cortical areas. Let us add, besides, that in the cerebrum, unlike in the cerebellum, neuronal segments arranged in layers or bands in contact with fixed kinds of nerve fibers do not exist; instead, the afferent and endogenous terminal fibers are intermingled and

seem to touch indifferently all parts of the pyramids; also, in spite of the persistent analyses [made] in recent years, the extent and precise connection of many endogenous fibers, such as the collaterals of the axons of the pyramids, the [axonal] arborizations of many cells with short axon, etc., are still unknown in the adult; this will give an approximate idea of how difficult and premature is our insistence on inquiring into the possible course of the impulses through the inextricable labyrinth of neurons with long and short axon that make up the cerebral gyri.

Consider what we are going to describe, then, as a rational conjecture based on the precarious present state of our knowledge about cortical fine structure, and by no means as a definitive architectonic and functional formula.

Cortical Sensory-Motor Arcs[NN]

The sensory-motor arc of the cortex includes three segments: the sensory or afferent fiber, coming from the thalamus and representing the portal of entrance of the impulses; the motor fiber or axon of the pyramids, forming the output pathway for cerebral impulses; and the intercalated nerve arc of the gray matter, formed by a very complicated chain of intermediary neurons. Of these three parts, the first two, that is to say, the pathways of reception and emission, are quite well known; not so the neuronal arc that links the extremities of these two pathways, and which probably includes an infinity of routes of very different length and trajectory, and at present indeterminable.

When a well-stained preparation of the human sensory cortex (method of Golgi) is examined, it is observed that the afferent or sensory fibers form extensive plexuses, inside which are included both pyramids and an infinity of neurons with short and semilong axon. The single channel represented by the afferent fiber is broken down thus into an infinity of secondary channels that traverse almost the whole gray matter of the hemispheres along variable radii. These channels, which can be considered schematically as arcs of variable extent joining the input and output fibers, are probably the following.

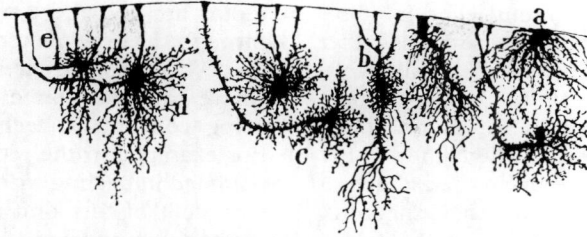

[FIG. 226]   Fig. 51. Neuroglial cells with tails and other neuroglial types in the first cerebral layer; cat of eight days. Golgi method. [This is fig. 80 of the first volume of the French version of the book.]

Short or Principal Arc

It is represented by two neurons: the thalamic sensory [neuron] whose axon [forms] an [intracortical] axonal arborization, and the giant and medium pyramids making up the pyramidal pathway or [pathway] of voluntary movements. The connection is established between the cited sensory arborizations and the somata and [apical] shafts of the pyramidal neurons. Thanks to this [direct] route, the sensory impulses would be rapidly transformed into reflex movement.

This communication of impulses is not individual but collective; that is to say, it is effected between a group of afferent fibers and a much more numerous constellation of neurons of projection. The avalanche of conduction still increases on descent of the impulses through the pyramidal axons, since a part of the impulse will shunt into the axonal collaterals which will lead the conduction to other homologous neurons of the same layer. Probably, this collateral connection takes place by initial contact between the terminal arborization of the [axonal] collaterals and the accessory dendrites of the soma and [apical] shaft of the adjacent cells.

Intragriseal Arc with Intercalation of Cells with Ascending Axons

A good part of the sensory arborizations enter also into contact with those cells called granules (small pyramids of the fourth layer and stellate cells), most of them furnished with an ascending axon, contacting the [dendritic] tufts of the pyramids in the plexiform layer, or at least [furnished] with important recurrent collaterals which enter into analogous relationships. The impulse transmitted to the re-ferred cells will be conducted then to groups of pyramids situated in the same gyrus but at a long distance from the territory of arborization of the sensory axons.

Intragriseal Arc with Intercalation of the Special or Horizontal Cells of the First Layer

The previous arc, which includes at least three neurons (sensory thalamic [cell], cell with semilong ascending axon, and distant pyramid), can be further extended by the contributions of other intercalated cells: the cell body and very long dendrites of the large horizontal [cells] of the first layer would receive the excitation of the terminal axonal arborization of the [cells] of Martinotti [which are excited by the sensory terminal arborization],[oo] and the [former cells] would act on the [dendritic] tufts of pyramids located at a great distance [from the sensory fibers][pp] in the same gyrus or perhaps outside its confines.

Interareal Intragriseal Arc

Among the pyramidal neurons in contact with the above-mentioned centripetal or sensory arborizations are many medium and small pyramids, whose axons do not enter the pyramidal pathway but, after traversing the white matter, terminate in the association areas of the same hemisphere. Here the arc is notably expanded, and the sensory residue, possibly in the form of a memory, could be preserved in a latent state in the new area, in order to [be] later discharged by the ideomotor neurons of this [area].

Interhemispheric Arc

That said above about the cells of [intrahemispheric] association must also be attributed to the callosal [neurons]. The impulses gathered by the pyramids whose axons either directly or indirectly (by means of collaterals) make up the corpus callosum will be propagated to the territories of association of the contralateral hemisphere, where they either remain in a latent state or are discharged at once by the corresponding ideomotor neurons.

Role of the Cells with Short Axon

Several authors, among them Monakow, have upheld the opinion that the cells with short axon represent short pathways of association or propagation inside the gray matter. According to Monakow, this role would be essential for the functioning of the gray matter, if the sensory or afferent fibers would never touch the cells with long axon but instead terminated exclusively on the soma and dendrites of the cells of Golgi, whose axonal arborization will have the duty to transmit the impulse to neurons of the motor type. We had expressed a similar opinion some time ago, although without the exclusivism of Monakow, considering that, if the said cells of Golgi are not the only place of termination of the centripetal fibers, at least they represent one of the connections of these, thus implying the possibility that the impulses collected by the soma and dendrites of such cells are transmitted to neurons with long axon lying at no great distance.

But, without rejecting this opinion at present, new observations made in the gray cortex of man and mammals, as well as in the cerebellar cortex, corpus striatum, and optic thalamus, have persuaded us that the main role performed by the cells with short axon is not merely that of distributors but in other still unknown [modes]. That the role of dispersing impulses and linking the extremities of the sensory-motor arc is not the essential [role] is confirmed by the following facts.

1. In the lower vertebrates, the junction between the motor and sensory neurons is made directly without intercalated cells with short axon. Even in the mammals, such cells are absent or very few in the spinal cord and medulla, which indicates that their collaboration is not essential for the closing of the sensory-motor arc and the transmission of impulses through the gray matter.

2. The cited cells are even found in organs where the diffusion of excitation, far from being convenient, seems highly prejudicial. For example, in the retina, as we already expounded in dealing with this [structure], there exist cells of this kind (small and large horizontal cells), situated at the level of the external plexiform layer, precisely in the place where the cones and rods enter into contact with the bipolar cells. If these cells with short axon would be constantly intercalated between these two elements of the nerve junction, the physiological effect would be to disturb or impede the special function of each retinal point.

3. As the result of our recent investigations on the cerebral cortex, small cells are known to exist with axons so short and with an arborization so exiguous and close to the parent cell [body] that it is not possible to grant them any efficacy as agents of diffusion of the impulses. And, although the said cells lie in the cerebrum and corpus striatum in places where afferent or sensory fibers are ramified, the arborizations of these [latter] are considerably more extensive than the dendrites of such cells.

4. No example is known of cells with short axon which receive special nerve fibers or that are connected exclusively with a particular category of cells with long axon; it is obvious that the axonal terminations from which they receive impulses are always the same as those of the cells with long axon. Besides, the cells with which the axonal arborizations [of the short axon cells] establish contact constantly possess more important and direct contacts with the afferent fibers. From this it is clear that the circuit followed by the nerve impulse in the cells with short axon is a useless detour, since the same nerve excitation has available, in order to reach its destination, another route of equal direction but much shorter and more logical.

In fig. 698, A, c, b [fig. 227], we show an example of the apparently useless detour followed by the afferent impulses on traversing the cells with short axon. The cerebrum presents innumerable cases of this kind. On account of this, the conjecture is suggested that

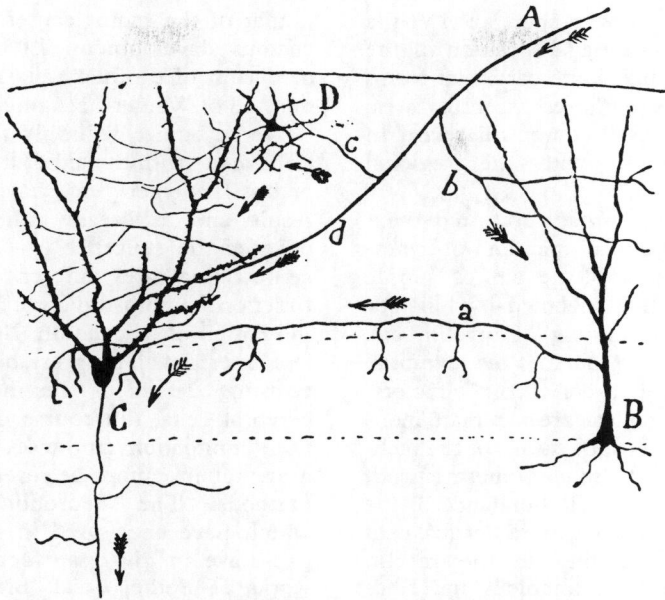

[*FIG. 227*]   Fig. 698. Scheme of the connections among the cells of the fascia dentata. *A,* afferent nerve fiber; *B,* cell with short axon whose terminations surround the granule [cells]; *C,* granule [cell]; *D,* small cell with short axon; *b, c, d,* branches of the afferent fiber. The direction of the connections is indicated with arrows.

the cells with short axon, without being excluded from performing other functions, are *condensers or accumulators of nervous energy.* The nature of the nerve [impulse] being not well known, it becomes difficult to understand how such cells increase the energy of the discharges. With the aim of not explaining but imagining the mechanism of their action, they could be compared to electric condensers or to [groups] of batteries charged up and joined by their extreme poles to fibers (afferent and efferent) of great length. The arrival of the impulse through a centripetal fiber would cause the discharge of the cells with short axon, which would contribute to increase the energy of the impulses that run through the chain of cells with long axon. The amount of latent energy in this way transformed into vital energy would depend on the intensity of the discharge received. In all the nervous actions that are undertaken a long time after the [arrival] of the excitation of external origin (memory, ideation, judgment, etc.), the [short-axon] cells would be diminishing their dynamic reserves until, exhausted, fatigue would follow.[62]

Historical Notes on the Structure of the Cerebral Cortex[QQ]

Finally, in recent years, the careful study of the regional cerebral cortex is beginning, an examination that was initiated by Meynert and Hammarberg but which has been somewhat forgotten, perhaps because of the prejudgment that the whole cerebrum has the same structural plan. Among those who have recently collected new facts in this difficult domain may be counted Henschen[63RR] (human visual cortex) and Schlapp (regional cortex of the monkey studied by the method of Nissl) and Calleja (olfactory cortex).[64]

Our investigations in the last four years have also revealed numerous details of organization of the motor, visual, acoustic, and olfactory cortices of the human cerebrum.[65SS] The consequences of this systematically undertaken labor, which is a long way away from reaching its conclusion, are the finding in the human cortex of new cellular types (the bitufted cells, the dwarf cells, etc.), the revelation of the morphology of the so-called *granule cells* and of the innumerable cells with short axon of the fourth layer, the terminal disposition of the sensory or afferent fibers, the particular forms that the pyramids show in each sensory area, and the other details that we will reveal in summary on dealing with the regional cortex.[TT]

Numerous authorities have preferred to examine the cerebral gyri of man and of gyrencephalic mammals with the aid of simple methods, such as that invented by Nissl or those used for the staining of myelin, etc. Schlapp,[66] for example, pursues his investigations on the several layers of the olfactory, motor, visual, and acoustic areas in man, monkey, horse, dog, cat, etc., by means of the technique of Nissl. Kaes[67] also continues his studies on the distribution and abundance of the medullated fibers in these various cortical centers of man by resorting to the myelin [staining] procedures. Hermanides and Köppen[68] analyze the cellular structure of several regions of the cortex of lissencephalic mammals by the method of Nissl. Köppen and Löwenstein[69] do the same in the cortex of carnivores and ungulates. Brodmann[70] uses simultaneously the technique of Nissl, the staining of myelin, and the impregnation of neurofibrils, indicating twenty-eight different types of cortex in the cerebrum of the monkey. O. Vogt[71] and Madame Vogt[72] investigate the value of the myelogenetic, myeloarchitectonic, and cytoarchitectonic methods, that is to say, the methods based on the development of myelin, on the distribution of myelinated fibers in the adult and the disposition of the layers and cells as shown by the appropriate techniques; they reach the conclusion that the former of these methods, or method of Flechsig, needs to be joined and complemented by the other two [methods] when one wants to distinguish unequivocally the cortical areas that differ in structure or function. Flechsig,[73] returning to his previous work, himself corrects his doctrines and distinguishes, thanks to his technique, thirty-five to forty physiologically different cortical territories in the child. Döllken[74] checks by the procedure of reduced silver nitrate the information furnished by the method of successive myelination and shows that the fibers of the areas of projection, in par-

ticular of the motor center, have a very precocious development. Livini[75] explores the cerebrum of the marsupials by means of the method of Weigert, etc., etc.

We recognize willingly that the investigations made with the aid of the simple methods of Nissl, Weigert, etc., have given important results and, as already indicated by us, demonstrate the existence of a great number of centers [that are] different in structure and function, in both the cortex of projection and the cortex of association. But that is more or less to restrict all progress, because the very interesting details of the morphology of the cerebral cells, the course of their processes, their connections in the several regions of the gray matter, cannot be revealed to us by such methods. The neurofibrillary procedures which have been used in order to fill these gaps have not given satisfaction, in spite of the works of Bethe, Cajal, Bielschowsky, Brodmann, van Gehuchten, Marinesco, and others. This is because of the considerable number of [cellular] elements that are impregnated, the necessary thinness of the sections, and their incapacity to reveal the final terminations of the dendrites emitted from the pyramidal cells or the axonal arborizations of the neurons with short axon. These defects, and still many others, more noticeable in the technique of Bielschowsky than in our own, oblige us to return to the method of Golgi. As long as no other procedure capable of providing isolated and selective stainings of the dendrites and of the final small axonal branches has been discovered, and as long as no more reliable and more consistent method has been invented, the method of Golgi remains, in effect, in spite of its inconsistency, [which has been] unreasonably exaggerated, the only method that can instruct us about the morphological types of cortical neurons and about their intercellular connections, on condition, of course, that we use as much as possible cerebra obtained from recently dead [humans] or sacrificed animals. To proceed in other ways is to condemn ourselves to ignore what is most interesting and most typical in the structure of the gray cortex; that is to delay and to interrupt the progress of our knowledge of the intimate mechanisms of the organ of thought.

Cajal's Notes

1. S. R. Cajal, Sobre la existencia de células nerviosas especiales en la primera capa de las circunvoluciones cerebrales. *Gaz. Méd. Catalana,* 15 December 1890. Textura de las circunvoluciones cerebrales de los mamíferos inferiores. *Nota Preventiva,* Barcelona, 30 November 1890.

2. S. R. Cajal, Las células de cilindro-eje corto de la capa molecular de cerebro. *Rev. Trim. Microgr.,* Vol. II, 1897.

3. K. Schaffer, Zur feineren Structur der Hirnrinde und über die funktionelle Bedeutung der Nervenzellenfortsätze, *Arch. f. Mikrosk. Anat.,* Vol. XLVIII, 1897.

4. S. R. Cajal, Sobre la existencia de células nerviosas especiales en la primera capa de las circunvoluciones cerebrales. *Gaceta Médica Catalana,* 15 December 1890. Structure de l'écorce cérébrale de quelques mammifères, *La Cellule,* Vol. VII, 1891.

5. S. R. Cajal, Las células de cilindro-eje corto de la capa molecular del cerebro. *Rev. Trim. Microgr.,* Vol. II, 1897.

6. Retzius, Die Cajal'schen Zellen der Grosshirnrinde beim Menschen und bei den Säugethieren, *Biol. Untersuch,* N.F., Vol. V, 1893, and Vol. VI, 1894.

7. Veratti, Ueber einige Struktureigenthümlichkeiten der Hirnrinde bei den Säugethieren, *Anat. Anzeiger,* no. 14, 1897.

8. S. R. Cajal, *Rev. Trim. Micrográf.,* Vols. IV, V, and VI, 1899, 1900, and 1901.

9. S. R. Cajal, *Le Cellule,* Vol. VII, 1891.

10. G. Retzius, Die Cajal'schen Zellen der Grosshirnrinde beim Menschen, etc., *Biol. Untersuch.,* Vol. V, 1893.

11. S. R. Cajal, Textura de las circunvoluciones cerebrales de los mamíferos inferiores, *Nota Preventiva,* 30 November 1890, and *Gaceta Médica Catalana,* 15 December 1890.

12. G. Retzius, Ueber den Bau der Oberflächenschicht der Grosshirnrinde beim Menschen und bei der Säugethieren, *Biologiska Föreningens Forhandlingar,* Vol. III, January–March 1891.

13. A. Kölliker, *Handbuch der Gewebelehre,* etc., 6th edition, Vol. II, [1896] p. 644 and following.

14. Schaffer, *Arch. f. Mikrosk. Anat.,* Vol. XLVIII, 1897.

15. Golgi, Sulla fina anatomia degli organi centrali del sistema nervoso, Pavia, 1886.

16. Mondino, Richerche macro-microscopiche sui centri nervosi, Milano, 1886, and Torino, 1887.

17. Martinotti, Su alcuni miglioramenti della tecnica della reazione al nitrato di argento, etc., *Annali di Freniatria e Scienze Affini,* Vol I, 1887.

18. S. Ramón y Cajal, La corteza visual, *Rev. Trim. Microgr.,* Vol. IV, 1899.

19. S. Ramón y Cajal, La corteza motriz, *Rev. Trim. Microgr.,* Vol. IV, 1899.

20. S. Ramón y Cajal, Estructura de la corteza visual, *Nota Preventiva, Rev. Ibero-Americana de Ciencias Médicas,* March 1899. See also our later works on the cerebral cortex in *Rev. Trim. Micrográf.,* Vols. IV, V, and VI, 1899, 1900, and 1901.

21. Retzius, Die Cajal'schen Zellen der Grosshirnrinde beim Menschen und bei den Säugethieren, *Biol. Untersuch.,* N.F., Vol. V, 1893. See in plate IV, figure 6, the cells labeled *kp.*

22. S. R. Cajal, Sur la structure de l'écorce cérébrale de quelques mammifères, *La Cellule,* Vol. VII, fasc. 1, 1891.

23. Estudios sobre la corteza humana. Especially see: Corteza acústica, *Rev. Trimestr. Micrográf.,* Vol. V, 1900.

24. Recent observations with our method of silver staining have persuaded us that in newborn mammals the neurofibrils form a mesh even in the dendrites, a mesh that is maintained with some variations in adulthood.

25. See our article: Consideraciones críticas sobre la teoría de Bethe acerca de la estructura y conexiones de las células nerviosas, *Trab. del Lab. de Investig. Biol.,* Vol. II, 1903, pp. 101–128. And the most recent: Un sencillo método de coloración del reticulo protoplásmico y sus efectos en diversos órganos nerviosos, *Trab. del Lab. de Investig. Biol.,* Vol. II, 1903, pp. 129–221.

26. Held, *Arch. f. Anat. u. Physiol.,* Anat. Abteil., 1902.

27. Donaggio, *Communication at the International Medical Congress in Madrid,* Vol. I, April 1903.

28. Bielschowsky, Die Silberimprägnation der Neurofibrillen, *Journal f. Psychologie und Neurologie,* Vol. III, 1904.

29. Schaffer, Ueber die Patho-histologie einer neuren Falles der Sachs'schen familliar-amaurotischer Idiotie, etc., *Journal f. Psychologie und Neurologie,* Vol. X, 1907.

30. Marinesco, Nouvelles recherches sur les neurofibrilles, *Revue Neurologique,* no. 15, 15 August 1904.

31. See, in the chapter on the cerebellum, the texture of the cells of Purkinje.

32. Soukhanoff, Sur le réseau endocellulaire de Golgi dans les éléments nerveux de l'écorce cérébrale, *Le Névraxe,* Vol. IV, 1903.

33. S. R. Cajal, Sobre la estructura del protoplasma nervioso, *Rev. Escolar de Medicina y Cirugía,* 1 November 1903. See also: *Trab. del Lab. de Invest. Biol.,* pt. 4, December 1903.

34. G. Retzius, *Biolog. Untersuch.,* N.F., Vol. IX, 1900.

35. E. Holmgren, Studien in der feineren Anatomie der Nervenzellen, from *Bonnet and Merkel anatomische Hefte,* Vol. XV, 1900.

36. Fixation in a mixture of equal parts of formol and acetone, then immersion in ammoniacal alcohol, impregnation of the pieces in the silver nitrate solution, and finally reduction.

37. S. R. Cajal, La red superficial de las células nerviosas centrales. *Rev. Trim. Micrográf.,* Vol. III, 1898.

38. S. R. Cajal, *Trabajos del Lab. de Investig. Biol.,* Vol. 2, 1903.

39. S. R. Cajal, Les conduits de Golgi-Holmgren du protoplasme nerveux et le réseau péricellulaire de la

membrane, *Trav. du Labor. de Rech. Biol.*, etc., Vol. VI, 1908.

40. S. R. Cajal, Sobre la existencia de bifurcaciones y colaterales en los nervios sensitivos craneales y sustancia blanca del cerebro, *Gaceta Sanitaria de Barcelona*, 10 April 1891. See also: Textura de las circunvoluciones cerebrales en los mamíferos inferiores, 10 December 1890.

41. S. R. Cajal, El azul de metileno en los centros nerviosos. *Rev. Trim. Micrográf.* Vol. I, 1896.

42. S. R. Cajal, Las células de cilindro-eje corto de la capa molecular del cerebro. *Rev. Trim. Micrográf.*, Vol. II, 1897.

43. S. R. Cajal, El azul de metileno en los centros nerviosos, *Rev. Trim. Micrográf.*, Vol. I, 1896.

44. S. R. Cajal, Un sencillo método para teñir las fibrillas interiores del protoplasma nervioso, *Archivos Latinos de Biología y Medicina*, no. 1, October 1903. Sobre la estructura del protoplasma nervioso, *Rev. Escolar de Medicina y Cirugía*, no. 3, 1 November 1903.

45. This formula, which stains much better than others the terminal nerve plexuses, consists of, first, fixation in 10 parts per 100 of formol, 6 hours; second, wash with water for some hours; third, hardening in 50 cc of 96 percent alcohol with 5 drops of ammonia, one day; fourth, [dip] in a solution of 1.50 parts per 100 of silver nitrate in the oven at 35°[C], five days; fifth, reduction as in the other formulae for impregnation of neurofibrils. See: S. R. Cajal, Quelques formules de fixation destinées à la méthode du nitrate d'argent, *Trav. d. Labor. d. Rech. Biol.*, etc., Vol. 5, 1907.

46. Semi Meyer, Ueber die Funktion der Protoplasmafortsätze der Nervenzellen, *Abhandl. d. Sächs. Ges. d. Wiss.*, 189[7]. Centrales Neuritenendigungen, *Arch. f. Mikros. Anat.*, Vol. 54, 1899.

47. Bethe, Ueber die Primitivfibrillen in den Ganglienzellen von Menschen und anderen Wirbelthieren, *Morphol. Arbeit. v. Schwalbe*, Vol. VIII, Part I, 1898.

48. F. Nissl, Nervenzellen und graue Substanz, *Münchener medicinische Wochenschrift*, nos. 31, 32, 33, 1898.

49. W. A[ldren] Turner and W. Hunter, On a form of nerve termination in the Central Nervous System, *Brain*, 1899.

50. Donaggio, *Riv. sperim. d. Freniatria*, Vol. XXIV, 1898–1899.

51. Held, Ueber den Bau der weissen und grauen Substanz, *Arch. f. Anat. u. Physiol.*, Anat. Abteil., 1902.

52. Simarro, Nuevo método histológico de impregnación por las sales fotográficas de plata, *Rev. Trimestr. Micrográf.*, Vol. V, 1900.

53. S. R. Cajal, Estructura de la corteza visual, *Rev. Trim. Micrográf.*, Vol. IV, 1899.

54. S. Ramón y Cajal, Sur la structure de l'écorce cérébrale de quelques mammifères, *La Cellule*, June 1891.

55. Kölliker, *Lehrbuch der Gewebelehre des Menschen*, 6th edition, Vol. II, 1896, p. 666.

56. With respect to this point, Flechsig has had to modify somewhat his point of view after his recent investigations and also because of the objections raised against his theory of the centers of association and projection; now he admits the existence, in small number, it is true, of radial or projection fibers in the centers of association. We will expose later his new conception of the cerebral structure.

57. S. Ramón y Cajal, El azul de metileno en los centros nerviosos. *Rev. Trim. Micrográf.*, Vol. I, 1896.

58. Kölliker, *Handbuch der Gewebelehre*, 1st edition, 1852.

59. Exner, Zur Kenntnis vom feineren Bau der Grosshirnrinde, *Sitzungsber. d. Kais. Akad. der Wissensch. in Wien*, 1881.

60. Martinotti, Beitrag zum Studium der Hirnrinde, etc., *Intern. Monatsschr. f. Anat. u. Physiol.*, Vol. VIII, 1890.

61. S. R. Cajal, Sobre las relaciones de las células nerviosas con las neuróglicas, *Rev. Trim. Micrográf.*, Vol. I, 1896. See also: Algo sobre la significación de la neuroglia, *Rev. Trim. Micrográf.*, Vol. II, 1897.

62. This opinion has been expounded in detail in our work entitled: Significación funcional de las células nerviosas de axón corto, *Trab. del Lab. de Invest. Biol.*, Vol. I, 1901–1902.

63. Henschen, Sur les centres optiques cérébraux, *Rev. Génér. d'Ophthlalm.*, 1894.

64. Calleja, La región olfativa del cerebro, Madrid, 1893.

65. S. R. Cajal, Estructura del asta de Ammon y fascia dentata, *Anal. d. l. Soc. Esp. d. Histor. Natur.*, 1893. Apuntes para el estudio experimental de la corteza visual del cerebro humano, *Rev. Ibero-Americana de Ciencias Médicas*, 1899. Estudios sobre la corteza humana, *Rev. Trim. Micrográf.*, 1899 and following.

66. Schlapp, The Microscopic Structure of Cortical Areas in Man and Some Mammals, *American Journal of Anatomy*, Vol. II, no. 2, 1903.

67. Kaes, *Die Grosshirnrinde des Menschen in ihren Massen und ihren Fasergehalt*, Jena, 1907.

68. Hermanides u. Köppen, Ueber die Furchen und über den Bau der Grosshirnrinde bei den Lissencephalen insbesondere über die Lökalisation des motorischen Centrums und der Sehregion, *Arch. f. Psychiatrie*, Vol. XXXVII, Part 2, 1903.

69. Köppen and Löwenstein, Studien über den Zellenbau der Grosshirnrinde bei Ungulaten und Carnivoren, etc., *Monatsschr. f. Psychiatrie u. Neurol.*, Vol. XVIII, Part 6, 1905.

70. Brodmann, Beiträge zur histologischen Lokalisation der Grosshirnrinde; III Mitteilung: Die Rindenfelder der niederen Affen, *Journ. f. Psychol. u. Neurol.*, Vol. IV, 1905.

71. O. Vogt, Der Wert der myelogenetischen Felder der Grosshirnrinde, *Anat. Anzeiger*, Vol. XXIX, nos. 11 and 12, 1906. Ueber strukturelle Hirncentra mit besonderer Berücksichtigung der Struktur der Felder des Cortex Pallii, *Verhandl. der Anatom. Gesellschaft*, twentieth meeting, Rostock, 1–5 June 1906.

72. Mme. Vogt, Sur la myélinisation de l'hémisphère cérébral du chat, *C. R. des Séances de la Société de Biol.*, 15 January 1898. Étude sur la myélinisation des hémisphères cérébraux, Paris, 1900.

73. Flechsig, Einige Bemerkungen über die Unter-

suchungsmethoden der Grosshirnrinde etc. aus der *Bericht. der math. phys. Klass, der königl. Säch, Gesellsch. der Wiss. Leipzig,* 11 January 1904.

74. Döllken, Beiträge zur Entwickelung der Säugergehirns, Lage und Ausdehnung des Bewegungscentrums der Maus, *Neurol. Centralbl.,* no. 2, 1907.

75. Livini, Il proencefalo di un Marsupiale, *Arch. di Anat. e di Embriol.,* Vol. VI, Part 4, 1907.

Editors' Notes

A. The text incorrectly says "633."

B. Figure added in the French edition of the book.

C. In the 1899 paper on the human visual cortex, Cajal says that these cells are more numerous in layers II and III.

D. The sentence in square brackets is in the French version of the book but not in the Spanish version.

E. Added in the French version.

F. Added in the French version.

G. The two paragraphs in square brackets are included in the French version of the book but not in the Spanish version. Figs. 677 and 678 are figs. 353 and 354 of the French work.

H. The paragraph in brackets is in the French version of the book but not in the Spanish version.

I. In the French version, the last sentence of this paragraph is modified to read: "[I]t is an error on which we have previously remarked: reticulum and arborizations are completely independent."

J. The two paragraphs in brackets are in the French version but not in the Spanish version. Fig. 357 is fig. 680 of the Spanish work. Fig. 358 is new.

K. Added in the French version.

L. The paragraph in square brackets is in the French version of the book but not in the Spanish version.

M. The paragraph in square brackets is in the French version of the book but not in the Spanish version.

N. The Spanish text says "fifth layer," which follows the designation of the layers in fig. 658. This layer, however, is designated the fourth layer in the introductory text to this chapter (page 794), layers 3 and 4 of fig. 658 being collectively referred to in the text as layer 3 (layer of medium and large external pyramids). The French text says "fourth layer" at this point.

O. The sentence in square brackets is in the French version os the book but not in the Spanish version.

P. The Spanish text says "fifth layer." See note N.

Q. The Spanish text says "fifth layer." See note N.

R. The Spanish text says "fifth layer." See note N.

S. Translated by Azoulay as "cellules à double bouquet protoplasmique."

T. Thus in the French.

U. The text incorrectly says "A."

V. The paragraph in square brackets is in the French version of the book but not in the Spanish version.

W. The Spanish text says "sixth." See note N.

X. The Spanish text says "fifth." See note N.

Y. The paragraph in square brackets is in the French version of the book but not in the Spanish version.

Z. Both Spanish and French versions of the text say "seventh layer." This stems from the same considerations outlined with respect to layers 4 and 5.

AA. The Spanish text says "motor." The French text omits the last part of the sentence.

BB. Both Spanish and French texts say "sensitive and sensory fibers."

CC. The phrase in square brackets is in the French version of the book but not in the Spanish version.

DD. The names in square brackets are in the French version of the book but not in the Spanish version.

EE. The white matter.

FF. The phrase in the square brackets is in the French version of the book but not in the Spanish version.

GG. The phrase in square brackets is in the French version of the book but not in the Spanish version.

HH. The phrase in square brackets is in the French version of the book but not in the Spanish version.

II. The phrase in square brackets is in the French version of the book but not in the Spanish version.

JJ. The phrase in square brackets is in the French version of the book but not in the Spanish version.

KK. The paragraph in square brackets is in the French version of the book but not in the Spanish version.

LL. Added in the French version of the book.

MM. This sentence is translated from the French version, where the sense is clearer than in the original Spanish.

NN. This title appears only in the French version.

OO. The phrase in square brackets is in the French version of the book but not in the Spanish version.

PP. The phrase in square brackets is in the French version of the book but not in the Spanish version.

QQ. What follows in the *Textura* is essentially a direct transcription of the section under this title in the work on the human motor cortex (Cajal, 1899b) and translated as part of chapter 16 in this volume. A few short passages that potentially might have offended Golgi or Kölliker are omitted, and the passage devoted to Hammarberg is abbreviated. The following concludes this section of the *Textura.*

RR. The reference is in the French version of the book but not in the Spanish version.

SS. The reference is in the French version of the book but not in the Spanish version.

TT. Azoulay's translation for the *Histologie* is a literal rendering of this section of the *Textura,* but where the Spanish version ends, he continues on as follows.

22

From: *Chapters 25–33* of *Histologie du Système Nerveux de l'Homme et des Vertébrés* (1911).

[Translated by L. Azoulay (Paris: Maloine, 1911), Vol. 2, pp. 599–823]

25. Continuing the Regions of the Cerebral Cortex: The Visual Cortex

The center of visual sensation according to the physiologists. Its structure in man and other mammals. Historical ideas relative to the constitution of the visual cortex.

The doctrine of cerebral localization, as created by Fritsch, Hitzig, and Ferrier, and as similarly enlarged and improved by Munk, Monakow, and Flechsig, of necessity has led the authorities to think that the diverse regions of the cerebral cortex possess a structure in which each differs somewhat [from the others]. Before the discovery of the centers of tactile, visual, and acoustic sensibility, one could remark, it is true, macroscopic and microscopic differences between certain gyri. However, these proofs were not given the importance that they merit because, thanks to Meynert, the neurologists had been preoccupied with a contrary hypothesis. This hypothesis, which Golgi and Kölliker have revived recently, although with certain reservations, is as follows. The special activity of an individual region of the cortex depends by no means on its structure; it depends only on the nature of the excitations which the peripheral sensory

apparatus conveys to it. Hence, according to this hypothesis, the visual sensation is born in the calcarine fissure and not elsewhere, simply because it is there that all the optic fibers terminate. All the works recently concerned with the regional structure of the cortex, works which have demonstrated that the differences between the sensory areas are greater than one imagined, rise up against this exaggerated hypothesis. Our researches, in particular, point out that it is not so. We are authorized to say with very great likelihood [of being correct] that the unique activities of each point of the cortex depend as much on the structure of the point as upon the quality of the sensory excitations which it receives. For the rest, the particular structural features of each region of the cortex are probably only a secondary phenomenon, the result of their adaptation to a function which, in order to serve them best, is perfected [for each of them].

Visual Cortex: The Cortical Localization of Visual Perception according to Physiological and Anatomicopathological Research

Experimentalists and clinicians [are always at odds] over the point in the human brain at which the central optic path of Gratiolet terminates and over its operation in mental vision. One of them, Henschen,[1] having studied and discussed all the cases of cortical lesions accompanied by more or less complete hemianopsia, without the least hesitation places the center of visual perception in the calcarine fissure. He goes so far as to localize visual impressions emanating from the superior sectors of the retina in the upper bank of the fissure; in the lower bank are those from the inferior sectors, and in the fundus those from the horizontal meridian, whereas the impressions carried in the macular bundle are diffused to the most anterior region of the fissure on the summit of the cuneus. Probst[2] and Tsuchida[3] also admit that the center of visual perception is the calcarine fissure. Of the others, the pathologists, such as Starr, Nothnagel, Vialet, Mauthner, Seguin, and Hun, and the histologists, such as Flechsig, O. Vogt, and Brodmann[4] are not so precise. The first attribute, in effect, mental vision to the whole surface of the occipital lobe or limit it, as in the work of Wilbrand and Dejerine, to the internal face and the extremity of this lobe; the second extend the visual area to convolutions bordering the calcarine fissure, to the cuneus, to the lingual lobule and the occipital pole. Ferrier, however, professes an opinion quite different, and much discussed; he places the seat of visual function in the *pli courbe* or angular gyrus of the parietal lobe. Finally, certain pathologists, such as Seppilli, Gowers, etc., in seeking to reconcile the most contrary viewpoints, admit to two localizations: one in the occipital lobe, the other in the parietal gyrus whose name we have just mentioned. In spite of all these disagreements, it is certain that in the majority of cases of hemianopsia due to cerebral lesion, one discovers the lesion to be either within the calcarine fissure or in its neighborhood, or among the optic fibers situated beneath the medial cortex of the occipital lobe. In certain cases, it is true, there proves to be at the same time an involvement of the parietal lobe, but only when the cerebral disorganization penetrates deeply and affects the subjacent optic radiations a little distant from the surface. This seems likely to be the case, since, with new highly demonstrative observations, assembled by Henschen, significant lesions of the parietal lobe, in the absence of this, do not give any visual problems; the lateral cortex of the occipital lobe is no longer the seat of mental vision, as proved in the series collected and skillfully discussed by the author we have cited. Monakow,[5] who accepts a localization in the calcarine fissure and in the cuneus, wrongly therefore supports the contrary.

Physiological experimentation agrees, in general, with the conclusions of the clinic, on condition that one recalls that the visual nuclei in animals, such as the dog and the monkey, have neither the same situation nor the same extent as in man. Munk, Steiner, and others have presented proof about where the visual area is localized in the rabbit, the cat, etc., on the lateral or dorsal face of the occipital lobe and, in the dog, upon the posterior extremity of the second occipital gyrus, as well as on the adjacent territories of the first and the third. When, following the examples of Munk, Goltz, Luciani, etc., one removes the cortex of one hemisphere in such regions from these animals, one obtains, in effect, a hemianopsia, that is to say, a blindness of the left or right parts of the two retinas, depending on which hemisphere is removed.

General Historical Idea of the Structure of the Visual Cortex

Gennari, Vicq d' Azyr, and Baillarger had already remarked that this cortex is distinguished from others by the presence of a white stripe, parallel to the surface and visible to the naked eye. To this, a macroscopic characteristic, Meynert[6] applied the microscope, and his study was so exact that, despite the imperfection of the methods, it is still the best that we possess. Here, according to this scientist, are the layers one finds in the visual cortex: first, *a molecular layer;* second, *a layer of small pyramidal cells;* third, *a layer of nuclei or granules, the layer corresponding to the fourth of the typical cortex;* fourth, *a layer of large pyramidal cells or of isolated cells;* fifth, *a layer of medium granules;* sixth, *a layer, similar to the fourth, made up of neuroglial nuclei and large, sparse nerve cells;* seventh, *a layer of nuclei or deep granules;* eighth, *a layer of fusiform cells corresponding to the fifth of the typical cortex.*

W. Krause,[7] Schwalbe,[8] Betz,[9] and other authorities after Meynert added next to nothing to his description. Similarly, Golgi,[10] in spite of employing his marvelous method, has scarcely advanced our understanding of the visual area, because, in following the convention of his times, he ignored the true location and studied instead an adjoining territory which was without doubt an association area.

The more recent work which Hammarberg[11] and Kölliker[12] have carried out with the aid of the methods of Nissl and Weigert does not represent much progress. As a result of these researches, Hammarberg, for example, has concluded that the visual cortex can be considered as a simple variety of what he calls *sensory cortex,* and among its characteristics are absence of pyramidal cells from the fourth layer; replacement of these cells by a large band of granule cells, the same divisible into three secondary laminae by the presence of two striae of a molecular character and poor in nervous elements; existence of a row of isolated pyramidal cells, noted previously by Meynert and situated under the third lamina of granule cells, between these and the layer of fusiform cells of that savant.

Henschen[13] has also examined the cortex of the calcarine fissure; he has found a particular structure characterized by large stellate cells and an intermediate nervous plexus corresponding to the stria of Gennari.

Schlapp,[14] who studied the brain of the monkey by the Nissl method, examining all its regions, ended up merely by substituting for the nomenclature of Meynert another which is no more fortunate. Hence: first, *layer of tangential fibers;* second, *layer of external polymorphic cells;* third, *layer of parapyknomorphic pyramidal cells;* fourth, *layer of granule cells;* fifth, *layer of small solitary cells;* sixth, *layer of deep granule cells;* seventh, *layer poor in cells;* eighth, *layer of internal polymorphic cells.* Apart from the third, fourth, sixth, and seventh layers, all the others correspond to the same numbering sequence as in the nomenclature of Meynert.

Finally, Brodmann, in research with the aid of the Nissl method, numbered the layers of the visual area in the cercopithecine [monkey]; he estimated them at eight, like Schlapp's. Of the structure of the layers, he does not furnish details.

This short historical résumé shows that, so far, only the superficial appearances of the visual cortex, the number of its layers, and the general outline of some of its cells are known. By contrast, complete ignorance reigns concerning the mode of termination of optic fibers and their relationships with the neurons, as well as about the morphology and other particulars of these elements. It is on account of these imperfect notions that we began, in our turn, the study of the visual cortex. We shall lay out here the most important results of our researches.

[*Editors' note:* What follows in both the *Textura* and the *Histologie* is a faithful, although abbreviated, rendition of the paper of 1899 on the human visual cortex. In one passage, however, Cajal changes his emphasis from that of the original paper. In referring to the layer of small stellate cells (layer V), he had originally stated that the majority of the cells in that layer were stellate cells with long axon (see chapter 15 in this volume). In the two versions of the textbook, he corrects this, as follows:

"*V. Layer of the small stellate cells with short axons (granules).* This layer also contains quite a number of stellate cells with long axon, completely similar to, although somewhat less voluminous than, those of the fourth layer; but the [granule] cells that dominate it, the ones that lend to the layer under study, [when] examined in preparations stained with carmine or hematoxylin, that appearance of a conglomeration of nuclei already noticed by Meynert, are certain diminutive spheroidal, fusiform, or stellate cells, whose size does not usually exceed 10 to 12 μm (fig. 383, *B*) [*fig. 72* in chapter 15].

In fig. 385 [*fig. 75* in chapter 15], we show some of these dwarf cells, whose impregnation is difficult in the adult human but which are from time to time stained in the child of a few days."]

26. Auditory Cortex

Auditory cortex of man. Auditory cortex in other gyrencephalic mammals. Insular cortex of man.

The Cortical Localization of Auditory Perception according to Physiological and Anatomicopathological Research

As with visual perception, we first ask physiology and pathological anatomy to indicate to us the place in the cerebral cortex that performs the perception of auditory sensations. According to Munk, Luciani, Ferrier, and Seppilli, it occupies in the monkey and other mammals a well-circumscribed region of the temporal lobe. The first of these physiologists specified it even more precisely in the dog, and fixed it more or less at the center of the two descending posterior gyri of the lobe. For the anatomists and anatomical pathologists, the auditory area would be found in man in the middle third of the first temporal gyrus. Among the more modern authors, Probst places it at the sylvian lip of this gyrus, that is to say, in the vicinity of the insula. As for Flechsig, O. Vogt, Mme. Vogt, and Campbell,[15] they have localized it at points that are little different.

Tied up with the auditory area is the *language area.* It extends, according to Dejerine, from the perimeter of the fissure of Sylvius, on the first temporal gyrus, to the gyri of the insula and as far as the base of the occipital lobe, forming a zone of rather considerable extent. This vast territory includes, as a consequence, a large part of the sensory-motor cortex and a rather important part of the association cortex, according to the terminology and the hypothesis of Flechsig.

Thus, there is more or less unanimity of opinion that the auditory area is properly situated in the first temporal gyrus of man. We have accordingly studied the structure of this gyrus without being preoccupied with the exact point at which a lesion produces mental deafness, since the question is still in dispute. We will also examine the insula, which many authorities number among the acoustic gyri.[16]

Historical Sketch of the Structure of the Auditory Cortex

The data one has possessed until now on the structure of the first temporal gyrus are rather few, because it has been regarded as identical to the typical cortex. Betz[17] and Schlapp[18] nevertheless note it in passing, while Hammarberg,[19] the only author who has made a systematic study of the whole cerebral cortex with the aid of the Nissl method, has given a more serious analysis, accompanied by a figure.

The first of these authors claims that the cortex of the three temporal gyri is characterized by the thickness of the fifth layer or layer of fusiform cells and by a layer of granule or small cells in the position of the third typical layer or layer of the large pyramidal cells.

Hammarberg recognizes in the first temporary gyrus; first, a *molecular layer,* or layer in which but rare cells are found; second, a *layer of small pyramidal cells,* with a diameter between 9 and 15 μm; third, a *layer of large pyramidal cells* from 20 to 30 μm, and corresponding to large and medium pyramidal cells of the motor cortex; fourth, a *layer of granule cells,* in which lie the small pyramidal cells and neurons of irregular shape; fifth, a *layer of ganglionic cells,* representing the seat of the large deep pyramidal cells of other regions of the cortex, the large pyramidal neurons being from 20–30 μm in diameter, others of medium size, and some small; sixth, a *layer of fusiform cells,* equivalent to the fifth layer of the typical cortex of Meynert, its great thickness reaching as much as 1.2 mm, and the fusiform cells which it contains varying from 9 to 30 μm. Finally, Brodmann[20] has described in the first temporal [gyrus] of the cercopithecus [monkey] a stratification almost identical to that which Schlapp indicated in the monkey. It corresponds to area 22 in the nomenclature of Brodmann, and it extends, according to him, throughout the whole gyrus.

Schlapp found that in the monkey the first temporal gyrus is identical to the *second cortical type* of his nomenclature, that is to say, to a cortex in which the layer of large pyramidal and polymorphic cells is subdivided into two strata, the one external, the other internal, by the interposition of a zone of granule cells. The cortex of the auditory gyrus would consist of seven layers, according to Schlapp. Save for the third or layer of medium pyramids included by Hammárberg in the layer of large pyramidal cells, these layers correspond rather well to those which the latter histologist distinguishes.

[*Editors' note:* The remainder of the text is, again, an abbreviated version of the paper of 1900 (chapter 17 in this volume). He does, however, provide a more extended account of certain aspects of the special giant cells of the auditory cortex. We translate the relevant section as follows.]

Cells Characteristic of the Acoustic Cortex

This is what we will call certain giant fusiform elements that we have discovered in the human auditory cortex[21] and so far not found in any other cortical region. The consistency with which such cells are observed in all our preparations of the human first [temporal] gyrus, and in the insula, inclines us to consider them as an important factor of acoustic function, although it is impossible at present to conceive the nature of the role that they perform in mental audition. [Cajal goes on to describe the cells in a more summarized form than in the original paper. Then he has the following to say about the axon.]

The axon is very thick, thicker than that of the giant pyramids; it often originates from a side of the cell, in its initial trajectory it runs either horizontally or obliquely, and, after tracing large curves that make following it difficult, it is incorporated into the white matter, where it is continuous with a robust myelinated nerve fiber. In the deepest cells, the axon can have a descending trajectory from the beginning. It is not the same with those located more superficially, where the trajectory is often steplike and uneven because of the great bends, a circumstance that allows us to distinguish, at first glance, these axons from those of the large pyramids of the fourth and sixth layers. Whatever its point of departure, the axon of these special cells of the auditory area gives off a multitude of collaterals, largely horizontal and repeatedly branched, which terminate at no very great distance. Some, particularly those belonging to the depeest specific cells, have a recurrent trajectory toward the surface of the cortex. The cell represented in fig. 397 at *a* [*fig. 130* in chapter 17] possessed

at least fourteen or fifteen of these collaterals; we have reproduced only six, because it has not been possible to represent the entire course of the axon. This interesting cell, which we show only at a magnification of 20x to 30x in the figure, was located in the layer of the medium pyramids, a place in which they are not very rare.

It is a great pity that we have not been able to determine the connections of these neurons, above all [their relations] with the terminations of the acoustic pathway. Whenever that is revealed, something we do not doubt, it will probably be found that the special cells of the auditory cortex have a great resemblance to the large stellate cells of the fourth layer of the visual cortex, since, as stated before, they are of large stature and do not possess the peripheral dendritic tuft.

27. Motor or Sensory-Motor Cortex

Sensory-motor cortex of man. Comparative structure of the principal motor convolutions. Structure of the precentral [gyrus]. Sensory-motor cortex of other mammals.

The Localization of the Sensory-Motor Area According to Physiological and Anatomico-pathological Research

Pathological anatomy accords with physiology in considering that the *precentral and postcentral gyri, the paracentral lobule, the posterior ends of the first, second, and third frontal gyri, with a neighboring portion of the parietal lobe,* make up the motor cortex in man. Within this vast region, which occupies the center of the vault formed by the cerebral cortex, are housed the three motor centers of the human body. The uppermost represents the lower limb; the intermediate corresponds to the upper limb; the lowest, finally, serves the face. It has been proven, among others, by Ferrier, Horsley, and Beevor, that the relative positions of the three centers persist, save for slight variations, in other gyrencephalic mammals such as the macaque and orangutan. One notices, meanwhile, that there is a tendency for them to be displaced dorsally and anteriorly, barely extending posterior to the fissure of Rolando.

In the dog, for example, Munk[22] demonstrated, in his physiological experiments, that the motor area is limited to the banks of the cruciate sulcus, that is to say, to the pre- and postcruciate marginal gyri of the frontal lobe.

The cortex we are going to study in this chapter is not only motor, it is also sensory, because, when lesions strike, particularly at the level of the two central gyri, one sees occurring at one and the same time motor paralyses and sensory defects. This is a fact well established from the observations of Luciani, Flechsig, Henschen, Dejerine, Mott, Schaffer, etc., as well as by the experiments of Munk and other scientists. Those authors who place terminations of the sensory fibers in other regions of the cortex, such as the parietal lobe, hippocampus, etc., such as Monakow, Ferrier, and Nothnagel, profess an opinion contrary to the teachings of the clinic and of physiology.

Thus, the motor cortex is simply the place in the brain in which arrive the terminals of the pathways which transmit tactile, painful, thermal, and muscular sensations from the whole organism. Thus, it is a sensory center differing only from the others merely in the considerable strength of its fibers of projection.

Comparative Structure of the Principal Motor Gyri

The precentral gyrus, with its upper end on the surface of the hemisphere, on the posterior ends of the first and second frontal [gyri], and in part also on the paracentral lobule, possesses a mode of lamination very different from that of the postcentral gyrus. One can understand, therefore, the great discrepancies that one encounters in the descriptions of authors relative to the number and extent of the layers of the motor area. Believing, unreservedly, that the structure of this area is uniform, he who studies only the precentral gyrus and he who studies only the postcentral [will, without doubt, for better or worse,] generalize his observations. Taking Meynert, for example, when he says that the motor cortex contains a true granule cell layer, he is probably, in fact, referring to the postcentral gyrus. Taking now Golgi, Edinger, Kölliker, and still others, it is extremely likely that they have based their researches on the precentral [gyrus], since they do not mention the existence of this layer of granule cells in the motor cortex. We have not wished to fall into the same error. We have accordingly subjected all regions of the sensory-motor cortex to a systematic study by the Nissl method. We have thus gained the conviction that the fissure of Rolando forms a limiting trench between the two central gyri. The structure of these two gyri is very different, as we have said, but not sufficiently to ascribe to each of them a particular [fine] structure.

We have reproduced in fig. 404 [*fig. 88* in chapter 16] a transverse section of these two gyri from a woman aged twenty-five years. It is easy to see that the difference rests principally on the thickness and the degree of development of certain layers rather than on the relative number of cells. The precentral [gyrus], seen to the right of the figure, does not show a well-marked layer of granule cells; by contrast, the two layers of large external and deep pyramidal cells are particularly evident, the number of Betz cells or giant pyramids is considerable, and the plexiform layer reaches a great thickness. It is otherwise with the postcentral [gyrus], which occupies the left of the figure; its layer of granule cells is clearly evident; it includes two distinct formations of large pyramidal cells, one external, the other internal, but customarily smaller than in the precentral gyrus; finally, the plexiform layer is somewhat thinner.[23]

If we compare now the postcentral gyrus with the [homo]typical cortex, which is probably a cortex of association, after the theory of Flechsig, we see in it the same number of layers. We see also that both do not possess the region of the plexus of thick afferent fibers coming from the white matter, a plexus that gives a unique character to the true motor area. All of these facts lead us to think that in man and the primates, the sensory-motor area is not present in this gyrus, but anterior to the fissure of Rolando. This assertion, we recognize, is contrary to the opinion professed by the physiologists and the pathological anatomists. But anything not proven is subject to error on their part. The physiologists may very well have ignored the phenomenon of diffusion of electrical excitation down to the fundus of the fissure of Rolando, and lesions of the postcentral gyrus in man may have destroyed the pathways originating from the true motor region, unnoticed by the neurologists.[24]

The ideas we are going to express on the subject of the diversity of structure and function of the gyri that bound the fissure of Rolando have received confirmation from various quarters. Monakow[25] and Flechsig[26] have come to its support, a little hypothetically, it is true, on the grounds that the pyramidal tract arises in man from the precentral gyrus. Sherrington[27] demonstrated also that a lesion of the postcentral gyrus is not followed, in the anthropoids, by degeneration in the pyramidal tract. These same facts have been verified by O. Vogt[28] in the same animals, with the aid of the degeneration method and that of electrical excitation of the cortex; this author verifies, in effect, in the orangutan, that stimulation applied to the postcentral gyrus does not provoke any movements. Finally, from the structural point of view, Brodmann[29] confirms, in the monkey, by use of the Nissl method, the difference we have previously indicated between the two gyri, pre- and postcentral. It is established, besides, that the true motor cortex, situated anterior to the fissure of Rolando and characterized by the presence of giant pyramidal cells and by the absence of a layer of granule cells, presents within its extent histological differences. It is permissible to admit the existence of four types of motor cortex, corresponding respectively to movements of the eyes, the head, the jaws, and the body.

Since the structure of the postcentral gyrus does not differ from that of the [homo]typical cortex which we have expounded in a preceding chapter, we will not describe it; we will limit ourselves to a study of the precentral gyrus whose motor character is no longer in doubt.

[Editors' note: What follows is a very abbreviated version of the paper of 1899 on the sensory-motor cortex, chapter 16 in this volume.]

[From Part of Chapter 33.] Association Cortex [(pp. 821–823)]

Flechsig was of the opinion that certain regions of the cortex of gyrencephalic mammals are not in direct relationship with the sensory fibers, and that these regions which become myelinated [late] and enter into activity late are particularly concerned with intellectual operations of the highest level. These regions, which one may call the *centers of memory,* because they probably include the sensory residues coming from the perceptive centers, spread over a very great part of the cerebral cortex, to an extent of almost four-fifths of the human [cortex].

Study of these cortical areas has hardly yet commenced. We have assayed, for our part, to contribute a study of their fine structure in infants aged a few months. Despite the rarity of the material and the inconsistency of the Golgi method, principal obstacles to this enterprise, [which is] of great breadth and bristling with difficulties, we have been able, in a number of very restricted cases, to impregnate the small, medium, and large pyramidal cells and also a small number of cells of the granule cell layer in the frontal and parietal gyri. Our impression resulting from this is that the fine structure of these gyri is quite similar to that of the postcentral gyrus, which we have dealt with as typical of the cerebral cortex in chapter 24 [chapter 21 of this volume].

The Nissl technique corroborates this impression; with it, we can appreciate that the association gyri include the same layers as the typical cortex, that is to say, first, *a plexiform layer;* second, *a layer of small pyramidal cells;* third, *a layer of medium pyramidal cells;* fourth, *a layer of large external pyramidal cells;* fifth, *a layer of granule or stellate cells;* sixth, *a layer of large deep pyramidal cells;* seventh, *a layer of medium and deep pyramidal cells;* and, finally, eighth, *a layer of triangular and fusiform cells.*[A]

Schlapp,[30] who has also studied the association areas, indicates that in man they cover the parietal lobe, a large part of the occipital and frontal lobes, excluding the motor area, the precuneus, and the insula of Reil, more or less completely. These areas would have in the monkey an identical but less extensive distribution. The number of layers that Schlapp lists in these areas is seven, in which our seventh and eighth layers are reduced to a single layer: *the internal layer of polymorphic cells;* it is the only difference between his nomenclature and ours.

Brodmann[31] has also presented a nomenclature of the layers of the association areas in the monkey and man, similar to that used for the postcentral gyrus.

Here is a concordance of our nomenclature with that of the layers which Brodmann differentiates in this cortex which constitutes his first type:

1. *Lamina zonalis* (plexiform layer).
2. *Lamina granularis externa* (layer of small pyramidal cells).
3. *Lamina pyramidalis* (layer of large and medium pyramids), subdivided into (a) *lamina mediopyramidalis* (layer of medium pyramidals) and (b) *lamina magnopyramidalis* (layer of large pyramidals).
4. *Lamina granularis interna* (layer of granule or small stellate cells).
5. *Lamina ganglionaris* (layer of large deep pyramidal cells).
6. *Lamina multiformis,.* subdivided into (a) *lamina triangularis* (layer of medium deep pyramidal cells, among which are the triangular cells) and (b) *lamina fusiformis* (our layer of the fusiform and triangular cells and layer of the fusiform cells of Meynert).

One can see that, apart from the different names, this nomenclature corresponds to that which Schlapp and we have presented.

The association areas are concerned, in all likelihood, with the phenomena of memory and hence are linked with the specific sensory areas. It is likely, therefore, that each of them presents, as we see it, a structure that varies somewhat in accord with the particular activity in which each is engaged. Thus, the area of visual ideation or area of memory phenomena accumulated from ocular sensations will not possess, in all likelihood, the same fine structure as the cortical regions destined to store auditory, tactile, or olfactory memories.

This concept has been confirmed by Brodmann in his view that in the cerebral cortex of the monkey, with its twenty-eight different structural types, the majority are found in the association or memory areas. Unfortunately, details about these different types are wanting,

for Brodmann employed neither the method of Golgi nor that of Ehrlich.

For certain of the association areas, namely those of olfaction, as represented by Ammon's horn, the subiculum, and the presubiculum, the demonstration is completely proven, nevertheless. We have seen, in effect, from what is presented by the Golgi preparations, a fine structure [that is] very specific and strongly different from that which is observed in the secondary olfactory area, that is to say, in the temporal olfactory cortex.

Cajal's Notes

1. Henschen, Sur le centres optiques cérébraux, *Rev. Génér. Ophthalm.*, 1894. Revue critique de la doctrine du centre corticale de la vision, 1900. *Klinische und anatomische Beiträge zur Pathologie des Gehirns,* Upsala, 1903.
2. Probst, Ueber zentralen Sinnesbahnen und die Sinneszentren des menschlichen Gehirnes, *Sitzber. Kaiser. Akad. Wiss. Wien. Math. - Natur. - Klasse,* Vol. CXV, part 3, 1906.
3. Tsuchida, Ein Beitrag zur Anatomie der Sehstrahlungen beim Menschen, *Arch. f. Psychiat.,* Vol. XLII, part 1, 1907.
4. Brodmann, Beiträge zur histologischen Lokalisation der Grosshirnrinde, *Journ. f. Psychol. u. Neurol.,* Vol. IV, 1905.
5. Monakow, Exper. u. pathol. anat. Untersuchungen über die optischen Centren u. Bahnen, etc., *Arch. f. Psychiatr.,* Vols. XX and XXV[II].
6. Meynert, Vom Gehirne der Säugetiere. *Strickers Handbuch d. Gewebelehre,* Vol. II, [1872].
7. Krause, *Allgemeine u. mikroskopische Anatomie,* Hannover, 1876.
8. Schwalbe, *Lehrbuch d. Neurologie,* Erlangen, 1881.
9. Betz, *Centralbl f. d. Mediz. Wissenschaft.,* nos. 11–13, 1881.
10. C. Golgi, Sulla fina anatomia degli organi centrali del sistema nervoso, Milano, 1886.
11. Hammarberg, *Studien über Klinik u. Pathologie d. Idiotie, etc.,* Upsala, 1895.
12. Kölliker, *Handbuch der Gewebelehre des Menschen,* 6th edition, Vol. II, Leipzig, 1896.
13. Henschen, *Pathologie d. Gehirns.,* Vol. III, 189[6].
14. Schlapp, Der Zellenbau der Grosshirnrinde des Affen Macacus, etc., *Arch f. Psychiatr.,* Vol. XXX, pt. 2., 189[8].
15. Campbell, *Histological Studies on the Localisation of Cerebral Function,* Cambridge, 1905.
16. S. R. Cajal, Corteza acústica, *Rev. Trim. Micrográf.,* Vol. V, 1900.
17. Betz, *Centralbl. f. d. Mediz. Wissenschaft.,* nos. 11–13, 18[8]1.

18. Schlapp, Der Zellenbau der Grosshirnrinde des Affen, etc., *Arch. f. Psychiatrie.*, Vol. XXX, pt. 2, 189[8].

19. Hammarberg, *Studien über Klinik. u. Pathologie d. Idiotie, etc.*, Upsala, 1895.

20. Brodmann, Beiträge zur histologischen Localisation der Grosshirnrinde, *Journal f. Psychologie u. Neurol.*, etc., Vol. IV, 1905.

21. S. R. Cajal, *Rev. Ibero-americana de Ciencias Médicas*, March 1889; and *Rev. Trim. Micrográf.*, Vol. V, 1900.

22. H. Munk, Ueber die Fühlsphären d. Grosshirnrinde, *Sitzungsber. d. Königl. Preussisch. Akad. d. Wissensch. zu Berlin*, Session of July 14, 1892.

23. Brodmann (Die Regio Rolandica, *Journal für Psychologie und Neurologie*, Vol. II, parts 2, 3, 4 1903) has also noted, after us, the differences between the two central gyri.

24. The majority of neurologists who in latter years have studied these cerebral gyri in man and gyrencephalic mammals seem not to know the history of this question and particularly our works that have dealt with this subject. We ourselves are obliged to call to mind that we were the first to indicate that the fundus of the fissure of Rolando forms, in man, a limiting trench between two cortical regions of absolutely distinct structure and probably with different functions (S. R. Cajal, Estudios sobre la corteza cerebral humana: Estructura de la corteza motriz del hombre y mamíferos, *Revista Trimestr. Micrográf.*, Vol. IV, 1899). We must recognize, however, that Schlapp had earlier demonstrated in 1898 that the fissure of Rolando forms, in the monkey, a line of demarcation between the two types of cortex of different structure (Schlapp, Der Zellenbau der Grosshirnrinde der Affen, etc., *Arch. f. Psychiatrie*, Vol. XXX, 189[8].

25. Monakow, *Gehirnpathologie*, 2nd edition, 1905.

26. Flechsig, Einige Bemerkungen über die Untersuchungsmethoden der Grosshirnrinde, *Arch. f. Anat.*, 1905.

27. Grünbaum and Sherrington, Observations on the Physiology of the Cerebral Cortex of Some Higher Apes, *Proceed. of the Royal Society*, Vol. 69, 1901. Observations on the Physiology of the Cerebral Cortex of the Anthropoid Apes, *Proceed. of the Royal Society*, Vol. [72], 1903.

28. Vogt, Ueber Strukturelle Hirncentra mit besonderer Berüchsichtigung der Strukturelle Felder des Cortex pallii, *Verhandl. der Anat. Gessellschaft.*, 20th Meeting in Rostock, 1–5 June 1906.

29. Brodmann, Beiträge zur histologischen Lokalisation der Grosshirnrinde; 1–5 Mitteilung, *Journal für Psychol. u. Neurol.*, 1903–1906.

30. Schlapp, The Microscopic Study of Cortical Areas in Man and Some Mammals, *American Journal of Anat[omy]*, Vol. II, no. 2, 1903.

31. Brodmann, Beiträge zur histologischen Lokalisation der Grosshirnrinde, etc., *Journal für Psychologie und Neurologie*, Vol. IV, 1905.

Editors' Notes

A. Most of the remaining paragraphs are additions to the original text of the *Textura.*

23

Comparative Structure of the Cerebral Cortex: Cortex of Small Mammals; Cortex of Birds, Reptiles, Batrachians, [and Fish]

[*From: Textura del sistema nervioso del hombre y de los vertebrados*, (Madrid: Moya, 1904),Vol. 2, pt. 2 chap. 46, pp. 1089–1109; also published in French as *Histologie du système nerveux de l'homme et des vertébrés*, Vol. 2, (Paris: Maloine, 1911), chap. 34, pp. 824–846.]

Man and gyrencephalic mammals substantially coincide in the architecture of the cerebral layers. Anatomical degradation or simplification begins especially in the rodents (rat, guinea pig, rabbit), it becomes more noticeable in the lower mammals, and it reaches its peak in the birds, reptiles, and batrachians. In the latter two classes of vertebrates, it can be said, as Edinger has demonstrated, that almost the whole cortex represents a series of centers of olfactory perception and association. [From this results a very rational division of the cortex into *archipallium* and *neopallium*. The former of these divisions, proposed by Elliot Smith, corresponds to the inferior region of the cortex and comprises almost exclusively the rhinencephalon or olfactory cerebrum; the second, which corresponds to the superior region of the cortex, includes the other sensory centers and reaches its full development only in the mammals. These two divisions are equivalent, more or less, to the *hypospherium* or inferior cerebrum and *epispherium* or superior cerebrum of Edinger.]^A

The structural simplification affects not only the number of differentiated centers or regions and layers of each area, but very especially the morphology of the neurons, which have a tendency, as the [phylogenetic] animal scale is descended, to become undifferentiated, to lose processes successively, and to reduce the points of contact with the nerve fibers from which they receive impulses. There are two anatomical features, however, that always persist, giving evidence of their great phylogenetic and functional significance: the radial orientation of the neurons, whose external pole constantly emits a peripheral [dendritic] tuft; and the existence beneath the pia of a plexiform layer, in which the [dendritic] tufts of the pyramids [enter into contact] with afferent nerve fibers. Recognizing the persistence of the orientation and form of the cerebral pyramid in all the vertebrates, as well as the elevated hierarchy of its functions, we dare to name it the *psychic cell*,[1] a designation by which we do not claim to exclude from so high a physiological task the monopolar ganglionic cells of the invertebrates, since structure represents only one of the conditions, and perhaps the less important, in the physiological hierarchy. Everything leads one to presume that superior functional capacity (memory, representation, association, consciousness, etc.) depends on both the chemical texture and composition of the protoplasm [of a cell] and the quality of the stimulus reaching it. With regard to the form, it can be considered as the conduit of the nervous activity, and so, the multiplicity of the cellular processes would have the function of multiplying associations and establishing the integration and continuity of nervous function.

Cortex of Small Mammals

We have already said that in rodents, and especially in the mouse, the cortex undergoes an important simplification. In effect, the thickness of the gray matter noticeably decreases; the cells shrink, and the number of layers is reduced to five because of the lack of a layer of granule cells; and the large pyramids form a single layer.

As shown in fig. 844, [fig. 228], the layers of the cerebral cortex of the mouse (and similarly of the rabbit) are five: first, *plexiform layer;* second, *layer of the small pyramids;* third, *layer of the medium pyramids;* fourth, *layer of the large pyramids;* fifth, *layer of the ovoid or polymorphic cells.* [Fig. 528 [*fig. 228*] gives an idea of this arrangement in the motor area, a region that is impregnated better by the Golgi method in the young mouse.

[We will say in advance that the neurofibrillary methods, [which are] more favorable for the determination of the course and termination of nerve fibers than for the recognition of the morphology of neurons in very young rodents, have allowed us, like other authors, to confirm the essential details of the description that follows. One of these methods, reduced silver nitrate, has especially helped Döllken[2] in his investigations on the location and extent of the motor area in rodents.][B]

Plexiform Layer

It is composed of the elements already studied, there being found in it both cells with short axon and horizontal cells, although in much smaller numbers than in gyrencephalic animals. In fig. 845, *A, B, C* [*fig. 32* in chapter 7], we show some horizontal cells of the cerebrum

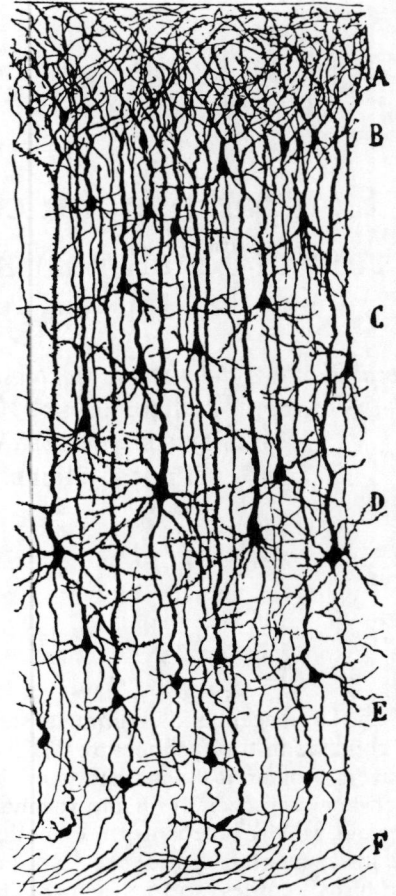

[*FIG. 228*] Fig. 844. Cerebral cortex; mouse of twenty days. Golgi method. *A,* plexiform layer; *B,* layer of the small pyramidal cells; *C,* layer of the medium pyramidal cells; *D,* layer of the large pyramidal cells; *E,* layer of the ovoid or polymorphic cells; *F,* white matter. [The captions for the figures have been translated from the French version of the book.]

of the rabbit of a few days. Notice their spindle or triangular shape, the enormous length of the processes, one of which is the axon, and the large number of ascending branches arising at right angles from the said processes. As a whole, the [axonal and dendritic] arborization is much weaker than in man. As a type of cell with short axon, we illustrate one with horizontal axon, also taken from the cerebrum of the rabbit (fig. 834, *D*) [*fig. 32*].

Layers of the Small and Medium Pyramids
(fig. 844, B, C) [fig. 228]

In comparison with man and other gyrencephalic animals, there is noticed [in the rodents] the relatively [larger size] of the cell body of the small pyramids, the thickness of their dendrites, and, above all, the scarcity of cells with short axon. Only in the rabbit have we been able to impregnate some; in the mouse, we have never seen them. Neither have we seen neurogliaform and bitufted cells (mouse and rat).

Layer of the Large Pyramids

These cells attract attention because of their elongated cell body, not so distinctly pyramidal or conical as that of the pyramids of the gyrencephalic animals; the robustness and spiny appearance of the radial dendrite, which can easily be followed to the first layer; and especially the behavior of the axon. This, on arriving at the white matter and before penetrating the corpus striatum, often (not always) gives off a collateral or sometimes a branch of bifurcation of an associative character.

This associative branch presents many variations in origin and direction, as we show in fig. 846 [fig. 229]. Sometimes, it arises from the bend described by the axon of projection on reaching the white matter (fig. 846, b, e) [fig. 229] and, after running horizontally for a certain distance, becomes ascending in distant cortical territories on the same side; at other times, it arises from the second bend, that is to say, from that described by the axon on penetrating the corpus striatum [fig. 846, d] [fig. 229], turning back to the white matter and getting lost in more medial cortical regions; finally, in others, the said branch originating from the first bend is incorporated, apparently, into the plane of the callosal fibers, running with them toward the midline.

All of these association branches were already seen by us in our first works on the subject;[3] but we thought at that time that the majority of the fine fibers of the white matter originating in this way represented commissural fibers, and we supposed, in addition (following the then current prejudice), the exis-

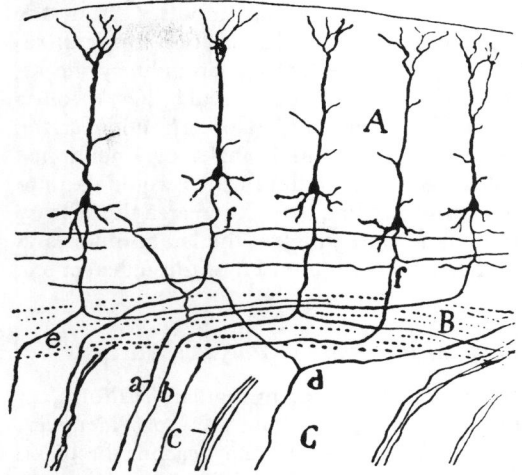

[FIG. 229] Fig. 846. Portion of a transverse section of the cerebral cortex of the mouse of fifteen days. Golgi method. A, cerebral cortex; B, white matter; C, corpus striatum; a, b, e, axons of projection furnished with a long collateral of association; c, axon devoid of this collateral; d, axon of projection giving off its collateral of association at the border of the corpus striatum; f, very long collaterals coming from giant pyramidal cells.

tence of a large number of axons of pyramids destined to form exclusively homolateral association fibers.

The new studies undertaken in the cortex of the rabbit, rat, and, above all, the mouse (from the seventh to the twentieth day [after birth]) have persuaded us of an important fact, namely that *the vast majority (perhaps all) of the homolateral fibers of association (anteroposterior, transverse, etc.) originating in the sensory areas of the cortex of the rodents represent, not direct fibers, but collaterals or branches of bifurcation of axons of projection.* Such is, at least, the habitual behavior of the association fibers in the following regions: motor, visual, sphenoidal olfactory,[c] interhemispheric cortices, etc. In the preceding study on the olfactory cerebrum, we have mentioned many examples of such an interesting disposition.

If this arrangement could be confirmed in the gyrencephalic mammals, its theoretical importance would be great, because it would allow us to forge a precise scheme of the course followed by the impulses, from the sense organs to the [association cortical] regions. So, each excitation brought by the afferent or sensory fibers would flow through the motor fiber or fiber of projection at the same time as through the above-mentioned collateral of association, which would carry to the corresponding association area the sensory residue destined to form the latent image and perhaps the memory itself of the act executed.

Layer of the Ovoid or Polymorphic Cells

It consists of ovoid, triangular, fusiform, or pyramidal cells with long axon, provided with a long [radial] dendrite that reaches the plexiform layer, few and varicose basal branches (fig. 844, *E*) [*fig. 228*], and a flexuous axon capable of being easily followed to the white matter. Among these cells appear some comparable to the granule cells of the gyrencephalic animals, since they possess robust and arciform recurrent collaterals (fig. 844) [*fig. 228*], as well as not a few globular cells, devoid of a radial [dendritic] shaft and possessing an ascending axon that goes up to the plexiform layer. There are also a small number of cells with short axon arborizing at a short distance [from the parent cell body].

White Matter

It consists of projection and association efferent fibers already described, callosal fibers also referred to in previous chapters, and thick afferent or sensory fibers. In fig. 844 [*fig. 228*], which represents a transverse section of the cortex of the mouse, the latter fibers appear in several layers, which, as we revealed earlier, engender very dense terminal plexuses, especially concentrated in the layers of the medium and large pyramids. The shortness of the course [of the afferent fibers] has frequently allowed us to follow the [parent fibers] back to the corpus striatum and observe that, on reaching the white matter, they usually bifurcate, engendering, thanks to the divergence of the initial branches, terminal arborizations of extraordinary extent.

Association Areas in the Cortex of Small Mammals

The thesis of the functional duality of the cortex has been maintained by Flechsig in man and primates; but in the carnivores and solipeds,[D] the centers of association would be but little developed; and in the rodents and other vertebrates, they would be completely lacking.

We have carefully examined the cortex of the rabbit and mouse to assure ourselves about the absence of the association areas, and the result has been to observe that in these animals there also exist cortical areas devoid of direct sensory pathways, but connected, apparently, by means of association branches, with the projection areas. In fig. 847 [*fig. 117* in chapter 16], in which the areas that possess plexuses made by fibers coming from the corpus striatum have been represented, it is observed that among the sensory areas there are territories of small extent, devoid or almost devoid of such fibers, although never lacking in fibers of projection. See, for example, the region *a*, located medial and superior to the visual area; the region *b*, located between the visual and acoustic areas; and the territory *E*, interposed between this and the olfactory area. Such intercalated areas seem to receive branches of bifurcation and collaterals of the axons originating in the adjoining sensory areas.

Would it be permissible to regard such intercalated gray areas as areas of association or memory? If the existence in the rodents of visual, motor, auditory, etc., association areas, separated from the sensory areas, seems probable, though not proven, the idea cannot be rejected that such special centers as Ammon's horn, and perhaps also the interhemispheric cortex, regions that do not receive direct sensory fibers but association fibers coming from sensory areas (centers of projection of Flechsig), may have an associative or memory function (in the sense of the theory of Flechsig.).

[Our point of view on the existence of centers of association in the rodents has been accepted by O. Vogt, Mme. Vogt, and, in general, by all the anatomists who have used the myelogenetic method of Flechsig in the rodents and other small gyrencephalic mammals. These authorities have seen, in effect, that the cerebrum of these animals includes zones with a precocious myelination and intermediate zones with late myelination, that is to say, sensory or projection centers and centers of association [respectively].

[In the last few years, the cerebrum of the lissencephalic mammals has been much studied with the aid of the methods of Nissl and Weigert. We shall give a summary of the results furnished by these investigations.

[Hermanides and Köppen[4] distinguish in the cerebrum of the rodents four different types of cortex, which they call the *motor type;* the *superior occipital type,* the *visual type,* and the *olfactory type.*

[Köppen and Löwenstein[5] have also differentiated in the ungulates and carnivores several cortical regions that correspond in large part to sensory areas.

[The work of Elliot Smith,[6] confirmed by Ziehen,[7] Zuckerkandl,[8] Kappers and Theunissen,[9] Livini,[10] and other authors has shown that in the marsupials and monotremes, the cerebral cortex considerably degenerates and shows arrangements that very much resemble those of the reptiles. Thus, the corpus callosum is lacking in the marsupials; in them, the commissural fibers destined to associate the several areas of the neopallium [of the two sides] are, therefore, completely lacking. They are replaced by the dorsal psalterium and the anterior commissure, commissural pathways belonging to the archipallium. In addition, the fascia dentata forms, in *Ornithorhynchus,* a protuberance on the medial face of the hemispheres and appears as a fascicle that goes around the thalamus from the frontal pole to the temporal extremity. Above the fascia denata, on the medial face of the hemispheres, is seen the *fissure of the hippocampus,* forming the inferior limit of a cortical region that is homologous to the hippocampal gyrus in the mammals. With regard to Ammon's horn, which lies adjacent to this region of cortex, it is also found on the internal face of the hemispheres, but hidden behind the fascia dentata. It results from this arrangement that the archipallium of *Ornithorhynchus* includes not only the inferior region of the cerebrum or piriform lobule but also the internal and superior faces of the hemispheres. The neopallium, of relatively little extent, is displaced, in this animal, to the lateral surface of the cerebrum; below, it is separated from the archipallium by the *external rhinal fissure,* [which is] extremely distinct.

[The marsupials possess an analogous cerebral organization, although a little less marked. Thus, in *Hypsiprymnus rufescens,* the fascia dentata does not form a protuberance into the interhemispheric fissure; it is a little displaced laterally, and it is covered, like Ammon's horn, by a cortex of gray matter that is probably homologous to the hippocampal gyrus.

[Also, in the marsupials, the olfactory centers become highly developed, to such an extent that a very distinct accessory lobe exists in their olfactory bulb, as Kappers and Theunissen have demonstrated.][E]

Cerebral Cortex of Birds

The cerebrum of the birds is characterized by the enormous size of the corpus striatum, the absence of an Ammon's horn or at least of a gray territory capable of being easily homologized with this center of the mammals, and the lack of a corpus callosum. With respect to the cortex in the strict sense, it is hardly more differentiated than that in the reptiles and batrachians, appearing dorsally and laterally adherent to the corpus striatum or basal ganglion, except on the medial face of the hemispheres, where a ventricular prolongation separates it from the [corpus striatum].

Only a limited description, which we are now going to summarize, has been made of this restricted cortical region, which could be called *interhemispheric or fissural cortex.*

Sala y Pons,[11] who studied the cerebrum of birds by means of the Golgi method, distinguishes in a perpendicular section of the above-mentioned region the following layers: first, *plexiform layer;* second, *layer of the small stellate cells;* third, *layer of the large stellate and pyramidal cells;* fourth, *layer of the deep stellate cells;* fifth, *epithelial layer.*

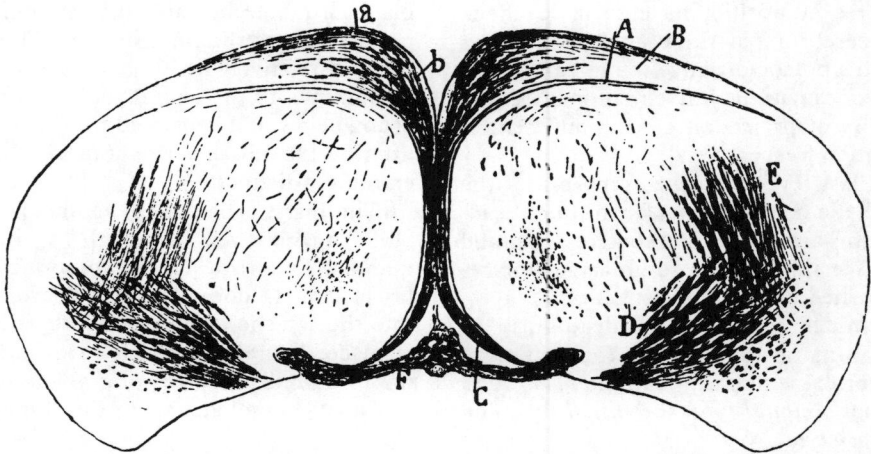

[*FIG. 230*]   Fig. 848. Frontal section through the middle region of the cerebrum; adult chicken. Weigert-Pal method. (Reproduced from Cl. Sala.) *A*, ventricle; *B*, supraventricular cerebral cortex; *C*, septomesencephalic fascicle; *D*, descending fibrillary bundles of the inferior fascicle of the cerebrum; *E*, superior descending bundles; *F*, tela choroidea; *a*, myelinated fibers; *b*, molecular layer.

1. Molecular or Plexiform Layer

It corresponds to the layer of the same name in the cerebrum of mammals, and in it are arborized the terminal dendrites of the cells with long axon of the underlying layers and not a few terminal nerve fibers.

The ascending dendrites distributed in the molecular layer do not originate from [apical] dendritic shafts but directly from the cell bodies of the stellate cells.[F]

With respect to the nerve fibers, [which are] mainly tangential, they represent either terminal branches of the cells with ascending axon, or collaterals originating along the course of ascending fibers, continuous, as we will see later, with the projection pathway, or, finally, superficial small axonal branches of cells with short axon. But the plexiform layer also exhibits a large number of medullated parallel fibers or fibers en passant, which originate from pyramidal cells and invade all layers of the cortex, including the plexiform layer.

The cited layer also contains special large fusiform cells, homologous to the horizontal cells of the cortex of mammals, and some cells with short axon.

2. Layer of the Small Stellate Cells

It consists of stellate or rarely fusiform cells provided with numerous dendrites that divide dichotomously and radiate in all directions: the ascending, in number two, three, or more, gain the plexiform layer; the descending can reach down beyond the third layer (fig. 849, *d*) [*fig. 231*]. With regard to the axon, after a variable descending course, it continues as a fiber of projection, entering the descending bundles of white matter that make up the *sagittal fascicle* or *septomesencephalic fascicle* of Edinger. Before entering the said bundles, it gives off three, four, or more collaterals, either ascending or descending, that by their ramifications help to form a dense nerve plexus in the upper half of the cortex. In some cells, the axon, after a short distance, seems to resolve itself into a free arborization of great extent, behaving like that of the so-called sensory [cells] of Golgi.

3. Layer of the Large Pyramidal and Stellate Cells

This layer contains the most voluminous cells of the cortex and those with the longest pro-

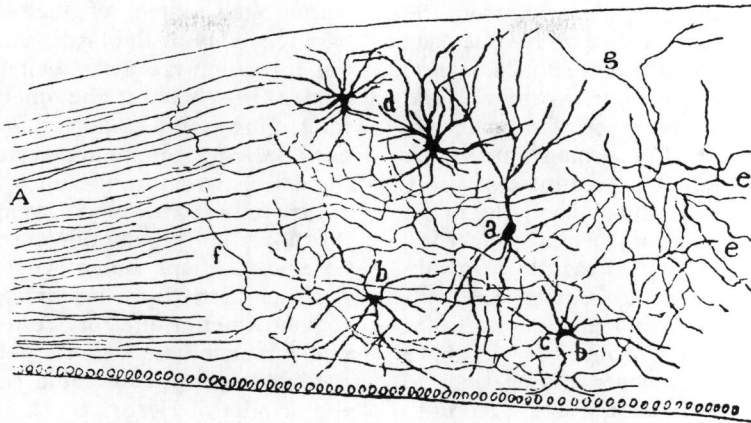

[*FIG. 231*]   Fig. 849. Frontal section of a part of the cerebral cortex; newborn chicken. The inferior portion is on the left. *A*, origin of the septomesencephalic fascicle; *a*, pyramidal cell; *b*, deep stellate cells; *c*, [*d*], superficial stellate cells; *e*, axons arising from pyramidal cells and destined for the septomesencephalic fascicle.

cesses. Regarding the shape, as can be seen in fig. 849, *a* [*fig. 231*], it is very variable; there are perfect pyramidal cells, resembling those of the cerebrum of mammals, since, like these, they have a thick ascending [dendritic] shaft and a triangular cell body provided with long descending processes, but a more or less vertically elongated stellate form is more common. In either case, these cells are distinguished by their long processes, of which the descending can approach the very epithelial [layer], after dividing dichotomously several times.

The axon behaves essentially as in the cells of the second layer; it is directed downward, giving off during its course two, three, or more collaterals, and after some bends, it becomes descending to enter the little bundles of the sagittal fascicle already mentioned. Sometimes, a collateral originating at the point of inflexion of the axon runs outward, that is to say, in the direction of the most lateral regions of the cortex; perhaps it represents a fiber of association.

4. Layer of the Deep Stellate Cells (fig. 849, *b*) [*fig. 231*]

It consists of small or medium stellate cells, which, on account of the behavior of the axon,

it is possible to classify as three types: (a) cells with an axon of projection that enters the septomesencephalic fascicle; (b) cells with short axon forming a broad nerve arborization; and (c) small cells with an axon resolving into a fine and dense arborization.

5. Epithelial Layer

As in the mammals, in young birds, the epithelial [layer] consists of elongated radial cells that extend from the ventricle to the cerebral surface. But this disposition is still embryonic, [and] it may be assumed that in the adult, as in the mammals, the peripheral epithelial extremity is atrophied. In addition to these cells, stellate neuroglial cells, which recall completely those of the plexiform layer of the mammals, are still seen dispersed throughout the gray matter, as well as certain elongated cells in the process of migration which represent the phases of transition between the ependymal cells and the adult neuroglial cells.

Pathways Originating in the Cortex

The axons coming from the external or inferolateral regions of the cortex gain, according to Edinger's observations,[12,13] the corpus striatum, in which their behavior is unknown.

With respect to the [axons] coming from the interhemispheric cortex that we have already described, they gather together in a sagittal fascicle, and are carried anteroposteriorly and downward with it to reach the midbrain, where, as Edinger has demonstrated, [the fascicle] bends laterally to terminate in a special thalamic ganglion and probably also in the cortex of the optic lobe (fig. 848, C)[G] [fig. 230].

The significance of this sagittal tract, observed some time ago by Bumm and confirmed by all the authors, is not known. Edinger, Wallenberg, and Holmes,[14] who have dedicated a careful and penetrating study to the cerebrum of birds, are not able to tell us to which pathway of mammals the septomesencephalic tract should correspond, nor do they dare compare it with the fornix, with which at first glance it shows some analogy. They are forced to this prudent reserve, on the one hand, by the absence of an Ammon's horn in birds and, on the other hand, by the lack of connections of the said septo[mesencephalic fascicle] with the mamillary apparatus. It seems to us more likely (although this homology is not certain either) that the above-mentioned *tractus* represents the projection portion of the cingulum of mammals, that is to say, the *fornix longus* of Forel, a pathway that, as we have noted, is none other than the ensemble of the axons of projection of the most inferior portion of the interhemispheric cortex.

A corpus callosum does not exist in the birds. There are, however, two commissural bundles probably belonging to the system of the anterior commissure. One of these, the *commissura pallii*, discovered by Meckel [and also] observed by Bumm, Osborn, Münzer and Wiener, and well described by Edinger, comes from the cortex of the most posterior portion of the cerebrum and appears to be destined to link the occipital portions of the cerebrum; the other, more robust, comes from a voluminous special nucleus of the corpus striatum (*epistriatum* or *nucleus rotundus*), visible in all the lower vertebrates and considered by Herrick as a rudiment of Ammon's horn.

According to Edinger, the *epistriatum*, together with three other very extensive gray nuclei, named *hyperstriatum* or superior, *mesostriatum*, and *ectostriatum*, would make up the complicated system of the *fundamental* or basal *ganglion* of the birds, animals in which this formation reaches a really colossal development in relation to the other cerebral territories. However, it could very well happen that not all the above-mentioned nuclei belong to the corpus striatum; the nucleus rotundus or epistriatum, from which a good proportion of the fibers of the anterior commissure originate, is perhaps homologous to Ammon's horn, or perhaps to the olfactory association region (superior olfactory cortex of the mammals). If such homology should be confirmed, the cited commissure could be compared, in the manner of Herrick, to the *ventral psalterium* or interammonic commissure of the mammals. Moreover, we must not forget that, in the mammals, the corpus striatum lacks a commissural system [which justifies this analogy.][H]

The other regions of the cortex, [which are] still not studied from the histological point of view, send their bundles of axons to the corpus striatum, where they intermingle and become confused with the striothalamic tracts and other striosagittal pathways discovered by Edinger in all vertebrates.

Cerebral Cortex of Reptiles

According to Edinger, the cerebral cortex of the reptiles resembles quite closely that of the mammals, although, as may be assumed, it possesses a notably simplified architecture. This similarity, which extends to the fine details of structure, as the investigations of my brother have shown beyond doubt, gives to the study of the cerebrum of the reptiles a capital importance for the elucidation of the fundamental plan of the organ of the mind in the higher vertebrates.[I]

Unfortunately, this analysis is not finalized, but we possess at present some valuable contributions to it, among which, because of their importance and thoroughness, we must cite those of Edinger[15] and my brother,[16] our own,[17] those of Neumayer,[18] Meyer,[19] Bottazzi,[20] and, above all, the older anatomists such as Stieda and Rabl-Rückhard,[21] who have also contributed not a little to promote the study.

The cerebral cortex of the reptiles includes several regions: the *supero-internal* [region] *(mediodorsal cortex)*, the *laterodorsal* [region], the *inferior or basal* [region], and the *internal or septal* [region]. It is not our intention to describe in detail such territories, but to point out briefly the main components of one of them, the supero-internal [region], which is so far the best analyzed.

A frontal section of this cerebral region shows the following layers: first, *superficial plexiform* [layer]; second, [layer] *of the pyramidal cells;* third, *deep plexiform* [layer]; fourth, *white matter;* and fifth, *ventricular ependyma* (fig. 850) [*fig. 232*].

1. Superficial Plexiform [Layer]

It forms a broad peripheral band perfectly demarcated from the underlying [layer] of the pyramidal cells [*fig. 232, A*]. Its structure, as we pointed out, coincides perfectly with the corresponding layer of mammals, since it is also made up of the interweaving of the following elements: (a) [dendritic] tufts of the pyramidal cells; (b) dendritic processes of intrinsic horizontal cells; (c) axonal arborizations coming from the axons of Martinotti; (d) recurrent [axon] collaterals. We should also add the arborizing terminal portions of the ependymal cells.

The cells of this layer, well studied by my brother, correspond to three different types: (a) cell with a long axon and a stellate or triangular shape, lying in the deeper third of the first layer and which can be considered as a displaced pyramid; (b) horizontal fusiform cells (fig. 850, *a*) [*fig. 232*], provided with long, smooth dendrites and with a tangential axon arborizing exclusively inside [the confines] of this layer; (c) dwarf stellate cells (discovered by my brother), furnished with fine and very short dendrites and a delicate axon [that is] rarely well stained and, on the whole, comparable to the dwarf cells described by us in the human cerebral cortex (fig. 850, *l*) [*fig. 232*].

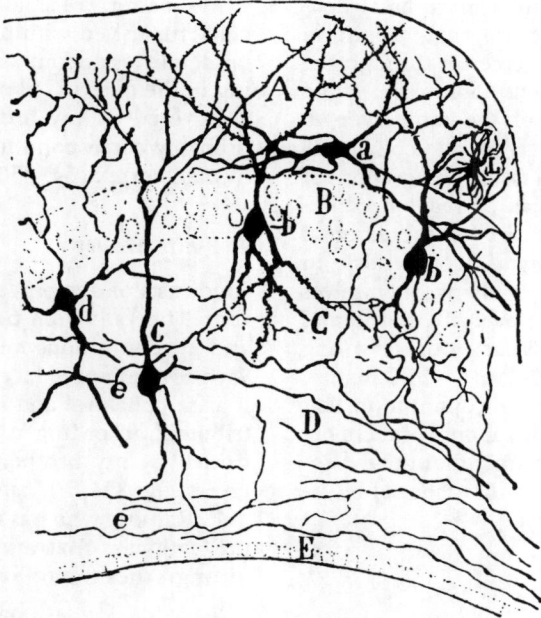

[*FIG. 232*] Fig. 850. Portion of a frontal section of the cerebral cortex of the chameleon *(Chamaeleo vulgaris)*. Golgi method. *A*, superficial plexiform layer; *B*, layer of the pyramidal cells; *C*, deep plexiform layer; *D*, white matter; *E*, ventricular ependyma; *a*, horizontal fusiform cells; *b*, pyramidal cell provided with a recurrent collateral to the molecular layer; *c*, pyramidal cell of the deep plexiform layer; *d*, neurons with ascending axon; *e*, branch of bifurcation of an axon running in the white matter.

With regard to the nerve fibers, there are three sources: some simply represent recurrent [axonal] collaterals of pyramids (fig. 850,b)[J] [fig. 232]; others are the terminal arborizations of the axons of Martinotti (fig. 850, d)[K] [fig. 232]; and, finally, the majority represent the terminal branches of [commissural] or association fibers arriving from the white matter (fig. 850, e) [fig. 232].

2. Layer of the Pyramidal Cells

It consists of an accumulation of cells arranged in three or four rows (fig. 850, B) [fig. 232], which resemble in their shape and packing density the cells of Ammon's horn of small mammals. Among them are observed spindle, triangular, and globular shapes and, above all, pyramidal shapes, which abound in the deeper parts of this layer. Except for the most superficial [cells], which are commonly furnished with two or more radial dendrites, the others show a thick [radial dendritic] shaft that breaks up into a tuft of spiny dendrites in the plexiform layer; one, two, rarely more basal dendrites aborizing in the internal plexiform layer; and an axon that descends through the underlying layers and gets lost in the white matter. Like the axon of the same type in mammals, this axon gives off collaterals, among which, according to the observations of P. Ramón, three kinds can be recognized: *recurrent* [collaterals] destined for the external plexiform layer; *horizontal* [collaterals], in number two or three, resolving themselves into arborizations at the level of the internal plexiform layer; and *association* or very long [collaterals], arising in the very white matter, where they run in directions opposite to that of the main axon or [main] axonal branch, because it is observed frequently that these association collaterals represent branches of bifurcation of the axonal trunk.

3. Deep Plexiform Layer (fig. 850, C) [fig. 232]

It could also be called *layer of the giant cells*, since in it are contained the most voluminous pyramids of the cortex, along with a very dense nerve plexus.

This plexus, [which is] very dense in the medial parts of this cortical region and less dense toward its outer borders, results from the interweaving of four kinds of fibers: collateral axonal arborizations coming from the axons of the pyramids; collaterals and terminal branches continuous with association fibers of the white matter; terminal and collateral branches belonging to commissural or callosal fibers; and, finally, extensive arborizations originating from thick fibers coming from the region of the septum, and which perhaps [are] continuous with sensory fibers.

Many of these fibers do not limit themselves to arborizing in the third layer and adding complexity to the plexus existing there, but they also furnish radial branches that, after crossing through the pyramids, finally terminate in the superficial plexiform layer.

With regard to the cells, they belong to two categories: (a) large pyramidal cells provided with a radial [dendritic] shaft [that reaches] the plexiform layer, some basal dendrites, and a robust axon continuous with a fiber of the white matter; (b) smaller globular or fusiform cells, furnished with descending and horizontal dendrites and an ascending axon terminating in the external plexiform layer. Such cells, discovered by my brother in *Lacerta agilis*,[L] probably correspond to Martinotti cells of the human cortex (fig. 850, d) [fig. 232].

4. White Matter

It consists of a supraventricular plane of horizontal fibers, which becomes denser medially and is continuous medially and downward with several nerve fascicles or pathways. From it arise collateral and terminal [branches], distributed, according to our observations, confirmed by my brother, in the two plexiform layers (fig. 851, E) [fig. 233].

P. Ramón, who has made a detailed study of the pathways that arise in this white matter, distinguishes the following pathways.

1. Homolateral Association Pathway

It consists of lateral branches of bifurcation of axons of pyramids which run laterally to terminate probably in the lateral cortical region (*laterodorsal cortex*).

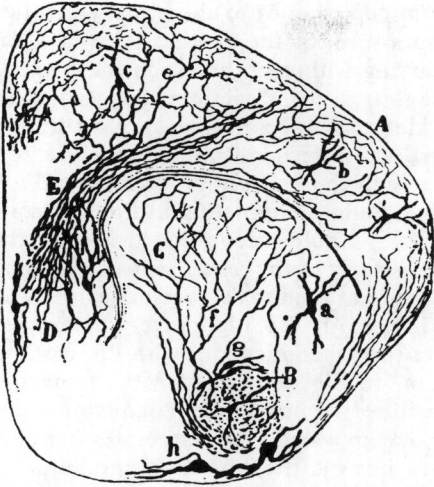

[FIG. 233]   Fig. 851. Frontal section of the cerebrum of the chameleon (Chamaeleo vulgaris). Golgi method. A, lateral region of the cortex; B, basal fascicle; C, fundamental ganglion or corpus striatum; D, region of the septum; E, white matter of the medial cortical region; a, cell of the fundamental ganglion; b, pyramidal cell of the external region of the cortex; c, pyramidal cell of the medial region of the cortex (fascia dentata of certain authors); d, collaterals of the white matter forming the molecular layer; e, terminal fiber coming from the white matter; f, fiber of the basal fascicle ramifying in the basal ganglion; g, cells enveloping the basal fascicle.

2. Longitudinal Association Pathway (Sagittal Bundle of P. Ramón)

This bundle, described by Edinger and located near the midline in the fundus of the interhemispheric fissure, gathers together a large proportion of the axons of the fissural cortex (fig. 852, FM) [fig. 234] and, running sagittally backward, terminates in the occipital region of the cerebrum. Because of its origin, position, and termination, it could be compared with the cingulum of mammals, from which also arises, as we have already said, a system of fibers destined to link the poles of the hemispheres.

3. Contralateral Association Pathway or Corpus Callosum

It consists of thick fibers originating both in the fissural cortical region and in lateral cere-

bral territories, and it describes an arch that inferiorly embraces the sagittal pathway (fig. 852, AC) [fig. 234]; [once] its fibers arrive on the contralateral side, they terminate by means of branches of such length that they embrace, in the opinion of P. Ramón, almost the whole dorsal cortex.

4. Direct and Crossed Pathway of Projection

As seen in fig. 852, FC and FD [fig. 234], a number of the fibers of the white matter arriving from the dorsomedial cortex are directed downward through the septum and reach the basal fascicle or main motor pathway, with which they descend to lower nuclei. It is seen that the said pathway consists of direct fibers (FD) and crossed fibers (FC). Such pathways, first distinguished by my brother and confirmed by Edinger, represent perhaps the for-

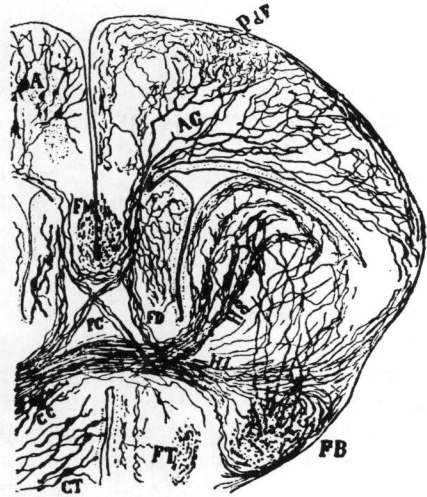

[FIG. 234]   Fig. 852. Frontal section of the cerebrum of the stump lizard (Lacerta stirpium). Golgi method. A, superomedial cortex; AC, callosal fibers arborizing in the opposite hemisphere; CC, cells whose axon is directed to the anterior commissure; CT, cells of the optic thalamus with horizontal axon; FM, sagittal or mesencephalic fascicle of Edinger; FC, crossed fascicles of the commissural system; FD, descending fascicles destined for the basal fascicle; FB, basal fascicle or bundle; FT, thalamic fibers; HI, inferior fascicle of the anterior commissure; HS, fascicle of the commissure destined for the spherical nucleus; PdF, terminal nerve plexus of the medial cellular region of the cortex.

nix longus of Forel of the higher vertebrates, that is, the projection portion of the *cingulum.*

Anterior Commissure

The cerebrum of the reptiles also has a true and very robust anterior commissure that is made up of two planes of fibers: *superior,* which represents a junctional bridge between the two rotundus nuclei (fig. 852, *HS*) [*fig. 234*]; and *inferior,* which contains fibers destined to join both olfactory or sphenoidal cortices (fig. 852, *HI*) [*fig. 234*].

Let us add also the *posterior pallial commissure,* which links the occipital extremities of the cortex and which could well correspond to the dorsal psalterium, especially if it should be proven that the said cortical region corresponds to the superior olfactory area of the cerebrum of mammals.

Other Regions of the Cortex

According to my brother, a similar histology is found in the laterodorsal cortex (fig. 851, *A*) [*fig. 233*], although without the regularity of the layers. Its pyramidal cells, of irregular shape, also send their axons to the white matter and in the directions of the sagittal bundle and corpus callosum.

Homology of the Superointernal Cortical Region

The general opinion put forward by Spitzka[22] and Edinger[23] and very ingeniously upheld by Meyer[24] and Smith[25] is that this cortical region represents the rudimentary Ammon's horn of the reptiles. According to Smith, the region would consist of two separate areas: one superolateral which corresponds to Ammon's horn, and the other medial or fissural, continuous with the preceding and made up of smaller and more close-packed pyramids, which represent the *granule cells* of the fascia dentata. This homology is based on [the appearances in] a mammal, *Ornithorhynchus,* in which the fascia dentata is found to be in continuity with Ammon's horn at certain places of the fissural or medial cortex, and in which, in those vertebrates that lack a corpus callosum, the position of the interammonic commissure or psal-

terium corresponds to the already-mentioned [commissure] of the reptiles. Mayer, without specifying with such precision the region homologous to the fascia dentata, also upholds the idea that in reptiles lacking a corpus callosum, the interhemispheric commissure has the role of the psalterium. With regard to the sagittal bundle originating in the said cortical region, it would [according to Meyer] correspond simply to the *fornix (anterior columns of the fornix* of mammals), a pathway that in the reptiles, as in the higher vertebrates, establishes special connections with the septum lucidum. In the opinion of Meyer, the fornix constitutes the first cerebral pathway of projection that appears in the vertebrates, just as Ammon's horn is the first differentiated cortex. The reptiles would still be bereft of an internal capsule, that is to say, of a projection pathway originating in the lateral portions of the cortex.

[Many others histologists, among them Kappers and Theunissen,[26] have accepted and upheld the concept of analogy in recent years.]^M

Without being unaware of the force of the reasons claimed by the authors in favor of the cited homologies, it is necessary to confess that the problem is not definitively solved, and that the topic is still open to other conjectures. Reasons as persuasive as those cited by Edinger, Meyer, and Smith, in our opinion, also argue in favor of the identification of the [superointernal] cortex [of the reptiles] with the *fissural or interhemispheric cortex* of the mammals, a cortex whose structure, in the mouse and guinea pig, is very similar, certainly, to that described in the reptiles (see fig. 832) [*fig. 188* in chapter 18].

In effect, this cortex occupies in the mammals the same place as in the reptiles and birds; it also possesses two plexiform layers; it likewise lies above the corpus callosum and, finally, gives origin to two systems of fibers: one sagittal and associative, the *cingulum,* and the other descending or projective, the *fornix longus* of Forel. Notice that the argument of Meyer (that the fornix is always connected with the septum) turns also in favor of our conjecture, since, like the *fornix longus* of Forel, the pathway of projection of the interhemispheric commissure is always connected with the septum. Finally, let us remember that in the reptiles and birds, in spite of the suppositions of Meyer, Smith, Brill, etc., nobody has proven the existence of a true fascia dentata. My brother, who has analyzed most carefully the fine structure of the fissural cortical region, has not been able to find any essential difference with respect to the cellular morphology and behavior of the axon between the pyramids of the superior and inferior portions of the supero-internal cortex. Never was it seen, for example, that the axons of the cells of the inferior [portion] are continuous with mossy fibers, terminating by means of free arborizations on the pyramids of the superior cortical portion; this feature is definitely known to be essential and characteristic of the granule cells of the fascia dentata, but it seems to me that Edinger, Meyer, Brill, and Smith have not paid attention to it.

Cerebral Cortex of Batrachians

The structure of the cerebral cortex of the batrachians is quite well known, thanks to the investigations of Oyarzun,[27] confirmed and extended in some points by ourselves,[28] Calleja,[29] and Berder,[30] and, above all, by my brother,[31] who is the one who has examined the subject most carefully. In regard to the general homology of the cerebrum of the amphibia, as well as the origin and course of the long pathways to which it gives rise, important contributions are also due to Stieda,[32] Osborn,[33] Edinger,[34] and Köppen.[35]

As Edinger, [Kappers, and the other authors][N] have noted, the construction of the cerebral gray cortex of the vertebrates begins in the amphibia. [There would be found, in effect, as in the reptiles, the olfactory centers of the three orders, because, according to Kappers, the fissural region of the cortex is in connection very particularly with the fibers coming from the secondary olfactory centers. This cortical region would thus represent a rudimentary Ammon's horn, very imperfect, it is true, since the cells there are not arranged in regular layers and since the fascia dentata is not differentiated.][O]

From the point of view of structure, this gray cortex displays naturally a more simple and elemental aspect. But this simplicity is rather related to the [smaller][P] number of cells and their processes than to the disposition or nature of the elements that form the *substratum* of higher[Q] nerve functions.

The cerebral cortex of the amphibia (frog, salamander, newt, etc.) is composed of three fundamental layers, which are, from deep to superficial; first, *epithelial* [layer]; second, [layer] of *the granule or pyramidal cells;* third, *molecular or plexiform* [layer]. The last is the thickest and contains an occasional nerve cell, as already recognized by Stieda.

1. Epithelial Layer

This layer, well described by Oyarzun, consists of a row of robust, triangular, or club-shaped cells that line the ventricular surface. Each cell gives off at its base one or perhaps several ciliated processes, which in our preparations are always folded back (fig. 853, *B*) [*fig. 235*]; and from its apex [arises] a thick and rough shaft directed toward the surface and complexly arborized; its final little branches [which are] velvety and varicose, reach the free surface where they expand in the form of a cone or cylinder (fig. 853, *B*) [*fig. 235*].

These epithelial cells make up the only supporting network of the cortex, and [the processes] form a large part of the plexiform layer, a circumstance first demonstrated by Oyarzun and confirmed by my brother.

2. Layer of the Granule Cells or Cerebral Pyramids

It is equivalent to the [layer] of the pyramids of reptiles and mammals. It contains triangular or elongated cells, whose base and apex give rise to two, three, or more [dendritic] shafts, notably branched and spiny, whose branches, as Oyarzun has well described, go up to the plexiform layer, where they end freely (fig. 853, *C*, *D*) [*fig. 235*].

The size of the cells decreases from deep to superficial, as occurs in the layers of the pyramids of mammals. The largest cells contact the cell bodies of the epithelial cells. The number of cells also decreases from deep to su-

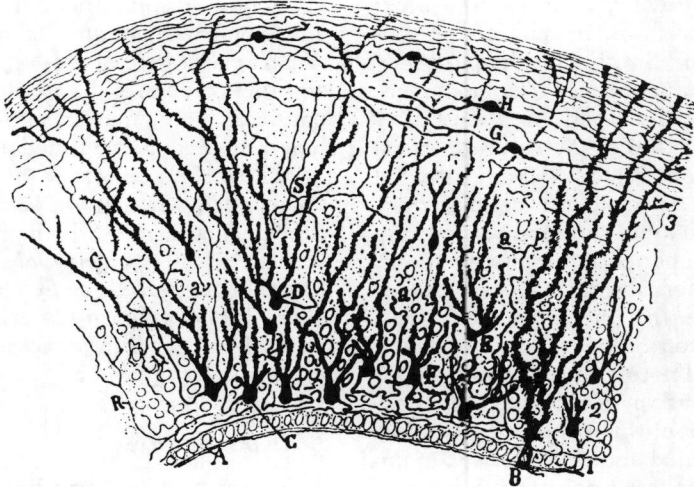

[*FIG. 235*]   Fig. 853. Transverse section of the superolateral region of the cerebral cortex of the frog *(Rana)*. Golgi method. *1*, ventricular epithelium; *2*, layer of the granules or pyramidal cells; *3*, molecular layer; *A*, ependymal layer; *B*, epithelial cell with in-curved cilium; *C*, cells whose axons ascend to the plexiform layer, where they ramify; *D*, cell whose axon ramifies in an S shape; *E*, cell whose axon first descends, then rapidly ascends and bifurcates in the superficial region of the layer of the granules; *F*, cell whose axon ascends to acquire rapidly an anteroposterior direction; *G*, horizontal cell of the molecular layer in which it was not possible to see the axon; *H, J*, other [horizontal] cells provided with an axon; *R*, collaterals of axons of pyramidal cells; *S*, axonal arborization of a cell with short axon, *D*. The letter *a* indicates anterior; the letter *p*, posterior.

perficial, until, by means of smooth gradations, a layer is reached in which only random, scattered, and rare cells are seen (plexiform layer).

The axon has been observed by Oyarzun, who claims that it is directed backward, forming anteroposterior bundles of nerve fibers. This fact is true, but we believe only for some cells commonly located in the upper part of the layer of the pyramids. In fact, the vast majority of the pyramids send their axons to the first layer, where they run tangentially over long distances. As is seen in fig. 853, *C* [*fig. 235*], this process arises from the base or lateral [side] of the soma, frequently descends for a short distance, and, after a variable horizontal course, bends to become radial and goes up to the plexiform layer, not without having provided in its course several collaterals distributed among the companion cells and at levels close to the plexiform [layer].

Where are the axons of these cells going to end? There is no doubt that while they course

in the first layer, they ramify prolixly, but their termination cannot be confirmed with certainty. In our opinion, the majority of such fibers make up a superficial pathway directed backward and downward and possibly incorporated into the basal fascicle. According to P. Ramón, many of these fibers would engender in the lateroventral region of the anterior [cerebral] vesicle a bundle, which he calls *lateral* [fascicle] and which, having arrived at the midbrain, would join with a peduncular pathway, originating, as is known, primarily in the basal or primordial ganglion.

The layer of the pyramids is inhabited by other cellular forms, well described by my brother, such as globular cells with ascending axon arborizing in the first layer (perhaps comparable to the cells of Martinotti) and globular or stellate cells furnished with numerous descending dendrites. Nor do cells with short axon seem to be lacking, according to what Calleja and my brother have indicated.

Plexiform Layer

It is thickest of all and is not as well delimited in the deeper part as in reptiles and mammals. It possesses the [cellular] elements so many times mentioned above, namely (a) terminal [dendritic] tufts of pyramids that extend sometimes to the free surface; (b) very numerous axonal arborizations; (c) tangential or en passant fibers and two kinds of cells with short axon: the horizontal fusiform type provided with a semilong axon distributed in the first layer, and the spheroidal type with short axon distributed at no great distance from its origin (fig. 853, *J. H. G*) [*fig. 235*]. P. Ramón also points out in this layer displaced pyramids, whose axon first descends and later goes up, and dwarf stellate cells of unknown character.

In short, and in order not to extend this description too greatly, the cortex of the batrachians corresponds in broad outline to that of the reptiles and mammals, but with the important exception that the first or plexiform layer is more complex than [in the reptiles and mammals], because it is composed of two formations: the axodendritic plexus characteristic of the first layer of man and higher vertebrates, and the white matter [made up] of projection and association [fibers]. As a consequence of this displacement of the white [matter], the axons of the pyramids are turned upside down and give rise to collaterals, not below but above the cell [body]. For the rest, this superficial position of the [white] matter, which calls to mind the situation of the tracts of the spinal cord, is also found, although not so accentuated, in certain regions of the cortex of the mammals (exogenous fibers distributed in Ammon's horn and fascia dentata, sphenoidal cortex covered by the lateral olfactory tract, etc.).

Cortex of Fish[R]

In general, the existence of a *pallium* or cerebral cortex in the strict sense is denied in fish. This important cerebral region, in which reside the higher mental activities, has in these animals still not left the primitive epithelial phase. It would possess, as a consequence, only the basal region of the cerebrum, the *hypo-spherium* of Edinger or *archipallium* of Smith, corresponding to the piriform lobe, to the paraolfactory regions, and to the corpus striatum of higher vertebrates. However, there are authors, such as Studnička,[36] who believe that in the cerebrum[S] of *Petromyzon* and *Protopterus* there exists a rudiment of gray matter formed by some little groups of nerve cells, which he considers homologous to pyramidal cells of the higher vertebrates. In the urodeles, which from this point of view more resemble the fishes than the batrachians, Nakagaba[37] also discovered, on the internal face of the hemispheres, a rudiment of gray matter. But to pronounce sentence definitively on this case, it would be necessary to apply the method of Golgi to the staining of the above-mentioned cells, both in the urodeles and in the fishes, and confirm with it the morphological features of pyramidal cells. So far, the silver chromate has been impotent to elucidate this point.

Cajal's Notes

1. S. R. Cajal, Les nouvelles idées sur la structure de système nerveux, etc., translation by Dr. L. Azoulay, Paris, 1894, p. 52.
2. Döllken, Beiträge zur Entwickelung des Säugergehirns; Lage und Ausdehnung des Bewegungscentrums der Maus, *Neurol. Centralbl.*, no. 2, 1907.
3. S. R. Cajal, Structure de l'écorce cérébrale de quelques mammifères, *La Cellule*, Vol. VII, 1891.
4. Hermanides and Köppen, Ueber die Furchen und über den Bau der Grosshirnrinde bei den Lissencephalen, insbesondere über die Lokalisation des motorischen Centrums und der Sehregion, *Arch. F. Psychiatrie*, Vol. XXXVII, pt. 2, 1903.
5. Köppen and Löwenstein, Studien über den Zellenbau der Grosshirnrinde bei den Ungulaten und Carnivoren, etc., *Monatschrift f. Psychiatrie u. Neurol.*, Vol. XVIII, pt. 6, 190[5].
6. Elliot Smith, A Preliminary Communication upon the Cerebral Commissures of the Mammalia with Special Reference to the Monotremata and Marsupialia, *Proceed. of the Linnean Society of New South Wales*, 2 Series, Vol. IX, 1894. The Origin of the Corpus Callosum; a Comparative Study of the Hippocampal Region of the Cerebrum of Marsupialia and Certain Cheiroptera, *Transact. of Linn. Society London*, Vol. VII, part 3, [1897]. The Fascia Dentata, *Anat. Anzeiger*, Vol. XII, 1896.
7. Ziehen, Das Zentralnervensystem der Monotremen und Marsupialier, *Denkschr d. Mediz Naturwiss. Gesellsch.*, Jena Vol. VI, 1901.
8. Zuckerkandl, Die Rindenbündel des Alveus bei Beuteltieren, *Anat. Anzeiger*, Vol. XXIII, 1903.

9. Kappers and Theunissen, Zur vergleichenden Anatomie des Vorderhirns der Vertebraten, *Anat. Anzeiger,* Vol. XXX, 1907. Die Phylogenese des Rhinencephalons, des Corpus striatum, etc., *Folia Neurobiologica,* Vol. I, no. 2, 1908.

10. Livini, Il proencefalo di un Marsupiale, *Arch. di Anat. e. di Embriologia,* Vol. VI, pt. 4, 1907.

11. Cl. Sala y Pons, La corteza cerebral de las aves, Madrid, 1893.

12. L. Edinger, Sur l'Anatomie comparée du corps strié (cerveau des oiseaux) [1903].

13. L. Edinger, Ueber die Herkunft des Hirnmantels in dem Tierreiche, *Berl. Klin., Wochenschr.,* no. 43, 1905. [This reference was added to the French version of the book.]

14. Edinger, Wallenberg, and Holmes, Das Vorderhirn der Vogel, *Abhandl. d. Senckenbergisch. Naturforsch. Gesellsch.,* Frankfurt a/M., Vol. XX, 1903.

15. Edinger, Untersuchungen über die vergleichende Anatomie des Gehirns. I. Das Vorderhirn, *Abhandl. d. Senckenbergisch. Naturforsch. Gesellsch.,* Frankfurt a/M., 188[9]. Neue Studien über das Vorderhirn der Reptilien, Frankfurt A/M., 1896.

16. P. Ramón, El encéfalo de los reptiles, Barcelona, 1891. Estructura del encéfalo del camaleón, *Rev. Trim Micrográf.,* Vol. I, 1896.

17. S. R. Cajal, Pequeñas contribuciones al conocimiento del sistema nervioso, 1891.

18. Neumayer, Die Grosshirnrinde der niederen Vertebraten, *Sitzungsber. d. Gesellsch. f. Morphol. u. Physiol.,* München, 1895.

19. A. Meyer, Zur Homologie der Fornixcommisur u. des Septum lucidum bei den Reptilien u. Säugern, *Anat. Anzeiger,* Vol. X, 1895.

20. Stieda, Ueber den Bau des centralen Nervensystems der Schildkröte. *Zeitsch. f.Wissensch. Zool.,* Vol. XXV, 1868.

21. Rabl-Rückhard, Das centrale Nervensystem des Alligators, *Zeitsch. f. Wissensch. Zool.,* [1878] Vol. XXX.

22. Spitzka, *Journ. of Nervous and Mental Diseases,* 1880.

23. Edinger, Riechapparat u. Ammonshorn, *Anat. Anzeiger,* Vol. VIII, no. 10, 1893.

24. A. Meyer, *Zeitsch. f. Wissensch. Zool.,* Bd. LV, 189[3]. Zur Homologie der Fornixcommissur und des Septum lucidum bei den Reptilien und Säugern, *Anat. Anzeiger,* Vol. X, no. 15, 1895.

25. E. Smith, The Fascia Dentata; *Anat.Anzeiger,* Vol. XII, nos. 4 and 5, 1896.

26. Kappers and Theunissen, Die Phylogenese des Rhinencephalon, des Corpus striatum, etc. *Folia Neuro-biologica,* Vols. 1 and II, 1908.

27. Oyarzun, Ueber den feineren Bau des Vorderhirns der Amphibien, *Arch. Mikrosk. Anat.,* Vol. XXXV, 1890.

28. S. R. Cajal, Pequeñas contribuciones al concocimiento del sistema nervioso, etc. II: Estructura fundamental de la corteza cerebral de los batracios, reptiles y aves. August 1891, Barcelona.

29. Calleja, La región olfatoria del cerebro, Madrid, 1893.

30. Berder, La cellule nerveuse et quelques recherches sur les cellules des hémisphères de la grenouille, Thesis, Lausanne, 1893.

31. P.Ramón, Investigaciones micrográficas en el encéfalo de los batracios y reptiles, etc., Zaragoza, 1894. L'Encéphale des amphibiens, *Bibliogr. Anatomique,* no. 6, 1896. Ganglio basal de los batracios y fasciculo basal, *Rev. Trim. Micrográf.,* Vol. V, 1900.

32. Stieda, Studien über das Centralnervensystem der Wirbelthiere, Leipzig, 1870.

33. Osborn, A Contribution to the Internal Structure of the Amphibian Brain, 1888.

34. Edinger, Untersuchungen über die vergleichende Anatomie des Gehirns. I, Das Vorderhirn, 188[9].

35. Köppen, Zur Anatomie des Froschgehirns, *Arch. f. Anat. u. Entwickelungsgeschichte,* 18[88].

36. Studnička, Zur Geschichte des Cortex cerebri, *Verhandl. d. Anat. Gesellsch., Versamml. Strassburg,* 13–16 May 1894.

37. Nakagaba, *Journ. of Morphol.,* 1891.

Editors' Notes

A. The sentences in brackets are in the French version of the book but not in the Spanish version.

B. The lines in brackets are in the French version of the book but not in the Spanish version.

C. "Temporal olfactory cortex" in the French version of the book.

D. Strictly, perissodactyla, but Cajal probably means ungulates generally.

E. The seven paragraphs in brackets are in the French version of the book but not in the Spanish version.

F. This sentence is omitted from the French text.

G. This figure is not referred to in the French version of the book, where it is fig. 532.

H. The phrase in brackets was added to the French version of the book.

I. This paragraph is considerably modified in the French version.

J. Both Spanish and French texts incorrectly say *"c."*

K. The French text incorrectly says *"b."*

L. *"Stirpium"* in the French version.

M. The sentence in brackets was added to the French version.

N. The phrase in brackets was added to the French version.

O. The lines in brackets were added to the French version.

P. This word was added to the French version.

Q. The French version says "rudimentary."

R. The greater part of this section has been translated from the Spanish version of the book, since it is more extensive than the corresponding paragraph of the French version.

S. "Pallium" in the Spanish version.

24

Histogenesis of the Cerebral Cortex

[*From: Textura del sistema nervioso del hombre y de los vertebrados*
(Madrid: Moya, 1904), vol. 2, part 2, chap. 47, pp. 1110–1120; also published in
French as *Histologie du système nerveux de l'homme et des vertébrés*,
Vol. 2 (Paris: Maloine, 1911), chap. 35, pp. 847–861]

Development of the cerebral cortex in rodents and man.[A] *[Morphological and cytological]*[B] *differentiation of the nerve cells. Differentiation of the neuroglia. Parallelism in ontogeny and phylogeny.*

Development of the Cerebral Cortex[C]

The cerebral cortex represents the vault of the primitive anterior vesicle, whose basal portion, which thickens very early and protrudes into the ependymal cavity, will give rise to the corpus striatum and sphenoidal lobe.

First Phases [of Development] in Rodents (Rabbit, Guinea pig, Mouse)

The first phases through which the said vault or cerebral pallium passes have been well studied by Kölliker[1] and His.[2] At first, this [mantle] consists exclusively of elongated epithelial cells, extending in parallel from the ventricle to the free surface, like the analogous [cells] in the primordium of the spinal cord. Later, two zones are differentiated: *internal,* where the elongated nuclei of the epithelial cells are lined up, and *external,* made up of an infinity of nuclei surrounded by little protoplasm. Such cells, the rudiment of the future gray matter, probably correspond to the *germinal cells* of His, [which are] still undifferentiated cells, capable of division by mitosis. However, the cells in the process of multiplication are preferentially found in the vicinity of the epithelium (rabbit embryo of eight to ten days).

From the tenth day onward (rabbit), the cells destined to form the gray matter multiply noticeably, becoming arranged in many irregular strata, in which the cell bodies are so close together that they barely allow us to distinguish certain radial appendages, [which are] perhaps rudiments of the axon and dendritic shaft. [One of these appendages is internal and more intensely stained than the other, which is peripheral. According to His, to whom we owe this observation, the former would become the axon, whereas the latter, which is somewhat inconstant, would subsequently disappear. This is not the opinion of Paton[3] and Hitaï,[4] for whom the appendage that first appears would be the peripheral dendrite.][D]

At this moment, the majority of the cells probably pass through the neuroblast phase of His, even though it cannot be affirmed with

453

certainty because of the impossibility of obtaining Golgi impregnations suitable for study.

On the fourteenth or fifteenth day, the cortex presents two new layers: a fibrillary, superficial or external [layer], [which is] poor in cells and outlines the plexiform layer; and another, [which is] deep or supra-ependymal, equally poor in neurons, and with a horizontally striated appearance. The latter represents the

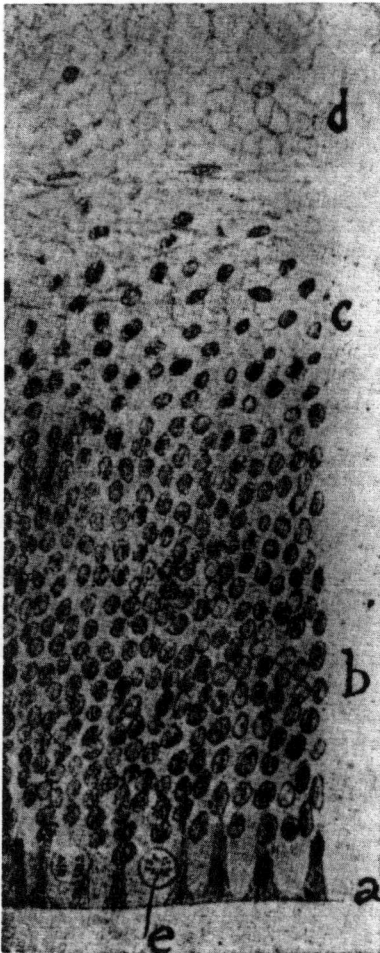

[FIG. 236] Fig. 854. Section of the wall of the anterior cerebral vesicle; human fetus of two months (taken from a picture of His). a, germinal layer; b, layer of the epithelial and neuroblast nuclei; c, intermediate layer; d, marginal veil; e, germinal cell.

first appearance of the white matter, [which is] still not medullated. Between both cell-poor zones lies the mass of elongated and very tight cells, destined to form the cerebral pyramids.

In the days that precede birth, the said intermediate gray zone has grown noticeably, already showing clear strata or planes of embryonic pyramidal cells. In it, it is possible to differentiate, besides the external plexiform layer, a *layer of deep fusiform and spheroidal cells* (polymorphic cells), another of *small ovoid cells* situated beneath the plexiform layer (medium and small pyramids), and, finally, an *intermediate layer* made up of well-differentiated *large pyramids*. The white matter appears very thick, but the majority of its fibers lack myelin.

Histogenetic Phases in the Cortex of the Human Fetus

According to His,[5] who has recently studied several human fetuses, cortical differentiation is initiated in the second month, with an appearance that is illustrated in fig. 854 [*fig. 236*]. At that time, the cerebral plate consists of the following layers: first, epithelial cell bodies or germinal zone, where germinal cells remain still in the process of mitosis (*e*); second, the zone of the nuclei, a thick formation in which reside many nuclei of epithelial cells and neuroblasts (*b*); third, intercalated layer of plexiform appearance with few nuclei; and fourth, the *marginal veil (Randschleier)*, a formation of reticulated appearance and which His considers as a true neuroglial network, although it is possible that the network appearance is merely due to the interweaving of collateral appendages of the radial or epithelial cells. In this period, white matter does not exist, nor is there differentiation of the gray matter.

These will happen later, that is to say, at the beginning of the third month. Notice in fig. 855, *c* [*fig. 237*] that many neuroblasts have migrated beneath the marginal veil, where they form a mass of bipolar cells, [which is] the first rudiment of the gray matter.

Such cells must have already passed the neuroblast phase, since beneath them is seen (fig. 855, b),[E] [*fig. 237*] a broad band of plexiform appearance, horizontally or obliquely

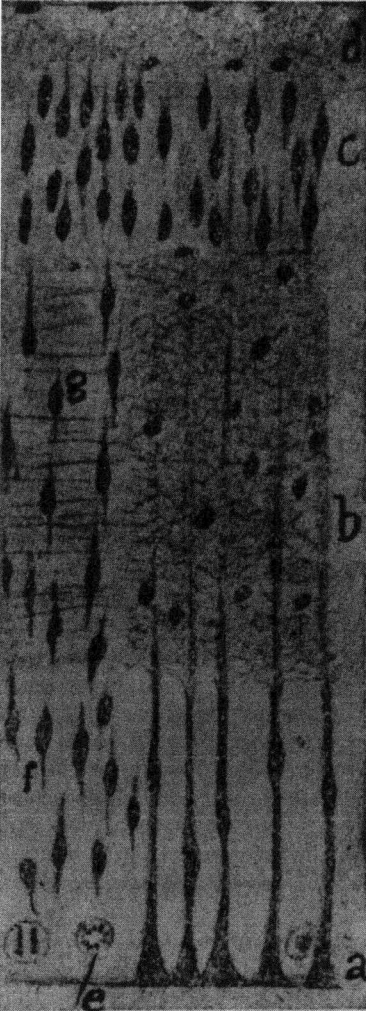

[*FIG. 237*] Fig. 855. Section of the cerebral cortex; human fetus at the beginning of the third month (taken with some modifications from a scheme of His). *a*, germinal layer; *b*, rudimentary white matter; *c*, rudimentary gray matter; *d*, marginal veil; *e*, mitotic epithelial nuclei; *g, f,* nuclei of epithelial cells and neuroblasts furnished with radial processes.

streaked with a large number of fibers, which are undeniably still immature axons, bereft of myelin. Observe also that the germinal zone continues elaborating neuroblasts, which immediately acquire the bipolar form (fig. 855, *e, f*) [*fig. 237*].

Differentiation of the Nerve Cells[F]

Morphological Differentiation

[The information that we have about morphological development varies a great deal in amount and in quality, depending on whether one considers neurons with long axon or neurons with short axon. Thus, it has seemed convenient to us to deal separately with these two kinds of neuron.

[*1. Morphological Differentiation of the Cells with Long Axon*][G]

The neurogenetic investigations of Vignal,[6] ourselves,[7] Retzius,[8] Kölliker,[9] Stefanowska,[10] etc., agree on an essential point, namely that the morphological differentiation of the pyramids is initiated in the deepest zones, especially in the intermediate or zone of the large cells, progressing subsequently toward the superficial or small pyramids to which the neurons of latest development belong. At the moment of birth, the giant pyramids are the most advanced in morphology and intraprotoplasmic differentiation.

In what order do the cellular processes appear?[H] Our investigations using the method of Golgi on the fetus of the mouse and rabbit and on these same animals a few days old have given the following results, in large part confirmed by Retzius, Kölliker, Berkley,[11] Thomas,[12] Stefanowska, etc.

[*a. Primitive Bipolar Phase.*] [In dealing with the histogenesis of the spinal cord (Vol. I, p. 596), we have learned that all nerve cells in the course of their development subsequent to the germinal and apolar phases very frequently pass through a bipolar phase that very rapidly gives way to a new stage, that of the neuroblast or piriform cell. The brief bipolar phase, demonstrated in the embryonic spinal cord of the chicken by our investigations and by those of Besta and Held, also occurs in the nerve cells of the chicken anterior cerebral vesicle, as we have observed at three and a half days of incubation in the embryo of this animal (fig. 540, B [*fig. 238*]. We have many reasons for believing that the same occurs in the earliest phases of development of the cerebral cortex in mam-

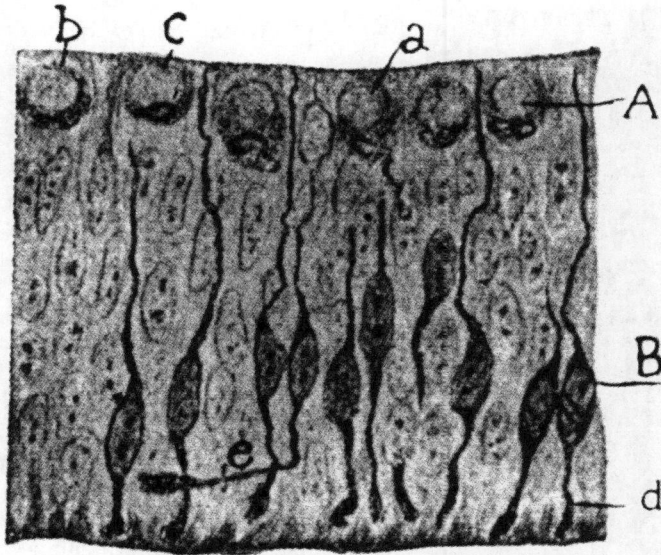

[*FIG. 238*]   Fig. 540. Section of the wall of the anterior cerebral vesicle; embryo of a chicken at three and a half days of incubation. Method of reduced silver nitrate. *A, a, b, c,* nerve cells in the apolar stage; *B,* bipolar nerve cells; *d,* growth cone; *e,* tangential axon. [This figure appears only in the French version of the book.]

mals and man, although we have no personal observations to support this assertion. Thus, it is very probable that the bipolar cells described by His and other authors in the human cerebral cortex after the germinal phase are merely the cells that have reached this primitive bipolar phase. Their external appendage, which Bonne[13] calls *preapex,* is destined to disappear, as His had already supposed, and there only remains the internal appendage which acquires the characteristics of an axon and has at its extremity a growth cone.][I]

b. Neuroblast Phase. [The first process to arise from the soma is the axon, and consequently, during the earliest phases, the neurons resemble the *neuroblast* of His.][J] [The neuroblast phase arises] as soon as the reabsorption of the peripheral appendage indicates the end of the preceding phase. It must also be very brief [as it is only observed in the very early periods of development, and][K] in newborn animals or in term fetuses, the cells that display this stage are very rare. The very few cells of this kind, found by us in term [fetuses of] the mouse and

rabbit, belong to the short-axon category of neurons that develop very late. In the human fetus, of the seventh to ninth month, the neuroblast phase is observed in some cells with short axon of the first layer. Even after birth, there exist in man cells that have not left this stage.

[*Different Opinions about the Primitive Position of the Axon*]. [The primitive position of the axon and the changes of direction that it undergoes during cellular development is a question regularly discussed in recent times. His, one of the protagonists in this dispute, admits that the axon originates from the deep side [of the cell] and that it turns off to form a fiber of the white matter. This is not the opinion of Paton, Hataï, and Hamilton. These histologists, according to their investigations on mammalian embryos, maintain that the processes of the nerve cells suffer a rotation and consequently a change of orientation. It is true that they do not agree about either the primitive direction of the processes or the direction of the rotation. The dendrite, which Hataï and Paton agree is the first process to appear, arises, according to Hataï, from the [upper] side of the cell, while, according to Paton, it arises from the deep side; consequently, this dendrite becomes deep for the first author and superficial for the second, after the movement of cellular rotation that both authors suppose occurs, although Hataï only attributes it to the cells of Martinotti; it goes without saying that the axon, generated subsequent to the dendrite, takes an opposite direction. The opinions of Paton, Hataï, and Hamilton rest on insufficient observations, as Bonne has justly pointed out; besides, they disregard entirely the initial existence of the two processes that His has for a long time demonstrated at the poles of neurons [that are] forming, and whose properties and roles are different, since the external [process] is destined to disappear.][L]

c. [Secondary][M] Bipolar Phase. From the third month of fetal life in man, and from the fourteenth or fifteenth [day] of gestation in the rabbit and mouse, the vast majority of the pyramids have the bipolar form, according to the investigations of Magini,[14] Vignal, and His. In the newborn mouse, rabbit, and dog, as we observed, almost all[N] the small pyramids (fig. 856, *c*) [*fig. 23* in chapter 5] still maintain this phase with slight variants.

During this period, the soma is ovoid, smooth, and radially elongated, and from its poles arise an external process, thick and strongly varicose,[15] as Magini has already observed, terminating at the cerebral surface or before reaching it by means of a varicosity that sometimes bifurcates; and a fine internal process, equally provided with varicosities although less voluminous than the above-mentioned, and deeply continuous with a fiber of the white matter. In this [bipolar] phase, basilar dendrites and axonal collaterals are lacking (fig. 857, *a, d*) [*fig. 239*].

d. Appearance of the Basilar Dendrites and Collaterals of the [Apical Dendritic] Shaft. Shortly after the [secondary][O] bipolar phase and some days before birth in the mouse and rabbit, a descending dendrite, originating near the axon or forming a common shaft with the latter, and some basilar dendritic branches can already be seen on the soma of the large pyra-

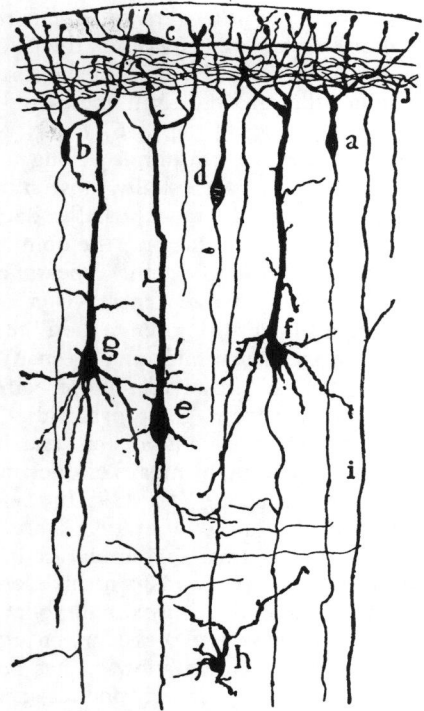

[*FIG. 239*]   Fig. 857. Portion of a frontal section of the cerebrum; mouse four days old. Method of Golgi. *a*, small pyramidal cell in the bipolar phase; *b*, cell of the same kind, already provided with a descending dendrite; *c*, horizontal cell of the plexiform layer; *d*, small pyramidal cell in the bipolar stage; *e, f, g*, pyramidal cells; *h*, cells of Martinotti; *i*, fiber coming from the white matter; *j*, terminal arborization of an ascending axon.

mids. Almost simultaneously, the lateral dendrites of the soma arise in the form of short spines, followed by the collaterals of the radial [dendritic] shaft, which develop from deep to superficial (fig. 857, *e, g*) [*fig. 239*], according to Stefanowska's observations. But before all these dendrites arise, the terminal [dendritic] tuft is differentiated; at the beginning, it is coarse and formed by two or three short, very varicose branches extending to near the pia (fig. 856, *c*) [*fig. 23*]. In the mouse, some days after birth, many small pyramids bereft of dendrites or with few rudimentary basal dendrites still exist (fig. 857, *a, b*) [*fig. 239*].

e. Appearance of the Axonal Collaterals.
According to what we discovered, the [axonal] collaterals arise from the axon in the form of short spines that grow at right angles and terminate in a varicosity (fig. 856, *d*) [*fig. 23* in chapter 5]. The first collaterals belong to the giant pyramids and are usually those situated closest to the soma; the more [distal] collaterals will only develop later (against the opinion of Stefanowska, who supposes the appearance of such branches in inverse order). After birth, the collaterals have still not arisen on the majority of the small pyramids and on many polymorphic cells; however, those already formed, coming from giant pyramids, have grown noticeably, dichotomizing and with their branches ending by means of thickenings or spherules (fig. 857, *g*) [*fig. 239*]. In the days following birth, the said branches are also emitted by many small pyramidal cells and reach in the large [pyramids] a notable length, especially the initial or [proximal] collaterals that already show several secondary or tertiary divisions. Finally, as Stefanowska has recognized, the spines or piriform appendages arise from the radial [dendritic] shaft and its terminal [dendritic] tuft. The late appearance of these appendages indicates the functional maturity of the neuron.

f. Formation of the Centripetal Nerve Fibers.
In the newborn mouse, the main axonal branches of the sensory, visual, and acoustic fibers are already outlined; their arborization will be completed over the next twenty or thirty days. The fibers of association are also very precocious, already appearing in the three or four days after birth, as is seen in fig. 857, *i* [*fig. 239*], in which a fiber of this kind was followed to the plexiform layer. Likewise, the fibers of the [cells] of Martinotti are also very early, so much so that in the mouse of one to two days a nerve plexus already exists in the deepest level of the plexiform layer (fig. 857, *j*) [*fig. 239*].

[2. Morphological Differentiation of the Cells with Short Axon][P]
We know little about the morphological development of this kind of cell, because of the extreme rarity with which they are impregnated in newborn animals or in newborn fetuses. A small number of observations made on the fetus of the mouse allow us to suppose that they also pass, like the neurons with long axon, through the neuroblast and bipolar phases, the thin branches of the axonal arborizations and the thin horizontal and descending dendrites appearing later. In the newborn child, some of these cells of the plexiform layer still show a certain radial orientation and the predominance of an ascending dendrite, which sometimes goes up to the pia.

In regard to the development of the special or horizontal cells of the first layer, we have already dealt in analyzing the typical cortex, on which occasion we have referred to the interesting embryonic phases of the same, discovered by Retzius and confirmed by Kölliker and ourselves.

Cytological[Q] *Differentiation*

Commonly, before birth, it is impossible to recognize the two main features of the protoplasm: the Nissl bodies and the neurofibrils of Bethe; but in the newborn rabbit, cat, and dog, the Nissl bodies and a neurofibrillar framework are already outlined in the giant pyramids, although small and poorly defined.

Differentiation of the Neurofibrils[R]

With respect to the neurofibrillar structural factor, the investigations that we have recently made[16] with reduced silver nitrate (fig. 858) [*fig. 240*] show that the nerve cell passes through these four successive phases.

a. Undifferentiated or Nonstainable Phase.
The protoplasm, which at this stage lacks avidity for staining of the neurofibrils, seems to be exclusively formed by a coarse spongioplasm of granular trabeculae strewn with very fine chromatic granules. All, or almost all, the cerebral pyramids are found in this state before birth, as well as the vast majority of the same in the first days after birth. The nucleus shows a nucleolus rich in spherules, and scattered through the [nucleoplasm] there are observed some granules that attract the silver nitrate.

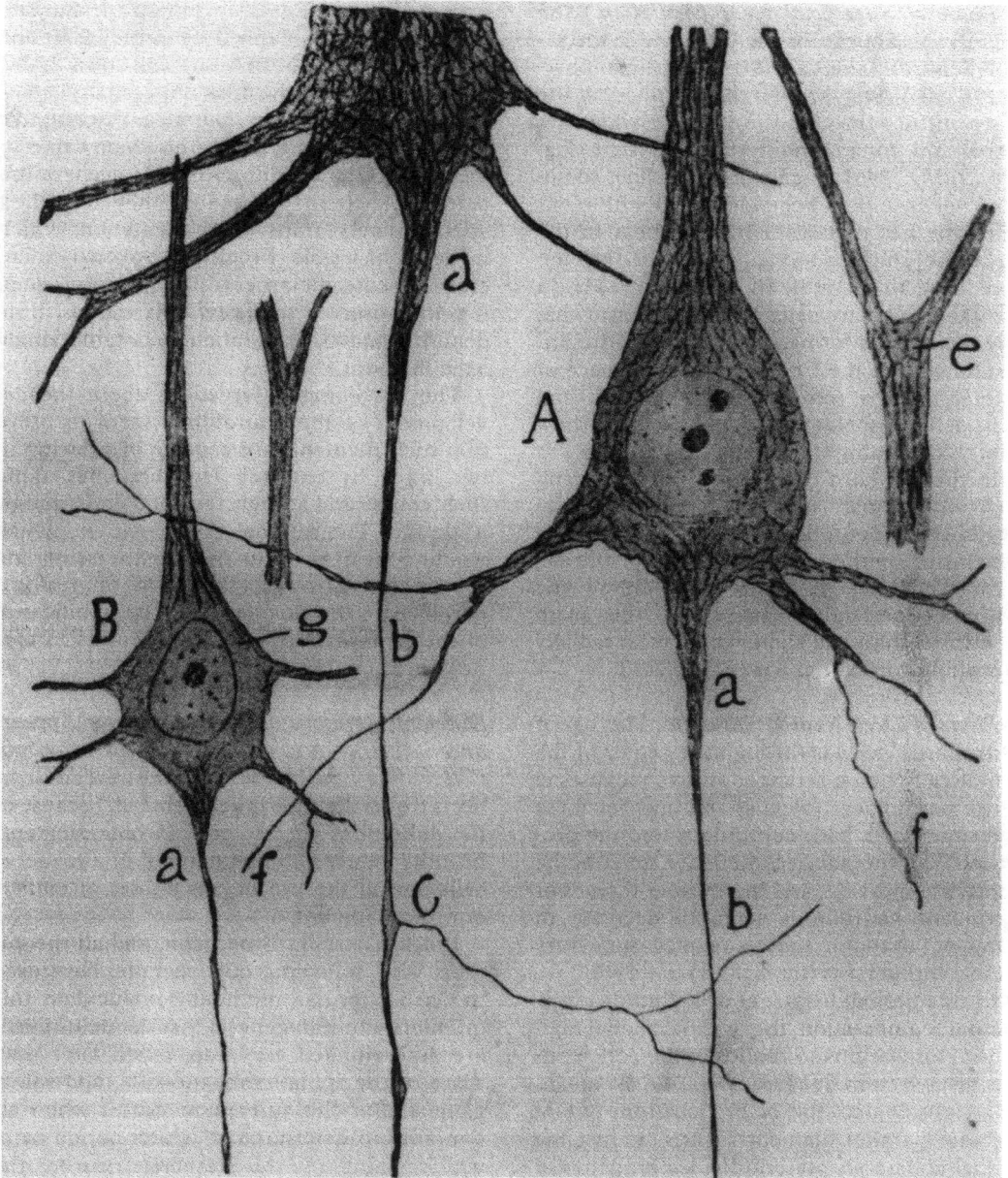

[*FIG. 240*]   Fig. 858. Large and medium pyramidal cells of a dog ten days old. Method of reduced silver nitrate. *A*, large pyramidal cells already provided with a perinuclear mesh of neurofibrils; *B*, medium pyramid with a still undifferentiated spongioplasm; *a*, axon; *b*, apex of the axonal cone; *c*, buds of collaterals; *f*, dendritic branches provided with a single neurofibril.

b. Phase of Superficial Neurofibrillation. The neurofibrils appear for the first time in the radial [dendritic] shaft and axon of the giant pyramids, extending through the periphery of the soma but not through the interior, which remains still in an undifferentiated state (fig. 858, *B*) [*fig. 240*]. Such fibrils are fine, somewhat varicose, and engender a net with elongated meshes that seems to disappear in the [dendritic] shaft and axon, where the skeleton is reduced to a bundle of parallel threads. In the axon of many cells, it could be said that [the skeleton] is formed by a single neurofibril resulting from the fusion and convergence of several threads coming from the shaft and basal dendrites. Not rarely, the said fibers show knotty thickenings (grumous state).

. In the newborn or few-days-old rabbit and dog, only the giant and some medium-size pyramids show neurofibrils. This circumstance, which our method [of reduced silver nitrate] shows very clearly, allows us to follow the processes perfectly, particularly the main [dendritic] shaft and axon, which cross radially the whole cortex (fig. 858, *b*) [*fig. 240*].

c. Phase of Deep Neurofibrillation. The net of neurofibrils extends through the center of the cell already being arranged in two plexuses: a dense perinuclear [plexus] and another loose and superficial, both continuous into the processes. The threads become more smooth, the knots disappearing, and the thinner threads or secondary neurofibrils seem to decrease in number, although the reticulated state very clearly still persists (fig. 858, *A*) [*fig. 240*].

In this period, by virtue of a kind of longitudinal segmentation, the original axonal neurofibril also begins to replicate, the collaterals arising as seen in fig. 858, *c* [*fig. 240*], by means of a right-angled bud or branch from one of the said parallel filaments. Thus, at first the axonal collaterals present divided branches of the main neurofibrils.

d. Fasciculated Phase. By five to thirty days (dog, rabbit), the neurofibrils become apparent in the medium pyramids and polymorphic cells, as well as in the large cells with short axon. In the large pyramids, in which they speed up their appearance, they now reach an extraordinary richness, forming little bundles that pass from the [apical dendritic] shaft and [other] dendrites to the soma and from this to the axon, which now does not contain one or two filaments as before, but a compact bundle distributed into the collaterals. Many fine or secondary filaments disappear or become imperceptible, perhaps because they lose their approximately transverse orientation which made them visible. Finally, the axonal collaterals increase their neurofibrillar contingent, it being observed that now only the last little dendritic and axonal branches contain a single axial filament.

The preceding observations about the development of the neurofibrils seem to prove that such filaments are capable of growing in two ways: by emitting true branches along their course and at their terminal ends, and by a kind of longitudinal segmentation, which would appear to occur in both the soma and the processes. Anyway, this point, of great importance for the elucidation of the significance of the protoplasmic skeleton, requires further new investigation.

Different Opinions about the Time of Appearance of the Neurofibrils in the Cerebral Cells.[5] The fibrillogenesis of the cerebral cortex is a question still much debated, because of the difficulties encountered in obtaining sufficiently intense impregnations of the nerve cells during the precocious phases of embryonic development.

Brock, Gierlich, Brodmann, and all the authors who, following our example, have used the neurofibrillar methods to elucidate this question, admit in general that the neurofibrils are differentiated very late, much later than those of the spinal cord, medulla, and spinal ganglia. But the agreement ceases when attempting to determine at which period or at which point of the cerebral neuron the [neurofibrils] make their appearance. After a few observations we had made[17] in the dog, rabbit, etc., we had supposed that the staining of the neurofibrils (and not their appearance, as some of us have said) takes place after birth, beginning in the large pyramidal cells. Brock,[18] whose investigations have been carried out on the fetus of the pig, thinks that the neurofibrils appear before birth, an opinion shared with Döllken, Brodmann, and Gierlich. Döllken,[19] who has studied the cerebral cortex of the mouse, maintains, in effect, that there is a perfect parallelism between fibrillogenesis and the myelination of the nerve fibers, which Brodmann refuses to accept, because neurofibrils are often seen, he says, in the tangential fibers before being seen in the radial or projection fibers, which, however, become myelinated earlier. Brodmann[20] claims, on the other hand, after his investigations on the cerebral cortex of man, that the intraprotoplasmic fibrils are already visible in human fetuses of four months; they would begin in the cells of Ammon's horn, and they would be formed later, though before birth, in a multitude of tangential and intrinsic fibers of the cortex. With respect to Gierlich,[21] he claims, to the contrary, that it is in the sixth-month fetus that the neurofibrils appear in the cerebrum of man; they would begin in the pyramidal pathway, progressing from the spinal cord and medulla toward the cortex, and would reach finally the cerebral neuron. This course of fibrillogenesis fits also with the theory of Apathy and of Bethe on the peripheral origin of the neurofibrils.

Let us remember on that score that the formation of the neurofibrils begins, according to us, in the cell body to propagate later to the processes. Let us also remember that, far from being a histological formation extraneous to ganglionic cells (*Ganglienzellen*), as Apathy claims, the neurofibrils are, for us, as well as for Held and Brodmann, the result of a differentiation of the protoplasm of the neuroblasts (see Vol. I, page 594 and following).

We have indicated in the generalites (Vol. I, page 596 and following) the great precocity of the neurofibrils in the cells of the retina, medulla, spinal cord, and dorsal root ganglia, a precocity brought to light by the works of Besta, Held,[22] and ourselves.

It would seem thus, after the works above summarized, that the neurofibrils of the cortex are distinguished from those of other centers by their late appearance, at a period when the neurons and nerve pathways have reached or almost reached their definitive development. However, nothing of that is true, as proved by our investigations on the course of fibrillogenesis in the cerebral cortex of mammalian embryos; the neurofibrils are as precocious in this cortex as in the rest of the central nervous system. If it has been thought to be different up to the present, it is due to a mistake that has been undetected by the neurologists. The cause of this mistake is the relative incapacity of the neurofibrillar skeleton of the cerebral cells to be impregnated during the intermediate phases of their development. This incapacity, which is not constant or absolute, since it varies depending on the formulas of impregnation and depending on environmental conditions, such as the cold, stems from the imperfection of the methods used at present and not from the absence of a neurofibrillar mesh at any period during the development of the cerebral cell. From the point of view of its affinity for colloidal silver, this cell seems to us, therefore, to pass through the following phases.

First Phase. The argentophilic substance is abundant, the neurofibrils are thick, and impregnation is easy but not constant; this phase includes the apolar, primitive bipolar, and neuroblast stages.

Second Phase. The argentophilic substance attracts little or no colloidal silver, perhaps because of the delicacy and dispersion of the neurofibrils; at most, some voluminous axons are stained brown. This second phase corresponds to the stage of the young nerve cell, already furnished with an axon and a definitive peripheral dendritic shaft, but still not completely formed.

Third and Last Phase. The neurofibrils again begin to be stained, especially in the axon. This recovery of stainability begins in the largest cells and in the thickest axons; it later slowly propagates to the cells of projection of medium size and to the large cells of association. This phase appears in the dog and rabbit a few days before birth; it progresses especially during the following days and reaches its highest point when the nervous system reaches the adult state. During this phase, there are often seen, especially in newborns and in term fetuses, cells whose axons are intensely impregnated, whereas the cell bodies and dendrites only contain a pale neurofibrillar framework, poorly loaded with reduced silver.

In short, the neurofibrils of the cerebral cells, as well as of the cerebellar cells, are formed from an early period of development, but their capacity to be stained in a regular and constant manner is late, in spite of the initial period of fleeting impregnation. In general, they begin to be stained in the most voluminous cells and fibers, irrespective of any differences in their function. We agree, therefore, with Brodmann when he denies any parallelism between fibrillogenesis and myelination of nerve fibers. We do not believe anymore that at present any relationship can be established between the moment of reappearance of stainability of the neurofibrils and the function of neurons.

Development of the Neuroglia

It is carried out according to the mechanism and steps already described in dealing with the histogenesis of the spinal cord. Let us remember that the neuroglial cells are nothing other than displaced epithelial cells, and, with respect to the cerebrum, the proofs of this doctrine are found in the appearance of the preparations of term embryos of mouse and rabbit. As is seen in fig. 859, c [fig. 25 in chapter 5], in the newborn mouse and rabbit, all the epithelial cells reach externally to the cerebral surface (as was observed some time ago by Magini and Vignal in the mammals and by Retzius and Kölliker in the human cortex), ending in a tuft of ascending branches. Each one of these branches, like the radial fibers of the cerebellum, present on terminating beneath the pia a pyramidal excrescence with an external base that, entering in contact with its companions, forms a general cuticle or covering for the gray matter. On their deep or undivided portion, the epithelial fibers possess, as recognized by Magini, certain ovoid thickenings, not corresponding to nuclei, as thought by this author, but to protoplasmic accumulations. About the eighth day after birth in the mouse, the radial or epithelial fibers become notably thinner, and the varicosities decrease in vol-

ume. Finally, within twenty or twenty-four days, the external prolongation of the ependymal cell, as well as the peripheral tuft, have been reabsorbed, only a relatively short, branched external process remaining, whose little branches do not penetrate even the deepest portions of the white matter.

In man, as Retzius has demonstrated, the radial fibers persist up to birth, disappearing afterward. In our preparations of the child of one month, it is already not possible to see epithelial shafts in the gray matter or remnants of the submeningeal terminal shaft. This atrophy occurs as the result of a progressive slimming of the process that becomes discontinuous, its fragments probably becoming absorbed.

Long before the epithelial cells disappear, a large number of them have already emigrated toward the periphery, in order to be transformed into neuroglial cells. In fig. 859, e [fig. 25 in chapter 5], from a rabbit of a few days, there are seen some epithelial cells that have abandoned the ventricular surface, stationing themselves at several levels in the white and gray matter. In the superficial layers and especially in the plexiform [layer], the displaced epithelial cells at a much earlier date already have numerous crinkly collateral processes, besides the internal and external radial [processes which are] testimony of their epithelial ancestry. Finally, near the [blood] vessels and adhering to the endothelium appear certain spidery cells, whose origin is doubtful. Since all of these phases of displacement and morphological differentiation of the epithelial cells, in order to be transformed into neuroglial cells, have been sufficiently detailed in other chapters of this book, we will not delay by referring to them in detail.

[New Opinions about the Origin of the Neuroglia and of the Ependymal Cells][T]

[Several opinions in relation to the development of the neuroglia of the cerebrum have appeared in recent years, almost all tending to modify the theory of His about the specific origin of the neuroglial and ependymal cells.

Paton, Hataï, Ziehen,[23] Bonome,[24] Bianchi,[25] and other neurologists are of the opinion that the germinal cells give origin by proliferation to a generation of special cells, which they call *indifferent cells* and from which would later come the neuroblasts, the spongioblasts, and the neuroglial cells. This can be seen as an opinion in accordance with the hypothesis of Schaper, an opinion that we have expounded on page 591 of Volume 1, with regard to the neuroglia of the spinal cord. Paton, for example, claims, without furnishing evidence or details, that the neuroglial cell has its origin in the spongioblast by a kind of degeneration or regression of the latter.

On the other hand, a certain number of investigators do not accept the unity of origin of the neuroglial cells. Capobianco,[26] Fragnito, and Hataï,[27] among others, distinguish, first, an ordinary neuroglia stemming from the epithelial cells and, second, a mesodermal neuroglia arriving in the cerebrum with the blood vessels; although for Capobianco this neuroglia derives from the connective tissue of the capillaries, Hataï attributes it, to a large extent, to the proliferation of the endothelial cells that later become detached from the vascular walls in order to be transformed into spidery cells. Certain dispositions described by Hataï with regard to this transformation recall somewhat the vascular thickenings we had observed a long time ago and which serve as a point of origin for the fascicles of spines simulating the neuroglial appendages still in a rudimentary stage.

Be that as it may, the endothelial or mesodermal origin of the neuroglia is still far from proven.]

Parallelism in the Phylogenic and Ontogenic Development [of the Cells of the Cerebrum][U]

From the study we have just concluded on the development of the cerebral cortex in the animal series and in the embryonic and youthful stages of mammals, it is deduced that ontogeny of the cerebral pyramid or *psychic cell* (as we have designated it in deference to the dignity of its activities)[V28] corresponds quite well to the stages of phylogeny. In fig. 860 [*fig. 34* in chapter 7], taken from a work of ourselves on the subject, the said similarity is displayed. Observe how the neuroblast phase reproduces,

grosso modo, the adult disposition of the neurons of invertebrates, and how the forms that the neuron goes through during human ontogeny closely resemble the adult [neurons] of batrachians and reptiles. In spite of everything, some ontogenetic phases remain without phylogenetic representation, such as the bipolar, but we already know that individual development is richer in transition forms than are existing species, because the former represents a continuous serial progression, while the latter represents a discontinuous process—on account of the elimination of intermediate forms?[W]

The same parallelism is observed in the neuroglial cells. In the fishes, batrachians, and reptiles, the only neuroglial framework is represented by the epithelial or ependymal cells, which, in the birds and mammals, correspond to a fleeting and very early ontogenetic phase.

Cajal's Notes

1. Kölliker, *Embryologie*, French translation, Paris, 1882, p. 585. *Handbuch der Gewebelehre des Menschen*, Vol. II, 6th edition, 1896.
2. W. His, Histogenese u. Zusammenhang der Nervenelemente, etc., *Verhandl. des X. Internation. Med. Congress*, Vol. II, 1891. See also: *Die Entwickelung des menschlichen Gehirns, etc.*, Leipzig, 1904.
3. Paton, The histogenesis of the cellular elements of the cerebral cortex, *Johns Hopkins Hospital Reports*, Vol. IX, 1900, p. 709.
4. Hataï, Observations on the Developing Neurones of the Cerebral Cortex of Foetal Cats, *Journ. of Compar. Neurology*, Vol. XII, no. 2, 1902.
5. W. His, *Die Entwickelung des menschlichen Gehirns, etc.*, Leipzig, 1904.
6. Vignal, Recherches sur l développement de la substance corticale du cerveau et du cervelet, *Arch. de Physiol. Norm. et Pathol.*, 4 series, Vol. II, 1888.
7. S. R. Cajal, Sur la structure d l'écorce cérébrale de quelques mammifères, *La Cellule*, Vol. VII, 1891.
8. Retzius, Ueber den Bau der Oberflächenschicht der Grosshirnrinde beim Menschen u. bei den Säugethieren, *Biol. Forening. Forhand.*, 1891. Die Cajal'schen Zellen der Grosshirnrinde beim Menschen u. bei den Säugethieren, *Biol. Unters.*, N.F., Vol. V, 1893.
9. Kölliker, *Handbuch der Gewebelehre*, 6th edition., Vol. II, 1896.
10. Stefanowska, Évolution des cellules nerveuses chez la souris après la naissance, Bruxelles, 1898.
11. Berkley, The Intracerebral Nerve-fibre Terminal Apparatus, etc., *Johns Hopkins' Hospit. Reports*, Vol. VI, 1896.
12. A. Thomas, Contribution a l'étude du dével-

oppement des cellules de l'écorce cérébrale par la méthode de Golgi, *Bull. Soc. de Biol.,* 27 January 1894.

13. Bonne, L'écorce cérébrale, etc., *Revue Générale d'Histologie,* Vol. II, pt. 6, Lyon-Paris, 1907.

14. Magini, Sur la névroglie et les cellules nerveuses cérébrales chez les foetus, *Arch. Ital. d. Biol.,* Vol. IX, 1888.

15. These varicosities have also been observed by Thomas, who attributes a certain importance to them in the development of the neurons. However, the extremely thick grains drawn by this author could very well be the result of some postmortem alteration of the cells.

16. S. R. Cajal, Un sencillo método de coloración selectiva del retículo protoplásmico y sus efectos en los diversos organos nerviosos. *Trab. d. Labor. de Invest. Biolog.,* Vol. II, 1903.

17. Cajal, Un sencillo método de coloración de las neurofibrillas, etc., *Trab. del Lab. de Invest. Biol.,* Vol. II, 1903.

18. Brock, Untersuchungen über die Entwicklung der Neurofibrillen der Schweinefoetus, *Monatschr. f. Psych. u. Neurol.,* Vol. XVIII, 1905.

19. Döllken, Beiträge zur Entwickelung des Säugergehirns, etc., *Neurol. Centralbl.,* no. 20, 1906.

20. Brodmann, Bemerkungen über die Fibrillogenie und ihre Beziehungen zur Myelogenie, etc., *Neurologisches Centralbl.,* no. 8, 1907.

21. Gierlich, Ueber die Entwicklung der Neurofibrillen in der Pyramidenbahn des Menschen, *Vortrag. auf der Versamml. Sudwestl. Neurolagen,* May 1906.

22. Besides the several reports of Held that we have cited in the first volume of this book, look up his general work, *Die Entwicklung des Nervengewebes bei den Wirbeltieren,* Leipzig, 1909, in which he maintained his ideas about the origin of the neurofibrils and progress of their formation, without giving, however, any more demonstrative argument.

23. Ziehen, Die Histogenese vom Hirn u. Rückenmark, etc., *Handbuch der vergleichenden Lehre der Wirbeltiere, Herausgegeben v. D. Hertwig,* Vol. 2, part III, Jena, 1906.

24. Bonome, Histogenese della nevroglia normale nei vertebrati, *Arch. Ital. de Biol. e Embriologia,* Vol. VI, pts. 1–2, 1907.

25. Bianchi, Sulle prime fasi di sviluppo dei centri nervosi, etc., *Annali di Neurologia,* year XXX, pts. 1–11, 1907.

26. Capobianco, De la participation mésodermique dans la genèse de la névroglie cérébrale, etc., *Arch. Ital. de Biol.,* Vol. XXXVII, 1902.

27. Hataï, On the origin of neuroglia tissue from the mesoblast, *Journ. of Comparative Neurol.,* Vol. XII, no. 4, 1902.

28. S. R. Cajal, les nouvelles idées sur la structure du système nerveux, etc., translation by Dr. Azoulay, Paris, 1894.

Editors' Notes

A. This title appears only in the French version.

B. The phrase in brackets is in the French version but not in the Spanish version.

C. This title appears only in the French version.

D. The sentences in brackets are in the French version but not in the Spanish version.

E. The French version incorrectly says *"d."*

F. This title appears only in the French version.

G. The preceding paragraph and the title are in the French version but not in the Spanish version.

H. This question appears only in the Spanish version.

I. This title and paragraph in brackets are in the French version but not in the Spanish version.

J. The phrase in brackets is in the Spanish version but not in the French version.

K. The phrase in brackets is in the French version but not in the Spanish version.

L. The paragraph in brackets is in the French version but not in the Spanish version.

M. Added in the French version.

N. The French version says "all."

O. Added in the French version.

P. This title appears in the French version of the book. In the Spanish version, the title is "Development of the Cells with Short Axon," and the text appears just before the item entitled "Development of the Neuroglia."

Q. "Structural" in the Spanish version.

R. This title appears only in the French version.

S. This title and the text that follows are only in the French version.

T. This title and the text that follows are only in the French version.

U. The phrase in brackets is in the French version but not in the Spanish version.

V. The phrase in parentheses is omitted in the French version.

W. The question mark was added in the French version.

25

Anatomicophysiological Considerations on the Cerebrum

[*From: Textura del sistema nervioso del hombre y de los vertebrados* (Madrid: Moya), Vol. 2, pt. 2, chap. 48, pp. 1121–1152; also published in French as *Histologie du système nerveux de l'homme et des vertébrés,* vol. 2 (Paris: Maloine, 1911), chap. 36, pp. 862–890]

Anatomical theories about the organization and functioning of the cerebrum. Theories of Flechsig and Monakow. Our hypothesis: centers of perception and primary and secondary centers of memory, unilaterality of the centers of memory, bilaterality and topographic symmetry of the perceptive centers, existence of centrifugal fibers in the perceptive and memory centers, sensory-memory and intermemory association pathways. Physiological postulates: unity of perception, [congruent] and continuous projection of the sensory [areas] in the cerebral cortex, intercrossings, economy of space and of protoplasm.

Histological theories of the functioning of the cerebrum: mechanism of sleep, of the association of ideas, etc. Cerebral adaptation. Improvement in the association of ideas, physiological compensations, etc. [A]

After the long and fatiguing analysis that we have just made of the structure of the cerebral cortex, it is now time to synthesize the more general results and to formulate, insofar as the still imperfect state of our knowledge permits us, a structural plan of the cerebrum. In this chapter, we will deal, naturally, with the examination of the most plausible theories, both anatomical and histological, passing then to expound the most acceptable provisional hypothesis, and the investigation ends by gathering together all the data that allow us to elaborate a definitive doctrine.

Anatomical Theories of the Organization and Function of the Cerebrum

Theory of Flechsig

In several chapters of this book, we have already alluded to the important anatomico-physiological doctrine of this author, but it is now convenient to present in more detail than we did previously the assemblage of ideas of the famous neurologist of Leipzig.

Flechsig[1] begins by declaring that the cerebral cortex is not a homogenous mass, but topographically, histologically, and physiologically consists of separate centers that he distinguishes as *projection or perception areas and association or intellectual areas.*

a. The *areas of projection* correspond to the sensory and motor areas indicated in the cerebrum by the work of Hitzig, Ferrier, Monakow, Munk, etc., who are largely in agreement with one another.

These areas have a structure that is different from that of the areas of association, and they also differ among themselves; they are characterized anatomically by being linked with deep nuclei (diencephalon, mesencephalon, medulla, and spinal cord) by two kinds of fibers of projection: *centripetal* and *centrifugal.* By means of the centripetal or sensory [fibers], they would receive excitations collected from the sense organs, and by means of the motor or centrifugal [fibers], the excitations would be reflected toward the peripheral motor nuclei.

The said centers of projection are four, namely *sensory-motor, visual, acoustic,* and *olfactory,* all of them located in the cortical regions that we have already indicated.

b. The *centers of association* possess a special structure that is common to all of them (cortex of five layers), and they are characterized anatomically by neither receiving nor emitting the said fibers of projection, and by being associated, by means of afferent and efferent fibers, with the areas of projection. Each area of association would thus collect, by means of its afferent fibers, all the excitations or sensory residues originating in the areas of projection, while simultaneously it would act on the sensory areas by means of centrifugal fibers, either to inhibit or to facilitate the impulses reflected [to the motor nuclei].

The areas of association in man occupy two-thirds of the cortex, and they are three: the *anterior,* extending through the anterior portion of the frontal lobe; the *middle,* corresponding to the *insula of Reil;* and the *posterior,* which includes a large portion of the occipital and temporal lobes and almost the whole parietal lobe.

The physiological hierarchy of the centers of association and projection is very different. The areas of projection are common to man and mammals and constitute the animal or vegetative cerebrum (perception and motor reflexes, etc.), whereas the areas of association, absent in rodents, scarcely developed in carnivores, somewhat more developed in monkeys, in which they already cover one-third of the cortex, and extremely extensive in man, in which they occupy two-thirds of the cortex, represent the *substratum* of the highest psychic activities (voluntary movement, memory, intelligence, aesthetic and moral senses, etc.). The lack of areas of association implies the lack of intellectual life; therefore, the rodents, which are bereft of these areas, and the newborn child, in which they are still not differentiated, are only capable of reflex actions. They see, feel, hear, and move, but they do not think, nor are they capable of acting on the projection or sensory areas in order to drive their activities and regulate their motor discharges.

Arguments Based on the Doctrine of Flechsig

The ideas we have just expounded are based on the results of the method of successive myelination (method of Flechsig) in the human embryo and newborn child. According to Flechsig, myelination of the nerve pathways proceeds from below up, [that is to say, going][B] from the spinal cord toward the medulla and telencephalon, and only when these regions are organized does myelin appear in the cerebral cortex. In the latter, myelination arrives in a series of differentiated physiological pathways, beginning in the areas of projection and invading the association areas a long time later. For example, in the newborn child, only the areas of projection of the cerebrum show their myelinated pathways (centripetal and centrifugal fibers), a circumstance that allows us to distinguish perfectly these areas, as well as to differentiate them from the association areas, [which are] still bereft of myelinated fibers. On beginning the second month, other myelinated fibers directed from the centers of projection appear in the adjacent association cortex. These would be nothing less than collaterals emitted from afferent or sensory projection fibers. Finally, some time later, the areas of association and the intermediate regions between these and the areas of projection become myelinated, long arciform or horizontal centripetal and centrifugal fibers, destined to link both kinds of area, appearing. In the opinion of Flechsig, no fiber originating in an area of association can be followed into the corona radiata, nor could it therefore reach the deep gray nuclei [of the diencephalon, medulla, and spinal cord].[C]

As evidence of the functional duality of the

cortex, Flechsig adduces (a) studies of comparative anatomy, confirming the lack of areas of association in rodents and lower vertebrates; (b) autopsies revealing that in men of superior talent the areas of association, especially the posterior, reach a notable development; (c) finally, autopsies in several clinical cases (cases of Heubner, Nothnagel, etc.) in which the loss, by cerebral lesion, of the visual or acoustic areas was not followed by the abolition of the corresponding memory or of ideation, an inexplicable fact if, as some suppose, the same cortical areas dedicated to perception (vision, hearing) would intervene [directly] in the respective memory function.

The important theory of Flechsig, introduced in a very stimulating and brilliant manner, when it became known to the neurologists, physiologists, and psychologists caused an excitement comparable only to that created previously by the cellular pathology of Virchow or the memorable bacteriological studies of Pasteur. It is not strange, therefore, that the new doctrine immediately gained many adherents in Germany (Kupffer, Kirschoff, etc.), and in Belgium and France won such clear talents as Van Gehuchten[2] and Jules Soury.[3]

Unfortunately, this phase of perhaps excessive excitement has now been followed by a no less excessive disenchantment, and the growing coldness threatens to ruin even the pluralist anatomicofunctional theory, the basis of the conceptions of the neurologist of Leipzig. Here are, in short, the main objections aimed at the cited theory, in the name of either pathological anatomy, methodological criticism, or psychology, by Monakow, Dejerine, Siemerling, Mahaim, Vogt, and others.

1. According to Monakow,[4] almost all the areas that Flechsig considers areas of association are related to deep nuclei by means of fibers of projection. Thus, the majority of the parietal gyri possess a descending pathway terminating in the pulvinar; the second temporal gyrus and the occipitotemporal gyrus are linked to the posterior nucleus of the thalamus; the second and third frontal gyri and a portion of the insula are connected to the internal thalamic nucleus, etc.

2. Dejerine[5] argues against Flechsig, declaring that the fascicle of Türck (an important

pathway of projection) comes from the second and third temporal gyri (*cortex of association* of Flechsig), that the corticorubral fibers originate in the parietal lobe, and that certain fibers originating in the anterior and medial areas of the frontal lobe, after running through the anterior segment of the internal capsule, gain the internal nucleus of the thalamus. And finally, he maintains with the greatest energy that all or almost all cortical regions give rise to fibers of projection terminating in several segments of the cerebrospinal axis, as a consequence of which the anatomical fact (absence and presence of fibers of projection) that serves as the basis of the concept of Flechsig lacks reality.

3. Ferrier and Turner[6] have found in the occipital cortex of the monkey two kinds of projection fibers: ascending and descending, destined to link the cerebrum with the optic thalamus and the superior colliculus. Rutishäuser[7] makes an analogous assertion, having observed in the frontal lobe of the monkey a descending system terminating partly in the thalamus and partly in the pons. Siemerling,[8] Vogt,[9] Mahaim,[10] etc., make similar objections.

Vogt especially brings against Flechsig not only anatomical but also physiopsychological reasons, declaring that present-day psychology demands a system of projection capable of connecting, in an immediate manner, the centers of ideation with the subcortical motor centers, in order to understand the emotional concomitants of intellectual acts. He adds that the anatomicophysiological doctrine of the areas of association is bereft of any psychological value, since the elucidation of the mechanism of psychic operations will only come from fine cortical histology, [it being urgent, therefore, to create a cellular psychology that responds to this purpose].[D]

No less expressive are the objections brandished against the embryological method of Flechsig.

Dejerine points out the error of logic that is committed by denying [the existence] of projection pathways in the association cortex, solely because they do not develop during the first two months after birth, as though such fibers could not appear later. But Siemerling, Vogt, and, above all, Monakow particularly insist on the inappropriateness of the method of progressive myelination as a basis for the concept of the [neurologist] of Leipzig.

Here are some observations.

a. In order for the conclusions of Flechsig to be true, it would be necessary that the projection pathways always develop before the association pathways, the peripheral before the central pathways, and the sensory pathways earlier than the motor pathways; but the investigations of Monakow, Vogt, and Siemerling, and in part also those of Righetti, Westphal, and others, prove that this rule has so many exceptions that it loses almost all its value. For example, in the cerebrum, at the same time that the radial fibers appear in the sensory areas, there are already observed numerous fibers of association whose course is impossible to follow, and further increasing this difficulty is the circumstance that myelination commences in any part of the course of the fibers and not in the direction of the impulses, as Flechsig claims.

b. In the spinal cord, where this study is easier than in the cerebrum, it is also incorrect that the projection fibers precede the fibers of association, and the sensory fibers the motor fibers. In this way, Monakow (and Trepinski, Giese, Westphal, etc.) cites cases in which the fibers of the anterior commissure and funiculi become myelinated in the spinal cord of the human fetus at the same time as the ventral root fibers, and this occurs before the true motor and sensory spinal nerves possess any trace of myelin.

c. As Westphal points out, it often occurs that the optic nerve (neuron of first order) becomes myelinated at the same time as and even later than the optic radiations (neuron of second order).

d. Monakow has found throughout the cerebrum [certain] gyri whose fascicles of association appear myelinated before the corresponding fibers of projection.

All of these facts bode very ill for the theory of Flechsig, because they tend to reduce the value of the rules of myelination on which the doctrine is based, rules that have as their general postulate that the myelin is formed according to the order of appearance of function.

Flechsig has modified his doctrine[11] in re-

sponse to these criticisms, some of which have too much strength to be denied. As a result of new embryological investigations, he now recognizes the existence of fibers of projection in the areas of association, although always in smaller numbers than in the sensory areas. In addition, he subdivides the areas of association, according to the time of their myelination, into two categories: first, late or terminal embryological areas that would be myelinated at least one month after birth; and [second,] intermediate embryological areas, situated between the previous ones and the areas of projection, and in which the myelin would appear at the time of birth. [With respect to the areas of projection themselves, they would have as common characteristics those of becoming myelinated before birth and of sending a multitude of nerve fibers into the corona radiata. There are twelve of these precocious areas. Seven of them seem to be sensory because they receive fibers from the sensory nuclei of the thalamus, etc.; the other five areas are still of an uncertain nature, but they could be unknown sensory areas (?). The fibers become myelinated in each area of projection in the following order: first the radiating sensory fibers, later the centrifugal radiating fibers, and finally the callosal and projection fibers.][E] Overall, the areas newly differentiated by Flechsig, including the projection areas, would amount provisionally to forty [a number that he later reduces to thirty-six[12]].[F]

Among the new areas of projection, he includes *Ammon's horn,* the *subiculum,* and a portion of the *gyrus fornicatus,* cortical regions that, as seen from my investigations, do not receive direct or first-order olfactory fibers but fibers of second order. This fact is interesting because it proves that organs that become myelinated at the same time do not always correspond to the same functional category. For the rest, Flechsig insists on the reality of the laws of myelination and attributes the main objections made against him to misinterpretations. To cite only an example: the *fascicle of Türck,* a pathway of sphenoidal projection, would not leave, as Dejerine declares, from the second and third temporal gyri, but from the first, thus representing the projection pathway of the acoustic area.

[It is more serious that the very principle of the myelogenetic method does not seem to be correct. O. Vogt[13] and C. Vogt[14] maintain, in effect, that areas are precociously or late myelinated, not with respect to their different functions, but because of the greater or lesser abundance and thickness of the fibers that enter or leave them. The process of successive myelination thus would not be as useful in distinguishing the cortical areas as Flechsig claims. Furthermore, there exist regions in the cortex that, from the point of view of the number, caliber, and time of myelination of their fibers, are transitional between the areas of precocious and late myelination. The existence of these regions of transition particularly reduces the precision of the myelogenetic method and obliges one to control the results by methods capable of revealing the arrangement of the cells and the course of the myelinated fibers. It is therefore impossible to dream of delimiting clearly, with the aid of the myelogenetic method, the specific cortical fields or islets and still less to fix the number at thirty-six, as Flechsig has recently done for the cerebrum of man. Finally, M. and Mme. Vogt object that primates are not the only mammals that possess areas of late myelination, that is to say, areas of association, in the sense used by Flechsig, because these areas also exist with identical charcteristics in the dog, cat, rabbit, etc.][G]

Theory of Monakow

The anatomicopathological investigations of this authority made primarily with the method of Gudden, have led him to consider the cortex divided into separate areas or centers, in accord with the physiological experiments of Hitzig, Munk, Ferrier, and the anatomicopathological [studies] of Beevor, Langley, etc. All of these areas (tactile, visual, auditory, and olfactory, as well as others with unknown functions) possess ascending and descending projection fibers, with the difference that some such corticopetal and corticofugal fibers would go to and from the spinal cord, and others would stop in the several thalamic nuclei, mesencephalon, pons, etc. For instance, the visual area is linked, by means of centripetal and cen-

trifugal fibers, with the lateral geniculate body; the auditory area with the medial [geniculate body]; the tactile or sensory area with the ventrolateral nuclei of the thalamus, etc.

But, in addition to these cortical areas which are phylogenetically the oldest, there would exist other, more recent [areas], characteristic only of mammals. The latter cerebral areas or fields which in part correspond to the areas of association of Flechsig, would receive the fibers of other thalamic nuclei, as well as fibers originating in the cerebellum, gray nuclei of the pons, substantia nigra, red nucleus, etc. whose physiological significance is little known.

Such accessory cortical areas would also present centrifugal and centripetal fibers, although the former, motor fibers in the broad sense, would be much more abundant in the areas that Flechsig calls areas of projection, and especially in the tactile area. But what, above all, characterizes [these new areas][H] is that the fibers of association, destined to link the several cerebral areas to one another, are the most numerous.

In short, the doctrine of Monakow, which essentially is in agreement with the opinion of Dejerine, approaches at many points the opinion of Flechsig, since the neurologist of Zürich admits more or less explicitly two kinds of cortical areas and affirms that the phylogenetically old areas possess more fibers of projection than the new areas, which correspond to the areas of association. A reconciliation of both doctrines is thus possible, above all since Flechsig has recognized the existence of projection fibers in the intellectual areas and has reduced the value of the fibers of projection as a differentiating criterion.[15]

[Monakow, in his more recent works,[16] brings to the usual doctrine of cerebral localization a certain number of restrictions. He does not accept, as Flechsig does, that cerebral functions are localized in a very specific manner at certain points in the cortex, because, for him, any psychic act is the result of the combination of a large number of elements, only some of which have their anatomical substratum in a rather precise region of the cerebral cortex; others have their substrata scattered through the whole extent of the cerebrum.

The elements clearly localized are those that are related to orientation in space and to movements performed in response to sensory excitation; the elements without a precise location are, on the other hand, those of sensory awareness, of memory, of judgment, in a word, the elements of the intellectual acts themselves.][I]

Our Hypothesis

In fact, in the present state of science, it is not possible to formulate a definitive theory about the architectonic and functional plan of the cerebrum. We still lack many precise histological data concerning the association or intellectual areas of Flechsig, as well as the anatomicophysiological determination of the cortical connections of numerous thalamic, mesencephalic, and pontine nuclei. It is possible, nevertheless, to profit from the positive materials, although incomplete, that we currently possess, forging with them a provisional anatomicofunctional synthesis, a sort of consensus of the opinions of Monakow, Dejerine, and Flechsig, while physiological experimentation, histology, and anatomicopathological investigation continue to collect all the necessary data.

In places where we were bereft of exact anatomicophysiological facts, we have resorted to the teachings of psychology in order to fill certain gaps; since, as Vogt correctly notes, at the present time the phenomena of consciousness are better known than cerebral architecture, and the science of the mind can more effectively aid the science of the cerebrum than the science of the cerebrum can aid that of the mind. It is idle to say that we do not seek to give to our conjectures the slightest dogmatic character; in science, hypotheses vary with the inexorable progression of facts that could not be anticipated, and ours would be very fortunate if, on being compared with future contributions, it were capable of maintaining some of the principles on which it is based.

Our theory is comprised of the following propositions: first, the existence of at least three kinds of cerebral areas; second, the bilaterality of the areas of perception and the unilaterality of the primary and secondary memory areas; third, the existence in all areas of fibers of centrifugal projection, [but the areas of perception would receive the sensory fibers from the thalamic nuclei, whereas the memory areas would receive their fibers from the areas of perception in the cortex];[J] fourth, the maintenance of [connections] between the sensory areas and the visual and tactile memory areas, [as well as between the latter areas themselves];[K] fifth, physiological and teleological postulates, etc.

1. The Existence of Three Kinds of Cortical Areas

That the cortical gray matter contains areas of different functional status is persuaded by numerous facts and reasons, some of them already invoked by Flechsig.

a. Science records an infinity of clinical cases in which the exclusive lesion of an area of perception (visual, auditory, tactile areas, etc.) abolishes for life the corresponding perception but not related memories and ideas.

b. It is also known that cases of lesions in gyri adjacent to the visual and auditory areas do not cause mental blindness or deafness but a weakness of memory and paralysis of the capacity for recognition of objects. Let us remember, for example, the cases reported by Wilbrand, in which the lesions of the lateral occipital gyri in man were followed only by a disturbance of visual memory and of the faculty of recognition. According to Gómez Ocaña and others, similar phenomena are observed in dogs when they have the parietal lobe partly removed.

c. The three areas of language respectively called *area for the motor images of speech* (gyrus of Broca), *area for auditory images of words* (posterior portion of the first temporal gyrus), and *area for visual images of symbols of language* (angular gyrus) are not areas of perception, but of memory and of recognition of images. As is well known, the individual who, as a consequence of lesions in any of those areas, has lost the memory of the acoustic or visual motor representations of words is not deaf, blind, or [mute]. He is only bereft of the understanding of verbal perception; the words represent for him completely new objects that he must learn like a child. This proves thus

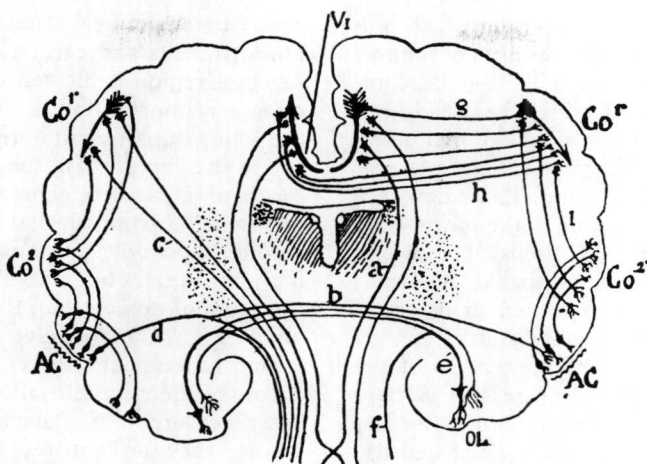

[*FIG. 241*]   Fig. 861. Scheme designed to show the three orders of areas of the cerebral cortex corresponding to each of the three senses. *VI*, visual perceptive center; *Co¹*, visual memory center of first order; *Co²*, memory center of second order in which are combined the elements of the several sensory categories; *AC*, acoustic perceptive center; *OL*, olfactory perceptive center; *a*, fibers of projection of the visual perceptive center; *c*, fibers of projection of the visual memory area; *b*, anterior commissure.

that there exist memory areas of three kinds: visual, acoustic, and sensory-motor, completely separate from their corresponding perceptive areas.

d. Histological investigation also comes to the support of this distinction, since it teaches us that the cortex of perception possesses a specific structure different from that of the memory cortex. This structure, which, as we have seen, varies noticeably in each perceptive area, very probably also varies in each memory area. An indication of this is found in Ammon's horn, a secondary memory area of olfaction, whose structure differs not only from that of the olfactory perceptive areas but also from all the other cortical memory areas.

e. Perception, while reflecting the external world, differs enormously from simple memory [function], making it difficult to believe that the same organ carries out two such dissimilar acts. In effect, the indirect representation or memory is not an attenuated copy of the percept, but a new mental event (as Wundt states), influenced and altered by volition, emotional state, sensation, and antecedent ideas, etc.; the evoked image appears to us vague and fragmentary, with simplifications and gaps that give to it a schematic and syn-

thetic character, something like those composite photographs of families. Besides, memory is usually a voluntary act preceded by an effort [of will]; it involves a character less individualized than generic (in fact, it copies a chronological series of impressions of the same object) and becomes joined to a sensation of intimacy, of consubstantiability with the subject (the *ego*), something of which a perception is completely bereft (the *nonego* of the philosophers), and is always presented to us as something unavoidable, extraneous to us, and independent of our will (fig. 861) [*fig. 241*].

f. Finally, it seems, a priori, little probable that nature, [usually] so faithful to the division of labor, abandons this principle in the most differentiated and perfect organ, entrusting such different activities as perception and memory to the same neuronal constellation.

Primary and Secondary Memory Areas. [Thus, there exist areas of perception and areas of memory, but]ᴸ the memory areas are probably of two kinds: *primary areas,* in which the residues of the perception of objects are deposited and in which takes place the recognition of new images and probably also the most simple intellectual and volitional operations (identification, differentiation, desire, etc.); and *secondary areas,* in which the residues of the residues are deposited, that is to say, the combined images, each of which is already not merely a simplified copy of an external object but a synthesis of elements belonging to several primary memory images. These new representations, corresponding to the *ideas* of the philosophers, have lost almost completely their representational and spatial character, for this reason being presented to us as divorced from external reality and as if they were the pure product of the actions of the ego. Within such [secondary] areas, or perhaps in others of an even higher order (tertiary memory areas?), there would be deposited also the fruits of the constructive scientific imagination and the creations of literary fantasy, that is to say, all those edifying complex and systematic ideas driven on by reflection, by study, and by experience (fig. 861, *Co²*) [*fig. 241*].

The reasons that suggest this duality of the memory areas are [as follows].

a. There are several known facts of anatomical and clinical observation that indicate differences and functional categories among the areas of association of Flechsig. For example, this author notes that [from the embryological point of view][M] each intellectual or association area includes areas of different anatomical order: the *intermediate areas,* situated in the vicinity of the areas of perception and whose development occurs relatively early; and the *terminal areas* [which are] the latest [in development] and typical of man and primates. The former could very well correspond to the primary memory areas, and the second, of late development, to the secondary memory areas.

b. Dejerine mentions cases of aphasia in which the language areas (memory areas of first order) have been destroyed without the loss of ideas. The patient, forced to think, thinks not with word images but with complex ideas, different from what occurs with the [patient] aphasic due to lesions of subcortical or association fibers and who thinks with symbols of language. These facts prove that ideas reside in cerebral places different from the simple verbal memory areas.

c. Our anatomical studies on the olfactory areas (rodents and carnivores) prove that the cerebral region dedicated to the reception of olfactory impressions is triple, consisting of the following areas, in order from the periphery to the center: first, the *inferior sphenoidal cortex* or area of olfactory perception (it receives fibers from the lateral olfactory tract); second, *superior sphenoidal cortex* and presubiculum (receives olfactory fibers originating in the areas of perception); third, *Ammon's horn* and *fascia dentata* (receives fibers from the superior sphenoidal cortex). According to the theory of Flechsig, the latter two cortical areas represent areas of association, but, on the whole, they do not resemble one another, since the superior sphenoidal cortex receives the olfactory impulses that have passed through only one cortical area, whereas Ammon's horn collects impulses passing sequentially through two gray areas. Therefore, is it not logical to think that these two superior olfactory areas represent, respectively, the primary and secondary olfactory memory areas? And could not such an arrangement perhaps be the key to the organization of the rest of the cortex?

d. Finally, since there exist areas for perception of the immediate image and areas for the representation of this perception, it is natural to suppose, according to the principle of the division of labor, that others also exist for combined ideas or sensory memories.

The Primary Memory Areas or Areas of Definite Images Are Located in the Vicinity of the Perception Areas.[N] This assertion is made probable by the following reflections.

a. The memory areas known so far in man (motor area of articulate language, area for visual images of words, area for acoustic images of words) reside in the vicinity of the corresponding sensory area.

b. Several authors have located, by means of clinical observations, the area of visual memories in the lateral occipital cortex, that is to say, in the surroundings of the visual perceptive area.

c. In the olfactory area, as we have set down, the probable primary memory area, or superior sphenoidal cortex, lies near and immediately after the perception area.

Concept of Cerebral Organization in the Gyrencephalic Mammals and in Lower Vertebrates.[O] The investigations of Edinger, my brother, and myself show that in small mammals, as well as in birds, reptiles, and batrachians, there exist very probably, beside the perceptive areas, others that correspond probably to the human memory areas. These accessory areas belong, in the batrachians and reptiles, almost exclusively to the olfactory system; but in the birds and mammals, whose cerebrum already possesses visual and acoustic perceptive areas, they perhaps pertain to the four main senses. The notable development of Ammon's horn and of other subordinate centers of the olfactory area in lissencephalic[P] mammals also makes probable the opinion that at least one or two sensory forms (olfactory and perhaps visual) of secondary memory centers have already appeared, although restricted in size. The fibers through which the sensory residues would be propagated from the perception to the memory areas are probably long collaterals or branches of bifurcation of projection axons. In fig. 863, *F, G* [*fig. 243*], we show schematically this arrangement for two hypothetical memory areas in the rodents (visual and olfactory).

As a consequence, the theory of Flechsig that denies in the lissencephalic[Q] mammals and lower vertebrates the areas of association seems to us inadmissible. In our opinion, the evolution of the sensory areas of the cerebrum in the animal series does not occur by parallel steps or stages, but by continuous, although unequal, advances of those sensory areas whose activity is the most advantageous for the necessities of the struggle for survival. By this we mean that in those animals whose predominant sense is, for example, smell, the [olfactory] cerebrum competes with, if it does not surpass in organization, that of man, showing the same hierarchy of olfactory areas as in man; although, with regard to other sensory specializations, it may be very inferior, being reduced to the perception areas and a few small primary memory areas.

2. The Perceptive Areas Are Symmetrical and Bilateral, Whereas the Primary and Secondary Memory Areas Are Unilateral[17]

All the known memory areas (area for motor images of words, area for word blindness, area for agraphia, area for verbal deafness, etc.) are unilateral, residing in right-handed individuals in the left hemisphere, and in left-handed individuals in the right hemisphere. As the three cited areas correspond to three very different sensory categories, that is, the tactile, the visual, and the auditory, it is extremely probable that the same occurs with all the other [memory areas]. In effect, it would be very strange if the visual and acoustic image of a letter or of a word were to be found wholly in one hemisphere and the image of a musical sound or of a geometrical figure in symmetrical areas of both hemispheres. Thus, we consider it very acceptable that the memory areas of one side, even though homologous to those of the opposite [side] in relation to the general function performed, do not lodge the same representations. In this way, the visual projection, for example, distributed as a perception in both hemispheres (the two calcarine fissures), is polarized or unilateralized on being transformed into a memory, diminishing its representational and spatial character, which is completely lost in the area for ideas or combined images. Such a disposition brings two economic advantages: increase of cerebral capacity, since each hemisphere files different memories; and a gathering in adjacent territories of the same side of those acquisitions of different sensory type (visual, acoustic, tactile, etc.) that, because they are related to the same external object, must be continuously associated in speech and thought, and require, as a consequence, short and vigorous pathways of connection.

Necessity of the Corpus Callosum. The preceding proposition, in our opinion, justifies the existence of the corpus callosum. In effect, the site of the perceptive image being bilateral and the area in which the integral remains of the same are registered being unilateral, it becomes absolutely necessary to have two kinds of fibers of association or at least two kinds of collaterals: *direct association* [fibers], which convey the homolateral half of the image to the memory area; and *commissural association or callosal* [fibers], which transmit to this same area the part of the projected image in the perceptive area of the other hemisphere. In fig. 861, *VI, Co¹* [*fig. 241*], where we draw schematically the two images—direct or perceptive image and indirect or memory image, respectively—we believe that we justify the callosal commissure and the homolateral perceptomemory bundle.

For the rest, the presence of callosal fibers in the areas of perception is a fact of positive observation. Accordingly, the anatomicopathologists have many times verified the presence of degeneration in the splenium of the corpus callosum of man, as a consequence of lesions of the calcarine fissure and adjacent areas, and we have had occasion to observe callosal fibers leaving (mouse, rabbit) two areas of projection: the visual and sensory-motor (fig. 863, *A*) [*fig. 243*]. With regard to the areas of olfactory perception (sphenoidal cortex, etc.), they possess, as is obvious, a robust commissure: the anterior commissure.[18]

Although we lack data about the places occupied by the secondary [memory]ᴿ images, it may be presumed that they are also unilateral. Besides, being made up of secondary images from primary memory elements scattered through the whole cortex, it seems likewise very probable that the cerebral areas that contain [the secondary images] maintain relations with all the primary memory areas of both hemispheres, by means of both homolateral association fibers and contralateral or callosal fibers. The still hypothetical character of these areas obliges us not to enter here into other considerations.

3. The Memory Areas As Well As the Perceptive Areas Possess Fibers of Projection, [but Their Afferent Fibers Are Thalamic for the Latter and Cortical for the Former]ˢ

This is a fact demonstrated by concordant clinical investigations, pathological experimentation, and normal anatomy, and recently admitted even by Flechsig himself, although with the reservation that the number of the

projection fibers is large in the perceptive areas and scanty in the areas of association (fig. 861, *c*) [*fig. 241*].

For our part, we can add to the concordant observations of Dejerine, Monakow, Siemerling, Vogt, etc., made in man and gyrencephalic mammals, the following two observations made in rodents:

a. In the rabbit, guinea pig, and mouse, all the cortical regions, without exception, emit descending fibers that traverse the corpus striatum and reach the spinal cord or stop in the thalamic, mesencephalic, pontine nuclei, etc. In some cases, such fibers of projection, as we said previously, represent branches of bifurcation of association fibers.

b. Even the cerebral areas [that are] evidently of association or memory (in the sense of not receiving direct sensory fibers), that is, the interhemispheric cortex and Ammon's horn, present motor pathways (*fornix longus* of Forel and *anterior columns* of the fornix).

The fibers of projection are of three kinds: first, *descending motor* fibers, that is to say, destined for the motor nuclei of the spinal cord or for the intermediate, motor nuclei of the thalamus, mesencephalon, medulla, etc.; second, *descending sensory* fibers (fig. 862, *a*) [*fig. 242*], terminating in the thalamic sensory nuclei (sensory nuclei, olfactory nuclei, medial and lateral geniculate bodies, etc.); third, *ascending sensory* or thalamocortical fibers that link the sensory nuclei of the thalamus and mesencephalon with the cerebral cortex (fig. 862, *b*) [*fig. 242*].

Differences between the Perceptive and Memory Areas in Relation to Their Radiating or Projection Fibers. It is very probable that both kinds of areas possess specific afferent and efferent fibers, but in the present state of science, the definite anatomical characteristic [that differentiates between the two kinds of areas]ᵀ deals only with afferent or ascending fibers.

In effect, according to what we believe to have been proven in the rodents,[19] the difference rests on the fact that the perceptive or projection areas receive sensory fibers originating in thalamic nuclei of the same category, whereas the association or memory areas lack thalamocortical fibers, these being replaced by

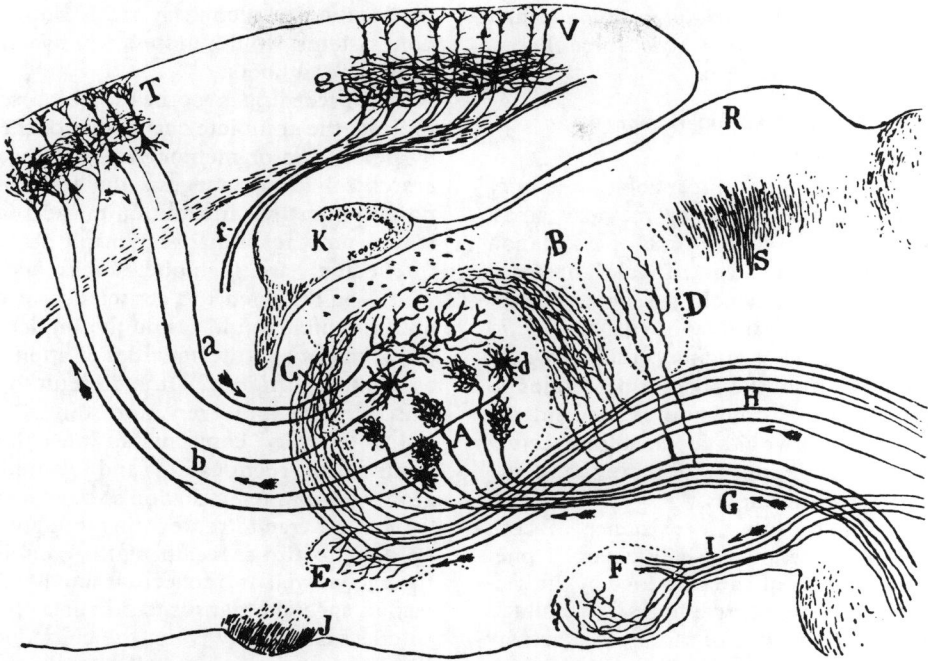

[*FIG. 242*]   Fig. 862. Scheme of the afferent and efferent pathways of the sensory-motor area of the cerebrum. *T*, sensory-motor area; *A*, sensory thalamic nucleus; *a*, corticothalamic fibers; *b*, thalamocortical or sensory fibers; *V*, visual area.

sensory-memory fibers, that is to say, fibers arising from the perception areas (fig. 861, *g*, *h*) [*fig. 241*].

We consider the following propositions regarding the descending fibers of projection probable but not proven: (a) The areas of perception are linked to the thalamic sensory nuclei by means of descending sensory fibers (fibers of expectant attention, as we have classified them on another occasion). Such connections would be lacking in the memory areas. (b) There would be two kinds of motor fiber: *long* or *direct* fibers (pyramidal and similar pathways), destined to link the cortical perception areas with the peripheral motor nuclei (perhaps by means of a funicular neuron of the spinal cord or medulla); and *short* or *indirect* fibers, arising from the memory areas and terminating in the intermediary motor nuclei of the thalamus, mesencephalon, and pons, whose neurons would transmit finally the cerebral impulse to the peripheral motor nuclei. The former corticomotor pathways

would have a reflex character; the second would represent the pathways of voluntary movement and of emotional phenomena; they would be, in short, the instrument of our ideas and of our deliberate volitions.

Between both kinds of motor pathways, there would exist transitions; that is to say, some direct or long motor fibers would also emit collaterals to the hypothalamic and pontine motor nuclei. Such mixed fibers, extremely developed in rodents and much less so in man (let us remember the establishment in man of an individual corticopontine pathway, different from the collateral pontine pathway of the rodents, etc.), would come to be the first phase in the anatomical and functional differentiation of the cortical motor pathways.

As examples of these two kinds of motor pathways, we will cite the *pyramidal pathway* originating in the tactile sensory cortex; and the *anterior columns of the fornix*, the [main] projection system of Ammon's horn (secondary memory area), whose fibers are linked with several lower nuclei (*septum lucidum,* small nucleus of the thalamic stria [medullaris], mamillary bodies, etc., etc.).

4. Sensory-Memory and Intermemory Association Pathways

Joining the areas of perception or sensory areas and the association or memory areas, Flechsig has supposed two kinds of association fibers: centripetal and centrifugal. Thanks to the former, about which we have already talked in previous paragraphs (fig. 861, *g, h*) [*fig. 241*], the visual or auditory residues would be transmitted from the areas of perception to the memory areas; by means of the second, the intellectual areas would be capable of acting by exciting, facilitating, or inhibiting the activity of the perceptive areas.

Tanzi, who accepts the existence of both kinds of fibers, explains hallucinatory phenomena by means of the existence of the second or memory-perceptive fibers.[20] If hallucinations were the result of the morbid activity of the perception areas (for example, the visual area), the projected image would be hemianopsic in the vast majority of cases, since it may not be presumed that chemical stimulants (toxins in infected fibers, alcohol in alcoholism) act at the same time and in a symmetrical manner in both hemispheres. [In a hallucination], the external image would suffer a sort of regression, moving along the memory-perception fibers toward the perceptive area (visual, acoustic, etc.), and reproducing again the sensation with its two essential attributes: the exteriorization or projection and the belief, illusory on this occasion, that the image is produced by a true object situated external to us.

In our opinion, the hallucinations of dreams whose images have all the prominence, energy, and coloring of a percept[21] could be explained in the same way.

But, besides these perceptomemory pathways, the laws of psychological association oblige us to admit the existence of fibers joining the several memory areas. These fibers must be of two kinds: (a) *secondary intermemory fibers,* devoted to the association of combined ideas or representations; (b) *primary-secondary intermemory fibers,* which serve to link the primary memory areas with the ideation or secondary areas. Both association systems would possess homolateral and contralateral fibers.

The preceding hypothesis, which seems to indicate the complete occupation of the cortex by perception or memory areas of diverse hierarchical levels, suggests the following important question. In addition to the said areas, would not the human cerebrum also possess intellectual areas, higher areas on which would be reflected the conscience of the ego and in which would reside the higher faculty of judgment and the activities of attention and association [of ideas]?[U] It is difficult to answer this question and even more difficult not to fall into risky conjectures, inevitably condemned to rectification and abandonment. However, on meditating on so deep a mystery, we are not free to repress this thought. In our opinion, to aim at localizing the conscience of the ego, as well as intellectual activity, the will, etc., in special organs is to pursue a chimera.[22] Intellectual activity is not the consequence of the activity of a privileged region, but the result of the combined action of a large number of primary and secondary memory areas. From the purely physiological point of view, intellectual activity lies in the creation of a functional connection between two images that are little or not related, whereas from the subjective point of view, there is the belief (formulated or not by symbols of language) that the functional link established in the cerebrum corresponds positively to a relation of succession, of coexistence, or of coherence between two or more phenomena of the external world. Attention, as well as emotion and conscience, represents collateral functional processes, and in a certain way these are accessories of the cited relationship, since both in animals and in man, there are numerous reflex reactions, perfectly suitable and directed to a purpose, that are not accompanied by such [psychic][V] epiphenomena.

By this we do not aim at identifying the reflex act or the instinct with an intellectual process. The former represents constant reactions, generally immediate, whose performance does not require volitional efforts of accommodation; whereas intellectual processes represent mediate reactions, almost specific for each individual, and accompanied by the awareness of an effort, of something like the sensation of a motor activity destined to join and put in order chains of weakly associated neurons.

The conscious or unconscious character of cerebral activity perhaps depends, as some claim, on the greater or lesser expenditure of vital force required by the propagation of the nerve impulse through the neuronal series, depending on whether the pathways are ample and well trodden or imperfect and little traveled.

5. Physiological Postulates Implicit in the Organization of the Cerebral Centers and Pathways

In our study of the pattern of visual projection to the cerebrum and of the decussations of the optic nerve and other pathways,[23] we have tried to demonstrate the incomprehensibility, from the utilitarian point of view, of the architectonic plan of the cerebrum, if we do not assume that Nature, in organizing the psychic centers, has obeyed these principles: unity of perception; congruent and continuous projection on the cortex of the retinal and tactile peripheral surfaces; economy of space and of conductor protoplasm.

a. Unity of the Perception of Visual [and Tactile Space, Smells,][W] and Sounds. Examining the

pattern of retinal projection on the cerebrum, according to the results of the investigations of the clinicians and the well-known dispositions of the optic chiasm, it is noticed that fibers originating from identical points of both retinas converge on a singular group of isodynamic pyramids of the cerebrum (fig. 571, *Rv*) [*fig. 244*].

The cerebral retinal unity seems to have no other aim than the substitution of the duality of the peripheral impression by the unity of central perception, so much so that the moment the ocular axes deviate from the position of convergence, the visual sensation becomes double, because the identical retinal points now correspond not to one but to two pleiades of isodynamic pyramids.

The unit of perception in the cerebral [somatic] sensory area is more simply achieved. Since each half of the impressionable tactile surface (and of the sensitivity of the muscles, tendons, etc.) concerns one side of space, and the central pathways related to it are exclusively contralateral, the unity of perception will result from the fact that any sensory afferent fiber furnishes a specific spatial sign and is in constant relation with a unique isodynamic group of pyramids.

In the nonspatial centers, such as the acoustic and olfactory, Nature has not had the necessity of being subjected to the above-mentioned demand in order to obtain unity of

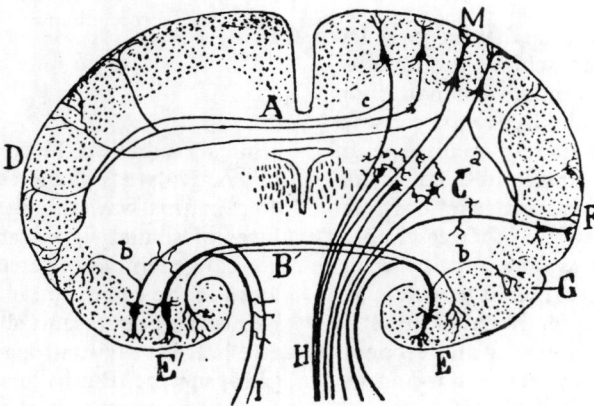

[FIG. 243] Fig. 863. Scheme of the projection and association fibers in the cerebrum of a rodent. A, corpus callosum; B, anterior commissure; C, corpus striatum; D, visual memory area; M, visual perceptive area; E, olfactory perceptive area; G, olfactory memory area.

sensation. Acoustic and olfactory sensations being merely qualitative or tonal, it was not so important that the impression of the same [excitation] should take place in both hemispheres. Even in the visual system, the duplication of perceptions becomes impossible when the peripheral impression is stripped of its analytical and spatial character[24] by means of any artifice.

Anatomically, the unity of acoustic and olfactory sensation, however, could be understandable by the projection in both hemispheres of the same qualitative impression, supposing that the isodynamic pleiad of pyramids is distributed in the two hemispheres, and that any afferent sensory fiber bifurcates, furnishing a direct branch destined for the homolateral half of the said cellular pleiad and another crossed branch (anterior commissure, etc.) destined for the contralateral half.[25]

This concept explains a very interesting property of the anterior commissure, namely that this transverse pathway joins homofunctional areas of both olfactory regions, in contrast to the corpus callosum which, as we have stated and as shown in fig. 863, A [fig. 243], links heterofunctional areas of both hemispheres. From this it is inferred that the said commissures are not homologous, since the corpus callosum contains mainly crossed fibers of spatial senses (vision and touch), whereas the anterior commissure contains crossed fibers of the merely qualitative senses (hearing and smell).

It is deduced from what has been stated that Nature, in order to achieve the unity of perception, acts differently, depending on whether the peripheral impression possesses a spatial character or is merely qualitative. In the former case, each sensory fiber conveying a peculiar spatial sign terminates on only one side of the cerebrum; in the other case, bilateral fibers conveying the same quality terminate in both hemispheres, thanks to which, besides increasing the perceptive intensity, it is possible to establish more easily and economically association pathways between the acoustic and visual memory areas.

b. *Concentric Symmetry*.[x] This principle, inferred from the results of physiological and

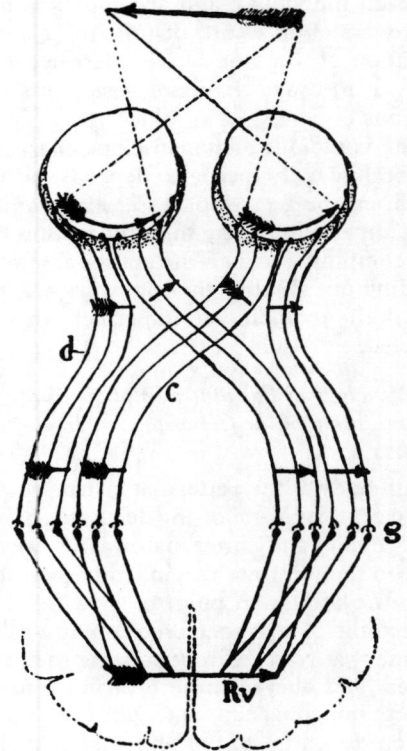

[*FIG. 244*] Fig. 245. Scheme of the decussation of the optic pathways and of the central visual projection in man. It is seen that a direct fascicle is necessary for animals with a single visual field. *c*, crossed fascicle of the optic nerve; *d*, voluminous direct fascicle; *g*, lateral geniculate body; *Rv*, projection of the mental image in the visual cortex of the cerebrum. [From Chapter 17 of the *Histologie*]

clinical studies on the relative positions of the perceptive areas of the cortex, can be enunciated in this way: the peripheral sensory surfaces of spatial significance (retina and skin) are congruently projected onto the perceptive areas of the cerebrum, in such a way that each hemisphere represents simultaneously the lateral halves of [visual] space and of the sensory [skin] surface. But by virtue of the crossing of the optic nerves and of the adaptive decussation of the central tactile and acoustic pathways, the right hemisphere represents the left side, and vice versa.

Such an arrangement embodies a postulate already enunciated in another chapter, namely that the correct perception of visual and tactile space requires a continuous and orderly cerebral projection (that is to say, with maintenance of the same spatial relations) of the peripheral sensory surface. Therefore, the central or peripheral destruction of an isodynamic group of neurons, as well as the disarrangement or transposition of the same, would produce necessarily and respectively a perceptive gap and a disorder of spatial reference. (Let us remember the cases of scotoma cited by Wilbrand and Henschen, and resulting from partial lesions of the calcarine fissure and visual afferent pathways.)

Furthermore, it is necessary to admit that an identical [topographical] projection exists in both the visual and tactile memory areas, with persistence of the spatial sign of the corresponding isodynamic cellular groups, since optic and sensory reminiscences present to us as congruent images [endowed with]^Y extent, outlined against space, and often exteriorized (dreams, hallucinations).[26]

c. Economy of Space and Protoplasm. Numerous anatomical arrangements are justified by this principle, namely the peripheral position of the gray matter, the folding of the gray matter (economy of space and of the trajectory of the nerve fibers), the proximity of areas that are joined by powerful and intimate functional relationships (let us remember, for instance, the proximity of the three areas of language), the establishment of the commissures at the points of shortest transverse distance, the proximity of the primary memory areas to the perceptive areas, etc. For economy of fibers, the [somatic] sensory and acoustic fibers became crossed once the fundamental decussation of the optic nerve was created, since it became necessary to have a homolateral concordance of the spatial signs of the visual, tactile, muscular, and tendinous perceptions, with the gathering in adjoining parts of the same hemisphere of all the areas corresponding to the same side of [external] space. [It is also a principle]^Z that economizes protoplasm and superfluous trajectory of the association pathways.

Hypotheses about the Histological Basis of Cerebral Function

We have already indicated that a topophysiological doctrine of the cerebrum, however excellent, and though capable of gathering important data relevant to the diagnosis and treatment of nervous diseases, leaves us in utter darkness regarding knowledge of the inner mechanism of psychic acts. The determination of the sequence of molecular processes that the neurons undergo during intellectual activity requires, like a previous question, an exact and complete histology of the cerebral areas and pathways, as well as precise ideas about those extremely complex changes or commutations of connection that must precede each dynamic, associative, emotional, or motor [behavior]. Even so, we will still not reach a mechanistic explanation of mental operations, if physiology, going deeply into the analysis of the nutritive metabolism of the cells, does not reveal to us the nature of the nerve impulse, the energy transformations that occur during the genesis and propagation of the impulse, as well as during the production of the concomitant phenomena of perception and thought, namely feelings, conscience, and volition.

This ideal is still very distant. But while chemistry, histology, and cytology slowly advance toward it, it will not be superfluous to introduce the histological conjectures that have been imagined in recent years for the understanding of certain relatively simple psychic and physiological processes.

Hypothesis of Duval [about the Mechanism of Sleep, Association of Ideas, Fatigue, Memory, Oblivion, etc.]^{AA}

It was many years ago that Rabl-Rückhard[27] raised the conjecture that some psychic acts could be explained mechanistically by a continuous ameboidism of the nerve cells; but as this author started from the hypothesis of the network theory of the gray matter, a network that everybody imagined as a solid and stable mesh, his idea did not awaken any echo. It is necessary to recognize that only Duval has had the merit of supporting the said hypothesis by exact anatomical data, applying them with the precision of concepts and language that are characteristic of the histologist of Paris, to the elucidation of the phenomena of wakefulness, sleep, hysterical paralysis, somnambulism, etc.

According to Duval,[28]

in man when sleeping, the cerebral arborizations of the [central[BB] sensory neurons are retracted like the pseudopods of an anesthetized leukocyte. The weak excitations produced in the sensory nerves lead in the sleeping human to reflex reactions, but they do not reach the cerebral cortex; stronger excitations cause the stretching or relaxation of the cerebral arborizations of the sensory neuron; the impulse, on passing to the cortical cells, leads to awakening, the successive phases of which clearly suggest the reestablishment of a series of [connections] previously interrupted by retraction and withdrawal of the pseudopodal arborizations.[29] Anesthesias and hysterical paralyses could be explained in the same way, as well as the increase in energy of the imagination, in memory, in the association of ideas, under the influence of various agents, such as tea and coffee, that could excite the ameboidism of nerve extremities that are in contiguity, in order to bring their arborizations closer and facilitate the passage of impulses.

In support of his hypothesis, Duval invokes [the following].

1. The morphology of the neurons, whose terminal nerve arborizations enter into contact, as shown in our works, with the cell body and dendrites of other neurons.

2. The investigations of Wiedersheim[30] on the ameboid movements of certain nerve cells of the *Leptodora hyalina.*

3. The observations of Pergens, demonstrating that the protoplasmic portion of the cones of the retina in fish shrink and shorten under the influence of light, a retraction that could also occur in the dendritic processes of the neurons of the ganglionic layer.

4. The discovery, by Ranvier, of movements in the terminal cilia of the olfactory cells of the frog.

5. The experiments with morphine, ether, and chloroform in animals, made by Demoor,[31] which seem to prove the retraction and disappearance, during pathological sleep, of dendritic spines and the shrinkage of the dendrites.

6. The conclusions of Stefanowska,[32] who, after numerous experiments in mice and guinea pigs involving electrification of the cerebrum, electrocution, inhalation of vapors of ether, chloroform, coal gas, etc., has seen the spines or piriform appendages of the dendrites become retracted and disappear with the formation on the dendrites of numerous varicosities. Since, for Stefanowska, the contact of the neurons is made between the axonal aborizations and the spines, as soon as these disappear, the passage of the impulses is suspended, and sleep and rest follow.

7. The works of Manouelian, made in the same laboratory as Duval, which testify that in mice subjected to continual exercise, and thus seized with extreme fatigue, the pyramidal cells have lost their spines, and their terminal dendrites acquire a moniliform state or ball-shaped local swellings. Such disconnection of the neuronal surfaces has been observed by Manouelian even in the olfactory glomeruli, where the dendritic tuft shrinks, becoming resolved into voluminous spheres.

8. The investigations of Odier[33] on the spinal cord, which show (although the interpretation of this author is unacceptable) that anesthetics make dendrites smaller and that induced impulses strongly shrink dendrites.

9. The confirmation by Querton[34] that during hibernation in the marmot, the piriform appendages of the cerebral dendrites are retracted, and the terminal [dendritic] tuft of the pyramids is modified, becoming dotted with varicosities.

10. The investigations of Havet,[35] who has confirmed some of the above-mentioned alterations in invertebrates, especially the varicose modification and the shrinkage and even disappearance of processes.

The hypothesis of Duval was severely combated by Kölliker,[36] who declared it unacceptable for the following reasons: first, the axons are not contractile under any kind of excitation; second, in those animals whose transparency allows one to observe the sensory nerve arborizations, no movement is observed (larvae of batrachians and siredons, etc.); third, the axon is composed of highly differentiated solid protoplasm, not of soft matter like leukocytes; fourth, psychic processes are stable acts, in large measure able to be regulated with respect to their intensity and duration, whereas ameboid movements are continuous, disordered, unavoidably obeying nutritive or thermal stimuli.[37]

To the a priori arguments of Kölliker in recent years have been added some negative observations of Azoulay,[38] Soukhanoff,[39] Lugaro,[40] and Reusz.[41]

Azoulay, who studied the cerebral pyramids of the mouse, subjected to the action of ether or to fatigue lasting one hour, was not able to find any morphological changes differing from the normal.

Soukhanoff, who in a former work confesses to be an enthusiastic supporter of the theory of Duval, in later works retreats from his resolution, declaring that the retraction of the spines and the varicose lesions of the dendrites in narcotized, fatigued, and anemic (by ligature of the aorta) animals are the result of a pathological process that has nothing to do with the functional physiological phases of the neurons (*varicose degeneration*).

Lugaro, after declaring that many of the neuronal modifications described by the authors are the consequence of bad fixation of the tissue, proposes, as the result of his investigations on the action of narcotics, a hypothesis that comes to be the antithesis of that of Duval. For Lugaro, the resting state corresponds to the presence of nonvaricose dendrites provided with numerous spines; the functional state [corresponds] to the normal dendritic arborization but bereft of these collateral appendages; and, finally, the varicose state [corresponds] to fatigue. In a previous work,[42] he had defended a somewhat different idea, since he claimed that a state of activity of the nerve protoplasm is accompanied by a swelling of the cell body, a swelling that, being propagated to the dendrites, would make the contact between the neuronal connections more intimate and efficacious and thus would expedite the passage of impulses.

With respect to Reusz, he declares the cited changes and especially the varicose state as artificial products that are found in normal tissue that is badly fixed, like that which comes from narcotized, cocainized, and fatigued animals, and therefore without any relation to

phases of neuronal physiology. However, recently, Narbut[43] believes he has seen a decrease and even a disappearance of dendritic spines in the cerebrum of the narcotized dog.

For his part, van Gehuchten[44] affirms the reality of the morphological changes produced by narcotics. In resting cells, the appendages (our spines) would be long and of uniform thickness, in agreement with the observations of Querton and Lugaro (filiform appendages).[45] Under certain experimental conditions, these appendages would become shorter, modify their form and become piriform, and possibly disappear completely, being later followed by a moniliform state of the dendrites. With regard to the significance of such changes, van Gehuchten makes no pronouncement, ignoring whether they are the result of a degenerative process or a state of physiological contraction of the neurons.

Although in a manner different from Duval, Renaut[46] has also imagined, based on his observations in the retina with the method of Ehrlich, a morphological explanation of functional activity and rest. In the opinion of the histologist of Lyon, the dendrites of the retina (plexiform layers) would enter into contact with each other, at the level of their varicosities. The resting state would be rendered by a weak development of the dendritic pearls or spheres, whereas a state of activity would be due to a rich absorption of matter in the said varicosities, with concomitant shortening of the dendritic processes.

[We had also presented a hypothesis[47] that we very rapidly abandoned and in which the neuroglial cells performed the main role. We had thought for a time that these cells were capable of lengthening their appendages and intervening between the neuronal connections, which would lead to inactivity in the latter. The neurons would return again to activity when they would enter into free contact with each other upon retraction of the neuroglial processes.][CC]

Of all the facts and arguments expounded in favor of and against the theory of Duval and similar [theories], one deduces that the question of neural ameboidism cannot yet be regarded as resolved, either positively or negatively. There is no truly positive evidence, because all the morphological modifications upon which the hypothesis rests (absorption of spines, varicosities, retraction of dendrites following the action of narcotics, fatigue, anemia, etc.) can be interpreted as pathological alterations independent of the functional state and even as [postmortem] disorders, according to what Soukhanoff declares and van Gehuchten implies. There is no cause either for definitively repudiating the hypothesis, because the negative observations held against it refer exclusively to the dendrites, that is to say, to only one of the elements of neuronal connection, ruling out the terminal axonal arborization, in which, perhaps during normal physiological activity, motor phenomena occur [that are] similar to ameboidism.[48] Also omitted has been examination of the soma and thick dendrites, at the level of which the more important axocellular contacts are made (pericellular baskets in the spinal cord, cerebellum, medulla, cerebrum, etc.), without any other reason for the exclusion than the difficulty of impregnating them, which leads to a mistake of logic similar to that famous one of Gall, who was against any important physiological localization in those cerebral gyri incapable of being explored by palpation.

Let us add, finally, that in spite of the precautions taken by Stefanowska, Demoor, and Soukhanoff in their contrary experiments, none of them seems to us to have taken into account sufficiently several grave causes of error which we have in vain pointed out for many years: (1) The retraction of the spines and the varicose state of the dendrites are the result of a postmortem cellular alteration, which is consistently observed in normal preparations of Ehrlich and Golgi when fixation is delayed.[49] (2) For the same reason, in the usual thick blocks, stained with silver chromate, the central zones always show cells without spines and strewn with varicosities. (3) When fixation is late and imperfect (slow method of Golgi), the spines do not appear. (4) Finally, the spines were actually discovered by us in preparations from mammals killed by chloroform. For many years, we have been in the habit of sacrificing animals by means of narcotics, and if the blocks are thin and the osmic acid rapidly penetrates, we have never been able to distin-

guish in the neurons varicosities or other changes that are not [also] present in animals dying by hemorrhage.

In short, we are not against the concept of Duval; rather, we feel for it a great attractiveness, easily excusable if it is considered that neural ameboidism not only fits well with the neuron theory but is almost a consequence of it (let us remember the ameboid phenomena of embryonic neurons). But we also think that the experimental proof has been obtained in a bad field, departing from that indicated by the cited illustrious histologist, who attributed motor phenomena to the axonal terminations and not to the dendrites. At the present time, it is necessary to confess that, although a harsh critic would reject as unfounded the facts, adduced by some authors, on retraction of dendrites, it could still be a possible histological explanation of sleep, distraction, forgetfulness, and many mental phenomena; and it could be defended favorably provided there did not appear against it precise and concordant observations made on the whole range of neuronal connections, that is to say, on the soma and dendrites on the one hand and on the axonal arborizations on the other, observations which [might] reveal the perfect stability of the surfaces of contact during the several physiological states capable of experimentation. And in spite of everything, a scrupulous mind could still raise hard-to-refute objections, because it is almost impossible to do experiments whose conditions approach the normal physiological state, during which the changes of position and form of the neuronal arborizations could be fleeting and erased, as occurs with active leukocytes before death.

Normal and Pathological Alterations of the Neurofibrils[DD]

We have just seen that the ameboidism of the cellular processes is a supposition for which definitive proof has still not been given. But there exists an internal ameboidism, that is to say, a series of changes of the protoplasmic reticulum correlating with some physiological states, which have just been revealed by the investigations of Tello[50] and ourselves,[51] and which perhaps may account for many dy-

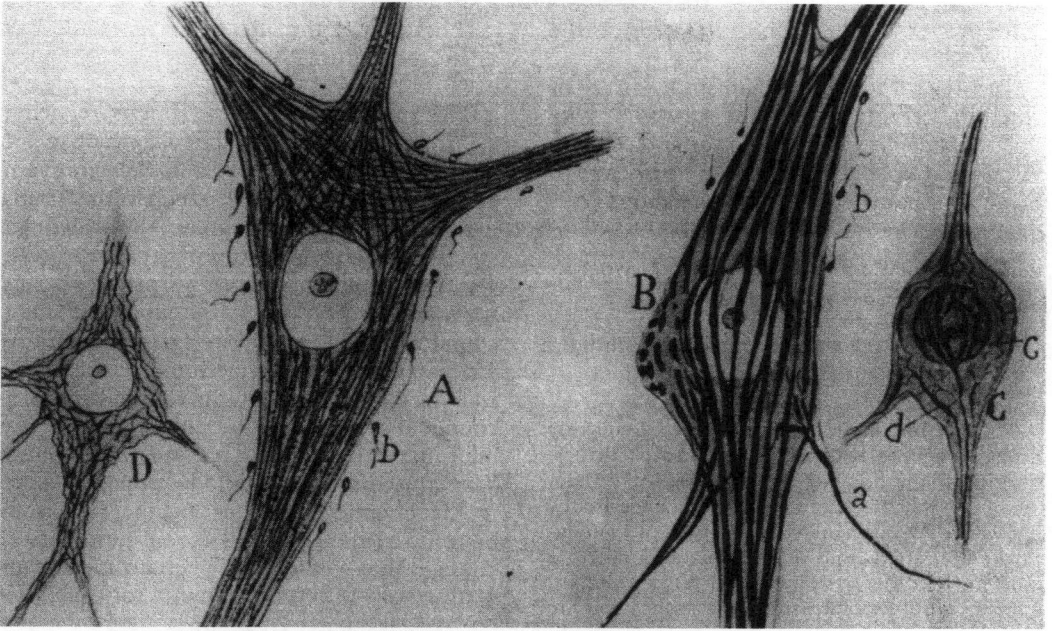

[FIG. 245] Fig. 864. Cells of the spinal cord of the lizard. A, D, motor and funicular cells in a state of activity (thirty hours in an oven at 30°[C]); B, C, motor and funicular cells of the spinal cord of a lizard maintained at ordinary temperature (12°[C]); a, axon; b, terminal nerve clubs; c, perinuclear network; d, thickened primary filament. [This is fig. 73 of the first volume of the French version.]

namic neuronal phenomena when we study them better.

As is seen in fig. 864, B [fig. 245], the neurofibrils of the neurons of reptiles, [inactive] due to the winter cold (temperature of 8° to 12° [C]), fuse together in colossal cords [that are] delicately granular, admirably impregnable with silver nitrate, and separated by large, clear spaces bereft of [contents]. The filaments of the axon are equally condensed into a single and homogenous thread, which branches on arriving at the [somal] protoplasm, and those resident in the dendrites suffer equal fusions and simplifications which lend them a singular appearance. This phenomenon is also presented, although with other characteristics, in the funicular cells (fig. 864, C) [fig. 245]. Only the neurons of the cerebrum, mesencephalon, and diencephalon, which remain active in spite of the action of the cold (the animal in wintertime [can] open the eyes and move the head), maintain a normal reticulum.

But as soon as springtime comes or the temperature of the cage in which the reptile lives is increased, or it is stimulated by any procedure that brings the spinal cord into play, the thin neurofibrils reappear, increasing enormously [in number], and the interfibrillar spaces, which now have a granular appearance, disappear. The recent investigations of Tello, made in our laboratory, prove that the passage of the B state to the A state (fig. 864, A, D) [fig. 245] is achieved by warming up the reptile for only half an hour.

On the left part of the figure, we show the state of activity and, on the right, the resting state. Notice the enormous difference in the reticulum in the two states, and bear in mind that in this experiment (absolutely consistent in its results in all reptiles) only perfectly normal conditions have been used in order to produce the cited variations.

Similar phenomena appear in nervous diseases, for example, in rabies, in which the inaction of the neurons comes from the disorganization of the nerve fibers that bring the impulses.

With regard to the mechanism by virtue of which the temperature or the state of activity produce such very interesting variations in the reticulum, our studies are still not sufficient to formulate a somewhat sure explanation.

Hypothesis of Tanzi about the Hypertrophy of Nerve Pathways by Exercise[52]

[Here is how the author himself formulates the hypothesis][EE]:

A nerve impulse that passes more frequently through a neuronal connection will provoke hypernutrition of the overexcited pathways, and as happens in the muscles, there will follow a hypertrophy that will result in an increase in length of the neuronal arborizations, and in consequence a decrease of the distance that separates the surfaces of contact. Since these spaces represent the resistance that the impulses must overcome, it will result that the conductivity of the nervous system will be inversely related to the interneuronal gaps. Exercise, tending to decrease these gaps, must thus increase the functional capacity of the neurons.

This theory, which is not based on any hypothetical factor but on the reality of neuronal connections, has the advantage, as Soury has pointed out, of showing us how habitual acts, by dint of being repeated, become easy and automatic, and how acts that we call conscious and voluntary movements, by contrast with reflex acts, from the physicochemical point of view, could depend on a state of resistance to the passage of nerve impulses.

Hypothesis of Lugaro about the Localization of the Dual Intellectual and Emotional Process

Lugaro,[53] starting from the concept of the inseparable intellectual and affective duality of any psychic operation, considers it probable that the elaboration of the phenomenon of consciousness takes place between the neurons, that is to say, in the connections of the afferent axonal terminations with the cell body

and dendrites of the pyramids, whereas the [elaboration] of the affective state would have as its substratum the interior of the neuron itself.

The intellectual process thus is related to the interneuronal connections, which would have been established during the embryonic period, by a chemotactic mechanism, similar to that invoked by us to explain the growth and connection of the neurons in the embryo. The very fact of the transmission of the impulse from one neuron to another would be due to chemical phenomena; in fact, the impulse causes a chemical change in the axonal arborizations which, acting in its turn as a physicochemical stimulus on the protoplasm of other neurons, would induce in these new impulses. The conscious state would be precisely linked to the chemical changes engendered in the neurons by the [afferent] axonal terminations, changes that would have a certain specific and qualitatively different character for each afferent axonal arborization.

There are no reasons for supporting or refuting this ingenious conjecture of Lugaro, which represents at the present time, and in the absence of objective physiological data, simply a possibility. Let us note, however, that the emotive tone that accompanies our perceptions and ideas could be linked also to the activity of other constituent elements of the gray matter (cells with short axon, cells and pathways of projection, etc.).

Our Theory on the Improved Growth of the Interneuronal Connections[54]

In several places in our works, based on the laws of development of neuronal morphology, we have expounded some conjectures destined to explain the improvement by repetition of certain psychic acts, as well as the originality and diversity of talents, logical memory, and even aberrations in the association of ideas.

We have just seen that the hypothesis of Tanzi gives an exact account of the facility and unconsciousness of certain psychic acts, but it does not explain to us the improved abilities created by [appropriate] exercise, which not only consists of making the [performance of a]^{FF} difficult act easy and prompt, but of performing [under certain conditions an act apparently]^{GG} impossible. Nobody ignores the fact that the work of a pianist, speaker, mathematician, thinker, etc., is absolutely unapproachable by the uneducated man, whose adaptation to such novelties (in cases in which such an individual meets favorable organic circumstances) is the work of many years of mental and muscular gymnastics. To understand this important phenomenon, it is necessary to admit, besides reinforcement of the preestablished organic pathways, the establishment of other new pathways, by means of the branching and progressive growth of the terminal dendritic and axonal arborizations. From such a supposition, acquired talent (leaving aside that which is related to cerebral capacity or organic memory, quantity of neurons, and other conditions that must also have an influence on the result) would have as its main conditions the presence of primary and secondary memory centers furnished with multiple and complicated connections joining groups or pleiades of neurons that are little or nonconnected in the cerebra of the uncultured. By virtue of that superior association, a slight sensory excitation, the [ghost] of an idea, or any other stimulus only capable of promoting vulgar or illogical associations in the uneducated individual would raise in a very cultivated and impressionable individual unexpected combinations of ideas that render schematically but accurately positive relations of external reality, and become condensed and expressed in general and fruitful formulae.

The above-mentioned hypothesis would also explain logical memory, that is to say, that concatenation and ordering of acquired information that is only achieved after a long effort of attention and consideration and by means of a reorganization of the memory centers; [and it would also explain] the creation of [organized] systems of ideas or complicated logical constructions (philosophical, religious, and political systems or creeds).

The observations and arguments that serve as support for this hypothesis are [as follows].

1. During embryonic development, the dendrites and axonal arborizations extend and branch progressively, entering into contact with an increasing number of neurons (see *Histogenesis of the Spinal Cord,* Vol. 1, chapter XXI, of this book).

2. It is also a fact that the definitive adjustment of these connections is only attained after some trials, since we observe that before the processes reach their destination and make stable contacts, numerous accessory [dendritic and axonal]^{HH} branches disappear; [these are] kinds of tentative associations [destined to persist or to disappear, depending on unknown circumstances],^{II} and their existence proves the great initial plasticity of the cellular arborizations.

3. In some areas, the processes go astray, acquiring abnormal connections (intra-epithelial branches, etc.). [We have shown many examples of false pathways when dealing with the histogenesis of the spinal cord];^{JJ} recently, we have found in the dog a few days old axons terminating by mistake in the ependymal cavity and in the process of reabsorption.

4. This adjustment in growth of the processes continues after birth, and there is a large difference with regard to the length and number of secondary and tertiary neuronal branches between the newborn child and an adult man.

5. It is also likely that such development is improved in certain areas by means of usage and, by contrast, is suspended and reduced in cerebral areas that are not cultivated.

6. The experiments on nerve sectioning prove that peripheral axons, both sensory and motor, are capable of growing and arborizing and, in restoring their connections with the skin and muscles, of becoming organized in a somewhat different manner.

7. Neuropathology knows of an infinite number of cases of functional restoration after grave lesions of differentiated cortical centers (reestablishment of the articulation of words in motor aphasia, disappearance of word deafness, reappearance of sensation in stroke, etc.). Such return to normality after the nerve fibers have been disorganized can only be understood by admitting that in the cerebrum, as in the sectioned peripheral nerves, the healthy cut end is capable of growing and emitting

new collaterals which, on running through the damaged regions, reestablish contacts with the disconnected neurons. When the latter neurons have been destroyed, the new-formed branches would go in search of other nerve cells [and, by entering into contact with them, give to their activity]^{KK} a new functional character.

The new processes would be oriented in the same direction as the predominant nerve impulses or in the direction of that intercellular association that is the object of the repeated solicitations of the will. This hypertrophy of the cellular processes could be accompanied by a certain active congestion that would provide nutritive materials. For the rest, according to what we expounded in another chapter (see histogenesis of the spinal cord), the mechanism of growth [of the new axonal branches]^{LL} could be understood as being under the influence of chemotactic actions.

[It results from the works made in recent years by Nageotte,[55] Marinesco and Minea,[56] ourselves,[57] Tello,[58] Guido Sala,[59] U. Rossi,[60] and other scientists that when an axon is interrupted in the spinal cord, cerebellum, cerebrum, and optic nerve, its central extremity or its collaterals are probably the site of the phenomenon of regeneration. However, nothing authorizes us to affirm in an irrefutable manner that these phenomena lead to the partial or total reestablishment of the injured pathways. It seems more probable, on the contrary, that degenerative phenomena follow it, causing the atrophy and reabsorption of the branches newly originated from the axon. Perhaps this result is due in large measure to the absence of Schwann cells which in the peripheral nerves serve to attract and orient by their secretions the new nerve shoots; perhaps it is even due to the rarity of the chemotactic substances elaborated by neurons that become adult and which are incapable for this reason of attracting the new-formed growth cones with sufficient energy. But the last word has not been said about these questions which one studies with a passion by means of the neurofibrillar methods.

One can, besides, explain the disappearance of certain physiological problems and the restoration of certain suspended functions in cerebral lesions that, for example, give rise to several kinds of aphasias without invoking necessarily the phenomenon of regeneration of the damaged pathways. This is what Monakow[61] has done in the following manner in his theory of *diaschisis*. When a specialized cortical area is injured, two kinds of disorders are seen to develop: *residual,* coming from the partial or total destruction of all the neurons that reside in this area or of those that send their axons to it; *initial* or *temporary,* which are caused by a sort of *shock* that interrupts the activity of areas that are nondamaged but which receive motor, commissural, or association fibers from the injured center. These paralyzed zones are the only ones that can recover their function, as soon as the cause of the disorder disappears.]^{MM}

If the acceptance of the capacity for growth and interconnection of neurons in the adult accounts for the talent of adaptation and for the capacity for varying our system of ideas, it is clear that the suspension of this activity in the old or rusty man (for absence of mental culture or other causes) could in some way explain the fixity of convictions, the unadaptability to the moral environment, and even the violent fear of the unknown; and when, by virtue of more or less pathological causes, a loosening of the connections takes place, I mean the atrophy and shrinkage of the [neuronal] processes and the partial disintegration of the memory systems, there will result amnesia, poverty in the association [of ideas], mental [slowness], and (carrying the disorder to extremes) even imbecility and madness. And it could be added yet that if in the madman, amnesiac, and aged man, old memories are more persistent than recent ones, it is due to the fact that the earlier created association pathways reached an unusual robustness, because they were formed during a period in which neuronal plasticity was at its peak.

With that we do not pretend to exclude, in the explanation of the adaptative and regressive phenomena to which we allude, other factors whose significance is at the present time indeterminate, for example, the changes occurring in the intraprotoplasmic pathways (cytoplasm and neurofibrils), the variations in the chemical composition of the cells, the richness in neurons with short axons, the varieties in the number and position of the neuroglial cells in the gray matter, etc.

Cajal's Notes

1. Flechsig, *Gehirn und Seele,* Leipzig, 189[6]. See also *Neurol. Centralbl.,* 189[6].
2. Van Gehuchten, Structure du télencéphale: Centres de projection et centres d'association, *Conférence faite à l'assemblée générale de la 66 session de la Société Scientifique de Bruxelles, tenue à Malines,* 1896.
3. J. Soury, *Système nerveux central: Structure et fonctions,* Paris, 1899.
4. Monakow, *Arch. f. Psychiatrie,* Vol. XXVII, 1895. Ueber den gegenwärtigen Stand der Frage nach der Lokalisation im Grosshirn, *Ergebn. d. Physiol.,* 1st year, Wiesbaden, 1902.
5. Dejerine, Sur les fibres de projection et d'association des hémisphères cérébraux, *Soc. d. Biologie,* 1897.
6. Ferrier and Turner, An Experimental Research upon Cerebro-cortical Afferent and Efferent Tracts, [*Phil. Trans.*] *of the Royal Soc.,* Vol. LVII [1894]; and *Neurol. Centralbl.,* 1898.
7. Rutishäuser, Experimenteller Beitrag zur Stabkranzfaserung im Frontalhirn des Affen, *Monatssch. f. Psychiatrie u. Neurol.,* Vol. V, 1899.
8. Siemerling, Ueber Markscheidenentwickelung des Gehirns und ihre Bedeutung für die Lokalisation, *Versamml. d. Vereins d. Deutsch. Irrenärzte zu Bonn,* 17 September 1898.
9. O. Vogt, Flechsigs Associationscentrenlehre, ihre Anhänger und Gegner, *Zeitsch. f. Hypnotismus,* etc., Vol. V, part 6, 189[7].
10. Mahaim, Centres de projection et centres d'association, etc., Liège, 1897.
11. Flechsig, Neue Untersuchungen über die Markbildung in den menschlichen Grosshirnlappen, *Neurol. Centralbl.,* 1 November 1898.
12. Flechsig, Weitere Mitteilungen über die entwicklungsgeschichtlichen (myelogenetischen) Felder in der menschlichen Gehirnrinde, *Neurol. Centralbl.,* 1903; and *Verhandlungen des Physiol. Kongresses,* Turin, 1901. Einige Bemerkungen über die Untersuchungsmethoden der Grosshirnrinde, *Königl. Sächs. Gesellsch. d. Wissensch. zu Leipzig,* 11 January 1904.
13. O. Vogt, Der Wert der myelogenetischen Felder der Grosshirnrinde, *Anat. Anzeiger,* Vol. XXIX, nos. 11–12, 1906. Ueber strukturelle Hirncentra mit besonderer Berücksichtigung der strukturellen Felder des Cortex Pallii, *Verhandl. der anatom., Gesellschaft,* 20 Versamml. in Rostock, 1–5 June 1906.
14. Mme Cécile Vogt, Sur la myélinisation de l'hémisphère cérébral du chat., *C. R. de la Soc. de Biol.,* 15 January 1898. Étude sur la myélinisation des hémisphères cérébraux, Paris, 1900.
15. In the expanded version of his doctrine (*Neurologisches Centralblat.,* 1898), Flechsig reveals that he never gave great importance to the radiating fibers in the anatomical differentiation of his two hierarchies of

areas, even having reached the point of conjecturing that the association [fibers] could be furnished with descending collaterals to the deep nuclei.
16. Monakow, Ueber den gegenwärtigen Stand der Frage nach der Lokalisation im Grosshirn, *Ergebnisse der Physiol.,* 3rd year, part 2, Wiesbaden, 1904. Neue Gesichtpunkte in der Frage nach Lokalisation im Grosshirn, *I Versamml, der Schweiz. Neurol. Gesellsch.,* in Bern, 13–14 March 1908 [1909].
17. The postulate, derived from the results of clinical investigations, has recently been accepted by Tanzi, who has applied it very ingeniously to the explanation of hallucinations. See E. Tanzi, Una teoria dell'allucinazione, *Riv. de patol. Nerv. e Mentale,* Vol. VI, part 12, December 1901.
18. Since the main primary memory areas seem to reside in the left hemisphere, it may be presumed that mnemonic and ideographic differentiation is initiated in the said hemisphere, passing later to the right hemisphere, in which there could exist, during youth, territorial reservations destined for later acquisitions. In left-handed individuals, the differentiation of the memory areas would occur in the reverse [fashion].
19. S. R. Cajal, La corteza motriz, *Rev. Trim. Microgr.,* Vol. IV, 1899.
20. Tanzi, Una teoria dell'allucinazione, *Riv. de Patol. Nerv. e Mentale,* Vol. VI, part 12, 1901.
21. Hypnotic experiences and self-observations, into the details of which we cannot enter here, have persuaded us that in dreams (discharges of the secondary and tertiary memory areas that are not fatigued by the work of the day), visual images possess perfect relief and exact coloring, although it is somewhat pale, in comparison with the sensation. He who dreams, irrespective of his position, perceives the objects in space as if he were awake, that is to say, within the prolongation of the visual axes, [which is] a clear indication that the perception areas come into play, by a sort of retrograde action, even though the imagined construct is formed in the memory areas. If, instead of the two kinds of aforementioned fibers, only the centripetal or sensory-memory fibers are admitted, the hallucinatory process, according to what Tanzi also implies, in this case would be explained by supposing a reversal of the law of dynamic polarization. For the rest, in dreams, a hallucinatory phenomenon would not result from a chemical excitation of external origin, but from the sheer overload of energy of all those ideographic territories associated by means of pathways developed long ago, and therefore very robust, [but whose] territories have remained inactive for a long time. For this reason, the events and preoccupations of daily work rarely encourage dreams, whereas the evocations of scenes and emotions from childhood and adolescence are very frequent, since they are located in areas that are not fatigued because of the lack of use of the memory. With regard to the incongruity of the [ideas] in dreams, it would result from the fact that the fatigued memory areas, and especially those that collaborate in the work of judgment, do not participate in the formation of the plastic or imagined construct.
22. Following Hitzig, Ferrier, and other physiolo-

gists, Flechsig has placed the higher psychic activities in the frontal lobe, that is to say, in the *anterior association area of the human cerebral cortex;* in this region there would exist, according to him, the point of departure for the acts of volition as well as the faculty of registering and associating all impressions. It seems to us really difficult to admit that a process as complex as self-awareness and the will can be located at a certain point in the cerebrum. But there are, besides, numerous facts that argue against this localization, supposed by Flechsig. On the one hand, the prefrontal cortex possesses a structure almost identical to that of the parietal and temporal regions; on the other, and according to the indications of Monakow, the frontal gyri are highly developed in the ungulates, which, however, are not the most intelligent of animals; finally, it is quite rare that intellectual disorders are revealed in individuals whose two frontal lobes are afflicted with considerable lesions, etc.

With regard to this, we particularly recommend reading the excellent criticism made by Monakow against the frontal theory of the cerebrum in his report entitled: Ueber den gegenwärtigen Stand der Frage nach der Lokalisation im Grosshirn, *Ergebn. d. Physiol.,* 3rd year, part 2, Wiesbaden, 1904. [This footnote was added to the French version.]

23. S. R. Cajal, Estructura del quiasma óptico y teoría general de los entrecruzamientos de las vías nerviosas, *Rev. Trim. Microgr.,* Vol. III, 1898.

24. For example, if one looks at the blue sky while deviating the ocular axes, one will not [see double], because one will have suppressed the lines and shadows that give the spatial value, only the same quality or tone remaining for both eyes (a uniform blue spot).

25. We reason here on the supposition that the two acoustic and olfactory perceptive areas possess exactly the same physiological value, according to what seems to result from the experiments of the physiologists and from clinical facts. It is clear that if, contrariwise, it should be proved that in each hemisphere there terminate sensory fibers [that are] qualitatively different, it will be necessary to imagine a sort of decussation with direct and crossed fibers, by means of which each unilateral isodynamic [cellular] group enters into connection with the equivalent receptor cells of the two cochleas and both nasal [mucous membranes]. This conjecture seems to us much less probable than the former, which rests, at least in regard to the olfactory apparatus, on well-observed anatomical facts.

26. Those blind for a long time, in whom the retina and the perceptive centers are more or less disorganized by disuse, are capable of dreams and visual hallucinations [that are] perfectly congruent and projected in space, which would not happen if the spatial and projective character of the reminiscences should necessarily depend on the collaboration of the perceptive areas. Needless to say, such dreams are always referred to acquisitions obtained during the period of visual health of the blind person.

27. Rabl-Rückhard, Sind die Ganglienzellen amöboid? etc., *Neurol. Centralbl.,* no. 7, 1890.

28. Duval, Hypothèse sur la physiologie des centres nerveux; théorie histologique du sommeil, *C.R. d. l. Soc. de Biol.,* nos. 3 and 5, 1895. See especially: Les neurones, l'amiboïdisme nerveux et la théorie histologique du sommeil, *Rev. d. l'École d'Anthropologie de Paris,* Vol. X, part II, 1900.

29. Lépine, independently of Duval, also reached a similar idea. See: Théorie mécanique de la paralysie hystérique, du somnambulisme, du sommeil naturel et de la distraction, *Revue de Médicine,* 1894; and *C.R. d. l. Soc. de Biol.,* no. 5, 1895.

30. Wiedersheim, *Anat. Anzeiger,* 1890.

31. Demoor, La plasticité morphologique des neurones cérébraux, *Arch. de Biol. de Bruxelles,* Vol. XIV, 1896.

32. Stefanowska, Les appendices terminaux des dendrites cérébraux et leurs différents états physiologiques, *Travaux du Labor. de l'Institut Solvay,* Bruxelles, 1897.

33. Odier, Recherches expérimentales sur les mouvements de la moelle épinière, Genève, 1898.

34. Querton, Le sommeil hibernal et les modifications des neurones cérébraux, *Travaux du Labor. de l'Institut Solvay,* Vol. 2, Bruxelles, 1898.

35. Havet, L'état moniliforme des neurones chez le invertébrés et quelques remarques sur les vertébrés, *La Cellule,* Vol. XXI, 1899.

36. Kölliker, Kritik der Hypothesen von Rabl-Rückhard u. Duval über amöboide Bewegungen der Neurodendren, *Sitzungsber. d. Wurzburg Phys. Med. Gesellsch.,* 9 March 1895.

37. Some of these objections are very weak; the fact that the axons do not move does not authorize us to deny the possibility of the contraction of central dendrites or cf pericellular [axonal] arborizations, neuronal elements never observable during life.

38. Azoulay, Psychologie histologique et texture du système nerveux, *Année Psychologique,* 1896.

39. Soukhanoff, Contribution à l'étude des modifications que subissent les prolongements dendritiques des cellules nerveuses sous l'influence des narcotiques, *La Cellule,* Vol. XIV, 1898. *Journal de Neurologie, 1898.* L'anatomie pathologique de la cellule nerveuse en rapport avec l'atrophie variqueuse des dendrites de l'écorce cérébrale, *La Cellule,* 1898.

40. Lugaro, Sulle modificazione morfologiche funzionali dei dendriti delle cellule nervose, *Rev. de Patol. Nerv. e Mentale,* 1898.

41. Reusz, Ueber Brauchbarkeit der Golgi'schen Methode in der Physiologie, u. Pathologie der Nervenzelle, *Magyar Sevoin Archivum,* Vol. III, 1902.

42. Lugaro, Sulle modificazione delle cellule nervose nei diversi stati funzionali, *Lo Sperimentale,* Vol. XLIX, 1895.

43. Narbut, Zur Frage des histologischen Schlafes, *Osobrenije Psich.,* no. 3, 1901.

44. Van Gehuchten, *Anatomie des centres nerveux,* 3rd edition, Vol. 1, 1900, p. 279; and 4th edition, 1906, p. 283.

45. This is a mistake which is easily rectified, simply by examining absolutely normal pieces with the 1.30

Zeiss apochromatic [lens]. In fact, in the normal cerebrum, as well as in all the nerve centers, the spines are constantly shown to be piriform, according to what we demonstrated in our former works on the cerebrum. The method of Ehrlich gives similar images.

46. Renaut, Sur les cellules nerveuses multipolaires et la théorie du neurone de Waldeyer, *Bull. d. l'Acad. d. Médec.*, Paris, 1895.

47. S. R. Cajal, Algunas conjeturas sobre el mecanismo anatómico de la ideación, asociación y atención, Madrid, 1895.

48. A priori, it seems more probable that the axonal arborizations are the seat of ameboidism, since the discharges go [toward them from] the dendrites and cell body.

49. For example, if an Ehrlich preparation of the cerebrum is fixed half an hour after commencing the action of the [methylene] blue, many spines are still seen, and the varicose state is little marked; one hour and a half later, the spines are completely lacking, and the pearled state of the protoplasm appears.

50. F. Tello, Sobre la existencia de neurofibrillas gigantes en los reptiles, *Trav. del Lab. de Inves. Biol.*, Vol. II, 1903.

51. S. R. Cajal, Variaciones normales y patológicas de las neurofibrillas, *Trav. del Lab de Inv. Biol.*, Vol. III, 1904.

52. Tanzi, I fatti e le induzioni nell'odierna istologia del sistema nervoso, *Rev. Sperim. d. Frenatria et d. Medic. Legal.*, Vol. XIX, 1893.

53. Lugaro, I recenti progressi dell'anatomia del sistema nervoso in rapporto alla psicologia et alla psichiatria, *Riv. d. Patol. Nerve. e Mentale.*, Vol. IV, parts 11–12, 1899.

54. S. R. Cajal, Consideraciones sobre la morfología de la célula nerviosa, Madrid, 189[4].

55. Nageotte, Note sur la présence de massues d'accroissement dans la substance grise de la moelle épinière, etc. *C.R. de la Soc. de Biol.*, 16 June 1906.

56. Marinesco and Minea, Note sur la régénérescence de la moelle chez l'homme, *C.R. de la Soc. de Biol.*, 16 June 1906. Marinesco, Sur la neurotisation des foyers de ramollissement et d'hémorragie cérébrale, *Revue Neurol.*, 30 December 1908.

57. Cajal, Note sur la dégénérescence traumatique des fibres nerveuses du cervelet et du cerveau, *Trav. du Lab. de Recherches Biol.*, Vol. V, 1907. Notas preventivas sobre la degeneración y regeneración de las vías nerviosas centrales, *Trav. del Lab.*, Vol. IV, 1905–1906.

58. F. Tello, La régénération dans les voies optiques, *Trav. du Lab. de Recher. Biol.*, Vol. V, 1907.

59. Guido Sala, Ueber die Regenerationserscheinungen im centralen Nervensystem, *Anatom. Anzeiger*, Vol. XXXIV, nos. 9–11, 1909.

60. U. Rossi, Per la rigenerazione dei neuroni, *Trav. du Lab. de Rech. Biol.*, Vol. VI, 190[8].

61. Monakow, Neue Gesichtspunkte in der Frage nach der Lokalisation im Grosshirn, *1 Versammlung der Schweiz. Neurol. Gesellschaft in Bern*, 13–14 March [1909].

Editors' Notes

A. These titles are translated from the French version of the book.

B. The phrase in brackets was added to the French version.

C. The phrase in brackets was added to the French version.

D. The phrase in brackets is not in the French version.

E. The sentences in brackets are only in the French version.

F. The phrase in brackets was added to the French version.

G. The paragraph in brackets is only in the French version.

H. The phrase in brackets is only in the French version.

I. The paragraph in brackets is only in the French version.

J. The phrases in brackets are only in the French version.

K. The phrase in brackets is only in the French version.

L. The phrase in brackets is added to the French version.

M. The phrase in brackets is added to the French version.

N. In the French version, the text accompanying this heading appears in the next-to-last paragraph of the item entitled "The Perceptive Areas Are Symmetrical and Bilateral, Whereas the Primary and Secondary Memory Areas Are Unilateral".

O. This title in the French version is "The Areas of Memory in Vertebrates Other Than Man." The corresponding text of the Spanish version appears just before the item entitled "Physiological Postulates following from the Organization of the Cerebral Areas and Pathways".

P. The Spanish version incorrectly says "gyrencephalic."

Q. The Spanish version incorrectly says "gyrencephalic."

R. Added to the French version.

S. The phrase in brackets was added to the French version.

T. The phrase in brackets was added to the French version.

U. Added to the French version.

V. Added to the French version.

W. Added to the French version.

X. In the French version, this title is "Reduced and Continuous Projection of the Peripheral Sensory Surfaces on the Cerebral Cortex."

Y. Added to the French version.

Z. The phrase in brackets was added to the French version.

AA. The words in brackets were added to the French version.

BB. The Spanish version says "cerebral."

CC. The paragraph in brackets is only in the French version.

DD. The title and the accompanying text are not in the French version.

EE. The phrase in brackets was added to the French version.

FF. Added to the French version.

GG. The phrase in brackets was added to the French version.

HH. Added to the French version.

II. The phrase in brackets was added to the French version.

JJ. The phrase in brackets was added to the French version.

KK. The phrase in brackets was added to the French version.

LL. Added to the French version.

MM. The two paragraphs in brackets appeared as a footnote added to the French version.

PART V

The Final Years (1921–1935)

The Cat and the Rodents; the Return to the Neuron Doctrine

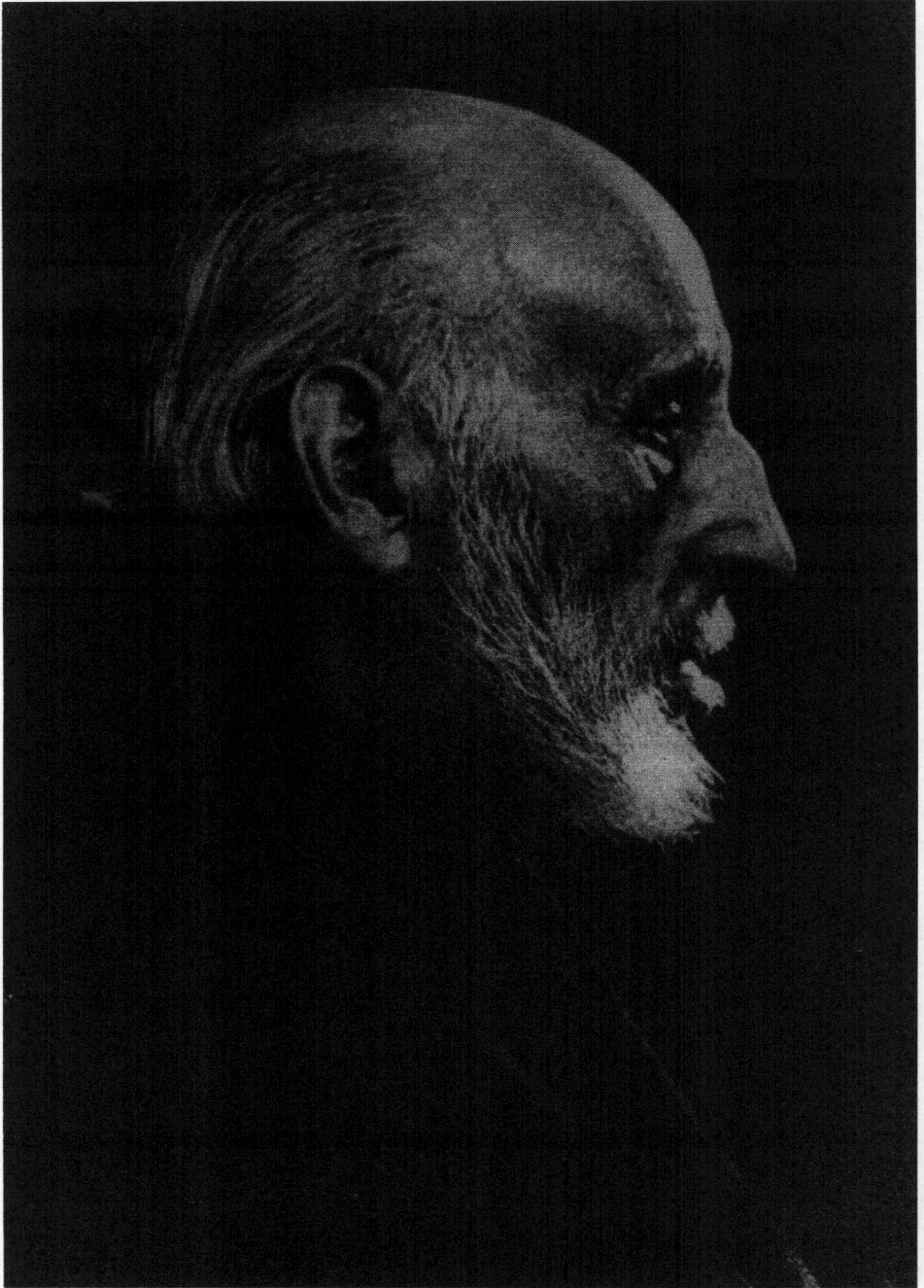

Santiago Ramón y Cajal at the age of eighty. Photograph in the Cajal Museum, from the frontispiece to the English translation of¿ *Neuronismo o Reticularismo?* by Ubeda-Purkiss and Fox (Cajal, 1954).

26

Introduction

After publication of the final volume of the *Histologie* in 1911, Cajal was to add little to his opus on the cerebral cortex for some years. Much of his scientific work in the period subsequent to publication of the great textbook was to be devoted to studies of neural degeneration and regeneration, as summarized in *Estudios sobre la degeneración y regeneración del sistema nervioso* (Cajal, 1913–1914, 1928). But he was concurrently working on the second volume of his autobiography *(Recuerdos de mi vida)*, dealing with the history of his scientific work. The first volume, covering his infancy and youth, had been published in 1901. In the second volume, which was finally published in 1917, he clearly had to reconsider his contributions on the cerebral cortex. We have translated his statements about what he felt was their significance in chapter 13, which serves to introduce the translations of the great works on the human cerebral cortex.

The second volume of the *Recuerdos* contained a large number of illustrations, including many figures taken from Cajal's published works. A few scientific illustrations, however, had not previously been published, including five accompanying the sections on the cerebral cortex. Because we have reproduced them in chapter 13, we will not repeat them in this chapter, although it would have been appropriate to do so, since at least three of them are in a style far more typical of Cajal's later period. They are stylistically very similar to those found in chapters 27 and 28 in this volume. A single forerunner of this style appeared in 1893 (see chapter 6) and was actually republished by Cajal in the paper translated in chapter 28. Since the cortical figures in the *Recuerdos* were apparently produced at this late period in Cajal's career, they presumably represent his definitive assessment of intracortical organization and the range of cortical cell types. Perhaps confirming this is their use in Cajal's final review works and in Tello's posthumous assessment of his master's contributions (Tello, 1935; see chapter 29 in this volume).

In 1921, Cajal returned to the cerebral cortex with a study of the visual area of the cat, a study that was to herald a new round of cortical Golgi studies from his laboratory. Most of these were to be the work of one of his pupils, R. Lorente de Nó. However, Lorente de Nó's first publication (1922b)—a still widely quoted study of what he took to be the auditory cortex of the mouse but which now appears to have been conducted on the first somatic sensory area—appeared in the same issue of the *Trabajos* as a paper by the master himself on the general cortex of rodents (Cajal, 1922b).

The studies of this period appear to have been initiated under the stimulus of the German cytoarchitectonic school, then at the peak of its influence, and there is an element of pique in Cajal's writing, perhaps stemming from the attention given to Nissl-and myelin-based architectonic studies—at the expense of those conducted with the Golgi methods. Indeed, on reading his opening paragraphs and the notes, one has the impression that he was conscious of a serious decline in the popularity of the Golgi technique by this time. It seems evident that he was not wrong, and apart from the work of Lorente de Nó, very little of consequence was to be added to our knowledge of the cortex from Golgi studies until they became popular again in the 1960s and 1970s.

Of the two cortical papers published by Cajal in this late period of his life, the first, on the visual cortex of the cat, seems to have brought him face to face with the realities of the peer review system, something to which, in publishing his works either at his own expense or by invitation, he was hitherto not ac-

customed. The German translation (Cajal, 1922a) of the 1921 paper on the cat visual cortex, which appeared in the *Journal für Psychologie und Neurologie,* contains numerous additions and emendations of a nature that seems to betray a referee's demands for clarification and justification. This interpretation is supported by Cajal's lengthy but uncharacteristically reserved interpolation of a rejoinder to criticisms he said had been made by the Swedish neurologist Henschen (see page 522.A, of chapter 27 in this volume). Perhaps Henschen was the reviewer and had insisted on a better indication of the cytoarchitecture of the area sampled (thus resulting in Cajal's earliest published cortical photomicrographs) and a clearer statement of how the Golgi impregnated cells were selected for illustration. Cajal's irritation with the cytoarchitectonic school, headed by Oskar Vogt, the editor of the *Journal für Psychologie und Neurologie,* and on whose reviewing board Henschen sat, is revealed in the 1922 paper on the general cortex of rodents (chapter 28). Perhaps his recognition that the cytoarchitectonic school had become preeminent is confirmed by the fact that, despite its translation into German (Cajal, 1923a), the last paper received virtually no attention then or subsequently.

27

Histology of the Visual Cortex of the Cat

[*Archivos de Neurobiología* 2:338–362, 1921]

In the year 1899, we commenced a series of investigations on the sensory cortex of certain animals, and particularly on that of man, with the methods of Nissl, Weigert, and Golgi.[1] These studies dealt mainly with animals of fifteen to thirty days (mouse, rabbit, cat, and dog), and they included almost all the sensory areas (the centers of projection of Flechsig). And with respect to the human, fetuses from the seventh month to birth and children from a few days up to half a year were used.

Limiting ourselves to the results obtained in the *visual region* of the fetuses and children of a few months, our analysis was quite fortunate. The precocity of development of the visual centers in man and the extraordinary abundance of fresh material available (we utilized more than two hundred still-warm dead bodies) allowed us to add to the classic descriptions of Gennari, Vicq D'Azyr, Meynert, Hammarberg, Henschen, Kölliker, Schlapp, etc., a considerable number of structural details not without interest and easily demonstrable by the Golgi methods of impregnation. Needless to say, the cortical region preferentially studied was the *calcarine sulcus,* in which

Meynert had already noted a specific fine structure. Fortunately, at that time and thanks to the works of the clinicians and anatomical pathologists (Henschen, Flechsig, Wilbrand, etc.), it was possible to establish with certainty that the sulcus mentioned above (and also the *cuneus, lingual gyrus,* etc., in accord with what Nothnagel, v[on] Monakow, Seguin, and others determined) represents the principal terminal projection field of the visual fibers, that is to say, of those originating particularly in the lateral geniculate body, the first subcortical relay of the optic impulses.

The numerous data obtained in some hundreds of excellent preparations obtained with the method of silver chromate, and the comparison with the results of the Nissl and Weigert-Pal procedures, led us to establish, on the basis of the cellular morphology and specific [arborization pattern] of the axon, the following nomenclature of the visual layers:

1. *Plexiform layer* (*molecular* of the authors).
2. *Layer of the small pyramids* (*external granules* of certain authors).
3. *Layer of the medium pyramids.*

4. *Layer of the large stellate cells.*
5. *Layer of the external granules or small stellate cells.*
6. *Layer of the external small pyramids with arched ascending axon.*
7. *Layer of the large pyramids (solitary cells of Meynert).*
8. *Layer of the deep small pyramids with arciform axon.*
9. *Layer of the fusiform cells.*

If nowadays we were to come back to the subject of the fine anatomy of the human calcarine sulcus, we would simplify somewhat this enumeration of layers, as subsequent investigations undertaken on animals close to man and on the carnivores require, in our opinion, the elimination of the sixth layer or [the layer] of the small pyramids with arched ascending axon, because it is partially juxtaposed and intermingled with the giant solitary cells of Meynert (our seventh layer), reserving such designation exclusively for the eighth layer, which is particularly dominated by that very singular cellular type. Thus, the eighth layer would become the seventh and the ninth the eighth, a stratum being removed.

With some variations in names and some more or less justified stratigraphical reductions,[2] the layers adopted by us were recognized in man and primates by Campbell, Brodmann, Mott, Monakow, etc., and in carnivores by these same authors and Minkowski.

When we enumerate below the stratification of the *visual area of the cat*, we will note the correspondence of the layers distinguished by us in the visual area of man and those easily recognizable in the cat and dog.

Let us remember that already in our extensive monograph on the human visual cortex, we noted many corresponding structures between both classes of mammals (man and carnivores), but our impartiality obliges us to recognize that the mentioned investigation, with respect to the cat and dog, suffered from an original sin, inevitable at that time. Trusting in the physiological experiments of Munk, our histological investigations concentrated exclusively on the *marginal gyrus* and on the *suprasylvian gyrus*, leaving without exploration the internal or interhemispheric surface and the whole cerebellar surface of the same. Now

then, the mentioned cytoarchitectonic studies of Campbell,[3] especially those made in the dog, and of Brodmann,[4] completely confirmed by Minkowski,[5] have demonstrated that the *area striata*, reputed by virtue of anatomical analogies and of anatomicopathological experiments to be the visual area of the cat, does not extend beyond the dividing sulcus between the marginal and suprasylvian gyri, stopping internally (interhemispheric fissure) in the territory of the cingulate gyrus or supracallosal gyrus. And still, within the marginal gyrus, the visual area would be confined, more or less, to the posterior two-thirds of the marginal gyrus. Figs. 1 and 2 [*figs. 246, 247*], taken from Brodmann, will give an idea to the reader of the localization of the visual area of the cat.

This localization, now very probable because of the mentioned cyto- and myeloarchitectonic analogies between the visual area of man and of primates and carnivore mammals, has been corroborated by means of the method of secondary degeneration by Minkowski in the dog and cat. This author, who has worked with the illustrious professor v[on] Monakow, has extirpated in the young cat either portions of or the whole striate area, and observing, months after the injury, the cellular atrophy produced in the *homolateral lateral geniculate body* in sections stained with the Nissl method, has not only confirmed the visual nature of the marginal gyrus but has also established the regions or areas of this, corresponding to special territories of the *lateral geniculate body, pulvinar,* and *lateral nucleus* of the thalamus. Such results are completely accepted by Monakow, as can be seen in his beautiful book on cerebral localization.[6]

We can then, fearless of grave errors and thanks to the confluence of the anatomicopathological results with those of the cytoarchitectonic investigations of the normal cortex, affirm that in the cat the visual area lies in the marginal gyrus (posterior two-thirds), especially on its internal side.

Methods

The cited investigations have been made, as we noted, with the aid of the staining procedures of Nissl and Weigert, procedures that in most cases are sufficient to distinguish the

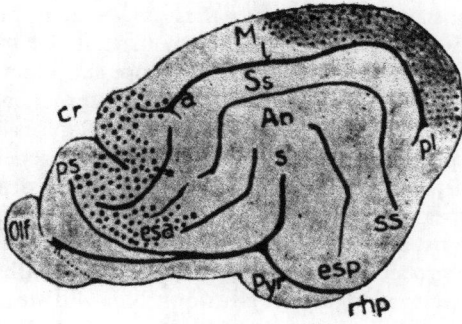

[*FIG. 246*] Fig. 1. Regions differentiated by Brodmann in the cortex of the cat, lateral surface.

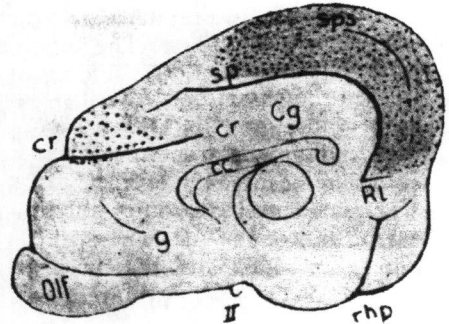

[*FIG. 247*] Fig. 2. Regions differentiated on the medial or interhemispheric surface of the cat. The gray area (*sps*) indicates the visual region.

physiologically different cortical areas. This is eloquently demonstrated on consulting the very patient and great work of Brodmann and his disciples, the previous work of Campbell, and, with respect to our present subject (visual cortex of the cat), the excellent atlas of C. Winkler and Ada Potter,[7] even though these authors did not pay particular attention to the problem of physiological localization.

But after accepting and applauding such outstanding and fruitful efforts, would it not also be beneficial to penetrate further, with the help of the silver methods,[8] particularly with those of Golgi and Cox, and the neurofibrillar methods into the labyrinth of visual cortical architecture in the cat and dog, determining as far as possible the form of the neurons and the behavior and termination of their axons? We are sure that such an analysis would complete in many ways the very simple and fragmentary picture revealed by the Nissl, Weigert, and similar procedures, and that the collected data about the fine structure would strengthen the histological and physiological basis of visual localization and, in general, of all cortical localizations. We believe, moreover, that such investigations will allow us perhaps to distinguish between those several and heterogeneous intrinsic elements of the optic cortex which are fundamental and in certain respects fixed—the ancient work of the phylogenetic evolution of higher vertebrates—and those that are *secondary* and of recent appearance, that is to say, the features of fine and delicate texture [that are] added to the primitive ones and which represent the latest perfections and ad-

aptations in optical function of man and primates.

Such is the principal object pursued in the present work. As the basis for our structural investigations, we have also used the classical methods of Nissl, Weigert-Pal (and those derived from them, such as the formula of Spielmeyer). With them, we have mainly looked at the *quantitative aspects* of the neurons, fibers, and layers that the methods of metallic impregnation, with their inevitable gaps, do not always allow us to determine.

As materials for study, young cats (fifteen to thirty days) have been especially chosen, plus fetuses and adults. The dog has been less investigated by us.

The structure of the visual area [of the dog] will be the subject of a separate work by us or by some of our disciples.

But a mere structural analysis is not sufficient to determine the origin and termination of the optic pathways. To fill this gap, we are preparing another paper, whose principal purpose will be to establish as far as possible, with the help of anatomicopathological methods, the origin of the fibers of the *stria of Gennari* and the probable connections that exist between the visual area and the corpus callosum.

Histology of the Visual Area of the Cat

Although our series of Nissl, Weigert, and reduced silver nitrate sections show some differences, depending on the portion of the marginal gyrus under study, it can be said that, in principle, the whole visual area or *striate cor-*

tex of the authors possesses the same structure throughout its gray matter. The differences depend on adaptations to the folding of the gyri. In fact, the lateral pressure that was experienced by the marginal gyrus during the embryonic and postfetal periods, dispersing the neurons in the direction of least resistance, led, as a consequence, to a compression with a decrease in numbers at the level of the sulci and to an enormous expansion in the radial direction, with an increase in numbers at the level of the most protuberant portions of the gyrus. The best and most representative preparations are obtained in the flat walls of the sulci and in the area of transition to the highest point of the *marginal gyrus.* Let us note also that from one radius to another, certain nervous types become rarefied or more numerous, leading sometimes, in the intermediate locations, to the laborious task of recognizing the specific architecture. Only in this way can we explain to ourselves the uncharacteristic [nature] of certain figures given by otherwise highly competent and prestigious modern authors; probably they took at random any radius of the visual cortex, without paying attention to considering whether or not that part contained the typical stratification. We exclude Campbell and Mott, who show the typical structure.[A]

It is prudent and discreet to flee, as did Henschen, Brodmann, Minkowski, and Monakow, etc., from the excessive *schematism* of certain representations, but it is also appropriate not to fall into the opposite extreme, that is to say, into that of *antischematism* at all cost or into obsequious objectivism that does not distinguish the typical from the atypical and which appears to forget that the presence of a thick radial artery is sufficient to alter noticeably the adjacent cytoarchitecture, and which, finally, does not take into account how frequent it is to observe in each layer groupings, perhaps isodynamic [groupings], of neurons separated by intercalary spaces with a somewhat different and difficult-to-classify [histological] texture.

The extent of the typical anatomical configuration of the visual cortex of the cat, in our series of sections [stained by] the methods of Golgi and Cox and silver nitrate, coincides al-

most completely with that assigned by Minkowski. Overall, it seems to us that the most characteristic territories are more abundant, or more easily recognizable, on the internal or interhemispheric side of the marginal gyrus and especially at its occipital angle and cerebellar surface.[3] Therefore, renouncing our former design of analyzing separately the several transverse segments of the gyrus, we are going to proceed with a synthetic exposition, without special topographic allusions. Nor will we separate in our descriptive picture the results obtained with each method. When we study the layers, we will describe together the structural revelations given by the procedures of Nissl, Weigert, Golgi, etc.[C]

Nomenclature of the Layers

Comparing the results of the various techniques used, in the gyrus marginalis of the cat can be distinguished the following layers, in large measure coincident with those recognized in man:

1. *Plexiform or molecular layer* (lamina *zonalis* of Brodmann).
2. *Layer of the small pyramids* (lamina *granularis* externa of B[rodmann]).
3. *Layer of the medium and large pyramids* (lamina *pyramidalis* of B[rodmann]).
4. *Layer of the large stellate cells* (superficial portions of the lamina *granularis* interna or layer IV of B[rodmann]).
5. *Layer of the small pyramids with arciform axon* (deep portion of the lamina *granularis* interna or layer IV of B[rodmann])
6. *Layer of the internal large pyramids or solitary cells* of Meynert (lamina *ganglionaris* of B[rodmann]).
7. *Layer of the polymorphic cells* (lamina *multiformis* of B[rodmann]).
8. *Layer of the white matter.*

These designations denote exclusively the morphological neuron type with long axon, which appears to dominate in each layer. I say *appears* because, although in the numerous excellent Golgi sections we observe certain kinds of cells to predominate and although we have tried to compare carefully the silver chromate images with those of the Nissl

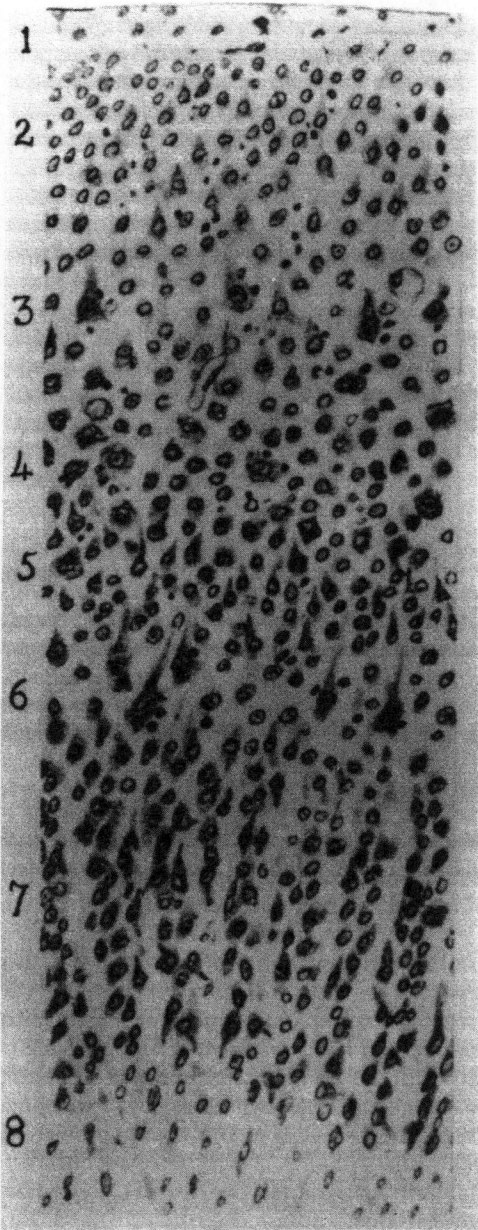

[FIG. 248] Fig. 3. Recognizable layers on the internal surface of the visual cortex of the adult cat. Nissl method. 1, plexiform layer; 2, layer of the small pyramids; 3, layer of the superficial large pyramids; 4, 5, layers of the granule cells with the two external and internal sublayers; 6, layer of the large solitary pyramids of Meynert; 7, layer of the polymorphic cells; 8, layer of the white matter and fusiform cells.

method, in order to integrate them reciprocally, it might happen that in some layers the neuron estimated as typical would not be represented on account of the inevitable lacunae in the staining but [would constitute] an important minority. In any case, whether the cell is in the majority of minority, it constitutes, in our opinion, the cellular variety most characteristic of each layer.

In figs. 3 and 13 [figs. 248, 258], we show the whole stratifications as they appear in a section [stained by] the methods of Nissl and Weigert-Pal. For these figures, the cortical regions in which the stratigraphic differentiation is shown most clearly and unequivocally (internal side of the marginal gyrus) have been chosen in accord with the preceding considerations. In the remaining illustrations, we show the morphological details of the neurons of each layer.

1. Plexiform Layer or Molecular Layer

In general, this layer has appeared to us somewhat thinner in the visual area than in other gyri. Important differences in thickness are also observed in the visual area, when comparing its several regions; thus, at the apex of the marginal gyrus, the layer is customarily half as thick as at the level of the sulci.

The general appearance and the fine anatomy of this layer differ in no particular way from those shown by other gyri. To this layer are applicable all the structural details collected in several of our works, either with the method of Golgi or with those of Ehrlich[9] or of Nissl, details that are unfortunately quite forgotten or unknown, [but which] nevertheless have been confirmed and extended by the distinguished Retzius, Kölliker, Veratti, and others.

The plexiform or molecular layer of the cerebrum constitutes, as is well known, the point of convergence and connection of enormous numbers of dendrites and of endogenous and exogenous axonal arborizations. Here are the main differentiable cellular elements [seen] with the methods of Golgi and Cox:

a. Small cells with short axon diffusely branched at a short distance. These cells are relatively scarce and show a triangular or polygonal shape (fig. 4, G)[D] [fig. 249].

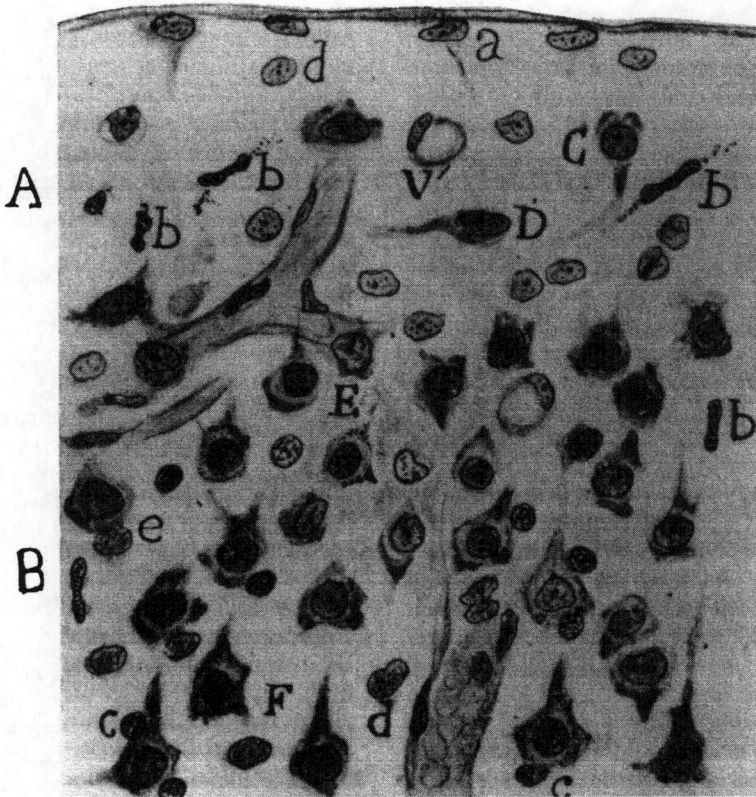

[*FIG. 249*]   Fig. 4. Plexiform layer and layer of the small pyramids. Nissl method. *a, d,* neuroglial cells; *b,* small rod cells; *D, C,* neurons of the plexiform layer; *E,* superficial small pyramids; *F,* somewhat larger deep pyramids.

b. Tangential cells with a fusiform or piriform soma and abundant protoplasm, very long horizontal dendrites, and an axon that runs, at a variable distance, parallel to the pia. As it appears in fig. 4 [*fig. 249*], the method of Nissl reveals that these specific cells (Cajal'schen Zellen of Retzius) inhabit the deep half of the layer under study (fig. 4, *D,C*) [*fig. 249*].

c. Terminal arborizations of the ascending fibers of Martinotti (fig. 6, *D*) [*fig. 251*].

d. Terminal tufts [of the apical dendrites] of all the cells with long axon of the underlying layers, excluding, as we will see below, the large stellate neurons of the fourth layer.

e. Ramifications of the recurrent collaterals of many small and medium pyramids (fig. 5, *b*) [*fig. 250*].

f. Fibrous neuroglia [of the glia limitans] (fig. 4, *a*) [*fig. 249*] characterized commonly by a triangular soma and descending tuft [of processes] and deep astrocytes, recognizable by their radial or cometlike configuration.

g. Small rod cells, [which are] well recognizable by their small size and the shape of their nuclei (fig. 4, *b*) [*fig. 249*]; these, according to what Achúcarro and [Del] Río-Hortega have demonstrated, and as confirmed by us, possess thin and very highly branched processes. And we do not include [in this description] the capillaries or the *limiting* membrane, well described by Held, or the connective tissue bundles that accompany the vessels of a certain caliber.

The enumerated cells—as already stated—are not unique to the visual area; they are

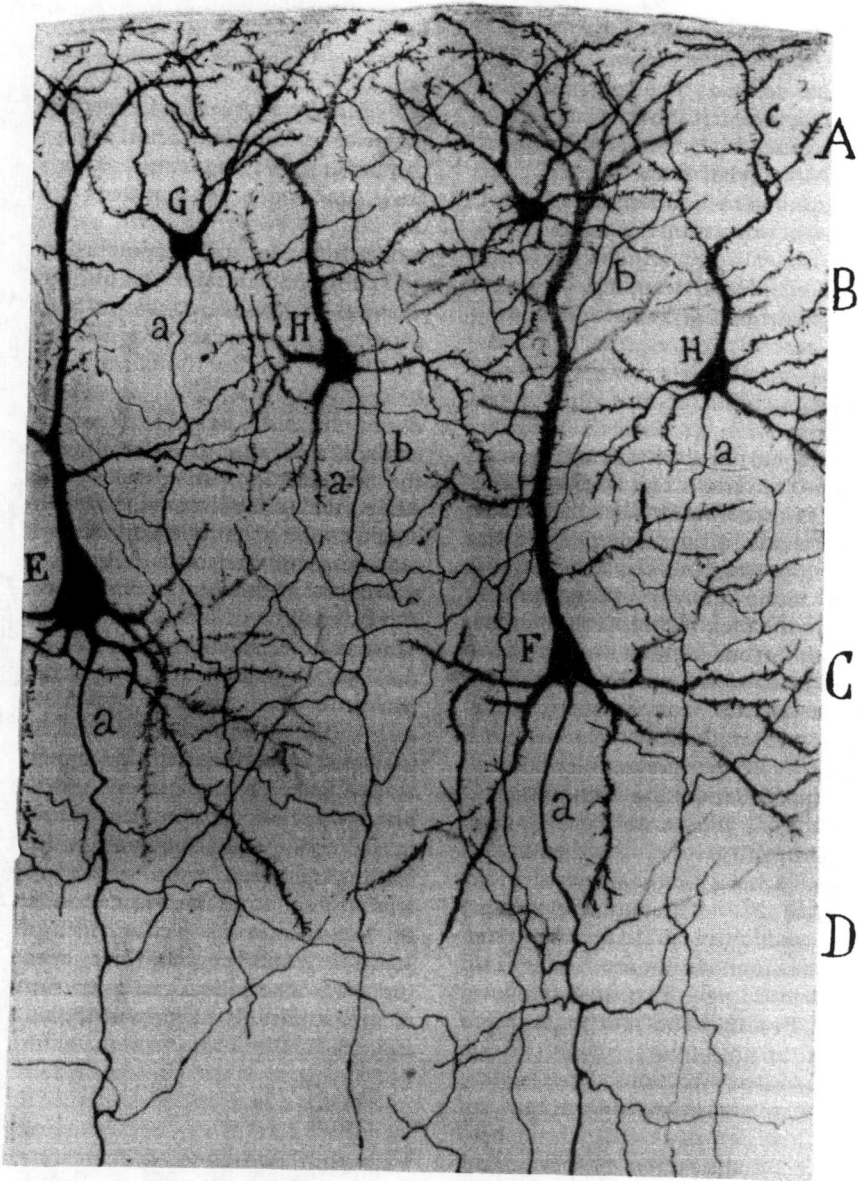

[*FIG. 250*] Fig. 5. Neurons of the second and third layers impregnated with the method of Golgi. *A*, plexiform layer; *B*, layer of the small pyramids; *C*, layer of the external large pyramids; *a*, axons; *b*, recurrent axonal collaterals.

found in the plexiform layer of the other gyri, where they are perhaps more abundant than in the region under study.

2. Layer of the Small Pyramids

We omit here the designation of *external granule cells (lamina granularis externa)* named[E] by Brodmann, because, in fact, the majority of the intrinsic nerve cells of the second layer show the configuration and arrangement of processes of genuine pyramids. If the most peripheral resemble polygons rather than cones or pyramids with the base deep, it depends on the fact that the ascending dendritic tuft destined for the plexiform layer comes directly from the soma, instead of arising, as in the deeper-situated neurons of the same type, from the extremity of an [apical] dendritic shaft. Of course, this pecularity cannot be well appreciated in the Nissl preparations used preferentially by Brodmann, Campbell, Bolton, Mott, v[on] Monakow, Henschen, Minkowski, etc.

With regard to the behavior of the terminal dendritic tuft in the plexiform layer and to the properties of the axon, nothing special is offered by these cells, which strictly conform to the descriptive picture exposed many years ago in other cortical regions by Golgi, us, Retzius, Martinotti, Kölliker, van Gehuchten, Schaffer, etc. (fig. 5, *H, G,*) [*fig. 250*]. With respect to the *axon,*[F] it will be sufficient to note that it is very thin and gives off a large number of collaterals, all arising almost at a right angle (fig. 5, *H, G*) [*fig. 250*]. Their numbers range between four and seven. It is observed frequently that the small secondary branches of the initial collaterals have a recurrent course, some of them invading the plexiform layer, whereas those arising lower down run in oblique or transverse directions. Each collateral, as the result of successive branchings, can generate four, five, or more small branches, generally varicose and sinuous. Their varicose appearance is accentuated in their terminal portions.

In fig. 5 [*fig. 250*], we present a reproduction of several small pyramids, taken from the cat of twenty-five days. Only four elements contained in the same region of two successive sections have been drawn. Those pyramids whose axon could be followed for a long distance have been chosen. In order to clarify the drawing, we have omitted the intermediate forms between the most superficial and the deep small neurons.

Cells with Short Axon. The second layer is also very rich in cells with short axon and in neurons with ascending axons, as we show in fig. 6 (*A, B, C*) [*fig. 251*]. In [fig. 251], *D*, has been reproduced a neuron with ascending axon. Notice the unusual smallness of the cells *A* and *B*, which resemble the minute types with short axon discovered by us in the human cerebral cortex (*arachniform cells*). The scarcity of their protoplasm permits the nucleus to be seen.

For the rest, the fact that the layer under study is rich in neurons is already evident in the Nissl sections in which regions are found where the somata are separated by distances smaller than a cell body (fig. 4, *E*) [*fig. 249*].

Comparing the silver chromate or Cox sections with those [stained by] the method of Weigert-Pal or the variant of Spielmeyer, it is at once observed that the axon collaterals of the small pyramids and, to a large extent, at least, the initial trajectory of the axon lack a myelin sheath. All of these processes inhabit, in fact, that extensive zone appearing as an empty space in preparations stained for myelin. This region of absent myelin corresponds to the second and also in part to the third layer of the visual area (fig. 13, *B, C*) [*fig. 258*]. Only from time to time is an ascending fiber or fiber of Martinotti observed crossing the white space to reach the plexiform layer (fig. 13, *c*) [*fig. 258*]. The plexiform layer in its deep half is almost entirely lacking in medullated fibers (fig. 13, *A*) [*fig. 258*].

3. Layer of the External Medium and Large Pyramids

Very thin and situated very superficially in comparison with other regions, it consists of one or two discontinuous rows of voluminous pyramids, as clearly shown by the Nissl method, and which are usually also stained by the methods of Bielschowsky and of reduced silver nitrate.

The name *lamina pyramidalis* given by

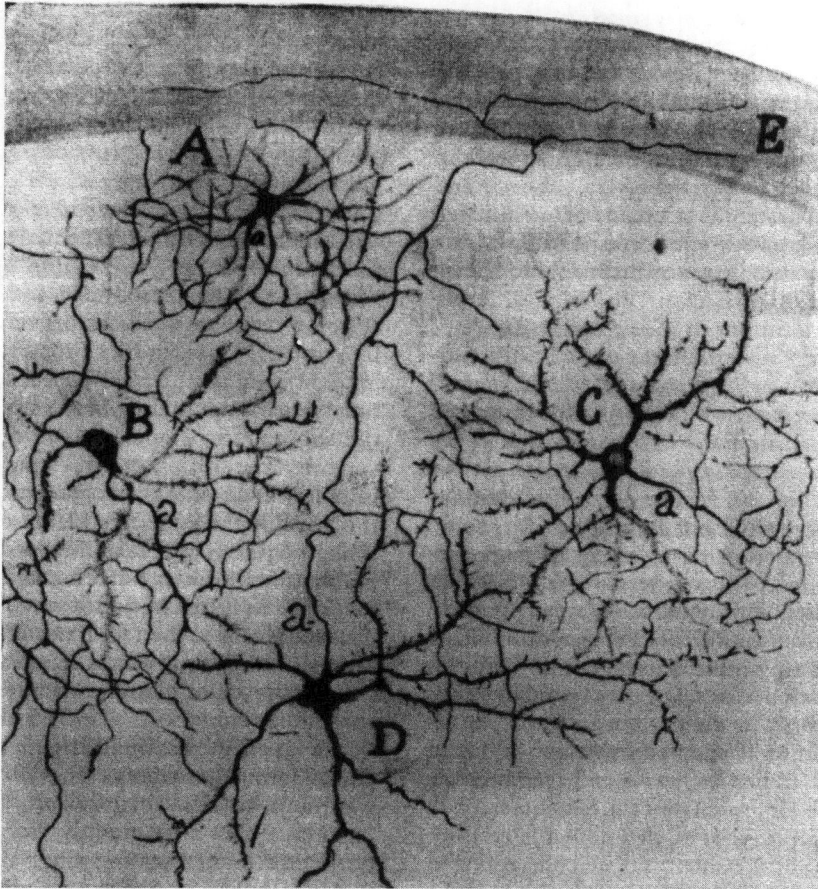

[*FIG. 251*] Fig. 6. Neurons with short axon of the layer of the small pyramids. *A,* minute cell of the arachniform type; *B, C,* other large types; *D,* cell with ascending axon, located near the layer of the superficial large pyramids; *E,* plexiform layer.

Brodmann to this layer is justifiable because the said cells suddenly emerge, without transitional changes in volume of the small pyramids (fig. 3, 3) [*fig. 248*]. There are, however, territories of the visual region in which there are intermediate shapes and sizes or which lack the cited elements, or in which these hardly surpass the diameter of the medium pyramids of other cortical areas.

The behavior of the aforesaid voluminous cells can be seen in fig. 5, *E, F* [*fig. 250*], in which we reproduce two of them. This figure excuses us from a meticulous description. We will only point out the richness in transverse and descending basal dendrites of the soma and the thickness of the axon from which arise five, six, or more copiously branched collaterals. In fortunate cases, it was possible to follow the axon to near the white matter. In its deeper trajectory, that is to say, when it has gone beyond the layer of the *stellate cells,* it does not give off collaterals or only does so very exceptionally.

4 [*and 5*]. Layer of the Stellate Neurons with Long Axon

Campbell, Brodmann, Minkowski, and other authors include under the general label of grains (*lamina granularis interna* of Brodmann) the whole robust band of generally small polygonal cells that lies between the layer of the *external pyramids* and [the layer] of the *solitary cells* of Meynert. According to Brodmann, this wide stratification appears in man divided into two sublayers, *external* and *internal,* separated by a plexus of medullated fibers, to a large extent corresponding to the *stria of Gennari.* It is thus justifiable to accept the three sublayers (IVa; IVb; IVc), differentiated by this author in the calcarine fissure of man and primate (*tristriated type*). In his opinion, the *sublayer of the superficial internal grains,* homologous to the formation described by Henschen and by us in man under the name of the *layer of the large stellate cells,* is lacking in the cat. In the persisting granular band, however, the cited author admits some structural heterogeneity, since he supposes that a relatively thick external portion would house the stria of Gennari, whereas the thinner deep level would enclose numerous close-packed and tiny cells. This disposition justifies the designation of *bistriate type* found by Brodmann not only in the cat but in the rabbit. A similar opinion is adopted by Minkowski. But for all that, in the cat, as we will see later, the layer of the large stellate cells is not lacking at all, although it is not as well demarcated from the stratum of the small stellate cells as it is in man. It is unquestionable that neither the method of Nissl nor that of Weigert is capable of differentiating clearly in the mammal mentioned the two divisions of the *lamina granularis interna,* except in some radii of the marginal gyrus, where, as we show in fig. 3, *4* [*fig. 248*], some polygonal or ovoid stellate cells of exceptional size can be seen. On the other hand, in good Golgi and Cox preparations, it is already possible to distinguish—never so well as in man and monkey—(a) a *superficial plane,* preferentially populated by stellate cells of regular size and large volume, and (b) a *deep plane,* where the majority of cells have the configuration of diminutive pyramids, endowed with an axon with recurrent branches.

a. Sublayer in Which the Stellate Cells with Long Axon Predominate. They have been described by us some time ago not only in the human visual cortex but in that of the same name in the cat;[10] they constitute one of the characteristics of the visual area of the higher mammals.

Variable in size and morphology, as can be seen in fig. 7 [*fig. 252*], it is possible to distinguish among them three kinds of configuration: (a) the *common star-shaped,* of regular size, endowed with divergent dendrites prolixly ramified (fig. 7, $C,^{G}D$) [*fig. 252*]; (b) the *mitral* or *semilunar,* rounded and free of processes at its upper pole but provided with prolixly ramified descending processes (fig. 7, *A*) [*fig. 252*]; and (c) the *star-shaped,* similar to the first type, except that from the superior side of the soma emerge one, two, or more thin ascending [dendritic] shafts, rapidly resolving into terminal branches that partially invade the layer of the superficial large pyramids, although without ever reaching—to judge by our preparations—the plexiform layer (fig. 7, *B*) [*fig. 252*]. Apart from their form, this peculiarity, that is to say, the fact that the soma has no representation in the first cerebral layer, constitutes the culminating attribute of the neurons under study.

The axon shows, in all the mentioned varieties, identical attributes. It is directed downward and, tracing an inflexion, gives off collaterals [that are] mainly ascending and transverse and, after crossing, almost always undivided, the layer of the solitary large pyramids, it is incorporated into the radial bundles and disappears in the white matter. With respect to the thickness and abundance of the axon collaterals of such neurons, there are many variants. The majority can be reduced to two: cells whose axon, impoverished by the superabundance and robustness of the collaterals emitted, becomes very thin when it reaches the underlying layers; and cells whose axon, little debilitated by the presence of collaterals, retains its original robustness down to the white matter.

In fig. 7 [*fig. 252*], we have put together the main types of stellate cells collected from the same region of several sections. Neurons have been chosen, of course, whose axons could be followed over a long distance. Preparations completely impregnated by the method of Cox show that the number of stellate cells per unit of thickness and surface is much larger than

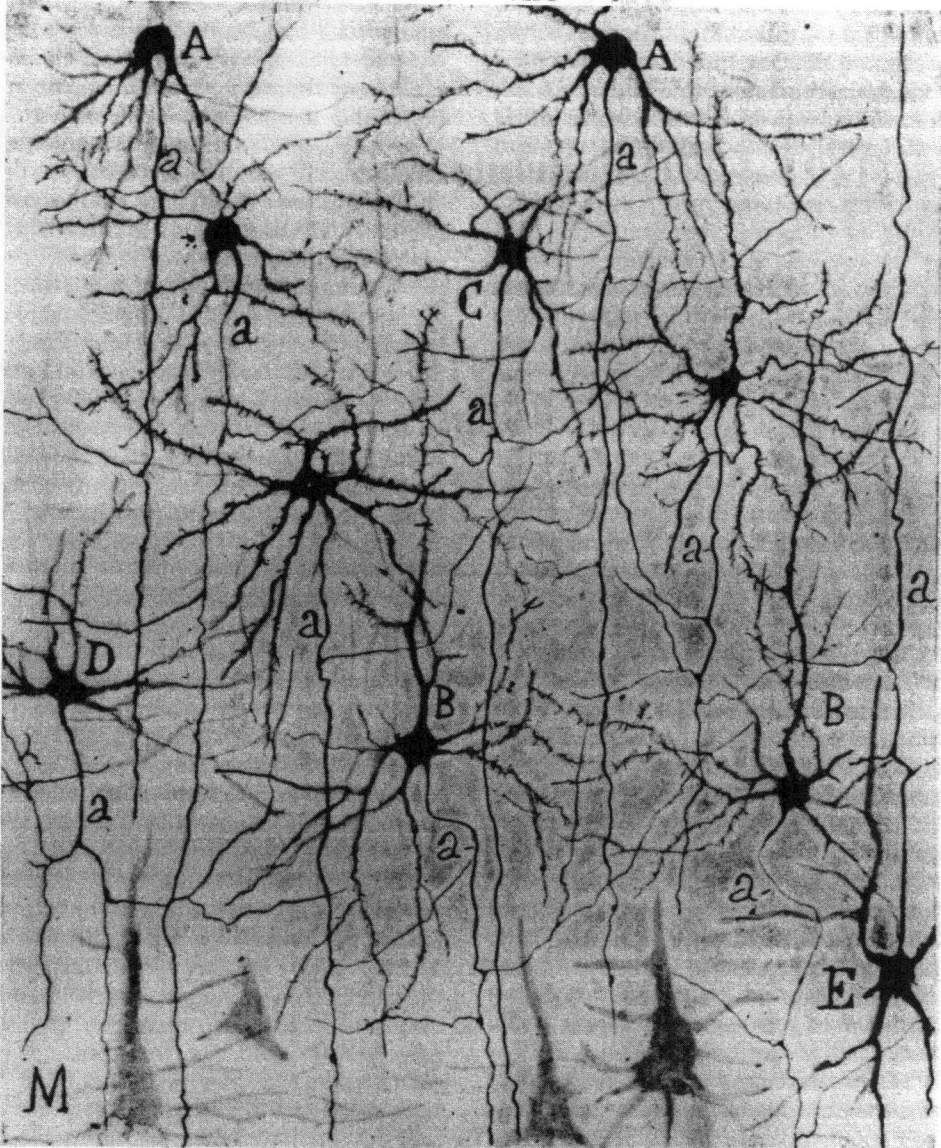

[*FIG. 252*]   Fig. 7. Layer of the stellate cells with long axon (cat of twenty-five days). *A*, mitral types; *C, D*, star-shaped type; *B*, types with rudimentary [apical] dendrite; *E*, neuron with ascending axon; *M*, layer of the large solitary pyramids.

that illustrated in the mentioned fig. 7 [*fig. 252*]. It is particularly true that in these sections, in which scarcely any cell with long axon is not impregnated, it is not always easy to distinguish a stellate cell with an axon of projection from a cell of a similar shape and size but provided with a short axon.

As we will see below, the layer under study constitutes the principal point of branching of the fibers of exogenous origin.

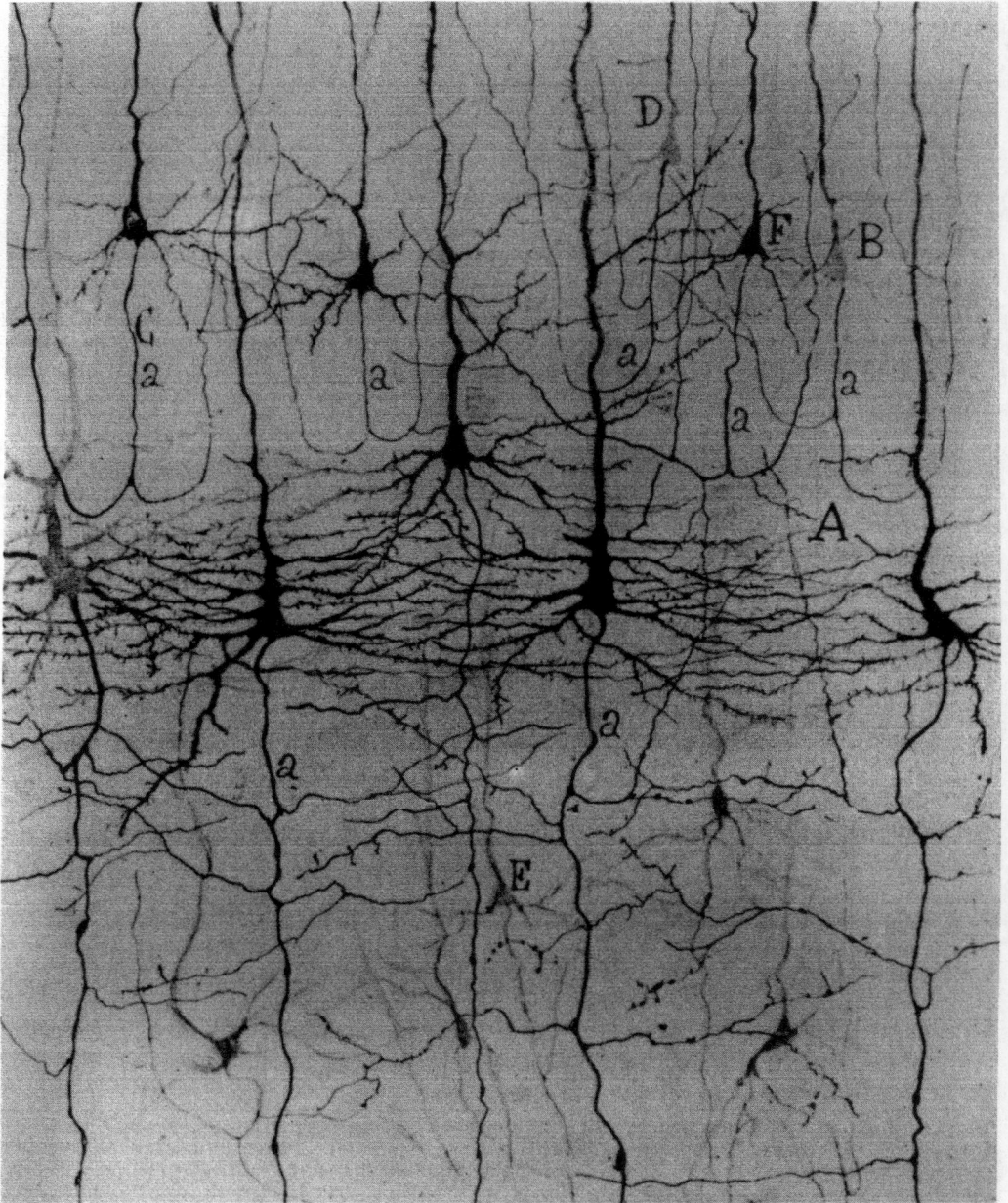

[*FIG. 253*] Fig. 8. Layers 5, 6, and 7 of the visual cortex of the cat of twenty-five days. Golgi method. *A*, layer of the large solitary cells of Meynert; *B, C, D, F,* neurons with arciform axon of the fifth layer (deep portion of the lamina granularis); *E*, neurons of the seventh layer; *a*, axons.

b. Sublayer of the Small Pyramids with Arciform Axon (Internal Half of the Lamina *Granularis* of Brodmann.) We designate it in this manner because it preferentially contains an extremely original type of neuron discovered by us in the calcarine sulcus of man and later confirmed in a part of the visual area of the cat, and characterized by showing, apart from the radial dendritic process prolonged up to the plexiform layer, a type of axon that, after running downward for a certain distance, divides itself into two or more arches (sometimes one) that continue as ascending retrograde branches. These minute cells extend across the lower part to the layer of the solitary giant pyramids and beyond, as we will indicate later; but their principal localization, or at least the territory in which they have been stained in greater numbers, is the sublayer under study. Needless to say, other cellular types are intermingled with them, especially quite a number of neurons with short axon and others with ascending radial axon, as we will expose later and as can be seen in fig. 9, *A, E* [*fig. 254*].

The principal varieties of cell with arciform axon have been reproduced in fig. 8, *D, F, G* [*fig. 253*]. Omitting the behavior of the radial [dendritic] shaft and basal dendrites, well appreciable in figs. 8 and 10 [*figs. 253, 255*], let us note that the axonal arch or arches show some differences worth mentioning:

a. Pyramid whose thin descending axon, after giving off some oblique or transverse collaterals, traces an arcade, to turn back and disappear into the external cortical layers (fig. 8, *B*) [*fig. 253*]. This variety is relatively rare.

b. Pyramid whose axon bifurcates, originating two arcades with opposite directions and situated at the same level (fig. 8, *C*)[H] [*fig. 253*]. This variety is very common.

c. Pyramid whose axon resolves itself into two or more arches situated in different planes (fig. 8, *D*) [*fig. 253*].

d. Pyramid whose axon resolves itself into two or more retrograde arches and gives off a thin descending collateral which sometimes crosses the underlying layer of the solitary pyramids [*fig. 253, F*].[1] We do not know if this collateral, which was already recognized by us in our work on the human visual cortex[11] and on the homologous region of the cat, continues as

a fiber of the white matter. We opt for the negative, noting the delicacy and frequent ramifications of such a delicate process.

Where in the upper part [of the cortex] are these robust arciform branches ending? Comparing our old analysis of the human calcarine sulcus with those made more recently on the young cat, we judge that, at least in the majority of cases, the final arborizations of the axonal arcades are distributed in the *external half of the layer of the granule cells or sublayer of the stellate cells*, where they transmit impulses probably of a visual nature. With this we do not exclude the possibility that such ramifications enter into relationships with several other cellular elements, including with the homonymous cells of the *sublayer of the small pyramids with arciform axon.*

Cells of Golgi and Cells with Ascending or Descending Axon. All the layers of the visual area are very rich in cells with short axons (*intercalary cells* of v[on] Monakow), but nowhere are they so concentrated as in the *layer of the stellate cells* (external and internal sublayers), as we demonstrated many years ago in the visual cortex of man.

Besides the *dwarf or arachniform type,* noted already by us in the visual area, and of a variety with short axon of regular size and arborization distributed in the vicinity of the soma (true type of Golgi), our preparations of the cat include, as an apparently dominant variety, certain cells with semilong ascending or descending axons, some of which we reproduce in fig. 9 [*fig. 254*].

These neurons have a starlike shape with divergent dendritic radiations, but their main characteristic is that the axon, besides being quite long, follows almost always a radial direction, gives off numerous branches that arise at a right angle, and is distributed in the several levels of the layer of the stellate cells. When the axon is descending, which happens frequently, it has its terminal territory in the *deeper sublayer* or [sublayer] of the *pyramids with arciform axon* (fig. 9, *B, C,*[1] *D*) [*fig. 254*].

If, on the contrary, the axon runs in an ascending direction, the place in which it preferentially arborizes is the *external sublayer,*

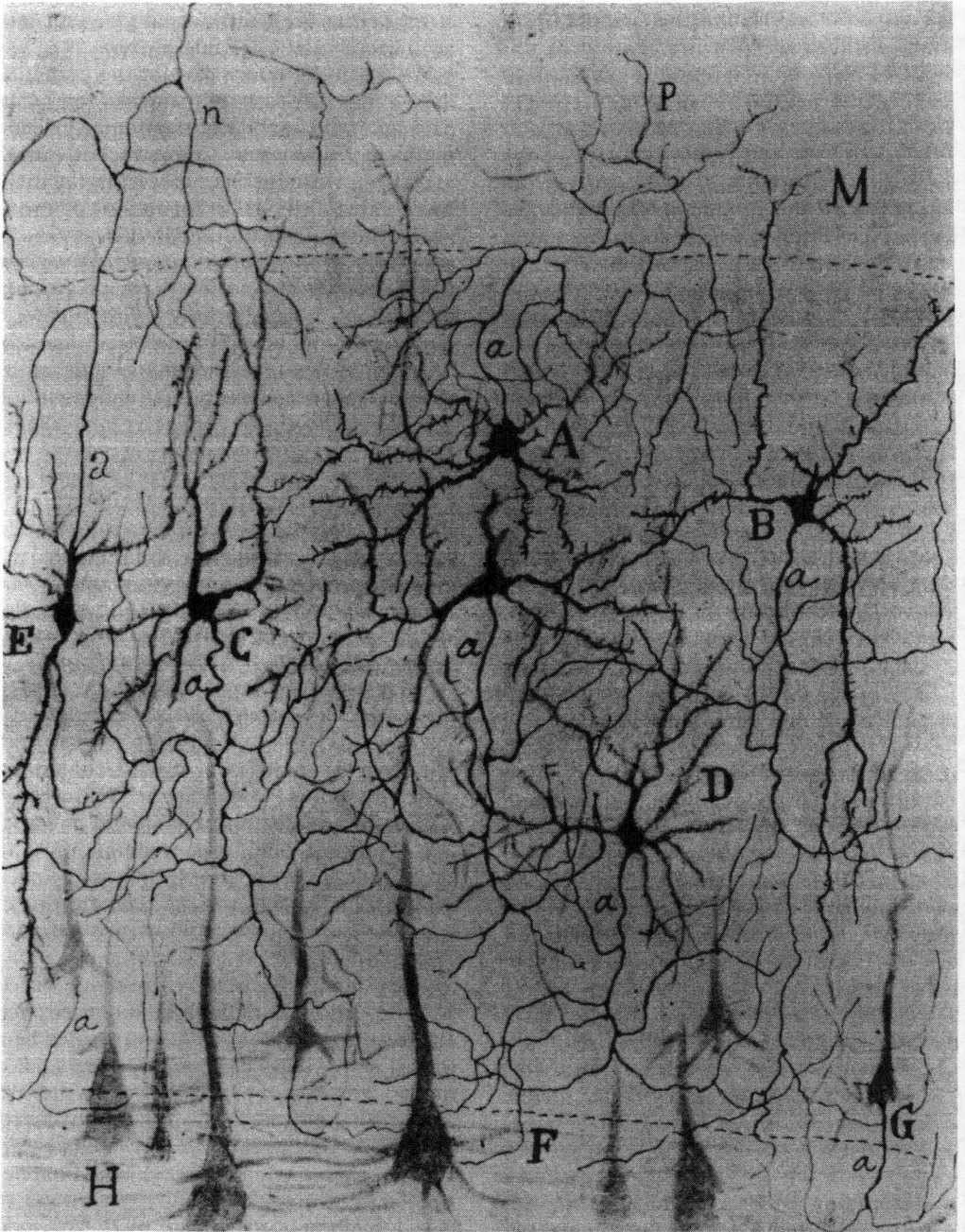

[*FIG. 254*]   Fig. 9. Some cells with short axon of the layer of the stellate cells (visual cortex of the cat of twenty days). *M*, layer of the superficial large pyramids; *F*, layer of the solitary pyramids of Meynert.

where the *large stellate cells with long axon* predominate (figs. 9, *A*; 11, *h, c*) [*figs. 254, 256*].

Some neurons with ascending axon can go beyond the limits of the layer of the stellate cells. Thus, the neurons *A* and *E* of fig. 9 [*fig 254*] provided axonal ramifications to the layer of the *superficial large pyramids,* whereas the cell *B,* with descending axon, sent terminal branches to the layer of the *solitary pyramidal cells* of Meynert (fig. 9) [*fig. 254*].

To be complete, let us still mention the existence in the sublayer of the pyramids with arciform axon (deep level of the layer of the stellate cells) of [an occasional] robust cell with ascending axon, which could be followed up to near the plexiform layer, where it probably ended. It is, as can be seen in fig. 7, *E* [*fig. 252*], a true *cell of Martinotti.*

About the nervous plexuses of the layer of the stellate neurons (stria of Gennari) we will deal later.

Let us mention still that in this sublayer there are observed [occasional] pyramids of common type and some stellate cells with long axon, similar to those noted in the preceding sublayer (fig. 7, *B*) [*fig. 252*].

[6]. Layer of the Deep Large Pyramids (Solitary Cells of Meynert)

With good reason, this layer has been considered, especially by Campbell, Mott, and others, as one of the most characteristic of the striate area of animals. Not only in man, where we had analyzed it in detail, but in the cat and dog, it shows up clearly as a definite band, situated between the layer of the granule cells, or [layer of] *small pryamids with arciform axon,* and [the layer] of the *polymorphic cells.*

It includes three main features: (a) the large and some medium pyramidal cells, (b) the transverse dendritic plexuses, and (c) a number of small neurons, among which those with arciform axon predominate.

a. The Giant Pyramidal Cells. [These] are clearly shown in Nissl preparations (fig. 10, *A*) [*fig. 255*]. They are cells rich in [Nissl granules, and are] arranged in discontinuous series, sometimes in clusters of three or four, separated by plexiform intervals poor in or devoid of voluminous cells. Where they constitute a

relatively uniform row is at the level of the sulci or intermediate territories [between the sulci] and the apex of the marginal gyrus; at the level of the apex, they usually undergo a change of plane, becoming more superficial, at the same time notably lengthening the chromophilic soma. In many sections of the apical region of the gyrus, the solitary pyramids are found almost in the central plane of the gyrus, whereas in the edges of the fissures, they inhabit the junction between the deep third and the superficial two-thirds. Particularly abundant, regular, and typical, they are present in the interhemispheric cortex (cerebellar surface), in the vicinity of that shallow fissure that several authors, and especially Winkler, call *sulcus suprasplenialis.*

Even in the Nissl sections, many variations can be observed in regard to the richness and position of the solitary pyramids. There are places where only a discontinuous row is found, as we show in fig. 10, *A* [*fig. 255*]; in other regions, two and even three rows are observed, the cells being packed in pleiades; finally, it is frequent to observe territories in which pyramids of smaller dimensions, although of the same character and inhabiting different planes, are intermingled with the colossal pyramids. For example, in fig. 8 [*fig. 253*], which represents a section of the cortex of the cat of twenty-five days, one of these relatively small solitary cells (*E*) is seen.

With respect to the structure [of the giant cells], there is nothing special to note, only the richness in [Nissl granules] and the exceptional size of the nucleus, whose nucleolus is customarily deflected toward the surface. With regard to the form, let us mention that the cellular contour often appears notched, from the sharp parts of which arise a dendrite. From the upper pole arises, as is shown in Golgi sections (fig. 8) [*fig. 253*], a robust, branched [apical dendritic] shaft that goes up to the plexiform layer, whereas from the base of the soma emerges the robust and flexuous axon, prolonged down to the white matter and provided with numerous collaterals (five, six, or seven), almost all with a transverse or oblique course and prolixly branched in the layer of the polymorphic cells. Some small axonal branches can also describe a recurrent trajectory

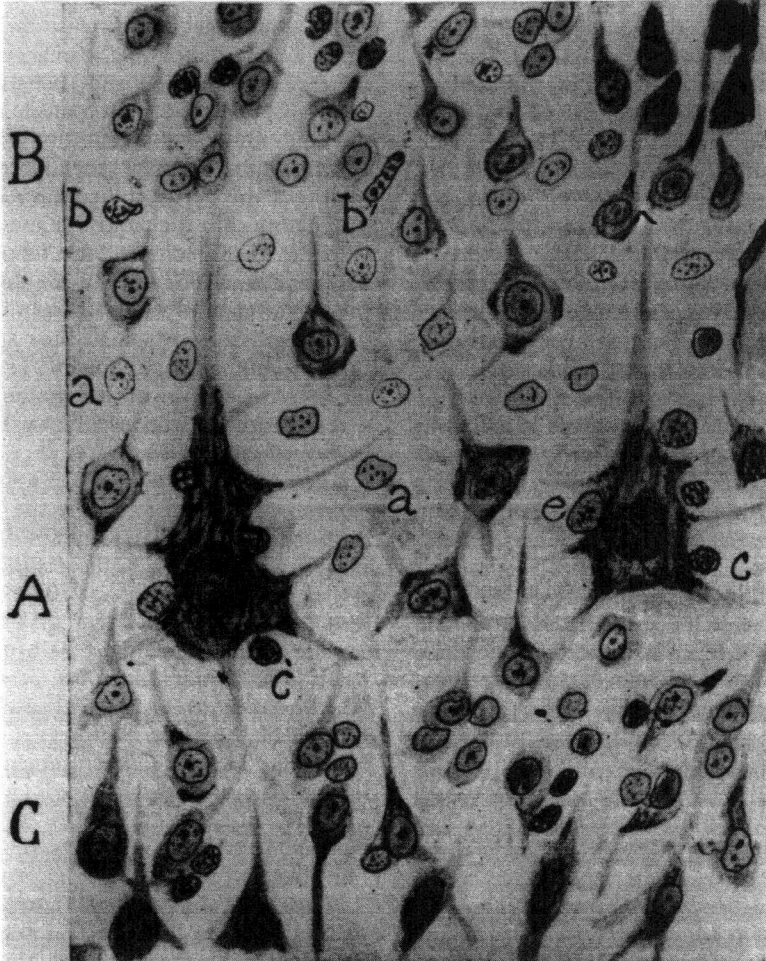

[*FIG. 255*] Fig. 10. Layer of the solitary pyramidal cells of Meynert and neighboring regions. Nissl method. *A,* large pyramids; *B,* layer of the cells with arciform axon (deep half of the lamina granularis); *C,* beginning of the layer of polymorphic cells; *a,* common glia; *b,* small rod cell and mesoglia.

and end either in the layer under study or in more superficial planes.

Although there is nothing special about the following peculiarity, let us record that the pyramids of Meynert are accompanied by satellite cells, of which some, to judge by the size and structure of the nucleus, correspond to what we called the *third* or *adendritic element* (*phagocytes* of certain authors), and others to the *pericellular glia,* characterized by the relative size of the nucleus and its poverty in chromatin. True *microglia* or *mesoglia,* like those described in the general cortex by Nicolás Achúcarro, Del Río-Hortega, and us, have not been clearly observed, although it is true that for this subject we have not applied the specific methods.

b. Horizontal Dendritic Plexus. As can be recognized in fig. 8, *A* [*fig. 253*], the existence of this plexus, whose processes run preferentially in a transverse or oblique direction, interweaving at acute angles, constitutes a characteristic as distinctive for the layer under study as the presence of the solitary pyramids themselves. Already the presence of such a dense feltwork can be guessed at in the Nissl sections, because of the large granular, pale, and neuron-poor spaces that separate the cited giant pyramids (fig. 10, A) [fig. 255]. The details of fig. 8 [fig. 253] excuse us from dwelling on the texture of so complicated a plexus, already described by us many years ago in the human cerebral cortex.

In the adult cat, the plexus only appears clearly at the level of the walls of the fissures; the apical portion of the marginal gyrus exhibits a thicker dendritic band, which is also more irregular and staircaselike. These alterations are influenced, without doubt, by the excessive number of the solitary pyramids as well as by the thinness and radial stretching of their somata.

c. Small Pyramids with Arciform Axon. They appear like advance elements of the same type as those in the fifth layer. We consider it probable that almost all the nerve cells revealed in the layer of the deep large pyramids with the Nissl method belong to this neuronal type (fig. 10, A) [fig. 255]. We have reproduced some of them in fig. 9, G and fig. 11, D and C [figs. 254, 256].

[7]. Layer of the Polymorphic Cells (Lamina *Multiformis* of Brodmann)

Of considerable thickness in the apical portions of the marginal gyrus, where it forms more than a third of the whole cortex, it becomes notably thinner in the floors and flat walls of the sulci. It is usually composed of rows of cells oriented in a radial direction and of similarly radial bundles of white matter that are none other than axonal bundles arising from the pyramids and stellate cells.

As is known, in man this layer is clearly differentiated in two levels or substrata: one tightly packed, made up of small pyramids with arciform axon (eighth layer); and the other looser, pale, and elongated, in which the triangular and fusiform cells with axon of projection (ninth layer) predominate.

In the cat, this distinction is less accentuated. However, in the appropriate territories, it is possible to distinguish also a *superficial*

zone rich in pyramidal or polyhedral neurons with an axon preferentially arciform and a *deep sublayer,* poor in cells, almost all of them fusiform and extended in the axis or axes of the marginal gyrus.

a. Superficial Sublayer or [Sublayer] of the Tightly Packed Neurons. Almost all the constituent cells have a soma of medium size, poor in [Nissl material] (fig. 10, C) [fig. 255], a long radial dendrite extending probably up to the plexiform layer, and an axon whose varied behavior allows us to classify such cells into the following kinds.

1. Small pyramids with arciform axon having single, double, or triple arcades, but apparently bereft of a collateral of projection invading the white matter. This type is very abundant, [although] it is so far impossible to determine its ratio to the rest of the cells (fig. 11, B, F, G) [fig. 256].

2. Neurons similar to the previous ones, but having a long descending collateral, continued as a thin fiber of the white matter. Such cells are very abundant in the human calcarine sulcus (eighth layer or layer of the deep granule cells). Figs. 11, E, and 12, A [figs. 256, 257] reproduce some of these neurons, whose descending axons could be followed down to the white matter (fig. 11, b) [fig. 256].

3. Pyramidal or triangular cells, relatively large and provided with collateral and basal dendritic processes, a radial [dendritic] shaft, frequently inflected near its origin (fig. 12, E, $C_i^K B$) [fig. 257], and, finally, a descending axon that, after giving off some thin collaterals with variable orientations, reaches the white matter. As we approach closer to the *deeper sublayer,* this kind of long axon appears to become more abundant.

4. Triangular, fusiform, or stellate cells with ascending axon, which can be followed across the superimposed layers up to near the plexiform layer in which it probably arborizes (fig. 12, D) [fig. 257].

5. Finally, from time to time, some neurons with short axons can be distinguished.

b. Sublayer of the Fusiform and Triangular Cells. It is quite thick, at the level of the most protuberant portion of the marginal gyrus; it

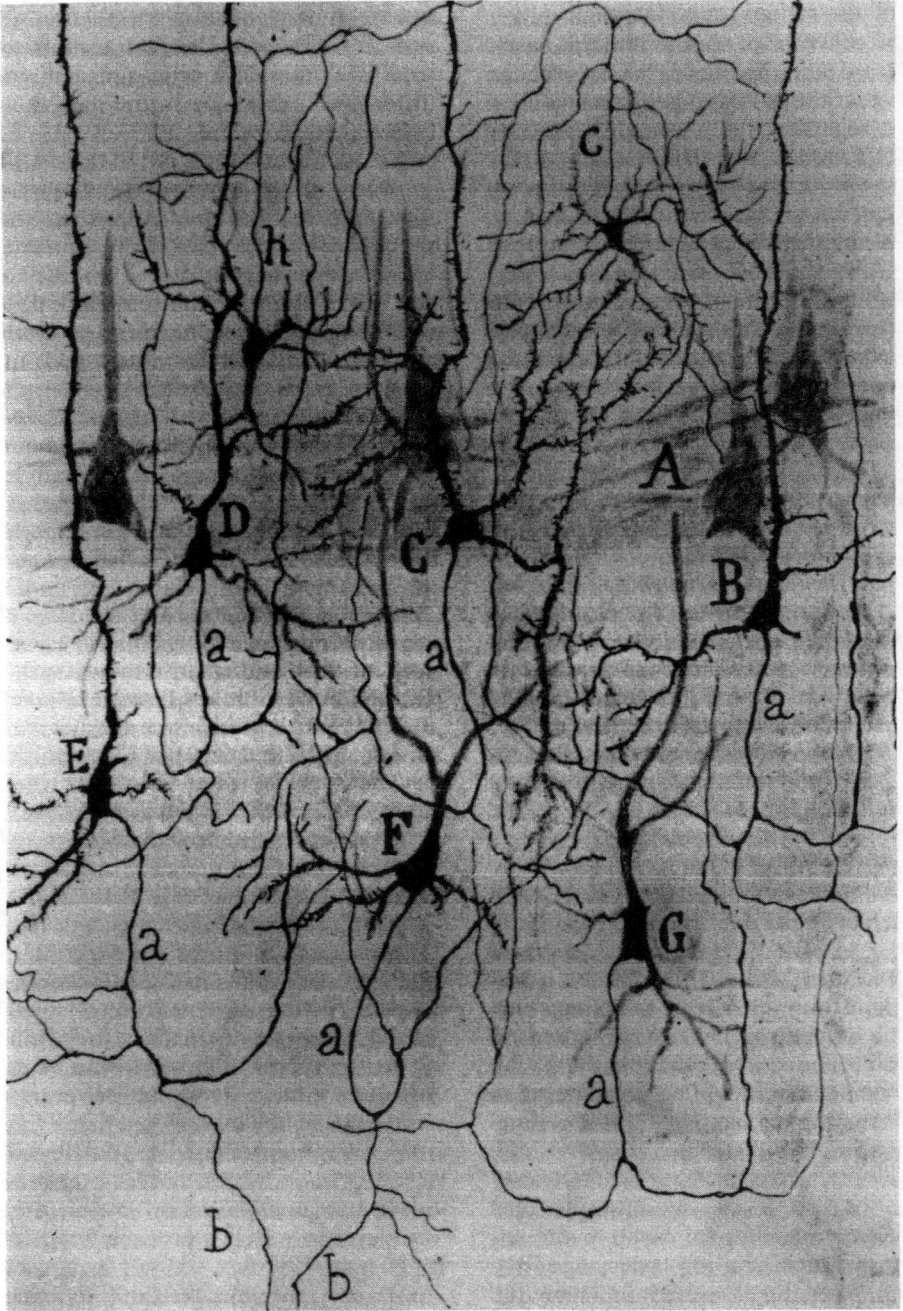

[*FIG. 256*] Fig. 11. Diverse neuronal types of layers 4, 5, and 6. *A*, layer of the solitary pyramids; *B, C, D, G*, pyramids with arciform axon; *E, F*, pyramids whose arciform axons gave off a branch to the white matter; *c, h*, neurons with ascending short axon of the fourth layer (deep sublayer).

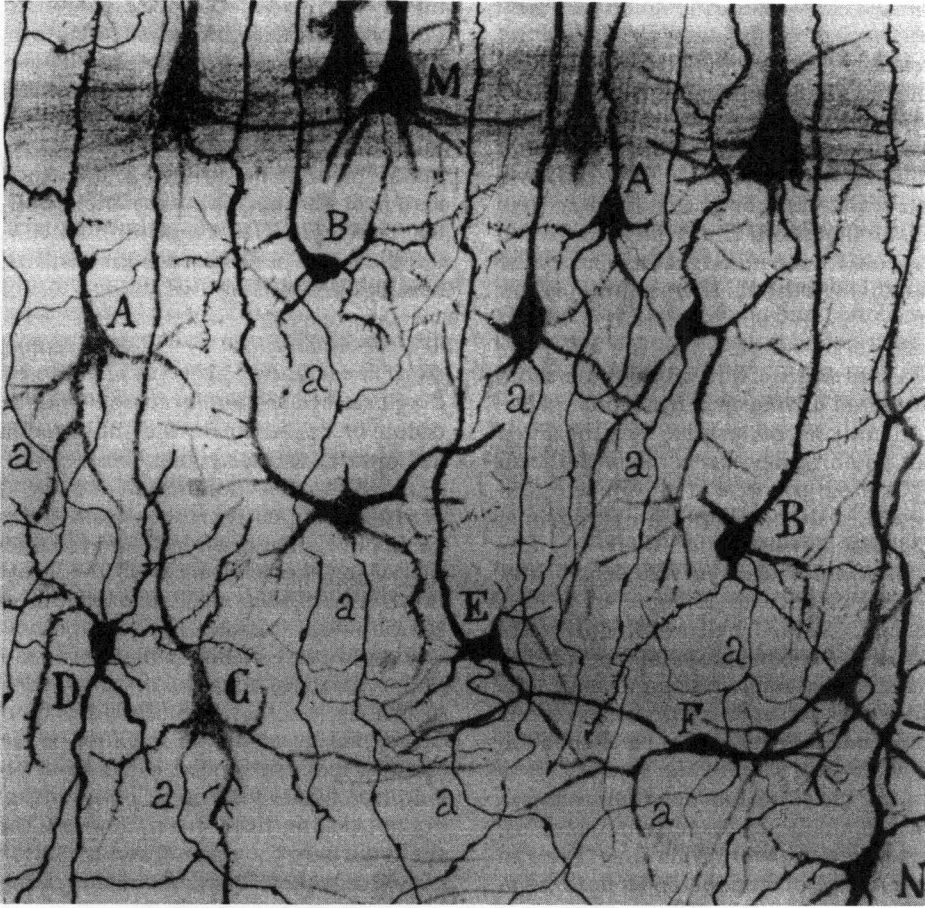

[*FIG. 257*]   Fig. 12. Neurons of the layer of the polymorphic cells. *M*, solitary pyramidal cells; *A, B*, pyramids whose axons were directed to the white matter; *D*, cell with ascending axon; *E, F, N*, triangular or stellate cells with long axon.

gets narrower and almost disappears at the level of the sulci, intimately intermingling with the bundles of white matter to whose directions the cells adapt. The Nissl method, and especially those of Golgi and Cox, allow us to differentiate two main varieties: the genuine fusiform type, with two thick, polar dendrites; and the triangular type which, in addition to the opposite-polar processes, shows frequently a short and thick lateral dendrite. It is impossible, given the deep localization of the somata of both varieties, to follow the apical [dendritic] shaft to its termination. We suspect, however, that, like the majority of the

neurons with long axon, it has a more or less thin dendritic representation in the plexiform layer. With regard to the axon, it is continuous, apparently without exceptions, with a fiber of the white matter. In the Nissl preparations, it is very frequent to observe dwarf satellite and glial cells around these neurons.

[8]. *Layer of the Fibers of the White Matter*

It is well known that any cortical sensory area enters into connection by means of systems of fibers with other more or less distant areas of the gray matter.

In spite of their abundance, the constituent

fibers of the visual white matter can be reduced to two large categories. The *endogenous or efferent fibers,* represented by the rich profusion of axons arising from the small and medium pyramids, the solitary pyramids of Meynert, stellate cells (fourth layer), and diverse types of the layer of the polymorphic cells; and the *exogenous or afferent fibers,* coming from the *secondary* or subcortical *visual foci (lateral geniculate body, pulvinar,* etc.) and perhaps, as some [authors] affirm, from other cortical regions.

a. Endogenous Fibers. We will say little about this category of axons, since they behave, during their intracortical course, like the fibers arising from any other cortical area. Suffice it to say that, after giving off a multitude of collaterals, almost all the fibers of this kind enter the radial bundles, in which there are thin, medium, and thick fibers, getting lost, finally, in the white matter.

In sections [stained by] the procedures of Weigert or of Spielmeyer, it is impossible to follow them individually inside the white core of the marginal gyrus, but in certain fortunate silver chromate sections, it was possible to follow them for long trajectories. Some of them were observed to form an ascending collateral, destined for widely separated radii of the superimposed gray matter. There are cases in which the above-mentioned collateral resembled, on account of this thickness, a branch of bifurcation, being distinguished in addition by not showing the least tendency to enter the visual cortex. Do such examples indicate association projections to some distant, homolateral cerebral territory or, instead, fibers destined for the corpus callosum?

This question is related to the still unelucidated problem of the significance of the *corpus callosum,* considered partially or totally by some authorities as a homotopical commissure, and regarded by others as a pathway of heterotopical association. Although the anatomical methods, even in small mammals, do not allow us to resolve definitively this point, guided by theoretical considerations, and as we conjectured many years ago,[12] we are inclined to admit that the fibers sent to the corpus callosum from the visual cortex have their termination in contralateral association areas (in the sense in which Meynert uses this term). And as far as I can judge, the observations made with anatomicopathological methods by Beevor[13] and Valkenburg[14] do not contradict this assertion, at least in principle. Anyway, the problem of the origin, course, and termination of the corpus callosum, about which Dr. Villaverde[15] has recently presented very interesting data and observations, still requires new and persevering studies.

b. Exogeneous Fibers or Fibers Arriving from Other Nervous Foci. It is sufficient to examine a well-stained section [prepared] with the procedure of Pal, of Spielmeyer, or of reduced silver nitrate, to notice that, besides the fibers grouped in radial bundles, in the deep planes of the visual cortex there exist fibers of a [distinctive] caliber almost always larger than that of the axons arising from the visual pyramids. These fibers are characterized, besides their unusual thickness, by their particular direction, almost always oblique or transverse with respect to the radial bundles (see fig. 13, *d,* and fig. 14) [*figs. 258, 259*]. Such collossal fibers, mainly related to the stria of Gennari, were already mentioned by us in the human calcarine fissure. Although less abundant, they are not lacking either from the visual cortex of the cat, where the silver chromate allows us to distinguish them easily from the endogenous fibers and to follow them up to their terminal arborizations.

Although the stria of Gennari is composed of many kinds of fibers, it is unquestionable that one of the principal sources of the components of the stria is represented by the above-mentioned robust exogenous fibers.

But before we examine the behavior of such fibers, let us say something about the *stria of Gennari,* which I would prefer to call the *plexus of Gennari.* Let us begin by affirming that in the cortex of the dog and cat, the cited stria does not stand out as clearly as in the human cerebrum. In general, except for the deep trajectory of its afferent fibers, the plexus outlined by myelin stains at the level of the layer of the stellate cells is composed of thin threads with varied orientations, frequently transverse and oblique, extremely close to-

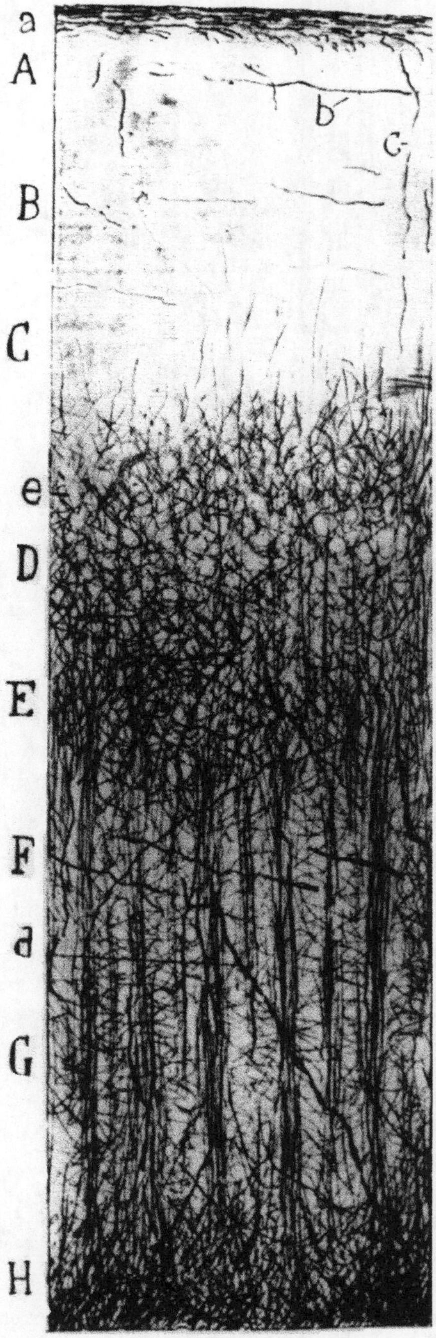

[FIG. 258] Fig. 13. Section of the internal or interhemispheric surface of the marginal gyrus (visual region) of the cortex of the adult cat. Staining of the myelinated fibers with the Weigert-Pal method. *a*,

gether, and enclosing meshes or rounded spaces in which are lodged the somata of the neurons (fig. 13, *D, e*) [*fig. 258*]. In these sections, the opinion of Brodmann is confirmed, according to which the main localization of the stria would correspond to the superficial or external portion of his *lamina granularis*, that is to say, to what we have designated the *external sublayer* of the said lamina, where the stellate neurons with long axon appear to predominate.

The good Golgi sections, besides corroborating this localization, reveal a plexus much denser and more intricate than the Weigert-Pal preparations. The same occurs with sections impregnated by the method of Bielschowsky, or with certain formulas of reduced silver nitrate. It indicates, obviously, that the terminal ramifications of the exogenous myelinated fibers lack a myelin sheath. The mentioned preparations allow us, besides, to observe that the *plexus of Gennari,* in fact, extends, although decreasing in the number of fibers, down to the fifth layer or [layer] of the large solitary pyramids.

In this plexus can be distinguished two main levels, not well demarcated because of the transitions [between them]:

a. *Superficial plane,* in which predominate thin medullated fibers and free, extensive, and varicose arborizations, oriented preferentially in the transverse direction (fig. 14, *B*) [*fig. 259*], although it is not rare to observe a quite robust horizontal or oblique fiber. This plane coincides almost exactly with the position of the *sublayer of the large stellate cells.* Some thin projections ascend, as illustrated in fig. 14 [*fig. 259*], up to the layer of the superficial large pyramids.

b. *The deep plane,* somewhat looser and with thicker fibers, is particularly localized in the

superficial portion of the plexiform layer; *A,* deep portion of the same, poor in medullated fibers; *B,* region of the small pyramids; *C,* layer of the large and medium external pyramids; *D,* sublayer of the stellate cells (layer 4); *E,* sublayer of the cells with arciform axon; *F,* layer of the solitary pyramids of Meynert; *G,* layer of the polymorphic cells; *H,* white matter; *d,* oblique colossal myelinated fibers to the stria of Gennari.

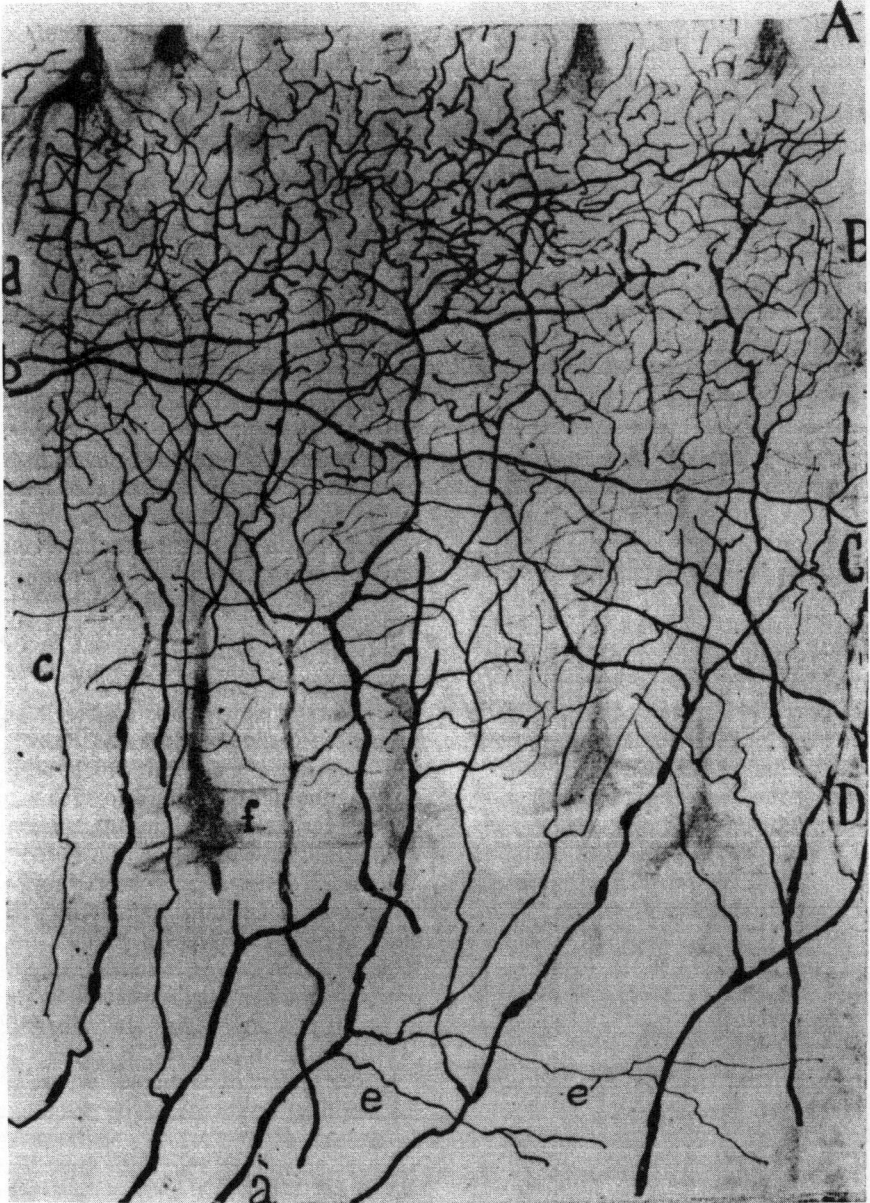

[*FIG. 259*]   Fig. 14. Exogenous fibers of large caliber impregnated by the Golgi method (visual cortex of the cat of twenty days). *A*, layer of the superficial large pyramidal cells; *B*, superficial portion of the plexus of Gennari; *a*, *D*, thick afferent fibers; *b*, horizontal arborizations.

sublayer of the pyramids with arciform axon (fig. [259], *C*). It does not lack thin branches and even hollows surrounded by tight arborizations, but especially prominent are a large number of thick, horizontal, and oblique fibers. In this plane, there are also numerous bifurcations of colossal afferent axons (fig. 14) [*fig. 259*].

To be complete, it is worth mentioning that the layers of the solitary pyramids of Meynert and of the polymorphic cells also have terminal ramifications of thick afferent fibers, although in small number (fig. 14, *e*) [*fig. 259*].

It is obvious, according to what has been said in the previous pages, that the stria or plexus of Gennari is not composed exclusively of the terminal arborizations of the colossal or medium-caliber exogenous fibers. In conformity with what the reader will have seen if he remembers the description of the third, fourth, and fifth layers, there are involved in the constitution of the mentioned feltwork, [which is] one of the most complicated presented by the nervous centers, numerous elements whose relative proportions are impossible to determine exactly at present.

Let us mention, among others, (a) the axonal collaterals of the superficial large pyramids (third layer); (b) the collaterals of the stellate cells (external portion of the lamina granularis); (c) the terminal arborizations of the numerous cells with short and semilong ascending and descending axons located in both sublayers of the fourth layer; (d) the terminal axon branches and extremely numerous collaterals arising from the small pyramids

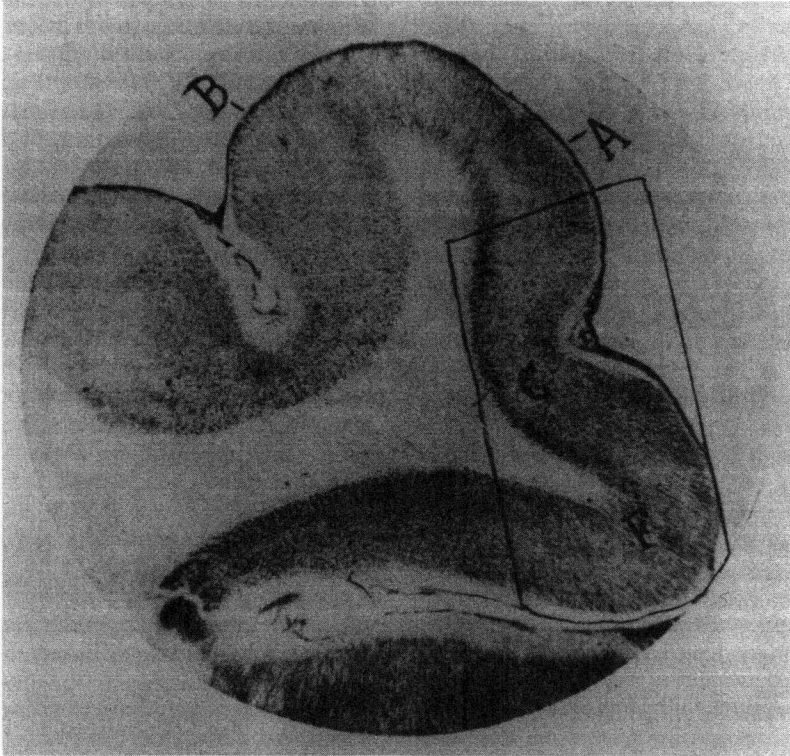

[*FIG. 260*] [Fig. 3 of the German translation.] Frontal section through the lower and upper part of the marginal gyrus of an adult cat (Nissl method). *A*, upper part of the gyrus; *B*, outer part; *C, F,* lower and inner parts of the same. Note: the square drawn in the lower region of the marginal gyrus yielded the best and most representative preparations with the chrome-silver method. This photomicrograph is bounded on the right by the interhemispheric fissure.

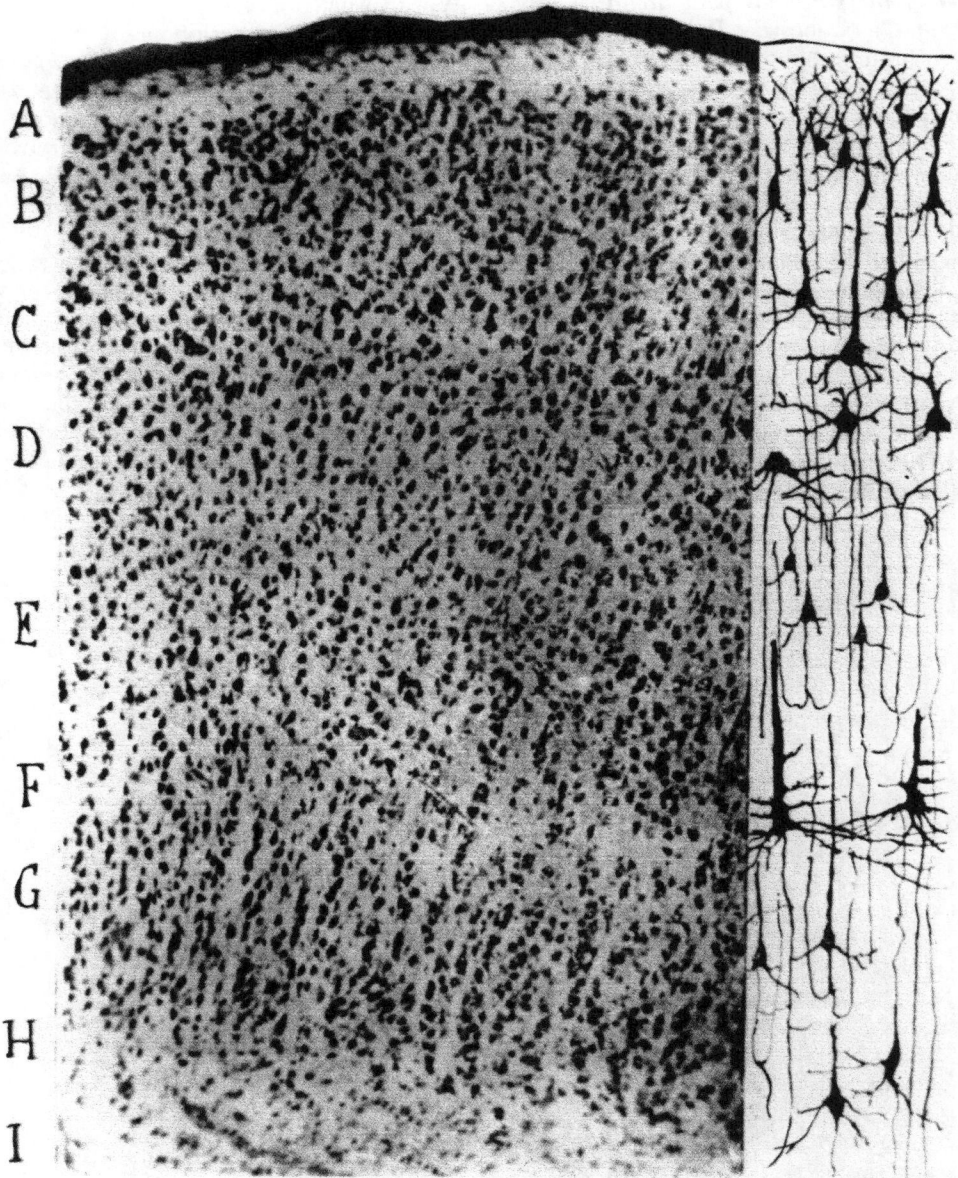

[*FIG. 261*] [Fig. 4, Plate 15 of the German translation.] Photomicrograph of the vicinity of the suprasplenial sulcus. The letters indicate the positions of the layers (adult cat). On the right, I have shown the neuronal types which appeared in the individual layers with the Golgi method.

with arciform axon located in the fourth layer (deep plane), layer of the solitary cells of Meynert, and external plane of the layer of the polymorphic neurons, etc.

This multiplicity of sources of the stria of

Gennari demands that the clinicians and anatomicopathologists exercise great caution in the interpretation of lesions of those cortical and subcortical foci which are supposed to be associated with the visual cortex and whose de-

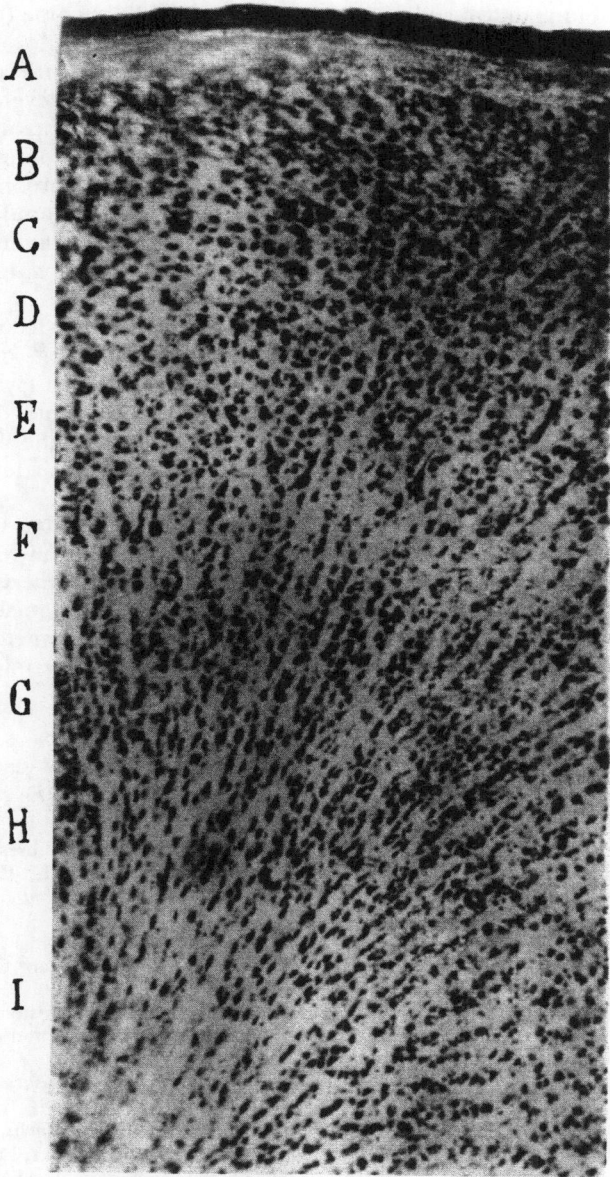

[*FIG. 262*] [Fig. 5, Plate 15 of the German translation.] Photomicrograph from the apex of a gyrus (region *F* in fig. 3 [*fig. 260*]). One notes the variability in layer *F* (solitary pyramids) and layer *E* (small cells with arciform axon). Furthermore, [one notes] the significant development of [layers] 8 and 9 (*G* and *H*). Adult cat, Nissl method.

generation or ablation is not followed to a predictable extent by the decrease or disappearance of the medullated plexus of the fourth layer (*lamina granularis* of Brodmann) and the double line of Baillarger.

Leaving aside the endogenous neural features of the stria of Gennari, there is no doubt that this contains a large number of exogenous fibers, according to what we supposed and as asserted by certain authors. It is for us unquestionable that at the level of the fourth and fifth layers (we do not exclude other layers), the visual cortex receives impulses coming from other nervous centers. These would be, especially, the preferred location of contact or of transmission between the neurons of the visual cortex and the fibers arriving from the subcortical visual centers. With a certainty perhaps greater than that permitted by the revelations of the methods, we have maintained the thesis that the colossal fibers arborizing in the stria [of Gennari] have their origin in the cells of the *lateral geniculate body, pulvinar,* and other visual regions of the thalamus.

Nowadays, despite the objection directed by Monakow[16] and others against this opinion, we continue to hold it, since the facts brandished against it can receive many different interpretations. We recognize, however, that the problem is not definitely resolved and that, [in order] to dispel doubts, it is necessary to resort to anatomicopathological methods. Such a task will be the subject of a future work, in which we will try (or some of our disciples will try) to elucidate, as far as allowed by the present methods, the origin of the exogenous fibers and the mode of termination of the endogenous fibers in laboratory animals.

And naught else for the present.

Conclusions

Until we study the visual cortex of carnivore and rodent mammals more rigorously and more carefully, let us be permitted to record here the most essential results:

1. Our cyto- and myeloarchitectonic investigations confirm in principle the localization and extent of the visual area of the cat, delineated by Brodmann, Campbell, and Minkowski.

2. There exists a great analogy, not only stratigraphic but also fine structural (cellular morphology, behavior of the axons, etc.), between the visual area of man and of the cat.

3. The main characteristics of the visual cortex, in part already mentioned by Meynert, Henschen, Campbell, Bolton, Mott, Brodmann, O. Vogt, Minkowski, etc., are:

a. The existence of a specific formation of *stellate cells with long axon* (external portion of the fourth layer).

b. The presence in the deep plane of the fourth layer and at the level of the sixth [layer] of certain cells whose axon, after tracing an arch, resolves itself into descending arborizations, distributed preferentially in the upper plane of the lamina granularis. Instead of an arched axon, these pyramidal cells show several axonal arcades, in which the [main] axon exhausts itself.

c. The existence of a deep layer of large pyramidal cells (*solitary cells* of Meynert), which at the level of the fifth layer generate a very dense plexus of horizontal dendrites.

d. The existence of the well-known stria of Gennari, located at the level of the lamina granularis.

e. Finally, the arrival at the said stria, such that it comes to be like the door of entrance to the visual area, of a large number of colossal exogenous fibers, distinguished from the efferent fibers by their diameter and oblique or staircaselike and sometimes transverse trajectory.

Consulted Bibliography[L]

Beevor. On the Course of Fibres of the Cingulum and the Posterior Parts of the Corpus Collosum, etc. *Phil. Trans. Roy. Society of London,* Vol. LXXXII, 1892, p. 135.

Bolton. The Exact Histological Localisation of the Visual Area of the Human Cerebral Cortex. *Phil Trans.,* Vol. CXCIII, 1900.

Brodmann. Beiträge zur histologischen Lokalisation der Grosshirnrinde. V. Mitteilung. *Journal f. Neurol. u. Psych.,* Vol. VI, 1906.

——. *Vergleichende Lokalisationslehre der Grosshirnrinde,* Leipzig, 1909.

——. *Allegemeinere Neurologie,* edited by M. Lewandowsky. Berlin, J. Springer, Part I, 1910. (Article by Brodmann, on cerebral localization.)

Cajal. La corteza visual. *Revista Trimestral Micrográfica,* Vol. VI, 1899.

——. *Histologie du système nerveux de l'homme et des vertébrés,* etc. Paris, Maloine, Vol. II, 1911, p. 599 and following.

Campbell. *Histological Studies on the Localisation of Cerebral Function.* Cambridge, 1905.

Flores. *A myceloarchitectura et a myelogenia do cortex cerebral do Erinaceus europeus.,* Lisbon, 1911.

Hammarberg. *Studien ueber Klinik u. Pathol. d. Idiotie,* etc., Upsala, 1895.

Henschen. Sur les centres optiques cérébraux. *Rev. Génér. d'Ophthalm.*, [1894.]

——. Ueber Sinnes und Vorstellungscentren in der Rinde des Grosshirns. *Zeitsch. f. die Gesamt. Neurol. u. Psychiatr.*, Vol. XLVII, parts 1–3, 191[9].

Kölliker. *Handbuch der Gewebelehre des Menschen*, etc., 6th edition. Vol. II, Leipzig, 1896.

Köppen and Löwenstein. *Monat. f. Psych. u. Neurol.*, Vol. XVIII, 190[5].

Mauss. Die Faserarchitektur Gliederung der Grosshirn bei niederen Affen. *Journ. f. Psychol u. Neurologie*, Vol. XIII, 1980, page 263.

Meynert. *Vom Gehirne der Säugethiere, Strickers Handbuch der Gewebelehre*, Vol. II, 1872.

——. *Vierteljahrschrift f. Psychiatr.*, 1867 and 1868.

Minkowski. Experimentelle Untersuchungen ueber die Beziehungen des Grosshirnrinde und der Netzhaut zu den primären optischen Zentren, etc. *Arbeiten aus dem Hirnanatomischen Institut in Zürich*, edited by Prof. Dr. C. v[on] Monakow., vol. VII, 1913.

Monakow. *Die Localisation im Grosshirn*, etc., Wiesbaden, 1914, p. 355 and following. See also: Exper. u. patho. anat. Unters, ueber die optischen centren u. Bahnen, etc. *Arch. f. Psychiatr.*, Vols. XX and XX[VII], [1889, 1895.]

F. W. Mott. The Progressive Evolution of the Structure and Function of the Visual Cortex in mammalia. *Arch. of Neurology of the Pathol[ogical] Labor[atory] of the London County Asylum*, Vol. III, 1907.

Munk. *Ueber die Funktion der Grosshirnrinde*, Berlin, 1889.

Schlapp. *Der Zellenbau der Grosshirnrinde des Idiotie*, Published by Dr. S. E. Henschen, Upsala, 1895.

——. Der Zellenbau der Grosshirnrinde des Affen. *Arch. f. Psychiatrie*, Vol. XXX, 189[8].

Sherrington and Grünbaum. Observations on the Physiol[ogy] of the Cerebral Cortex of the Higher Apes. *Proc. Roy. Society*, Vol. CXXXIX [1901].

Soury. Le cerveau. *Dictionnaire de Physiol.*, Vol. II, 1896.

Tsuchida. Ein Beitrag zur Anat. der Sehstrahlungen bei Menschen. *Arch. f. Psychiatr.*, Vol. XLII, part 1, 1907.

[Van] Valkenburg. Researches on the Corpus Callosum. *Brain*, 1913.

Villaverde. Estudios anatómico-experimentales sobre el curso y terminación de las fibras callosas. *Trabajos del Lab. de Investig. Biol.*, Vol. XIX., [1921].

Vogt. (Cécil et Oskar). *Atlas*, Jena, 1904.

C. Winkler and Dr. Ada Potter. *An Anatomical Guide to Experimental Researches on the Cat's Brain*, Amsterdam, 1914.

Cajal's Notes

1. La corteza visual, *Revista Trimestral Microgr.*, Vol. IV, 1899. See also *Histologie du système nerveux des vertébrés*, etc., Paris, Maloine, Vol. II, 1911, p. 599 and following.

2. The disagreements existing between different authors and ourselves regarding the number and structure of the layers, differences which are attributable to the different techniques used, will be discussed in other work.

3. Campbell, *Histological Studies on the Localisation of Cerebral Function*, Cambridge, 1905.

4. Brodmann, *Beiträge zur histologischen Lokalisation der Grosshirnrinde*, V. Mitteilung *Journal f. Neurol. u. Psych.*, Vol. VI, 1906. See also: *Vergleichende Lokalisationslehre der Grosshirnrinde*, Leipzig, 1909.

5. Minkowski, *Experimentelle Untersuchungen ueber die Beziehungen der Grosshirnrinde u. der Netzhaut zu der primären optisches Zentren*, etc. *Arbeiten aus dem Hirnanatomischen Institut in Zürich*, edited by Prof. Dr. C. V[on] Monakow, Vol. VII, 1913.

6. V. Monakow, *Die Lokalisation im Grosshirnrinde*, etc., Weisbaden, 1914, p. 335 and following.

7. C. Winkler and Dr. Ada Potter, *An Anatomical Guide to Experimental Researches on the Cat's Brain*, Amsterdam, 1914.

8. I take well the point that the method of Golgi has the misfortune to be unfashionable nowadays. This is testified to satiety in the little representation given to its marvelous revelations (if they are not systematically disdained) in the recent works of neurology and in multitudinous monographs on the visual cortex, thalamus, geniculate bodies, etc.

But does there, by chance, exist any method like the Golgi that permits us to determine the morphology of the cerebral neurons and to ascertain the behavior of the axon? And, until an equivalent or better method for exactly differentiating the terminal ramifications is discovered, are we going to eliminate from the undivided estate of neurological science all the thousands of facts collected in thirty years of tenacious and indefatigable labor, limiting all our scientific ambition to a tedious and very arduous catalogue of layers and the distribution of sizes and forms of neuronal somata? If it should occur, such a repudiation would be equivalent to suppressing the noble curiosity directed at elucidating the great problem of interneuronal connections and that of the pathways followed by the nervous impulse inside the gray matter, sacrificing the purest ideal of neurohistology to the mere task—whose importance we recognize—of physiological localization from the applied point of view.

Someone will allege, without doubt in order to cover up their silence or their disdain, that the methods of Golgi and [other] similar [methods], besides frequently giving artificial images, are very inconsistent. The inconsistency is true, unfortuantely; but it has been enormously exaggerated. And with respect to the *artifacts*, has it not been proven thousands of times that methods as different as dissociation, Ehrlich's, Cox's sublimate, that of Bielschowsky, and our reduced silver nitrate formulae [give results] coinciding essentially with the revelations of the silver chromate? Very appropriate to dispel the lack of confidence and prejudices against the metallic impregnations are the modern techniques proposed for neuroglia (procedures of gold-sublimate and formol-uranium of Cajal; of the tannin and ammoniacal silver of Achúcarro; of [Del] Río-Hortega, in his variants of this procedure, and in his own silver carbonate method, etc.), which give extraordinarily similar if not identical images to those obtained with the classical and important formulas of Weigert and of Golgi. And I do not insist on the modifications of the method of Bielschowsky, which in the hands of several authors have shown equal concordances with respect to the staining of the glia. See, among many other known formulae, the one recently published by us: Una modificación del método de Bielschowsky para la coloración de la neuroglia, etc., *Trabajos del Laboratorio de Investigaciones Biológicas,* Vol. XVIII, 1920.

9. Cajal, Sobre la existencia de células nerviosas especiales en la primera capa de las circunvoluciones cerebrales, *Gaz. Méd. Catalana,* December 189[0]. See *La Cellule,* Vol. VII, 1891; and Las células de axón corto de la capa molecular del cerebro, *Rev. Trim. Microgr.,* Vol. II, 1897. El azul de metileno en los centros nerviosos, idem, Vol. I, 1896.

10. Cajal, *Histologie du système nerveux de l'homme et des vertébrés,* Vol. II [1911].

11. Cajal, *Histologie du système nerveux,* Vol. II, 1911. See fig. 398 [*fig. 128*] and 387, A, B, C [*fig. 78*], taken from the cerebrum of the cat, and fig. 388 [*fig. 80*], taken from man.

12. Cajal, La corteza visual, *Revista Trimestral Microgr.,* Vol. IV, 1899.

13. Beevor, On the Course of Fibres of the Cingulum and Posterior Parts of the Corpus Callosum, etc., *Phil. Trans Roy. Society of London,* Vol. LXXXII, 189[1], p. 135.

14. [Van] Valkenburg, Researches on the Corpus Callosum, Brain, 1913. This author is the most adamant against the relationships of the visual cortex with the corpus callosum. And although, from the adduced pathological features, and even from his own affirmations, it does not necessarily follow that there is an absence of commissural fibers ("No callosal fibers originate or terminate in the striate cortex," he says), but because such fibers could come from the several layers of small pyramids and polymorphic cells or from collaterals of axons of projection (in the very white matter), and terminate in the form of unmyelinated thin branches in different cerebral layers, perhaps in the plexiform layer, the conclusions of Valkenburg leave the problem intact.

15. Villaverde, Estudios anatómico-experimentales sobre el curso y terminación de las fibras callosas, *Trabajos del Laboratorio de Investigaciones Biológicas,* Vol. XIX [1921]. According to this author, who has worked in our laboratory, both with anatomicopathological methods and with anatomical ones, certain cerebral areas (*area gigantocellularis* of Brodmann) corresponding to the sensori-motor localizations, would probably have a homotopical callosal representation; but Villaverde does not exclude the possibility of the existence of callosal fibers arising from the same area and distributed to heterotopical regions of the contralateral side.

16. V[on] Monakow, *Die Lokalisation im Grosshirn,* etc., Wiesbaden, 1914.

Editor's Notes

A. At this point in the German translation of his paper—made by Ernst Fischer-Franz and Clara Karl and published in the *Journal für Psychologie und Neurologie* 29:161–181 (1922a)—Cajal inserts the following paragraphs and several new figures:

These differences in the layers depend on whether one speaks of the most prominent part of the marginal gyrus or the vicinity of its sulci. This can be seen very well in the photomicrographs of Nissl sections (figs. 4 and 5, plate 15) [*figs. 260, 261*].

I recently received a reproach from Professor Henschen, especially to the effect that my drawings of the cells that occur in the human calcarine fissure are too sketchy. As far as the Nissl sections of the human visual cortex which illustrate the beginning of my previous work are concerned, Henschen is absolutely correct. My intention was to show as clearly as possible the distinctive features used in classifying this area.

But the remarks of the Swedish neurologist about the illustrations of the results of Golgi staining are unjustified. All of these figures are true and exact representations of excellent preparations.

One does not need to mention first that every author who makes the effort to examine the calcarine fissure of fetuses of eight to nine months and children of one to three months by the above-mentioned finer anatomical methods can easily confirm all the neuron types [that I] indicated. The only liberty taken was the artistic grouping of cells from various serial sections. Because the results of the Golgi procedures are very incomplete, it was unquestionably necessary to make use of this device. Otherwise, a very large number of figures would have been necessary, resulting in an essential loss of exact and clear representation.

There are also, however, certain illustrations, particularly of nervous tissue, from single sections.

B. At this point in the German translation, Cajal inserts the following lines and another new figure:

The particular area examined and from which I obtained the best preparations is shown in the photomicrograph fig. 3 [*fig. 260*], by the rectangle. The photomicrographs figs. 4 and 5, plate 15 [*figs. 261, 262*], are also taken from there, and are portions of [the regions labeled] C and F, the inner side of the marginal gyrus (fig. 3) [*fig. 260*]. In the foregoing figure, which can be regarded as a typical region of the visual area, one notices the great laminar variation in the layer of the solitary pyramids. This variation in layering depends on whether the section has caught the apex of the gyrus as in fig. 3, F, and fig. 5, plate 15 [*figs. 260, 262*], or the vicinity of a sulcus (fig. 3, C and fig. 4, plate 15) [*figs. 260, 261*]

Finally, for better orientation of the reader, and easier recognition of the morphological types [of neurons] which form the layers and which can be demonstrated by the Nissl method, I have sketched in fig. 4, right [*fig. 261*], the neurons that are most frequently impregnated by the Golgi-Cox methods.

C. The last three sentences are omitted from the German translation.

D. The cells do not appear in this figure and cannot be readily identified in others.

E. Cajal says "baptized."

F. Here and subsequently in this paper, Cajal tends to use "neurite" instead of "axon."

G. The original text incorrectly says "B."

H. The original text incorrectly says "G."

I. Our insert.

J. The original text gives "G."

K. The original text gives "G."

L. Not all of these works are cited by footnotes or mentioned in the text.

28

Studies on the Fine Structure of the Regional Cortex of Rodents 1: Suboccipital Cortex (Retrosplenial Cortex of Brodmann)

[Trabajos del Laboratorio de Investigaciones Biológicas de la Universidad de Madrid 20:1–30, 1922]

A. Introduction

It is our purpose, after fifteen years of activity devoted to the study of other neurological subjects (fine structure of neurons, central nervous terminations, structure of ganglia, neurogenesis, regeneration of nerves and of the gray matter, analysis of the neuroglia and of the Golgi apparatus, technical explorations, etc.), to undertake a series of works directed at completing, if possible, the already old investigations of Flechsig, Golgi, Edinger, Hammarberg, Kölliker, Retzius, Henschen, etc., and the more recent ones of Campbell, Mott, the Vogts, Watson, Brodmann (and his pupils Zunino, Rose, Flores, etc.), Hermanides and Köppen, Isenschmid, Fortuyn, Ariëns Kappers, etc., with respect to the structure of the regional cortex.

Abandoning, as inaccessible to our tools, the problem of the mechanism of origin and intracentral propagation of the nervous impulse, the immediate purpose of all histological investigation must be concentrated at present on indicating the interneuronal connections of each cortical area, and, especially, to form a

base for and to extend as much as possible the doctrine of functional localization, without prejudging, of course, either the essence or the mode of physiological activity. All regional anatomical explorations implicate this postulate: a common functional identity [is determined by] the same type of structure and connections, whatever the mammal examined.

In accord with Brodmann, we consider that, in this anatomicofunctional evaluation, the *structural criterion* must prevail over the topographic. If one does not wish to risk falling into grave mistakes, the latter must only be applied to mammals belonging to the same species or to very close genera.

It is important to explain what we understand by the structural norm or criterion. In our opinion, stratigraphic analogy, grossly appreciated in Nissl or Weigert preparations, constitutes a valuable data point, but [it is] not completely decisive or infallible. In corroboration of this assertion, it is enough to remember that there exist in rodents several cerebral areas provided with legitimate *striae of Gennari* and even of layers of *granule cells* (small neurons), as in the visual area, but which have nothing to do with the visual impulse. For example, in the lissencephalic mammals, five regions endowed with the mentioned stria can be seen: the *visual,* the *suboccipital (retrosplenial area),* the *supracallosal,* the *presubiculum,* and our *spheno-occipital focus* (pole of the *piriform lobe).* And some of these centers also possess granule cell formations, even though the morphology of their elements is very different. But about the vague and equivocal concept of the granule cell we will deal on another occasion.

There is little value, therefore, in dealing with the differentiation of cortical areas based exclusively on the revelations of the Nissl and Weigert methods, because they show an insignificant portion of the constituent features of the gray matter.[1] Strictly speaking, the physiological and even the anatomical specificity of the cortical areas must result from the convergence of three categories of data: first, of the fine structure obtained from preparations revealing not only the gross stratification of the gray matter but the true neuronal morphology (including, if possible, the origin, trajectory, and terminations of axons); second, the data obtained by physiological experiments and the methods of experimental pathological anatomy, the only methods capable of elucidating the great problem, [which is the] obsessive preoccupation of the clinics, of the connections at a distance; and third, that derived from the ontogenic method of the progressive myelination of the axons.

Let us hasten to declare that this ideal is not completely attainable at present. Nevertheless, in spite of the progress of neurological technique, we do not possess a staining method able to supply, in a constant manner, isolated and absolutely complete images of the neurons, [in order to face] the inextricable meshwork of the gray matter, a sort of feltwork in which everything appears to be in contact and to be intimately connected, an obstacle that is all the greater because of the necessity of exploring thin sections, in which fibers and cells necessarily appear mutilated. It is possible, however, to get somewhat close to the said ideal, if in our analysis we make use of all the neurological methods known at present, particularly those that exquisitely reveal neuronal

morphology, that is, the Golgi and the neurofibrillar [stains] and eventually that of Ehrlich. Certainly, the Golgi and neurofibrillar formulae have been applied already to the argument of many authors and of ourselves; but, judging by the publications of the last fifteen years relating to the cerebral cortex, the employment of these has been made on a small scale and with little confidence of success. This distrust is justified when dealing with the adult human; but if we make use of more favorable conditions by using animals fifteen to thirty days [old], particularly the cat, the dog, the rabbit, and the mouse, sections [that are] very well impregnated and extremely impressive are easily obtained with the silver chromate, Golgi-Cox, and neurofibrillar methods.

As we have already said elsewhere,[2] such studies, if they are conducted with method and perseverance, will enrich and consolidate the doctrine of cerebral localization. Even so, needless to say, the work will be fragmentary and unidimensional. Because the complete and enlightened anatomicofunctional notion of the functional centers of the gray matter constitutes a remote and future ideal, which will only be achievable when, having collected all the objective material, it will be possible to integrate and fuse the partial data, arrived at in different ways, into a supreme synthesis.

To contribute analytically and to collect from the histological field the facts for this scientific desideratum will constitute the end point of our investigations and that of our pupils and collaborators.

To initiate the exploration, we are going to reveal the structure of the *suboccipital focus (retrosplenial field)* of rodents, adding some new details to our old inquiries, [which are] a little forgotten by the neurologists at present.

The starting point of our exposition will be the cyto- and myeloarchitectonic analysis of the cerebral cortical fields differentiated in lower mammals by Brodmann and the scientists of his school. We will also be inspired by the works on localization of the English authors Campbell, Mott, Fortuyn, etc., and in those of the Dutch, Ariëns Kappers, Ernst de Vries, and Winkler, etc., investigators whose conclusions do not always agree with the results of the Berlin school.

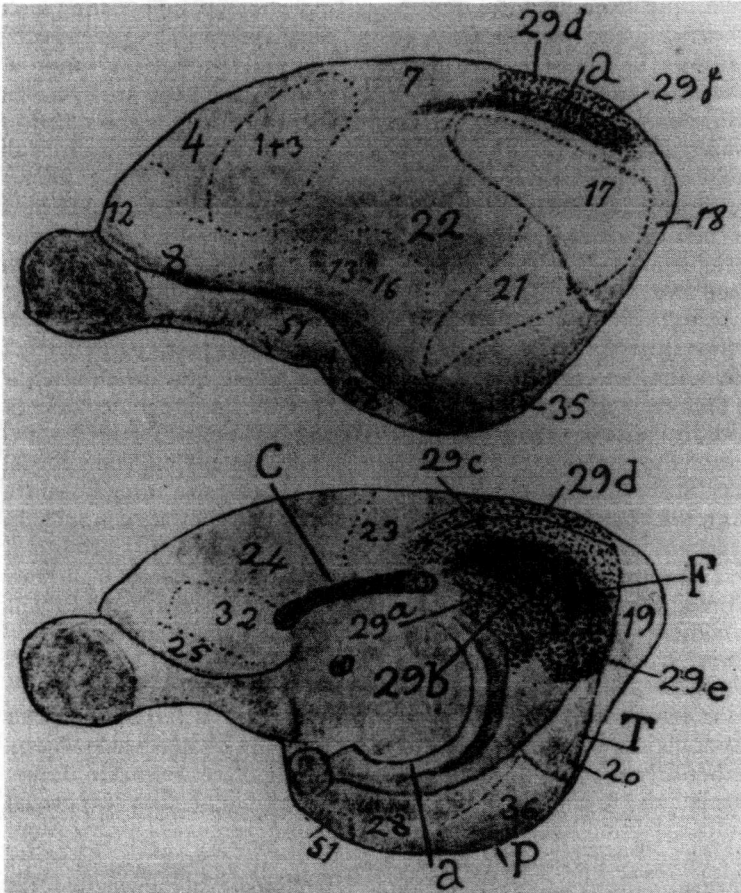

[FIG. 263] Fig. 1ᵃ. Areas delimited in the cortex of the rabbit by Brodmann and his pupils. The granular region (*29a, 29h, 29c, 29d, 29f*) represents the retrosplenial area or suboccipital focus. The upper figure shows the external surface of the cortex; the lower, the internal [surface].

Suboccipital Cortex of the Rabbit (Retrosplenial Field of Brodmann)

As a little-known background to this type of cortex, studied by us in 1893, we will reproduce here the more significant paragraphs of our old work.[3] In this transcription, we will restrict ourselves exclusively to the structural details characteristic of the said retrosplenial center. Here is the text to which we allude.

"As is known, not all the cerebral cortex exhibits exactly the same structure. For some time, the neurologists have mentioned that in the cerebrum of the higher mammals, certain regions show structural variations, either in the number of layers or in the volume and abundance of cells and nerve fibers."

Our purpose, in the present work, consists of the study of the *inferior occipital cortex*, that is to say, the territory located underneath the occipital pole, not far from the subiculum [*fig. 263*].

The more notable changes in comparison with the typical cortex that the inferior suboccipital region presents affect the molecular layer and the second and third layers.

Here are the layers of the suboccipital cortical region: first, *molecular;* second, *layer of the vertical fusiform cells;* third, *middle fibrillar layer or layer of the small pyramids;* fourth, *layer of the large pyramids;* fifth, *layer of the polymorphic cells.*

[*Editors' note:* What follows is an almost verbatim transcription of the greater part of chapter 6 of this volume (Cajal, 1893e) which Cajal essentially only modified to the extent that he removed all of his 1893 allusions to this area of cortex as having visual connotations.]

To date, there is this note published by us in 1893, which was translated by Kölliker, together with our monograph on *Ammon's horn* and reproduced in summarized form in the French version of our work on the *Histology of the Nervous System.*[4]

We do not consider [our] preceding work and the figure that illustrated it (fig. 1, plate 1) [*fig. 264*] as irreproachable. To be sure, the facts related are exact; the later investigations of Brodmann in the rabbit and other rodents, those of Zunino made with the method of Weigert in [the rabbit], the cytoarchitectonic studies of Isenschmid in the mouse, of Rose made in several lissencephalic animals, particularly the guinea pig, of Fortuyn also made in the rabbit, mouse, and other rodents, etc., confirm [our studies] in principle, even though these authors have used techniques different from ours.

But our old description was too incomplete. It did not mention the second layer or [layer] of *stellate cells,* well appreciable in Nissl stained sections. It suffered also from a mistake shared with several authors (Mott, Hermanides and Köppen, etc.), excusable at the time it was published, of hypothetically considering the region as a visual area. The presence of a deep white band located in the layer of the granule cells and which resembles the stria of Gennari, and the localization of the visual area, by then already fixed for man and primates on the internal face of the occipital lobe, were the arguments of analogy that induced us to make [an incorrect] statement, rectified years later in our work on the nervous system as a whole,[5] in which the visual region of the rodents is seen to be situated on the external face of the occipital lobe. We were led to make this correction especially by a peculiarity observed in the cerebrum of the mouse

a few days old, in which the *suboccipital focus* receives fibers from the arcuate or supracallosal fascicle. And as we could not demonstrate the arrival of fibers from the thalamic ganglia, the question of the significance of this center, of large extent in the rodent, remained undecided.

Many years after us, Brodmann,[6] in making patient and sagacious cytoarchitectonic studies on the cerebrum of many species of mammals, confirmed our suboccipital focus in the rabbit and other rodents and gave to it the name of *retrosplenial area (Typus retrosplenialis granularis).* This cortical variety, indicated by the number *29* in his map of the cerebrum of the rabbit, consisting of anteroposterior areas with a somewhat different structure (*29d, 29b, 29a, 29e*), was considered by him as a heterotypical type, characterized by the rudimentary development of the second layer (our layer of small pyramids), the relative development of the first (plexiform) and third (of the medium pyramids) layers, and the exceptional extent of the fourth layer or [layer] of the granule cells. He described also the *layer of the large pyramids,* which he subdivided into fifth and sixth sublayers, and, finally, near the white matter, he observed cells of smaller size corresponding to our *stratum of polymorphic cells.* For the rest, to Brodmann belongs the credit for having outlined with considerable precision the borders of this area in the rabbit and in many other mammals.

After Brodmann, we find in his disciple Zunino[7] explicit confirmation of area *29* or *retrosplenial cortex* in the rabbit, which he explored with the method of Weigert. Both authors appear to ignore our work of 1893 on the suboccipital cortex. Without descending to the analytical study of the cells, Zunino gives a good reproduction of the plexuses, particularly of the horizontal [plexus] located at the level of the *granule cells (layer IV* of Brodmann), a plexus already drawn by us in the rabbit and guinea pig; [our] sections were stained with the procedures of Weigert and of Golgi. A good representation of the cyto- and myeloarchitectonics of area *29* of the rabbit is also found in the *Atlas* of Winkler.[8] Finally, Fortuyn,[9] who has made a good cytoarchitectonic study of the areas of the cortex of the rabbit and of other rodents, also describes the retrosplenial cortex, to which he gives the name *group of areas Z,* which do not coincide exactly with the subdivisions of area *29* distinguished by Brodmann. To these discrepancies we will allude later.

With respect to the mouse, we find also in the work of Isenschmid[10] a correct description and localization of the retrosplenial cortex, which he studied with the method of Nissl. He called it *formation S,* and he places it behind the corpus callosum and underneath the *formation Q,* corresponding to what we have called in the mouse by the name of *interhemispheric* or *supracallosal cortex.*

In other mammals, several authors, among them Mott, Watson, and Köppen and Löwenstein[11] (carnivores and ungulates), have seen and localized, more or less precisely, the suboccipital focus. Plate 15, fig. 4, of the latter authors seems to us to reproduce the retrosplenial focus, even though they have not given it this name or detailed its structure.

Another disciple of Brodmann, M. Rose,[12] comes back to the arguments, analyzing the myelo- and cytoarchitectonics of many lissencephalic mammals. In the cerebrum of the mouse, an animal he has studied with special care, he indicates several of the centers distinguished by us many years before, such as the *temporo-occipital* (pole of the piriform lobe), the *presubicular,* the *visual,* the *supracallosal,* and, finally, the *suboccipital* or *retrosplenial,* which he designates, like Brodmann, *area 29.* Later, when we deal with this focus in the mouse, we will give an account of the stratigraphy revealed by Rose and Fortuyn.

After this background, let us reveal here briefly the results of our new studies on the *suboccipital* or *retrosplenial* focus (*area 29* of Brodmann).

Localization

In our first explorations of the cortex of the rabbit, guinea pig, and mouse, we placed this variety of gray matter underneath the occipital lobe, in a fossa this possesses for lodging the mesencephalon, not far from the presubiculum.

Thanks to Brodmann and his disciples, we now know better the limits of this region in the rodents. Our new investigations, made with the methods of Nissl and Spielmeyer (rabbit, mouse, guinea pig), confirm in principle the borders indicated by Brodmann and the structural diversity of the areas *29a, 29b, 29d,* etc., within a generic structural plan that is revealed, especially, in Golgi sections.

The microphotographs 2, 3, and 4 [*figs. 265–267*] and the scheme in text fig. 1 [*fig. 263*] excuse us from entering here into details about the extent of area *29* and of its variations in structure. We will point out only that in our preparations of the rabbit, this type of cortex is quite prolonged forward, getting close to the supracallosal cortex, the representative in rodents of the gyrus fornicatus; behind, it does not reach the occipital pole, as Brodmann and Zunino have well represented; on the outside, it goes up to the superior border of the interhemispheric fissure, extending further up the external cerebral face, as the sections become more anterior. As we show in fig. 1 [*fig. 263*], and in disagreement with the descriptions and representations of Brodmann, Zunino, Rose, and Fortuyn, we extend area *29* somewhat more laterally. In effect, in the most frontal sections that pass through the *visual area,* it is observed that the *retrosplenial area* borders on this, having for its frontier the *lateral sagittal sulcus (sulcus lateralis;* fig. 1, *a)* [*fig. 263*], a rudiment of one of the fundamental fissures indicated by Elliot Smith in the cerebrum of mammals. Let us note, however, that, although in this region close to the cited sulcus, the same zones of the area *29* are found, the morphology of the neurons of the second and third layers are modified, imprinting on this cerebral region a particular stamp, as we will see later. Finally, medially, the retrosplenial area descends close to the subiculum.

In accord with Brodmann, Zunino, and Fortuyn, our Nissl and Weigert preparations reveal, in this extensive cortical territory, anteroposterior bands or areas with a somewhat different structure (*areas 29a, 29b, 29c, 29d,* etc., of Brodmann; areas $z^1, z^2, z^3, z^4,$ etc., of Fortuyn). The field near the sagittal lateral sulcus, which we mentioned earlier, could be designated, to avoid confusion, *area 29f* (fig. 1) [*fig. 263*]. Such regional diversity, perfectly appreciable in the microphotographs (figs. 2 and

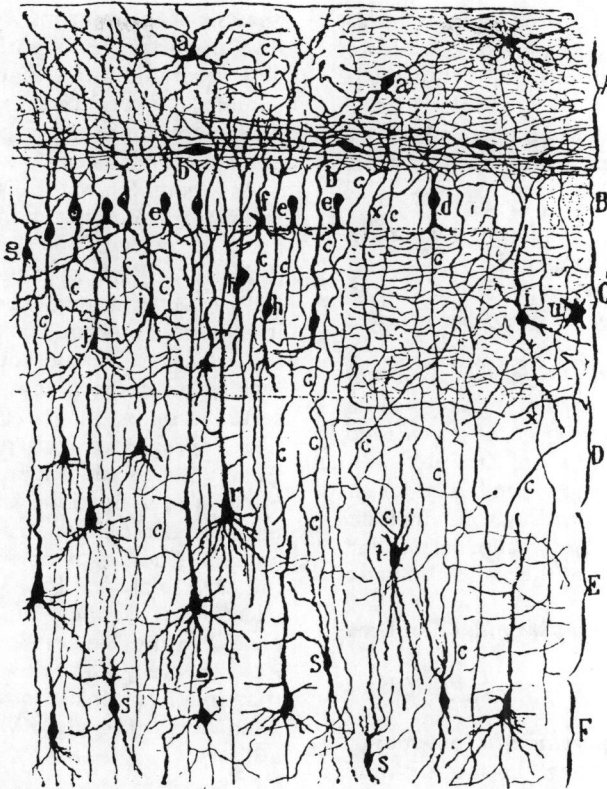

[*FIG. 264*] Plate I. Fig. 1. It reproduces the illustration published in our work of 1893. The letters in the margin indicate the order of the layers. *A*, plexiform layer; *B*, [layer] of the vertical fusiform neurons; *C*, deep plexiform [layer]; *D*, [layer] of the medium pyramids; *E*, [layer] of the large pyramids; *F*, [layer] of the polymorphic cells; *a*, neurons with short axon of layer I; *b*, large horizontal fusiform cells; *d*, vertical fusiform cells; *i*, *u*, neurons with ascending axon, etc.

This figure, made up of cells found in several successive sections, corresponds to the inferior or concave portion of the retrosplenial cortex of the rabbit of a few days, which is the one that possesses the more characteristic structure. [We have taken our figure from the 1893 paper, since the lettering reproduced better than the (modified) lettering on the figure reproduced in 1922.]

3, plate I) [*figs. 265, 266*], is seen also in the Golgi and neurofibrillary sections; but the divergence does not reach the point of diminishing the fundamental structural plan, as is observed in fig. 5, plate III [*fig. 268*], in which are reproduced two distant anteroposterior areas: one corresponding to area *29f* and the other to area *29c*. Later we will say something about these little stratigraphic deviations, also observed by Zunino in his myeloarchitectonic studies and by Rose in his cytoarchitectonic studies of the guinea pig and mouse.

For the rest, these structural variants linked by smooth transitions are observed in almost all the cortical areas, whatever their physiological significance.

Structure of the Suboccipital or Retrosplenial Focus (Retrolimbic Area of Zunino)

After the summary of our work of 1893, we will restrict ourselves here to completing the old description with some additional details.

Let us begin by exposing the differentiable layers in the region under study. The scheme of six typical layers of Brodmann is hardly applicable to this case, not precisely because of the number but because of the cellular type that the neurologist of Berlin binds to each layer. In our opinion, the strata easily separable in the said cortex of the rabbit are the following:

1. *Plexiform or molecular layer (lamina zonalis of Brodmann or layer I).*
2. *Layer of the stellate cells with long axon (layer II or layer of the superficial pyramids of Brodmann).*
3. *Layer of the vertical fusiform neurons* (corresponding only in part to *layer IV* of Brodmann or his *layer of the granule cells* and to *layers II and III* of Zunino).
4. *Internal plexiform layer* and layer of the deep vertical fusiform neurons. Included also in *layer IV* of Brodmann, corresponding equally to that of the same number of Zunino.
5. *Layer of the medium pyramids (V* of Brodmann).
6. *Layer of the large pyramids (VI* of Brodmann).
7. *Layer of the polymorphic cells* (not counted by Brodmann, although he shows it in his figures).

As can be seen from the preceding enumeration, we have added beneath the plexiform layer a neuronal layer unnoticed in our preparations of 1893 (the layer of the stellate cells), well observed by Brodmann and his disciples, although they did not determine the shape of its cells; we suppress the layer II of Brodmann or layer of the superficial granule cells, corresponding to our small pyramids, because [the granule cells] do not exist [there], not even in rudimentary form, as Fortuyn noticed; and, finally, we divide the layer IV of Brodmann into two strata clearly differentiable in the Weigert and neurofibrillary preparations. Following our custom, the designations express the neuronal form as it is shown in the Golgi preparations.

1. Plexiform Layer

We can add nothing essential to our old description, in which we made a meticulous

analysis of the neurons with short axon inhabiting the first layer. We will only say, in accord with several authors, that this plexiform layer exhibits an exceptional thickness, and contains thus many more nerve cells than any congeneric layer of the cerebral cortex.

As a complement to fig. 1, plate I [*fig. 264*] taken from our first monograph, we show in fig. 6, *A*, plate IV [*fig. 269*] a large horizontal fusiform cell whose tangential axon could be followed over a long trajectory, during which it gave off numerous collaterals arborizing in the first layer. The nervous plexus of this layer reaches an unusual complexity, as can be observed in fig. 7, *A* [*fig. 270*], which copies a section impregnated with reduced silver nitrate. Finally, let us add a type of fiber that escaped our first investigations: the presence of terminal axonal ramifications originating from exogenous fibers arriving from the white matter (fig. 8, *p*, plate VI) [*fig. 271*]. For the rest, the exceptional richness of the plexus is shown clearly in the Weigert-Pal sections, as Zunino has observed, and who has noticed besides, that area *29a* consists of two planes of medullated fibers (see plate V of the work of this author).

2. Layer of the Stellate Cells

These neurons, arranged in several very tight, irregular rows, show up by their larger size than the cells of the third layer, and exhibit a variable shape, triangular, polygonal, or stellate. Because they have little affinity for the silver chromate, they passed unnoticed in our first studies. Insisting recently on their impregnation, we have been able to stain them both with the method of Golgi and with that of the reduced silver. The latter procedure, as well as that of Bielschowsky, only sporadically impregnates some occasional cells (fig. 7, *B*, plate V) [*fig. 270*].

In fig. 5, *B*, plate III, and fig. 6, *A*, plate IV [*figs. 268, 269*], we show some of these robust cells which are in no way similar to the small pyramids of other regions of the cortex. Notice the thickness of the soma, with a stellate form, from whose contours arise ascending and descending dendrites: the ascending (figs. 6, *B*; and 8, *a*) [*figs. 269, 271*] are several, disseminating and branching through the whole thickness of the first or superficial plexiform layer. The axon, relatively thick, arises from the deep side of the soma, gives off collaterals in its trajectory to the deep plexiform layer, and, finally, in the more favorable cases, can be followed into the white matter. Evidently, this stellate cell belongs to [the class of] cells with long axon.

Not all the cells of this layer have the same form and dimensions; in it lie some of more reduced size and with thinner dendrites. The axon, however, behaves in the same way as that of the voluminous stellate types (fig. 6, C) [fig. 269].

3. Layer of the Vertical Fusiform Cells (Part of Layer IV or Layer of the Granule Cells of Brodmann)

The morphological details showing the notable characteristics of this neuronal variety are indicated in our transcription of the work of 1893 and in the illustrations that accompany it (fig. 1, Bd, plate I) [fig. 29 in chapter 6, fig. 264].

Our new studies on the rabbit of twenty-five to thirty days confirm completely the old description, as can be seen by examining figs. 6 and 8 [figs. 269, 271]. Notice that all these fusiform cells possess a bipolar soma, in which is glimpsed the nucleus (an indication of the thinness of the layer of protoplasm), a radial [dendritic] shaft destined for layer I, a descending process resolving into a moderate tuft of spiny dendrites distributed in the deep plexiform layer, and, lastly, a thin axon, arising almost always far away from the soma, from the bend formed by a secondary dendritic process when it separates from the ascending shaft. Here is a case in which the law of dynamic polarization, such as was formulated by Van Gehuchten and ourselves, does not have a strict application. However, this mode of axon origin harmonizes well with our formula of *axipetal polarization*. It is very common to notice that the said axon originates low down, in the very deep plexiform layer (figs. 6 and 8) [figs. 269, 271].

The very thin axon of the said vertical fusiform cells has been followed sometimes into the thickness of the white matter. It is not possible thus to doubt that one is dealing with a long axon, comparable to that of the small pyramids of other cerebral territories. During its trajectory to the deep plexiform layer, it gives off three or more collaterals destined to ramify in this layer. More deeply, when the axon reaches the layers of the pyramids, the emissions of collaterals become rare.

We will not insist on the description of these original cells, whose details appear clearly in fig. 1, plate I, and figs. 6 and 8 [figs. 264, 269, 271]. We will only point out for now, first, that such cells are not comparable, neither in their shape nor in the behavior of their axon to the true granule cells (*layer IV* of Brodmann); second, that the monopolar or spongioblastic forms described and illustrated in our first communication (fig. 1, e, plate I) [fig. 264] are not present in the rabbit whose age exceeds twenty-five days, having thus to be considered as early phases of the development of the bipolar type; such young neurons, which resemble neuroblasts, show us that the radial [dendritic] shaft is a late formation, preceded always by the axon and the descending dendrite; third, finally, that such bipolar forms remain in the adult or almost adult rabbit. In effect, the cells of this type, impregnated in the rabbit of two or more months, have not experienced more changes other than a certain axial slenderness of the soma and a notable elongation of the [dendritic] shafts.

Finally, to end with layer III, let us note that it is crossed, as the neurofibrillar preparations clearly show (fig. 7, C) [fig. 270], by a multitude of perforant fibers and bundles destined for the superficial plexiform layer, in addition to the descending axons of the stellate cells and the [apical dendritic] shafts of the pyramids of the deep layers.

4. Layer IV or Deep Plexiform Layer

Identified by us, and well described and drawn by Zunino (the *layer IV* of this author), Winkler, and all those who have explored the focus under study with the Weigert method, it appears in the neurofibrillar and Spielmeyer preparations as a concentric plexus of tight fibers, perfectly separated from the bordering

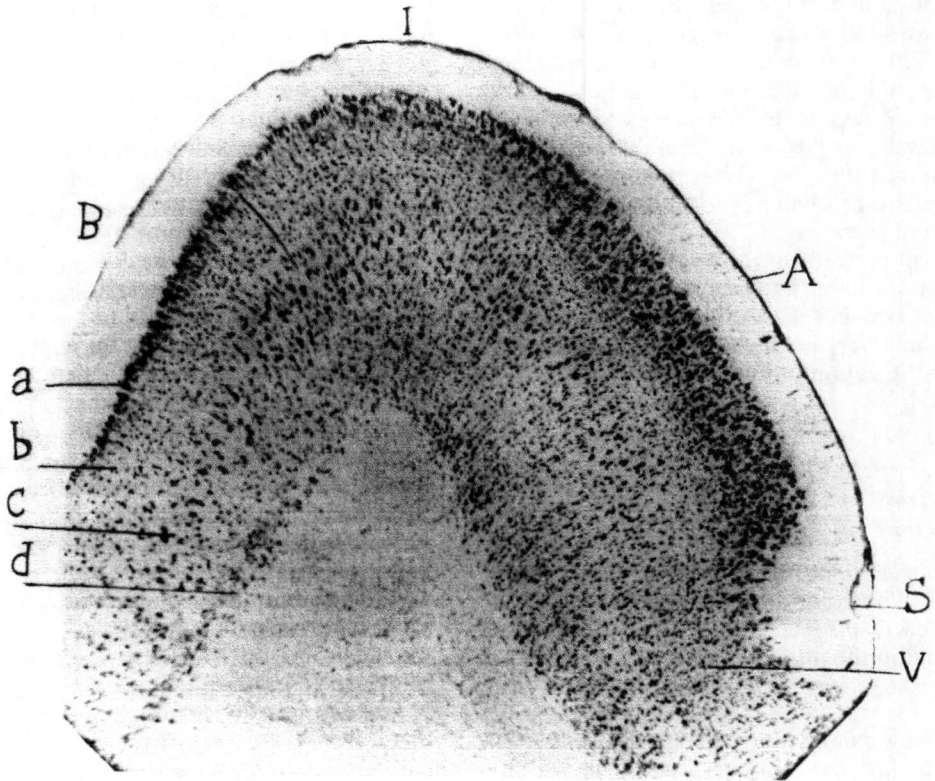

[FIG. 265]   Fig. 2. Frontal section of the superior portion of area 29. In *A* is reproduced area *29f,* situated near the sagittal sulcus (*S*); in *B,* area *29d,* with its prolongation toward the interhemispheric fissure (*a*); *a,* layer of the stellate cells; *b,* layer of the vertical fusiform cells; *c,* layer of the large pyramids; *d,* polymorphic cells.

Plate II.   It contains several microphotographs, obtained at low magnification, of the retrosplenial cortex of the rabbit. (Method of Nissl.)

layers (fig. 7, *C'*) [*fig. 270*]. The predominant direction of the fibers is parallel to the layer, being arranged in tight bundles that, in some places, are separated [in order] to lodge a multitude of diminutive cells. The Golgi preparations, consequently, reveal two kinds of factors: the nerve cells and the endogenous and exogenous axonal arborizations.

a. Fusiform Neurons

They are the most abundant cells of this layer, in which they are arranged frequently in concentric levels. In the Nissl sections, it is impossible to discover their form, since only the nuclei appear, which, because of their smallness and abundance, suggest the idea that layer IV or the deep plexiform layer is inhabited exclusively by granule cells or diminutive cells in continuity with the preceding layer (figs. 4, *D*; 5, *C'*, plate III) [*figs. 267, 268*]. Without the help, therefore, of procedures that stain the myelin or the axons, layers III and IV appear to fuse together as one. There is something to this [idea], since the vertical

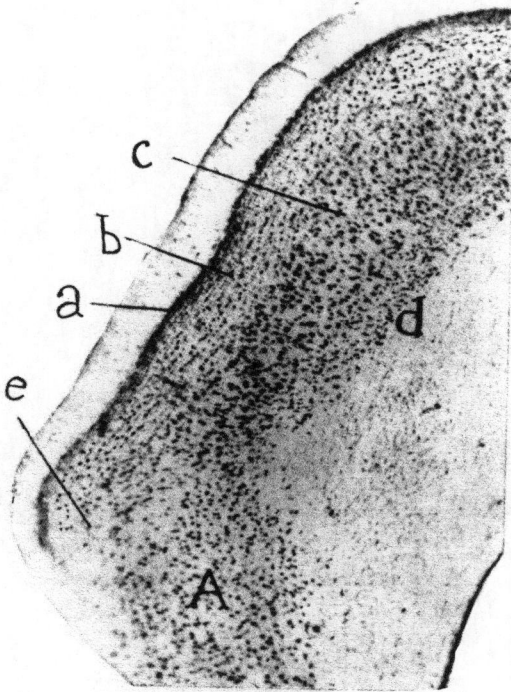

[FIG. 266] Fig. 3. It reproduces another frontal section corresponding to the occipital fossa, that is to say, to areas 29c, 29b, and 29a. The letters indicate the same layers as in the previous figure [a, b, c, d].

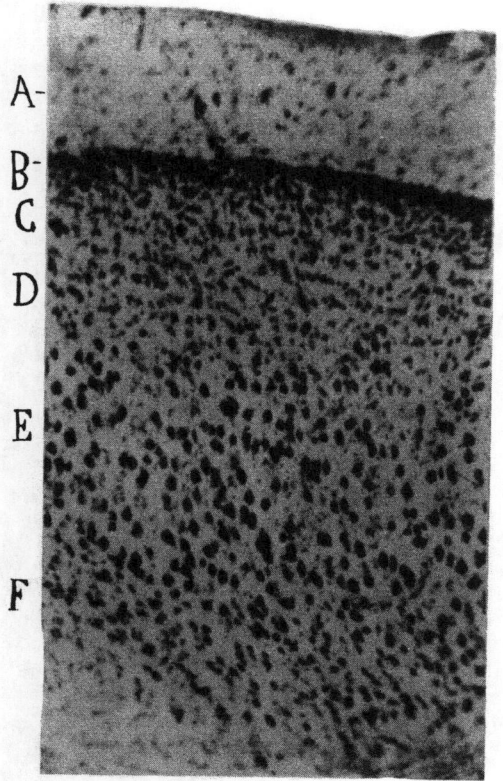

[FIG. 267] Fig. 4. Microphotograph at higher magnification of a frontal section of area 29c. A, plexiform layer; B, [layer] of the stellate cells; C, [layer] of the vertical fusiform cells; D, [layer] of the deep fibrillar plexus; E, [layer] of the large pyramids; F, [layer] of the polymorphic cells.

fusiform cells, as we indicated some time ago and as demonstrated in figs. 6, 7, and 8, d [figs. 269, 271], are exceedingly abundant, having more or less the form, size, and general behavior of the diminutive cells of layer III. Thus, there is a thin axon originating from the starting point of the terminal shaft of the descending [dendrite], and an external [dendritic] shaft sent to layer I, where it is resolved into another tuft of dendrites. Our recent studies confirm also the existence of some genuine pyramids and of some voluminous cells with ascending axon already observed in our first exploration (fig. 1, i, plate I) [fig. 264]. It is very possible

also that the large cells presented in fig. 7, C' [fig. 270] belong to the latter cellular type, indicated already by us in 1893.

Apart from the morphology of the several kinds of neurons, what really lends a special physiognomy to layer IV, distinguishing it perfectly from layer III, is the configuration of the territory in which the inferior terminal [dendritic] tufts of all the fusiform cells of layers III and IV and the thick and divergent descending dendrites of the stellate cells (layer II) exclusively meet, as can be observed in figs. 6 and 8 [figs. 269, 271] taken from Golgi sections. All of these dendrites generate very

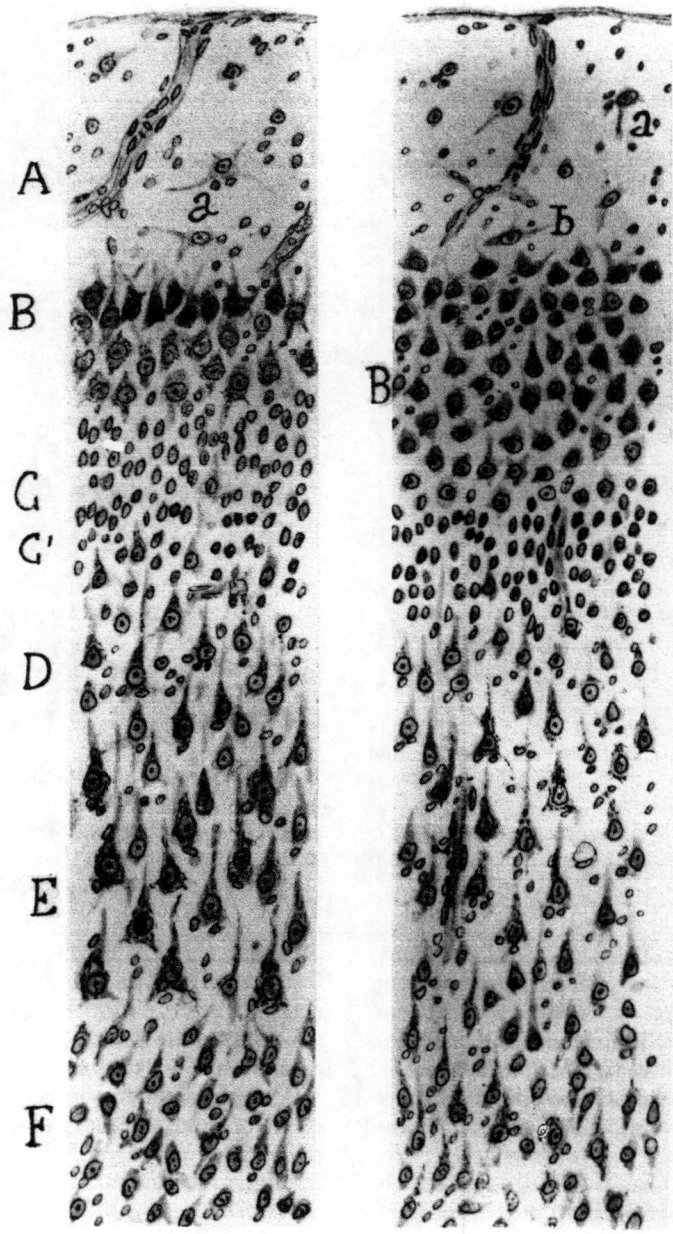

[*FIG. 268*] Plate III. Fig. 5. It reproduces, at high magnification, two somewhat separate areas of the retrosplenial cortex of the rabbit, stained with the method of Nissl. The figure at the left corresponds to area *29d* (more medial part), whereas that at the right copies a section of area *29f*. The letters indicate the numerical order of the layers.

complicated horizontal plexuses, separating the pleiades or small islands of neurons. Coming to join such plexuses, and with the aim of establishing connections of contact, are an infinity of prolixly divided nerve fibers.

b. Nerve Fibers

It is convenient to distinguish them as *endogenous* and *exogenous*.

The *endogenous,* indicated in our first work, represent nervous collaterals of the cells of layers II and III, or other collateral arborizations of cells with ascending axons located in layers V and VI. Fig. 1, *s, t* (plate I) and figs. 6 and 8 [*figs. 264, 269, 271*] excuse us from insisting on this important integrative factor of the plexus of layer IV.

Exogenous fibers were suspected in our first communication, were demonstrated in a study, unfortunately somewhat incomplete, on the suboccipital focus of the mouse[13] and guinea pig, and have been completely confirmed by our recent investigations in the rabbit. We reproduce several of them in fig. 8, plate V [*fig. 271*], in which has been gathered those observed in several successive sections.

One of the most typical is that reproduced at *f* (fig. 8) [*fig. 271*]. Coming from the white matter, this quite thick fiber crossed undivided the layers of the pyramids, but when it reached the deep plexiform layer, it bifurcated, each branch giving off several more or less parallel collaterals, which complicated the concentric plexus of the said layer. From one of these tangential projections emerged a small ascending branch (*P*) [left] which, after crossing the layer of the fusiform cells, was resolved into a tuft of thin threads, distributed to layer I. The area of distribution of the projection of the fiber *e,* fig. 8 [fig. 271], was no less extensive. In other exogenous fibers, it was not possible to discover but part of the final arborization distributed in the deep plexiform layer (*h, g*). Finally, some fibers of this kind gave off, before assailing layer IV, collaterals destined for the layer of the medium pyramids.

We consider that a good part of the medullated fibers revealed in the fourth layer by the Weigert and neurofibrillary methods undoubtedly represent branches of exogenous fibers.

With regard to the origin of these fibers, it is not possible at present to affirm anything definite. In our old works on the cerebral focus under study, we demonstrated the entry of the axons coming from the *arcuate fascicle* (mouse, guinea pig), situated, as is known, underneath and on the sides of the supracallosal cortex, homologous to the *gyrus fornicatus* of the gyrencephalic animals. But because this anteroposterior pathway possesses a heterogeneous composition, we are not very sure that the fibers [attached] to the same would be identical to the ones we have just described in the rabbit. This point requires still more meticulous and patient investigation.

5. Layer V or [Layer] of the Medium Pyramids

Of short extent and well visible in fig. 7, *D*, plate V, and fig. 1, *D*, plate I [*figs. 270, 264*], we can add nothing essential to our old description. It will be enough to remember that from the point of view of the size, morphology, behavior of the axon, etc., the [cells] are identical to the small and medium pyramids of other cortical areas. In the neurofibrillar preparations, they are recognized either by their reduced size or by the presence of a reticulated soma of pale and not always well-stained threads (fig. 7, *D*, plate V) [*fig. 270*]; however, the bipolar cells of layers III and IV escape the silver impregnation, showing a completely unstained cell body.

6. Layer VI or [Layer] of the Large Pyramids

They attract the colloidal silver with great affinity, as can be seen in fig. 7, *E* [*fig. 270*]. Their thick apical shafts cross almost the whole cortex, bifurcating often when they reach layer III, to be distributed finally in the superficial plexiform layer. Finally, it is possible to follow the axon, which is well perceptible in Bielschowsky and reduced silver nitrate sections, into the white matter. With regard to the axon collaterals, they can be seen in fig. 1, plate I [*figs. 29, 264*], taken from our work of the year 1893. In this same illustration are observed, among other neural varieties, cells

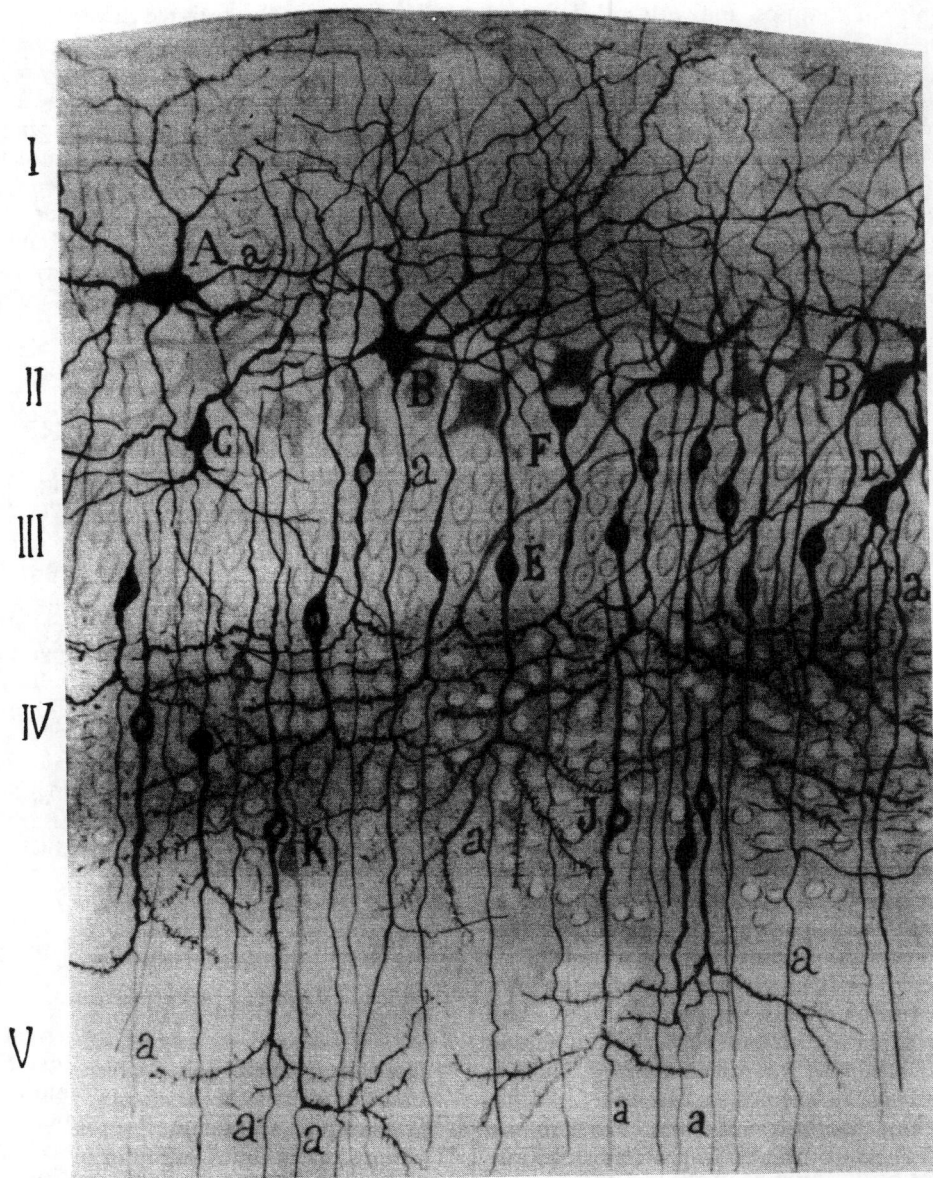

[FIG. 269] Plate IV. Fig. 6. It copies the structure of area 29c, impregnated by the method of Golgi. Rabbit of twenty-five days. In the figure, cells collected from four successive sections have been gathered:

  I. Plexiform layer with a neuron with horizontal axon (A).
  II. Layer of the large stellate cells (B).
  III. Layer of the vertical fusiform cells (E).
  IV. Deep plexiform layer and [layer] of the more internal fusiform cells (F).
  V. Layer of the medium pyramids. The axon is labeled with an a.

with ascending axon distributed in layer I (plate I, fig. 1, *s, t*) [*fig. 264*].

7. *Layer VII or [Layer] of the Polymorphic Cells*

Our recent explorations of this layer, with its relatively tiny cells, have not revealed any new details. Let us remember only that in it are typical medium pyramids, triangular and fusiform cells with descending axons lost in the white matter, and, finally, fusiform cells with ascending axon, distributed to layers VI, V, IV, and I. The axon of the cell *s*, fig. 1, plate I [*fig. 264*], gives an idea of the dilated axonal ramification. Sometimes, some neurons with short axon are also found.

Structural Differences Appreciated in the Several Anteroposterior Areas or Bands of the Retrosplenial Region

We have already indicated that all those authors who have analyzed the myelo- and cytoarchitecture of this cerebral area divide it into areas with a somewhat different structure (Brodmann, Rose, Zunino, Fortuyn, etc.). In our preparations, likewise, as we have exposed above, the existence of these areas is confirmed; their stratigraphy offers important modifications, mainly affecting layers II, IV, VI, and VII.

Such variability, whose range could be increased still further by exploring meticulously the borders of the retrosplenial field and its transitions with bordering areas, shows up preferentially in frontal sections examined at low magnification. It can be said that in these sections each cortical radius exhibits some stratigraphic peculiarities. Beginning from outside to inside, there is noticed, for example, in fig. 5 [*fig. 268*], right (areas *29d* and *29f*), the enormous thickness of the formation of the stellate cells (layer II) and the loose and lax disposition of the same, whose size is also rather smaller than that of the congener neurons of areas *29a* and *29b*. The details of field *29f* have been reproduced in fig. 5 [*fig. 268*] (right), where it is observed, besides, that layer III is relatively thin and the pyramids of layer VI less voluminous.

The Golgi sections corresponding to the area *29f* (territory close to the *lateral sagittal sulcus*) reveal an interesting transition between the retrosplenial cortex and a band that precedes the appearance of the visual cortex. As we show in fig. 9, plate VII [*fig. 272*], layer II or [layer] of the *stellate cells* (*B*) exhibits a multitude of large, triangular, fusiform, and star-shaped cells, some with a tendency to adopt a conical or pyramidal configuration, whereas in layer III, the diminutive fusiform type is converted progressively into a small pyramid, with ovoid soma and thin lateral and basal dendrites (*C*). Most of the neurons of layer II and of layer III are provided with a long axon, which can be followed to the white matter. The axon collaterals of these small cells are distributed preferentially in the layer of the large pyramids. In sum, examination of this field near the lateral sulcus, and which embraces nearly two-thirds of the exterior portion of the retrosplenial cortex, gives us the impression of an inversion of the first two pyramidal layers; the smaller ones, which should be superficial, adopt a deep position, and the external medium and large ones (layer of the stellate cells), which should be deep, become superficial. A plexus less rich in nerve fibers than that observed in the dense regions of area *29* inhabits layer III (*C*).

As we explore more medial areas and get close to the interhemispheric fissure, passing from field *29d* to *29b* and *29c*, layer II becomes narrower, while at the same time its constituent neurons become closer together and increase in size (fig. 5, left, and figs. 6 and 7*B*) [*figs. 268–270*]. Also, layer VII or [the layer] of the polymorphic cells progressively loses thickness. The section reproduced on the left of fig. 5 [*fig. 268*] makes evident those mutations, which correspond to the area called by Brodmann, Zunino, and Rose area *29c*. Figs. 6 and 8 [*figs. 269, 271*], copied from good Golgi preparations, also belong to this territory.

Finally, the area (area *29a*) situated in the inferior fossa of the occipital lobe has these structural features still more accentuated. Layer I reaches a maximum thickness, as well as layer III, or [the layer] of the fusiform cells, whereas layer II exaggerates its thinning until the point where, in proximity to the presubi-

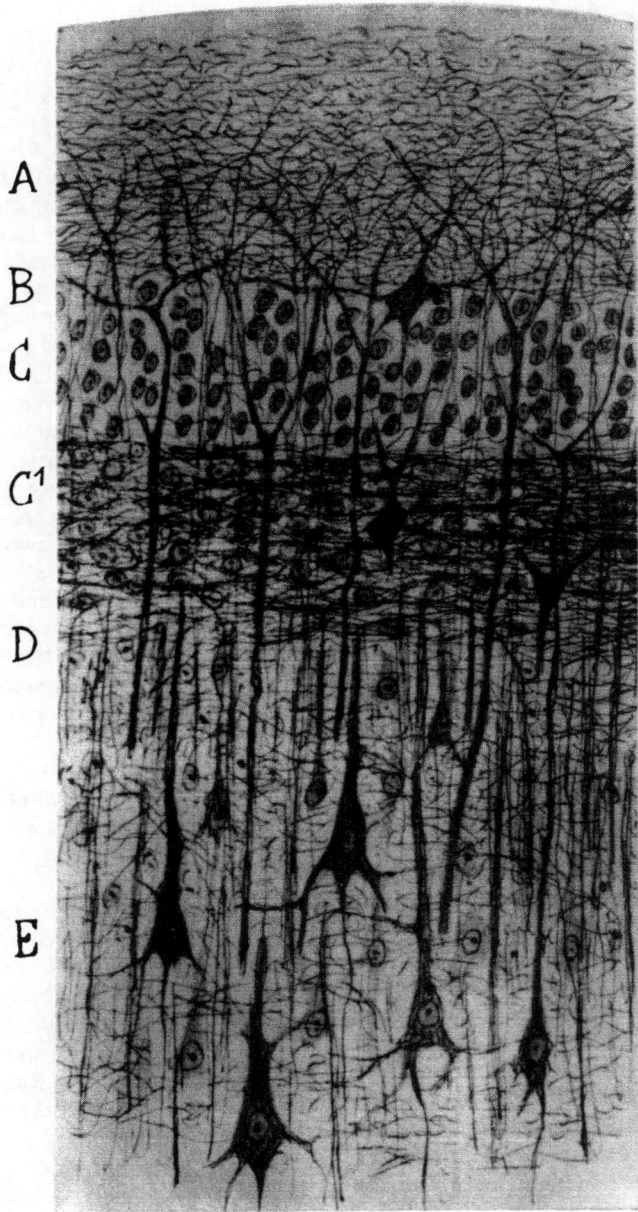

[*FIG. 270*] Plate V. Fig. 7. Frontal section of the same field *29c*, impregnated with the method of reduced silver nitrate. Note the superficial plexus *A* and deep plexus *C'*, exceptionally rich in medullated and un-medullated fibers. The letters indicate the succession of the layers.

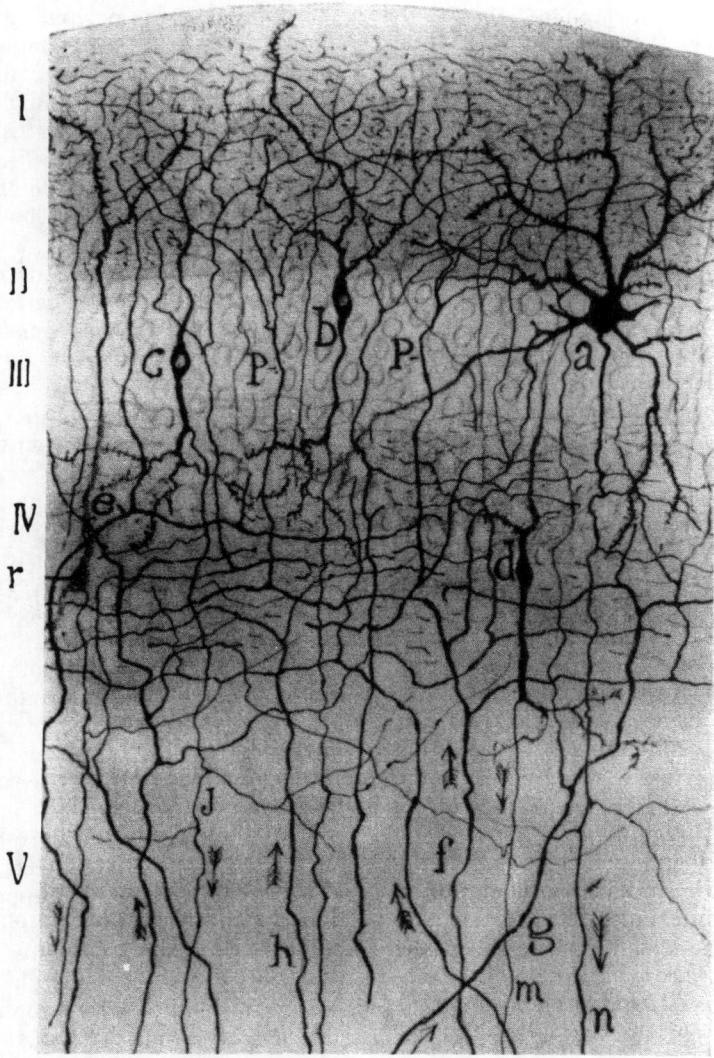

[*FIG. 271*] Plate VI. Fig. 8. Another section of the suprathalamic region of the retrosplenial cortex of the rabbit. In this figure, fibers and cells collected in several successive sections have been gathered. The numbers label the layers in order. *a*, stellate cell (layer II) with an axon that gave off collaterals to the deep plexus and also to the layer of the medium pyramids; *b*, *c*, vertical fusiform cells; *d*, fusiform cell of the deep plexus; *r*, *f*, *g*, *h*, exogenous fibers distributed to both plexiform layers; *p*, perforant fibers of exogenous origin destined for layer I.

culum, it only consists of one or two rows of tight neurons (fig. 3, *a*, plate II, and fig. 5,[A] plate II) [*figs. 266, 268*]. In its turn, layer VII decreases noticeably. In this place, as drawn well by Zunino, the medullated plexus of layer IV reaches its maximum tightness and differ-

entiation, and the large pyramids (layer VI) are of the largest stature. The section in fig. 7, plate V [*fig. 270*], which reproduces a reduced silver nitrate preparation, corresponds to this place or near to it.

Finally, near Ammon's horn, the suboccipital cortex (fig. 3, plate II) [*fig. 266*] abruptly stops, forming a layer II like a hook. Further on begins another type of cortex, devoid of granule cells, which corresponds to the superior end of the presubiculum, a cortex that acquires its full differentiation and extent only in more inferior sagittal sections.

Retrosplenial Cortex of the Mouse (*Mus musculus*)

Noted for its peculiar structure in several passages of our monographs[14] and in our work as a whole,[15] it has been the subejct of systematic and precise observations by Isenschmid, Maximilian Rose, and Fortuyn. We owe to Rose[16] the most meticulous analysis of the retrosplenial cortex of the mouse, in which he also differentiates several other areas already studied by us during the years 1901 and 1902. This author has taken advantage of both the Weigert and Nissl methods.

In his description of *area 29*, Rose adopts the same nomenclature as Brodmann; that is to say, he distinguishes the sagittal areas *a*, *b*, and *c*, with the exception of *29d*, which is not observed or not clearly recognized in the mouse. Also, Fortuyn gives less relative extent to this suboccipital region, in the [mouse], and he includes it in what he called *group Z*. In fig. 22, page 261 of the work of the latter author, it is observed that the most typical portion, that is to say, the one that reproduces best the [structure of the] retrosplenial field of the rabbit, is that entitled *Z II* and located behind the corpus callosum. This not very extensive cerebral region corresponds more or less to area *29a* of M. Rose. The field Z of Fortuyn appears to us to belong to the presubiculum (since it lacks the layer of granule cells), whereas Z III coincides with the one we described some time ago under the name of *interhemispheric* or supracallosal *cortex*. In other animals, for example, in the hedgehog (*Erinaceus europaeus*) and in the bat (Rose [1912]), the region under study is still more restricted. Watson (1907) indicates it also in the insectivores.

In the mouse, the typical retrosplenial region also reaches little extent, inhabiting the

thalamic fossa of the occipital pole, as can be observed in the microphotograph in plate VIII (fig. 10) [*fig. 273*]. Forward, however, it is rather more extensive, invading the supracallosal region. Evidence on that is given by the microphotograph in fig. 12 [*fig. 275*], which represents a horizontal section of the occipital lobe of the mouse, passing above the corpus callosum.

It is difficult in these sections to separate the field *29* from that which we had designated some time ago as *interhemispheric cortex*, for they appear to be continuous by smooth transitions. In any case, the layer of the granule cells (layer III) becomes thinner and progressively disappears as more frontal regions are explored (fig. 12) [*fig. 275*].

The retrosplenial cortex of the mouse is distinguished, at first glance, by these three characteristic features: enormous thickness of the plexiform layer (fig. 10, *A*) [*fig. 273*]; existence of a layer of very close-packed stellate cells (layer II, fig. 10, *B*) [*fig. 273*]; and, finally, a perfect differentiation of a layer of small fusiform neurons (*granule cells* of the authors; fig. 10, *C*) [*fig. 273*]. Underneath this emerges a stratum identical to the layer of the large pyramids (fig. 10, *D*) [*fig. 273*], not clearly separated, deeply, from the polymorphic cells.

The internal or interhemispheric portion (area *29b³*) appears less characteristic (fig. 10, *F*) [*fig. 273*]; in it there still appears a formation of stellate neurons, although little dense, but layer III or the granular layer is seen to be thin, discontinuous, and little demarcated. Also, layer I appears to be atrophic.

Finally, above, that is to say, on the external face of the occipital lobe (*E*), the granule cells do not form a separate stratum, and the superficial plexiform layer becomes notably thinner. These and other stratigraphical peculiarities make one doubt that area *29* is extended further upward than the interhemispheric fissure.

It is not our purpose to explore meticulously the extent of the retrosplenial region of the mouse or to discuss the data, which we judge to be well interpreted, as collected by Rose and other neurologists. Here we are going to limit ourselves to listing briefly some unfortunately very incomplete observations, made in chrome-silver sections of the inferior portion,

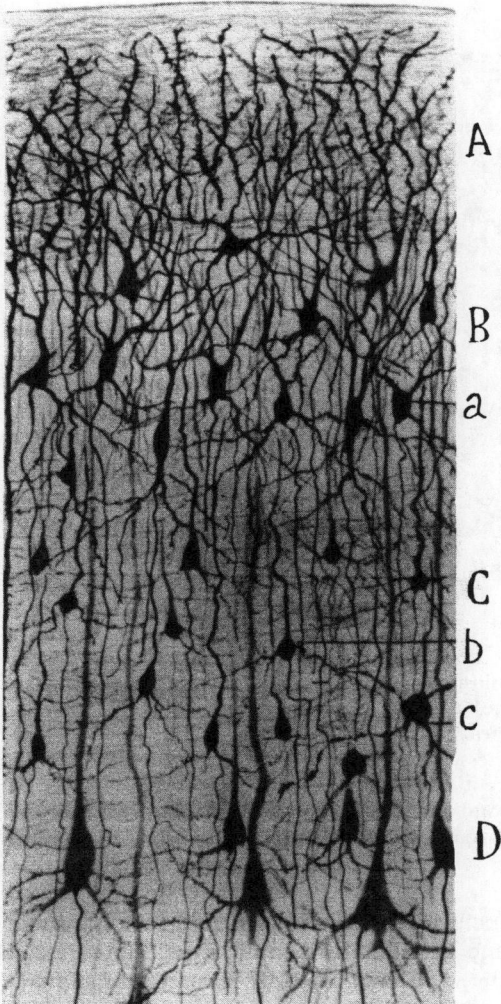

A

B

a

C

b

c

D

[*FIG. 272*] Plate VII. Fig. 9. It reproduces a frontal section of area *29f* of the rabbit, not far from the lateral sagittal sulcus. Notice the thickness of layer II or [the layer] of the stellate cells, among which already are seen large or medium pyramidal cells (*B*) and the transformation of the fusiform cells (*C*) into small pyramidal cells.

that is to say, of the most typical area of this region in the mouse (*Mus musculus*) of fifteen to twenty-five days.

Let us begin by declaring that the same stratifications are perceptible, although not as clearly as in the cortex of the rabbit. We will

not make of them a meticulous study; the imperfect nature of the impregnations imposes on us a laconic [style].

[*Layer I or Plexiform Layer*]

The *plexiform* layer or [*layer*] *I*, reaches great development, exhibiting an exceptionally rich nervous plexus equal to that of the rabbit, besides numerous cells with short axon (fig. 11, plate IX) [*fig. 274*].

[*Layer II or Layer of the Stellate Cells*]

In *layer II* or the [layer] of the *stellate cells*, we have only been able to impregnate some cells, which we show in fig. 11, *d* [*fig. 274*]. Notice that they coincide, in this way, with respect to the somatic form and distribution of the dendrites and axon, to those mentioned in the comparable cortex of the rabbit. Probably their number is fewer than in the rabbit.

Layer III or [*Layer*] *of the Small Fusiform Cells* (figs. 10; 12, *c*) [figs. 273, 275]

They possess, as in the rabbit, an ovoid soma and two polar dendrites (fig. 11, *a, b*) [*fig. 274*]; but, if we have to judge by the cells that have attracted the silver chromate, the typical disposition has suffered some changes, which are attributable perhaps to the narrowness of layer III. Of course, in some cells, the axon arises from the descending [dendritic] shaft (fig. 11 *a, b*) [*fig. 274*]; in others, perhaps in the majority, it arises from the soma or near it; also, cells are not rare that, instead of exhibiting a [single] descending [dendritic] shaft, exhibit two dendrites with the same direction. For the rest, the axon gives off projections to the plexus of layer IV and to the layers of the medium and large pyramids.

Layer IV or Deep Plexiform [*Layer*]

It also encloses a meshwork of nerve fibers with a preferentially tangential course and numerous fusiform cells (fig. 11, *D*) [*fig. 274*], similar to the ones described in the rabbit, besides others more similar to small pyramids.

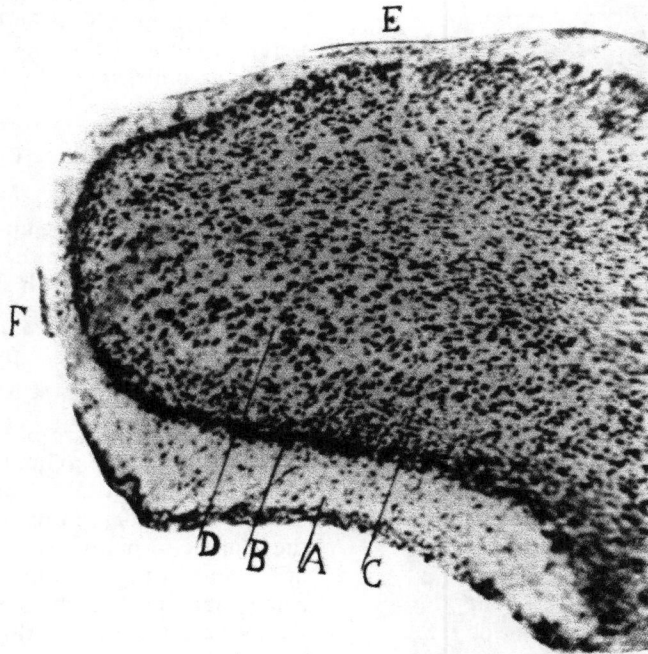

[FIG. 273] Plate VIII. Fig. 10. Frontal section of the most posterior portion of the occipital lobe of the cerebrum of the adult white mouse. The upper part of the figure (E) corresponds to the superior surface of the hemisphere; the vertical line (F), to the interhemispheric fissure, touching the occipital lobe of the other side; and, finally, the deep part of the same, which possesses a plexiform layer of exceptional thickness, touches the optic thalamus. Only it exhibits a well-differentiated layer of vertical fusiform cells (layer III). A, plexiform layer; B, layer of the stellate cells, very tight and obscure; C, layer of the fusiform cells; D, layer of the large pyramids. Method of Nissl. Microphotograph taken with a 0.65 objective and the Zeiss compensation ocular 8. Green monochromatic light.

Layers V, VI, and VII

They coincide with those exposed in previous pages, except for their smaller size and [indistinct] differentiation. In relation to the large pyramids, the ovoid form of the soma is to be noticed. For the rest, the [apical dendritic] shafts of the cells with long axon of these deep layers also reach layer I, where they resolve into spiny dendritic tufts.

In sum, with some variations in cellular morphology and some tectonic simplifications, area 29 of the mouse duplicates quite well the cortex of the same name of the rabbit and of other rodents.

General Considerations and Conclusions

The preceding descriptions of the tectonics of area 29 in the rabbit and mouse allow us to include this cortex, in accord with Brodmann and his disciples Zunino, Rose, Flores, etc., in the type designated by [Brodmann] as *fundamental type or* [*type*] *of six layers* (*homogenetic cortex, isocortex* of O. Vogt).

What characterizes this cortex with six strata, individualizing its distinctiveness, are these [four] features:

a. The enormous development of the plexiform layer or layer I, which encloses a very rich number of neurons with short axon and those with very long tangential axon.

b. The presence underneath the same of a specific layer of large stellate cells morphologically distinct both from the pyramids and from the cells included by Brodmann in the *lamina granularis* (*small pyramids* of other authors).

c. The appearance of a layer III, formed by vertical fusiform cells, whose thin axon comes

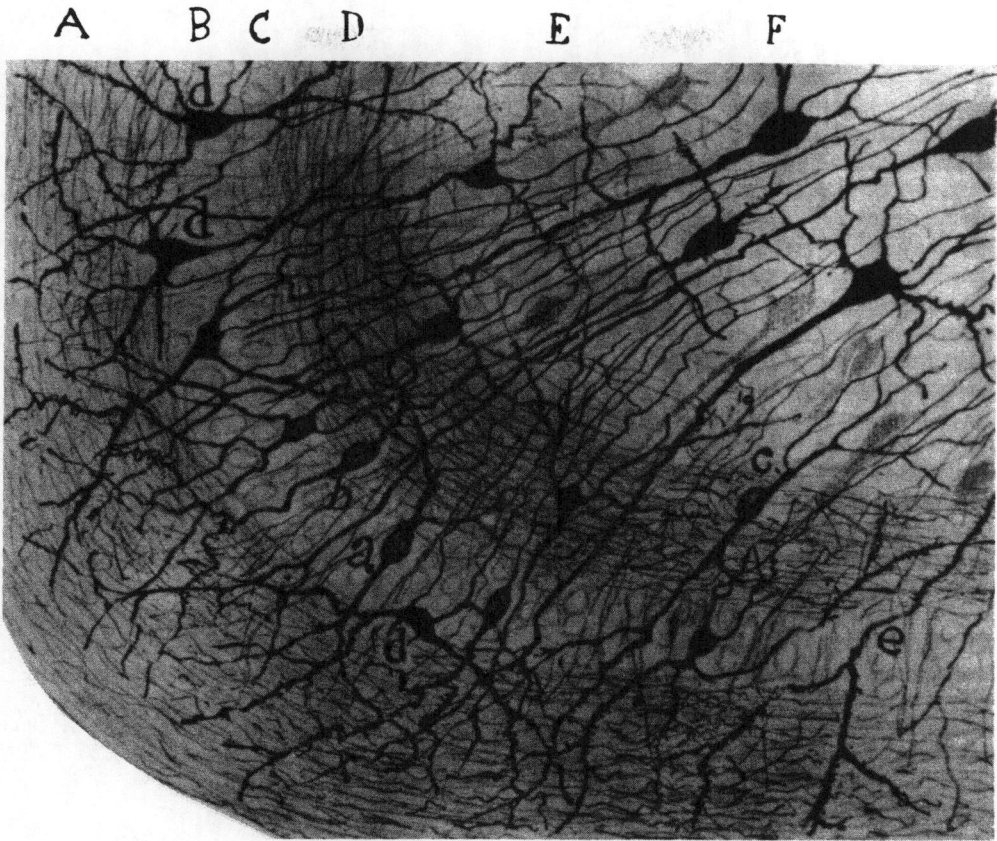

[*FIG. 274*]   Plate IX. Fig. 11. Infero-internal region of the retrosplenial cortex of the mouse of fifteen days (preparation of Lorente de Nó). In it are observed, more or less, the same layers as in the rabbit, except for some variations of detail. The letters in the margin indicate the order of the layers I to VI. The cells included in the figure have been collected from several successive sections. *d,* stellate cells; *a, b,* vertical fusiform cells (layer III); *c,* fusiform cell of the deep plexiform layer (*D*); *F,* large pyramids.

from the inferior extremity of the descending dendrite.

d. The existence, beneath layer III, of a very dense nervous plexus, in large part composed of exogenous fibers, among which reside numerous fusiform cells, similar to the preceding.

In regard to the homology of the specific layers of this type of gray matter, that is, layers II and III, nothing secure can be affirmed. Morphologically, layer II is not comparable to that of the small or large pyramids, nor can layer III *(fusiform cells)* be identified, as Brodmann does, with a *lamina granularis interna (layer IV* or [layer] of granule cells in the strict sense). However, if we abandon the strict mor-

phological criterion as well as the consideration of the relative neuronal size, and we attend exclusively to the trajectory and behavior of the axons and dendrites, we could homologize layer II with the *layer of the external medium and large pyramids* of other cortical territories and [layer] III or [layer] of the fusiform cells with the *[layer of the] small pyramids.* To accept such a homology, one might have to abandon the *prejudgment of rigorous tectonic ordination* and admit that, in the retrosplenial field, as in other regional cortices, the respective position of the layers are inverted, in such a way that the one that should be [layer] II *(fusiform cells)* becomes III, and the one that should occupy [layer] III or IV *(stellate cells*

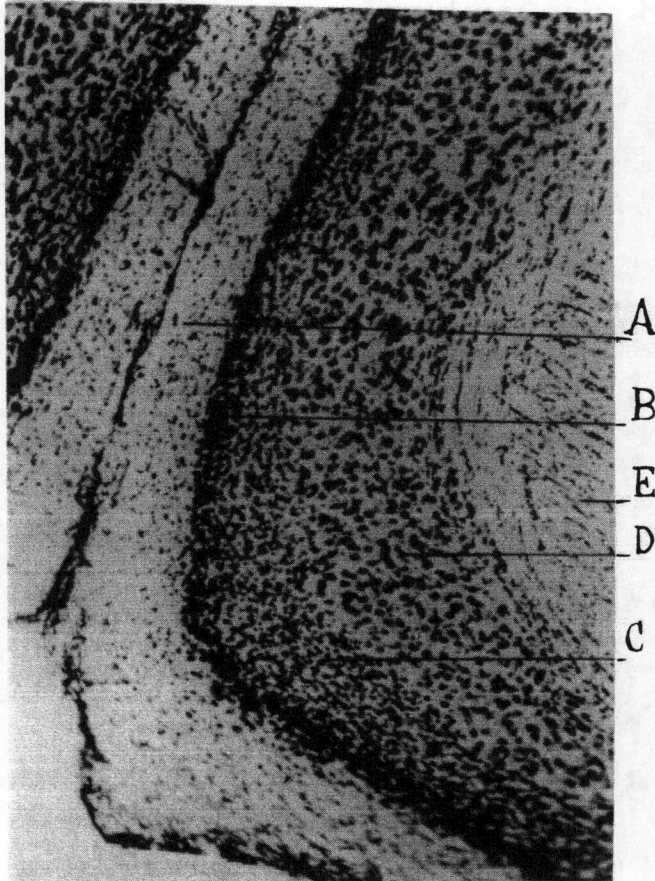

[*FIG. 275*]   Plate X. Fig. 12. Horizontal section of the retrosplenial region of the adult mouse. The section passes somewhat above the corpus callosum. To the left is seen the interhemispheric fissure; at the right, a piece of corpus callosum (*E*). The letters label the successive layers. Notice how the fusiform cells (layer III), which have their maximum size in *C*, become progressively more slender anteriorly. Notice, finally, the enormous thickness of the plexiform layer in the postero-inferior part of the occipital cortex, that is to say, in the suprathalamic region. (Nissl preparation made by Dr. Lorente [de Nó].)

similar to external large pyramids) becomes layer II. This interpretation harmonizes well with what we know about the structure of area *29f,* in which the continuity of the fusiform cells with a layer of small pyramids and the progressive transformation of the stellate neurons (layer II) into pyramids of medium size are observed. Let us note, however, that the mentioned inversion of layers II and III is confined to the territory bordering the *sulcus sagittalis lateralis.*

With regard to the physiological significance of this cortical region, nothing categor-ical can be affirmed. It is known that, for Henschen,[17] the *retrosplenial field* constitutes the terminal relay for gustatory stimuli. Basing [his view] on an interesting clinical case, the Swedish neurologist localized the perception of taste, not only in area *29* of man but in part of the bordering suboccipital gyri. For his part, Ariëns Kappers,[18] relying on systematic studies in comparative neurology, considers the mentioned field as attached to the olfactory system.

We lack proper clinical data and works of anatomicopathological experimentation to evaluate the referred opinions. We consider probably, however, in accord with Ariëns Kappers, that area *29* is the seat of a psychic activity similar or very close to that of olfaction. In favor of the intimate similarity between the retrosplenial cortex and the areas with an undoubted olfactory function, the following facts militate:

1. The suboccipital or retrosplenial cortex is found to be notably developed and differentiated in the macrosmatic animals (dog, guinea pig, rabbit, cat, etc.).

2. It resides constantly in proximity to the presubiculum, spheno-occipital focus (area *28* of Brodmann), and Ammon's horn, as though denoting the exercise of an equal or parallel function with the olfactory.

3. It appears very early in the phylogenetic series of the mammals, as noted by Ariëns Kappers.

4. It coincides surprisingly in texture and tectonic ordination with regions surely related to secondary or tertiary pathways of an olfactory character; for example, to the *sphenoidal cortex,* situated underneath the termination of the *external root* of the olfactory [tract], which, besides showing a layer II of voluminous stellate neurons, contains a layer III of small vertical fusiform cells, equal to those indicated in the retrosplenial region; and to our *spheno-occipital center* or center at the pole of the piriform lobe (*area 28* or *entorhinal* area of Brodmann and Rose), in which there is also a layer II of large stellate cells and a layer III of small pyramidal cells.

But to include area *29* definitively in the system of olfactory centers and to exclude completely a gustatory character, or any other psychic activity, it is necessary to undertake anatomicopathological experiments (not bereft, unfortunately, of difficulty, given the deep position of the said region), with the aim of observing the centrifugal pathways, whose degeneration is provoked by the ablation of the same, and the thalamic center or centers consequently affected by degeneration; because it is a fact stated by several authors and confirmed anatomically by us that all sensory areas of the cortex (except Ammon's horn and secondary olfactory foci [19]) send descending fibers precisely arborized in the thalamic center in which they meet the afferent sensory pathways. (This fact has been demonstrated by

us in the mouse for the thalamic foci and superior colliculus in the visual system and for the sensory nucleus of the thalamus.) If the said experiments would be undertaken with skill and good fortune, it would perhaps be possible to determine at one stroke the subcortical secondary relay of the sensory pathway related to area *29,* and the cerebral area from which the corticothalamic fibers, which perhaps are not lacking from any of the nuclei of the [diencephalon], arise. A lack of connections with the thalamus could be considered as another indication that the mentioned field represents a tertiary olfactory relay.

Bibliography Consulted

Cajal. Estructura de la corteza suboccipital de los pequeños mamíferos. *Anales de la Sociedad Española de Historia Natural,* Vol. XX, 1893.

——. Beiträge zur feineren Anatomie des grossen Hirns II: Ueber den Bau der Rinde des unteren Hinterhauptslappens der kleinen Säugethiere. *Zeitschrift f. Wissensch. Zool,* Vol. LVI, Part 4, 1893 (translation of A. v. Kölliker).

——. Histologie du système nerveux de l'homme et des vertébrés, etc., Vol. II, 1911, p. 807.

——. Textura de la corteza visual del gato. *Trabajos,* etc., Vol. XIX, October 1921.

Hermanides and Köppen. Ueber die Furchen und den Bau der Grosshirnrinde bei den Lissencephalen, etc. *Arch. Psychiatrie,* Vol. XXXVII, 1903.

O. Vogt. Zur anatomischen Gliederung des Cortex cerebri. *Journal für Psychol. u. Neurologie,* Vol. II, 1903.

Cécile and Oskar Vogt. Allgemeiner Ergebnisse unserer Hirnforschung. *Journ. für Psychol. u. Neurologie,* Vol. XXV, 1919.

Watson. The Mammalian Cerebral Cortex with Special Reference to the Comparative Histology I: Order Insectivora. *Arch. of Neurology,* Vol. III, London, 1907.

K. Brodmann. Feinere Anatomie des Grosshirns. *Handbuch der Neurologie,* edited by M. Lewadowsky, Vol. I, 19[10].

——. *Vergleichende Lokalisationslehre der Grosshirnrinde,* Leipzig, J. A. Barth, 1909.

Haller. Beiträge zur Phylogenese des Grosshirn der Säugethiere. *Arch f. Mikros. Anat.,* Vol. 69, 190[6].

——. Die Mantelgebiete des Grosshirn vom den Nagern aufsteigend bis zum Menschen. *Arch f. Mikros. Anat.,* Vol. 76, 1910.

A. Kappers and W. Theunisen. Die Phylogenese des Rinencephalon, des Corpus striatum und der Vorderhirnkommisure. *Fol. Neurobiol.,* Vol. I, 1908.

[Kappers, A.] The Phylogenesis of the Palaeo-Cortex and Archi-Cortex Compared with the Evolution of the Visual Neo-Cortex. *Arch. of Neurol and Psych.,* Vol. 4, 1909.

——. *Folia Neurobiologica,* Vol. IV, 1910. In it, an excellent criticism of the ideas of Brodmann is made.

———. *Die vergleichende Anatomie des Nervensystems der Wirbelthiere und des Menschen,* Part II, Haarlem, 1921, section II, pp. 1176 and 1185.

Isenschmid. Zur Kenntniss der Grosshirnrinde der Maus. *Aus den Anhang zu den Abhandl. d. Königl. Preuss. Akademie der Wissensch. vom Jahre 1911,* Berlin, 1911.

C. Zunino. Die myeloarchitektonische Differenzierung der Grosshirnrinde bei Kaninchen. *Journal f. Psych. u. Neurol.,* Vol. XIV, 1909.

Flores. Die Myeloarchitektonik, u. die Myelogenie des Cortex cerebri beim Igel. *Journ. f. Psychol. u. Neurol.,* Vol. XVII, 1911.

C. Winkler and Ada Potter. *An Anatomical Guide to Experimental Researches on the Rabbit's Brain,* Amsterdam, 1911.

M. Rose. (Krakau) Histologische Lokalisation der Grosshirnrinde bei kleinen Säugethieren *(Rodentia, Insectivora, Chiroptera). Journal für Psychol. und Neurologie,* Vol. XIX, 1912.

S. E. Henschen. Ueber die Geruch- und Geschmackszentren. *Monatschrift. f. Psychiatr. u. Neurologie,* Vol. XLV, Part 3, Berlin, 1918.

Th. Ziehen. *Anatomie des Centralnervensystems,* Jena, G. Fischer, 1920 (in press).

Cajal's Notes

1. The said methods are unable to stain the dendrites of the neurons or the formidable number of nonmedullated fibers or the cells with short axon. And even within the domain of their revelations, the data yielded by the said methods are sometimes difficult to appreciate. This serves to cause the discrepancies with respect to the number and extent of the areas or cortical fields presented in the works of the English school and in those of the school of Brodmann.

2. Cajal, Estructura de la corteza visual del gato, *Trabajos,* etc., Vol. XX, 1921.

3. Cajal, Estructura de la corteza occipital inferior de los pequeños mamíferos, *Anal. de la Socied. Españ. de Historia Natural,* Vol. XXII, 1893. See also: Cajal, Beiträge zur feineren Anatomie des grossen Hirns II: Ueber den Bau der Rinde des unteren Hinterhauptslappens, *Zeitschrift f. Wissench. Zool.,* Vol. LVI, Part 4, 1893.

4. Cajal, *Histologie du système nerveux de l'homme et des* [*vertébrés*], Vol. II [1911], p. 807, figs. 519, 520, and 521 [*figs. 190, 191, 168*].

5. Cajal, *Histologie du système nerveux de l'homme et des* [*vertébrés*], Vol. II, [1911], p. 807, figs. 519, 520, and 521 [*figs. 190, 191, 168*].

6. Brodmann, *Allgemeine Neurologie,* Part 1, edited by M. Lewandowsky, Berlin, J. Springer, 1910, p. 244.

7. Zunino, Die myeloarchitektonische Differenzierung der Grosshirnrinde beim Kaninchen, *Journ. f. Psychol. u. Neurol.,* Vol. XIV, Parts 1–2, 1909.

8. Winkler, C., and Ada Potter, *An Anatomical Guide to Experimental Researches on the Rabbit's Brain,* Amsterdam (Plates XV and XVI), 1911.

9. R. Droogleever Fortuyn, Cortical Cell Lamina-

tion of the Hemispheres of Some Rodents, *Arch. of Neurol. and Psychiatry,* etc., Vol. VI, 1914.

10. Isenschmid, Zur Kenntnis des Grosshirnrinde der Maus, *Aus dem Abhand. zu den Königl. Preuss. Akad. der Wissensch.* Berlin, 1911. Among all those who studied the cerebrum of the rodents, this is the person who best knows our monograph of 1893, the German translation of which he mentions.

11. Köppen and Löwenstein, Studien über den Zellenbau der Grosshirnrinde bei Ungulaten u. Carnivoren, etc., *Monatsch. f. Psychiatrie u. Neurol.,* Vol. XVIII, 19[05].

12. Maximilian Rose, Histologische Lokalisation der Grosshirnrinde bei keinen Säugethieren (Rodentia, Insectivora, Chiroptera), *Journ. f. Psychol. u. Neurol.,* Vol. IX, 1912.

13. Cajal, *Histologie du Système Nerveux de l'Homme et des* [*Vertébrés*], Vol. II, [1911].

14. Cajal, Estructura de la corteza olfativa, etc., *Trabajos del Lab. de Investig. Biol.,* Vol. I, 1901–1902. (There is a German translation of this and other monographs published by the firm of J. A. Barth of Leipzig.)

15. Cajal, *Textura del sistema nervioso del hombre y de los vertebrados,* Vol. II, 1904. See also: *Histologie du système nerveux de l'homme et des vertébrés,* Vol. II, p. 706 and following. Much expanded French translation of Dr. L. Azoulay, Maloine, Paris, 1911.

16. It is surprising how a neurologist so well oriented and so knowledgeable of the literature as Rose (and we could say the same of Zunino, Flores, and even of Brodmann) should indicate and name in the mouse and other rodents, without citing us, centers *described widely and in detail* by us before 1900, and published besides in our overall work (French translation of Dr. Azoulay) on the histology of the nervous system. To mention just one example: the center at the pole of the piriform lobe, called by us *spheno-occipital* and called by Rose, following Brodmann, *area entorhinalis* (areas *28a* and *28b*), has many pages (forty-eight) and twenty-four figures devoted to it in our monographs and in the cited book, in which are elucidated not only the fine structure (methods of Nissl and Golgi) but the important connections of the said focus with the *dorsal psalterium and Ammon's horn of both sides.*

17. Henschen, Ueber die Geruchs- und Geschmackszentren, *Monatschr, f. Psychiatrie u. Neurologie,* Vol. XLV, Part 3, Berlin, 191[9].

18. Ariëns Kappers, *Die vergleichende Anatomie des Nervensystems der Wirbeltiere,* parts I and II, Haarlem, 1921.

19. The fornix, originating from Ammon's horn, seems to us to represent a motor pathway. In any case, it is not comparable to the mentioned corticothalamic pathways, which enter into contact with the same thalamic neurons that receive the impulses of the ascending sensory fibers. [This footnote is not indicated by a number in the text.]

Editors' Note

A. Probably *fig. 267.*

29

The Final View

After 1922, Cajal, now in his seventies, continued to publish, but his output was confined to technical notes, contributions to Festschriften in honor of distinguished fellow scientists, republications in French of some of his older Spanish works, and compilations of earlier papers. Many of these appeared in parallel French versions of the *Trabajos,* published, with separate volume numbers, under the title *Travaux du Laboratoire de Recherches Biologiques de l'Université de Madrid.* This has proved to be a great source of confusion to copy editors of scientific works ever since. Among the reissued works, there appears to be an emphasis on the neuroglia—one of his late interests and perhaps also resulting from his conflict with Del Río Hortega on the subject—and on the retina (probably because he had not published on this subject for many years). One compilation, however, contains material relating to the cerebral cortex.

Funded by a group of professors at the University of Montevideo and by Uruguayan scientific and cultural organizations, in 1929, Cajal published in French his *Études sur la neurogenèse de quelques vertébrés.* This was subsequently translated into English by Guth under the title *Studies on Vertebrate Neurogenesis* (1960). The volume is a compilation of previously published works on neural development, the earliest dating back to 1890. A relatively short section devoted to the development of cells in the cerebral cortex draws primarily on the *La Cellule* paper of 1891 (see chapter 5 in this volume) but with additions from the paper of 1893 on the structure of the inferior occipital cortex in small mammals (see chapter 6), from chapter 47 of the *Textura* (see chapter 24), and from the paper on the human motor cortex (see chapter 16). A significant proportion of the figures are enlargements of those appearing as parts of composite plates in the *La Cellule* paper. The work deals with the development of neuroglial cells and of pyramidal cells, along much the same lines as the accounts appearing in *La Cellule* and in the *Textura* and the *Histologie,* and the figure legends are identical to those in the earlier works. There is also a lengthy description of the development of the special cells of layer I, in the course of which Cajal emphasizes that in the adult animal the special cells never possess more than a single axon. He attributes his earlier accounts of multiple axons on these cells (see chapters 4–8 in this volume) to his exclusive focus on the embryonic phases of the special cells. He therefore now definitively regards the special cells as a form of cell with short axon.

Cajal's final four works (1933; 1934 a, b; 1935) were devoted to raising the banner of the neuron doctrine which he felt was again under attack. In *fig. 276*, we reproduce one of Cajal's handwritten notes, preserved in the Museo Cajal and dating from the period when

he was preparing these works. The better known of the later publications is *¿Neuronismo o Reticularismo? Las Pruebas Objetivas de la Unidad Anatómica de las Células Nerviosas* (1933). This was translated into English in 1954 under the title *Neuron Theory or Reticular Theory? Objective Evidence of the Anatomical Unity of Nerve Cells,* by Ubeda-Purkiss and Fox. A literal French translation appeared almost simultaneously (1934) with the original publication in the *Travaux du Laboratoire de*

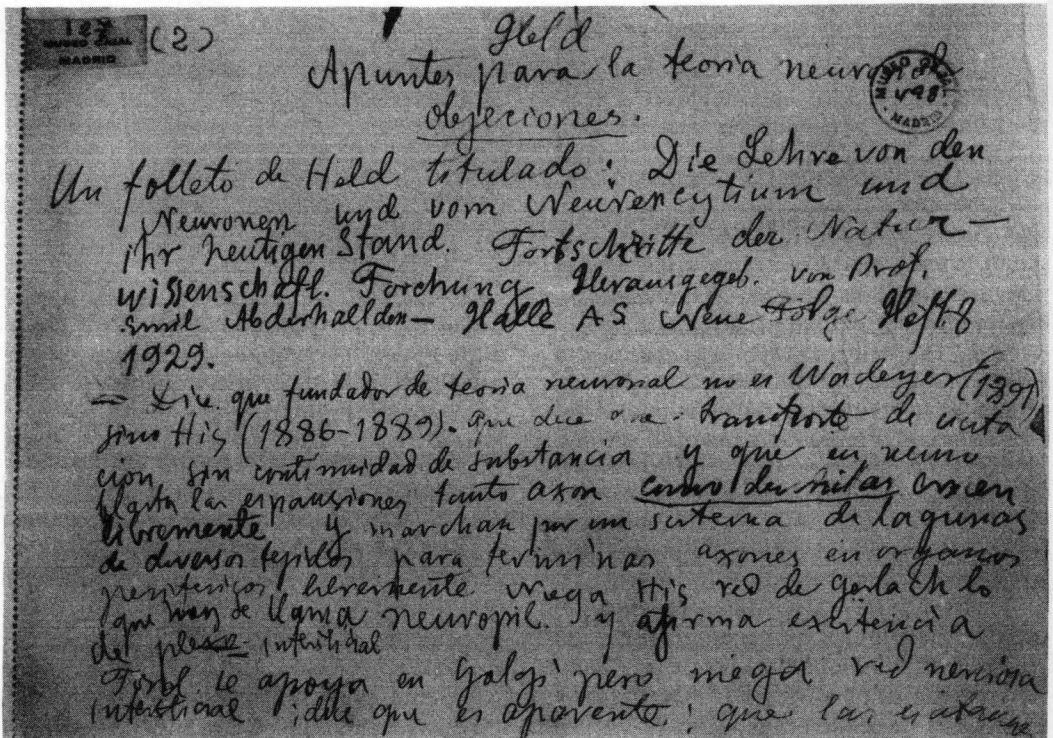

[*FIG. 276*]   A note by Cajal made during the preparation of his last great work. The text reads: "Held. Notes for the neuronal theory. *Objections.* A pamphlet of Held entitled: Die Lehre von den Neuronen und vom Neurencytium und ihr heutigen Stand. Fortschritte der Naturwissenschaft. For[s]chung Herausgegeb. vom Prof. Emil Abderhalden. Halle A. S. Neue Folge Heft 8 1929. [The Neuron Theory and the Neurencytial Theory and Their Present Status, *Fortschritte der Naturwissenschaft. Forschung,* edited by Professor Emil Abderhalden, Halle, New Series, Part 8, 1929.] He says that the founder of the neuronal theory is not Waldeyer (1891) but His (1886–1889), who says that transmission of excitation [occurs] without continuity of substance and that in neuroblasts the processes, either axon or *dendrites,* grow freely and run through a system of lacunae in several tissues, the axons terminating freely in peripheral organs. His denies the network of Gerlach, which nowadays is called neuropil, and affirms the existence of an interstitial plexus. Forel follows Golgi but denies the interstitial nervous net; he says that it is apparent: that the excitations . . . " [From the Museo Cajal].

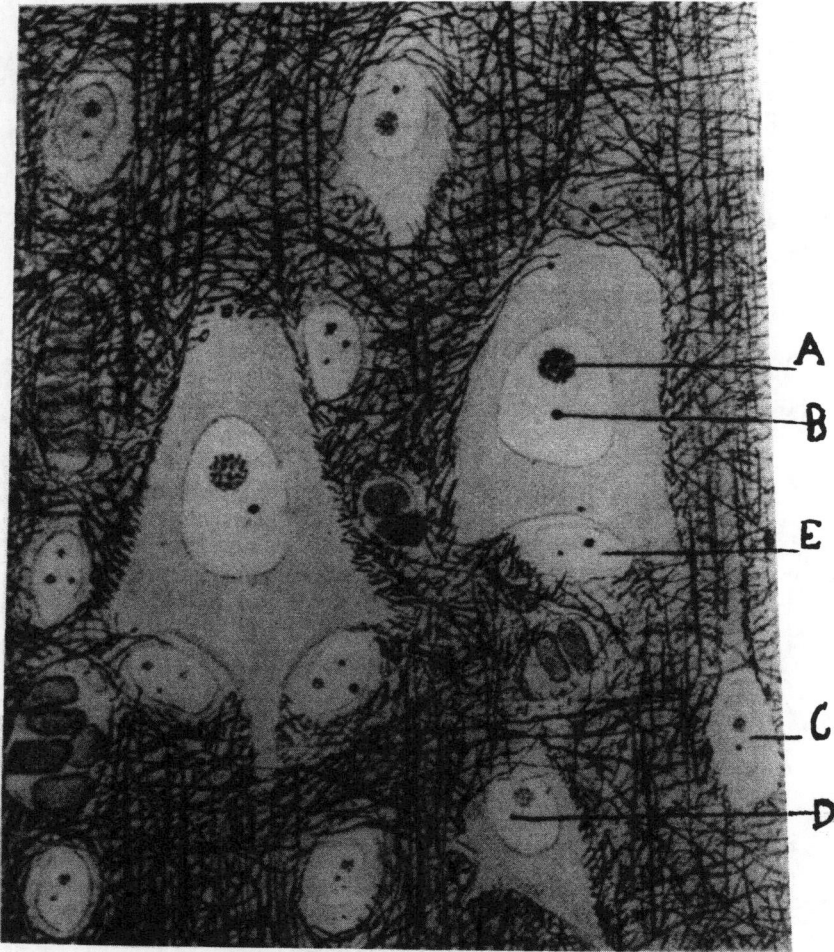

[*FIG. 277*] [Fig. 47 of *¿Neuronismo o Reticularismo?* (Cajal, 1933).] Terminal plexus about the pyramids. Cerebral cortex of an adult dog [reduced silver preparation]. *A*, nucleolus of a giant pyramid; [*B, D,* intranuclear bodies]; *C*, small pyramid; *E*, basal neuroglial cell.

Recherches Biologiques de l'Université de Madrid. The second 1934 paper was a short work in German, taken from one section of the *¿Neuronismo o Reticularismo?* and attacking the periterminal fibrillar network described by Boeke. The final work, published posthumously in Bumke and Foerster's *Handbook of Neurology* (1935), is a German translation by Miskolczy of the *¿Neuronismo o Reticularismo?* with numerous additions and modifications, particularly in the figures used to illustrate the work.[A] Whether these modifcations are by Cajal or the translator is unknown to us. However, certain of the additional figures are taken from those reproduced in Tello's (1935) work, *Cajal y su Labor Histológica.* We may therefore conjecture that Tello, described by Cajal as his most beloved pupil, had a hand in the new version.

On page 184 of his eulogy of Cajal's work, Tello remarks:

Cajal's collaboration having been requested in the preparation of the second edition of the great treatise of Lewandowsky,[B] he forwarded (1932) an extensive article on the neuron. Later, he published in

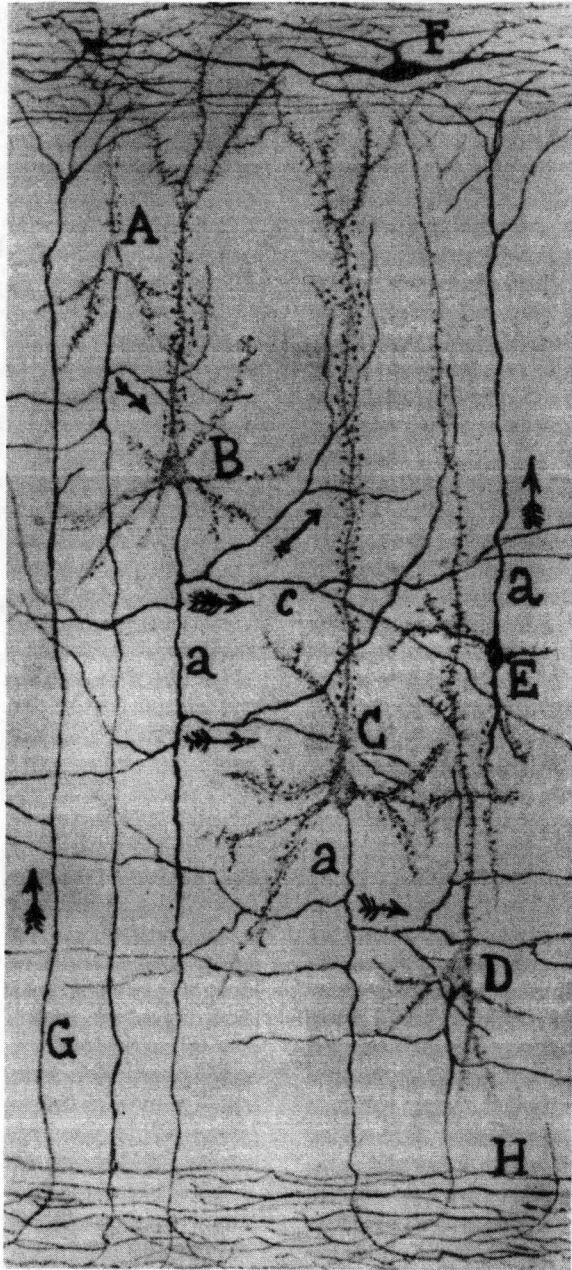

[*FIG. 278*] [Fig. 48 of *¿Neuronismo o Reticularismo?* (Cajal, 1933).] *A*, small pyramid; *B*, *C*, medium and giant pyramids; *a*, axon; *b*, [not shown] axon collaterals which appear to cross the basal and apical dendrites of the pyramids; *H*, white matter; *F*, special cells of the first layer of the cerebral cortex; *G*, fiber coming from the white matter. The arrows indicate the supposed direction of nerve impulses.

Spanish in the *Archivos de Neurobiología* (1933) an expanded version of that work, and finally, in 1934, after he died, a posthumous French version appeared in the *Travaux du Laboratoire de Recherches Biologiques*. The early proofs of this work were corrected by him, but, already suffering from the illness that would put an end to his glorious existence, he gave me the final proofs so that I could make the ultimate corrections and take care of publication.

Tello does not mention the chapter for the Bumke and Foerster *Handbuch*, but we deduce that he was a major contributor to it.

The original Spanish version of the *¿Neuronismo o Recticularismo?* and the German translation that succeeded it are of relevance to us, since a relatively long section of each draws on Cajal's cerebral cortical studies for data in further proof of the neuron doctrine. Moreover, several drawings of cortical preparations are presented, among them four that appear nowhere else [*figs. 277–280*]. His chief concern in referring to the cerebral cortex in these works is to illustrate the complex nature of axon terminations therein. He dwells on the complexity of the neuropil, the pericellular baskets, dendritic spines, and the connections between afferent fibers and the various forms of neurons in the cortex.

Cajal, in the section of *¿Neuronismo o Reticularismo?* on the cerebral cortex, is concerned with the elucidation of interneuronal connections in the cerebral cortex, which he regarded as an extremely difficult problem on account of the extraordinary length, widespread branching, and variety of orientations of the afferent nerve fibers and of the collaterals of the pyramidal cell axons. After considering the merits of the neurofibrillar [*fig. 277*] and methylene blue methods, he again concludes that only the Golgi method, though often incomplete, still furnished the most satisfactory images of these processes. He reproduces *fig. 229* to illustrate this point. He then goes on to discuss synapses between the various components of the interstitial axonal plexus of the cortex and the somata and dendritic shafts of pyramidal cells. It is to be noted that, by now, he is regularly using the term *synapse*, introduced by Sherrington in 1897 but for some time after that not entering into Cajal's publications. In the course of this exposition, Cajal introduces a new scheme of probable connections based on the assumption that the main connected elements are axon collaterals and dendrites [*fig. 278*]. He felt it likely that most of the collaterals made their contacts on dendritic spines, with some also on somata.

Cajal takes great pains to demolish a recent concept of Held's (1929) that the dendritic spines are no more than terminal boutons

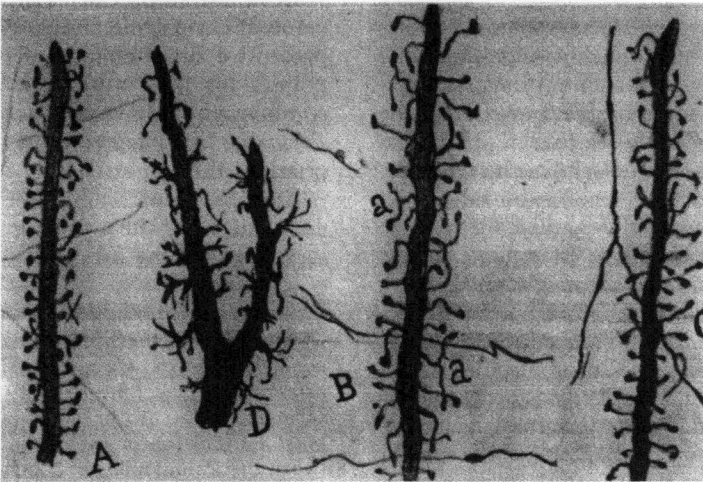

[*FIG. 279*] [Fig. 5Ő of *¿Neuronismo o Reticularismo?* (Cajal, 1933).] Types of collateral spines of cerebral pyramids. *A*, rabbit; *B*, child of two months; *C*, spines of a one-month-old cat (visual region); *D*, portion of a dendrite of a spinal motor neuron of a cat in a phase before end feet are formed.

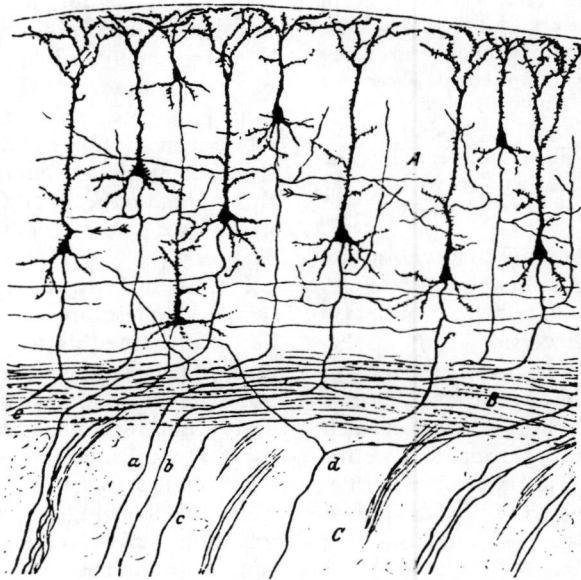

[*FIG. 280*] [Fig. 40 of *Die Neuronlehre* (Cajal, 1935).] Several pyramidal cells in the cerebral cortex (*A*) of the young mouse. In this figure, we have several cells, whose side branches (*f*) can be followed over a great extent, schematic drawing. [This figure is an extended version of fig. 48 bis from *¿Neuronismo o Reticularismo*, fig. *229* in the present volume.]

(*Endfüssen*) serving to link pyramids with one another and with the interstitial nerve plexus, and which Cajal implies is an atavistic return to Bethe's (1903) idea that the spines represented protoplasmic continuities as part of a general *neurencytium*. He says that no one has ever seen the spines' continuity with axons and that Held's preparations do not illustrate typical spines. In a long footnote, as well as in the text itself, Cajal details his part in the discovery of the spines and how it was he who promoted them at a time when most others, including Golgi himself, regarded them as an artifactual silver chromate precipitate. In fig. 50 [*fig. 279*], he shows drawings of spines from several preparations that had not been published elsewhere, and he reproduces fig. 1 [*fig. 43*] from his 1896 paper on the spines (Cajal, 1896e). A second, briefly discussed topic on the cerebral cortex is the terminations of centripetal fibers from the thalamus in the sensory cortex, and a third deals with the terminations of short axon neurons. In illustrating these, he reproduces *figs. 85* and *105,* plus an additional figure of interneuronal connections in the fascia dentata. Finally, there is brief mention of

Martinotti cells with their axons forming terminal nests about the special cells of layer I, still lovingly referred to as the *"Cajal'schen Zellen* of Retzius."

In summing up Cajal's final feelings on the cerebral cortex, the concluding paragraph represents a slight change of perspective and a pointer for the future. Having in his earlier summarizing comments, as expressed in the *Recuerdos* (see chapter 13 in this volume), emphasized the importance of the cortical interneurons, he now comes to see the input-output connections of the cortex as being the necessary focus for the future:

In summary, the little that is currently known about the types of neuroneuronal connections in the cerebral cortex confirms in principle the mode of synaptic contact in the other brain regions. However: clarification of the mode of connection between the innumerable endogenous and exogenous [elements], terminal and collateral branches arising from the thalamic, callosal, and association fibers at present constitutes an insuperable problem. In it many generations of future neurologists will put their sagacity and their patience to the test.

Editors' Notes

A. There are ninety-two figures in the German version, compared with seventy-two in the original. But many of the originals are also exchanged for others.

B. *Handbuch der Neurologie,* edited by M. Lewandowsky, Berlin, Springer, 1910–1914, 5 vols. in 6. [Our assumption, but we have not been able to identify a later edition or any contribution by Cajal. It is possible that Tello is referring to the chapter for the Bumke and Foerster *Handbook.*]

PART VI

Conclusion

A Modern View

30

The Functional Histology of the Cerebral Cortex and the Continuing Relevance of Cajal's Observations

Historical Background

Cortical histology had had approximately a fifty-year history before Santiago Ramón y Cajal commenced his initial studies on the small mammals in 1890. The earliest studies, carried out on unfixed, dissociated, and unstained material, had served to establish the existence of nerve cells in the cortex (Ehrenberg, 1833, 1836; Valentin, 1836; Remak, 1841); the possible continuity of some of these with myelinated fibers of the white matter had been suggested (Remak, 1841). Further advances, however, depended on the introduction of fixation of neural tissue in chromic acid (Hannover, 1840) or chromic salts and the even later introduction of carmine as a histological stain (Gerlach 1858, 1872). In 1849, Kölliker had been able to detect differences in the morphology of unstained neurons dissociated from the fixed human cerebral cortex, referring to pyramidal, triangular, round, and spindle forms (Kölliker, 1849, 1852). It was Berlin (1858), however, who first stained sections of the cortex with carmine and was able to discern not only the arrangement of its cells into layers but also the presence of three types

of cells that he called pyramidal, fusiform or spindlelike, and grains or granules. These terms were to predominate in Cajal's day and far beyond.

After Berlin's discoveries, the laminar patterns of cell aggregation dominated studies of the cerebral cortex for a time, starting with Meynert (1867–68, 1872) and leading directly to the great German school of cytoarchitectonics that was to have such a profound influence over cortical neuroanatomy in the first three decades of the twentieth century. (See Jones, 1984a, and Kemper and Galaburda, 1984, for recent reviews.) The layering schemes of the early contributors to this field— Meynert (1872), Lewis (1878), Lewis and Clarke (1878), Hammarberg (1895), Schlapp (1898), and Bolton (1900)—are all considered at length by Cajal in his great works on the human cortex (see chapters 13–19 in this volume). The schemes of the later contributors— Campbell (1905), Brodmann (1903a, b; 1905a, b; 1906)—were to receive consideration in the *Histologie* and in the late works. Studies of myeloarchitectonics, made possible by the introduction of the Weigert stain in 1882—notably those of Kaes (1893), Bechterew (1894),

Edinger (1896b), and Flechsig (1898)—also received close attention from Cajal.

Cajal's immediate predecessor in his approach to the cortex, however, was Golgi, since the focus of both investigators was on the cells themselves rather than on layering patterns. Several other authors were singled out by Cajal for special mention in the introduction to his *La Cellule* paper of 1891 (see chapter 5 in this volume). Among these, we should probably recognize Deiters, who in 1865 was to confirm conclusively that the axons of cortical cells were continuous with fibers of the white matter, and Kölliker, the later editions of whose textbook of histology were to carry the results of Cajal's early labors into general circulation (Kölliker, 1896). However, it was the discovery of the Golgi technique (Golgi, 1873) and Golgi's early exploitation of it in the cerebral cortex (Golgi, 1883a, b, 1884, 1885, 1886, 1894) that were to provide the stimulus to Cajal's own work. For the first time, the application of the Golgi technique permitted the staining of individual cortical neurons in their entirety—soma, dendrites, and axon. For a time, in these early days, Retzius (1891, 1893a, b, 1894) was paralleling Cajal's work in Golgi studies of the cerebral cortex. Having been "scooped" by Retzius in applying the stain to the human cortex, Cajal was to keep a wary eye on the publications of this talented Swedish worker. Martinotti (1889, 1890), the pupil of Golgi, also strongly influenced Cajal's early studies, primarily on account of his description of the axons that Cajal, more than anyone, was responsible for linking permanently with his name.

Golgi, who, at the time of Cajal's entry into the field, had largely given up research, described in detail and illustrated pyramidal cells and large, star-shaped cells in the cerebral cortex of man and animals, making clear distinctions between axons and dendrites and demonstrating, in his bicolored drawings, extensive systems of axon collaterals. No dendritic spines were illustrated or described, and although he was committed to the reticularist viewpoint, few if any of his drawings show anastomoses between the processes of different cortical cells. In general, he considered pyramidal cells a form of his type I or "motor" cell with a principal axon that left the cortex, while the star-shaped cells had highly local axonal ramifications that anastomosed in a nervous network throughout all layers of the gray matter. These constituted a form of his type II or "sensory" cell. To Golgi, dendrites represented a special nourishing element of the nerve cell, designed to bring the cell into intimate contact with blood vessels, and he considered that the apical dendrites of the pyramidal cells were a special adaptation enabling them to be brought into contact with the blood vessels entering the cortex through the molecular layer, either directly or through the numerous neuroglial cells which he considered the sole inhabitants of layer I. Golgi made little attempt to relate cortical cell morphology to the layers of the cortex and was not concerned with potential histological differences between cortical areas, mainly because he had adopted what Cajal was to call (see chapters 14 and 15 in this volume) a unicist theory of cortical organization. That is, he believed that all areas and the cellular layers of the cerebral cortex were fundamentally similar and that any functional differences they displayed would be based on their input-output connections. Golgi's drawings, therefore, while excellent representations of cortical nerve cells, have relatively little localizing value. In Golgi's defense, it should probably be pointed out that most of his work was carried out before the heyday of studies of cerebral localization. It is indicative of Cajal's greatness that he could perceive the fundamental similarity in cortical structure while seeking differences in cell type and patterns of connections that would serve as differentiating factors among individual cortical areas. These two attitudes were to dominate his work.

Cajal's Material and His Method of Analysis

Cajal's material, at least that which remains and which we have examined in the Cajal Museum, is not, comparatively speaking, extraordinary or superlative. In our opinion, he was working with Golgi-stained sections of a caliber comparable to the best being produced today, but they are not unique in their high quality [*figs. 281–285*]. Hence, what he saw

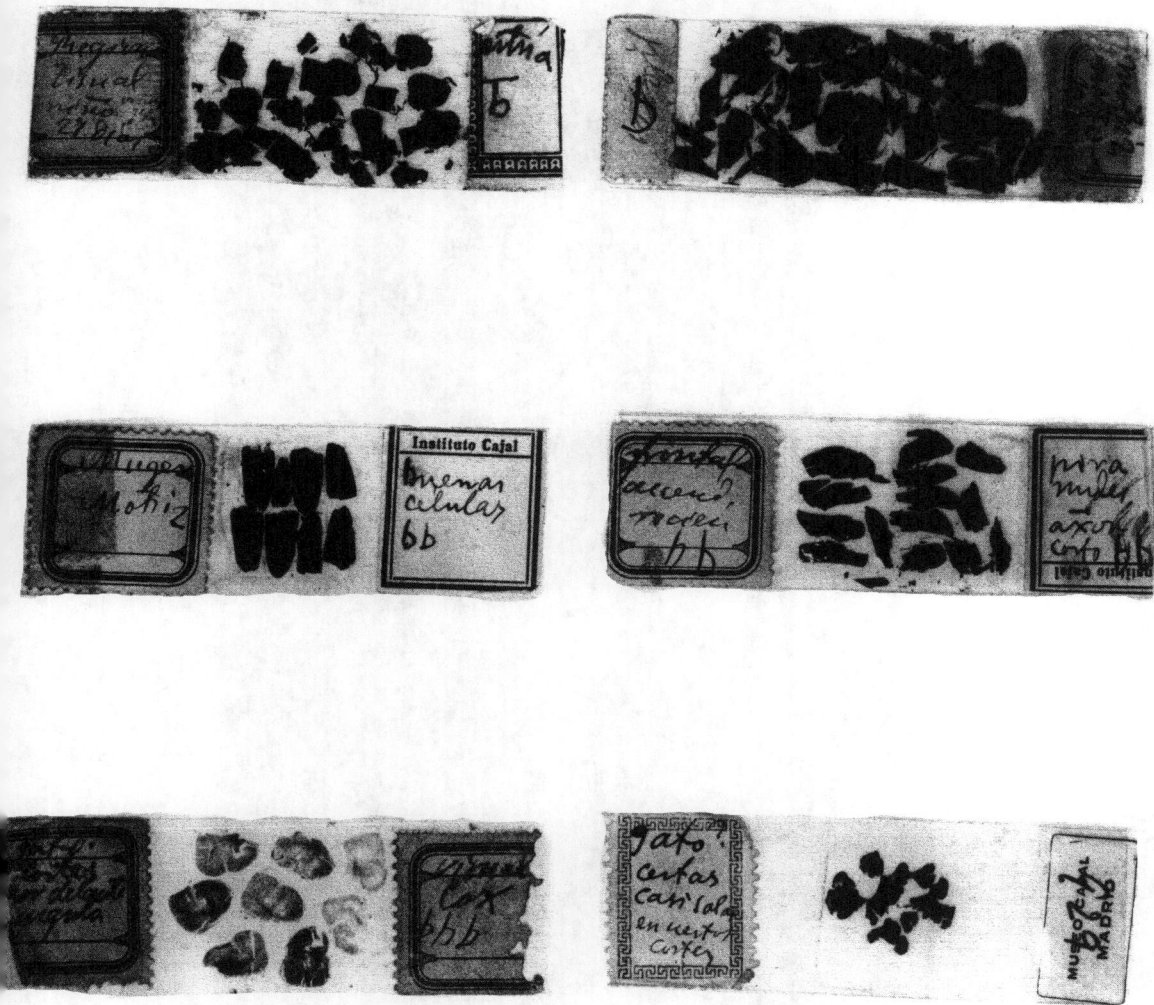

[*FIG. 281*]   Photograph of typical Cajal preparations currently housed in the Museo Cajal and labeled in Cajal's handwriting. Five of the slides contain sections from blocks of cerebral cortex. The upper four are rapid Golgi preparations; the one at lower left is a Golgi-Cox preparation, and the one at lower right (with cover slip) is a reduced silver preparation from the cerebellum. The *b*'s on the labels stand for "buena." One *b* indicates an average preparation, two *b*'s a very good preparation, and three an excellent one. Our photomicrographs [*figs. 282–285, 288, 291, 294, 295, 300, 304, 307, 319, 322, 328, 331–334*] are all taken from preparations rated with three *b*'s.

The labels read as follows. *Left column, top,* "visual region, child 27 days, stria, b"; *left middle,* "woman, motor [cortex], good cells, bb"; *left bottom,* "cat, sections in front . . . visual [cortex], Cox, bbb"; *right column, top,* "plexuses, b, motor [cortex], child 19 days"; *right middle,* "precentral gyrus, newborn [child], pyramids, short axon, bb"; *right bottom,* "cat? baskets, almost isolated in certain sections."

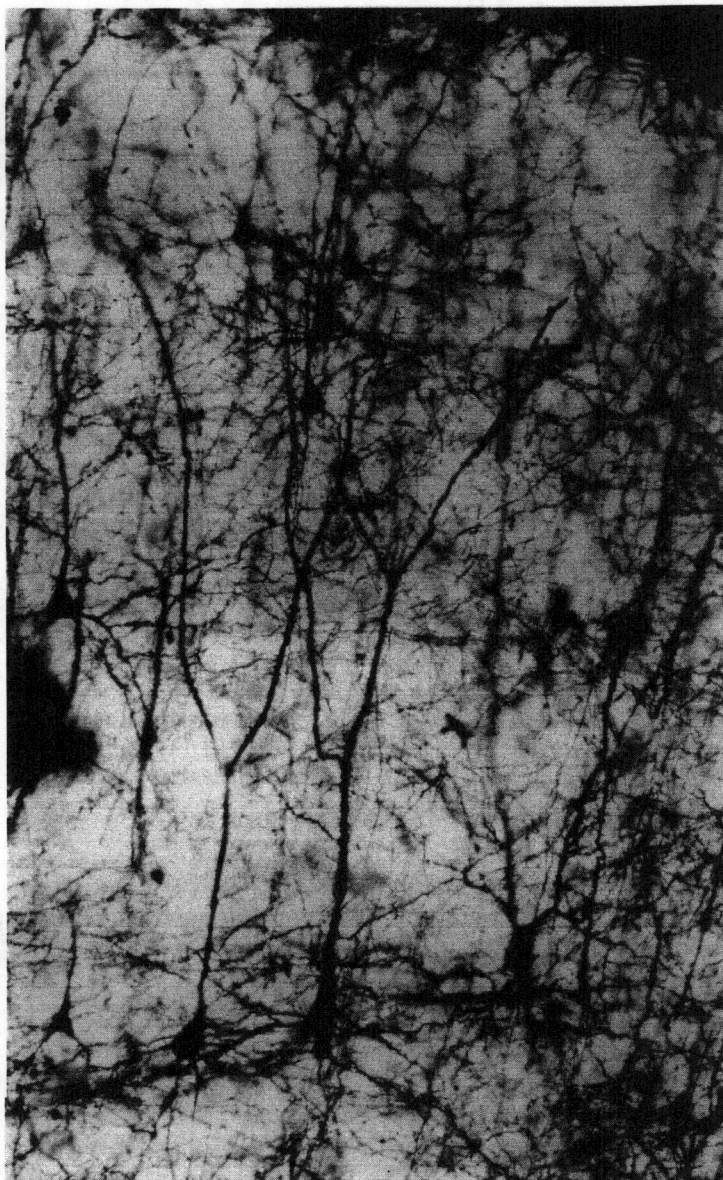

[*FIG. 282*]   Photomicrograph from a typical rapid Golgi preparation by Cajal showing pyramidal neurons in layers II–V of the cat visual cortex. × 420.

could also have been visualized by any other skilled worker of the same period. Cajal himself obviously realized this and, like any modern researcher, was frequently irritated by claims of other authors that were clearly based on material inferior to his own. It is also clear that while he was confident that the revelations of the Golgi technique, as practiced by him, were not artifactual, he was always prepared to control for potential artifacts through the use of a complementary stain. It is for this reason that he seized on the methylene blue method soon after its introduction (see chapters 9–12). Indeed, Cajal himself tacitly acknowledges in his autobiography (see chapter 1) that it was the realization that most other scientists were unwilling to venture beyond the techniques of their particular school that gave him a certain competitive edge. And, as emerges clearly throughout the preceding pages, Cajal was as competitive as any modern scientist.

Cajal's methods and his mode of working are little known to us. Only in the 1891 *La Cellule* paper (see chapter 5) does he give us any indications of his application of the Golgi technique, and this is eminently practical, with such novel procedures as painting the cortex with blood to ensure satisfactory impregnation of layer I. The great works on the human cortex and the late works on the cat and rodent cortex contain no technical details. More details are forthcoming concerning his applications of methylene blue and reduced silver stains, where he was obviously experimenting with the techniques (e.g., Cajal 1896c, 1903b–e).

Cajal's most successful Golgi preparations were those made with the rapid method (Golgi, 1875). The blocks, after fixation and silvering, were not embedded but were usually cut on a sliding microtome [*fig. 281*], though preliminary sections might be cut freehand. After dehydration and clearing, they were mounted, without coverslips, in balsam, which would have been applied in layers over many weeks. Many of these preparations retain their freshness to this day [*figs. 282–285, 288, 291, 294, 295, 300, 304, 307, 319, 322, 328, 331–334*].

It is popularly believed today that Cajal exercised a considerable degree of artistic license in making his drawings of nerve cells, and from Cajal's comments in his introduction to the German version of his paper on the cat visual cortex (Cajal, 1922a, see chapter 27 in this volume), it seems this charge was also leveled against him in his own lifetime. The only statements by Cajal about his methods of analysis are made in the *La Cellule* paper (1891d; see chapter 5 in this volume), in which he

clearly states that he used a camera lucida [*fig. 2*] for drawing his cells. We cannot, of course, rule out the possibility that he put finishing touches to the drawings while sitting up in bed, as Penfield's comments (see chapter 1) seem to imply.

Cajal certainly arranged cells from different sections artistically and in a manner pleasing to the eye, and he admits this in his rebuttal of Henschen's criticisms (see chapter 27). This, however, is part of Cajal's genius, for his choices of cells for juxtaposition were always clearly designed to make interpretive points about patterns of laminar organization of cells and fibers and about interconnections between cells and layers. It is further indicative of Cajal's genius that these interpretations nearly always remain valid to this day, and it is their placement in an artistic setting that invites the modern reader of Cajal to pay careful attention to them.

Another potential criticism that should probably be discounted is the view that Cajal's drawings of individual cells may have been composites derived from portions of several cells. We can find no evidence of this in correlating Cajal's drawings with his Golgi preparations, indeed, in several instances we feel confident that we have identified the actual cell he drew for a particular figure. Further evidence for his probity in this regard is his unwillingness to identify the pericellular baskets of layers III and V as positively arising from large stellate neurons (chapters 15, 16) and his frequently expressed frustration at not being able to follow certain long axons, particularly those of the special cells of layer I (chapters 4, 15, 16), to their destinations. It is our opinion that all of Cajal's composite figures are combinations of cells that were individually fully impregnated and that the excellence of his material and his confidence that he could use actual preparations to make generalizing statements undoubtedly account for the fact that only rarely did he resort to schematic figures.

Cajal's naming of cortical neurons and their processes was always systematic, although his common use of one or more synonyms for a particular element, such as *nests* for *baskets* and *arachniform* for *neurogliaform,* has led to

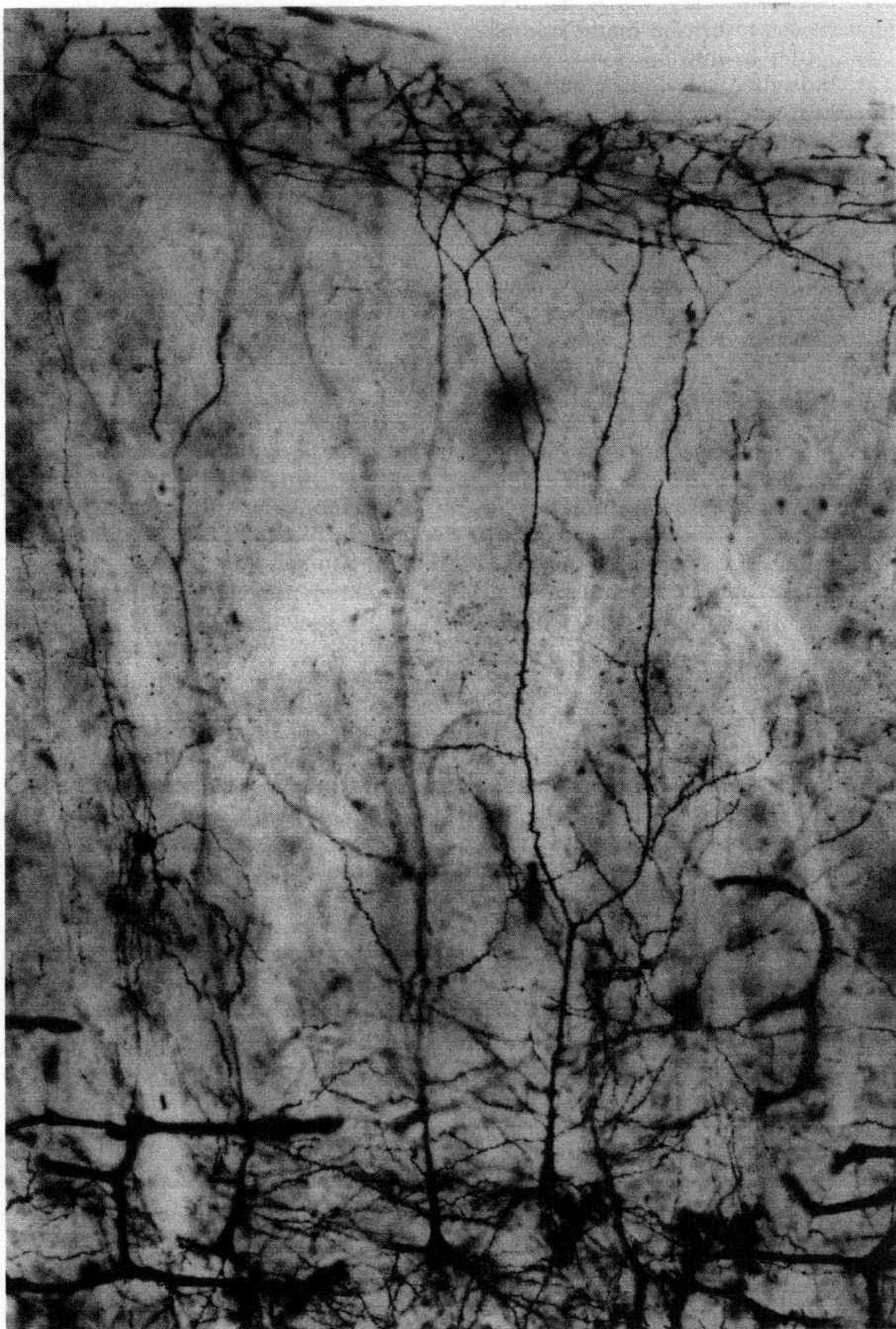

[*FIG. 283*] Photomicrograph from one of Cajal's preparations of the postcentral gyrus of a newborn human, showing layer V pyramids with their apical dendritic tufts in layer I. At left is a small nonpyramidal neuron. × 160.

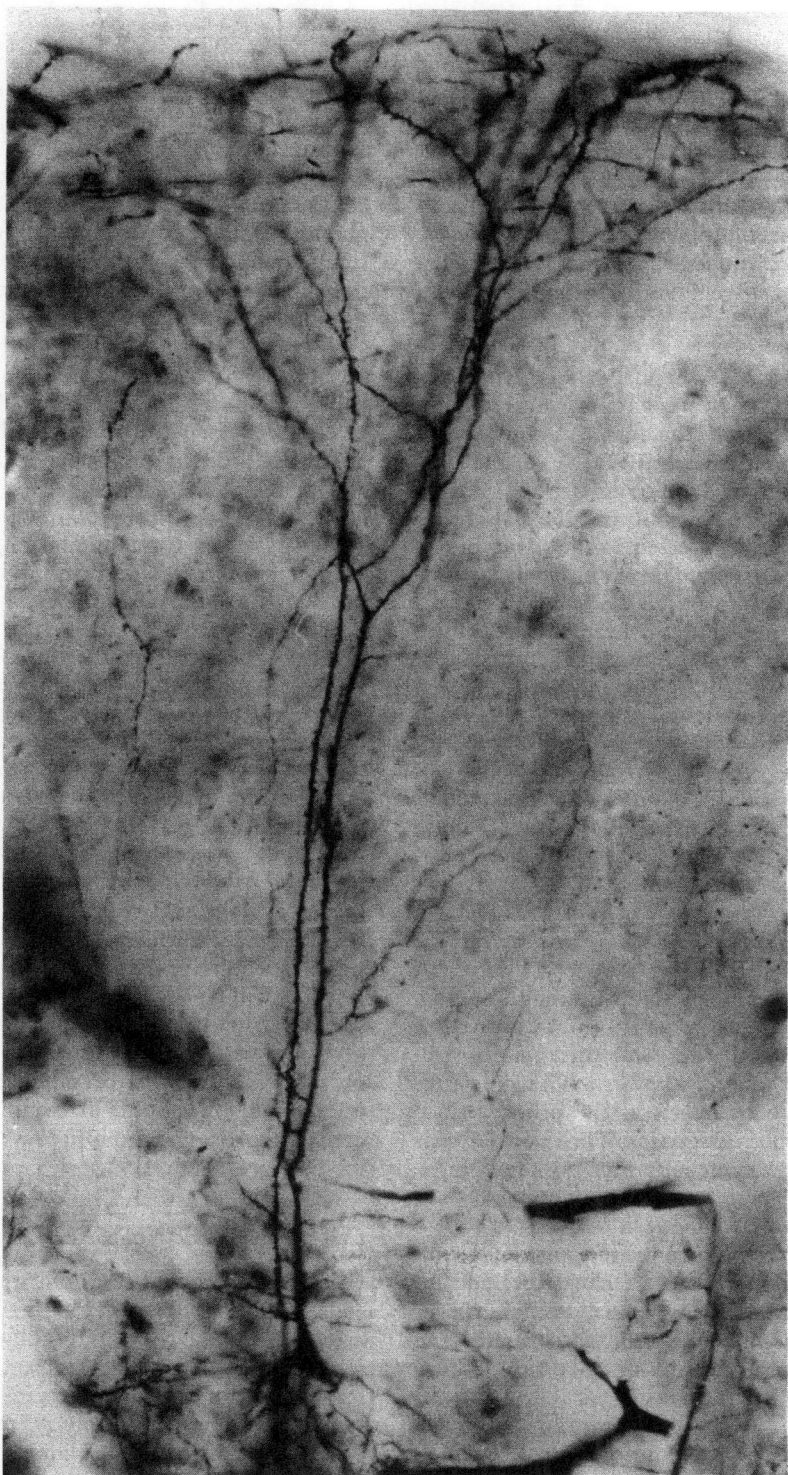

[*FIG. 284*] Photomicrograph from one of Cajal's preparations of the postcentral gyrus of a newborn child, showing the pronounced dendritic tuft formed in layer I by a layer V pyramid. × 170.

confusion in later years. A certain amount of confusion has also been introduced as a result of certain new words used by Azoulay in his otherwise faithful translation of the *Textura*, the *Histologie du système nerveux* (Cajal, 1911). Nowhere could this be more evident than in Azoulay's use of the phrase *cellule à double bouquet protoplasmique* for what Cajal called the *bitufted cell* (chapters 15, 16). Cajal was usually careful to refer to the processes of nerve cells by Deiters' (1865) terms: *protoplasmic processes* for dendrites and *axis cylinder* for axon, sometimes alternatively referring to the latter as the *functional expansion*, following van Gehuchten (1891a, b). Azoulay was thus, appropriately, referring to the bitufted nature of the dendrites. In our translation, we have consistently referred to the two types of processes as *dendrites* and *axon*, avoiding all alternatives. The bitufted cells of Cajal, regarded by him as one of the hallmarks of the human cortex, in addition to a bitufted dendritic appearance, have strongly vertical, often bidirectional bundles of axon collaterals that have been erroneously interpreted in modern times as the reason for Azoulay's appellation. Perhaps here is a case for a new term, such as *bipannacled cell*, as used felicitously for these cells by the translators of Cajal's lectures at Clark University (Cajal, 1899c).

Cajal's Contributions

Sometimes the major trends in, and scientific highlights of, Cajal's contributions to the understanding of the cerebral cortex are lost in the sheer volume of his work. This plus a reliance on the *Histologie* as the primary Cajal source and, perhaps, unfamiliarity with modes of scientific expression, such as those mentioned above but now long superseded, have sometimes caused modern workers to fail to recognize the continuing relevance of Cajal's observations on cortical cell structure and intracortical connectivity. Thus, it is not uncommon to see a "new" cell "discovered" and named without recognition that the identical cell appears in the pages of Cajal.

Cajal's genius was for description and for ordering his descriptions into rational schemes. This is why his work on the cerebral cortex re-

mains relevant in our time, since modern analyses of the cortex, whether anatomical, physiological, or chemical, are still in the descriptive phase. In the publications we have translated, Cajal emerges as no great theorist, being content to. accept the principles of dynamic polarization of the nerve cells, their functional linkages by contact, and the functional plurality of the cortical areas. He simply gets down to the business of describing cells and layers, while seeking circuits and organizational features specific for each functional cortical area. In regard to cortical function, he usually reflected the prevailing neurological dogmas of his day on associationism, learning and memory, and functional localization. Periodically, however, there are flashes of genuine insight of a fundamental neurobiological nature that were often not only far ahead of his own time but also ahead of that of succeeding generations of scientists. Now, when many of these same ideas are being resurrected, it is not generally realized that, as with so many other concepts of general neurobiological import, Cajal had been among the first to raise them. Among these we may list his ideas on dendritic growth and plasticity, on functionally regulated plasticity of connections, and on circuits for the successive elaboration of afferent activity, manifested today in receptive field analyses of neurons in the visual cortex. We will not dwell further on the more speculative aspects of Cajal's work. Readers will be able to analyze these for themselves, particularly in chapter 25. In what follows, we will select a number of anatomical observations and interpretations that are unquestionably highlights of Cajal's work on the cerebral cortex and attempt to place them in a modern perspective.

Cell Types in the Neocortex

Cajal's fundamental division of cortical neurons (chapter 7) is into long-axon cells (pyramidal cells) and short-axon cells, although he tended to split Martinotti cells off from the latter as a sort of intermediate group with semilong axons. His eye was always on two aspects of neuronal structure: fundamental similarities in morphology that transcended individual differences between neurons, and the position occupied by a particular cell class in the wiring of the cortex. He could thus (chapter 21) see that layer VI neurons, though rarely possessing a triangular soma, send an apical dendrite toward layer I and an axon into the white matter, and as a consequence have strong affinities with the more typical pyramidal cells. This is a point of view that has acquired renewed popularity today. Similarly, Cajal could see that the large spiny stellate cells in the middle layer of the visual cortex, with axons that leave the cortex, are so similar to pyramidal neurons that he felt they must have lost their apical dendrites. The usual absence of such cells from other areas of the cortex, as revealed by Cajal and in modern studies of primates, indicates that they are probably unique to the striate area. One possibility that might account for their unique structure is the high cell-packing density and thinness of this area relative to other cortical areas in primates. Cajal was also able to see the fundamental similarity between small spiny cells of layer IV with ascending axons and pyramidal neurons, in fact referring to them as small pyramids with arciform axons. In modern parlance, comparable cells are more commonly referred to as spiny stellate neurons. It is coming to be recognized, however, that a symmetrical, star-shaped form is unusual for these cells, except in the visual cortex. Elsewhere, they have a more elongated dendritic field (Jones, 1975; Lund, 1984) and can come to resemble very closely a pyramidal cell. Lorente de Nó (1922b, 1949) attempted to pursue a middle course by referring to pyramids, star cells, and star pyramids in his studies of spiny neurons in the mouse cortex.

Among the short-axon cells, Cajal also tended to generalize and, unlike his successors, made little attempt at finer classifications. He was ready, nevertheless, to point out a singular type of cell, such as the special cells of layer I or the giant cells in the auditory cortex, when he encountered it. It is Cajal's capacity for generalization that can make a cursory reading of his works unsatisfactory, if the reader is seeking to determine what are Cajal's fundamental classes of neuron with short axon in the cortex. Instead of giving a basic classifica-

tion, he describes the cells as he sees them in each layer. Although some, such as the small pyramids with arciform axon, are restricted to a particular layer, others are not, and their forms may be modulated from layer to layer.

Leaving aside the special cells of layer I and the giant cells that he thought, erroneously, to be unique to the auditory cortex, Cajal's basic subdivision of cortical neurons is as follows. Cells with long axon included pyramidal cells and certain other forms, usually referred to as triangular or fusiform, which he saw as modified pyramids, plus the large stellate cells described mainly in layer IV of the visual cortex but also mentioned in the motor cortex. These he also tended to regard as a modified form of pyramid. In the group of cells with short axon, he usually distinguished neurogliaform or arachniform cells, bitufted cells, small pyramids with arciform axon, cells giving rise to pericellular nests, cells with ascending axon (usually but not invariably regarded as synonymous with Martinotti cells), and cells with rather vaguely defined, locally ramifying axons ("short-axon cells," not otherwise specified).

Apart from the pyramidal cells and the bitufted cells, Cajal paid little attention to dendritic morphology or somal shape as means of cell classification. To him, it was the distribution of the axon that was the all-important criterion to be used in classifying short-axon cells, and his classification of pyramidal cells and what he saw as their modified forms also depends to a considerable extent on axonal (including collateral) distribution patterns. In this, his work has a decidedly modern flavor.

Pyramidal Cells

A modern definition of a pyramidal cell would unquestionably incorporate all of the following elements: substantial apical and basal dendritic systems covered in dendritic spines and an axon that leaves the cortex for other cortical areas or subcortical sites (see Feldman, 1984). Such a definition obviously incorporates Cajal's recognition that a cell need not have a pyramidal cell body in order to be incorporated in the definition. In this modern usage, however, the term *pyramidal cell* has tended to become a shorthand way of saying *long-axon*

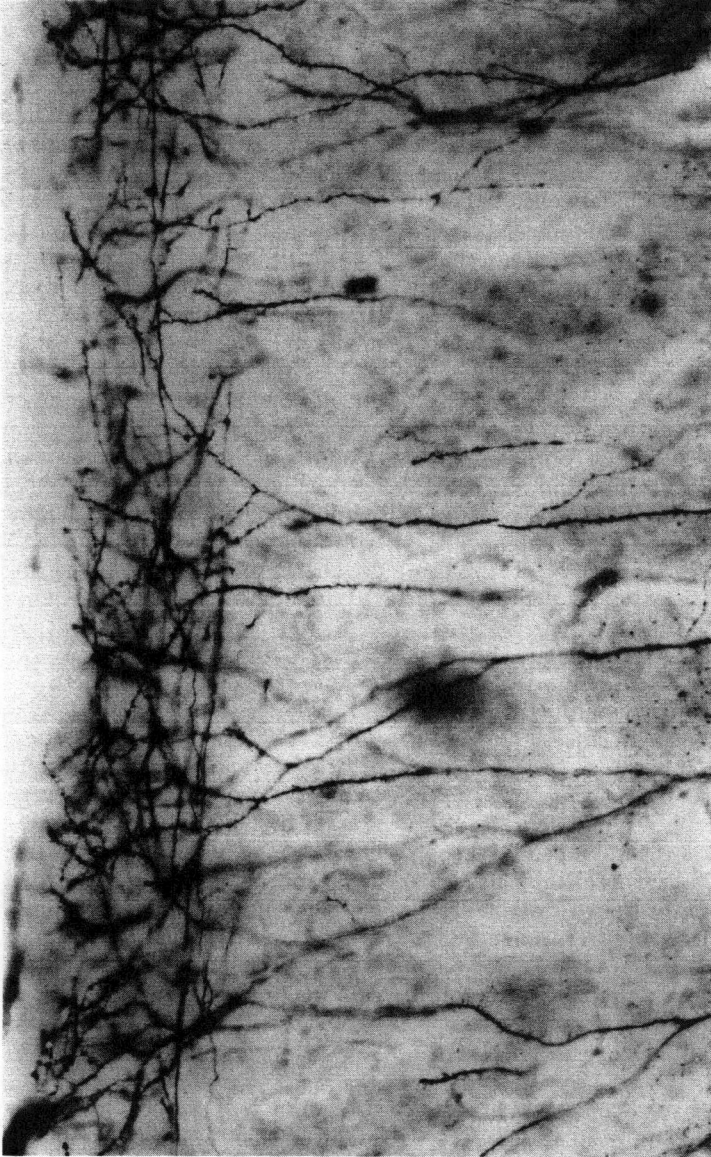

[*FIG. 285*]   Photomicrograph from one of Cajal's preparations of the postcentral gyrus of a newborn child, showing layer I apical dendritic tufts, some of which could be traced to apical dendrites of layer V pyramidal cells. Note horizontal axons of layer I. × 200.

---→

[*FIG. 286*]   Camera lucida drawing by F. Valverde, showing large pyramidal neurons of layer V, spiny non-pyramidal neurons with arciform axons, and certain other forms of neuron in the visual cortex of a monkey. *From:* Valverde (1985).

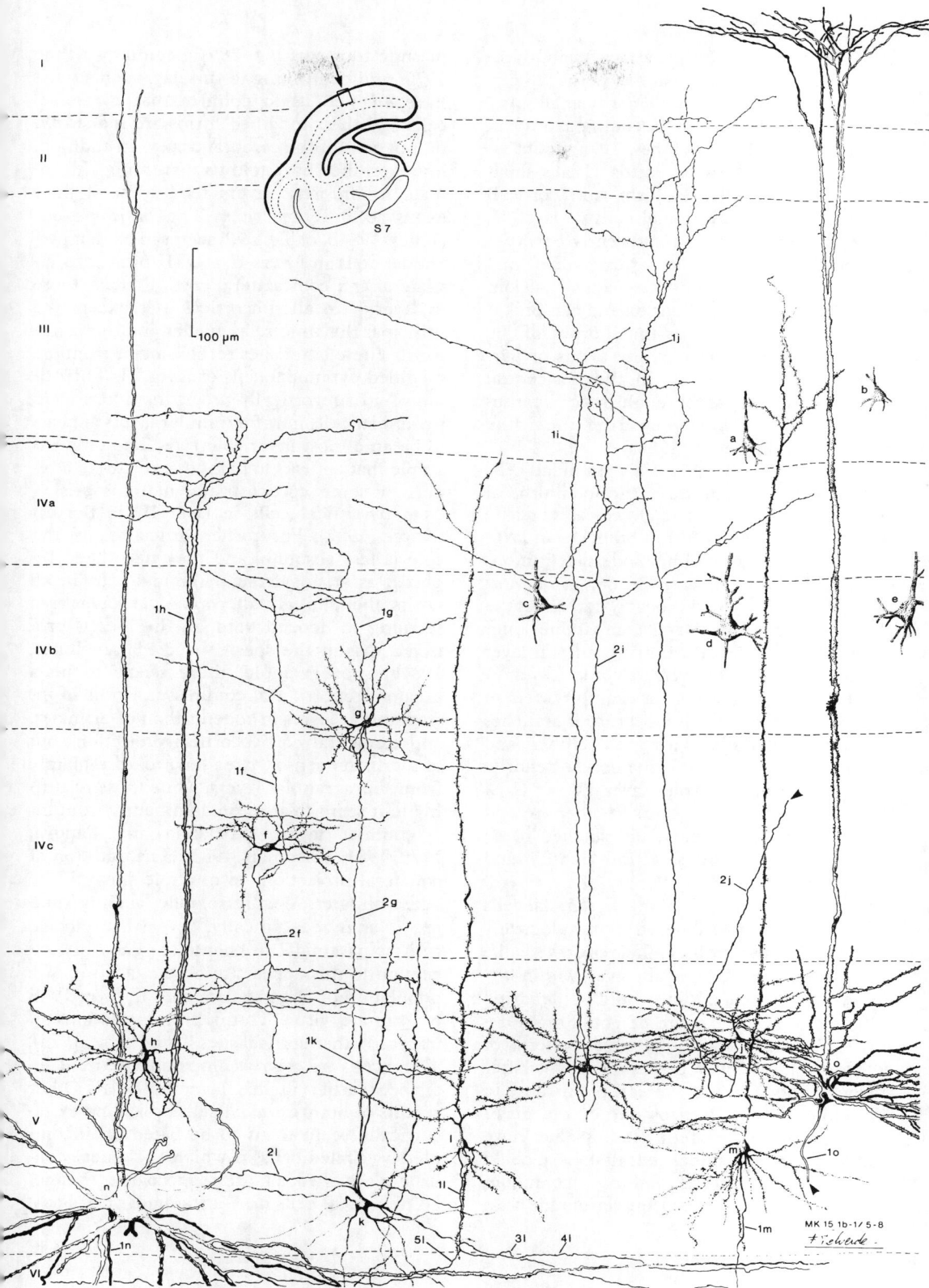

I

II

III

100 µm

IVa

IVb

IVc

V

VI

S 7

1j

1i

1h

1g

1f

g

f

2f

2g

c

2i

a

b

d

e

2j

h

1k

i

o

2l

n

l

1l

m

1o

k

1n

5l

3l

4l

1m

MK 15 1b-1/ 5-8

Fichwede.

cell. The emphasis on the extracortical projection of pyramidal neurons has perhaps been overstated when one considers that small spiny neurons of layer IV with ascending axons can in many cortical areas (Jones, 1975) adopt an elongated form, thus becoming Cajal's small pyramidal cells with arciform (intracortical) axons. The small pyramidal cells of layer II, some of whose axons have recently been described as not leaving the cortex (Gilbert and Wiesel, 1983), certainly have axons that join quite distant patches of cortex and can probably still be considered as the shortest of the long-axon cells. Moreover, the axons of pyramidal cells of layer III in the postcentral gyrus can clearly pass through large expanses of cortex before finally entering the white matter (DeFelipe et al., 1986a).

Cajal's insistence that all pyramidal cells and their fusiform brethren in the entorhinal and piriform cortex had an apical dendrite forming a substantial tuft of branches in layer I does not always enter into modern definitions of pyramidal cells [*figs. 282–288, 290*]. Most modern workers would probably agree that the majority of pyramidal and comparable long-axon cells have apical dendritic tufts in layer I. Certain forms, however, may not. Layer VI corticothalamic neurons, for example, seem to end their apical dendrites as a tuft of branches in layer IV of the visual cortex (Gilbert and Wiesel, 1979), and even if the parent dendrite continues onward beyond layer IV, as Cajal had recognized and as occurs in other areas, it usually ends as a solitary, unbranched trunk (Valverde, 1971; Jones, 1975; Hendry and Jones, 1983a).

Cajal clearly recognized that pyramidal cells in animals and man differed morphologically [*fig. 288*]. At the very least, their sizes were different from layer to layer and even within layers. Allied with this, there could be dendritic differences, but, above all, he could often detect variations in the intracortical patterns of collateral branching of their axons as the latter traversed the layers of the cortex en route to the white matter. Perhaps one of the major contributions of modern studies that have added data on pyramidal cells that Cajal could not provide are those derived from techniques of cellular labeling based on retrograde axo-

plasmic transport [*fig. 289*]. Beginning in the 1970s and continuing to this day, such studies have enabled us to confirm that pyramidal cells and their modified forms are indeed *the* output cells of the cerebral cortex. In addition, however, they have told us that those with somata in different layers tend to send their axons to different sites. The basic pattern (Jones, 1984b, c) [*fig. 290*] seems to be that pyramidal cells in layers II and III project to ipsilateral and contralateral cortical areas, those in layer V to all subcortical sites except the principal thalamic relay nuclei and the claustrum. These latter sites receive axons from the modified pyramidal cells of layer VI. The origin of all subcortically projecting axons from pyramidal cells in infragranular layers appears to be an almost invariable rule. The only example that appears to gainsay it relates to a report of some corticostriatal neurons arising from pyramidal cells in layer III in the cat (Royce, 1982). For corticocortical axons, the rule is less absolute, and they have been reported as arising from pyramidal cells in all layers, the laminar pattern in a particular area seeming to depend both on the area(s) projected to and the species studied (see Jones, 1984b). For example, there seems to be a greater proportion of commissural cells in infragranular layers of rodents than of primates, and ipsilateral corticocortical projections out of a primary sensory area tend to arise mainly from supragranular layers, while those returning to it seem to arise predominantly from infragranular layers (Rockland and Pandya, 1979, 1981; Friedman, 1983). The question of collateral projections to multiple sites will be taken up later. Most retrograde labeling studies, if analyzed critically, reveal the labeled cells as pyramidal in character. The only exception to this appears to be the labeling of a population of large stellate cells in layer IV B of primate visual cortex from injections of tracer in other cortical sites (Lund et al., 1975). These cells are clearly comparable to those described earlier in this layer by Cajal. Other reports of nonpyramidal cells projecting extracortically seem to us to be based on incompletely labeled cells in which the apical dendrite is not filled, a failure to recognize that not all pyramidal cells have a triangular cell body,

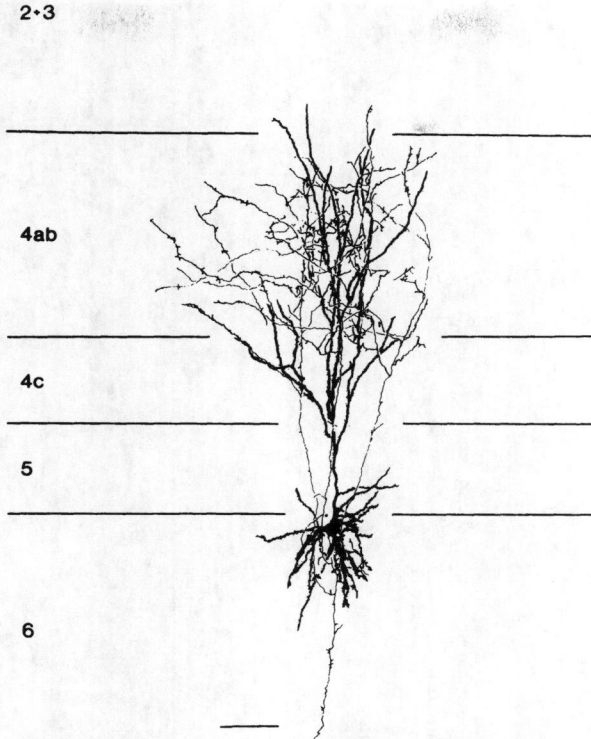

[FIG. 287]   Intracellularly injected layer VI neuron in cat visual cortex. The cell is typical of the modified pyramids of that layer and has strongly recurrent axon branches to layer IV, in which its dendritic tuft receives thalamocortical axon terminals. The primary axon projects subcortically, commonly to the thalamus. *From:* Gilbert and Wiesel (1979).

and the labeling of the modified ("fusiform") pyramids of layer VI.

Apart from their differential connections, the morphologies of different classes of pyramidal cells have also received attention in recent studies, especially those involving intracellular recording and injection of tracers into the cells, with subsequent histological recovery. While many aspects of these studies can be seen as generally confirming Cajal's earlier descriptions, such as the peculiar, foreshortened nature of layer II pyramids [*fig. 291*], others present interesting new sidelights. At the dendritic level, Deschênes et al. (1979) have shown that in a population of layer V pyramids of the cat, positively identified as projecting into the pyramidal tract, those having the functional characteristics of "slow" pyramidal tract neurons possess small somata

and quite restricted systems of basal dendritic branches and few side branches of the apical dendrite, but an extensive tuft of very spiny dendritic branches in layer I. By contrast, those characterized as "fast" pyramidal tract neurons have larger somata and apical and basal dendritic systems that are more widespread in the tangential plane, but a relatively less extensive tuft of relatively aspiny branches in layer I.

On the axonal side, pyramidal neurons of the same layer in cat visual cortex but with different types of receptive field can have quite different patterns of intracortical axon collaterals [*fig. 292*]. Layer V cells with standard complex receptive fields and projecting to the superior colliculus have very extensive collaterals in layer VI, while those with special complex receptive fields have few (Gilbert and

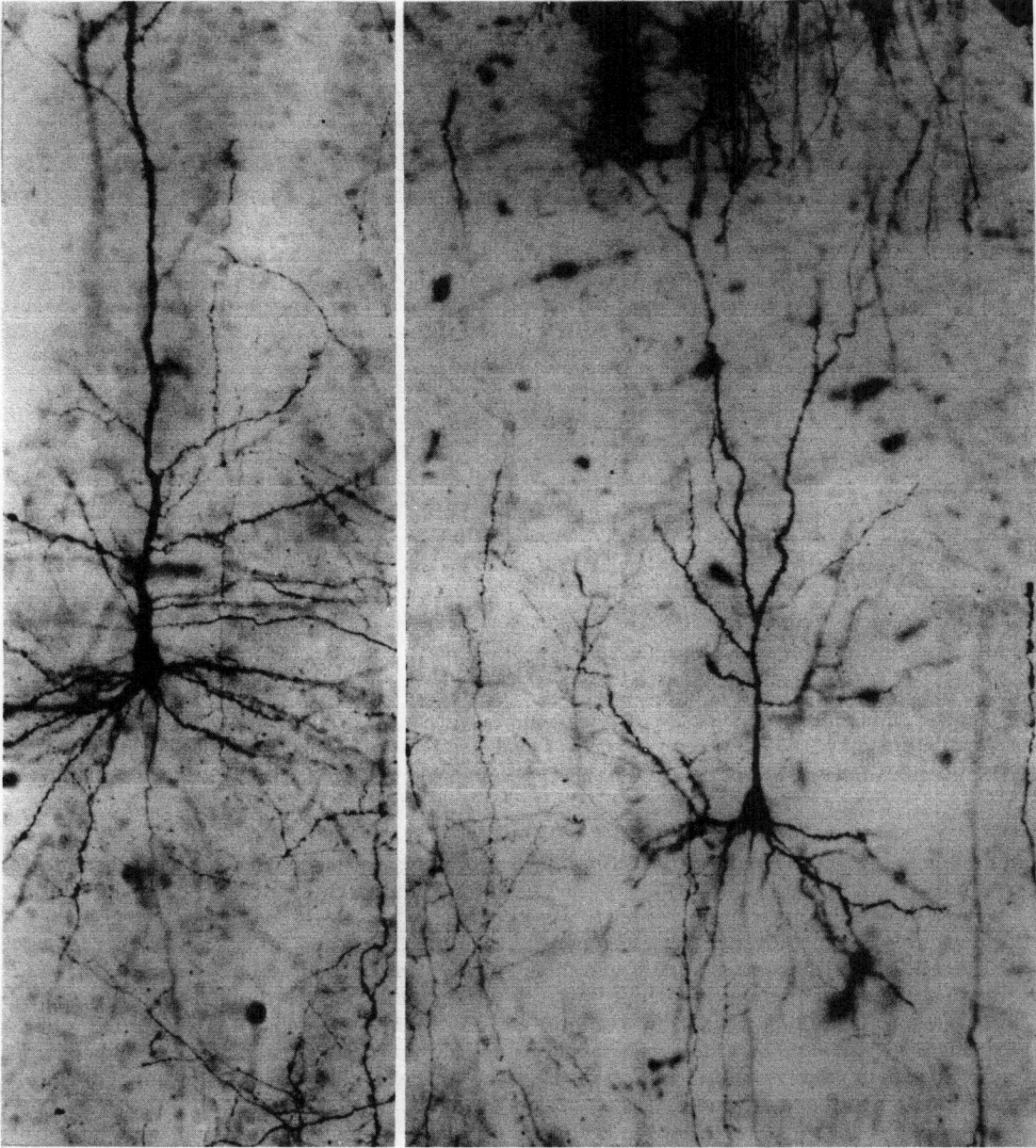

[*FIG. 288*]   Photomicrographs from Cajal's preparations, showing deep layer III pyramids in the precentral gyrus of a fifteen-day-old child (left) and in the visual cortex of a one-month-old cat. Both × 250.

Wiesel, 1979, 1981). These two kinds of layer V pyramidal cells, themselves, appear to be differentially affected by connections descending from layer III and which consist, at least in part, of the collaterals of the axons of layer III

pyramids [*fig. 293*] (Gilbert and Wiesel, 1979, 1983). After deactivating the supragranular layers by cooling, corticotectal cells with standard complex properties become silent, while those with special complex properties remain unaffected (Schwark et al., 1986; Weyand et al., 1986). It now appears that pyramidal cells of different receptive field types and/or with cell bodies in different layers can have quite unique patterns of intracortical axonal collateralization—another modern verification of Cajal's earlier intimations—and these have quite important implications for tracing intracortical circuitry, as will be discussed below.

Dendritic Spines

Cajal made much of the dendritic spines of pyramidal cells (chapters 9–12 and 29 in this volume), although for a time even his usually most ardent supporter, Kölliker, was inclined to view them as artifacts of the Golgi procedure [*fig. 294*]. Golgi professed to never having observed them. It was with some glee, therefore, that Cajal seized on methylene blue as a method for independently verifying their existence. There seems to be little question that Cajal saw the dendritic spines as major sites of synaptic connection, a point that had to await the early days of electron microscopy for final verification (Gray, 1959). Even then, it came as some surprise that the vast majority of synapses on pyramidal cells were on dendritic spines, large areas of the somal and dendritic shaft surfaces being free of synapses (Colonnier, 1968; Jones and Powell, 1970a; Peters and Kaiserman-Abramof, 1969). The biophysical workings of the spine synapse continue to be sources of considerable theorizing (Jack et al., 1975 Shepherd et al., 1985). Cajal also clearly had intimations of the functional plasticity of dendritic spines, as expressed here in chapter 25, and also a subject of many inter-

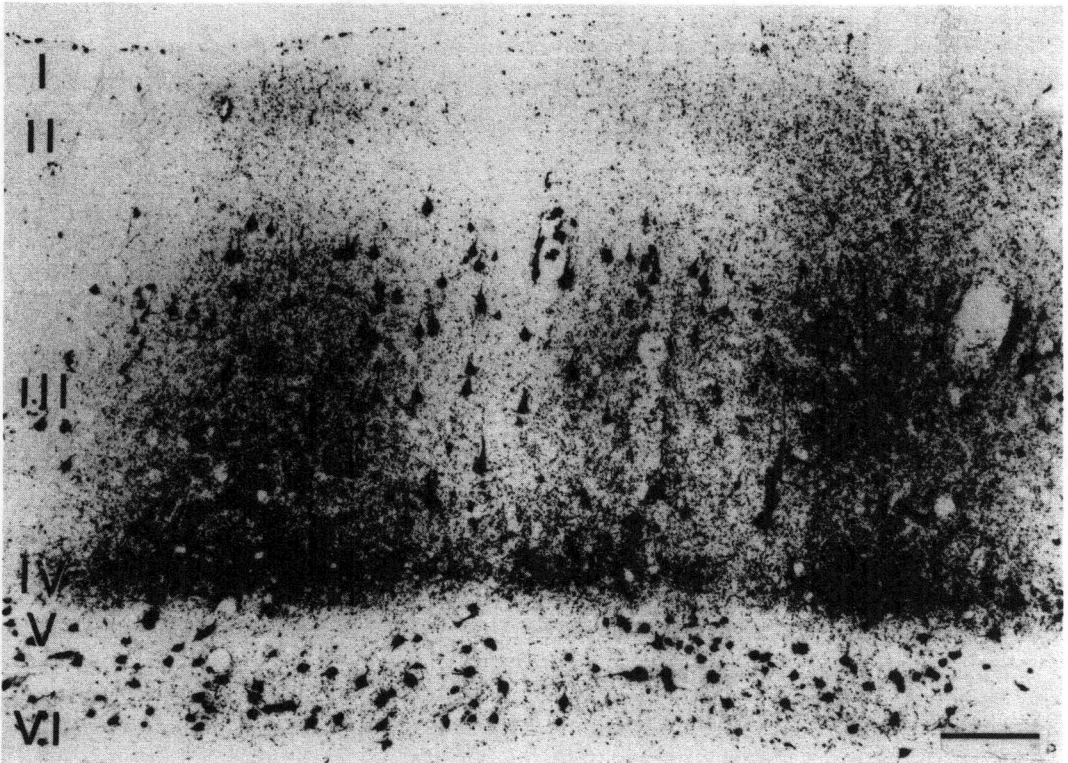

[*FIG. 289*] Retrograde labeling of pyramidal cells, primarily in layers III and VI, and anterograde labeling of axon terminations, primarily in layers II–IV, in the second somatic sensory area of a monkey in which horseradish perixodase had been injected into the first somatic sensory area two days previously. Bar 500 μm. *From:* Friedman et al. (1980).

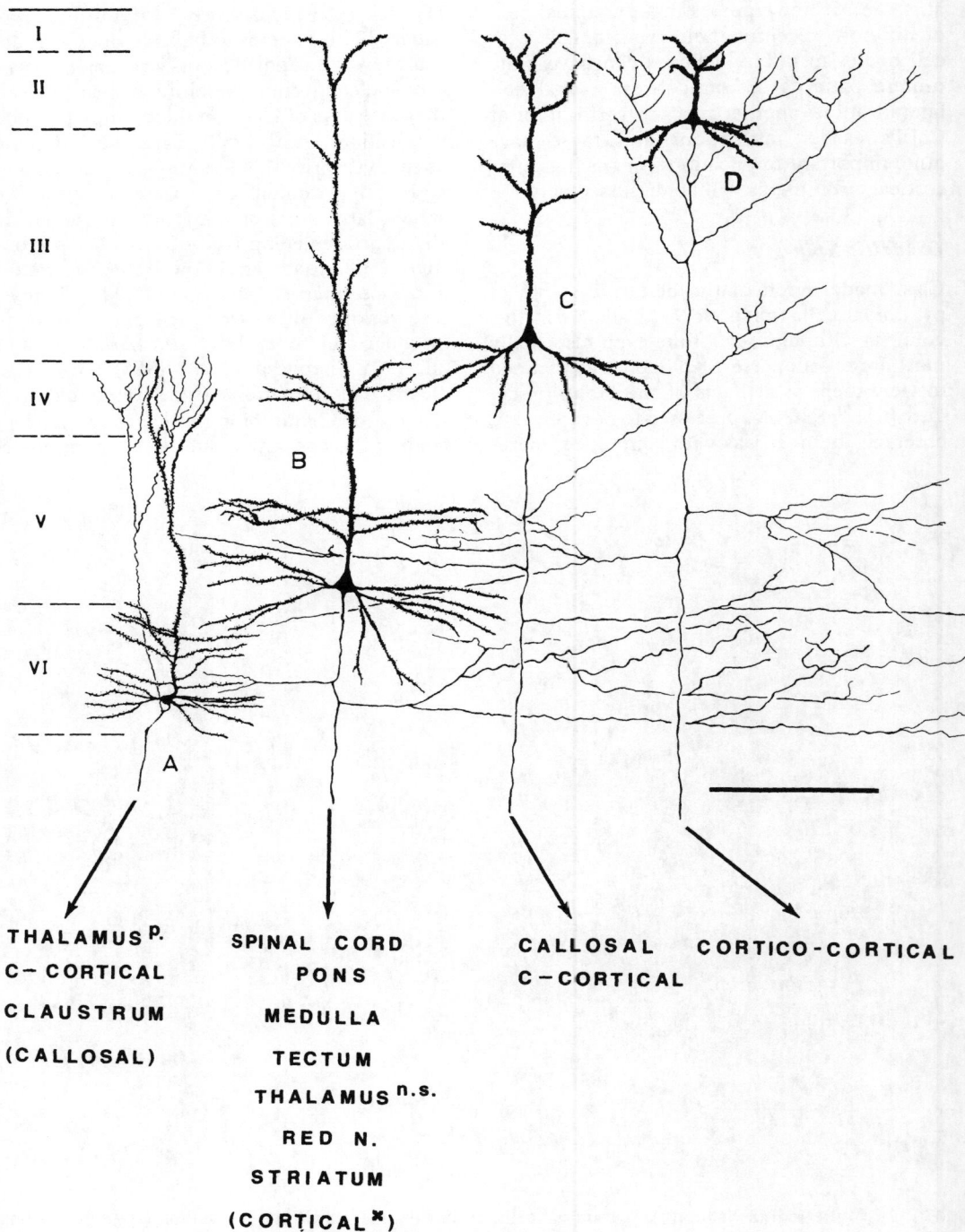

[*FIG. 290*] Schematic summary of the major targets of pyramidal neurons in layers II, III, V, and VI of the monkey cortex. *n.s.*, nonspecific thalamic nuclei; *p*, principal thalamic relay nuclei; *x*, from some cortical areas only. *From:* Jones (1984b).

esting recent conjectures (e.g., Crick, 1982) and experimental studies (e.g. Valverde and Esteban, 1968; Valverde, 1968).

Although clearly recognizing their predominance on pyramidal neurons, Cajal made little attempt to use the presence or absence of dendritic spines as a defining characteristic of cortical neurons, pyramidal or nonpyramidal. One reason for this may lie in the fact that his material, as revealed in his drawings, seemed to demonstrate considerable populations of spines on most forms of cortical neuron—even on forms that are usually recognized today as being essentially aspiny. The customary explanation of this difference between Cajal's material and that produced in modern Golgi studies is his consistent use of immature and even fetal brains. In these, as shown in a number of later studies (Marin-Padilla, 1969; Jones, 1975; Lund et al., 1977), there seems to be a transient hyperproduction of dendritic spines on neurons that will subsequently become largely or wholly spine-free.

Spiny Stellate Cells

This small, spine-laden intrinsic neuron, apparently exclusively localized in the middle layers of the cortex (especially layer IV), and the subject of much modern research (see Lund, 1984), was apparently never described by Cajal. It is our opinion, however, that he would have seen the spiny stellate neuron of modern descriptions as belonging to his category of small pyramidal neurons with arciform axons [figs. 296–298].

The spiny stellate neuron—a small layer IV cell, with a round soma, a radiating perisomatic rather than a basal system of dendrites, and lacking a pronounced apical dendrite—has been extensively described in the visual cortex of many species (Lund, 1973; Le Vay, 1973; Gilbert and Wiesel, 1979; Lund et al., 1979; Martin and Whitteridge, 1984). In the visual cortex, the cell has acquired a certain prominence on account of its correlation, in intracellular staining studies, with cortical neurons having simple receptive fields and because of the distribution of its axon. The axon can have a relatively slender descending branch to layers V and VI, but the greater part of the axonal

ramification is formed by a series of recurrent, "arciform" collaterals, given off shortly after the origin of the axon and ascending vertically into layers III and II. As a consequence, they are often seen as representing a major relay in the circuit linking simple cells at the heart of the layer of thalamic terminations to complex cells in the supervening layers (e.g., Gilbert, 1983).

Outside the primary visual cortex, exactly comparable spiny stellate neurons are difficult to find. Cells similar to those in the primary visual area can be observed where the cortical layers are compressed in the floor of a sulcus (Jones, 1975) or in special situations such as the "barrels" of the rodent somatic sensory area (Woolsey et al., 1975). Elsewhere, however, the spiny stellate neuron appears to be drawn out into an elongated form, with a pronounced ascending dendritic system that may even approach layer I (Jones, 1975). The radiating perisomatic system of dendrites is usually retained, as are the strongly recurrent axon collaterals that are often more obviously bundled than in the striate area and contribute an ascending element to the radial fasciculi (Szentágothai 1970, 1973; Jones, 1975) [figs. 296–298]. In these, they seem to enfold the apical dendrites of pyramidal cells. There seems to be little doubt that the small spiny cells are Cajal's small pyramids with arciform axon, but in morphology, as indicated above, and in spine distribution (Jones, 1975; Peters and Jones, 1984), they also appear to be the more widely distributed version of the spiny stellate neuron. Even in the visual cortex itself, some authors, such as Valverde (1971) [fig. 286], show the spiny stellate neurons with substantial ascending dendrites. Recognition of the commonality caused Lorente de Nó (1949) to call the elongated form of the cell a "star pyramid." Others, identifying the cell more with the pyramidal cells, have been led to believe that no spiny stellate neurons occur in particular areas of the cortex (Ramón-Moliner, 1961a–c; Lund et al., 1981). It seems to us that a small spiny cell resident among the main layer of thalamic terminations, and with strongly recurrent axon collaterals, is, indeed, a feature of all cortical areas, irrespective of its precise appellation. Cajal's emphasis on axonal

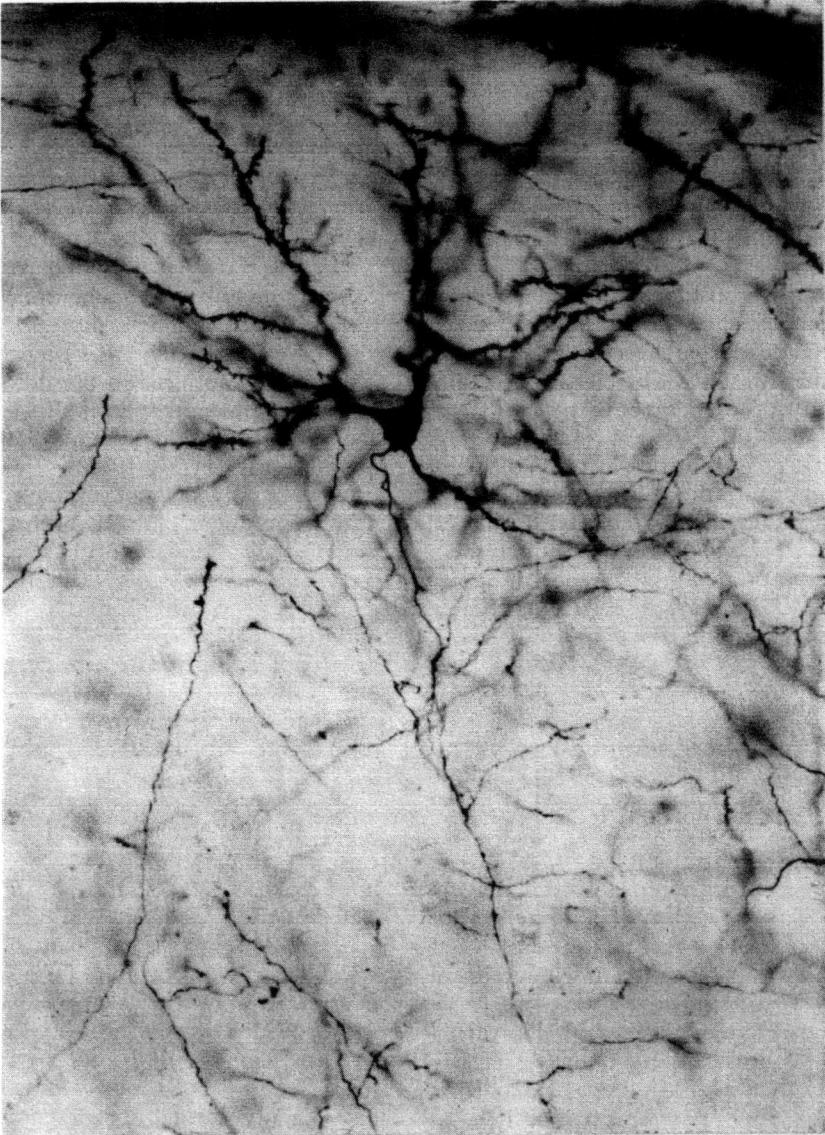

[*FIG. 291*] Photomicrograph from one of Cajal's preparations of the visual cortex of a one-month-old cat, showing a typical layer II pyramid with its bifid apical dendritic system, its axon, and axon collaterals. × 500.

distribution as the chief morphological condition of cell type is more than amply justified in this case.

These small spiny cells with ascending axons have the features of an excitatory cortical interneuron. Their axon collaterals make asymmetric synapses, predominantly on the dendritic spines of other spiny cells (LeVay, 1973; Saint Marie and Peters, 1985; White, 1978; White and Rock, 1980). They are evidently not GABAergic (Houser et al., 1983b; Hendry et al., 1983a), but, in staining positively for glutamate (Conti et al., 1987), they may use an excitatory amino acid transmitter.

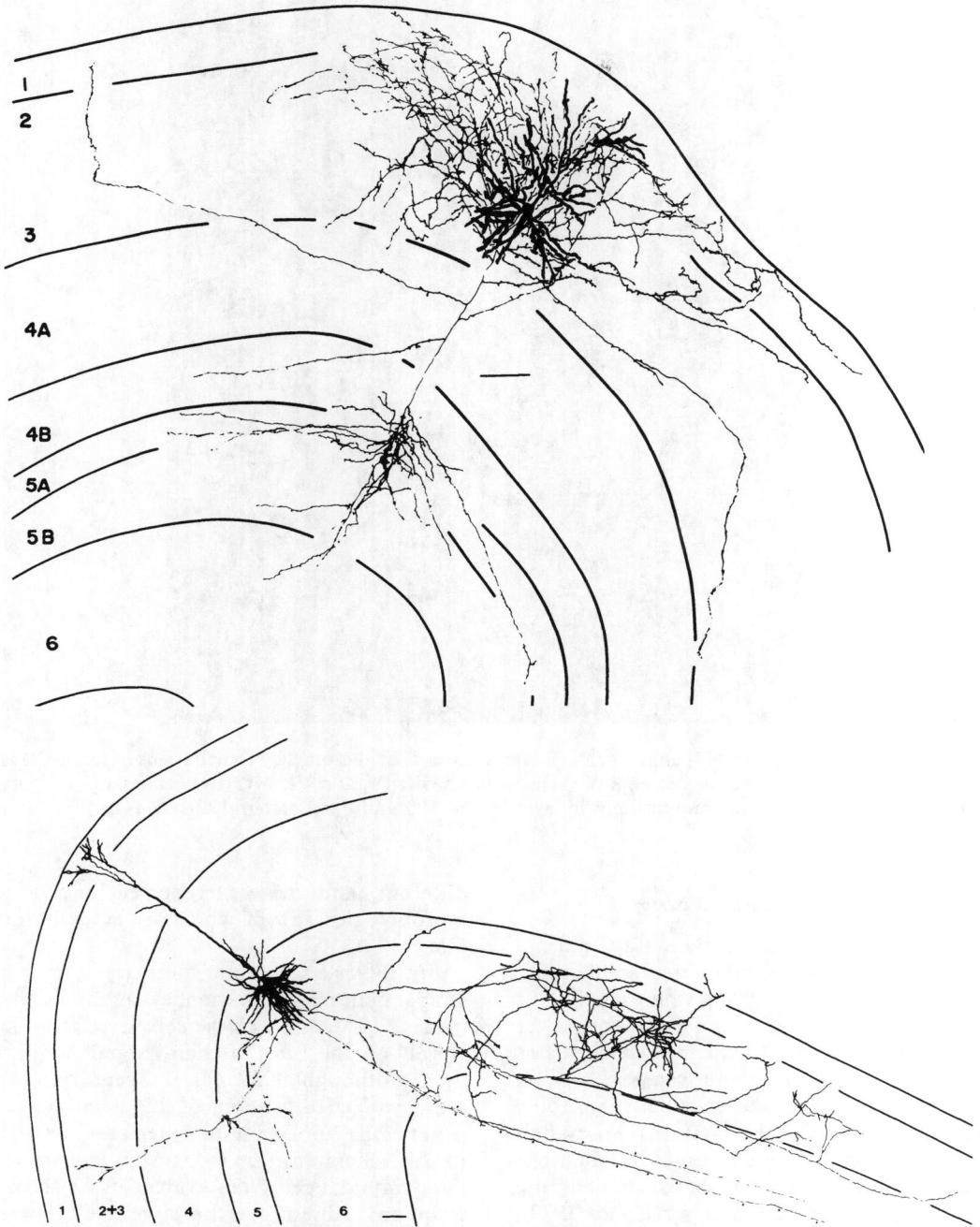

[*FIG. 292*] Intracellularly injected pyramidal neurons in layers III (*above*) and V (*below*) of the visual cortex of the cat, showing the differential laminar distributions of the intracortical collaterals of their axons. Bars 100 μm. *From:* Martin (1984, *above*) and Gilbert and Wiesel (1979, *below*).

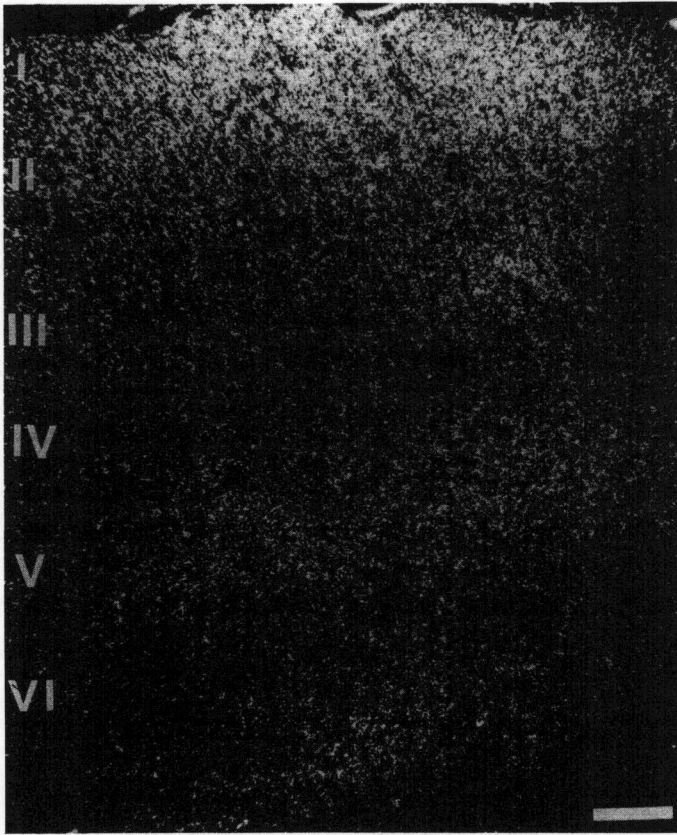

[*FIG. 293*]   An injection of [³H] amino acids in layers I and II of the monkey somatic sensory cortex leads to autoradiographic labeling of descending axons in layers III, IV, and VI, with an accumulation of label indicative of terminal axonal ramifications in layer V. Bar 100 μm. *From material described in:* Jones et al. (1978).

Nonspiny, Nonpyramidal Neurons

For reasons mentioned earlier, Cajal did not use dendritic spine population as an identifier for cell class. However, with the exception of the small pyramid with arciform axon, all of his short-axon neurons can be recognized as belonging to one or another category of what are now recognized as essentially nonspiny neurons. The distinction between "spiny stellate" neurons and intrinsic cortical neurons that lacked significant populations of dendritic spines was first emphasized by Lund (1973), while Jones (1975) advocated the use of the term *nonpyramidal* as an alternative to *stellate* for all intrinsic neurons, because most showed

different, and quite stereotyped, individual morphologies, few of which are actually star-like.

Fig. 299 is a schematic summary of nonpyramidal neurons in the monkey cerebral cortex (Jones, 1975), in which the cells were classified largely on the basis of their axonal ramifications. Although made for the sensory-motor areas, with modifications of fine detail only, it is generally applicable to other areas as well. In this scheme can be recognized most of the nonpyramidal cell types evident in Cajal's descriptions. Absent are the large stellate neurons of layer IV B in the visual cortex whose axons pass to other cortical areas (chapters 15 and 27 in this volume). Also absent are the special cells of layer I, probably because the classification was derived from adult specimens (see below), and the giant cells thought by Cajal to be specific for auditory cortex, although these were later found in small numbers in the sensory-motor areas (Jones, 1975). Classical Martinotti cells are also not shown (see below).

In the scheme can be seen very large neurons (A) with a short vertical axon giving off long horizontal collaterals ending in nests or baskets. The deeper of these cells, in layers III and V, have a very large soma that in motor cortex can approach in size that of the Betz cells (DeFelipe et al., 1986b). They are clearly the progenitors of the pericellular baskets of Cajal, as initially confirmed by Marin-Padilla (1969, 1970a, b). Hence their current name, *basket cells*. The horizontal axon collaterals are myelinated (DeFelipe et al., 1986b) and can be several millimeters in length, especially in the sensory-motor areas of primates, where they are preferentially oriented in the sagittal direction (Marin-Padilla, 1969; Jones, 1975). They terminate in symmetric synapses on the somata and proximal dendrites of pyramidal cells and of other basket cells (Somogyi et al., 1983b; DeFelipe et al., 1986b). The basket cells and their terminals, from immunocytochemical studies, indubitably appear to be GABAergic (Freund et al., 1983; Houser et al., 1983b, 1984; Hendry et al., 1983a; DeFelipe et al., 1986b) [*figs. 300–303*].

The *double bouquet cell* (H) is clearly identical to Cajal's bitufted or bipannacled cell (Azoulay's *cellule à double bouquet protoplasmique* or *dendritique*). It was first demonstrated again in its entirety in modern times by Jones (1975), possibly because most intervening studies were not carried out on the primate cortex. The double bouquet of the modern cell is clearly the tightly bundled set of thick, un-

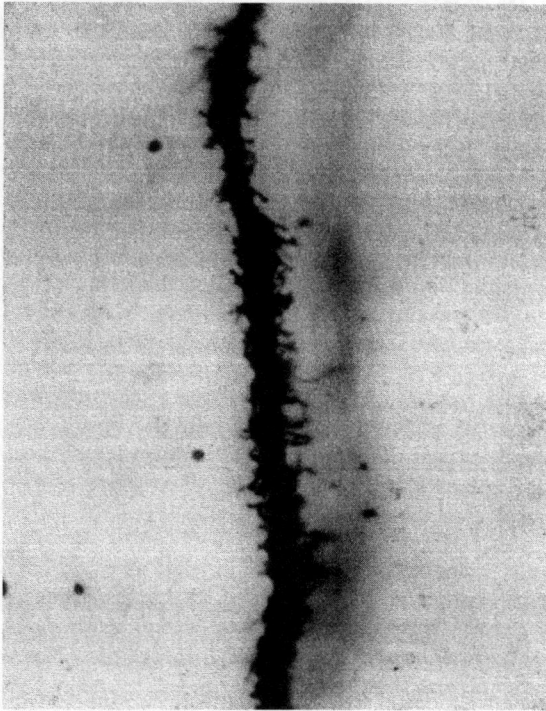

[*FIG. 294*]   Photomicrograph from one of Cajal's preparations, showing dendritic spines on the apical dendrite of a large layer V pyramid in the visual cortex of a one-month-old cat. × 960.

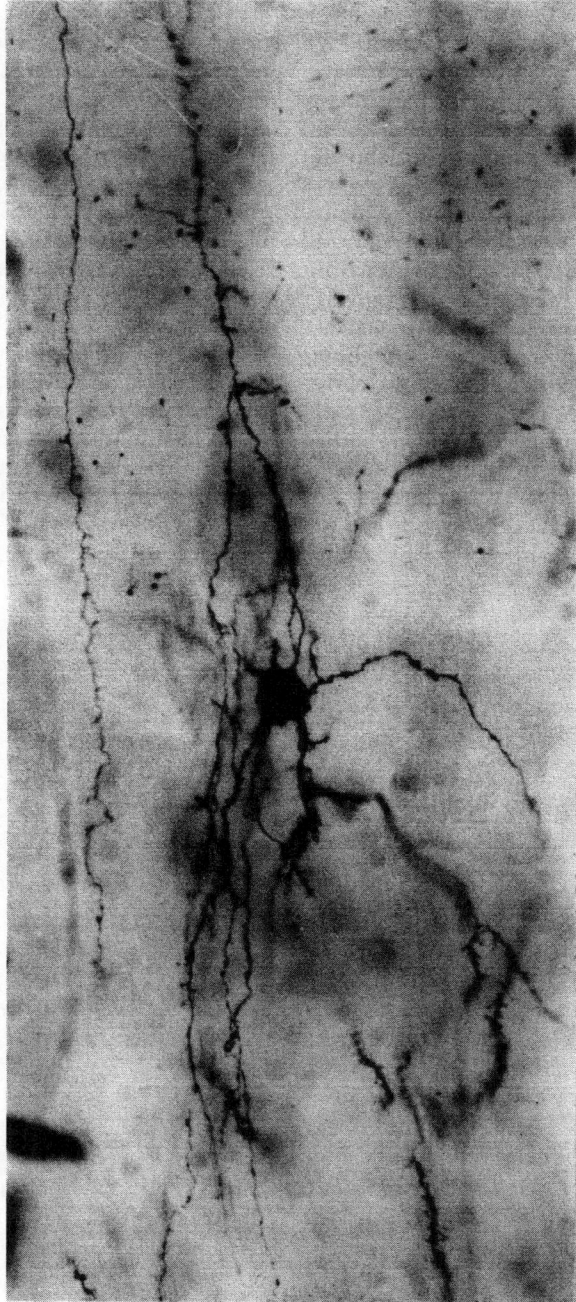

[*FIG. 295*]   Photomicrograph from one of Cajal's preparations, showing a small sparsely-spiny cell with axonal arcades in the postcentral gyrus of a newborn child. × 425.

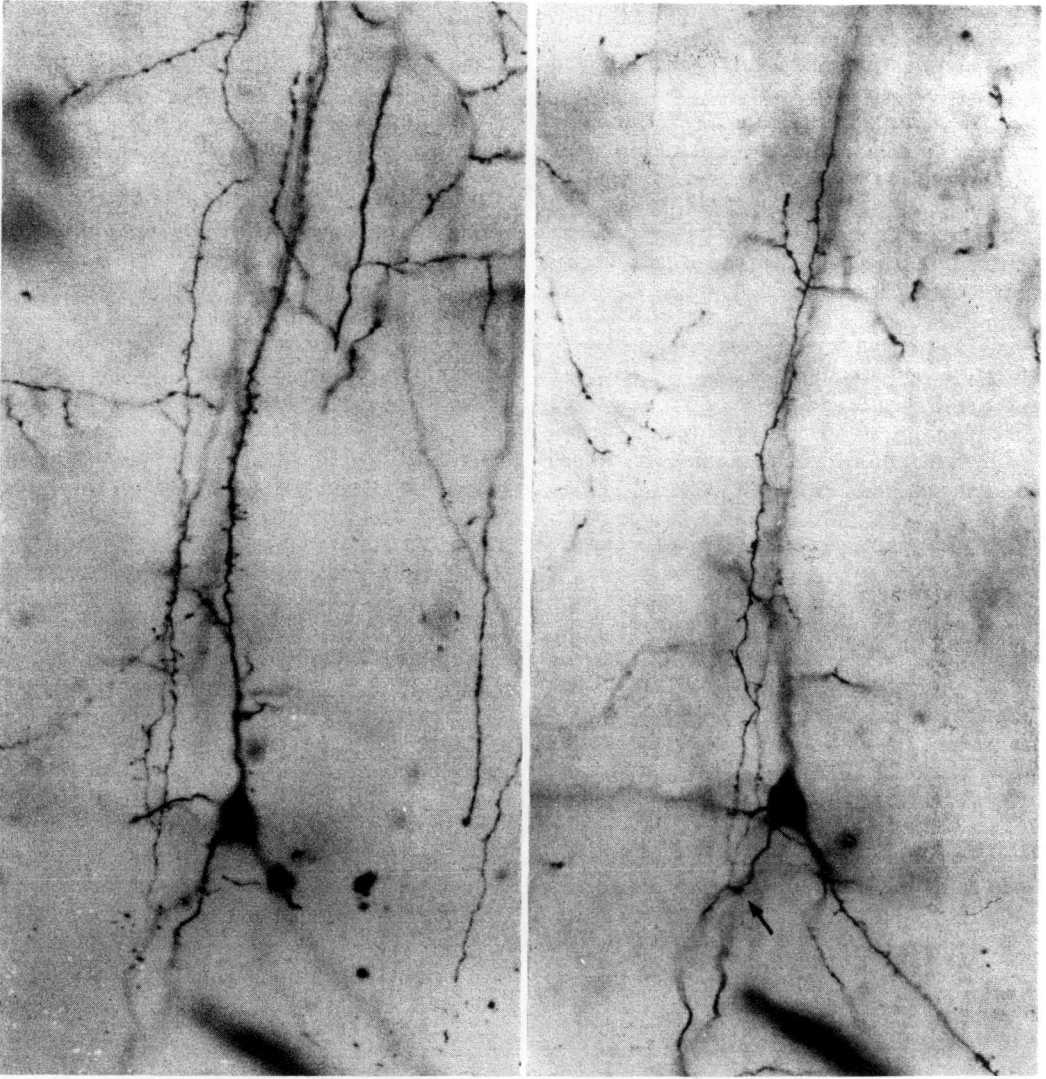

[*FIG. 296*] Photomicrographs at two planes of focus, showing a small spiny cell (a "star pyramid") with arciform axon collaterals in layer IV of area *3b* in a monkey. The parent axon and the origins of two recurrent branches are seen at right *(arrow)*. *From:* material of J. DeF. × 600.

myelinated, descending, and sometimes ascending axon collaterals [*figs. 304–306*]. These give rise to many knoblike terminals along the branches of apical dendritic shafts of pyramidal cells caught in the bundle. The terminals form symmetric synapses (Somogyi and Cowey, 1981). The final spray of the descending axon bundle ends in the inner band of Baillarger (Jones, 1975). The double bouquet cells are likely, though not definitively proven, to be GABAergic (Cowey et al., 1981; Houser et al., 1983a; DeFelipe and Jones, 1985). It is also likely that double bouquet cells, most of whose somata are situated in layers II and III, belong to the population of cells specifically and selectively labeled by high-affinity uptake and retrograde transport of [³H] GABA injected into layer V of the cortex (Cowey et al., 1981; Somogyi et al., 1981; DeFelipe and Jones, 1985) [fig. 324].

Neurogliaform cells (*C*) are clearly the same as the cells called this or "arachniform" by Cajal. Attention was first drawn to them in modern times by Valverde (1971, 1985), who called them "clewed" cells, on account of their tightly intertwined, unmyelinated, local axonal ramification [figs. 307, 308]. They are clearly the same as the "clutch" cells of Kisvárday et al. (1986), are apparently GABAergic (Houser et al., 1983b; Kisvárday et al., 1986), and end in symmetric synapses (Mates and Lund, 1983).

The rather nonspecific-looking aspiny cell with its axon branches distributed in *short ar-* *cades* (*E*) is fairly typical of what Cajal generally simply called a cell with short axon [fig. 295]. Peters and Saint Marie (1984) include them in the group of "smooth and sparsely spinous nonpyramidal cells forming local axonal plexuses." Various forms of this cell have been studied by Valverde (1976), Fairén and Valverde (1979), and Fairén et al. (1984), and several have now been stained by intracellular injection (Gilbert, 1983). For an individual cell, the major axonal ramifications can be above, below, or around the soma, as Cajal indicated. Peters and Fairén (1978) and Peters and Proskauer (1980) have shown that the axon, which is unmyelinated, terminates in symmetrical synapses on somata and dendrites of seemingly any type of neuron within the domain of the axon. The terminals of the axon of this rather

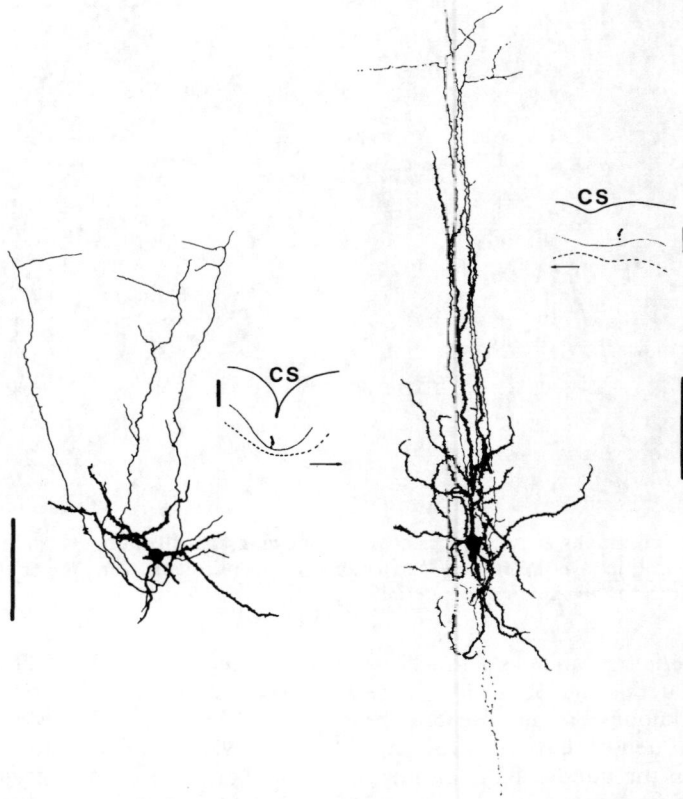

[*FIG. 297*] Small spiny neurons with arciform axon collaterals from layer IV of area *3b* of a squirrel monkey. Cell at left is a "spiny stellate cell," that at right a "star pyramid." Bars 1 mm, 100 μm. *CS*, central sulcus. *From:* Jones (1975).

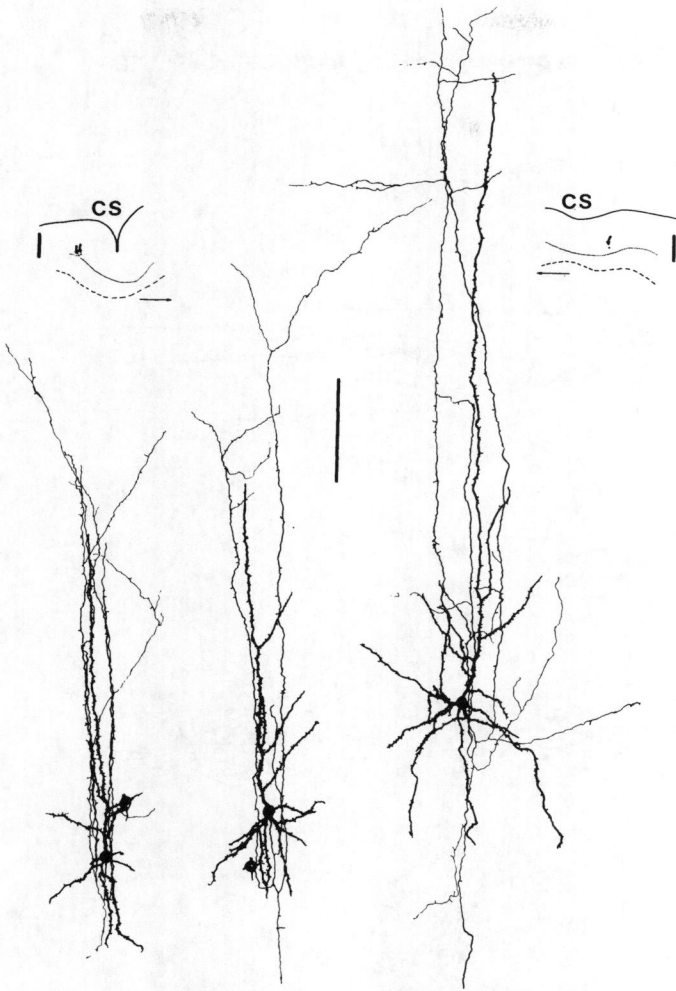

[*FIG. 298*] Small spiny neurons with arciform collaterals from layer IV of areas *1* and *2* of the squirrel monkey cortex. Cells at left are "star pyramids"; that at right resembles a small pyramid. Bars 1 mm, 100 μm. *From:* Jones (1975).

"generalized" form of cortical neuron may account for the greatest proportion of symmetric synapses in the cortex (Peters and Saint Marie, 1984). This may well be correct for layers II–IV in which this cell type is concentrated. They are probably also GABAergic (Houser et al., 1983b, 1984) [*figs. 309, 310*].

The long, stringy *bitufted* or *fusiform cells* (*F*), commonly found in layers II–III and in layer VI and the underlying white matter, are the same as those identified by Cajal, although

they should not be confused with the fusiform cells of the piriform and entorhinal areas which he saw as modified forms of extrinsically projecting pyramidal neuron. The bitufted or fusiform neurons more obviously have the form drawn in *fig. 299* in monkeys and cats. In rodents, they tend to be narrower, with fewer processes, and are often genuinely bipolar (Peters, 1984a), although this form can occur in primates as well [*fig. 311*]. In early studies, the axons of these types of cell were

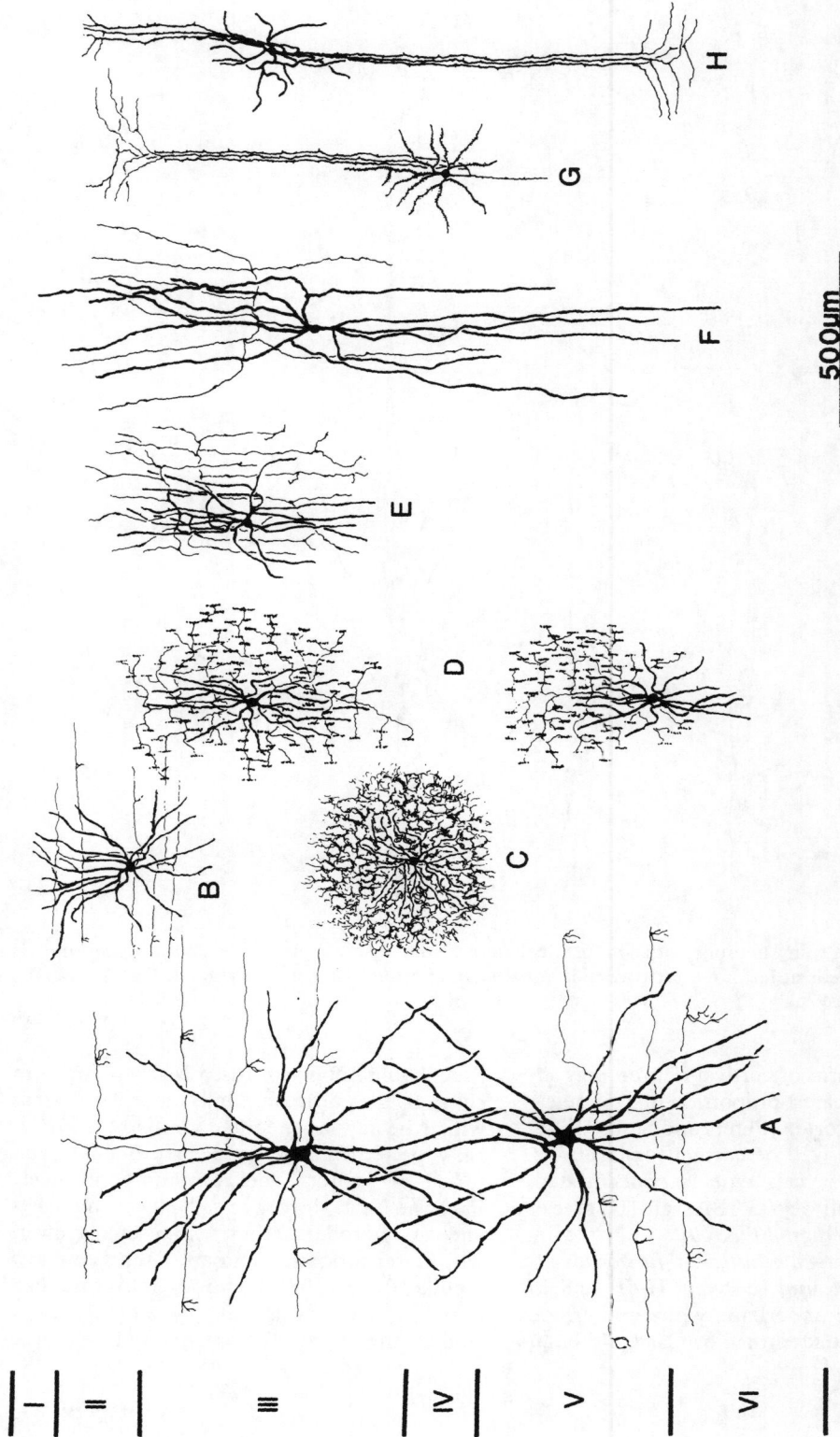

[FIG. 299] Semischematic summary of the major types of nonpyramidal neurons found in the primate cerebral cortex (after Jones, 1975). The small spiny cell with arciform axon (*G*) is the only nonpyramidal neuron with a significant population of dendritic spines. Cells *A–F* and *H* are essentially aspiny in adults. *A, B,* basket cells; *C,* neurogliaform or arachniform cell; *D,* chandelier cells; *E,* cell forming axonal arcades; *F,* bitufted or bipolar cell; *H,* double bouquet cell (Cajal's "bitufted" cell).

described as ending in asymmetrical synapses (Peters and Kimmerer, 1981; Fairén et al., 1984). In more recent studies, this population of neurons has been shown to be the group immunoreactive for virtually all of the known cortical neuropeptides (Jones and Hendry, 1986; Jones et al., 1988) [*fig. 312*] and commonly for glutamate decarboxylase (GAD) or GABA as well (Hendry et al., 1984a; Somogyi et al., 1984; Schmechel et al., 1984) [*fig. 313*]. The synapses of the peptide immunoreactive cells are almost invariably symmetric, in keeping with a synapse that is also GABAergic [*fig. 314*] (Hendry et al., 1983b, 1984b; Freund et al., 1986; Jones et al., 1987, 1988; Peters et al., 1987). Cells of very similar appearance have been shown in rats to be immunoreactive for choline acetyltransferase (Houser et al., 1983a), which is commonly colocalized with immunoreactivity for vasoactive intestinal polypeptide (Eckenstein and Baughman, 1984). Other bitufted or bipolar neurons, not

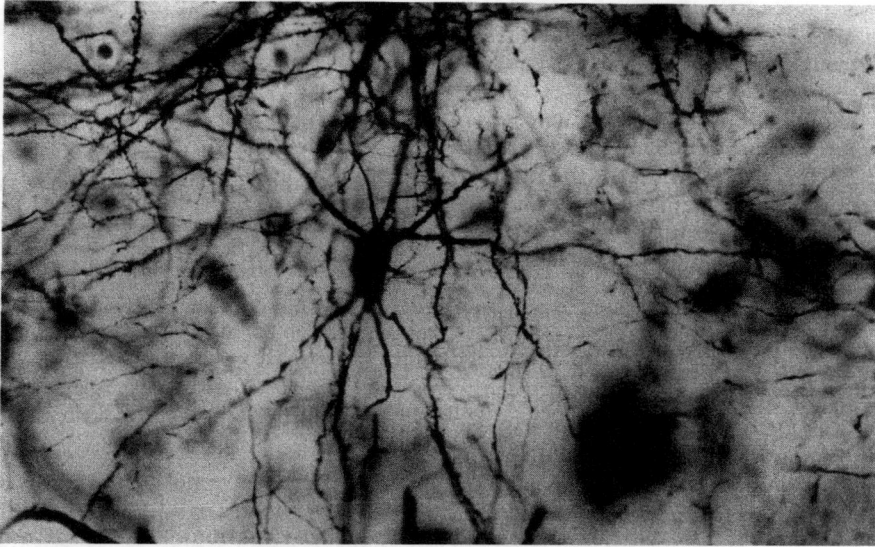

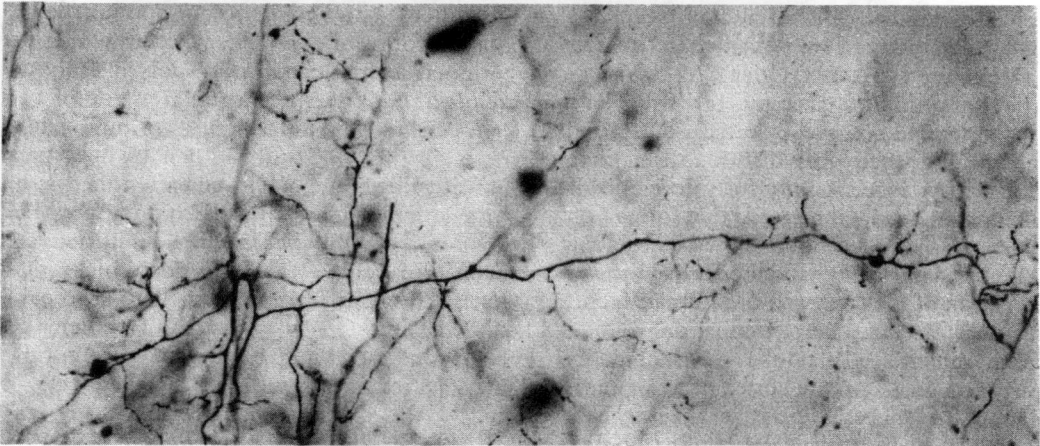

[*FIG. 300*]   Photomicrographs from Cajal's preparations, showing: *Top,* a large, basket cell in layer V of the precentral gyrus of a newborn child, × 460; *Bottom,* a probable basket cell axon [cf. *fig. 83*] from the visual cortex of a one-month-old cat, × 380.

immunoreactive for known peptides, can have axons that clearly indicate their belonging to the chandelier or double bouquet cell classes.

The one nonspiny, nonpyramidal cell type in *fig. 299* clearly not described by Cajal is the *chandelier cell (D)*, first described by Szentágothai and Arbib (1974; Szentágothai, 1975) and the subject of several subsequent light and electron microscopic studies (Jones, 1975; Somogyi, 1977; Somogyi et al., 1982; Fairén and Valverde, 1980; Lund et al., 1979, 1981; Peters et al., 1982; Peters and Regidor, 1981; DeFelipe et al., 1985; Marin-Padilla, 1987). It appears that chandelier cells are ubiquitously distributed through the neocortex of virtually all mammals (Peters, 1984b; Fairén et al., 1984). They may be found in all layers except layer I but are most prominent in the supragranular layers. It is the axon that is the most distinctive feature of the chandelier cell, for it devolves into a series of vertical rows of boutons reminiscent of the candles of a chandelier. These rows of boutons end exclusively on the initial segments of the axons of pyramidal neurons in symmetric, GABAergic synapses (Somogyi et al., 1982; Peters et al., 1982; DeFelipe et al., 1985). A single chandelier cell can contribute single or multiple rows of boutons to a single axon initial segment, and there is considerable variation in the numbers of chandelier cell boutons that a given pyramidal axon initial segment may receive. In monkeys, layer V pyramidal cell initial axon segments, on average, receive fewer than those in layer III (DeFelipe et al., 1985) [*figs. 315–318*].

In attempting to account for why Cajal never described chandelier cells, we can only conclude that their only distinguishing characteristic, the axon, was not fully developed in the fetal and neonatal material that formed the greater part of his collection. Marin-Padilla (1987) has described chandelier cells in the visual cortex of eight-month-old human brains, but there are no descriptions of younger human material. Chandelier cells could be clearly recognized in the cortex of five-month-old monkeys (Jones, 1975). It has recently been reported by DeCarlos et al. (1985) that there is a certain amount of postnatal maturation of chandelier cell axons in the auditory cortex of cats.

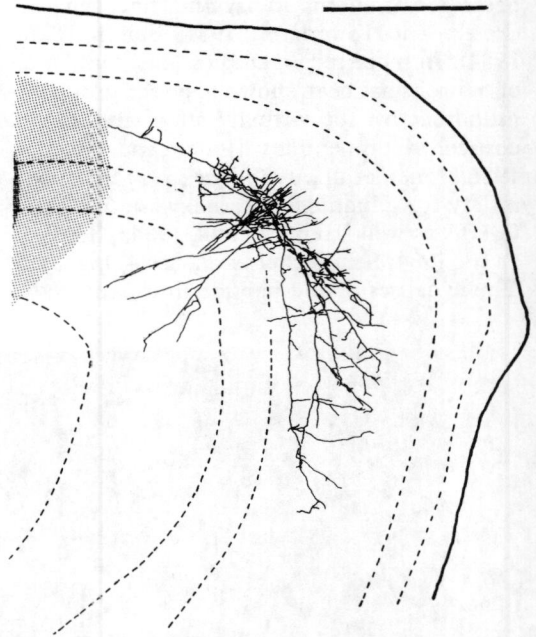

[*FIG. 301*]   Camera lucida drawing of a large basket cell, labeled through one of its axon collaterals which entered an injection of horseradish peroxidase in the monkey postcentral gyrus, sagittal section. Bar 1 mm. *From:* DeFelipe et al. (1986b).

We ourselves have not been able to identify chandelier cells in any of Cajal's extant material. However, a number of cells otherwise identified by him could, in our opinion, be immature forms of chandelier cells in which the terminal axonal candles are not yet fully developed. This seems particularly true of certain cells that he described as forming axonal nests [*figs. 56, 70, 96*] and which are not typical basket cells. Some of these he identified as bitufted (double bouquet) cells, but these [*fig. 96*] do not have the characteristic bitufted cell axon. We believe that our photomicrograph [*fig. 319*] taken from one of Cajal's preparations is likely to be an immature chandelier cell axon, and it may be the actual cell drawn by Cajal for *fig. 96* (see also *fig. 70*).

Cajal-Retzius Cells

Cajal first described what he called the special cells of layer I in 1890 (chapter 2), in the cortex of neonatal rodents, rabbits, and cats. They were described almost simultaneously in the fetal human cortex by Retzius (1891) [*fig. 320*], who called them *Cajal'sche Zellen.* Cajal obviously took great delight in this appellation, never failing to use it when the occasion presented itself. Retzius (1893a, b, 1894) was unable to stain the cells in postnatal humans, but this was later achieved by Cajal (chapters 7, 14, 15). Kölliker (1896) drew a fine distinction between Cajal's cells and Retzius's cells, both of which he thought might be a form of neuroglial cell, but because he described them together, they acquired subsequently the joint eponym *Cajal-Retzius cell.*

Cajal-Retzius cells, although described at in-

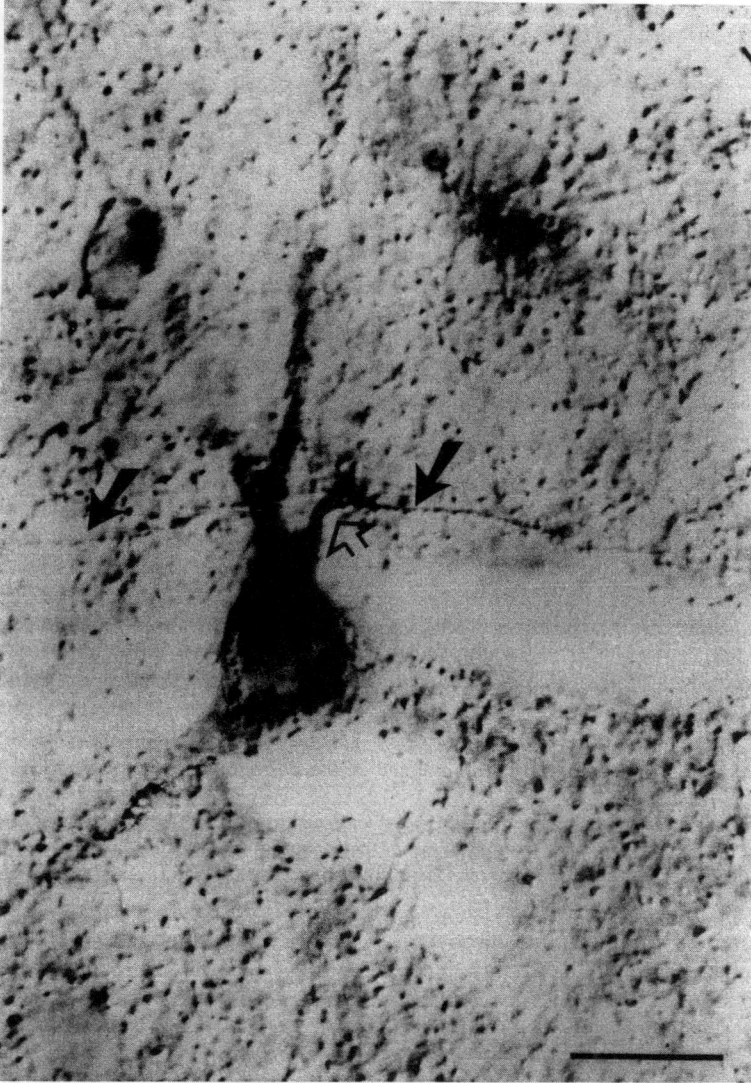

[*FIG. 302*]   Large multipolar neuron, probably a basket cell, with ascending axon (*open arrow*) and horizontal collaterals (*filled arrows*), immunocytochemically stained for glutamic acid decarboxylase in layer V of the motor cortex of a macaque monkey. Bar 25 μm. *From:* Houser et al. (1983b).

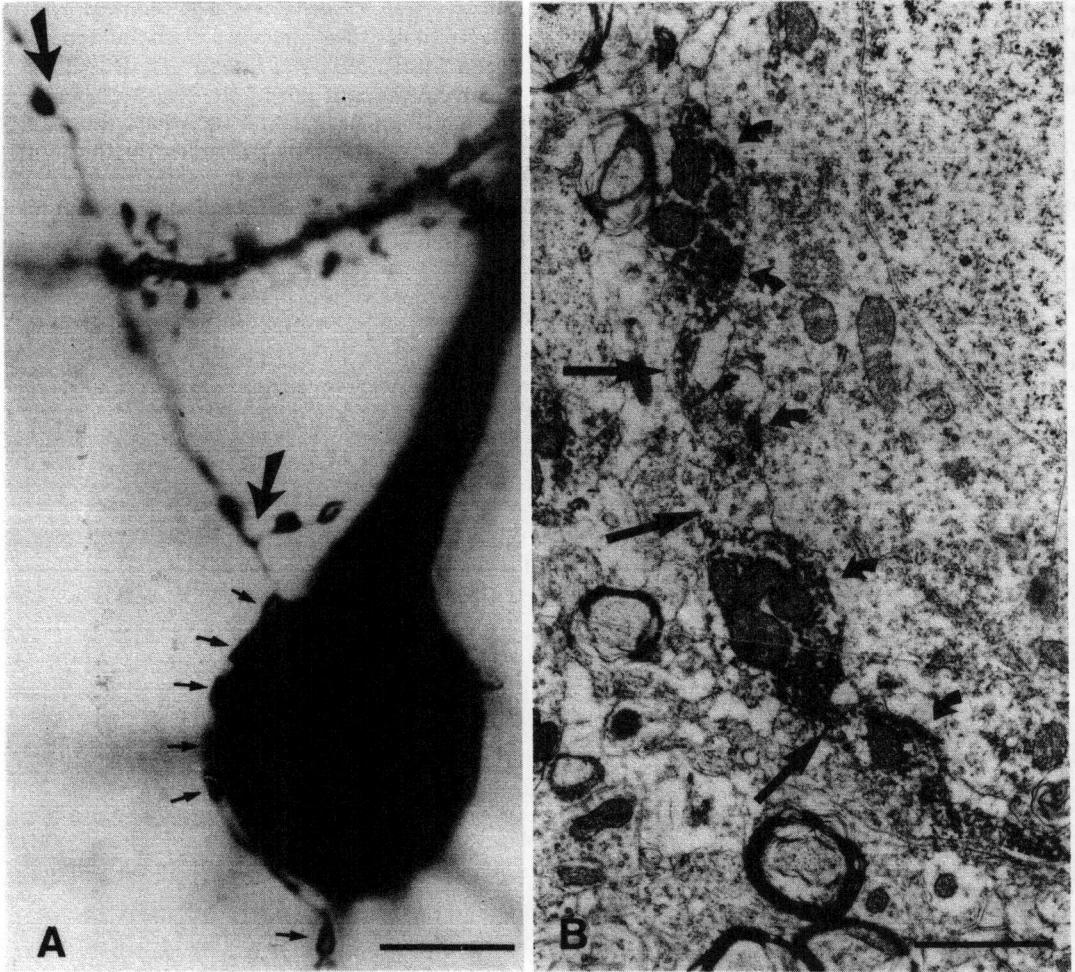

[FIG. 303] A, Golgi-Kopsch impregnated basket cell axon branch (large arrows), branching and forming a multiterminal ending on the soma of a pyramidal cell in the postcentral gyrus of a squirrel monkey. Bar 5 μm. From: Jones (1975).

B, Electron micrograph of a similar multiterminal ending immunocytochemically stained for glutamic acid decarboxylase, making synapses (curved arrows) on the soma of a pyramidal neuron in layer V of the somatic sensory cortex of a macaque monkey. Bar 1 μm. From: Hendry et al. (1983a).

tervals subsequent to their original discovery by Cajal and Retzius, have not been the subject of many recent studies, and there is a general opinion that they are a transient cell form that may disappear as the cortex matures. According to Marin-Padilla, who has conducted the most extensive recent study on the human cortex (Marin-Padilla and Marin-Padilla, 1982; Marin-Padilla, 1984), such cells [fig. 321] do

not disappear but, as a small, fixed population, simply become more widely separated from one another as the cortex enlarges. He sees them remaining and as major contributors to the axonal plexus of layer I. The fine structure of Cajal-Retzius cells has been described recently (Larroche and Houcine, 1982; König and Marty, 1981).

It is important to emphasize that the vast

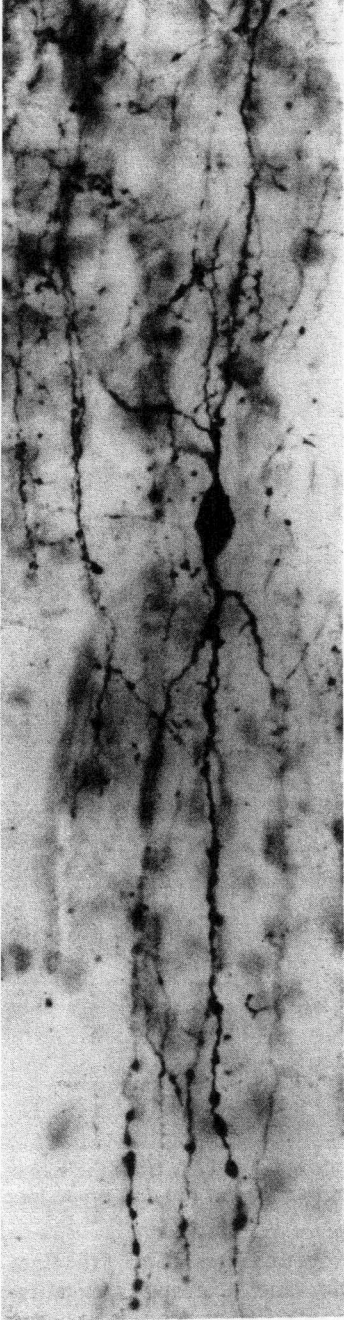

[*FIG. 304*] Photomicrograph from one of Cajal's preparations, showing a bitufted ("double bouquet") cell in layer III of the visual cortex of a fifteen-day-old human brain. × 430.

majority of the small neuronal population residing in layer I of the adult cortex consists, as recognized by Cajal (chapter 12), of conventional short-axon neurons. These are 100 percent GABAergic (Hendry et al., 1987). Whether the Cajal-Retzius cells should also be considered GABAergic is not yet known. Their synaptic relations also need to be explored. We could not identify any Cajal-Retzius cells in the extant preparations of Cajal (but see *fig. 322*).

Martinotti Cells

Martinotti's (1890) original description focused primarily on thick, myelinated axons ascending vertically to layer I from deeper layers of the cerebral cortex. In layer I, they either turned horizontally or branched in a T and extended tangentially over long distances. Martinotti was not particularly specific about the cells from which these axons arose, and his drawing suggests pyramidal cells as the source. Cajal, in his earlier studies (chapters 5–8), felt that he had discovered their origin in a form of large fusiform neuron resident in layers III–V [*fig. 33, c* in chapter 7]. Cajal supposed that the terminal axonal arborizations of Martinotti cells formed pericellular nests about the cell bodies of the special cells of layer I (chapter 17). With time, his descriptions of the cells of origin became less restrictive, and he tended to refer to any nonpyramidal cell with an axon ascending vertically to layer I as a *Martinotti cell,* or he omitted the eponym altogether. In his summarizing statements about Martinotti cells in the *Textura* and the *Histologie* (chapter 21, page 392, in this volume), Cajal says he regards them as globular, ovoid, or fusiform cells, found in all layers but most common in the deeper layers. Many of these deeper cells he draws as large stellate cells which look suspiciously like modern basket cells in which the full extent of the horizontal collaterals is not stained [e.g., *fig. 102, F*]. In many instances, Cajal does not show the vertical axon shaft even reaching layer I.

The term *Martinotti neuron* has essentially dropped out of modern descriptions of the cerebral cortex, probably because of the imprecision with which such cells can be de-

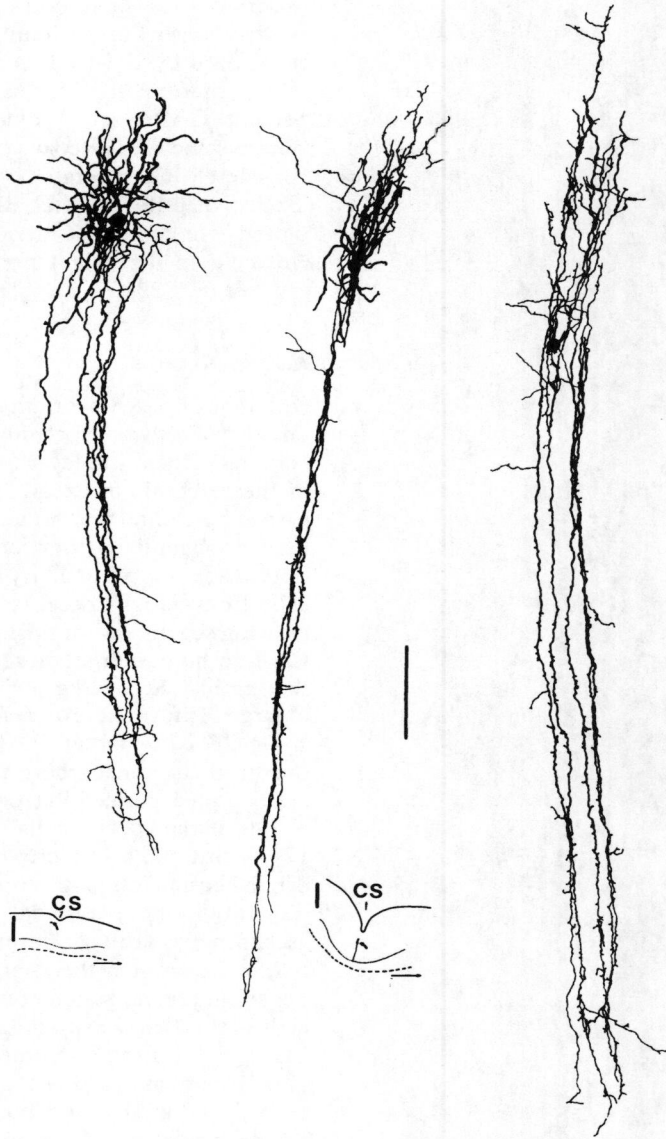

[*FIG. 305*]   Camera lucida drawings of Golgi-impregnated double bouquet cells from the somatic sensory cortex of a squirrel monkey. Axon, only, is drawn on cell at right. Bars 1 mm, 100 μm. *From:* Jones (1975).

fined. Indeed, they may not be a single type of cell. We believe that the cells shown in *fig. 323* may be of a type that Cajal would consider a Martinotti neuron.

It seems possible that neurons of this type, with somata situated at several cortical levels, send axons to layer I. Others may send axons selectively to layers II or III. Both laminar specificity and a strong verticality in these types of interlaminar connections are revealed in experiments in which [³H] GABA, injected into superficial layers of the cortex, is transported retrogradely to cell somata situated only in certain subjacent layers and only im-

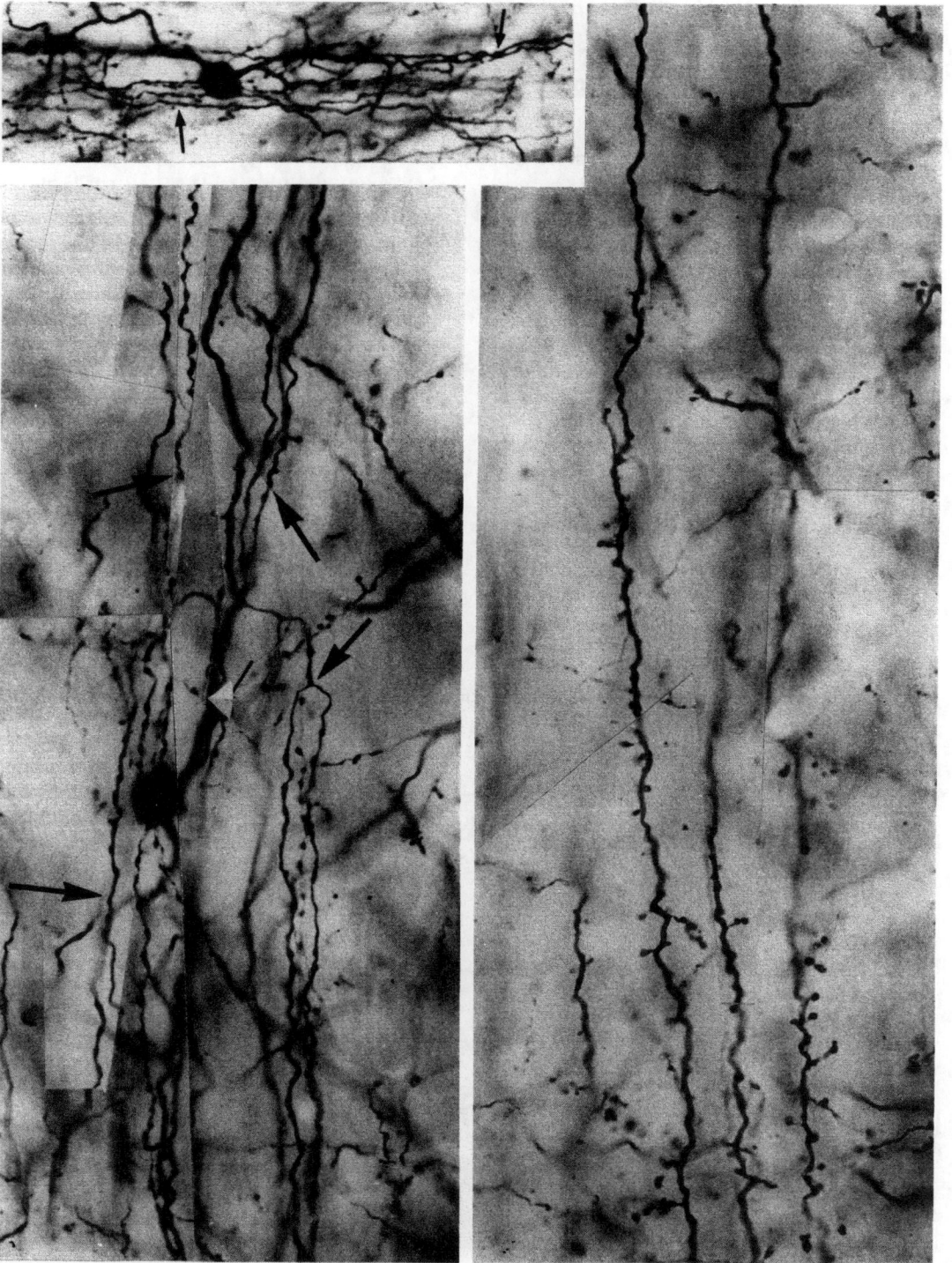

[*FIG. 306*]   Photomicrographs of a Golgi-impregnated double bouquet cell from layer III of the somatic sensory cortex of a squirrel monkey. Low-powered photomicrograph *(top left)* is turned on its side. Arrows indicate ascending and descending axon branches. Those in right figure are continuous with the descending branches seen in left figure. × 140 (*A*); × 775 (*B*); × 875 (*C*). *From:* Jones (1975).

mediately deep to the injection site [fig. 324] (Somogyi et al., 1983a; DeFelipe and Jones, 1985). If the labeled neurons can be considered Martinotti cells, then the specificity of GABA uptake and transport may imply that they, like most cortical nonpyramidal neurons, are GABAergic. Excitatory, vertical, interlaminar connections are probably mediated to a large extent by collaterals of pyramidal cell axons (Gilbert and Wiesel, 1979, 1983; Martin and Whitteridge, 1984).

Thick, Martinotti-type axons continue to be described entering layer I (e.g., Marin-Padilla, 1984). Marin-Padilla [fig. 325] shows them to have a form different from that of cortical afferents arising from brainstem sites and which also terminate in extended branches in layer I (e.g., Morrison et al., 1982) [fig. 326].

Short-Axon Neurons and Phylogeny

At several places in his works (e.g., chapters 13 and 17 in this volume), Cajal specifically mentions his belief that the increasing functional capacity of the cerebral cortex in phylogeny is associated with a great increase in the number of neurons with short axon, that is, in those that we would now call nonpyramidal cells. According to Cajal, a large percentage of short-axon neurons is the hallmark of the human cortex, and he singled out the bitufted or double bouquet neurons for special mention in this regard (e.g., chapter 14).

The Golgi method, which was, of course, Cajal's primary method, does not readily lend itself to quantification, although most workers seem to agree that, overall, it stains neurons randomly and more or less in proportion to their actual population. Hence, Cajal's statements are undoubtedly qualitative assessments based on the frequency with which he observed short-axon neurons and pyramidal neurons in his material.

Until recently, modern attempts to quantify cortical neurons have suffered from similar drawbacks. Although total cell numbers in a cortical area can be readily assessed from Nissl stains (Bok, 1929; Conel, 1947; Sholl, 1956;

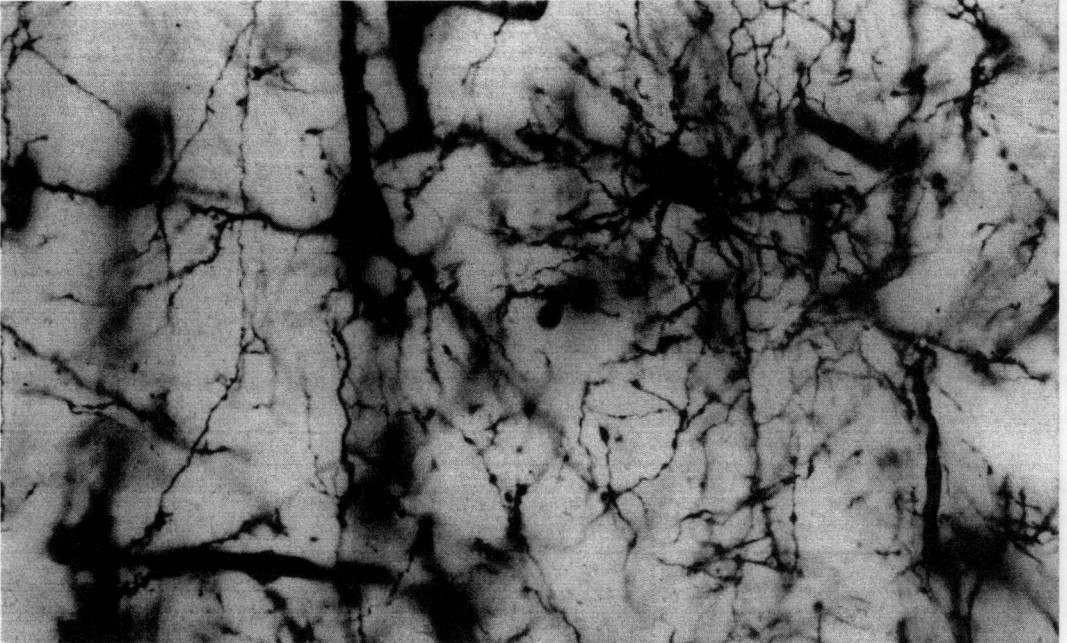

[FIG. 307] Photomicrograph from one of Cajal's preparations of the "occipital pole" of an eighteen-day-old cat, showing the soma of a pyramidal cell (left) and a neurogliaform cell (right). × 550.

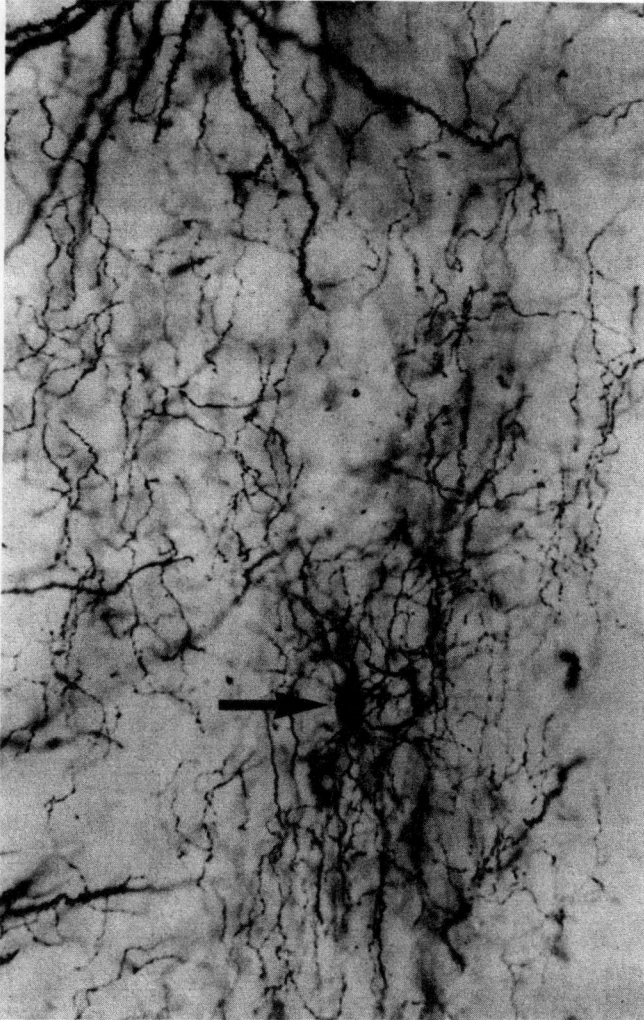

[*FIG. 308*] Neurogliaform cell and part of its extensive axonal plexus in layer IV of the somatic sensory cortex of a squirrel monkey. $\times$ 375. *From:* Jones (1975).

Rockel et al., 1980), these stains do not permit ready identification of cell types. Combined Nissl and Golgi staining could only yield significant results regarding the proportions of cells of different types, if it could be assumed that these are stained by the Golgi method in proportion to their actual numbers. There is no guarantee of this, especially insofar as most Golgi methods result in quite patchy staining. Sholl (1956) made an attempt at quantification based on a number of rather tenuous assumptions which resulted in his concluding that the nonpyramidal cell population was at its lowest in layer IV of the visual cortex—a somewhat counterintuitive conclusion.

Most neuroanatomists who have attempted quantitative or semiquantitative analyses of the cerebral cortex, however unsatisfactory the available methods, have concluded that the pyramidal cell is all-predominant, accounting

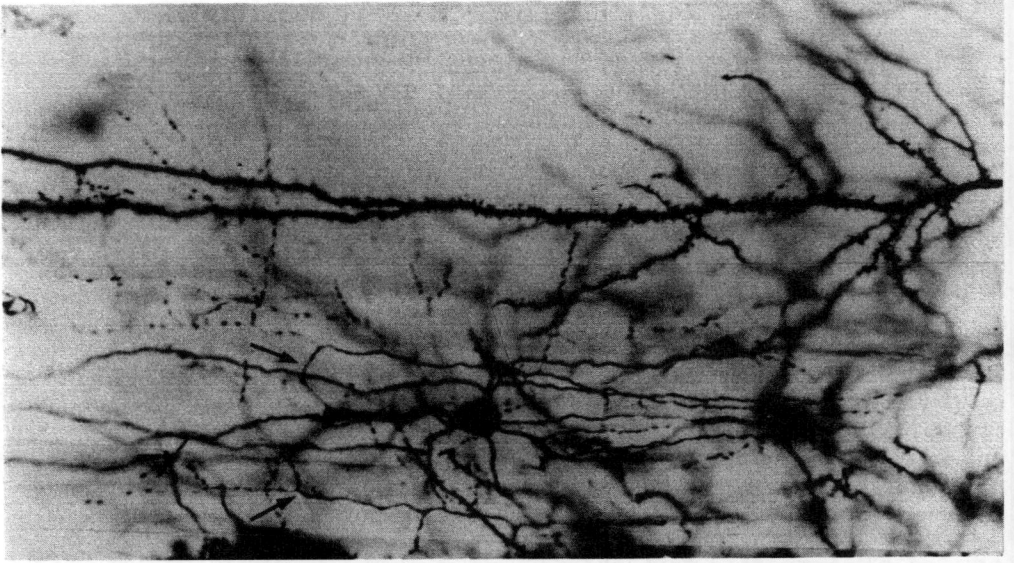

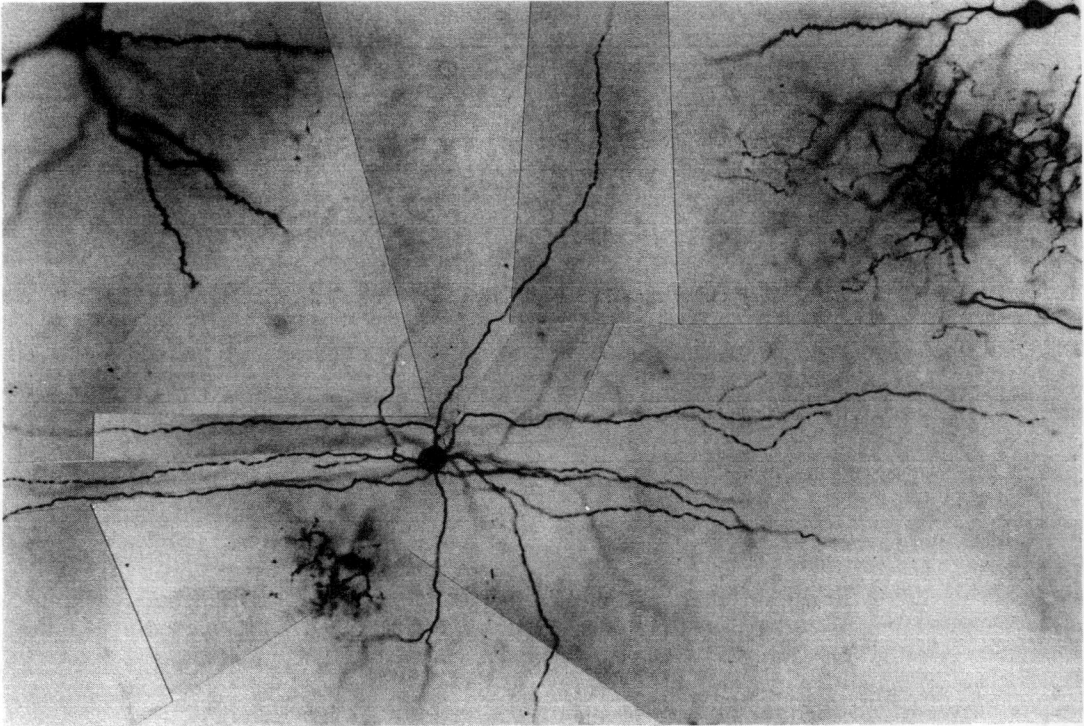

[*FIG. 309*] Aspiny cells that form axonal arcades (Cajal's short-axon cells not otherwise specified), in the somatic sensory cortex of a squirrel monkey. × 250 (*lower*), × 375 (*upper*). *From:* Jones (1975).

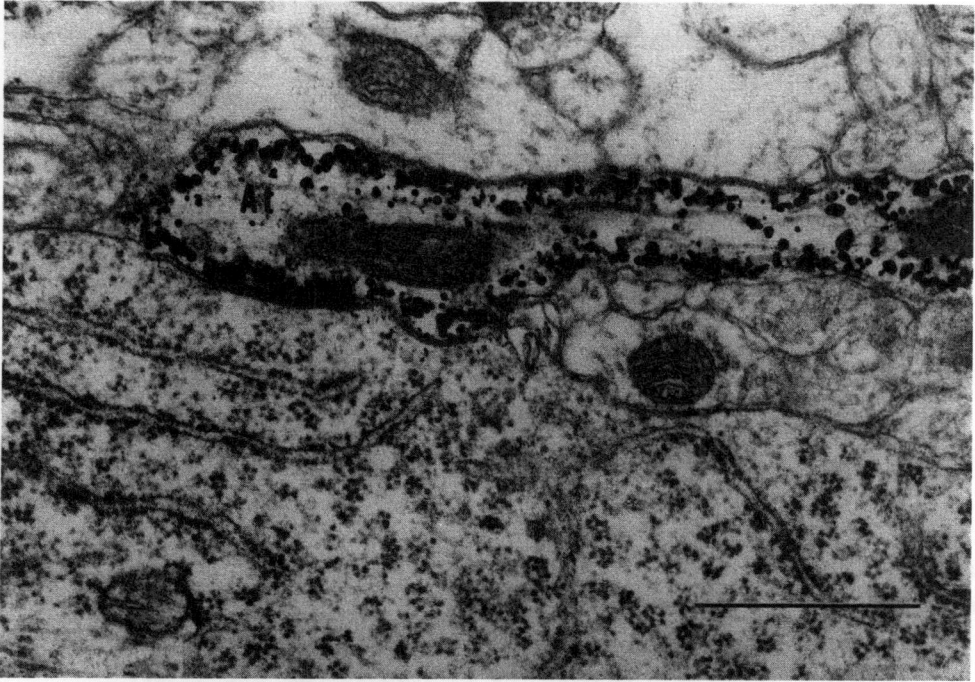

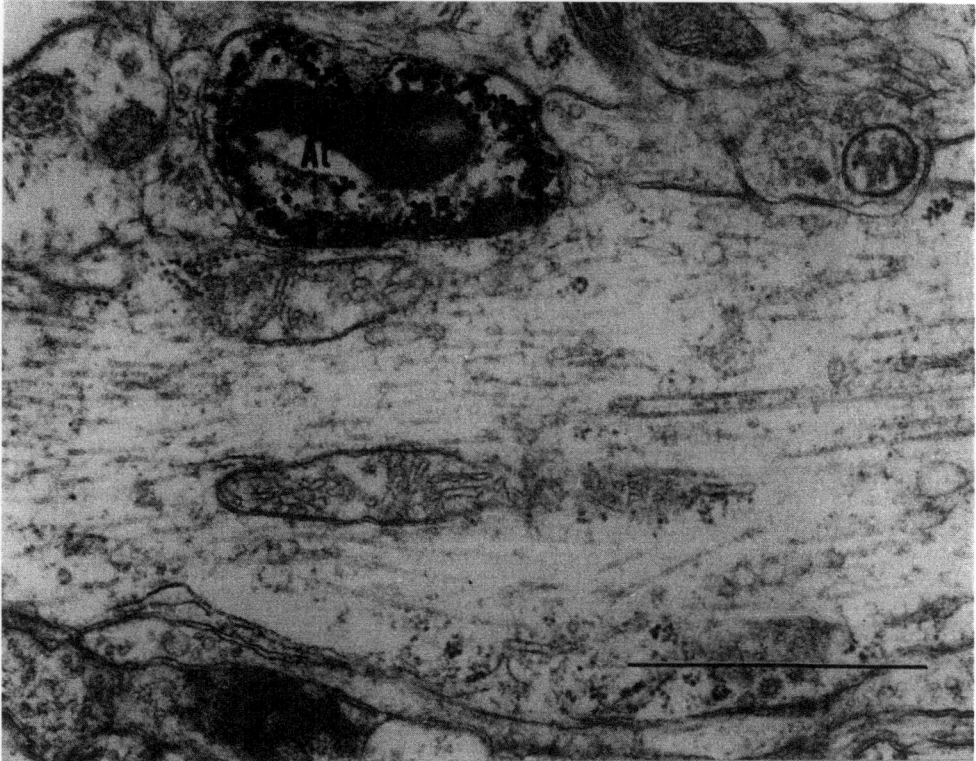

[*FIG. 310*]   Electron micrographs, showing gold-toned axon terminals of a previously Golgi-impregnated aspiny cell with local axonal arcades in layer III of the visual cortex of a rat. The terminals are forming symmetrical synapses on a nonpyramidal cell soma (*above*) and on the apical dendrite of a pyramidal cell (*below*). *From:* Peters and Saint Marie (1984).

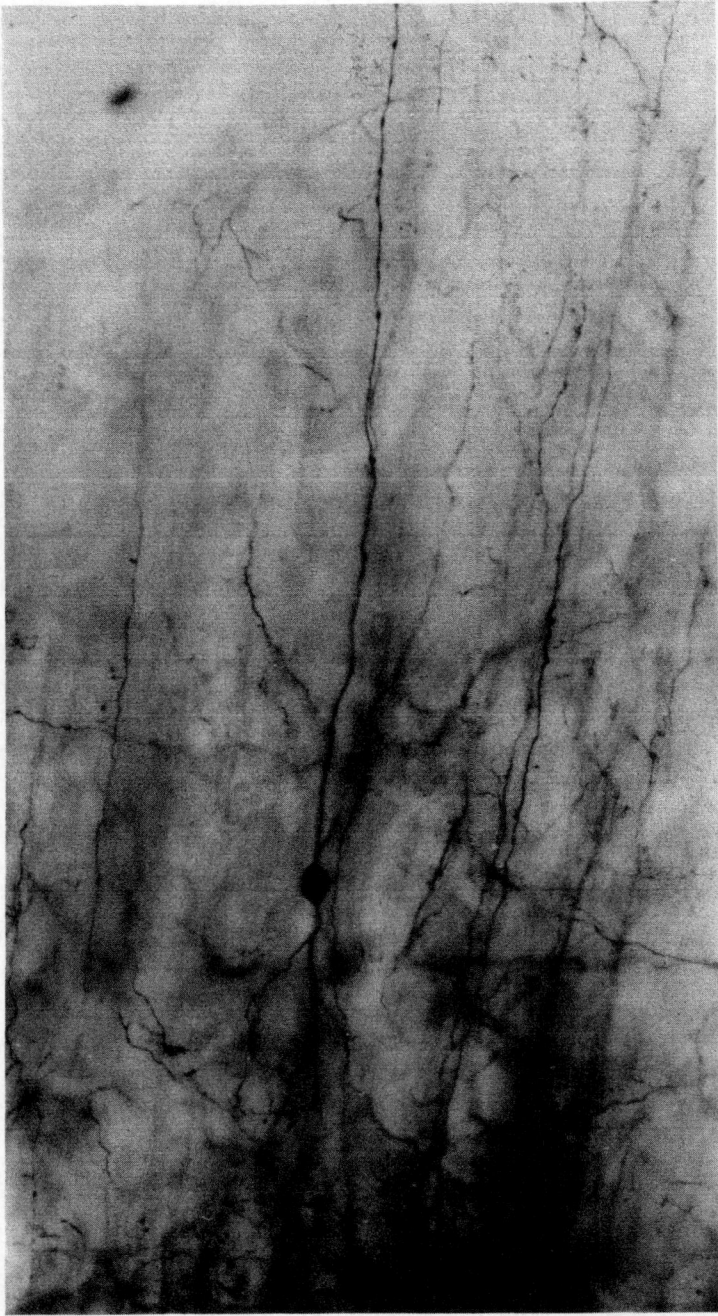

[*FIG. 311*]   Golgi-impregnated bipolar neuron from deep layer III in area *1* of the cortex in a macaque monkey. × 400. *From:* material of J. DeF.

for 75 percent or more of the neuronal population in the cortex of experimental animals (Shkol'nik-Yarros, 1971; Braitenberg, 1978; Sloper et al., 1979; Winfield et al., 1980). In rodents, a recent study (Peters, 1987), based on morphological features that are usually thought to distinguish pyramidal from non-pyramidal neurons at the electron-microscopic level (Colonnier, 1968; Peters and Kaiserman-Abramoff, 1969; Jones and Powell, 1970; Peters, 1971), has placed the nonpyramidal cell population at 10–15%.

With the introduction of immunocytochemical markers, it is now possible to assess accurately the proportions of cortical neurons expressing a particular transmitter or transmitter-related enzyme [fig. 327]. When GABA neurons were quantified in this manner in ten areas of the monkey cortex, it was found that in all areas except the striate area, they account for at least 25 percent of the total neuronal population. In the primary visual cortex, despite a total neuronal population nearly double that in other areas and a corresponding

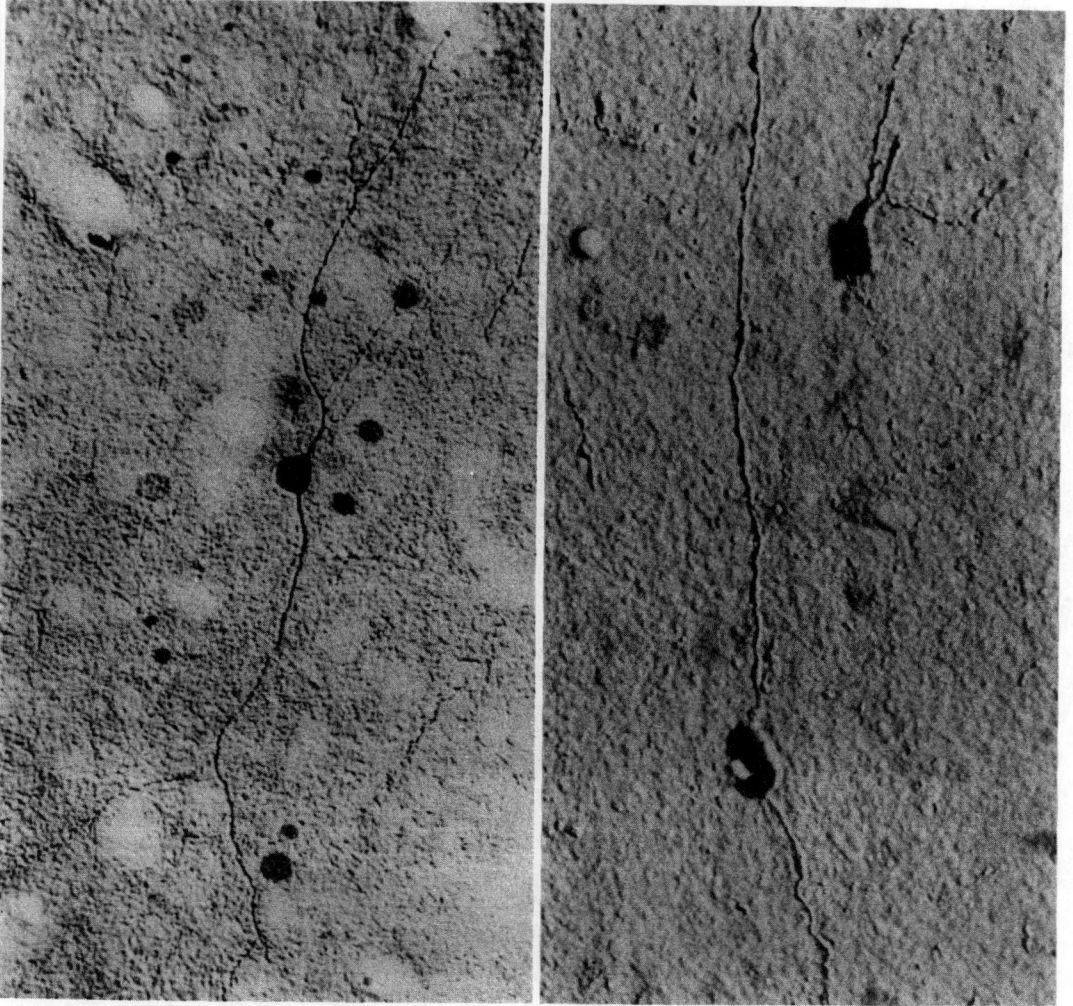

[FIG. 312]   Bipolar neurons immunoreactive for cholecystokinin (left) and neuropeptide Y (right) in the cerebral cortex of a rat. × 500. From: Hendry (1987).

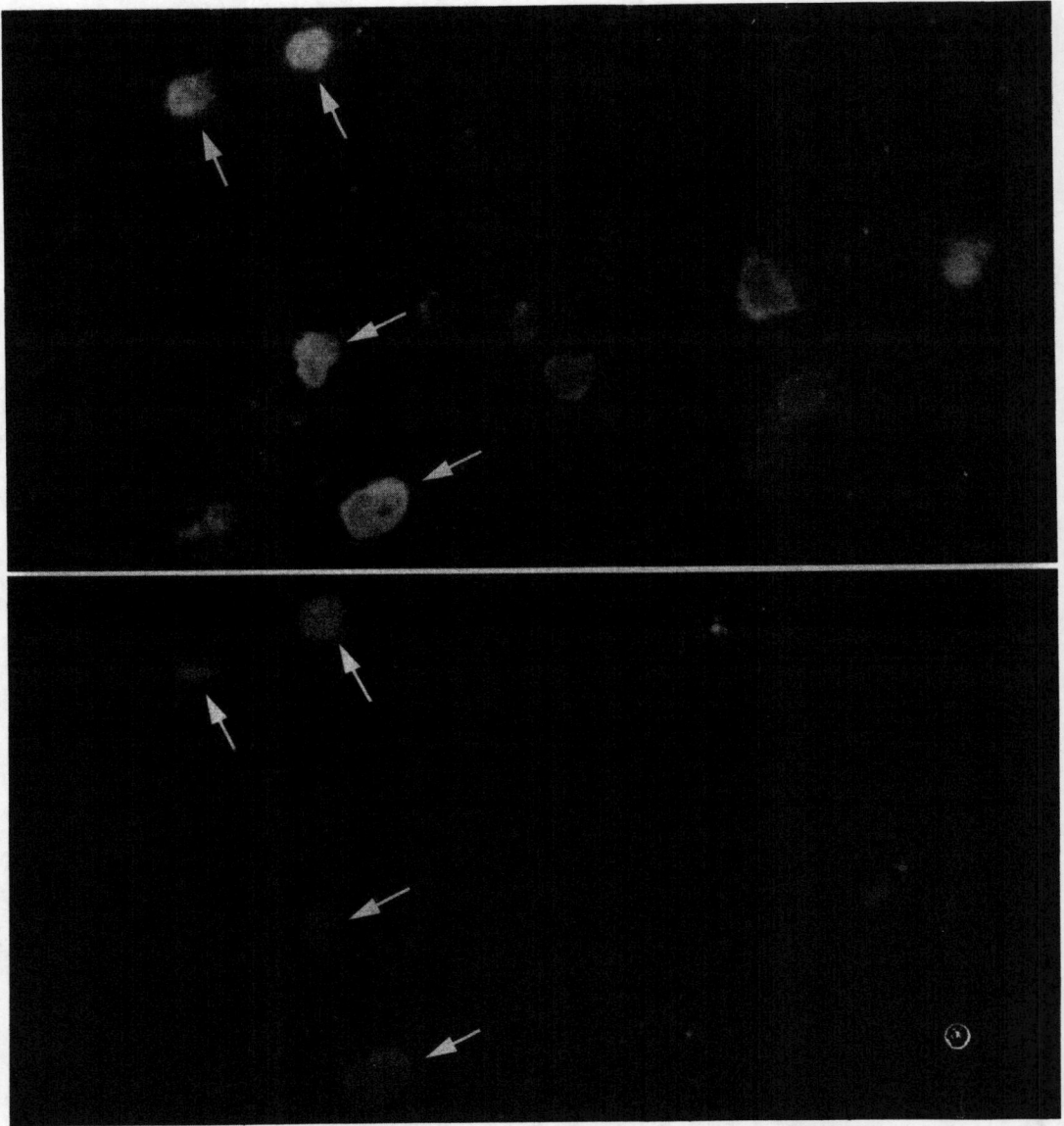

[*FIG. 313*]   Fluorescence photomicrographs from the same field of layer V in area *17* of a monkey, showing several cells *(above)* immunocytochemically stained for gamma aminobutyric acid. Four of the cells *(arrows)* are double stained for substance P *(below)*. ×650. *From:* Jones et al. (1988).

increase in the density of GABA-immuno-reactive cells, the proportion of the latter falls to less than 20 percent (Hendry et al., 1987). If we assume that GABA neurons probably account for all the nonspiny, nonpyramidal cells in the cortex, then a significant proportion of the 70–75 percent non-GABA-immunoreactiveneurons must consist of the spiny, putatively excitatory form of intrinsic neuron (Cajal's small pyramidal neuron with arciform axon or the modern spiny stellate cell and its variants). Possibly, it is an increased number of

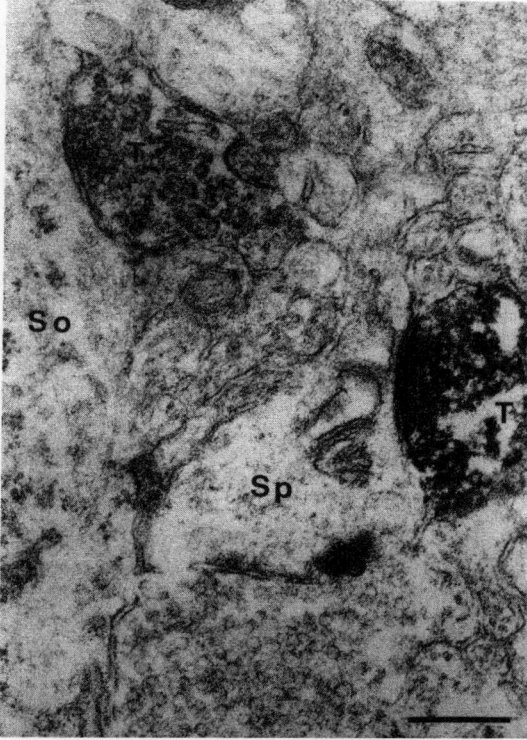

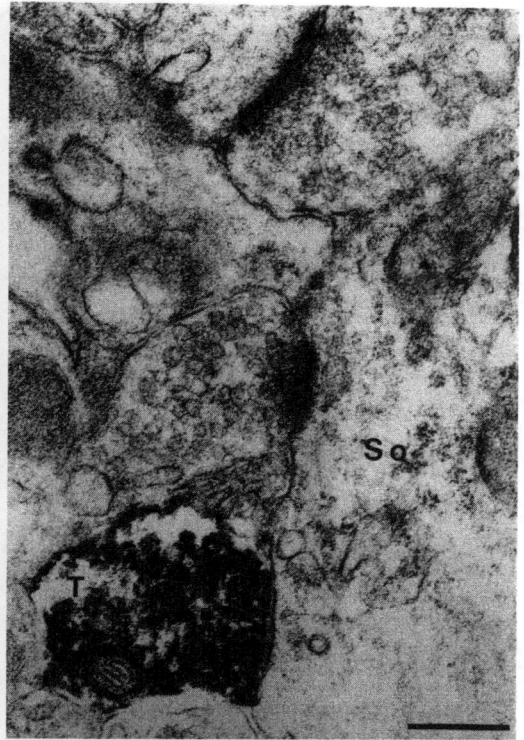

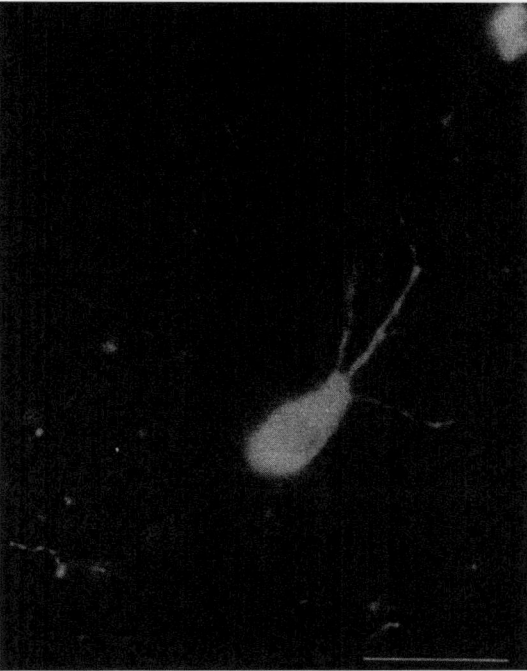

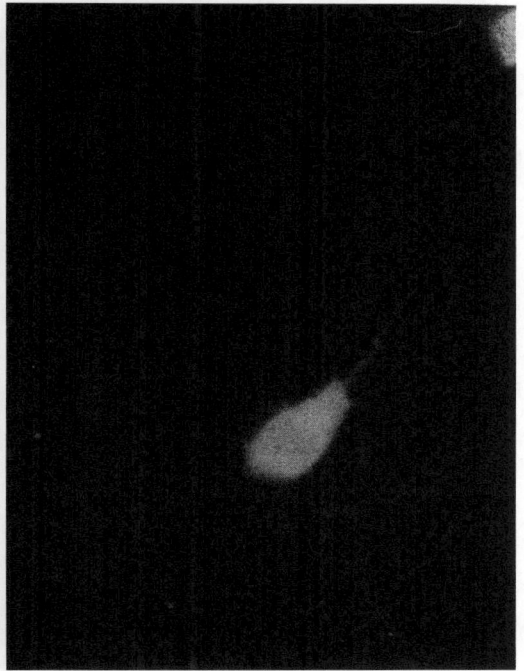

[*FIG. 314*] *Top pair:* Electron micrographs of substance P immunoreactive axon terminals (*T*) in the somatic sensory cortex of a macaque monkey, making symmetric synaptic contacts on cell somata (*So*) and on a dendritic spine (*Sp*). Bar 0.25 μm. *From:* Jones et al. (1988).

Bottom pair: Fluorescence photomicrographs from area *4* of the cortex of a macaque monkey, showing a single cell in layer VI, immunoreactive for both neuropeptide Y (*left*) and substance P (*right*). Bar 100 μm. *From:* Jones et al. (1988).

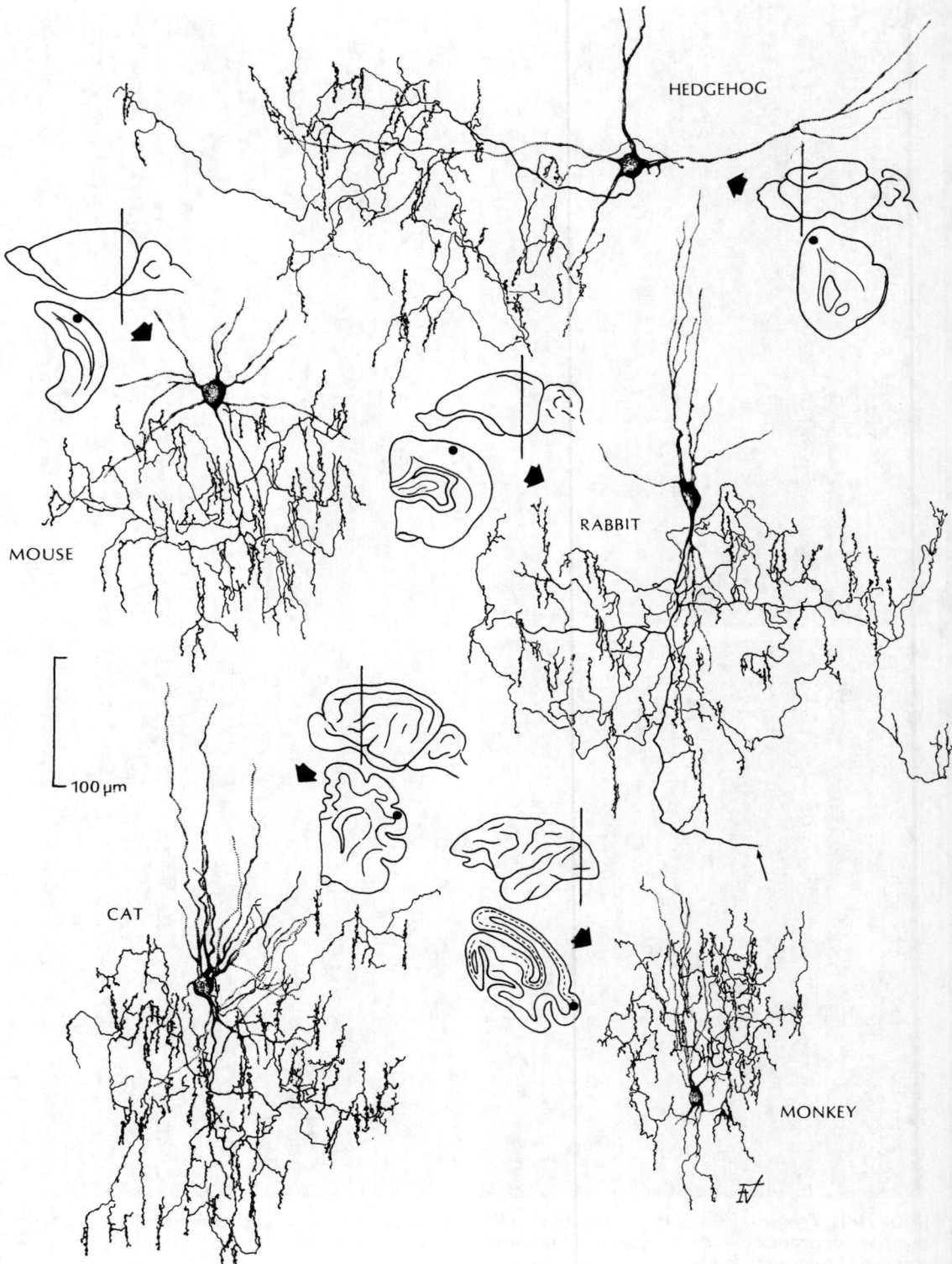

[*FIG. 315*]   Camera lucida drawings of chandelier neurons from the cerebral cortex of several species. *From:* Valverde (1983).

these latter that accounts for the "dilution" of the GABA cells in the visual cortex.

If these quantitative immunocytochemical results in monkeys are compared with the results of similar studies in rodents, then Cajal's suggestion of a trend toward increasing numbers of short-axon neurons with the increasing functional complexity of the cortex may be justified. Thus, Meinecke and Peters (1987) and Fairén et al. (1986) report that only 10 to 15 percent of rat and mouse cortex neurons are GABA immunoreactive. However, by contrast, Conti et al. (1987) report 31 percent of such neurons in rat cortex.

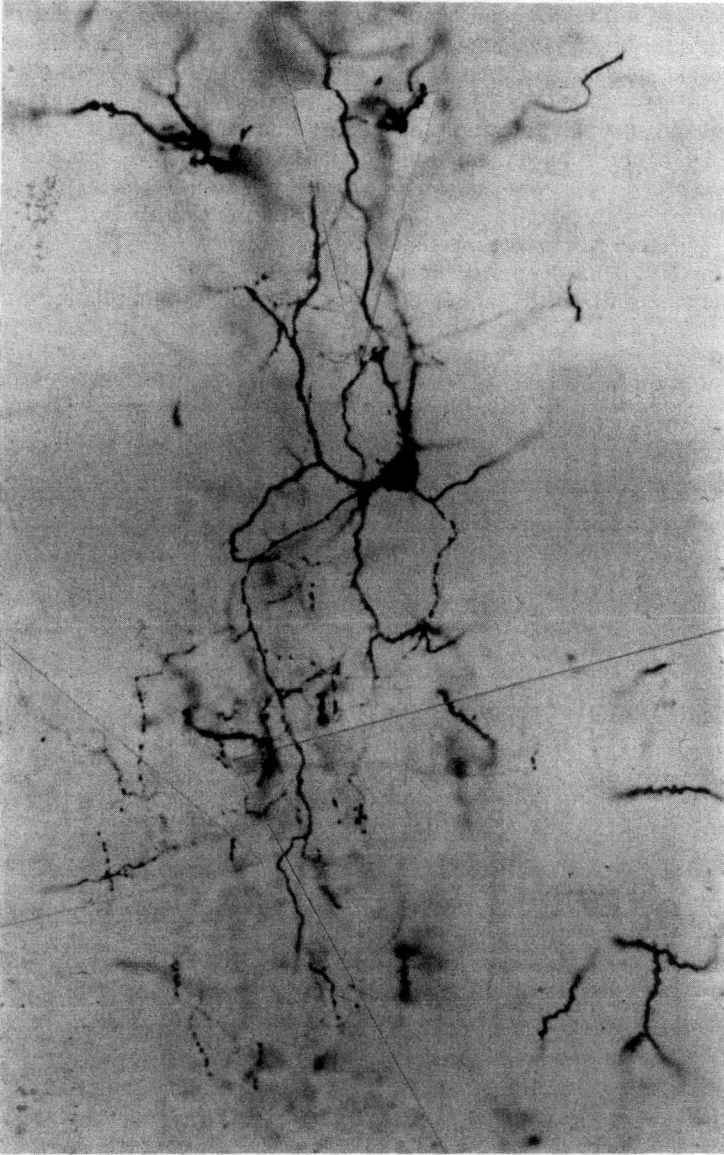

[*FIG. 316*]   Photomicrograph of a chandelier cell and part of its axonal ramification in the somatic sensory cortex of a squirrel monkey. × 250. *From:* material of E.G.J.

Afferent Fibers to the Cortex

Cajal, more than anyone, is responsible for the first clear recognition of the fact that afferent fibers from subcortical structures terminate in every neocortical area, and for making a distinction between these and commissural fibers of the corpus callosum (chapters 5, 14–17, 21, 25 in this volume). He was less certain about the identification of ipsilateral associational fibers, although he clearly accepted their existence. So convinced was Kölliker (1896) of Cajal's contributions on the identification of subcortical afferents that he dubbed them "Ramón's fibers" [fig. 328].

Cajal was initially hesitant about the exact sites of subcortical origin of the large myelinated fibers that traversed the deeper cortical layers obliquely and terminated in masses of branches in the middle layers (see chapter 13), but, following the experimental work of Monakow (1882, 1885, 1889) on thalamocortical connectivity, Cajal quickly accepted their thalamic origin. It may be noted that one of the regions he particularly used in order to portray these fibers was the motor area which lacks an internal granular layer. Also noteworthy is the fact that Cajal did not restrict the terminal ramifications of thalamic afferents to layer IV in any cortical area, although this idea still dominates much thinking on the cortex. Modern studies, however, are in agreement with Cajal, and it is probable that in the monkey brain thalamic afferents terminate largely in layer III in cortical areas outside the three primary sensory areas (Jones and Burton, 1976) [fig. 329].

The topographic relationships between tha-

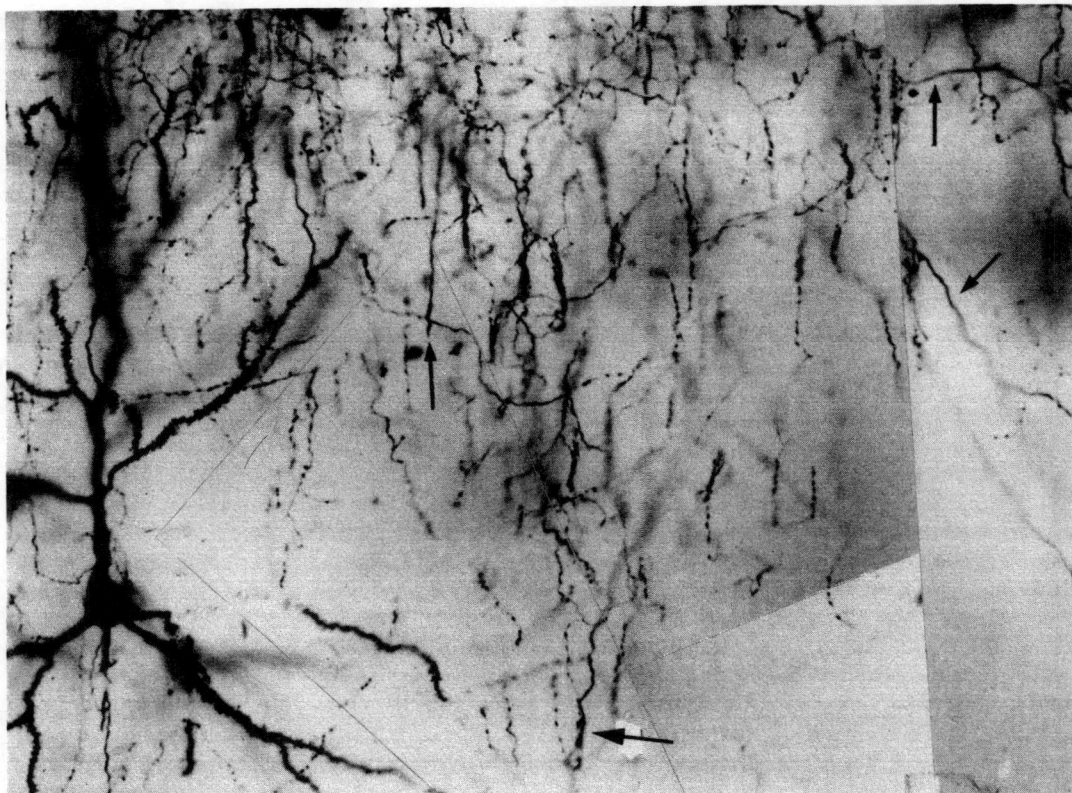

[FIG. 317] Chandelier cells' axonal plexuses (arrows) in layer II of the somatic sensory cortex of a squirrel monkey. × 250. From: Jones (1975).

lamic nuclei and cerebral cortex are not immediately relevant to the theme of this book. The history of studies designed to elucidate them and a modern consensus can be found in Jones (1985).

Perhaps where we have advanced most beyond Cajal's studies of thalamocortical fibers is in the recognition that these can have varying morphologies and distributions and that they can arise from functionally and morphologically different forms of thalamic neuron [*fig. 330*]. The basic morphology of a thalamocortical axon is much as Cajal described it, but in the visual cortex of the cat, at least two and possibly three different forms of the axon can be identified. These form the central projections of thalamic neurons innervated selectively by the physiological classes of retinal ganglion cells known as X, Y, and W (Ferster and LeVay, 1978; Gilbert and Wiesel, 1979; Martin and Whitteridge, 1984) and appear also to be represented in other species (Blasdel and Lund, 1983). The parent cells in the dorsal lateral geniculate nucleus have quite different morphologies (Friedlander et al., 1981), and comparable distinctions may exist in other thalamic nuclei (Yen et al., 1985). In monkeys, color-specific lateral geniculate neurons appear to form yet another separate channel to particular, localized foci in visual cortex (Livingstone and Hubel, 1982, 1983).

The new results on the differential laminar projections in the cortex of specific classes of thalamic neuron have led to recognition of the likelihood that there are separate channels of information flow through the sensory nuclei of the thalamus to the cortex that may not interact with one another in the thalamus and may, indeed, interact but little in the cortical area at which they first arrive (reviewed in Jones, 1985). To this must be added the fact that other populations of cells situated in the intralaminar and other thalamic nuclei, and even in a relay nucleus itself, can have diffuse projections on the cortex, the axons often ending in layers I and/or VI (Jones, 1985; Herkenham, 1986). Apparently, many of these are involved in the control of cortical excitability and the regulation of state (Jasper, 1960; Steriade and Deschênes, 1984). Finally, there are a series of types of afferent fiber that arise from

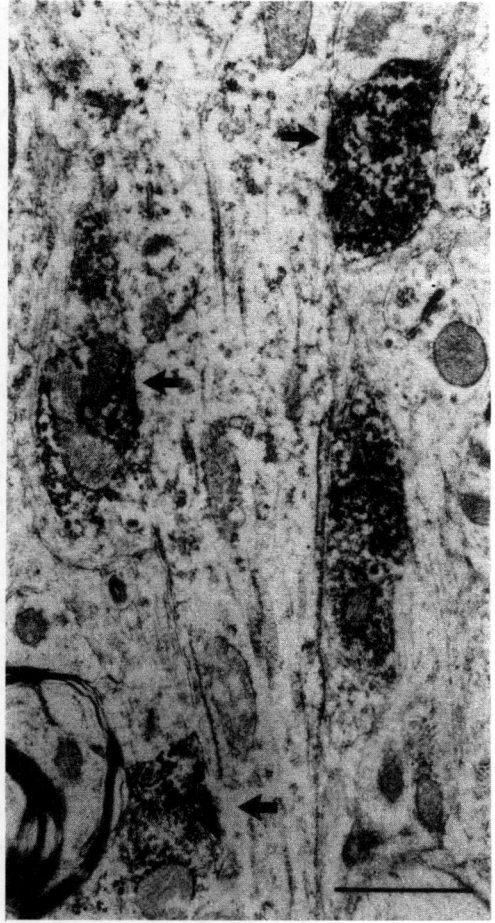

[*FIG 318*]   Axon terminals, immunoreactive for glutamic acid decarboxylase and presumed to arise from a chandelier cell axon, ending (*arrows*) on the initial segment of the axon of a pyramidal neuron in layer V of the monkey motor cortex. Bar 1 μm. *From:* Hendry et al. (1983a).

basal forebrain and brainstem sites, that bypass the thalamus and mostly terminate diffusely in the cortex, in varied laminar patterns. Most have substantial projections to layer I [*fig. 326*] and include cholinergic (Rye et al., 1984), serotoninergic (Kosofsky et al., 1984), noradrenergic (Morrison et al., 1978, 1982), and dopaminergic (Fuxe et al., 1974) fibers. All these were unknown to Cajal, and their function is little known to us today.

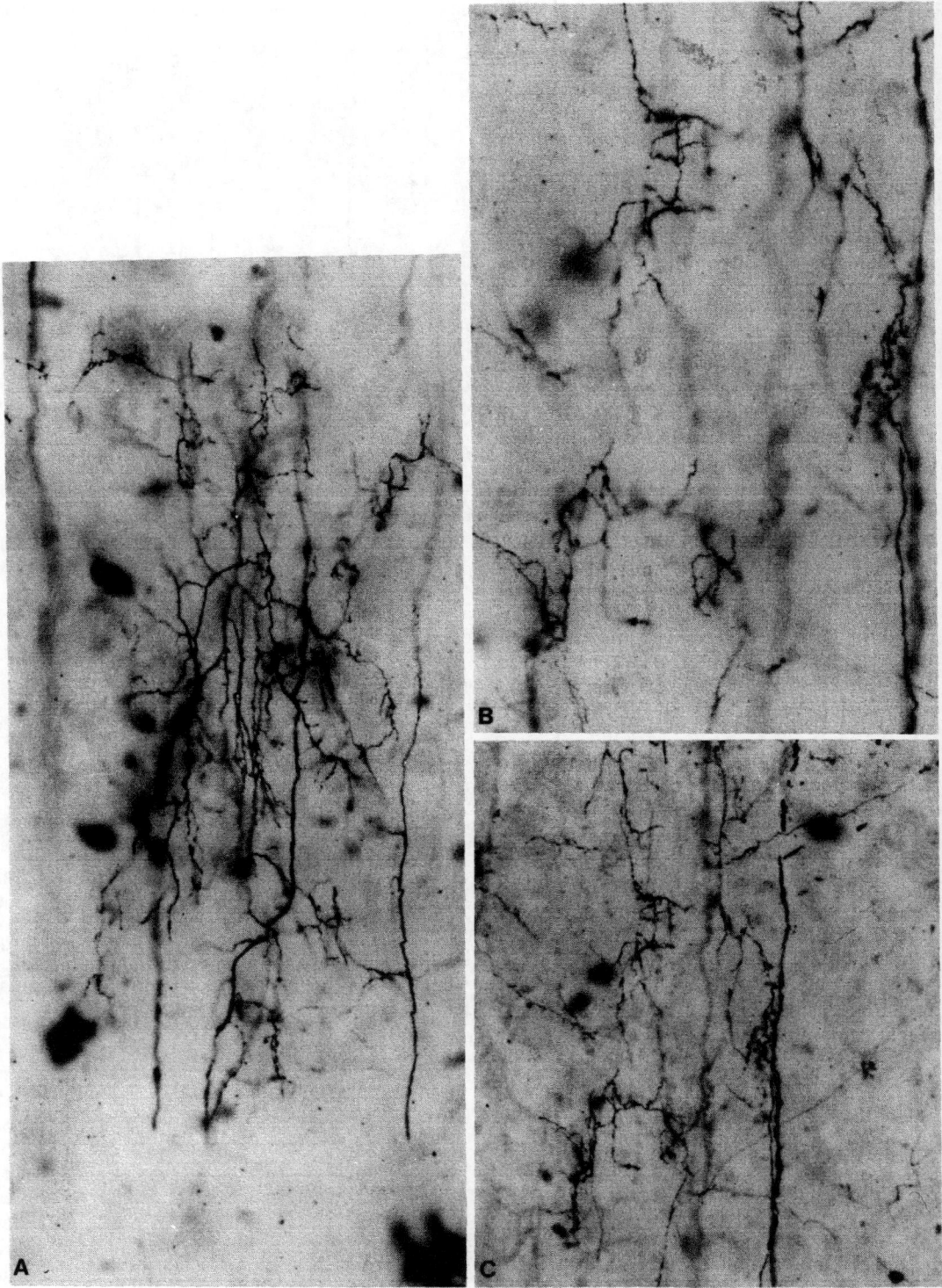

[*FIG. 319*]   Photomicrographs from one of Cajal's preparations of the visual cortex of a one-month-old cat. The axonal plexuses illustrated are from layers II–III and suggest immature axonal ramifications of chandelier cells. Cajal appears to have drawn these or similar ramifications for [*figs. 70* and *96*]. *B* and *C* are the same plexus at different magnifications. × 275 (*A*), × 550 (*B*), × 400 (*C*).

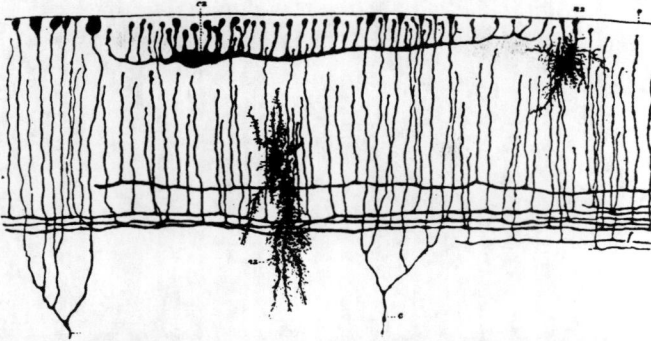

[*FIG. 320*]   Layer I of the cerebral cortex of a human fetus, as drawn by Retzius (1893b), showing a special cell, the horizontal and vertical processes of other special cells, glial cells, and radial glial processes.

Intracortical Circuits

In the final chapter on the cerebral cortex in the *Textura* and the *Histologie* (chapter 25 in this volume), Cajal devoted several pages to consideration of the arcs of connection leading from thalamic afferent fibers to pyramidal cell output. Contrary to the opinion that seems to have prevailed until quite recently, he did not perceive cortical circuitry as being fundamentally based on thalamic inputs to "stellate cells" in layer IV followed by a relay from these to the pyramidal cells. This rather simplistic view tended to dominate cortical anatomy and physiology until a few years ago and still maintains a hold on cortical theorizing. Cajal had a much more modern view of cortical circuitry, seeing it as multidimensional. He accordingly detected three fundamental loops of connections: one in which thalamic fibers terminate directly on pyramidal neurons, a second in which one or a few short-axon neurons intervene, and a third in which there may be a sequence of interlaminar connections, including those formed both by short-axon cells and by the axon collaterals of pyramidal neurons.

In perceiving these different types of cortical circuit, all of which have been justified by modern anatomical and physiological research (Jones and Powell, 1970b; Ruiz-Marcos and Valverde, 1970; Toyama et al., 1974, 1977; Gilbert and Wiesel, 1979, 1983; Bullier and Henry, 1979; White, 1979; Sloper and Powell, 1979; Hornung and Garey, 1981; White and Rock, 1980; Winfield et al., 1982; Hendry and Jones, 1983b; Martin et al., 1983; Benshalom and White, 1986; Martin and Whitteridge, 1984; Valverde, 1986), Cajal was well ahead of his time. It is these different types of intracortical circuit that now form the basis for the analysis of intracortical processing in the sensory areas. Extensive reviews are available for the visual cortex regarding the increasing complexity in receptive field structure of neurons that occurs as a microelectrode moves from the main layer of thalamic terminations into layers superficial and deep to it (Hubel and Wiesel, 1977); the types of cell whose interlaminar connections may mediate the convergence that the increase in receptive field complexity implies (Gilbert, 1983; Martin, 1984); and the relative roles of direct, monosynaptic thalamic connections and inputs from intracortical neurons in shaping the receptive field structure of a particular cell type (Bullier and Henry, 1979; Malpeli et al., 1986; Schwark et al., 1986). The role of inhibitory, GABAergic cortical neurons is also being explored (Sillito, 1977, 1979, 1984; Dykes et al., 1984). As might be expected from the large population of cortical GABA neurons (Hendry et al., 1987), the effects of GABA on neurons in the visual and somatic sensory areas, as judged by selective blockade by bicuculline, is quite profound, leading in the visual cortex to uncovering of previously nondetectable binocular inputs to a neuron and to a loss in its selectivity for specifically oriented stimuli and for stimuli moving in a particular direction

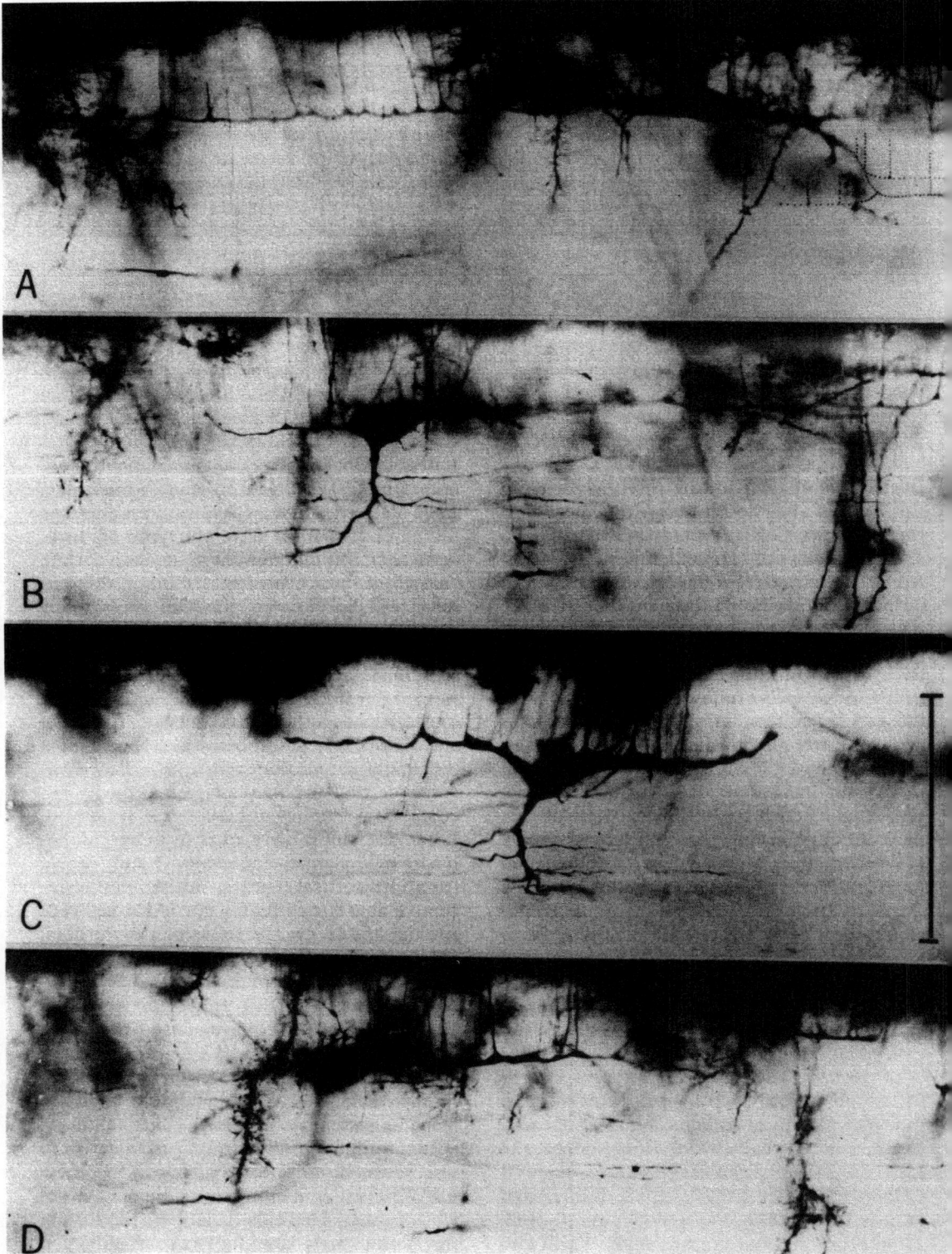

[*FIG. 321*] Photomicrographs of Golgi-impregnated Cajal-Retzius cells from a thirty-week-old human fetus. Bar 100 μm. *From:* Marin-Padilla and Marin-Padilla (1982).

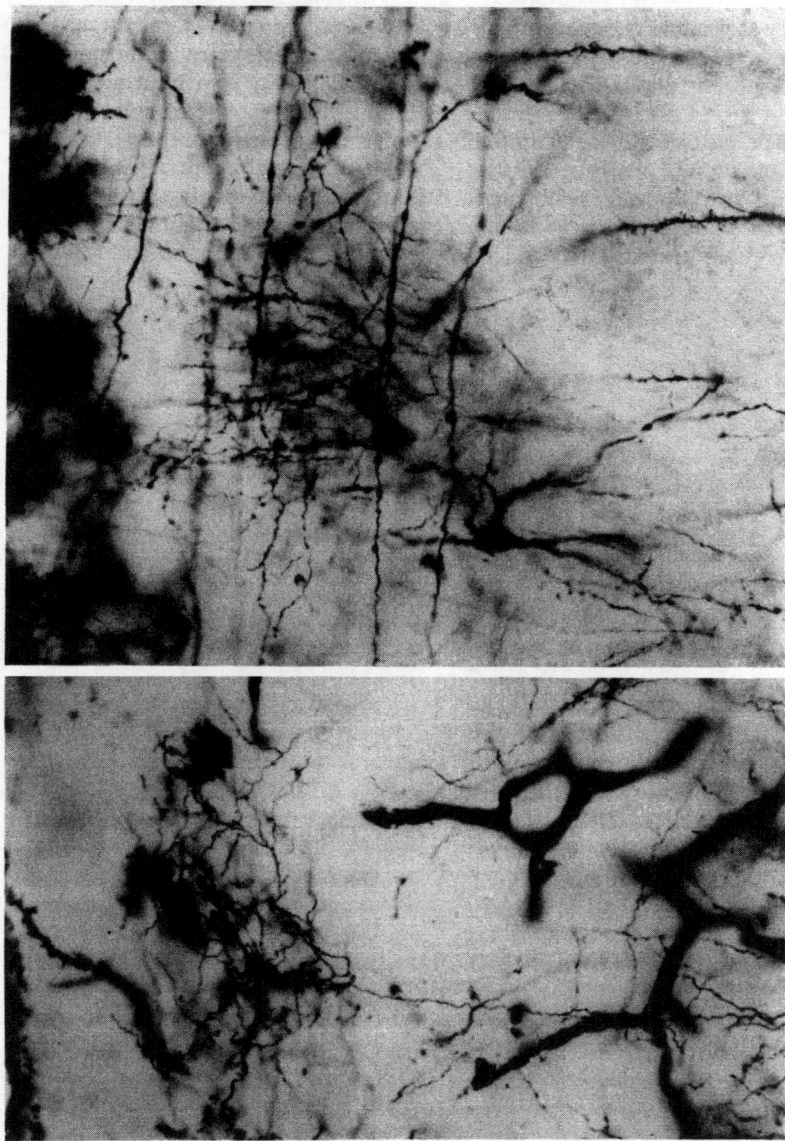

[*FIG. 322*] Photomicrographs from Cajal's preparations, showing (*left*) an ascending axon ending in ramifications in layer I at the "occipital pole" of a fourteen-day-old cat; (*right*) large horizontal axons in layer I of the motor cortex in a fifteen-month-old human brain. × 400 (*left*), × 430 (*right*).

(Sillito, 1977, 1979, 1984). Some disagreement does, however, remain about the exact role of inhibition in the shaping of the receptive fields of visual cortical neurons (Ferster, 1986).

One aspect of cortical circuitry that Cajal did not emphasize was verticality or columnarity, something that was to come to the fore in the later anatomical work of Lorente de Nó (1922b, 1949) and which has tended to dominate modern cortical studies since the initial physiological observations of Mountcastle (1957), Mountcastle and Powell (1959), and Hubel and Wiesel (1962). Cajal was certainly aware of the interlaminar circuitry that under-lies the functional columnarity of the cortex, but he did not recognize the focal nature of the thalamic input in which the column must have its fundamental basis (Hubel and Wiesel, 1977; Jones, 1981). This is not surprising in view of the apparently enormous extent of the thalamocortical axons as he saw them. In addition, Cajal was clearly impressed by the horizontal plexuses of the cortex as revealed in Golgi and Weigert preparations (chapter 16), and he had no concept of inhibition in the cortex which presumably serves to focus further afferent input and the interlaminar flow of activity [*figs. 331–333*].

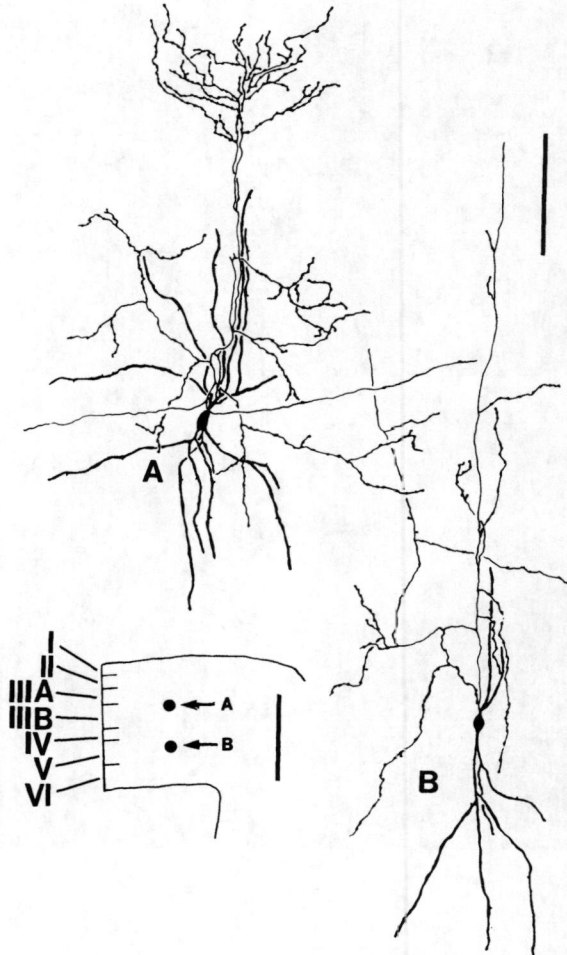

[*FIG. 323*] Golgi-impregnated cells, possibly conforming to what Cajal would have called Martinotti cells in the somatic sensory cortex of the monkey. Bars 1 mm, 100 μm. *From:* DeFelipe and Jones (1985).

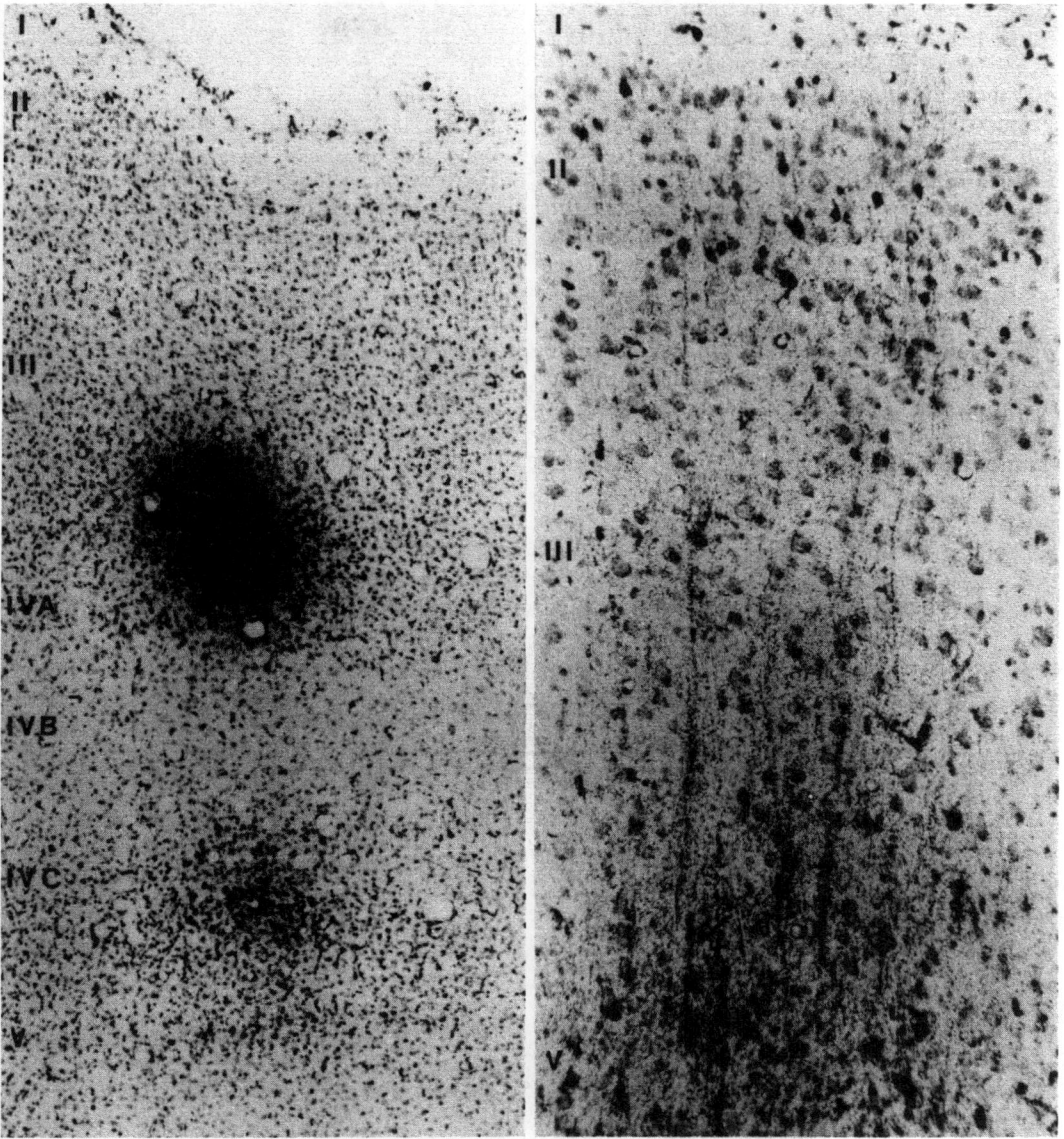

[FIG. 324]   Left: [³H] gamma aminobutyric acid injected into layer III of area 17 in a monkey leads to selective retrograde labeling of neurons in layers IVC and V immediately beneath the injection site. Right: A similar injection in layer V of the monkey motor cortex leads to selective retrograde labeling of cells in layer II immediately above the injection site. × 75 (A), × 125 (B). From: DeFelipe and Jones (1985).

Intracortical Collaterals of Pyramidal Cell Axons

Cajal saw the intracortical collaterals of pyramidal cell axons as major elements in cortical circuitry [fig. 334]. He was impressed by two major aspects of their organization: first, their obvious relevance in transmitting activity of groups of neurons in a particular layer to other neurons of the same type ("congener neurons") in the same layer; second, the significance of specifically distributed ascending or descending collaterals in transferring activity from one cortical layer to another. It is this second aspect of intracortical axonal collateralization that has achieved some prominence in modern studies of intracortical circuitry, as mentioned above.

It is doubtful that Cajal, despite the high quality of his preparations, demonstrated the full extent of axonal collateralization of any pyramidal neuron. Modern studies of cortical cells recovered histologically after the intracellular injection of horseradish peroxidase have generally revealed far more extensive and longer collateral branches than hitherto demonstrated, although Cajal suspected that they might be longer than evident in his preparations. The collaterals of a layer V pyramid

in layer VI of the visual cortex of the cat, for example, can extend for several hundred microns (Gilbert and Weisel, 1983) [*fig. 292*], and collaterals of layer III corticocortical neurons in the monkey somatic sensory areas have been shown to extend over 6–10 mms (DeFelipe et al., 1986a) [*figs. 335, 336*].

It is noteworthy that in all these labeling studies, the long collaterals give off highly focused, dense concentrations of terminal ramifications at intervals, with long intervening stretches virtually devoid of terminal branches [*figs. 292, 335*]. This could form the basis for communications between widely separated functional columns of the same or different types.

The morphology of the terminals of pyr-

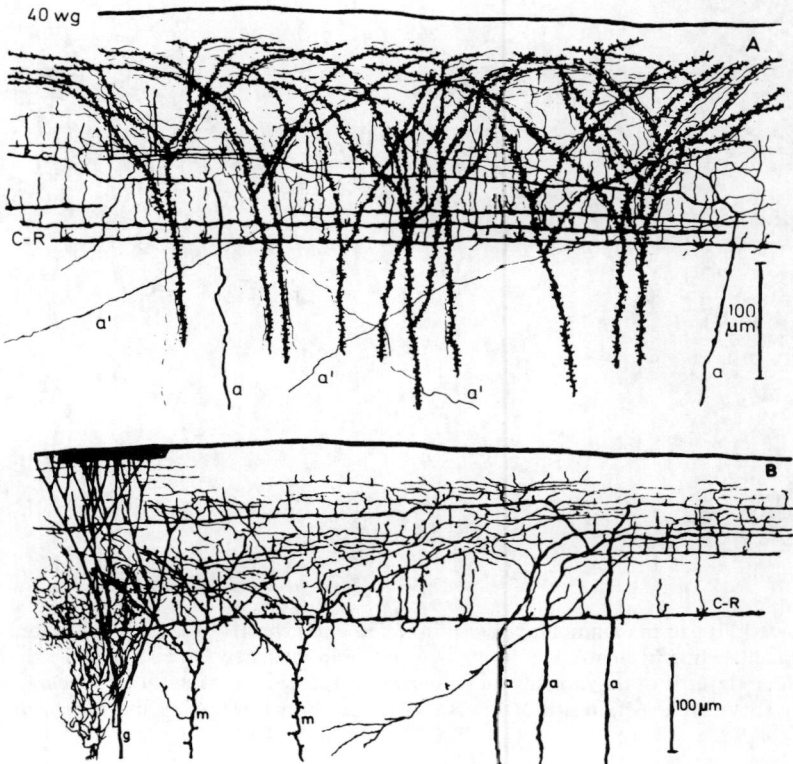

[*FIG. 325*] Camera lucida drawings from layer I of the motor cortex of newborn human brains. *Above:* Apical dendritic tufts of pyramidal cells showing their relationships to extrinsic afferent fibers (*a*), fibers from deeper layers (*a'*), and the processes of Cajal-Retzius cells (*C-R*). *Below:* Martinotti axons (*m*), processes of Cajal-Retzius cells (*C-R*), extrinsic afferents (*a*), and radial glial processes (*g*). *From:* Marin-Padilla and Marin-Padilla (1982).

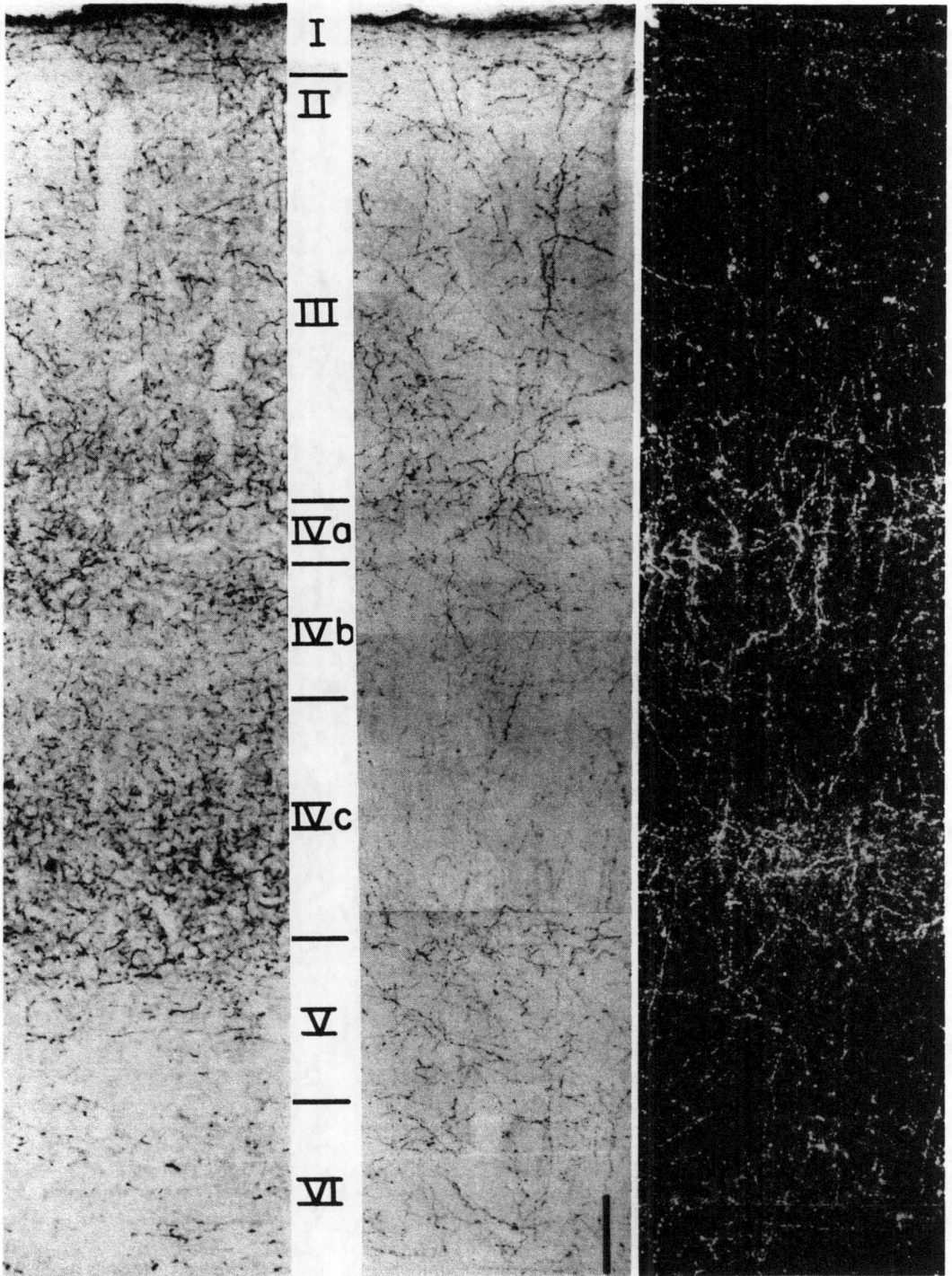

[*FIG. 326*]   Immunocytochemically stained sections through the visual cortex of macaque monkeys, showing the distribution of extrinsic afferent fibers immunoreactive for serotonin (*left*) and noradrenaline (*middle*), and of intrinsic processes immunoreactive for neuropeptide Y (*right*). Bar 100 μm. *Left and middle from:* Morrison et al. (1982); *right from:* Hendry et al. (1984).

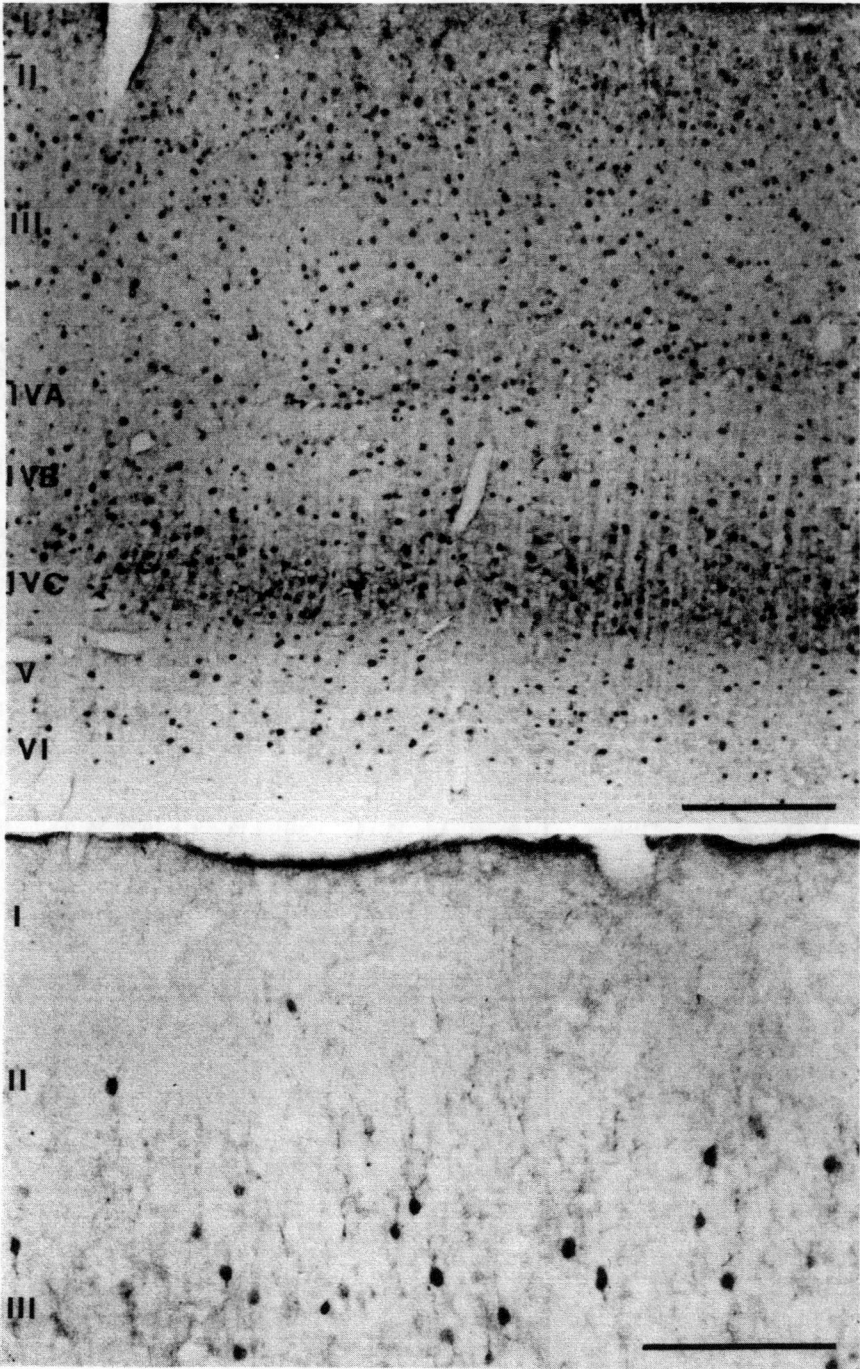

[*FIG. 327*]   *Above:* Neurons immunoreactive for gamma aminobutyric acid in the visual cortex of a monkey. Bar 250 μm. *From:* Hendry et al. (1987). *Below:* Neurons immunoreactive for cholecystokinin in the auditory cortex of a 140-day macaque monkey fetus. Bar 100 μm. *From:* material of S.H.C. Hendry and E.G.J.

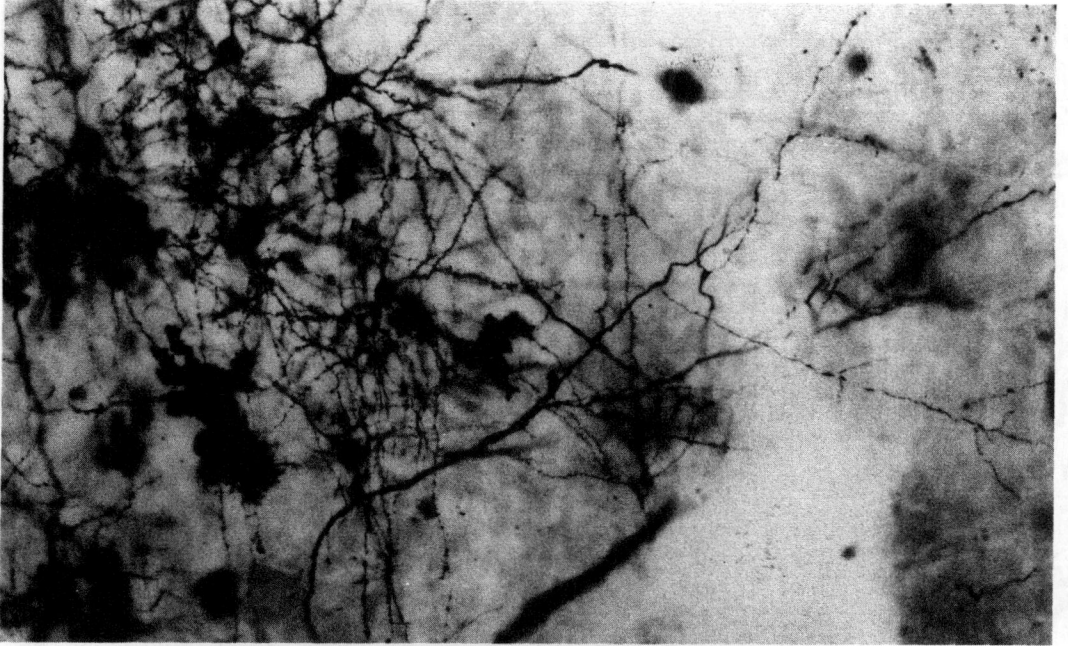

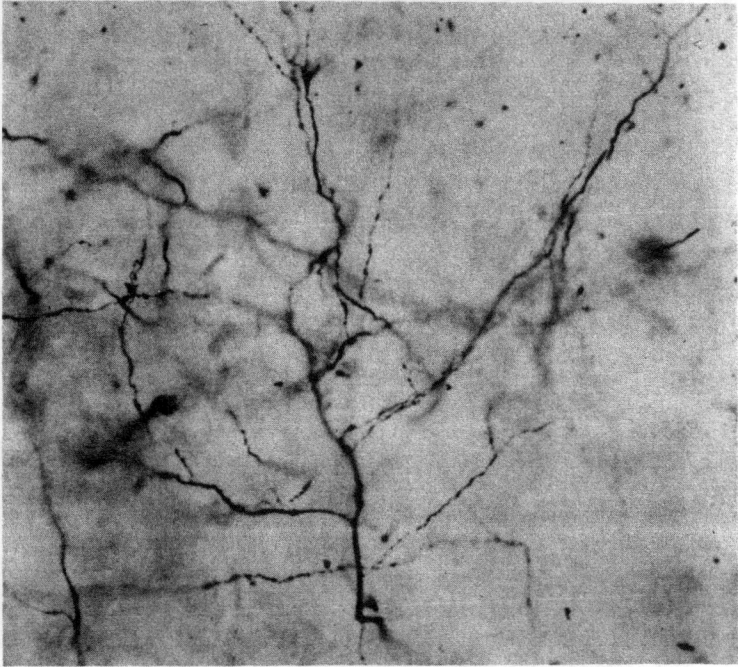

[*FIG. 328*]   Photomicrographs from Cajal's preparations of the cat visual cortex, showing parts of two large afferent fibers of the type that he interpreted (correctly) as arising from the thalamus and arborizing in layer IV. Note spiny cells in upper figure. × 250 *(upper)*, × 450 *(lower)*.

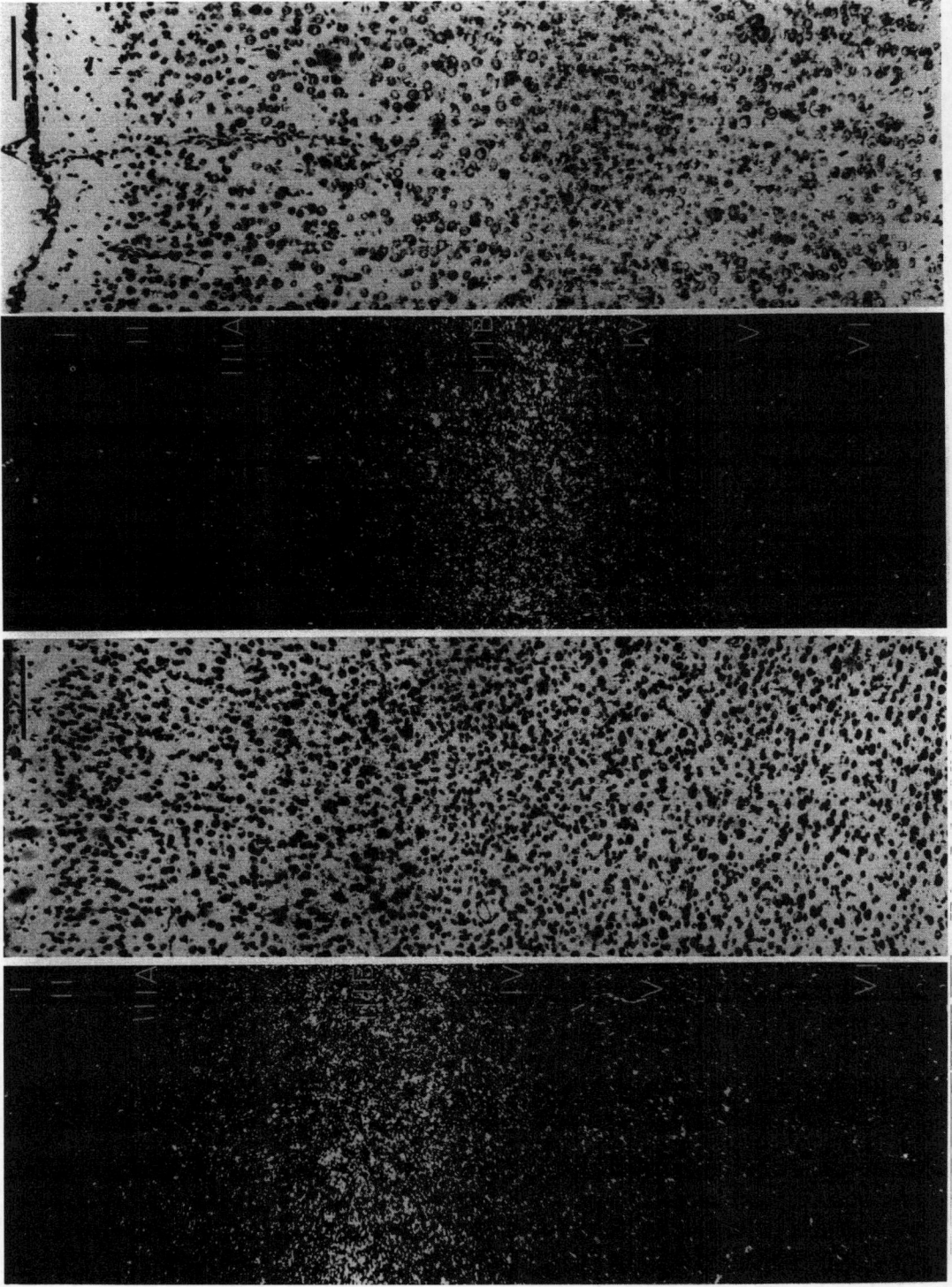

[FIG. 329] Pairs of alternate dark-field and bright-field photomicrographs of portions of areas 5 (*left pair*) and 7 (*right pair*) in a rhesus monkey, showing the laminar distribution of autoradiographically labeled thalamocortical fibers × 115. *From:* Jones and Burton (1976).

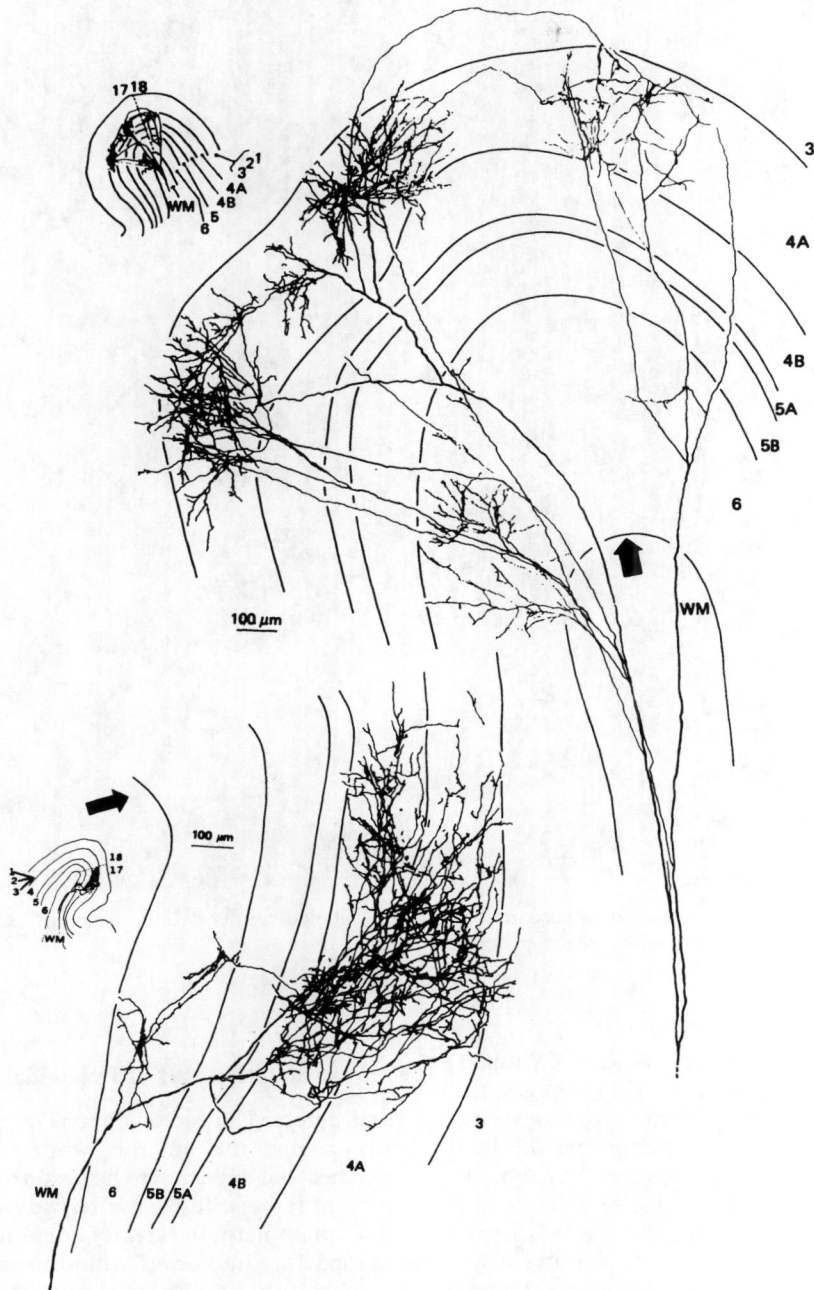

[*FIG. 330*] Identified X-type *(left)* and Y-type *(right)* geniculocortical axons, injected with horseradish peroxidase and ending in the visual cortex of the cat. *From:* Martin (1984).

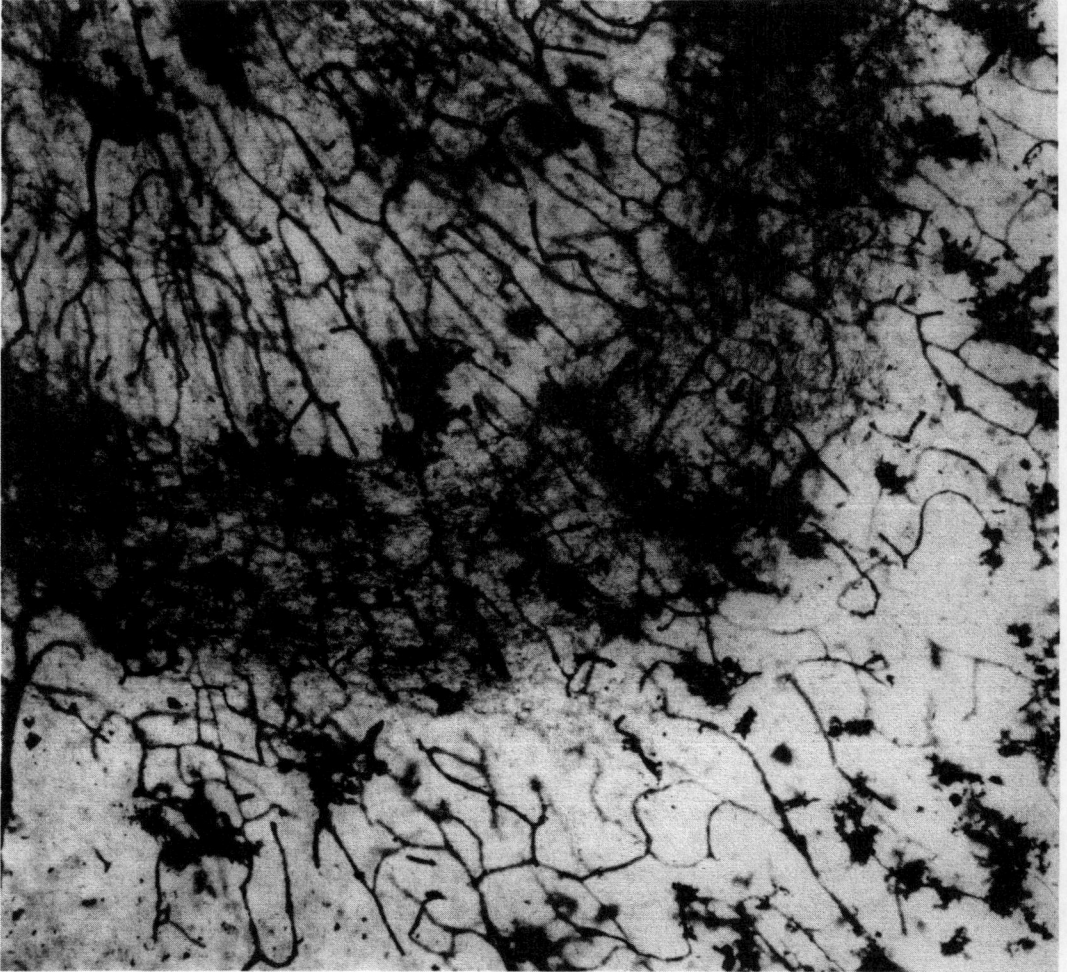

[*FIG. 331*]   Photomicrograph from a preparation of Cajal, labeled simply "child, Gennari," showing the dense plexus in the middle layers of the visual cortex. × 90.

amidal cell collaterals is asymmetric (Winfield et al., 1981; McGuire et al., 1984), suggesting an excitatory synapse, and there is a large body of physiological data indicating that the terminals of both collaterals and parent axon are excitatory (e.g., Phillips, 1959; Ts'o et al., 1986). Neurochemical and immunocytochemical studies suggest that the transmitter is an acidic amino acid, probably glutamate (Donoghue et al., 1985; Conti et al., 1987; see Jones, 1986, for a review).

Subcortical Collaterals of Pyramidal Cells

Cajal detected numerous axons of pyramidal cells giving rise in the white matter to branches that appeared to be destined for quite different targets. In his earliest studies on the small mammals, he clearly identified axons destined for the corpus callosum which had branches either returning to the cortex locally or apparently projecting to more distant cortical areas ipsilaterally (chapter 5 in this vol-

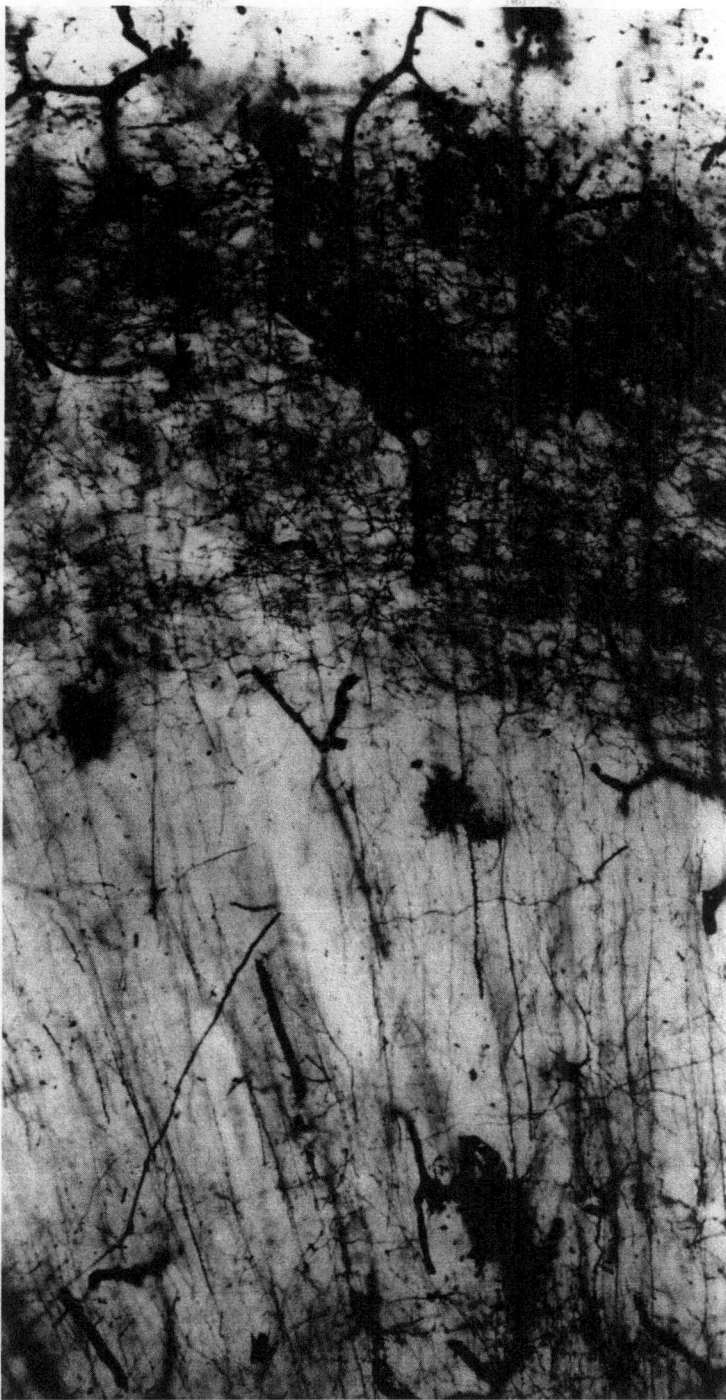

[*FIG. 332*]   Photomicrograph from a preparation of Cajal, labeled "Gennari, Golgi, child." Note oblique afferent fiber in lower part of figure. × 200.

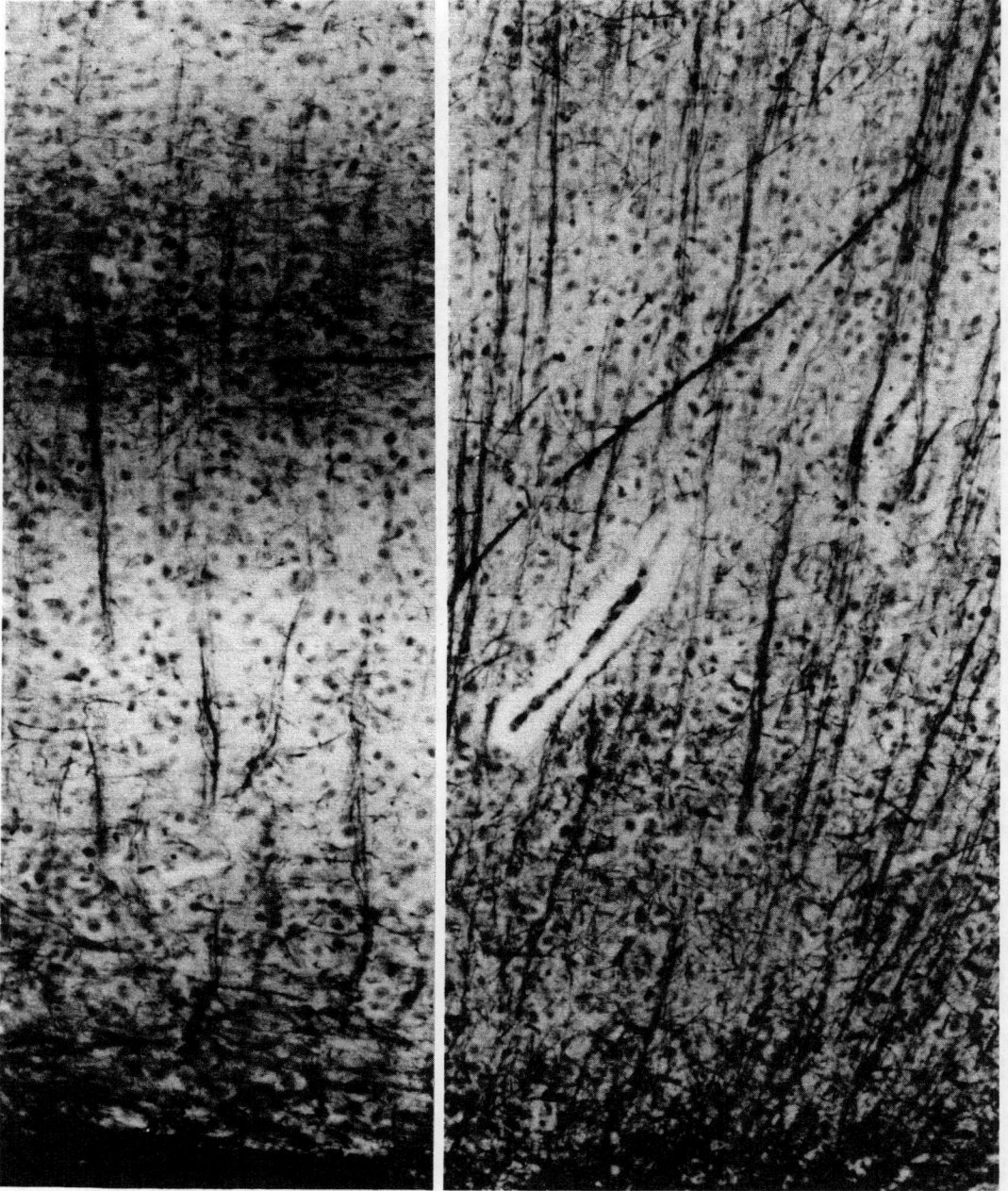

[*FIG. 333*] Photomicrographs from Weigert preparations made by Cajal of the adult human visual cortex, showing the radial fasciculi and stria of Gennari *(left)* and the radial fasciculi and an obliquely oriented thalamic afferent *(right)*. × 220 *(left)*, × 250 *(right)*.

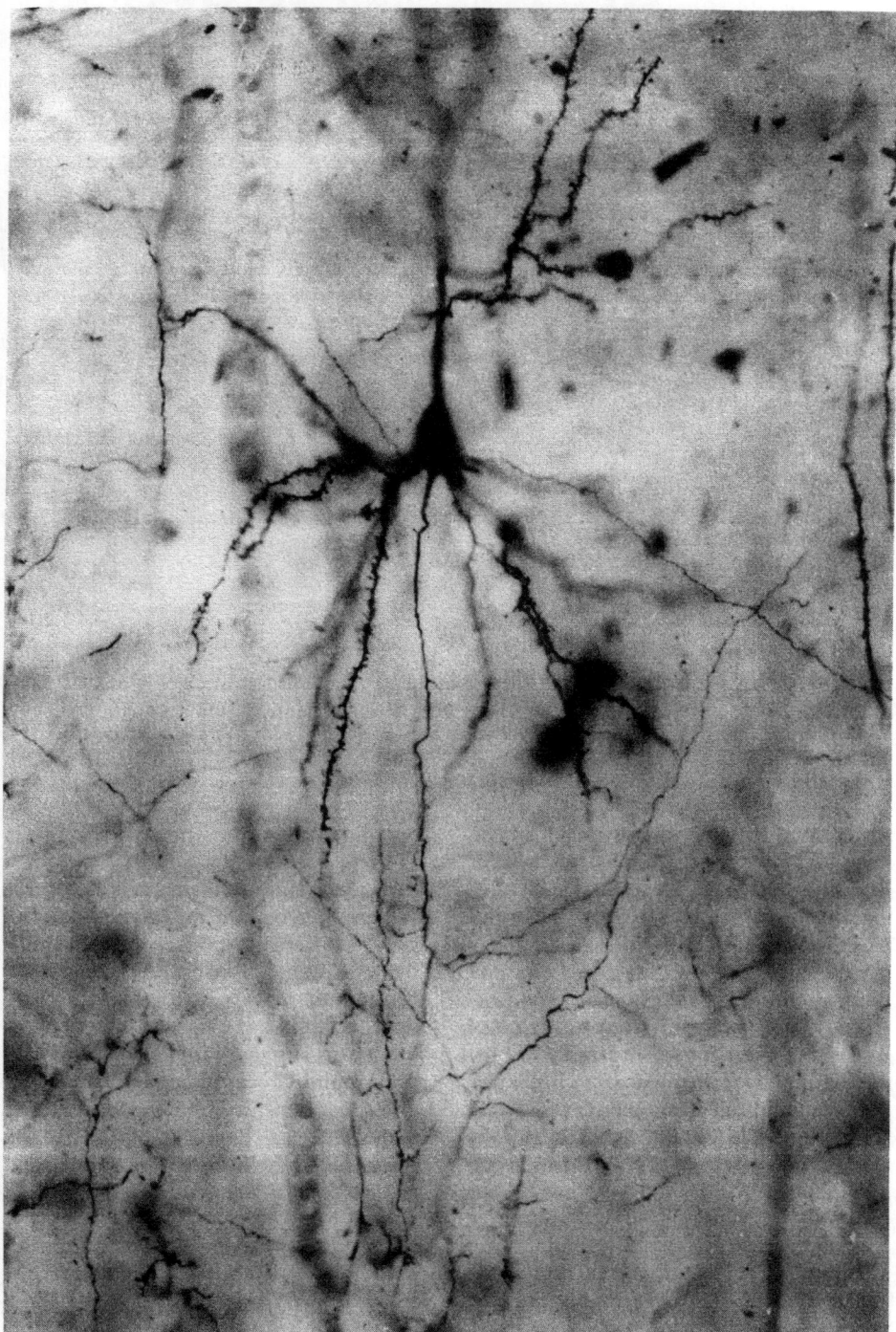

[*FIG. 334*] Photomicrograph from a preparation of Cajal, showing a layer III pyramidal neuron with its axon and axon collaterals in the human motor cortex. × 400.

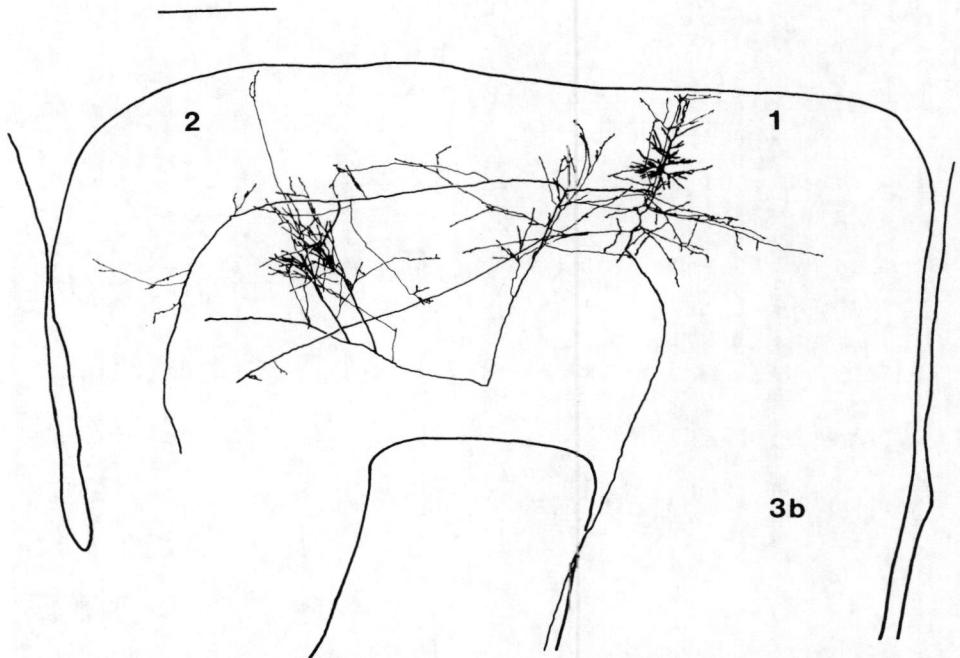

[*FIG. 335*]   Pyramidal neuron of layer III in area *1* of the somatic sensory cortex of a monkey, labeled with horseradish peroxidase injected into its main axon projecting (*to right*) to motor cortex, and showing the columnlike terminations of its collateral projection to area 2. Bar 500 μm. *From:* DeFelipe et al. (1986a).

ume). In a few cases, he also observed subcortically projecting axons giving rise to what were almost certainly callosal or ipsilateral corticocortical fibers [*figs. 5, 6, 20*]. But in this study, he also mentioned a significant population of especially commissural axons that projected into the corpus callosum without branching. As he came to study the human cortex, he was even more impressed by the presence of dual populations of commissural and subcortically projecting axons, some with branches to other sites and specific populations without (chapters 15–17, 21). In subcortical sites (chapter 25, p. 465, in this volume; *Histologie*, Vol. 1, p. 969), Cajal noted in man the appearance of a substantial population of pyramidal tract fibers that passed directly to the pontine nuclei, unlike in animals in which virtually all such fibers were collaterals of axons continuing on in the pyramidal tract. Collateral fibers were also present in man, but Cajal perceived the direct, presumably corti-

copontine fibers as a newly evolved feature of the human brain.

Modern studies have made use of tracer substances retrogradely transported in axons, some of them of different colors and thus capable of being used to demonstrate collateral projections from a single cortical cell to multiple sites. The earlier studies in primates tended to suggest rather limited collateralization, mainly because cells projecting to different sites were stratified into different layers and sublayers (Lund et al., 1975; Jones and Wise, 1977) [*fig. 290*]. For subcortically projecting cells, this tended to conflict with the results of electrophysiological studies in cats that reported extensive collateralization (Endo et al., 1973). Where multiple tracers have been used, the results have been varied and the subject of different emphasis. Cortical cells with axons projecting to two or more subcortical sites or to ipsilateral and contralateral cortical areas have definitely been reported (Rustioni and Hayes, 1981; Goldman-Rakic and Schwartz, 1982; Andersen et al., 1985; Ugolini and Kuypers, 1986). Some sites appear privileged, however. Axons projecting to claustrum and thalamus, for example, always arise from separate cells in layer VI (LeVay and Sherk, 1981), and axons projecting from the cortex to the thalamic relay nuclei are not collaterals of those projecting to other subcortical sites (Catsman-Berrevoets and Kuypers, 1981), and

corticospinal neurons in the adult rat do not have commissural collaterals (Catsman-Berrevoets et al., 1980). Where collateralization has been positively reported by double-retrograde-labeling strategies, the number of double-labeled cells has commonly been small, especially in primates where 5 percent or less of a cell population labeled from one site can be double labeled from another (e.g., Andersen et al., 1985) [fig. 337].

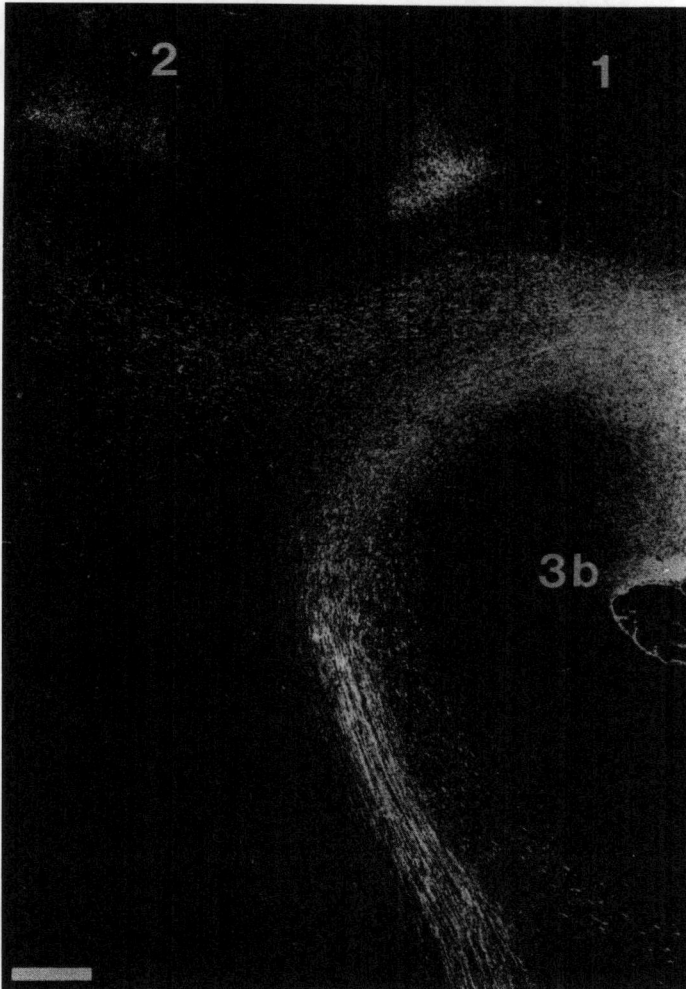

[FIG. 336]   Dark-field photomicrograph showing columnlike patterns of axonal terminations in areas 1 and 2 of a monkey, demonstrated by autoradiography following injection of [³H] amino acids in area 3b. Bar 500 μm. From: DeFelipe et al. (1986a).

It is possible, therefore, that the increasing trend toward laminar and sublaminar segregation of output cells in the cortex of primates, in comparison with rodents and carnivores (Jones, 1984b), is accompanied by an increasing trend toward reduced collateralization. This is, in a sense, a restatement of Cajal's interpretation, which suggested the appearance of a totally new set of uncollateralized fibers. It seems possible that fibers projecting only to a particular site and those projecting to the same site as collaterals of other projections may have different functional properties. This has been confirmed in monkeys for the parent cells in the motor cortex of direct corticorubral fibers and for those arising as collaterals of pyramidal tract axons (Fromm et al., 1981).

The two types have different temporal patterns of discharge in relation to movement onset.

Retrograde tracing studies in fetal and neonatal brains have demonstrated that the axons of cortical cells have the capacity during development to send branches to multiple target sites, for example, into the pyramidal tract and to another cortical area (Stanfield and O'Leary, 1985). Others may send branches into the corpus callosum and to ipsilateral cortical areas (Innocenti et al., 1977; Innocenti, 1981). Eventually, one of these major branches is lost. For example, cells of the developing visual cortex invariably lose any pyramidal tract axon they may have (O'Leary and Stanfield, 1986; Schreyer and Jones, 1988), and cells in

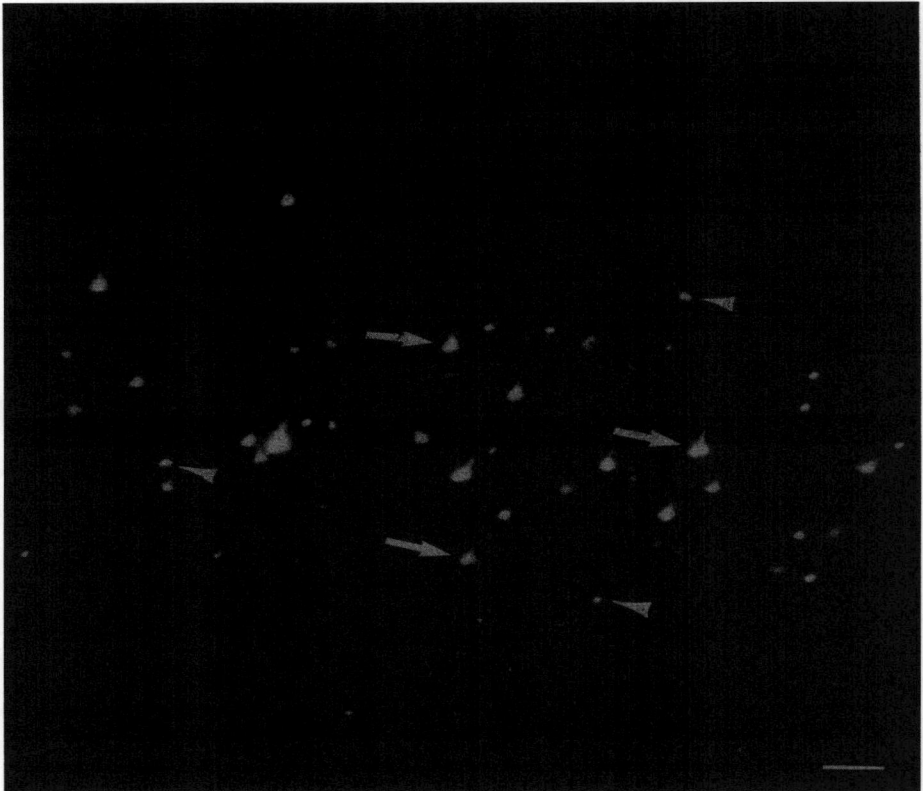

[*FIG. 337*] Fluorescence photomicrograph of retrogradely labeled pyramidal cells in area 7 of a monkey following injection of fast blue into contralateral area 7 and of nuclear yellow into ipsilateral prefrontal cortex. Arrows show examples of fast-blue-labeled cells and arrowheads of nuclear-yellow-labeled cells. No cells in this field are double labeled. Courtesy of Dr. C. Asanuma (see Andersen et al., 1985).

many regions of cortex lose callosally projecting axon branches (Innocenti, 1981; O'Leary et al., 1981) while retaining branches to the ipsilateral cortex. Conceivably, this pruning phenomenon progresses even further in the primate brain and results in a more selective form of cortical projection than that found in rodents and other nonprimates. The presence of extensive collateralization of pyramidal cell axons in immature animals may account for the readiness with which Cajal observed them, since he almost invariably used material from fetal or young postnatal brains.

Conclusions

It would be possible to extend this analysis of Cajal's contributions and how they continue to impinge on concepts and experimental studies of the present age. Among the subjects we have not touched on are some for which he has been given little or no credit, such as his recognition some years before Brodmann of the differential cytoarchitecture of the pre- and postcentral gyri in man (chapter 16 in this volume) and of the limbic cortex in rodents (chapters 6, 18, 28). Other contributions, such as the analysis of the connectivity of the hippocampal formation and related areas (chapter 18), are such fundamental anatomy that it is difficult now to conceive of them as being the work of one person. His contributions to the development and comparative structure of the cortex (chapters 23, 24) were relatively superficial, but they, too, contain a number of basic facts. Finally, there are his speculations about the plasticity of dendrites and of interneuronal connections in the cortex (chapter 25). Similar concepts have only recently reappeared, and they, in particular, show not only how far ahead of his time Cajal was but also how his thoughts continually ran in the direction of fundamental neurobiological principles. In this, he differed greatly from many of his contemporaries who commonly saw the study of brain structure merely as a means of understanding the symptomatology of human neurological disease. It is his capacity to look beyond the obvious that is the secret of Cajal's genius and the reason why his observations retain their freshness and relevance to this day.

Bibliography

In this section, we have gathered full bibliographic details of all the works to which Cajal made reference in the course of his writings, plus those alluded to in our own commentary. Cajal's referencing, although typical of his day and incomplete by modern bibliographic standards, is, on the whole, remarkably accurate. Only in his very last papers did we discover significant errors. As a consequence, we have had little difficulty in identifying the vast majority of the works to which he referred. Those we have not been able to verify are largely privately printed monographs or proceedings of conferences that had a limited circulation. In some instances, we have been able to consult a later, published version of the same work and have referenced that. The few that we could not verify are so indicated in the following list.

Albarracín, A. (1982). *Santiago Ramón y Cajal o la pasión de España*. Barcelona: Editorial Labor.

Andersen, R. A., Asanuma, C., and Cowan, W. M. (1985). Callosal and prefrontal associational projecting cell populations in area 7A of the macaque monkey: A study using retrogradely transported fluorescent dyes. J. comp. Neurol. *232*:443–455.

André-Thomas (1894). Contribution a l'étude du développement des cellules de l'écorce cérébrale par la méthode de Golgi. Compt. rend. Soc. Biol. Paris *46*:66–68.

Andriezen, W. L. (1893). The neuroglia elements in the human brain. Brit. med. J. *2*:227–230.

Arnstein, C. (1887). Die Methylenblaufärbung als histologische Methode. Anat. Anz. *2*:125–135.

Athias, [M.] (1897a). Recherches sur l'histogenèse de l'écorce du cervelet. J. Anat. Physiol. Paris. *33*:372–404.

Athias, M. (1897b). Structure histologique de la moelle épinière du têtard de la grenouille (Rana temporaria). Bibliogr. Anat., Paris, *5*:58–89.

Azoulay, L. (1896). Psychologie histologique et texture du système nerveux. L'Année Psychologique *2*:255–294.

Ballet [F.], and Faure, [M.] (1899). Atrophie des grandes cellules pyramidales dans la zone motrice de l'écorce cérébrale, après la section expérimentale des fibres de projection, chez le chien. Soc. méd. Hôp., Paris, *16*:361–365.

Bechterew, W. (1891). Zur Frage über die äusseren Associationsfasern der Hirnrinde. Neurol. Centralbl. *10*:682–684.

Bechterew, W. (1894). *Die Leitungsbahnen im Gehirn und Rückenmark. Ein Handbuch für das Studium des Nervensystems* (translated by V. Weinberg). Leipzig: Besold.

Bechterew, W. (1895). Über die Schleifenschicht. Arch. Anat. Physiol., Anat. Abt. *1895*:379–395.

Beevor, C. E. (1891). On the course of the fibres of the cingulum and the posterior parts of the corpus callosum and fornix in the marmoset monkey. Phil. Trans. roy. Soc., London, *82*:135–199.

Benshalom, G., and White, E. L. (1986). Quantification of thalamocortical synapses with spiny stellate neurons in layer IV of mouse somatosensory cortex. J. comp. Neurol. *253*:315–341.

Berder, [?] (1893). La cellule nerveuse et quelques recherches sur les cellules des hémisphères de la grenouille. Thesis, Lausanne [not verified].

Berkley, H. J. (1895). Studies on the lesions produced by the action of certain poisons on the cortical nerve cell. I. Alcohol. Brain 18:473–496.

Berkley, H. J. (1896). The intra-cerebral nerve-fibre terminal-apparatus, and modes of transmission of nervous impulses. Johns Hopkins Hospital Reports 6:89–108.

Berlin, R. (1858). Beiträge zur Strukturlehre der Grosshirnwindungen. Erlangen: Junge.

Besser, [L.] (1866). Zur Histogenese der nervösen Elementartheile in den Centralorganen des neugeborenen Menschen. Virchows Arch. path. Anat. 36:305–334.

Bethe, A. (1894–95). Studien über das Centralnervensystem von Carcinus maenas nebst Angaben über ein neues Verfahren der Methylenblaufixation. Arch. mikr. Anat. 44:579–622.

Bethe, A. (1896). Eine neue Methode der Methylenblaufixation. Anat. Anz. 12:438–446.

Bethe, A. (1898). Über die Primitivfibrillen in den Ganglienzellen von Menschen und anderen Wirbelthieren. Morphol. Arbeiten. 8:95–116.

Bethe, A. (1903). Allgemeine Anatomie und Physiologie des Nervensystems. Leipzig: Thieme.

Betz, [W.] (1874). Antomischer Nachweis zweier Gehirnzentra. Centralbl. med. Wiss. 12:578–580, 595–599.

Betz, W. (1881). Ueber die feinere Struktur der Grosshirnrinde des Menschen. Centralbl. med. Wiss. 19:193–195, 209–213, 231–234.

Bianchi, V. (1907). Sulle prime fasi di sviluppo dei centri nervosi nei vertebrati. Annali Nevrol. 25:1–16.

Bielschowsky, M. (1902). Die Silberimprägnation der Axencylinder. Neurol. Centralbl. 21:579–584.

Bielschowsky, M. (1903). Die Silberimprägnation der Neurofibrillen. Neurol. Centralbl. 22:997–1006.

Bielschowsky, M. (1904). Die Silberimprägnation der Neurofibrillen. J. Psychol. Neurol., Leipzig, 3:169–198.

Blasdel, C. G., and Lund, J. S. (1983). Termination of afferent axons in macaque striate cortex. J. Neurosci. 3:1389–1413.

Blumenau, L. (1891). Zur Entwicklungsgeschichte und feineren Anatomie des Hirnbalkens. Arch. mikr. Anat. EntwMech. 37:1–15.

Bok, S. T. (1929). Der Einfluss der in den Furchen und Windungen auftretenden Krümmungen der Grosshirnrinde auf die Rindenarchitektur. Z. ges. Neurol., Psychiat. 121:682–750.

Boll, F. (1874). Die Histologie und Histiogenese der nervösen Centralorgane. Arch. Psychiat., Nerv-Krankh., 4:1–138.

Bolton, J. S. (1900). The exact histological localisation of the visual area of the human cerebral cortex. Phil. Trans. roy. Soc., London, 193:165–222.

Bonne, C. (1906–1907). L'écorce cérébrale. Rev. gén. Histol. 2:291–581.

Bonne, C. (1910). L'écorce cérébrale. Part 2. Rev. gén. Histol. 12:351–380.

Bonome, A. (1907). Istogenesi della nevroglia normale nei vertebrati. Arch. ital. Anat. Embriol. 6:157–345.

Bottazzi, F. (1893). Intorno alla corteccia cerebrale e spezialmente intorno alle fibre nervose intracorticali dei vertebrati. Richerche lab Anat. norm. Univ. Roma 3:241–316.

Boyd, I. A. (1958). The methylene-blue technique for staining muscle spindles. J. Physiol., London, 144:10–11P.

Braitenberg, V. (1978). Cortical cytoarchitectonics: General and areal. In: Architectonics of the Cerebral Cortex. M.A.B. Brazier and H. Petsche (eds.). New York: Raven, pp. 443–465.

Broca, P. (1861). Sur le principe des localisations cérébrales. Bull. Soc. Anthropol., Paris, 2:190–204, 309–321.

Brock, G. (1905). Untersuchungen über die Entwicklung der Neurofibrillen des Schweinefötus. Mschr. Psychiat. Neurol. 18:467–480.

Brodmann, K. (1903a). Beiträge zur histologischen Lokalisation der Grosshirnrinde. Erste Mitteilung: Die Regio Rolandica. J. Psychol. Neurol., (Leipzig), 2:79–107.

Brodmann, K. (1903b). Beiträge zur histologischen Lokalisation der Grosshirnrinde. Zweite Mitteilung: Der Calarinatypus. J. Psychol. Neurol., (Leipzig), 2:133–159.

Brodmann, K. (1905a). Beiträge zur histologischen Lokalisation der Grosshirnrinde. Dritte Mitteilung: Die Rindenfelder der niederen Affen. J. Psychol. Neurol., (Leipzig), 4:177–226.

Brodmann, K. (1905b). Beiträge zur histologischen Lokalisation der Grosshirnrinde. Vierte Mitteilung: Der Riesenpyramidentypus und sein Verhalten zu den Furchen bei den Karnivoren. J. Psychol. Neurol., (Leipzig), 6:108–120.

Brodmann, K. (1906). Beiträge zur histologischen Lokalisation der Grosshirnrinde. Fünfte Mitteilung: Über den allgemeinen Bauplan des Cortex pallii bei den Mammaliern und Zwei homologe Rindenfelder im besondern. J. Psychol. Neurol., (Leipzig), 6:275–400.

Brodmann, K. (1907). Bemerkungen über die Fibrillogenie und ihre Beziehungen zur Myelogenie mit besonderer Berücksichtigung des Cortex cerebri. Neurol. Centralbl. 26:338–349.

Brodmann, K. (1909). Vergleichende Lokalisationslehre der Grosshirnrinde in ihren Prinzipien dargestellt auf Grund des Zellenbaues. Leipzig: Barth.

Brodmann, K. (1910). Feinere Anatomie des Grosshirns. In: Handbuch der Neurologie. M. Lewandowsky (ed.). Vol. 1. Allgemeinere Neurologie. Berlin: Springer, pp. 206–307.

Bullier, J., and Henry, G. H. (1979). Laminar distribution of first-order neurons and afferent terminals in cat striate cortex. J. Neurophysiol. 42:1271–1281.

Burckhardt, K. R. (1889). Histologische Untersuchungen am Rückenmark der Tritone. Arch. mikr. Anat. 34:131–156.

Cajal, S. Ramón y (1888a). Estructura de los centros nerviosos de las aves. Rev. trim. Histol. norm. patol. 1:1–10.

Cajal, S. Ramón y (1888b). Sobre las fibras nerviosas de la capa molecular del cerebelo. Rev. trim. Histol. norm. patol. *1:*33–49.

Cajal, S. Ramón y (1889a). *Manual de Histología Normal y Técnica Micrográfica.* Valencia: Aguilar.

Cajal, S. Ramón y (1889b). Estructura del lóbulo óptico de las aves y origen de los nervios ópticos. Rev. trim. Histol. norm. patol. *1:*65–78.

Cajal, S. Ramón y (1889c). Contribución al estudio de la estructura de la médula espinal. Rev. trim. Histol. norm. patol. *1:*79–106.

Cajal, S. Ramón y (1889d) Sobre las fibras nerviosas de la capa granulosa del cerebelo. Rev. trim. Histol. norm. patol. *1:*107–118.

Cajal, S. Ramón y (1889e). Sur l'origine et la direction des prolongations nerveuses de la couche moléculaire du cervelet. Internat. Mschr. Anat. Physiol. *6:*158–174.

Cajal, S. Ramón y (1889f). Sur la morphologie et les connexions des éléments de la rétine des oiseaux. Anat. Anz. *4:*111–121.

Cajal, S. Ramón y (1889g). Conexión general de los elementos nerviosos. La Medicina Práctica *2:*341–346.

Cajal, S. Ramón y (1890a). Sur l'origine et les ramifications des fibres nerveuses de la moelle embryonnaire. Anat. Anz. *5:*85–95, 111–119.

Cajal, S. Ramón y (1890b). Sur les fibres nerveuses de la couche granuleuse du cervelet et sur l'évolution des éléments cérébelleuse. Internat. Mschr. Anat. Physiol. *7:*12–31.

Cajal, S. Ramón y (1890c). A quelle époque apparaissent les expansions des cellules nerveuses de la moëlle épinière du poulet? Anat. Anz. *5:*21–22, 609–613, 631–639.

Cajal, S. Ramón y (1890d). Sobre la existencia de células nerviosas especiales en la primera capa de las circunvoluciones cerebrales. Gac. méd. Catalana *13:*737–739. (Republished 1924 in Trabajos Escogidos *1:*625–628. Madrid: Jimenez and Molina.)

Cajal, S. Ramón y (1890e). A propos de certains éléments bipolaires du cervelet avec quelques détails nouveaux sur l'évolution des fibres cérébelleuse. Internat. Mschr. Anat. Physiol. *7:*447–468.

Cajal, S. Ramón y (1890f). Textura de las circunvoluciones cerebrales de los mamíferos inferiores. Nota preventiva. Gac. méd. Catalana *1:*22–31.

Cajal, S. Ramón y (1890g). Pequeñas comunicaciones anatómicas II: Sobre la existencia de colaterales y de bifurcación en las fibras de la sustancia blanca de la corteza gris del cerebro. *Pequeñas Comunicaciones Anatómicas,* Barcelona, Privately printed, pp. 6–8.

Cajal, S. Ramón y (1891a). Sur la fine structure du lobe optique des oiseaux et sur l'origine réelle des nerfs optiques. J. internat. Anat. Physiol. *8:*337–366.

Cajal, S. Ramón y (1891b). Sobre la existencia de bifurcaciones y colaterales en los nervios sensitivos craneales y sustancia blanca del cerebro. Nota preventiva. Gac. san. Barcelona *3:*282–284.

Cajal, S. Ramón y (1891c). Pequeñas contribuciones al conocimiento del sistema nervioso I: Estructura y conexiones de los ganglios simpáticos. II: Estructura fundamental de la corteza cerebral de los batracios, reptiles y aves. III: Estructura de la retina de los reptiles y batracios. IV: Estructura de la médula espinal de los reptiles. Trabajos del Laboratorio Histológico de la Facultad de Medicina, Barcelona, August 1891, pp. 1–56.

Cajal, S. Ramón y (1891d). Sur la structure de l'écorce cérébrale de quelques mammifères. La Cellule *7:*125–176.

Cajal, S. Ramón y (1892a). El nuevo concepto de la histología de los centros nerviosos. Rev. Ciencias Méd. *18:*457–476.

Cajal, S. Ramón y (1892b). Observaciones anatómicas sobre la corteza cerebral y asta de Ammon. Anal. Soc. Española Historia natural *21:*192–204.

Cajal, S. Ramón y (1893a). *Nuevo concepto de la histología de los centros nerviosos.* Barcelona: Henrich.

Cajal, S. Ramón y (1893b). Neue Darstellung vom histologischen Bau des Centralnervensystems. Arch. Anat. Physiol., Anat. Abt., Supplement *1893:*319–428.

Cajal, S. Ramón y (1893c). Estructura del asta de Ammon y fascia dentata. Anal. Soc. Española Historia natural *22:*53–114.

Cajal, S. Ramón y (1893d). Beiträge zur feineren Anatomie des grossen Hirns I: Über die feinere Struktur des Ammonshornes. Trans. by A. [von] Kölliker. Z. wiss. Zool. *56:*615–663.

Cajal, S. Ramón y (1893e). Estructura de la corteza occipital inferior de los pequeños mamíferos. Anal. Soc. Española Historia natural *22:*115–125.

Cajal, S. Ramón y (1893f). Beiträge zur feineren Anatomie des grossen Hirns II: Über den Bau der Rinde des unteren Hinterhauptslappens der kleinen Säugetiere. Trans. by A. [von] Kölliker. Z. wiss. Zool. *56:*664–672.

Cajal, S. Ramón y (1894a). The Croonian lecture: La fine structure des centres nerveux. Proc. roy. Soc., London, *55:*444–467.

Cajal, S. Ramón y (1894b). The minute structure of the nervous centres. Brit. med. J. *98:*141.

Cajal, S. Ramón y (1894c). *Les nouvelles idées sur la structure du système nerveux chez l'homme et chez les vertébrés.* Edition française revue et augmentée par l'auteur. Translated by L. Azoulay, Preface by M. Duval. Paris: Reinwald.

Cajal, S. Ramón y (1894d). Estructura íntima de los centros nerviosos. Rev. Ciencias Méd., Barcelona, *20:*145–160.

Cajal, S. Ramón y (1894e). Histología. Consideraciones generales sobre la morfología de la célula nerviosa. La Veterinaria Española *37:*257–260; 273–275; 289–291.

Cajal, S. Ramón y (1894f). Algunas contribuciones al conocimiento de los ganglios del encéfalo. Anal. Soc. Española Historia natural *23:*195–237.

Cajal, S. Ramón y (1895a). Algunas conjeturas sobre el mecanismo anatómico de la ideación, asociación y atención. Rev. Med. Cir. Prac. Madrid: Moya, pp. 1–14.

Cajal, S. Ramón y (1895b). Corps strié. Bibliogr. Anat. *3:*58–62.

Cajal, S. Ramón y (1896a). Las colaterales y bifurcaciones de las raíces posteriores de la médula espinal demostrados con el azul de metileno. Rev. clin. Térapéut. Farm. *10*:1–8.

Cajal, S. Ramón y (1896b). Nouvelles contributions à l'étude histologique de la rétine et à la question des anastomoses des prolongements protoplasmiques. J. Anat. Physiol., Paris, *33*:481–543.

Cajal, S. Ramón y (1896c). Estructura del protoplasma nervioso. Anal. Soc. Española Historia natural, 2nd series, *5*:10–46.

Cajal, S. Ramón y (1896d). Sobre las relaciones de las células nerviosas con las neuróglicas. Rev. trim. Micrográf., Madrid, *1*:38–41. (Reprinted 1931.)

Cajal, S. Ramón y (1896e). Las espinas colaterales de las células del cerebro teñidas con el azul de metileno. Rev. trim. Micrográf., Madrid, *1*:123–136. (Translated as: Les épines collatérales des cellules du cerveau colorées au bleu de méthylène; republished 1931.)

Cajal, S. Ramón y (1896f). El azul de metileno en los centros nerviosos. Rev. trim. Micrográf., Madrid, *1*:151–203. (Translated as: Le bleu de méthylène dans les centres nerveux; republished 1931.)

Cajal, S. Ramón y (1896g). Beitrag zum Studium der Medulla Oblongata des Kleinhirns und des Ursprungs der Gehirnnerven. Translated by J. Bresler. Leipzig: Barth.

Cajal, S. Ramón y (1897a). Algo sobre la significación fisiológica de la neuroglia. Rev. trim. Micrográf., Madrid, *2*:33–47.

Cajal, S. Ramón y (1897b). Las células de cilindro-eje corto de la capa molecular del cerebro. Rev. trim. Micrográf., Madrid, *2*:105–127.

Cajal, S. Ramón y (1897c). Leyes de la morfología y dinamismo de las células nerviosas. Rev. trim. Micrográf., Madrid, *2*:1–12.

Cajal, S. Ramón y (1898a). Estructura del kiasma óptico y teoría general de los entrecruzamientos de las vías nerviosas. Rev. trim. Micrográf., Madrid, *3*:15–65.

Cajal, S. Ramón y (1898b). La red superficial de las células nerviosas centrales. Rev. trim. Micrográf., Madrid, *3*:199–204.

Cajal, S. Ramón y (1899, 1904). *Textura del sistema nervioso del hombre y de los vertebrados*. Madrid: Moya, 2 vols. in 3.

Cajal, S. Ramón y (1899a). Estudios sobre la corteza cerebral humana I: Corteza visual. Rev. trim. Micrográf., Madrid, *4*:1–63.

Cajal, S. Ramón y (1899b). Estudios sobre la corteza cerebral humana II: Estructura de la corteza motriz del hombre y mamíferos superiores. Rev. trim. Micrográf., Madrid, *4*:117–200.

Cajal, S. Ramón y (1899c). Comparative study of the sensory areas of the human cortex. *In: Clark University 1889–1899 Decennial Celebration*. W. E. Story and L. N. Wilson (eds.). Worcester, MA: Clark Univ., pp. 311–382.

Cajal, S. Ramón y (1899d). Apuntes para el estudio estructural de la corteza visual del cerebro humano. Rev. Ibero-Americana Cienc. Méd. *1*:1–14.

Cajal, S. Ramón y (1900a). Estudios sobre la corteza cerebral humana II: Corteza motriz (conclusión). Rev. trim. Micrográf., Madrid, *5*:1–11.

Cajal, S. Ramón y (1900b). Estudios sobre la corteza cerebral humana III: Corteza acústica. Rev. trim. Micrográf., Madrid, *5*:129–183.

Cajal, S. Ramón y (1900c). Contribución al estudio de la vía sensitiva central y estructura del tálamo óptico. Rev. trim. Micrográf., Madrid, *5*:185–198.

Cajal, S. Ramón y (1900–1903). Studien über die Hirnrinde des Menschen. Parts I–IV. Die Sehrinde (1900); Die Bewegungsrinde (1900); Die Höhrrinde (1902); Die Riechrinde beim Menschen und Säugetier (1903). Translated by J. A. Bresler. Leipzig: Barth.

Cajal, S. Ramón y (1901a). Estudios sobre la corteza cerebral humana IV: Estructura de la corteza cerebral olfativa del hombre y mamíferos. Trab. Lab. Invest. biol. Univ. Madrid *1*:1–140.

Cajal, S. Ramón y (1901b). Significación probable de las células nerviosas de cilindro-eje corto. Trab. Lab. Invest. biol. Univ. Madrid *1*:151–157.

Cajal, S. Ramón y (1902a). Estructura del septum lucidum. Trab. Lab. Invest. biol. Univ. Madrid *1*:159–188.

Cajal, S. Ramón y (1902b). Sobre un ganglio especial de la corteza esfeno-occipital. Trab. Lab. Invest. biol. Univ. Madrid *1*:189–206.

Cajal, S. Ramón y (1902c). Die Endigung des äusseren Lemniscus oder der sekundären akustichen Nervenbahn. Deutsche med. Wschr. *16*:275–278.

Cajal, S. Ramón y (1903a). Consideraciones críticas sobre la teoría de A. Bethe, acerca de la estructura y conexiones de las células nerviosas. Trab. Lab. Invest. biol. Univ. Madrid *2*:101–128.

Cajal, S. Ramón y (1903b). Sobre la estructura del protoplasma nervioso. Revista Escolar de Medicina y Cirugía *1*:81–89.

Cajal, S. Ramón y (1903c). Un sencillo método de coloración del retículo protoplásmico y sus efectos en los diversos centros nerviosos de vertebrados e invertebrados. Trab. Lab. Invest. biol. Univ. Madrid *2*:129–221.

Cajal, S. Ramón y (1903d). Sobre un sencillo proceder de impregnación de las fibrillas interiores del protoplasma nervioso. Arch. Lat. Med. Biol., Madrid. *1*:1–6.

Cajal, S. Ramón y (1903e). Über einige Methoden der Silberimprägnierung zur Untersuchung der Neurofibrillen, der Achsencylinder und der Endverzweigungen. Z. wiss. Mikrosk., *20*:401–408.

Cajal, S. Ramón y (1904a). Algunos métodos de coloración de los cilindros-ejes, neurofibrillas y nidos nerviosos. Trab. Lab. Invest. biol. Univ. Madrid *3*:1–7.

Cajal, S. Ramón y (1904b). Variations morphologiques du reticulum neurofibrillaire à l'état normal et pathologique. Comp. Rend. Assoc. Anat. 6th session, Toulouse, pp. 191–198. [Translated from: Trab. Lab. Invest. Biol. Univ. Madrid *3*:9–15.]

Cajal, S. Ramón y (1904c). Variaciones morfológicas, normales y patológicas del reticulo neurofibrilar. Trab. Lab. Invest. biol. Univ. Madrid *3*:9–15.

Cajal, S. Ramón y (1906a). Notas preventivas sobre la

degeneración y regeneración de las vías nerviosas centrales. Trab. Lab. Invest. biol. Univ. Madrid 4:295–301.

Cajal, S. Ramón y (1906b). Studien über die Hirnrinde des Menschen V: Vergleichende Strukturbeschreibung und Histogenesis der Hirnrinde. Anatomisch-physiologische Betrachtungen über das Gehirn. Struktur der Nervenzellen des Gehirns. Translated by J.A. Bressler. Leipzig: Barth.

Cajal, S. Ramón y (1907a). Note sur la dégénérescence traumatique des fibres nerveuses du cervelet et du cerveau. Trav. Lab. Rech. biol. Univ. Madrid 5:105–116.

Cajal, S. Ramón y (1907b). Quelques formules de fixation destinées à la méthode au nitrate d'argent. Trav. Lab. Rech. biol. Univ. Madrid 5:215–226.

Cajal, S. Ramón y (1908). Les conduits de Golgi-Holmgren du protoplasme nerveux et le réseau péricéllulaire de la membrane. Trav. Lab. Rech. biol. Univ. Madrid 6:123–135.

Cajal, S. Ramón y (1909, 1911). Histologie du système nerveux de l'homme et des vertébrés. Trans. by L. Azoulay. Paris: Maloine, 2 vols.

Cajal, S. Ramón y (1913–1914). Estudios sobre la degeneración y regeneración del sistema nervioso. Madrid: Moya, 2 vols.

Cajal, S. Ramón y (1917). Recuerdos de mi vida, Vol. 2: Historia de mi labor científica. Madrid: Moya.

Cajal, S. Ramón y (1920). Una modificación del método de Bielschowsky para la impregnación de la neuroglia común y mesoglia y algunos consejos acerca de la técnica del oro-sublimado. Trab. Lab. Invest. biol. Univ. Madrid 18:129–141.

Cajal, S. Ramón y (1921a). Textura de la corteza visual del gato. Trab. Lab. Invest. biol. Univ. Madrid 19:113–146.

Cajal, S. Ramón y (1921b). Textura de la corteza visual del gato. Arch. Neurobiol., Madrid, 2:338–362.

Cajal, S. Ramón y (1922a). Studien über die Sehrinde der Katze. J. Psychol. Neurol., Leipzig, 29:161–181.

Cajal, S. Ramón y (1922b). Estudios sobre la fina estructura de la corteza regional de los roedores. Trab. Lab. Invest. biol. Univ. Madrid 20:1–30.

Cajal, S. Ramón y (1923a). Studien über den feineren Bau der regional Rinde bei den Nagetieren. J. Psychol. Neurol., Leipzig, 30:1–28.

Cajal, S. Ramón y (1923b). Recuerdos de mi vida, 3rd edition. Madrid: Pueyo.

Cajal, S. Ramón y (1928). Degeneration and Regeneration of the Nervous System. Translated and edited by Raoul M. May. London: Oxford University Press, 2 vols.

Cajal, S. Ramón y (1929). Études sur la neurogenèse de quelques Vertébrés: Recueil de mes principales recherches concernant la genèse des nerfs, la morphologie et la structure neuronale, l'origine de la névroglie, les terminaisons nerveuses sensorielles, etc. Madrid: Tipografía Artística.

Cajal, S. Ramón y (1933). ¿Neuronismo o Reticularismo? Las pruebas objetivas de la unidad anatómica de las células nerviosas. Arch. Neurobiol. Madrid 13:1–144.

Cajal, S. Ramón y (1934a). Les preuves objectives de l'unité des cellules nerveuses. Trav. Lab. Rech. biol. Univ. Madrid 29:1–137.

Cajal, S. Ramón y (1934b). Die Neuronenlehre und die periterminalen Netze Boekes. Arch. Psychiat. Nervenkrh. 102:322–332.

Cajal, S. Ramón y (1935). Die Neuronenlehre. Translated by D. Miskolczy. In: Handbuch der Neurologie, Vol. 1. O. Bumke and O. Foerster (eds.). Berlin: Springer, pp. 887–994.

Cajal, S. Ramón y (1937). Recollections of My Life. Translated by E. H. Craigie with the assistance of J. Cano. Philadelphia: American Philosophical Society. (Reprinted, without date, Cambridge, MA: MIT Press.)

Cajal, S. Ramón y (1954). Neuron Theory or Reticular Theory? Objective Evidence of the Anatomical Unity of the Nerve Cells. Translated by M. Ubeda Purkiss and C. A. Fox. Madrid: Consejo Superior de Investigaciones Científicas.

Cajal, S. Ramón y (1955). Studies on the Cerebral Cortex (Limbic Structures). Translated by L. M. Kraft. London: Lloyd-Luke.

Cajal, S. Ramón y (1960). Studies on Vertebrate Neurogenesis. Translated by Lloyd Guth. Springfield, IL: Thomas.

Cajal, S. Ramón y, and Olóriz, F. (1897). Los ganglios sensitivos craneales de los mamíferos. Rev. trim. Micrográf. Madrid, 2:129–152.

Cajal, S. Ramón y, and Tello y Muñoz, J. F. (1928). Elementos de histologiá normal y de técnica micrográfica, 9th edition. Madrid: Tipografía Artística.

Calleja, C. (1893). La región olfatoria del cerebro. Madrid: Moya.

Campbell, A. W. (1905). Histological studies on the localisation of cerebral function. Cambridge: Cambridge Univ. Press.

Capobianco, F. (1902). De la participation mésodermique dans la genèse de la névroglie cérébrale. Arch. ital. Biol. 37:152–155. (Author's summary of a paper published in 1901 in Monitore Zool. Ital. 12.)

Catsman-Berrevoets, C. E., and Kuypers, H.G.J.M. (1981). A search for corticospinal collaterals to thalamus and mesencephalon by means of multiple retrograde fluorescent tracers in cat and rat. Brain Res. 218:15–33.

Catsman-Berrevoets, C. E., Lemon, R. N., Verburgh, C. A., Bentivoglio, M., and Kuypers, H.G.J.M. (1980). Absence of callosal collaterals derived from rat corticospinal neurons: A study using fluorescent retrograde tracing and electrophysiological techniques. Exp. Brain Res. 39:433–440.

Colonnier, M. (1968). Synaptic patterns on different cell types in the different laminae of the cat visual cortex: An electron microscope study. Brain Res. 9:268–287.

Conel, J. L. (1939, 1941, 1947). The postnatal development of the human cerebral cortex. 3 vol. Cambridge, MA: Harvard Univ. Press.

Conti, F., Rustioni, A., Petrusz, P., and Towle, A. C. (1987). Glutamate-positive neurons in the somatic sensory cortex of rats and monkeys. J. Neurosci. 7:1887–1901.

Cowey, A., Freund, T. F., and Somogyi, P. (1981). Organization of [³H] GABA-accumulating neurones in the visual cortex of the rat and the rhesus monkey. J. Physiol. London, *320:*15–16P.

Cramer, A. (1898). Beitrag zur Kenntnis der Optikuskreuzung in Chiasma und des Verhaltens der optischen Centren bei einseitiger Bulbusatrophie. Arb. anat. Inst., Wiesbaden, *10:*415–484.

Crick, F. (1982). Do dendritic spines twitch? Trends. Neurosci. *5:*44–46.

DeCarlos, J. A., Lopez-Mascaraque, L., and Valverde, F. (1985). Development, morphology and topography of chandelier cells in the auditory cortex of the cat. Dev. Brain Res. *22:*293–300.

DeFelipe, J., Hendry, S.H.C., Jones, E. G., and Schmechel, D. (1985). Variability in the terminations of GABAergic chandelier cell axons on initial segments of pyramidal cell axons in the monkey sensory-motor cortex. J. comp. Neurol. *231:*364–384.

DeFelipe, J., Conley, M., and Jones, E. G. (1986a). Long-range focal collateralization of axons arising from corticocortical cells in monkey sensory-motor cortex. J. Neurosci. *6:*3749–3766.

DeFelipe, J., Hendry, S.H.C., and Jones, E. G. (1986b). A correlative electron microscopic study of basket cells and large GABAergic neurons in the monkey sensory-motor cortex. Neurosci. *17:*991–1009.

DeFelipe, J., and Jones, E. G. (1985). Vertical organization of γ-amino butyric acid-accumulating intrinsic neuronal systems in monkey cerebral cortex. J. Neurosci. *5:*3246–3260.

Deiters, O.F.K. (1865). *Untersuchungen über Gehirn und Rückenmark des Menschen und der Säugetiere.* M. Schultze (ed.). Braunschweig: Vieweg.

Dejerine, J. (1895, 1901). (With the collaboration of Mme. Dejerine-Klumke.) *Anatomie des centres Nerveux.* 2 Vols. in 3 (Vol. 1, 1895; Vol. 2, parts 1 and 2, 1901). Paris: Rueff.

Dejerine, J. (1897). Sur les fibres de projection et d'association des hémisphères cérébraux. Comp. Rend. Soc. Biol., Paris, *49:*178–181.

Demoor, [J.] (1896). La plasticité morphologique des neurones cérébraux. Arch. Biol., Paris, *14:*723–755.

Deschênes, M., LaBelle, A., and Landry, P. (1979). Morphological characterizations of slow and fast pyramidal tract cells in the cat. Brain Res. *178:*251–274.

Dogiel, A. S. (1889). Eine neue Imprägnations-methode der Gewebe mittelst Methylenblau. Arch. mikrosk. Anat. EntwMech. *33:*440–445.

Dogiel, A. S. (1896). Die Nervenelemente in Kleinhirne der Vögel und Säugethiere. Arch. mikrosk. Anat. EntwMech. *47:*707–719.

Döllken, [A.] (1907). Beiträge zur Entwickelung des Säugegehirns: Lage und Ausdehnung des Bewegungscentrums der Maus. Neurol. Centralbl. *26:*50–59.

Donaggio, [A.] (1898). Nuove osservazioni sulla struttura della cellula nervosa. Riv. sperim. freniatr. med. leg. Alien. ment. *24:*772–798.

Donaggio, A. (1903). Le fibrille nella cellula nervosa dei mammiferi. Bibliogr. Anat. *12:*197–199.

Donoghue, J. P., Wenthold, R. J., and Altschuler, R. A. (1985). Localisation of glutaminase-like and aspartate aminotransferase-like immunoreactivity in neurons of cerebral neocortex. J. Neurosci. *5:*2597–2609.

Dotto, [?], and Pusateri, [?] (1897). Sulle alterazioni degli elementi della corteccia cerebrale secondari a focali emorragici intracerebrali e sulla connessione della corteccia dell'insula di Reil colla capsula esterna nell'uomo. Riv. Pathol. nerv. ment. *2:*8–14.

Droogleever Fortuyn. See Fortuyn.

Duval, [M.] (1876). Sur le sinus rhomboïdal des oiseaux. Gaz. Méd., Paris, 4th series, *5:*409–410.

Duval, M. (1877). Recherches sur le sinus rhomboïdal des oiseaux et sur la névroglie périépendymaire. J. Anat. Physiol., Paris, *13:*1–17.

Duval, M. (1895). Hypothèse sur la physiologie des centres nerveux: Théorie histologique du sommeil. Compt. Rend. Soc. Biol., Paris (series 10), *2:*74–113.

Duval, M. (1900). Les neurones, l'amiboïsme nerveux: La théorie histologique du sommeil. Rev. École Anthropol., Paris, *10:*37–71.

Dykes, R. W., Landry, P., Metherate, R., and Hicks, T. P. (1984). Functional role of GABA in cat primary somatosensory cortex: Shaping receptive fields of cortical neurons. J. Neurophysiol. *52:*1066–1093.

Eckenstein, F., and Baughman, R. W. (1984). Two types of cholinergic innervation in cortex, one co-localized with vasoactive intestinal polypeptide. Nature *309:*153–155.

Edinger, L. (1889a). Untersuchungen über die vergleichende Anatomie des Gehirns I: Das Vorderhirn. Abh. Senckenb. naturforsch. Gesellsch., Frankfurt, *15:*91–119.

Edinger, L. (1889b). *Zwölf Vorlesungen über den Bau der nervösen Centralorgane,* 2nd edition. Leipzig: Vogel.

Edinger, L. (1893) Vergleichend-entwickelungsgeschichtliche und anatomische Studien im Bereiche der Hirnanatomie, 3, Reichapparat und Ammonshorn. Anat. Anz. *8:*305–321.

Edinger, L. (1896a). Untersuchungen über die vergleichende Anatomie des Gehirns 3:Neue Studien über das Vorderhirn der Reptilien. Abh. Senckenb. naturforsch. Gesellsch., Frankfurt, *19:*313–386.

Edinger, L. (1896b). *Vorlesungen über den Bau der nervösen Zentralorgane des Menschen und der Thiere,* 5th ed. Leipzig: Vogel.

Edinger, L. (1899). *Vorlesungen über den Bau der nervösen Zentralorgane des Menschen und der Tiere,* 6th edition. 2 vols. Leipzig: Vogel.

Edinger, L. (1903). Sur l'anatomie comparée du corps strié (cerveau des oiseaux). Compt. Rend. Assoc. Anat., Paris, *5:*187–192.

Edinger, L. (1905). Ueber die Herkunft des Hirnmantels in der Tierreihe. Berl. klin. Wochenschr. *42:*1357–1361.

Edinger, L., Wallenberg, A., and Holmes, G. (1903). Untersuchungen über die vergleichende Anatomie des Gehirns 5: Untersuchungen über das Vorderhirn der Vögel. Abh. Senckenb. naturforsch. Gesellsch., Frankfurt, *20:*343–426.

Ehrenberg, C. G. (1833). Notwendigkeit einer feineren mechanischen Zerlegung des Gehirns und der Nerven. Poggendorffs Ann. Phys. Chem. *28:*449–465.

Ehrenberg, C. G. (1836). Beobachtung einer bisher unbekannten auffallenden Struktur des Seelenorgans bei Menschen und Tieren. Abh. Akad. Wiss., Berlin (Phys. Math. Kl.), *1836*:665–723.

Ehrlich, P. (1881). Über das Methylenblau und seine klinisch-bacterioskopische Verwerthung. Z. klin. Med. *2*:710–713.

Ehrlich, P. (1886). Über die Methylenblau-reaktion der lebenden Nervensubstanz. Dtsch. med. Wochenschr. *12*:49–52.

Eichorst, [H.] (1875). Ueber die Entwickelung des menschlichen Rückenmarkes und seiner Formelemente. Virchows Archiv. path. Anat. *64*:425–475.

Endo, K., Araki, T., and Yagi, N. (1973). The distribution and pattern of axon branching of pyramidal tract cells. Brain Res. *57*:484–491.

Exner, S. (1881). *Untersuchungen über die Localisation der Functionen in der Grosshirnrinde des Menschen.* Wien: Braumüller.

Exner, S. (1881). Zur Kenntnis der motorischen Rindenfelder. Sitzungsb. Kaiserl. Akad. Wiss. Wien, Math.-Naturw. Cl. *84*:185–190.

Exner, S. (1881). Zur Kenntnis vom feineren Bau der Grosshirnrinde. Sitzungsb. Kaiserl. Akad. Wiss. Wien, Math.-Naturw. Cl. *83*:151–153.

Exner, S. (1881–1882). Zur Frage nach der Rindenlokalisation beim Menschen. Arch. Ges. Physiol., Bonn, *27*:412–421.

Fairén, A., Cobas, A., and Fonseca, M. (1986). Times of generation of glutamic acid decarboxylase immunoreactive neurons in mouse somatosensory cortex. J. comp. Neurol. *251*:67–83.

Fairén, A., DeFelipe, J., and Regidor, J. (1984). Non-pyramidal neurons: General account. *In: Cerebral Cortex*, Vol. 1: *Cellular Components of the Cerebral Cortex.* A. Peters and E. G. Jones (eds.). New York: Plenum, pp. 201–254.

Fairén, A., and Valverde, F. (1979). Specific thalamocortical afferents and their presumptive targets in the visual cortex: A Golgi study. *In:* Development and Chemical Specificity of Neurons. Progress in Brain Research, Vol. 51 (M. Cuénod, G. W. Kreutzberg, and F. E. Bloom, eds.). Amsterdam: Elsevier, pp. 419–438.

Fairén, A., and Valverde, F. (1980). A specialized type of neuron in the visual cortex of cat: A Golgi and electron microscope study of chandelier cells. J. Comp. Neurol. *194*:761–779.

Falzacappa, [E.] (1888). Genesi della cellula specifica nervosa e intima struttura del sistema centrale nervoso degli uccelli. Bolet. Soc. Nat., Napoli, Ser. I, *2*:185–193.

Feldman, M. L. (1984). Morphology of the neocortical pyramidal neuron. *In: Cerebral Cortex*, Vol. 1: *Cellular Components of the Cerebral Cortex.* A. Peters and E. G. Jones (eds.). New York: Plenum, pp. 123–200.

Ferrier, D., and Turner, W. A. (1894). A record of experiments illustrative of the symptomatology and degenerations following lesions of the cerebellum and its peduncles and related structures in monkeys. Phil. Trans. roy. Soc., London, *185*:719–778.

Ferrier, D., and Turner, W. A. (1898). An experimental research upon cerebro-cortical afferent and efferent tracts. Proc. roy. Soc. Lond. *72*:1–3. (Abstracted by M. Rothmann.) *In:* Referate.Anatomie, Neurol. Centralbl. *17*:67–68.

Ferster, D. (1986). Orientation selectivity of synaptic potentials in neurons of cat primary visual cortex. J. Neurosci. *6*:1284–1301.

Ferster, D., and LeVay, S. (1978). The axonal arborizations of lateral geniculate neurons in the striate cortex of the cat. J. Comp. Neurol. *182*:923–944.

Flechsig, P. E. (1886). Zur Lehre vom centralen Verlauf der Sinnesnerven. Neurol. Centralbl. *5*:545–551.

Flechsig, P. (1889). Ueber eine neue Färbungsmethode des centralen Nervensystems und deren Ergebnisse bezüglich des Zusammenhanges von Ganglienzellen und Nervenfasern. Arch. Anat. Physiol., Physiol. Abt., *1889*:537–538.

Flechsig, P. (1895). Weitere Mittheilungen über die Sinnes- und Associationscentren des menschlichen Gehirnes. Neurol. Centralbl. *14*:1118–1124, 1177–1179.

Flechsig, P. (1896a). Die Lokalisation der geistigen Vorgänge. Neurol. Centralbl. *15*:999–1000, 1003.

Flechsig, P. (1896b). *Gehirn und Seele,* gehalten am 31 Oktober 1894 in der Universitätskirche zu Leipzig. Leipzig: Veit. (Reviewed 1896 in Neurol. Centralbl. *15*:661–662.)

Flechsig, P. (1896c). *Ueber die Lokalisation der geistigen Vorgänge insbesondere der Sinnesempfindungen des Menschen.* Leipzig: Veit.

Flechsig, P. (1898). Neue Untersuchungen über die Markbildung in den menschlichen Grosshirnlappen. Neurol. Centralbl. *17*:977–996.

Flechsig, P. (1901). Ueber die entwickelungsgeschtliche (myelogenetische) Flächengliederung der Grosshirnrinde des Menschen. Arch. ital. Biol. *36*:30–39.

Flechsig, P. (1903). Weitere Mittheilungen über die-entwickelungsgeschichtlichen (myelogenetischen) Felder in der menschlichen Grosshirnrinde. Neurol. Centralbl. *22*:202–206.

Flechsig, P. (1904). Einige Bemerkungen über die Untersuchungensmethoden der Grosshirnrinde, insbesondere des Menschen. Bericht der Königl. sächs. Gessellsch. Wiss. Leipzig, Math.-Phys. Klasse *56*:177–214. (Reprinted 1905 in Arch. Anat. Entwickl. *1905*:337–444.)

Flores, [A.] (1911a). A myeloarchitectura e a myelogenia do cortex cerebral do Erinaceus europaeus. Lisbon: Da Silva.

Flores, A. (1911b). Die Myeloarchitektonik und die Myelogenie des Cortex cerebri beim Igel, Erinaceus europaeus. J. Psychol. Neurol., Leipzig, *17*:215–247.

Forel, A. (1887). Einige hirnanatomische Betrachtungen und Ergebnisse. Arch. Psychiat., Berlin, *18*:162–198.

Fortuyn, A. B. Droogleever (1914). Cortical cell lamination of the hemispheres of some rodents. Arch. Neurol. Psychiat., London, *6*:221–354.

Freund, T. F., Martin, K.A.C., Smith, A. D., and Somogyi, P. (1983). Glutamate decarboxylase-immunoreactive terminals of Golgi-impregnated axoaxonic cells and of presumed basket cells in synaptic contact with pyramidal neurons of the cat's visual cortex. J. comp. Neurol. *221*:263–278.

Freund, T. F., Maglóczky, Z., Soltész, I., and P. Somogyi (1986). Synaptic connections, axonal and dendritic patterns of neurons immunoreactive for cholecystokinin in the visual cortex of the cat. Neuroscience, *19*:1133–1159.

Friedlander, M. S., Lin, C.-S., Stanford, L. R., and Sherman, S. M. (1981). Morphology of functionally identified neurons in the lateral geniculate nucleus of the cat. J. Neurophysiol. *46*:80–129.

Friedman, D. P. (1983). Laminar patterns of termination of cortico-cortical afferents in the somatosensory system. Brain Res. *273*:147–151.

Friedman, D. P., Jones, E. G., and Burton, H. (1980). Representation pattern in the second somatic sensory area of the monkey cerebral cortex. J. comp. Neurol. *192*:21–41.

Fromm, C., Evarts, E. V., Kroller, J., and Shinoda, Y. (1981). Activity of motor cortex and red nucleus neurons during voluntary movement. *In: Brain Mechanisms and Perceptual Awareness*. O. Pompeiano and C. Ajmone Marsan (eds.). New York: Raven Press, pp. 269–294.

Fusari, [R.] (1887). Untersuchungen über die feinere Anatomie des Gehirnes der Teleostier. Intern. Mschr. Anat. Physiol. *4*:275–300.

Fuxe, K., Hökfelt, T., Johansson, O., Jonsson, G., Lidbrink, P., and Ljungdahl, A. (1974). The origin of the dopamine nerve terminals in limbic and frontal cortex: Evidence for meso-cortico-dopamine neurons. Brain Res. *82*:349–355.

Ganser, S. (1878). Ueber die vordere Hirncommissur der Säugethiere. Arch. Psychiat. Neurol. *9*:286–299.

Ganser, S. (1882). Vergleichend-anatomisch. Studien über das Gehirn des Maulwurfs. Morphol. Jahrb. *7*:591–725.

Gerlach, J. von (1858). Ueber die Einwirkung von Farbstoff auf lebende Gewebe. Wiss. Mitt. Phys. med. Soc., Erlangen, *1*:5–12.

Gerlach, J. von (1872). Über die struktur der grauen Substanz des menschlichen Grosshirns. Zentralbl. med. Wiss. *10*:273–275.

Giacomini, C. (1882–1883). Sezioni microscopiche dell'intero encefalo umano adulto. Giorn. Accad. Med. Torino, third series, *30*:939–954.

Giacomini, C. (1883a). Nuovo microscopio per l'esame delle lezioni dell'intero encefalo umano adulto. Giorn. Accad. Med. Torino, third series, *31*:210–214.

Giacomini, C. (1883b). Fascia dentata del grande hippocampo nel cervello humano. Giorn. Accad. Med. Torino, third series, *31*:674–742.

Giacomini, C. (1883c). Nuovo microscopiche dell'intero encefalo umano adulto e nuovo microscopio per esaminarle. Osservatore Torino *19*:421–449, 457–529.

Gierke, H. (1885–1886). Die Stützsubstanz des Centralnervensystems. Arch. mikrosk. Anat., EntwMech. *25*:441–554.

Gierlich, N. (1906–1907). Ueber die Entwicklung der Neurofibrillen in der Pyramidenbahn des Menschen. Deutsch. Z. NervHeilk. *32*:97–107.

Gilbert, C. D. (1983). Microcircuitry of the visual cortex. Ann. Rev. Neurosci. *6*:217–248.

Gilbert, C. D., and Wiesel, T. N. (1979). Morphology and intracortical projections of functionally characterised neurones in the cat visual cortex. Nature *280*:120–125.

Gilbert, C. D., and Wiesel, T. N. (1981). Laminar specialization and intracortical projections in cat primary visual cortex. *In: The Cerebral Cortex*. F. O. Schmitt, F. G. Worden, G. Adelman, and M. G. Dennis (eds.). Cambridge, MA: MIT Press.

Gilbert, C. D., and Wiesel, T. N. (1983). Clustered intrinsic connections in cat visual cortex. J. Neurosci. *3*:1116–1133.

Goldman-Rakic, P. S., and Schwartz, M. L. (1982). Interdigitation of contralateral and ipsilateral columnar projections to frontal association cortex in primates. Science *216*:755–757.

Golgi, C. (1873). Sulla sostanza grigia del cervello. Gaz. med. Ital. Lombardia *6*:244–246. (Verified from *Opera Omnia*, 1903, Vol. 2, pp. 91–98. Milan: Hoepli.)

Golgi, C. (1875). Sui gliomi de cervello. Riv. sper. Freniat. Med. leg. ment. *1*:66–78.

Golgi, C. (1883a). Recherches sur l'histologie des centres nerveux. Arch. ital. Biol. *3*:285–317.

Golgi, C. (1883b). Sulla fina anatomia degli organi centrali del sistema nervoso. Riv. sper. freniat. Med. leg. Alien. ment. *9*:1–17, 161–192, 385–402. (Verified from *Opera Omnia*, 1903, Vol. 1, pp. 295–375. Milan: Hoepli.)

Golgi, C. (1884). Recherches sur l'histologie des centres nerveux. Arch. ital. Biol. *4*:92–123.

Golgi, C. (1885). Sulla fina anatomia degli organi centrali del sistema nervoso. Riv. sper. freniat. Med. leg. Alien. ment. *11*:72–123, 193–220.

Golgi, C. (1886a). Sulla fina anatomia degli organi centrali del sistema nervoso. Milan: Hoepli.

Golgi, C. (1886b). Sur l'anatomie microscopique des organes centraux du système nerveux. Arch. ital. Biol. *7*:15–47.

Golgi, C. (1894). Untersuchungen über den feineren Bau des centralen und peripherischen Nervensystems. Translated by R. Teuscher. Jena: Fischer.

Golgi, C. (1907). La doctrine du neurone, théorie et faits. *In: Les Prix Nobel 1904–1906*. Stockholm: Norstedt. (Translated, 1967, as: The neuron doctrine-theory and facts. *In: Nobel Lectures, Physiology or Medicine (1901–1921)*. Amsterdam: Elsevier.)

Gray, E. G. (1959). Axo-somatic and axo-dendritic synapses of the cerebral cortex: An electron microscope study. J. Anat. *93*:420–433.

Greppin, L. (1889). Weiterer Beitrag zur Kenntnis der Golgi'schen Untersuchungsmethode des centralen Nervensystems. Archiv. Anat. Physiol, Suppl., pp. 55–78.

Grünbaum, A.S.F., and Sherrington, C. S. (1901). (See Sherrington and Grünbaum, 1901.)

Grünbaum, A.S.F., and Sherrington, C. S. (1903). Observations on the physiology of the cerebral cortex of the anthropoid apes. Proc. roy. Soc., London, 72:152–155.

Gudden, B. von (1870). Experimentaluntersuchungen über das peripherische und centrale Nervensystem. Arch. Psychiat., Berlin, 2:693–723.

Haller, B. (1906). Beiträge zur Phylogenese des Grosshirns der Säugetiere. Arch. mikrosk. Anat. Entw-Mech. 29:117–222.

Haller, B. (1910). Die Mantelgebiete des Grosshirns von den Nagern aufsteigend bis zum Menschen. Arch. mikrosk. Anat. EntwMech. 76:305–321.

Hammarberg, C. (1895). Studien über Klinik und Pathologie der Idiotie nebst Untersuchungen über die normale Anatomie des Hirnrinde. Translated by W. Berger and edited by S. E. Henschen. Upsala: Berling.

Hannover, A. (1840). Die Chromsäure, ein vorzügliches Mittel bei mikroskopischen Untersuchungen. Arch. Anat. Physiol., Physiol. Abt. 1840:549–558.

Hataï, S. (1902a). On the origin of neuroglia tissue from the mesoblast. J. comp. Neurol. 12:291–296.

Hataï, S. (1902b). Observations on the developing neurones of the cerebral cortex of fetal cats. J. comp. Neurol. 12:199–204.

Havet, J. H. (1899). L'état moniliforme des neurones chez les invertébrés avec quelques remarques sur les vertébrés. La Cellule 16:37–46.

Held, H. (1891). Die centralen Bahnen des Nervus acusticus bei der Katze. Arch. Anat. Physiol., Anat. Abt., 1891:271–291.

Held, H. (1893). Die centrale Gehörleitung. Arch. Anat. Physiol., Anat. Abt., 1893:201–248.

Held, H. (1902). Über den Bau der grauen und weissen Substanz. Arch. Anat. Entwickl. 1902:189–224.

Held, H. (1909). Die Entwicklung des Nervengewebes bei den Wirbeltieren. Leipzig: Barth.

Held, H. (1929). Die Lehre von den Neuronen und vom Neurencytium und ihr heutiger Stand. In: Fortschritte der naturwissenschaftl. Forschung. N. F. Heft 8. E. Abderhalden (ed.). Berlin: Urban and Schwarzenberg, pp. 1–72.

Hendry, S.H.C. (1987). Recent advances in understanding the intrinsic circuitry of the cerebral cortex. In: Higher Brain Functions: Recent Explorations of the Brain's Emergent Properties. (S. P. Wise, ed.) New York: Wiley, pp. 241–283.

Hendry, S.H.C., Houser, C. R., Jones, E. G., and Vaughn, J. E. (1983a). Synaptic organization of immunocytochemically identified GABA neurons in the monkey sensory-motor cortex. J. Neurocytol. 12:639–660.

Hendry, S.H.C., and Jones, E. G. (1983a). The organization of pyramidal and non-pyramidal cell dendrites in relation to thalamic afferent terminations in the monkey somatic sensory cortex. J. Neurocytol. 12:277–298.

Hendry, S.H.C., and Jones, E. G. (1983b). Thalamic inputs to identified commissural neurons in the monkey somatic sensory cortex. J. Neurocytol. 12:299–316.

Hendry, S.H.C., Jones, E. G., and Beinfeld, M.C.

(1983b). Cholecystokinin-immunoreactive neurons in rat and monkey cerebral cortex make symmetric synapses and have intimate associations with blood vessels. Proc. Natl. Acad. Sci. USA 80:2400–2404.

Hendry, S.H.C., Jones, E. G., DeFelipe, J., Schmechel, D., Brandon, C., and Emson, P. C. (1984a). Neuropeptide-containing neurons of the cerebral cortex are also GABAergic. Proc. Natl. Acad. Sci. USA 81:6526–6530.

Hendry, S.H.C., Jones, E. G., and Emson, P. C. (1984b). Morphology, distribution and synaptic relations of somatostatin- and neuropeptide Y-immunoreactive neurons in rat and monkey neocortex. J. Neurosci. 4:2497–2517.

Hendry, S.H.C., Schwark, H. D., Jones, E. G., and Yan, J. (1987). Numbers and proportions of GABA immunoreactive neurons in different areas of monkey cerebral cortex. J. Neurosci. 7:1503–1519.

Henle, J. (1879). Handbuch der systematischen Anatomie des Menschen. Vol. 3, part 2, Handbuch der Nervenlehre des Menschen, second edition. Braunschweig: Friedrich.

Henschen, S. E. (1890–1930). Klinische und anatomische Beiträge zur Pathologie des Gehirns. 6 volumes in 8 parts. Upsala: Almqvist and Wiksell (Vols. 1–4, parts 1–4, 1890, 1892, 1896, 1911); Stockholm: Nordiska Bokhandeln (Vol. 5, parts 5 and 6, 1920); privately printed (Vol. 6, parts 7 and 8, 1922, 1930).

Henschen, S. E. (1894). Sur les centres optiques cérébraux. Rev. gén. Ophthalm. 13:337–352.

Henschen, S. E. (1900). Sur le centre cortical de la vision. Compt. Rend. 13th Internat. med. Congress, Paris, 12, Ophthalmology section, pp. 232–249.

Henschen, S. E. (1919a). Über Sinnes- und Vorstellungscentren in der Rinde des Grosshirns. Zugleich ein Beitrag zur Frage des Mechanismus des Denkens. Z. ges. Neurol. Psychiat. 47:55–111.

Henschen, S. E. (1919b). Ueber die Geruchs- und Geschmachszentren. Mschr. Psych. Neurol. 45:121–165.

Herkenham, M. (1986). New perspectives on the organization and evolution of nonspecific thalamocortical projections. In: Cerebral Cortex, Vol. 5, Sensory-Motor Areas and Aspects of Cortical Connectivity. E. G. Jones and A. Peters (eds.). New York: Plenum, pp. 403–445.

Hermanides, S. R., and Köppen, M. (1903). Ueber die Furchen und über den Bau der Grosshirnrinde bei den Lissencephalen, insbesondere über die Lokalisation des motorischen Centrums und der Sehregion. Arch. Psychiat., Berlin, 37:616–634.

Hill, A. (1896). The chrome-silver method, a study of the conditions under which the reaction occurs and a criticism of its results. Brain 19:1–42.

His, W. (1886). Zur Geschichte des menschlichen Rückenmarkes und der Nervenwurzeln. Abhandl. Math.-Phys. Class. Königl. säch. Gesellsch. Wiss., Leipzig, 13:147–209, 477–513. (Reprinted with same title, 1886. Leipzig: Hirzel.)

His, W. (1889). Die Neuroblasten und deren Entstehung im embryonalen Marke. Abhandl. Math.-Phys.

Class. Königl. säch. Gesellsch. Wiss., Leipzig, 15:313–372. (Republished in Arch. Anat. Entwickl. 1889:249–300.)

His, W. (1890). Histogenese und Zusammenhang der Nervenelemente. Abh. Internat. Med. Congress, Berlin, Anat. section, 7 August 1890. (Published in Arch. Anat. Entwickl. Suppl., pp. 95–117.)

His, W. (1904). Die Entwickelung des menschlichen Gehirns während der ersten Monate. Leipzig: Hirzel.

Holmgren, E. (1900). Studien in der feineren Anatomie der Nervenzellen. Arb. anat. Inst., Wiesbaden, 15:1–89.

Honegger, J. (1890). Vergleichend-anatomische Untersuchungen über den Fornix und die mit ihm in Beziehung stehenden Gebilde. Rec. Zool. suisse 5:201–434.

Hornung, J. P., and Garey, L. J. (1981). The thalamic projection to cat visual cortex: Ultrastructure of neurons identified by Golgi impregnation or retrograde horseradish peroxidase transport. Neurosci. 6:1053–1068.

Houser, C. R., Crawford, G. D., Barber, R. P., Salvaterra, P. M., and Vaughn, J. E. (1983a). Organization and morphological characteristics of cholinergic neurons: An immunocytochemical study with a monoclonal antibody to choline acetyltransferase. Brain Res. 266:97–119.

Houser, C. R., Hendry, S.H.C., Jones, E. G., and Vaughn, J. E. (1983b). Morphological diversity of immunocytochemically identified GABA neurons in monkey sensory-motor cortex. J. Neurocytol. 12:617–638.

Houser, C. R., Vaughn, J., Hendry, S.H.C., Jones, E. G., and Peters, A. (1984). GABAergic neurons in the cerebral cortex. In: Cerebral Cortex, Vol. 2; Functional Properties of Cortical Cells. E. G. Jones and A. Peters (eds.). New York: Plenum, pp. 63–89.

Hubel, D. H., and Wiesel, T. N. (1962). Receptive fields, binocular interaction and functional architecture in the cat's visual cortex. J. Physiol., London, 160:106–154.

Hubel, D. H., and Wiesel, T. N. (1977). Functional architecture of macaque monkey visual cortex. Proc. roy. Soc., London, B., 198:1–59.

Huguenin, G. (1873). Allgemeine Pathologie der Krankheiten des Nervensystems: Ein Lehrbuch für Ärzte und Studierende. Zürich: Zurcher and Furrer.

Innocenti, G. M. (1981). Growth and reshaping of axons in the establishment of visual callosal connections. Science 212:824–827.

Innocenti, G. M., Fiore, L., and Caminiti, R. (1977). Exuberant projection into the corpus callosum from the visual cortex of newborn cats. Neurosci. Lett. 4:237–242.

Isenschmid, R. (1911). Zur Kenntnis der Grosshirnrinde der Maus. Abhandl. Königl. preuss. Akad. Wiss., Berlin, 3:1–46.

Jack, J.J.B., Noble, D., and Tsien, R. W. (1975). Electric Current Flow in Excitable Cells. Oxford: Oxford Univ. Press.

Jasper, H. H. (1960). Unspecific thalamocortical rela-

tions. In: Handbook of Physiology, Section 1: Neurophysiology, Vol. 2. J. Field, H. W. Magoun, and V. E. Hall (eds.). Washington, D.C.: American Physiological Soc., pp. 1307–1321.

Jones, E. G. (1975). Varieties and distribution of nonpyramidal cells in the somatic sensory cortex of the squirrel monkey. J. comp. Neurol. 160:205–268.

Jones, E. G. (1981). Anatomy of cerebral cortex: Columnar input-output relations. In: The Cerebral Cortex. F. O. Schmitt, F. G. Worden, G. Adelman, and S. G. Dennis (eds.). Cambridge, MA: MIT Press, pp. 199–235.

Jones, E. G. (1984a). History of cortical cytology. In: Cerebral Cortex, Vol. 1: Cellular Components of the Cerebral Cortex. A. Peters and E. G. Jones (eds.). New York: Plenum, pp. 1–33.

Jones, E. G. (1984b). Laminar distribution of output cells. In: Cerebral Cortex, Vol. 1: Cellular Components of the Cerebral Cortex. A. Peters and E. G. Jones (eds.). New York: Plenum, pp. 521–553.

Jones, E. G. (1984c). Identification and classification of intrinsic circuit elements in the neocortex. In: Dynamic Aspects of Neocortical Function. G. Edelman, E. Gall, and W. M. Cowan (eds.). New York: Wiley, pp. 7–40.

Jones, E. G. (1985). The Thalamus. New York: Plenum.

Jones, E. G. (1986). Neurotransmitters in the cerebral cortex. J. Neurosurgery 65:135–153.

Jones, E. G., and Burton, H. (1976) Areal differences in the distribution of thalamocortical fibers in cortical fields of the insular, parietal and temporal regions of primates. J. comp. Neurol. 168:197–248.

Jones, E. G., Coulter, J. D., and Hendry, S.H.C. (1978). Intracortical connectivity of architectonic fields in the somatic sensory, motor and parietal cortex of monkeys. J. comp. Neurol. 181:291–348.

Jones, E. G., DeFelipe, J., Hendry, S.H.C., and Maggio, J. E. (1988) Tachykinin neurons in monkey cerebral cortex. J. Neurosci. 8:1206–1224.

Jones, E. G., and Hendry, S.H.C. (1986). Co-localization of GABA and neuropeptides in neocortical neurons. Trends Neurosci. 9:71–76.

Jones, E. G., Hendry, S.H.C., and DeFelipe, J. (1987). The peptide neurons of the cerebral cortex: A limited cell class. In: Cerebral Cortex, Vol. 6: Further Aspects of Cortical Function, including Hippocampus. E. G. Jones and A. Peters (eds.). New York: Plenum, pp. 237–266.

Jones, E. G., and Powell, T.P.S. (1970a). Electron microscopy of the somatic sensory cortex of the cat I: Cell types and synaptic organization. Phil. Trans. roy. Soc., London, B., 257:1–11.

Jones, E. G., and Powell, T.P.S. (1970b). An electron microscopic study of the laminar pattern and mode of termination of afferent fibre pathways to the somatic sensory cortex of the cat. Phil. Trans. roy. Soc., London, B., 257:45–62.

Jones, E. G., and Wise, S. P. (1977). Size, laminar and columnar distribution of efferent cells in the sensory-motor cortex of monkeys. J. comp. Neurol. 175:391–438.

Kaes, T. (1893). Beiträge zur Kenntnis des Reichtums der Grosshirnrinde des Menschen an markhaltigen Nervenfasern. Arch. Psychiat., Berlin, 25:695–758.

Kaes, T. (1907). Die Grosshirnrinde des Menschen und ihre Massen und ihr Fasergehalt. Jena: Fischer.

Kahler and Toldt. See Toldt and Kahler.

Kappers, C. U. Ariëns (1909). The phylogenesis of the palaeocortex and archicortex compared with the evolution of the visual neocortex. Arch. Neurol. Psychiat., London, 4:161–173.

Kappers, C. U. Ariëns (1910). Review of: Brodmann, K. (1909). Vergleichende Lokalisationslehre der Grosshirnrinde in ihren Prinzipien dargestellt auf Grund des Zellenbaues. Leipzig: Barth. In: Folia Neurobiol. 4:152–167.

Kappers, C. U. Ariëns (1921). Die vergleichende Anatomie des Nervensystems der Wirbeltiere und des Menschen. 2 Vols. Haarlem: Bohn.

Kappers, C. U. Ariëns, and Theunissen, W. F. (1907). Zur vergleichenden Anatomie des Vorderhirns der Vertebraten. Anat. Anz. 30:496–509.

Kappers, C. U. Ariëns, and Theunissen, W. F. (1907–1908). Die Phylogenese des Rhinencephalons, des Corpus striatum, und der Vorderhirnkommissuren. Folia Neurobiol., Amsterdam, 1:164–172.

Kappers, C. U. Ariëns, and Theunissen, W. F. (1908). Die Phylogenese des Rhinencephalon, de Corpus striatum, und der Vorderhirnkommissuren. Folia Neurobiol. Amsterdam 1:173–288.

Kemper, T. L., and Galaburda, A. M. (1984). Principles of cytoarchitectonics. In: Cerebral Cortex, Vol. 1: Cellular Components of the Cerebral Cortex. A. Peters and E. G. Jones (eds.). New York: Plenum, pp. 35–58.

Kisvárday, Z. F., Cowey, A., and Somogyi, P. (1986). Synaptic relationships of a type of GABA-immunoreactive neuron (clutch cell), spiny stellate cells and lateral geniculate nucleus afferents in layer IVC of the monkey striate cortex. Neurosci. 19:741–761.

Kölliker, A. von (1849). Neurologische Bemerkungen. Z. wiss. Zool. Abt. A. 1:135–163.

Kölliker, A. von (1852). Handbuch der Gewebelehre des Menschen, 2nd edition. Leipzig: Engelmann.

Kölliker, A. [von] (1882). Embryologie ou traité complet du développement de l'homme et des animaux superieurs. Trans. by A. Schneider from the second German edition (Entwicklungsgeschichte des Menschen und der höheren Thiere. 1879. Leipzig: Engelmann.) 2 Vols. Paris: Reinwald.

Kölliker, A. von (1887). Die Untersuchungen von Golgi über den feineren Bau des centralen Nervensystems. Anat. Anz. 2:480–483.

Kölliker, A. [von] (1890a). Zur feineren Anatomie des centralen Nervensystems. Erster Beitrag. Das Kleinhirn. Z. wiss. Zool. 49:663–689.

Kölliker, A. [von] (1890b). Zur feineren Anatomie des centralen Nervensystems. Zweiter Beitrag. Das Rückenmark. Z. wiss. Zool. 51:1–54.

Kölliker, [A] von (1892). Ueber die Entwickelung der Elemente des Nervensystems contra Beard und Dohrn. Verhandl. anat. Gesellsch., Jena, 1892:76–78.

Kölliker, A. von (1894). Ueber den Fornix longus von Forel und die Riechstrahlungen im Gehirn des Kaninchens. Verhandl. anat. Gesellsch. 8:45–52.

Kölliker, A. von (1895). Kritik der Hypothesen von Rabl-Rückhard und Duval über amoeboide Bewegungen der Neurodendren. Sitzungsb. Würzburger Phys. med. Gesellsch. 6:38–42.

Kölliker, A. [von] (1896). Handbuch der Gewebelehre des Menschen, 6th ed., Vol. 2: Nervensystem des Menschen und der Thiere. Leipzig: Engelmann.

König, N., and Marty, R. (1981). Early neurogenesis and synaptogenesis in cerebral cortex. Bibliogr. Anat. 19:152–162.

Köppen, M. (1888). Zur Anatomie des Froschgehirns. Arch. Anat. Entwckl. 1888:1–33.

Köppen, M., and Löwenstein, S. (1905). Studien über den Zellenbau der Grosshirnrinde bei den Ungulaten und Karnivoren und über die Bedeutung einiger Furchen. Mschr. Psychiat. Neurol. 18:480–509.

Kosofsky, B. E., Molliver, M. E., Morrison, J. H., and Foote, S. L. (1984). The serotonin and norepinephrine innervation of primary visual cortex in the cynomolgus monkey (Macaca fascicularis). J. comp. Neurol. 230:168–178.

Krause, W. (1876–1880). Allgemeine und mikroskopische Anatomie, 3rd edition. Hannover: Hahn.

Lachi, P. (1891). Contributo alla istogenesi della nevroglia nel midollo spinale del pollo. Atti Soc. tosc. sci. nat. Mem., Pisa. 11:267–310.

Lahousse, E. (1886). La cellule nerveuse et la névroglie. Anat. Anz. 1:114–128.

Larroche, J.-C., and Houcine, O. (1982). Le néo-cortex chez l'embryon et le foetus humain: Apport du microscope électronique et du Golgi. Reprod. Nutr. Dev. 22:163–170.

La Villa, I. (1898). Algunos detalles concernientes a la oliva superior y focos acústicos. Rev. trim. Micrográf., Madrid, 3:75–83.

Lenhossék, M. von (1891a). Zur Kenntnis der ersten Entstehung der Nervenzellen und Nervenfasern beim Vogelembryo. Verhandl. X. internat. med. Congr., Berlin, 1890, 2:115–124.

Lenhossék, M. von (1891b). Die Entwickelung der Ganglienanlagen bei dem menschlichen Embryo. Arch. Anat. Entwckl. 1891:1–25.

Lenhossék, M. von (1895). Der feinere Bau des Nervensystems im Lichte neuester Forschungen, 2nd edition. Berlin: Fischer.

Lépine, R. (1894). Sur un cas d'hystérie à forme particulière. Rev. méd., Paris, 14:713–728.

Lépine, R. (1895). Théorie mécanique de la paralysie hystérique, du somnambulisme, du sommeil naturel et de la distraction. Compt. Rend. Soc. Biol., Paris, 47:85–86.

LeVay, S. (1973). Synaptic patterns in the visual cortex of the cat and monkey: Electron microscopy of Golgi preparations. J. comp. Neurol. 150:53–86.

LeVay, S., and Sherk, H. (1981). The visual claustrum of the cat I: Structure and connections. J. Neurosci. 1:956–980.

Lewandowsky, M. (1907). Die Funktionen des zentralen Nervensystems: Ein Lehrbuch. Jena: Fischer.

Lewandowsky, M. [Ed.] (1910–1914). *Handbuch der Neurologie.* 5 vols. in 6. Berlin: Springer.

Lewis, W. B. (1878). On the comparative structure of the cortex cerebri. Brain *1:*79–96.

Lewis, W. B. (1880). Researches on the comparative structure of the cortex cerebri. Phil. Trans. roy. Soc., London, *171:*33–64.

Lewis, W. B. (1889). *A Textbook of Mental Diseases: With Special Reference to the Pathological Aspects of Insanity.* London: Griffin.

Lewis, W. B. (1897). The structure of the first or outermost layer of the cerebral cortex. Edinburgh Med. J. New Series, *1:*573–592.

Lewis, W. B., and Clarke, H. (1878). The cortical lamination of the motor area of the brain. Proc. roy. Soc., London, *27:*38–49.

Livingstone, M. S., and Hubel, D. H. (1982). Thalamic inputs to cytochrome oxidase-rich regions in monkey visual cortex. Proc. Natl. Acad. Sci. USA *79:*6098–6101.

Livingstone, M. S., and Hubel, D. H. (1983). Specificity of cortico-cortical connections in monkey visual system. Nature *304:*531–534.

Livini, F. (1907). Il proencefalo di un marsupiale (*Hypsiprymnus rufescens*). Arch. ital. Anat. Embriol. *6:*549–584.

Lorente de Nó, R. (1922a). Estudios sobre el cerebro posterior (Protruberancia y bulbo raquídeo). Trab. Lab Invest. Biol. Univ. Madrid. *20:*101–112. (Republished 1924 as: Études sur le cerveau posterieur. Trav. Lab. Rech. biol. Univ. Madrid *22:*51–65.)

Lorente de Nó, R. (1922b). La corteza cerebral del ratón. (Primera contribución—La corteza acústica). Trab. Lab. Invest. biol. Univ. Madrid *20:*41–78.

Lorente de Nó, R. (1949). Cerebral cortex: Architecture, intracortical connections, motor projections, *In: Physiology of the Nervous System,* 3rd edition. J. F. Fulton (ed.). London: Oxford Univ. Press, pp. 288–313.

Löwe, L. (1880). *Beiträge zur Anatomie und zur Entwickelungsgeschichte des Nervensystems,* Vol. 1: *Die Morphogenesis des centralen Nervensystems der Säugethiere und des Menschen.* Berlin: Springer.

Löwenthal, N. (1897). *Über das Riechhirn der Säugetiere.* Braunschweig: Vieweg.

Lugaro, E. (1895). Sulle modificazioni delle cellule nervose nei diversi stati funzionali. Lo Sperimentale, Sezione Biologica, no. 2, *49:*1–35.

Lugaro, E. (1897). Sulla genesi delle circunvoluzioni cerebrali e cerebellari. Riv. Patol. nerv. ment. *2:*97–116.

Lugaro, E. (1898). Sulle modificazioni morfologiche funzionali dei dendriti delle cellule nervose. Riv. Patol. nerv. ment. *3:*337–359.

Lugaro, E. (1899). I recenti progressi dell'anatomia del sistema nervoso in rapporto alla psicologia ed alla psichiatria. Riv. Patol. nerv. ment. *4:*481–514, 537–547.

Lund, J. S. (1973). Organization of neurons in the visual cortex, area 17, of the monkey (*Macaca mulatta*). J. Comp. Neurol. *147:*455–496.

Lund, J. S. (1984). Spiny stellate cells. *In: Cerebral Cortex, Vol. 1: Cellular Components of the Cerebral Cortex.* A. Peters and E. G. Jones (eds.). New York: Plenum, pp. 255–308.

Lund, J. S., Boothe, R. G., and Lund, R. D. (1977). Development of neurons in the visual cortex of the monkey (*Macaca nemestrina*): A Golgi study from fetal day 127 to postnatal maturity. J. Comp. Neurol. *176:*149–188.

Lund, J. S., Hendrickson, A. E., Ogren, M. P., and Tobin, E. A. (1981). Anatomical organization of primate visual cortex area 17. J. comp. Neurol. *202:*19–46.

Lund, J. S., Henry, G. H., MacQueen, C. L., and Harvey, A. R. (1979). Anatomical organization of the primary visual cortex (area 17) of the cat: A comparison with area 17 of the macaque monkey. J. comp. Neurol. *184:*599–618.

Lund, J. S., Lund, R. D., Hendrickson, A. E., Bunt, A. H., and Fuchs, A. F. (1975). The origin of efferent pathways from the primary visual cortex, area 17, of the macaque monkey as shown by retrograde transport of horseradish peroxidase. J. comp. Neurol *164:*287–304.

McGuire, B. A., Hornung, J.-P., Gilbert, C. D., and Wiesel, T. N. (1984). Patterns of synaptic input to layer 4 of cat striate cortex. J. Neurosci. *4:*3021–3033.

Magini, G. (1887a). Nevroglia e cellule nervose cerebrali nei feti. Atti. 12 Congress. Med. Ital., Pavia, *1:*281–291. (Also appeared as: Sur la névroglie et les cellules nerveuses cérébrales chez les foetus. Arch. ital. Biol. *11:*59–60 [1888].)

Magini, G. (1887b). Sur la névroglie et les cellules nerveuses cérébrales chez les foetus. Arch. ital. Biol. *11:*59–60.

Magini, G. (1888). Nouvelles recherches histologiques sur le cerveau du foetus. Arch. ital. Biol. *10:*384–387.

Mahaim, A. (1897). Centres de projection et centres d'association du cerveau. Ann. Soc. méd-chir., Liège, *36:*142–149.

Malpeli, J. G., Lee, C., Schwark, H. D., and Weyand, T. G. (1986). Cat area 17, I: Pattern of thalamic control of cortical layers. J. Neurophysiol. *56:*1062–1073.

Marchi, V. (1887). Sulla fina struttura dei corpi striati e dei talami ottici. Reprinted from: Rev. Speriment. Freniatr. *12.* Reggio Emilia: Calderini, pp. 28. (English translation in Alienist and Neurologist, St. Louis, MO, *9:*1–23 [1888].)

Marinesco, G. (1899). Sur les altérations des grandes cellules pyramidales consécutives aux lésions de la capsule interne. Rev. Neurol., Paris, *7:*358.

Marinesco, G. (1904a). Étude sur les troubles de la sensibilité vibratoire dans les affections du système nerveux. Compt. Rend. Soc. Biol., Paris, *56:*333.

Marinesco, G. (1904b). Lésions des neuro-fibrilles consécutives à la ligature de l'aorte abdominale. Compt. Rend. Soc. Biol., Paris, *56:*600.

Marinesco, G. (1904c). Lésions des neuro-fibrilles produites par la toxine tétanique. Compt. Rend. Soc. Biol., Paris, *57:*62.

Marinesco, G. (1904d). Nouvelles recherches sur les neurofibrilles. Rev. Neurol., Paris, *12*:813–826.

Marinesco, G. (1904e). Recherches sur la structure de la partie fibrillaire des cellules nerveuses à l'état normal et pathologique. Rev. Neurol., Paris, *12*:405–428.

Marinesco, G. (1904f). Sur deux cas de paralysie flasque dans la compression du faisceau pyramidal sans dégénérescence de ce dernier, avec signe de Babinski et absence des réflexes tendineux cutanés. Rev. Neurol., Paris, *12*:210–218.

Marinesco, G. (1908). Sur la neurotisation des foyers de ramollissement et d'hémorragie cérébrale. Rev. Neurol., Paris, *16*:1293–1305.

Marinesco, G. and Minea, J. (1906). Note sur la régénérescence de la moelle chez l'homme. Compt. Rend. Soc. Biol., Paris, *60*:1027–1028.

Marin-Padilla, M. (1969). Origin of the pericellular baskets of the pyramidal cells of the human motor cortex: A Golgi study. Brain Res. *14*:633–646.

Marin-Padilla, M. (1970a). Prenatal and early postnatal ontogenesis of the human motor cortex: A Golgi study, I: The sequential development of the cortical layers. Brain Res. *23*:167–183.

Marin-Padilla, M. (1970b). Prenatal and early postnatal ontogenesis of the human motor cortex: A Golgi study, II: The basket-pyramidal system. Brain Res. *23*:185–191.

Marin-Padilla, M. (1984). Neurons of layer I: A developmental analysis. *In: Cerebral Cortex*, Vol. 1: *Cellular Components of the Cerebral Cortex*. A. Peters and E. G. Jones (eds.). New York: Plenum, pp. 447–477.

Marin-Padilla, M. (1987). The chandelier cell of the human visual cortex: A Golgi study. J. Comp. Neurol. *256*:61–70.

Marin-Padilla, M., and Marin-Padilla, M. T. (1982). Origin, prenatal development and structural organization of layer I of the human cerebral (motor) cortex: A Golgi study. Anat. Embryol. *164*:161–206.

Martin, K.A.C. (1984). Neuronal circuits in cat striate cortex. *In: Cerebral Cortex*, Vol. 2: *Functional Properties of Cortical Cells*. A. Peters and E. G. Jones (eds.). New York: Plenum, pp. 241–283.

Martin, K.A.C., Somogyi, P., and Whitteridge, D. (1983). Physiological and morphological properties of identified basket cells in the cat's visual cortex. Exp. Brain Res. *50*:193–200.

Martin, K.A.C., and Whitteridge, D. (1984). Form, function and intracortical projections of spiny neurones in the striate visual cortex of the cat. J. Physiol. London. *353*:463–504.

Martinotti, C. (1887). Su alcuni miglioramenti della tecnica della reazione al nitrato d'argento nei centri nervosi. Ann. Freniatr. Sci. affini, Torino, *1*:34–35. (Republished 1888 in Arch. ital. Biol. *9*:24–25.)

Martinotti, C. (1888–1889). Contributo allo studio della corteccia cerebrale, ed all'origine centrale dei nervi. Ann. Freniatr. Sci. Affini, Torino, *1*:314–332.

Martinotti, C. (1890). Beitrag zum Studium der Hirnrinde und der Centralursprünge der Nerven. Intern. Mschr. Anat. Physiol. *7*:69–90.

Mates, S. L., and Lund, J. S. (1983). Neuronal composition and development in lamina 4C of monkey striate cortex. J. comp. Neurol. *221*:60–90.

Mauss, T. (1908). Die faserarchitektonische Gliederung der Grosshirnrinde bei den niederen Affen. J. Psychol. Neurol., Leipzig, *13*:263–325.

Meinecke, D., and Peters, A. (1987). GABA immunoreactive neurons in rat visual cortex. J. comp. Neurol. *261*:388–404.

Merk, [L.] (1887). Die Mitosen im Centralnervensystem: Ein Beitrag zur Lehre vom Wachsthume desselben. Denkschr. Kaiserl. Akad. Wiss. Wien, Math.-natur. Cl. *53*:79–118.

Meyer, A. (1893). Ueber das Vorderhirn einiger Reptilien. Z. wiss. Zool. *55*:63–133.

Meyer, A. (1895). Zur Homologie der Fornix-commissure und des Septum pellucidum bei den Reptilien und Säugern. Anat. Anz. *10*:474–482.

Meyer, S. (1895). Die subcutane Methylenblauinjektion ein Mittel zur Darstellung der Elemente des Centralnervensystems von Säugethieren. Arch. mikrosk. Anat. EntwMech. *46*:282–290.

Meyer, S. (1896). Ueber eine Verbindungsweise der Neuronen, nebst Mittheilungen über die Technik und der Erfolge der Methode der subcutanen Methylenblau-Injection. Arch. mikrosk. Anat. EntwMech. *47*:734–748.

Meyer, S. (1897). Ueber die Funktion der Protoplasmafortsätze der Nervenzellen. Bericht. Math.-Phys. Cl. Königl. sächs. Gesells. Wiss., Leipzig. October 25, 1897, pp. 475–495.

Meyer, S. (1899). Ueber centrale Neuritenendigungen. Arch. mikrosk. Anat. EntwMech. *54*:296–311.

Meynert, T. (1867–1868). Der Bau der Grosshirnrinde und seine örtliche Verschiedenheiten, nebst einem pathologisch-anatomischen Corollarium. Vierteljahrschrift für Psychiatrie *1*:77–93, 125–217; *2*:88–113, 381–403. (Reprinted 1872, Neuwied: Heuser.)

Meynert, T. (1872). Vom Gehirne der Säugethiere. *In: Handbuch der Lehre von den Geweben des Menschen und der Thiere*. S. Stricker (ed.), 694–808. Leipzig: Engelmann, Vol. 2, pp. 694–808.

Meynert, T. (1874). Skizze des menschlichen Grosshirnstammes nach seiner Aussenform und seinem inneren Bau. Arch. Psychiat., Berlin, *4*:387–431.

Meynert, T. (1884). *Psychiatrie: Klinik der Erkrankungen des Vorderhirns*. Vienna: Braumüller.

Minkowski, M. (1913). Experimentelle Untersuchungen über die Beziehungen der Grosshirnrinde und der Netzhaut zu den primären optischen Zentren, besonders zum Corpus geniculatum externum. Arb. Hirnanat. Inst. Zürich *7*:259–362.

Monakow, C. von (1882). Weitere Mitteilungen über durch Extirpation circumscripter Hirnrindenregionen bedingte Entwickelungshemmungen des Kaninchengehirns. Arch. Psychiat. Nervenkrh. *12*:141–156, 535–549.

Monakow, C. von (1885). Experimentelle und pathologisch-anatomische Untersuchungen über die Beziehungen der sogenannten Sehsphäre zu den infracorticalen opticus centren und zum N. opticus. Arch. Psychiat. Nervenkrh. *16*:151–199, 317–352.

Monakow, [C. von] (1888). Rôle des diverses couches de cellules ganglionnaires dans le gyrus sigmoïde du chat. Arch. Sci. phys. nat. 20:358–360.

Monakow, C. von (1889). Experimentelle und pathologisch-anatomische Untersuchungen über die optischen Centren und Bahnen, nebst klinischen Beiträgen zur corticalen Hemianopsie und Alexie. Arch. Psychiat. Nervenkrh. 20:714–787.

Monakow, C. von (1895). Experimentelle und pathologisch-anatomische Untersuchungen über die Haubenregion, den Sehhügel und die Regio subthalamica, nebst Beiträgen zur Kenntnis früh erworbener Gross- und Kleinhirndefecte. Arch. Psychiat. Nervenkrh. 27:1–128, 386–478.

Monakow, C. von (1897). Gehirnpathologie. Vienna: Hölder.

Monakow, C. von (1902–1904). Ueber den gegenwärtigen Stand der Frage nach der Lokalisation im Grosshirn. Ergebn. Physiol. 1:534–583; 3:100–172.

Monakow, C. von (1905). Gehirnpathologie, 2nd edition. Vienna: Hölder.

Monakow, C. von (1909). Neue Gesichtspunkte in der Frage nach der Lokalisation im Grosshirn. Cor.-Bl. Schweiz. Aerzte, Basle, 39:401–415.

Monakow, C. von (1909–1910). Der rote Kern, die Haube und die Regio subthalamica bei einigen Säugetieren und beim Menschen: Vgl. anatomische, normal-anatomische, experimentelle und pathologisch-anatomische Untersuchungen. Arb. Hirnanat. Inst., Zürich, 3:51–267; 4:103–225.

Monakow, C. von (1914). Die Lokalisation im Grosshirn und der Abbau der Funktion durch kortikale Herde. Wiesbaden: Bergman.

Mondino, C. (1887). Ricerche Macro-microscopiche sui Centri Nervosi. Turin: no publisher.

Mondino, C. [and Minto, G.] (1897). Contributo allo studio della epilessia psichica; perizia psichiatrica. Ann. nevrol. Napoli 15:319–339.

Monti, A. (1895). Sur l'anatomie pathologique des éléments nerveux dans les processus provenant d'embolisme cérébral: considérations sur la signification physiologique des prolongements protoplasmiques des cellules nerveuses. Arch. ital. Biol. 24:20–33.

Morrison, J. H., Foote, S. L., Molliver, M. E., Bloom, F. E., and Lidov, H.G.W. (1982). Noradrenergic and serotonergic fibers innervate complementary layers in monkey primary visual cortex: An immunohistochemical study. Proc. Natl. Acad. Sci. USA 79:2401–2405.

Morrison, J. H., Grzanna, R., Molliver, M. E., and Coyle, J. T. (1978). The distribution and orientation of noradrenergic fibers in neocortex of the rat: An immunofluorescence study. J. comp. Neurol. 181:17–40.

Mott, F. W. (1895). Experimental enquiry upon the afferent tracts of the central nervous system of the monkey. Brain 18:1–20.

Mott, F. W. (1907). The progressive evolution of the structure and function of the visual cortex in the mammalia. Arch. Neurol., London, 3:1–48.

Mountcastle, V. B. (1957). Modality and topographic properties of single neurons of cat's somatic sensory cortex. J. Neurophysiol. 20:408–434.

Mountcastle, V. B., and Powell, T.P.S. (1959). Neural mechanisms subserving cutaneous sensibility, with special reference to the role of afferent inhibition in sensory perception and discrimination. Bull. Johns Hopkins Hosp. 105:201–232.

Munk, H. (1889). Ueber die Funktion der Grosshirnrinde; gesammelte Mittheilungen mit Anmerkungen, 2nd edition. Berlin: Hirschwald.

Munk, H. (1892). Ueber die Fühlsphäre der Grosshirnrinde. Sitzunsgsber. d. Königl, preuss. Akad. Wiss. Berlin. (Reprinted 1896 in Ueber die Funktionen von Hirn und Rückenmark. Berlin: Hirschwald.)

Nageotte, J. (1906). Note sur la présence de massues d'accroissement dans la substance grise de la moelle, et particulièrement dans les cornes antérieures, au cours de la paralysie générale et du tabes. Compt. Rend. Soc. Biol., Paris, 60:811–812.

Nakagaba, I. (1891). The origin of the cerebral cortex and the homologies of the optic lobe layers in the lower vertebrates. J. Morph. 4:1–10.

Nansen, F. (1887a). Nerve-elementerne, deres struktur og sammenhäng i centralnevensystemet. Nord. med. Ark., Stockholm, 19:1–24. (Republished 1888: Anat. Anz. 3:157–169.)

Nansen, F. (1887b). The Structure and Combination of the Histological Elements of the Central Nervous System. Bergen: Bergens Mus. Aarsberetning, pp. 29–214.

Narbut, [?] (1901). (Summary by Stieda of an article originally in Russian: Stieda, L. [1903] Zur Frage der histologischen Theorie des Schlafes. Neurol. Centralbl. 20:729–730.)

Neumayer, L. (1895). Die Grosshirnrinde der niederen Vertebraten. Sitzungsber. Gesells. Morphol. Phys., München, 1:61.

Nissl, F. (1894–1895). Der gegenwärtige Stand der Nervenzellenanatomie und Pathologie. Allgem. Zeitschr. Psych., Berlin, 51:981–986.

Nissl, F. (1895). Ueber die Nomenklatur in der Nervenzellenanatomie und ihre nächsten Ziele. Neurol. Centralbl. 14:66–75, 104–110.

Nissl, F. (1898). Nervenzellen und graue Substanz. München. med. Wochenshr. 31:988; 32:1023; 33:1060.

Nissl, F. (1913). Die Grosshirnanteile des Kaninchens. Arch. Psychiat. Nervenkrh. 52:867–953.

O'Leary, D.D.M., and Stanfield, B. B. (1986). A transient pyramidal tract projection from the visual cortex in the hamster and its removal by selective collateral elimination. Dev. Brain Res. 27:87–99.

O'Leary, D.D.M., Stanfield, B. B., and Cowan, W. M. (1981). Evidence that the early postnatal restriction of the cells of origin of the callosal projection is due to the elimination of axonal collaterals rather than to the death of neurons. Dev. Brain Res. 1:607–617.

Obersteiner, H. (1888). Anleitung beim Studium des Baues der nervösen Centralorgane in gesunden und kranken Zuständen. Vienna: Toeplitz, Leipzig: Deuticke. [second edition 1892; third edition, 1897].

Obregia, A. (1890a). Fixierungsmethode der

Golgi'schen Präparate des centralen Nervensystems. Virch. Archiv. Path. Anat. *122*:387.

Obregia, A. (1890b). Über Augenbewegungen auf Sehsphärenreizung. Arch. Anat. Physiol., Physiol. Abt., *1890*:260–279.

Odier, R. (1898). Recherches expérimentales sur les mouvements de la cellule nerveuse de la moelle épinière. Basle and Geneva: Revue med. Suisse Romande, Georg, pp. 8–36.

Osborn, H. F. (1888). A contribution to the internal structure of the amphibian brain. J. Morph. *2*:51–96.

Oyarzun, A. (1890). Ueber den feineren Bau des Vorderhirns der Amphibien. Arch. mikrosk. Anat. EntwMech. *35*:380–388.

Paton, S. (1900). The histogenesis of the cellular elements of the cerebral cortex. Johns Hopk. Hosp. Rep. *9*:709–741.

Peters, A. (1971). Stellate cells of the rat parietal cortex. J. comp. Neurol. *141*:345–374.

Peters, A. (1984a). Bipolar cells. *In: Cerebral Cortex*, Vol. 1: *Cellular Components of the Cerebral Cortex*. A. Peters and E. G. Jones (eds.). New York: Plenum, pp. 381–407.

Peters, A. (1984b). Chandelier cells. *In: Cerebral Cortex*, Vol. 1: *Cellular Components of the Cerebral Cortex*. A. Peters and E. G. Jones (eds.). New York: Plenum, pp. 361–380.

Peters, A. (1987). Number of neurons and synapses in primary visual cortex. *In: Cerebral Cortex*, Vol. 6: *Further Aspects of Cortical Function, including Hippocampus*. E. G. Jones and A. Peters (eds.). New York: Plenum, pp. 267–294.

Peters, A., and Fairén, A. (1978). Smooth and sparsely-spined stellate cells in the visual cortex of the rat: A study using a combined Golgi-electron microscope technique. J. comp. Neurol. *181*:129–172.

Peters, A., and Jones, E. G. (1984). Classification of cortical neurons. *In: Cerebral Cortex*, Vol. 1: *Cellular Components of the Cerebral Cortex*. A. Peters and E. G. Jones (eds.). New York: Plenum, pp. 107–122.

Peters, A., and Kaiserman-Abramof, I. R. (1969). The small pyramidal neuron of the rat cerebral cortex. The synapses on dendritic spines. Z. Zellforsch. *100*:487–506.

Peters, A., and Kimerer, L. M. (1981). Bipolar neurons in rat visual cortex: a combined Golgi-electron microscopic study. J. Neurocytol. *10*:921–946.

Peters, A., Meinecke, D. L., and Karamanlidis, A. N. (1987). Vasoactive intestinal polypeptide immunoreactive neurons in the primary visual cortex of the cat. J. Neurocytol. *16*:23–38.

Peters, A., and Proskauer, C. C. (1980). Synaptic relationships between a multipolar stellate cell and a pyramidal neuron in the rat visual cortex: a combined Golgi-electron microscope study. J. Neurocytol. *9*:163–184.

Peters, A., Proskauer, C. C., and Ribak, C. E. (1982). Chandelier cells in rat visual cortex. J. comp. Neurol. *206*:397–416.

Peters, A., and Regidor, J. (1981). A reassessment of the forms of non-pyramidal neurons in area 17 of cat visual cortex. J. comp. Neurol. *203*:685–716.

Peters, A., and Saint Marie, R. L. (1984). Smooth and sparsely spinous non-pyramidal cells forming local axonal plexuses. *In: Cerebral Cortex*, Vol. 1: *Cellular Components of the Cerebral Cortex*. A. Peters and E. G. Jones (eds.). New York: Plenum, pp. 419–445.

Petrone, L. M. (1887). Intorno allo studio della struttura della nevroglia dei centri nervosi cerebrospinali. Gazz. Med. Ital. Lomb., Milano, *47*:301–307.

Phillips, C. G. (1959). Actions of antidromic pyramidal volleys on single Betz cells in the cat. Qt. Jl. exp. Physiol. *44*:1–25.

Probst, M. (1898). Experimentelle Untersuchungen über das Zwischenhirn und dessen Verbindungen, besonders die sogenannte Rindenschleife. Dtsch. Z. NervHeilk., *13*:384–408.

Probst, M. (1900a). Physiologische, anatomische und pathologisch-anatomische Untersuchungen des Sehhügels. Arch. Psychiat. Nervenkrh. *33*:721–817.

Probst, M. (1900b). Experimentelle Untersuchungen über die Anatomie und Physiologie des Sehhügels. Mschr. Psychiat. Neurol. *7*:387–404.

Probst, M. (1901a). Ueber den Bau des vollständig balkenlosen Grosshirns sowie über Mikrogyrie und Heterotopie der grauen Substanz. Arch. Psychiat. Nervenkrh. *34*:709–786.

Probst, M. (1901b). Zur Kenntnis des Bindearmes, der Haubenstrahlung und der Regio subthalamica. Mschr. Psychiat. Neurol. *10*:288–309.

Probst, M. (1903). Über die Leitungsbahnen des Grosshirns mit besonderer Berücksichtigung der Anatomie und Physiologie des Sehhügels. Jb. Psychiat. Neurol. *23*:18–106.

Probst, M. (1906). Über die zentralen Sinnesbahnen und die Sinneszentren des menschlichen Gehirns. Sitzungb. Akad. Wiss. Wien, math.-nat. Kl. *115*:103–176.

Querton, L. (1898). Le sommeil hibernal et les modifications des neurones cérébraux. Trav. Lab. Inst. Solvay, Brussels, *2*:1–58.

Rabl-Rückhard, [H.] (1878). Das Centralnervensystem des Alligators. Z. wiss. Zool. *30*:336–373.

Rabl-Rückhard, H. (1890). Sind die Ganglienzellen amöboid? Eine Hypothese zur Mechanik psychischer Vorgänge. Neurol. Centralbl. *9*:199.

Ramón, P. (1889). Trabajos de la sección de técnica anatómica de la Facultad de Medicina de Zaragoza. [Not verified]

Ramón, P. (1890). Investigaciones de histología comparada en los centros ópticos de distintos vertebrados. Thesis, Zaragoza.

Ramón, P. (1891). El encéfalo de los reptiles. Barcelona: [no publisher identified].

Ramón, P. (1894). Investigaciones micrográficas en el encéfalo de los batracios y reptiles. Zaragoza: La Derecha.

Ramón, P. (1896a). Estructura del encéfalo del camaleón. Rev. trim. Micrográf., Madrid, *1*:46–83.

Ramón, P. (1896b). L'encéphale des amphibiens. Bibliogr. Anat., Paris, *4*:232–252.

Ramón, P. (1900). Ganglio basal de los batracios y fascículo basal. Rev. trim. Micrográf., Madrid, *5*:23–35.

Ramón-Moliner, E. (1961a). The histology of the

postcruciate gyrus of the cat I: Quantitative studies. J. comp. Neurol. *117:*43–62.

Ramón-Moliner, E. (1961b). The histology of the postcruciate gyrus of the cat II: A statistical analysis of the dendritic distribution. J. comp. Neurol. *117:*63–76.

Ramón-Moliner, E. (1961c). The histology of the postcruciate gyrus of the cat III: Further observations. J. comp. Neurol. *117:*229–249.

Ranvier, L. (1875–1886). *Traité technique d'Histologie.* Paris: Savy.

Ranvier, L. (1883). De la névroglie. Arch. Physiol. norm. pathol., Paris, 3rd series, *1:*177–185.

Rauber, A. (1885–1886). Die Kerntheilungsfiguren im Medullarrohr der Wirbelthiere. Arch. mikrosk. Anat. EntwMech. *26:*622–644.

Remak, R. (1841). Anatomische Beobachtungen über das Gehirn, das Rückenmark und die Nervenwurzeln. Müllers Arch. Anat. Physiol. Wiss. *1841:*506–522.

Renaut, J. (1895). Sur les cellules nerveuses multipolaires et la théorie du "neurone" de Waldeyer. Bull. Acad. méd., Paris, March 5, 1895. [Quoted from Bonne, 1910.]

Retzius, G. (1890). Zur Kenntnis des Nervensystems der Crustaceen. Biol. Unters., Neue Folge, *1:*1–99.

Retzius, G. (1891). Ueber den Bau der Oberflächenschicht der Grosshirnrinde beim Menschen und bei den Säugethieren. Biol. Unters., Neue Folge, *3:*90–102.

Retzius, G. (1892a). *Biologische Untersuchungen von Gustav Retzius, Neue Folge,* Vol. 3. Stockholm: Samson and Wallin.

Retzius, G. (1892b). Die nervösen Elemente der Kleinhirnrinde. Biol. Unters., Neue Folge, *3:*17–24.

Retzius, G. (1892). Die Endigungsweise der Riechnerven. Biol. Unters., Neue Folge, *3:*25–28.

Retzius, G. (1893a). *Biologische Untersuchungen von Gustav Retzius, Neue Folge* Vol. 5. Stockholm: Samson and Wallin.

Retzius, G. (1893b). Die Cajal'schen Zellen der Grosshirnrinde beim Menschen und bei Säugethieren. Biol. Unters., Neue Folge, *5:*1–8.

Retzius, G. (1894). Weitere Beiträge zur Kenntnis der Cajal'schen Zellen der Grosshirnrinde des Menschen. Biol. Unters., Neue Folge, *6:*113–173.

Retzius, G. (1900). Weiteres zur Frage von den freien Nervenendigungen und anderen Strukturverhältnissen in den Spinalganglien. Biol. Unters., Neue Folge, *9:*69–76.

Reusz, F. von [1903]. Über Brauchbarkeit der Golgischen Methode in der Physiologie und Pathologie der Nervenzellen. Neurol. Centralbl. *21:*17. (Originally published 1902 in a Hungarian journal.)

Rockel, A. J., Hiorns, R. W., and Powell, T.P.S. (1980). The basic uniformity in structure of the neocortex. Brain *103:*221–244.

Rockland, K. S., and Pandya, D. N. (1979). Laminar origins and terminations of cortical connections of the occipital lobe in the rhesus monkey. Brain Res. *179:*3–20.

Rockland, K. S., and Pandya, D. N. (1981). Cortical connections of the occipital lobe in the rhesus monkey: Interconnections between areas 17, 18, 19 and the superior temporal sulcus. Brain Res. *212:*249–270.

Rose, M. (1912). Histologische Lokalisation der Grosshirnrinde bei kleinen Säugethieren (Rodentia, Insectivora, Chiroptera). J. Psychol. Neurol., Leipzig, *19:*391–479.

Rossi, V. (1908). Per la rigenerazione dei neuroni. Trav. Lab. Rech. biol. Univ. Madrid *6:*227–241.

Rottenberg, D. A., and Hochberg, F. H. (eds.) (1977). *In: Neurological Classics in Modern Translation.* New York: Hafner, pp. 7–29.

Royce, G. J. (1982). Laminar origin of neurons which project upon the caudate nucleus: A horseradish peroxidase investigation in the cat. J. Comp. Neurol. *205:*8–29.

Ruiz-Marcos, A., and Valverde, F. (1970). Dynamic architecture of the visual cortex. Brain Res. *19:*25–39.

Rustioni, A., and Hayes, N. L. (1981). Corticospinal tract collaterals to the dorsal column nuclei of cats: An anatomical single and double retrograde tracer study. Exp. Brain Res. *43:*237–245.

Rutishäuser, F. (1899). Experimenteller Beitrag zur Stabkranzfaserung im Frontalhirn des Affen. Mschr. Psych. Neurol. *5:*161.

Rye, D. B., Wainer, B. H., Mesulam, M. M., and Saper, C. B. (1984). Cortical projections arising from the basal forebrain: A study of cholinergic and noncholinergic components employing combined retrograde tracing and immunohistochemical localisation of choline acetyltransferase. Neurosci. *13:*627–643.

Saint Marie, R. L., and Peters, A. (1985) The morphology and synaptic connections of spiny stellate neurons in monkey visual cortex (area 17): A Golgi-electron microscopic study. J. comp. Neurol., *233:*213–235.

Sala, G. (1909). Ueber die Regenerationserscheinungen im zentralen Nervensystem. Anat. Anz. *34:*193–199.

Sala y Pons, C. (1892). Estructura de la médula espinal en los batracios. Trab. Lab. Histol. Facultad Med., Barcelona, February *1892:*1–22.

Sala y Pons, C. (1893). La corteza cerebral de los aves. Madrid: [publisher not identified]. (Republished 1899 as L'écorce cérébral des oiseaux, translated by L. Azoulay. Compt. Rend. Soc. Biol., Paris, 9th series, *5:*974–976.)

Schäfer, E. A. (1893). The spinal cord and brain. *In: Quains' Elements of Anatomie,* 10th edition, Vol. 3, Part 1. E. A. Schäfer and G. D. Thane (eds.). London: Longmans, Green.

Schaffer, K. (1892). Beitrag zur Histologie des Ammonshornformation. Arch. mikrosk. Anat. EntwMech. *39:*611–632.

Schaffer, K. (1897). Zur feineren Struktur der Hirnrinde und über die funktionelle Bedeutung der Nervenzellenfortsätze. Arch. mikrosk. Anat. EntwMech. *48:*550–572.

Schaffer, K. (1903). Über Markfasergehalt eines normalen und eines paralytischen Gehirns. Neurol. Centralbl. *17:*802–818.

Schaffer, K. (1907). Ueber die Pathohistologie eines neueren Falles (VIII) von Sachs'schen familiär-amaurotischer Idiotie mit einem Ausblick auf das Wesen der sogenannten Neurofibrillen. J. Psychol. Neurol., Leipzig, *10*:121–144.

Schaper, A. (1895). Einige kritische Bermerkungen zu Lugaros Aufsatz: Über die Histogenese der Körner der Kleinhirnrinde. Anat. Anz. *10*:422–426. (A review of: Lugaro, E. (1894). Über die Histogenese der Körner der Kleinhirnrinde. Anat. Anz. *9*:710–713.)

Schlapp, M. (1895). Der Zellenbau der Grosshirnrinde der Idiotie, Publié par le Dr. S. E. Henschen. Upsala, 1895. (Not identified. Possibly in: Henschen, S. E. *Beiträge zur Pathologie des Gehirns,* Vol. 3, 1896, Stockholm: Almqvist and Wiksell.)

Schlapp, M. (1898). Der Zellenbau der Grosshirnrinde des Affen, Macacus cynomolgus. Arch. Psychiat. Nervenkrh. *30*:583–607.

Schlapp, M. G. (1903). The microscopic structure of cortical areas in man and some mammals. Amer. J. Anat. *2*:259–281.

Schmechel, D. E., Vickrey, B. G., Fitzpatrick, D., and Elde, R. P. (1984). GABAergic neurons of mammalian cerebral cortex: Widespread subclass defined by somatostatin content. Neurosci. Lett. *47*:227–232.

Schreyer, D. J., and Jones, E. G. (1988). Axon elimination in the developing corticospinal tract of the rat. Dev. Brain. Res. 38:103–119.

Schwalbe, G. (1881). Lehrbuch der Neurologie. *In: Lehrbuch der Anatomie des Menschen,* Vol. 2, part 2, 3rd section. C.E.E. Hoffmann (ed.). Erlangen: Besold, pp. 287–1026.

Schwark, H. D., Malpeli, J. G., Weyand, T. G., and Lee, C. (1986). Cat area 17, II: Response properties of infragranular layer neurons in the absence of supragranular layer activity. J. Neurophysiol. *56:*1074–1087.

Sehrwald, E. (1889). Zur Technik der Golgischen Färbung. Z. wiss. Mikros. *6:*443–456.

Shepherd, G. M., Brayton, R. K., Miller, J. P., Segev, I., Rinzel, J., and Rall, W. (1985). Signal enhancement in distal cortical dendrites by means of interactions between active dendritic spines. Proc. Natl. Acad. Sci. USA *82:*2192–2195.

Sherrington, C. S. (1897). The central nervous system. *In: Textbook of Physiology,* 7th edition, Vol. 3. M. A. Foster, (ed.). London: Macmillan.

Sherrington, C. S., and Grünbaum, A-S.F. (1901). Observations on the physiology of the cerebral cortex of some of the higher apes. Proc. roy. Soc., London, 69:206–209.

Shkol'nik-Yarros, E. G. (1971). *Neurons and Interneuronal Connections of the Central Visual System.* New York: Plenum.

Sholl, D. A. (1956). *The Organization of the Cerebral Cortex.* London: Methuen.

Siemerling, E. (1898). Ueber Markscheidenentwickelung des Gehirns und ihre Bedeutung für die Lokalisation. München. klin. Wochenschr. *45:*1395.

Sillito, A. M. (1977). Inhibitory processes underlying the directional specificity of simple, complex and hy-percomplex cells in the cat's visual cortex. J. Physiol., London, *271:*699–720.

Sillito, A. M. (1979). Inhibitory mechanisms influencing complex cell orientation selectivity and their modification at high resting discharge levels. J. Physiol., London, *289:*33–53.

Sillito, A. M. (1984). Functional considerations of the operation of GABAergic inhibitory processes in the visual cortex. *In: Cerebral Cortex,* Vol. 2: *Functional Properties of Cortical Cells.* E. G. Jones and A. Peters (eds.). New York: Plenum, pp. 91–117.

Simarro, L. (1900). Nuevo método histológico de impregnación por las sales fotográficas de plata. Rev. trim. Micrográf., Madrid, *5:*45–71.

Sloper, J. J., Hiorns, R. W., and Powell, T.P.S. (1979). A qualitative and quantitative electron microscopic study of the neurons in the primate motor and somatic sensory cortices. Phil. Trans. roy. Soc. London B, *285:*141–171.

Sloper, J. J., and Powell, T.P.S. (1979). Ultrastructural features of the sensori-motor cortex of the primate. Phil. Trans. roy. Soc. London *285:*123–139.

Smith, G. E. (1894). A preliminary communication upon the cerebral commissures of the Mammalia with special reference to the Monotremata and Marsupialia. Proc. Linn. Soc. N.S.W., 2nd Series, *9:*635–657.

Smith, G. E. (1896a). The fascia dentata. Anat. Anz. *12:*111–126.

Smith, G. E. (1896b). The morphology of the true "limbic lobe," corpus callosum, septum pellucidum and fornix. J. Anat. *30:*157–167, 185–205.

Smith, G. E. (1897). The origin of the corpus callosum; a comparative study of the hippocampal region of the cerebrum of *Marsupialia* and certain *Cheiroptera.* Trans. Linn. Soc., London, 7:47–69.

Smith, G. E. (1898). Further observations upon the fornix, with special reference to the brain of *Nyctophilus.* J. Anat. *32:*231–246.

Smith, G. E. (1907). A new topographical survey of the cerebral cortex: Being an account of the distribution of anatomically distinct cortical areas and their relationship to the cerebral sulci. J. Anat. *41:*237–254.

Somogyi, P. (1977). A specific axo-axonal interneuron in the visual cortex of the rat. Brain Res. *136:*345–350.

Somogyi, P., and Cowey, A. (1981). Combined Golgi and electron microscopic study on the synapses formed by double bouquet cells in the visual cortex of the cat and monkey. J. Comp. Neurol. *195:*547–566.

Somogyi, P., Cowey, A., Halász, N., and Freund, T. F. (1981). Vertical organization of neurones accumulating [³H]-GABA in visual cortex of rhesus monkey. Nature *294:*761–763.

Somogyi, P., Cowey, A., Kisvárday, Z. F., Freund, T. F., and Szentágothai, J. (1983a). Retrograde transport of γ-amino [³H]-butyric acid reveals specific interlaminar connections in the striate cortex of monkey. Proc. Natl. Acad. Sci. USA *80:*2385–2389.

Somogyi, P., Freund, T. F., and Cowey, A. (1982). The

axo-axonic interneuron in the cerebral cortex of the rat, cat and monkey. Neurosci. 7:2577–2607.

Somogyi, P., Hodgson, A. J., Smith, A. D., Ninzi, M. G., Gorio, A., and Wu, J.-Y. (1984). Different populations of GABAergic neurons in the visual cortex and hippocampus of the cat contain somatostatin- or cholecystokinin-immunoreactive material. J. Neurosci. 4:2590–2603.

Somogyi, P., Kisvárday, Z. F., Martin, K.A.C., and Whitteridge, D. (1983b). Synaptic connections of morphologically identified and physiologically characterized large basket cells in the striate cortex of cat. Neurosci. 10:261–294.

Soukhanoff, S. (1898a). Contribution à l'étude des modifications que subissent les prolongements dendritiques des cellules nerveuses sous l'influence des narcotiques. La Cellule 14:387–395.

Soukhanoff, S. (1898b). L'anatomie pathologique de la cellule nerveuse en rapport avec l'atrophie variqueuse des dendrites de l'écorce cérébrale. La Cellule 14:399–415.

Soukhanoff, S. (1898c). Contribution à l'étude des modifications des cellules nerveuses de l'écorce cérébrale dans l'anémie expérimentale. J. Neurol. Hypnol., Paris, 3:173–179.

Soukhanoff, S. (1903). Sur le réseau endocellulaire de Golgi dans les éléments nerveux de l'écorce cérébrale. Nevraxe 4:45–53.

Soury, J. (1892). Cerveau. In: Dictionnaire de Physiologie, Vol. 2. C. Richet (ed.). Paris: Alcan.

Soury, J. A. (1899). Le système nerveux central: Structure et fonctions; Histoire Critique des Theories et des Doctrines. Paris: Carré and Naud., 2 vols.

Spitzka, E. C. (1880). Contributions to encephalic anatomy, Part VII: The brain of Iguana. J. nerv. ment. Dis. 7:461–464.

Stanfield, B. B., and O'Leary, D.D.M. (1985). The transient corticospinal projection from the occipital cortex during the postnatal development of the rat. J. comp. Neurol. 238:236–248.

Stefanowska, M. (1897). Sur les appendices terminaux des dendrites cérébraux et leurs différents états physiologiques. Trav. Lab. Inst. Solvay, Brussels, 1:1–58.

Stefanowska, M. (1898). Évolution des cellules nerveuses corticales chez la souris après la naissance. Trav. Lab. Inst. Solvay, Brussels, 2:1–44.

Steiner, I. (1888). Les fonctions du système nerveux et leur phylogenèse. Compt. Rend. Soc. Biol., Paris, series 8, 5:566–569.

Steiner, I. (1890). Die Funktionen des Centralnervensystems der wirbellosen Thiere. Sber. preuss. Akad., Berlin, 1890:39–49.

Steiner, J. (1891). Sinnessphären und Bewegungen. Pflügers Archiv. ges. Physiol. 1:603–614.

Steriade, M., and Deschênes, M. (1984). The thalamus as a neuronal oscillator. Brain Res. Rev. 8:1–63.

Stieda, L. (1868). Studien über das centrale Nervensystem der Vögel und Säugethiere. Z. wiss. Zool. 19:1–94.

Stieda, L. (1870). Studien über das centrale Nervensystem der Wirbelthiere. Z. wiss. Zool. 20:273–456.

Stieda, L. (1875). Ueber den Bau des centralen Nervensystems der Schildkröte. Z. wiss. Zool. 25:361–406.

Stirling, W. (1893). Outlines of Practical Histology: A Manual for Students, 2nd edition. London: Griffin.

Studnička, F. K. (1894). Zur Geschichte des "Cortex cerebri." Verhandl. Anatom. Gesellsch., Strassburg, 8:193–198.

Szentágothai, J. (1970). Les circuits neuronaux de l'écorce cérébrale. Bull. Acad. Roy. Méd. Belgique, 7th series, 10:475–492.

Szentágothai, J. (1973). Synaptology of the visual cortex. In: Handbook of Sensory Physiology, Vol. 7/3. "Central Processing of Visual Information, Part B." Visual Centers of the Brain. R. Jung (ed.). Berlin: Springer.

Szentágothai, J. (1975). The "module-concept" in cerebral cortex architecture. Brain Res. 95:475–496.

Szentágothai, J., and Arbib, M. A. (1974). Conceptual models of neural organization. Neurosci. Res. Progr. Bull. 12:307–510.

Tanzi, E. (1893). I fatti e le induzioni nell'odierna istologia del sistema nervoso. Rev. Sperim. frenatr. Medic. legal. 19:419–472.

Tanzi, E. (1901). Una teoria dell'allucinazione. Riv. Patol. nerv. ment. 6:529–549.

Tartuferi, F. (1877). Sull'anatomia microscopica e sulla morfologia cellulare delle eminenze bigemine dell'uomo e degli altri mammiferi. Gazz. med. ital., Series 8, 3:1–14.

Tello, [J.] F. (1903). Sobre la existencia de neurofibrillas colosales en las neuronas de los reptiles. Trab. Lab. Invest. biol. Univ. Madrid 2:223–225.

Tello, [J.] F. (1907) La régénération dans les voies optiques. Trav. Lab. Rech. biol. Univ. Madrid 5:237–248.

Tello, J. F. (1935). Cajal y su labor histológica. Madrid: Universidad Central.

Terrazas, R. (1897). Notas sobre del cerebelo y el crecimiento de los elementos nerviosos. Rev. trim. Micrográf., Madrid, 2:49–65.

Toldt, [C.], and Kahler, [O.] (1888). Lehrbuch der Gewebelehre. (Toldt, C. [1888]. Lehrbuch der Gewebelehre mit vorzugsweiser Berücksichtigung des menschlichen Körpers: Mit einer topographischen Darstellung des Faserverlaufes im Centralnervensystem von Prof. O. Kahler, 3rd edition. Stuttgart: Enke, pp. 172–325.)

Toyama, K., Maekawa, K., and Takeda, T. (1977). Convergence of retinal inputs onto visual cortical cells I: A study of the cells monosynaptically excited from the lateral geniculate body. Brain Res. 137:207–220.

Toyama, K., and Matsunami, K. (1976). Convergence of specific visual and commissural impulses upon inhibitory interneurones in cat's visual cortex. Neurosci. 1:107–112.

Toyama, K., Matsunami, K., Ohno, T., and Tokashiki, S. (1974). An intracellular study of neuronal organization in the visual cortex. Exp. Brain Res. 21:45–66.

Ts'o, D. Y., Gilbert, C. D., and Wiesel, T. N. (1986). Relationships between horizontal interactions and functional architecture in cat striate cortex as revealed by cross-correlation analysis. J. Neurosci. 6:1160–1170.

Tsuchida, U. (1907). Ein Beitrag zur Anatomie der Sehstrahlungen beim Menschen. Arch. Psychiat. Nervkrh. 42:212–248.

Tuczek, F. (1882). Anordnung der markhältigen Nervenfasern in der Grosshirnrinde und über ihr Verhalten bei Dementia paralytica. Neurol. Centralbl. 1:315–337.

Turner, W. A., and Hunter, W. (1899). On a form of nerve termination in the central nervous system, demonstrated by methylene blue. Brain 22:123–124.

Ugolini, G., and Kuypers, H.G.J.M. (1986). Collaterals of corticospinal and pyramidal fibres to the pontine grey demonstrated by a new application of the fluorescent fibre labelling technique. Brain Res. 365:211–227.

Unger, L. (1880). Untersuchungen über die Entwickelung des cerebralen Nervengewebes. Sitzungsb. Kais. Akad. Wiss. Wien, math.-naturw. Cl., 1879, 80:137–157.

Valentin, G. G. (1836). Über den Verlauf und die letzten Ende der Nerven. Nova Acta Phys.-Med. Acad. Leopoldina, Breslau, 18:51–240.

Valentin, G. G. (1841). Hirn und Nervenlehre. In: (S. T. Soemmering's) Vom Baue des menschlichen Körpers. Revised and completed by W. Th. Bischoff et al. (1839–1845, 8 Vols.), Vol. 6, Leipzig: Voss.

Valverde, F. (1968). Structural changes in the area striata of the mouse after enucleation. Exp. Brain Res. 5:274–292.

Valverde, F. (1971). Short axon neuronal subsystems in the visual cortex of the monkey. Intern. J. Neurosci. 1:181–197.

Valverde, F. (1976). Aspects of cortical organization related to the geometry of neurons with intra-cortical axons. J. Neurocytol. 5:509–529.

Valverde, F. (1983). A comparative approach to neocortical organization based on the study of the brain of the hedgehog (Erinaceus europaeus). In: Ramón y Cajal's Contribution to the Neurosciences. S. Grisolía, C. Guerri, F. Samson, S. Norton, and F. Reinoso-Suárez (eds.). Amsterdam: Elsevier, pp. 149–170.

Valverde, F. (1985). The organizing principles of the primary visual cortex in the monkey. In: Cerebral Cortex, Vol. 3: Visual Cortex. A. Peters and E. G. Jones (eds.). New York: Plenum, pp. 207–257.

Valverde, F. (1986). Intrinsic neocortical organization: Some comparative aspects. Neurosci. 18:1–23.

Valverde, F., and Esteban, M. E. (1968). Peristriate cortex of mouse: Location and the effects of enucleation on the number of dendritic spines. Brain Res. 9:145–158.

Van Gehuchten, A. (1891a). Le bulbe olfactif chez quelques mammifères. La Cellule 7:203.

Van Gehuchten, A. (1891b). La structure des centres nerveux: La moelle épinière et le cervelet. La Cellule 7:79–122.

Van Gehuchten, [A.] (1896). Structure du télécéphale: Centres de projection et centres d'association. Conférence faite à l'assemblée générale de la 66 session

de la Société Scientifique de Bruxelles, Malines. (Published as: Van Gehuchten, A. (1897). Les centres de projection et les centres d'association de Flechsig dans le cerveau terminal de l'homme. J. Neurol. Hypnol., Paris, 2:2–15, 18–20.)

Van Gehuchten, A. (1900). Anatomie du système nerveux de l'homme, 3rd edition. Louvain: Uystpruyst-Dieudonné.

Van Gehuchten, A. (1906). Anatomie du système nerveux de l'homme, 4th edition. Louvain: University Library.

Van Valkenburg, C. T. (1913). Experimental and pathologico-anatomical researches on the corpus callosum. Brain 36:119–165.

Veratti, E. (1897). Ueber einige Struktureigenthümlichkeiten der Hirnrinde bei den Säugethieren. Anat. Anz. 13:377–389.

Vignal, W. (1884). Développement des éléments de la moelle épinière des mammifères. Arch. Physiol. Norm. Path., Paris, 3rd series, 4:364–426.

Vignal, W. (1888). Recherches sur le développement des éléments des couches corticales du cerveau et du cervelet chez l'homme et les mammifères. Arch. Physiol. Norm. Path., Paris, 4:228–254, 311–338.

Villaverde, J. M. de (1921). Estudios anatómico-experimentales sobre el curso y terminación de las fibras callosas. Trab. Lab. Invest. biol. Univ. Madrid 19:37–68.

Vogt, C. (1898). Sur la myélinisation de l'hémisphère cérébrale du chat. Compt. Rend. Soc. Biol., Paris, 50:54–56.

Vogt, C. (1900). Étude sur la myélinisation des hémisphères cérébraux. Paris: Steinheil.

Vogt, (Cecil et Oskar) (1904) Atlas. Jena. (Not identified. Possibly: Vogt, O. [Ed.] [1902–1904]. Neurobiologische Arbeiten. Series 1: Beiträge zur Hirnfaserlehre; Series 2: Weitere Beiträge zur Hirnanatomie. Denkschriften der med.-natur. Gesells. Jena: Fischer, Vols. 9, 10, 12 [6 parts].)

Vogt, C., and Vogt, O. (1919). Allgemeine Ergebnisse unserer Hirnforschung. J. Psychol. Neurol., Leipzig, 25:279–462.

Vogt, O. (1897). Flechsigs Associationscentrenlehre, ihre Anhänger, und Gegner. Z. Hypnotism., Psychother., psychophysiol. psychopathol. Forsch., Berlin, 5:347–361.

Vogt, O. (1903). Zur anatomischen Gliederung des Cortex cerebri. J. Psychol. Neurol., Leipzig, 2:160–180.

Vogt, O. (1906a). Der Wert der myelogenetischen Felder der Grosshirnrinde (Cortex pallii). Anat. Anz. 29:273–287.

Vogt, O. (1906b). Ueber strukturelle Hirncentra mit besonderer Berücksichtigung der Struktur der Felder des Cortex Pallii. Verhandl. Anat. Gesellsch. Rostock. 1–5 June 1906. Anat. Anz. Suppl. 29:74–114.

Vulpius, O. (1892). Über die Entwicklung und Ausbreitung der Tangentialfasern in der menschlichen Grosshirnrinde während verschiedener Altersperioden. Arch. Psychiat. Nervkrh. 23:775–798.

Waldeyer, W. (1891). Über einige neuere Forschungen

im Gebiete der Anatomie des Centralnervensystems. Deutsch. med. Wschr. *17*:1213–1218; 1244–1246; 1267–1269; 1331–1332; 1352–1356.

Wallenberg, A. (1900). Secundäre sensible Bahnen im Gehirnstamme des Kaninchens, ihre gegenseitige Lage und ihre Bedeutung für den Aufbau des Thalamus. Anat. Anz. *18*:81–105.

Wallenberg, A. (1905). Sekundäre Bahnen aus dem frontalen sensibeln Trigeminuskern des Kaninchens. Anat. Anz. *26*:145–155.

Watson, G. A. (1907). The mammalian cerebral cortex with special reference to its comparative histology I: Order insectivora. Arch. Neurol., London, *3*:48–117.

Weigert, C. (1882). Über eine neue Untersuchungsmethode des Zentralnervensystems. Zentralbl. med. Wiss. *20*:753–757, 772–774.

Weyand, T. G., Malpeli, J. G., Lee, C., and Schwark, H. D. (1986). Cat area 17, IV: Two types of corticotectal cells defined by controlling geniculate inputs. J. Neurophysiol. *56*:1102–1108.

White, E. L. (1978). Identified neurons in mouse SmI cortex which are postsynaptic to thalamocortical axon terminals: A combined Golgi-electron microscopic and degeneration study. J. comp. Neurol. *181*:627–662.

White, E. L., and Rock, M. P. (1980). Three-dimensional aspects and synaptic relationships of a Golgi-impregnated spiny stellate cell reconstructed from serial thin sections. J. Neurocytol. *9*:615–636.

Wiedersheim, R. (1890). Bewegungserscheinungen im Gehirn von *Leptodora hyalina.* Anat. Anz. *5*:673–679.

Wilson, A. (1894). Science jottings. Illustrated London News *104*:430.

Winfield, D. A., Brooke, R.N.L., Sloper, J. J., and Powell, T.P.S. (1981). A combined Golgi-electron microscopic study of the synapses made by the proximal axon and recurrent collaterals of a pyramidal cell in the somatic sensory cortex of the monkey. Neurosci. *6*:1217–1230.

Winfield, D. A., Gatter, K. C., and Powell, T.P.S. (1980). An electron microscopic study of the types and proportions of neurons in the cortex of the motor and visual areas of the cat and rat. Brain *103*:245–258.

Winfield, D. A., Rivera-Domínguez, M., and Powell, T.P.S. (1982). The termination of geniculocortical fibres in area 17 of the visual cortex in the macaque monkey. Brain Res. *231*:19–32.

Winkler, C., and Potter, A. (1911). *An Anatomical Guide to Experimental Researches on the Rabbit's Brain.* Amsterdam: Versluys.

Winkler, C. and Potter, A. (1914). *An Anatomical Guide to Experimental Researches on the Cat's Brain.* Amsterdam: Versluys.

Woolsey, T. A., Dierker, M. A., and Wann, D. F. (1975). Mouse SmI cortex: Qualitative and quantitative classification of Golgi-impregnated barrel neurons. Proc. Natl. Acad. Sci. USA *72*:2165–2169.

Yen, C.-T., Conley, M., and Jones, E. G. (1985). Morphological and functional types of neurons in cat ventral posterior thalamic nucleus. J. Neurosci. *5*:1316–1338.

Zacher, T. (1887). Ueber das Verhalten der markhaltigen Nervenfasern in der Hirnrinde bei der progressiven Paralyse und bei anderen Geisteskrankheiten. Arch. Psychiat. Nervkrh. *18*:60–97.

Ziehen, G. T. (1897–1901). Das Centralnervensystem der Monotremen und Marsupialier. Denkschr. med.-nat. Gesellsch., Jena, 6 (part 1):1–188, 677–728.

Ziehen, G. T. (1906), *In: Handbuch der vergleichenden und experimentellen Entwicklungslehre der Wirbeltiere.* 3 vols. O. Hertwig (ed.). Jena: Fischer.

Ziehen, G. T. (1920). *Anatomie des Centralnervensystems.* Jena: G. Fischer (in press). (Published as: Ziehen, G. T. [1921]. *Makroskopische und mikroskopische Anatomie des Rückenmarks und Gehirns. In: Handbuch der Anatomie des Menschen,* Vol. 4, parts 1–3. K. von Bardeleben [ed.]. Jena: Fischer.)

Zuckerkandl, E. (1903). Die Rindenbündel des Alveus bei Beuteltieren. Anat. Anz. *23*:49–60.

Zunino, G. (1909). Die myeloarchitektonische Differenzierung der Grosshirnrinde beim Kaninchen (Lepus cuniculus). J. Psychol. Neurol., Leipzig, *14*:38–70.

Index

Acetylcholine, 583
Ameboidism, neuronal, 479–482
Ammon's horn, 137, 294, 316, 320, 330–334, 337, 338, 341, 344, 351, 355, 360, 414, 415, 441, 545
Ammon's horn, afferent pathways, 360. *See also* Bundle, angular; Pathway, spheno-ammonic
Ammon's horn, perforant bundles, 334. *See also* Pathway, perforant
Ammon's horn, as tertiary olfactory center, 373–375
Ammon's horn and fascia dentata, exogenous fibers, 330–332
Amphibians. *See* Batrachians
Amygdala, 329, 360
Aphasia, 472
Apparatus of Golgi-Holmgren, 396, 398
Archipallium, 437, 441
Area, angular or spheno-occipital, 333, 334, 351, 363–364, 371. *See also* Focus, angular or spheno-occipital; Ganglion, angular or spheno-occipital
Area, association or ideational, 147. *See also,* Cortex, association
Area, entorhinal, 545
Area, entorhinal, medial, 375n. *See also* Focus, spheno-occipital
Area, motor
  extent of in the mouse, rat and rabbit, 239. *See also* Cortex, motor or sensory-motor
Area, olfactory, 302–314. *See also* Cortex, olfactory
  cells with short axon and nervous plexuses of the deeper layer, 312–313
  double pyramids, 310
  giant polymorphic cells, 305
  layer of the deep polymorphic cells or layer of the fusiform/triangular cells, 311–312

layer of the giant polymorphic cells, 304–306
layer of the semilunar and horizontal triangular cells, 304
layer of the tasseled pyramids, 304, 308–311, 313
nervous plexuses and cells with short axon of the second layer, 306–308
plexiform layer, 303–304
pyramidal cells, 306
white matter, 312
Area, retrosplenial, 526. *See also* Cortex, retrosplenial
Area, sensory-motor. *See also* Cortex, motor
  comparative structure, 239, 433
  localization, 432
  motor and sensory components, 432–434, 436n, 621
Area, spheno-occipital, 337, 338. *See also* Cortex, spheno-occipital
Area, suboccipital, 525
Area, visual, 134. *See also* Cortex, visual
  in the cat, rabbit, and other mammals, 183, 374–375, 495–523. *See also* Cortex, visual, of cat. *See* Cortex, visual, human
Areas, association, 131, 136, 146, 147, 185, 440, 441, 466–468. *See also* Cortex, association
Areas, association in small mammals, 440–441, 473
Areas, association in smooth cerebra, 239–240
Areas, language, 431, 470
Areas, memory, 471–473, 474
Areas, olfactory, primary, 137, 185
Areas, olfactory, secondary, 137, 360
Areas, olfactory, tertiary, 137
Areas, perceptive, 473, 474
Areas, perceptive and memory, 474–476
Areas, projection, 136, 147

Areas, sensory-afferent and motor, 81, 185–186. *See also* Cortex, motor

Aspiny cells with local axonal arcades, 592, 593. *See also* Cells with short axon

Association, centrifugal or moderator fibers of, 181, 476–477. *See also* Cells, association; Fibers, association

Attention, 476

Axons, free terminations, 24, 84, 87

Axons, multiple, 21, 30. *See also* Cells with multiple axons

Baillarger, external stria of, 39

Basket cells, 174–176, 401, 583–586. *See also* Cells, basket

Baskets, pericellular, 176, 402, 403

Batrachians, cerebral cortex of, 77–78, 449–451

Betz cells, 190, 192, 409

Bipolar neurons, 594, 595

Birds, cerebral cortex of, 78–79, 441–444

Bitufted cells, 202, 209, 212, 235, 587. *See also* cells, bitufted and Double bouquet cells

Body, lateral geniculate, 134, 181, 520

Bulb, olfactory, 289, 290

Bundle, alvear spheno-ammonic, 345

Bundle, angular or crossed, 333–336, 338–339

Bundle, angular or crossed spheno-ammonic, 335, 336, 339, 341, 344, 345, 351

Bundle, corticothalamic, 184

Bundle, crossed angular, 331

Bundle, crossed angular or spheno-ammonic, 355, 371

Bundle, crossed spheno-ammonic, 137

Bundle, perforant, 345

Bundle, spheno-ammonic, 137

Bundle, superior longitudinal, 327

Bundle, suprafimbrial, 337

Bundles, inferior perforant, 341

Bundles, perforant spheno-ammonic, 336

Bundles, spheno-alvear, 371

Bundles, spheno-ammonic, superior perforant, 339–341

Cajal
  autobiography, 493
  cell classifications of, 564–565
  cells of, 6, 12, 99, 113, 119, 121, 136, 146, 153, 198
  contributions of, 564
  definitive assessment of intracortical organization, 493
  fibers of, 7, 142, 181
  fundamental neurobiological principles, 621
  and German cytoarchitectonic school, 494, 546n
  and Golgi method, 3, 494–497, 521n
  last works, 548–550
  lectures of 1892, 7
  material and method of analysis, 5, 558–561
  method of drawing cells, 4
  methods of staining, 4
  methylene blue studies, 107–111, 113–127
  nomenclature, 561–564
  and peer review, 494, 522n
  photomicrographs, 494, 517, 519, 533, 542, 544
  reduced silver method, 380, 387, 393, 399, 411, 425n, 426n
  referencing, 622
  technique, 25

Cajal-Retzius cells, 584–587, 604, 608. *See also* Cajal, cells of

Capsule, extreme, 284

Caudate nucleus, 287

Cell, basilar neuroglial, 402, 403

Cell, giant with horizontal axon, 145–146

Cells, arachniform, 154, 167, 169, 177, 186, 385, 407, 502, 507, 590–591. *See also* Cells, neurogliaform

Cells with arciform axon, 176, 184, 515, 517

Cells with ascending axons, 37, 142, 421. *See also* *layers of individual areas*

Cells, association, 21, 51, 118, 146

Cells, basket, 174–176, 401–403, 583–586. *See also* Basket cells

Cells, bitufted, 134, 144–145, 159–160, 202, 209, 212, 235, 407–408, 587. *See also* Bitufted cells

Cells, callosal, 45–48, 51. *See also* Corpus callosum

Cells, cerebral, morphological types of, 75–76, 564, 565, 582

Cells of the cerebrum
  parallelism in phylogenetic and ontogenetic development, 463

Cells, chandelier, 584, 598, 602

Cells, Deiters', 50, 198, 384

Cells, dwarf, 430, 507. *See also* Cells, arachniform

Cells, endothelial, 50

Cells, ependymal, 462

Cells, epithelial, 6, 14
  as guides to developing axons, 49
  development, 48–49

Cells, excitomotor, 82

Cells, giant pyramidal, 71, 184, 190, 192, 409

Cells, giant stellate, 157, 177

Cells, Golgi, 76, 125. *See also* Golgi

Cells, granule, 246, 253

Cells with long axon, 9, 76. *See also individual areas*
  appearance of the axonal collaterals, 458
  appearance of the basilar dendrites and collaterals of the apical dendritic shaft, 457
  axon, 456–457
  development, 455–462
  neuroblast phase, 456
  primitive bipolar phase, 455
  secondary bipolar phase, 457

Cells, motor, 24, 36, 39, 45, 58–59, 70–71, 125

Cells with multiple axons, 12, 76, 31, 32, 66, 119, 379, 421. *See also* Cells, special of layer I

Cells, nerve
  development, 50–51
  form and structure of, 24

Cells, neurogliaform 226, 263–264, 270–276, 385, 590–591. *See also* Cells, arachniform

Cells, neuroglial with vascular pedicles, 419

Cells, pyramidal. *See also* Pyramidal cells; *layers of individual areas*
  development, 15
  diversity of processes, 80
  evolution of, 69
  general morphological characteristics, 7, 24, 68
  phylogeny, 86

Cells, sensory, 24, 36
Cells, sensory and motor, 9, 24, 36
Cells with short axon, 5, 9, 36, 70–71, 76, 113, 166, 184. *See also* layers *of individual areas*
  development, 458
  functional role, 422–423
Cells, specific acoustic, 266. *See also* Cortex, auditory, specific cells
Cells, special of layer I, 10–12, 21, 201–206, 379, 385–387, 547, 603
  axons, 203–204
  collaterals, 204
  dendrites, 203–204
  development, 120, 154, 205–206, 385, 386
  types, 204–205
Cells, special of the molecular layer, 5, 9, 11, 20, 51, 56–58, 65–66, 66–68, 99, 113, 119–124, 153
Cells, special or horizontal of the first layer, 65, 119–124, 421
Cells, stellate, with long axons
  auditory cortex, 432
  motor cortex, 219
  visual cortex, 140, 367, 373, 430, 504, 505, 514, 520
Cells, stellate, of the stria of Gennari, 140. *See also* Cortex, visual
Cells of vertical association, 118
Centers, association and projection, 181, 185, 465–469. *See also* Cortex, association
Centers, olfactory, secondary, 360
Centers, projection or sensory-motor, 136, 147, 465–469
Cerebellum, granule cells of, 121
Cerebrum
  anatomicophysiological considerations, 465–490
Cerebrum, organization and function, anatomical theories, 465–479
Chandelier cells, 584, 598–603
Chemotaxia, 121
Cingulum, 138, 325, 327, 331, 332, 334, 336–339, 346–349, 351, 353–359, 360, 414
  bundles destined for the subiculum, 358
  components, 353–354
  connections, 354–359
  fibers, 354–356
  fibers destined for the focus of the occipital pole, 357–358
  history, 346–348
  layer of the focus of the occipital pole, 358
  perforant fibers destined for the plexiform layer, 358, 383–387
  posterior terminations of the fibers, 357–358
  termination of the anterior branches, 356–357
Circuits, intracortical, 24, 74–75, 83–86, 420–422, 603–606
Clark University, 130–133
Claustrum, 284–286
  affinities, 285–286
  cells, 285
Clubs, terminal, 402–403
Collaterals, olfactory, 294
Columns of axonal terminations, 618, 619
Commissura pallii, 444
Commissure, anterior, 19, 42, 48, 75, 294, 322–323, 325, 327, 334, 414, 478

  anterior or bulbar portion, 323–324
  connections of bulbar portion, 324
  connections of sphenoidal portion
  sphenoidal portion, 324–326
Commissure of the fornix, 414
Concentric symmetry, 478
Conduction, avalanche of, 180
Connections between cortical cells, 32, 81, 603–606. *See also* Circuits, intracortical
Connections by contact, 8, 86–87
Connections, cortico-ammonic, 346
Connections, intercortical, growth of, 81, 87
Connections, neuronal, plasticity of, 81, 87, 484–486
Consciousness, act of, 81, 475
Corpus callosum, 14, 18, 42–45, 243, 325, 331, 333–335, 337, 339, 355, 414, 473, 474, 514, 522n
  collateral axons, 414
  direct axons, 414
  fibers, 39, 44–45, 84
  splenium of the, 352
  terminal fibers, 415
Corpus striatum, 286–287, 334
  cells, 286–287
  fibers, 287
Cortex, acoustic, 185, 251. *See also* Cortex, auditory
Cortex, association, 147, 239–240, 433, 434–435
  layers, 434–435
  memory, 435
  olfactory, 435
Cortex, auditory, 136, 430–432
  arciform collaterals, 262
  axons of Martinotti, 261
  bitufted cells, 259–260, 264, 270
  evolution, 280
  exogenous fibers destined for the plexiform or first layer, 274
  exogenous fibers terminating in the plexus of the layer of the granule cells, 272–274
  fibers of Martinotti, 256, 258, 270
  giant specific cells, 267
  giant stellate cell, 279
  granule cells, 265, 271
  historical sketch of the structure, 431
  interradial plexus, 271
  large bitufted cell, 227
  layer of the deep medium pyramids, 264–266
  layer of the fusiform cells, 269–270
  layer of the giant pyramids, 260
  layer of the granule cells, 261–264
  layer of the medium pyramids, 257–260
  layer of the small pyramids, 257
  layers, 253–254
  localization, 251–252
  medullated fibers and plexuses, 270–272
  nervous plexuses, 270–275
  neurogliaform cells, 263–264, 270, 276
  plexiform layer, 254–258
  special cells, 266–268, 432
  special cells of the first layer, 270
  specific cells, 266–268, 432
  tangential fibers, 270

Cortex, auditory (*continued*)
    thin fibers distributed to the second, third, and
        fourth layer, 274–275
    upside-down pyramidal cell, 279
Cortex, auditory, layer I
    axons, 255–256
    cells, 254–255
Cortex, auditory, layer II
    cells, 257
Cortex, auditory, layer III
    cells with short axon, 258–260
    pyramids, 258
Cortex, auditory, layer IV, 260–262
Cortex, auditory, layer V
    cells with short axons, 262–264
    large and displaced medium pyramids, 262
    recurrent collaterals, 262
    small pyramids, 261–262
Cortex, auditory, layer VI
    ascending short axon cells, 266
    cells of Golgi or colossal cells with short axon, 266
    fusiform cells with ascending axon, 265
    medium and large pyramids, 265
    minute neurogliaform cells, 266
    pyramidal or triangular cells, 266
    triangular cells with descending axon, 265
    triangular or stellate cell of medium size and with
        ascending short axon, 266
Cortex, auditory, layer VII, 269
Cortex, auditory, mechanism of propagation of nerve
    impulses, 273–274
Cortex, auditory, of nonhuman mammals
    layer of the granule cells, 276
    layer of the large pyramids, 278
    layer of the small and medium pyramids, 276
    layer of the triangular and fusiform cells, 279
    plexiform layer, 276
    seventh or fibrocellular layer, 279
Cortex, auditory, in other gyrencephalic mammals
    cells, 275–280
    layers, 275–280
Cortex, auditory, sensory fibers, 271
Cortex, cerebral. *See also individual areas*
    afferent fibers, 237–241
    of amphibia. *See* Batrachians
    anatomicophysiological considerations, 79
    association areas, 382, 440–441
    batrachians, 77–78, 449–451
    circuitry, 549–551
    collaterals, 43
    comparative structure, 437–451
    concepts of, 139
    connections of, 24, 74–75, 83–86, 420–422, 603–
        606
    development of, 15
    fibers and nerve plexuses, 413
    general plan of the structure, 382
    historical notes on the structure, 423–424
    input-output connections, 420–422
    intercalated plexuses, 194
    layer of the deep large pyramids, 408–410
    layer of the fusiform and triangular cells, 13

layer of the fusiform cells, 412
layer of the globular cells, 12
layer of the large pyramids, 12
layer of the medium and large pyramids, 392
layer of the medium pyramids and triangular cells,
    410–412
layer of the polymorphic cells, 35
layer of the small pyramids, 12, 32, 387
layer of the small stellate and pyramidal cells, 404–
    408
layers, 191, 383
medullated plexuses of the gray matter, 416–418
methylene blue studies, 107–111, 113–127
nerve plexuses of the gray matter, 39–40
neuroglia, 418–420
projection or perception areas and association or
    intellectual areas, 237–238, 465
reptiles, 444–449
sensory areas, 382
small mammals, 23–53, 437–441
terminal plexuses, 418
theories of functional localization, 189–190
Cortex, cerebral, of batrachians
    connections, 450–451
    epithelial layer, 449
    layer of the granule cells or cerebral pyramids, 449
    layers, 449–451
    plexiform layer, 451
Cortex, cerebral, of birds, 441–444
    epithelial layer, 443
    homologies, 444
    layer of the deep stellate cells, 443
    layer of the large pyramidal and stellate cells, 442
    layer of the small stellate cells, 442
    layers, 441
    molecular or plexiform layer, 442
    pathways originating in the cortex, 443–444
Cortex, cerebral, of fish, 451
Cortex, cerebral, layer I, 383–387. *See also* Cortex,
    cerebral, molecular layer; Cortex, cerebral,
    plexiform layer
    ascending nerve fibers, 387
    neurogliaform cells, 385
    special cells, 385–387
    superficial polymorphic cells, 384
    tangential fibers, 385
    tufts of pyramids, 387
Cortex, cerebral, layer II
    bitufted fusiform cells, 391
    cells, 387–392
    cells with axons ascending to the first layer, 392
    cells with short axon, 390
    dwarf of neurogliaform cells, 390
    small cells with ascending axons resolving
        themselves into very dense arborizations, 391
    voluminous stellate cell, 390
Cortex, cerebral, layer III
    cells with short axon, 400–404
    large and medium pyramidal cells, 392
Cortex, cerebral, layer IV
    bitufted cells with axon resolved into vertical tiny
        bundles or threads, 407–408

cells whose axon goes up to the plexiform layer and second layer, 407
cells with ascending axon distributed to the fourth layer, 407
cells with long axon, 404
cells with short axon, 407–408
diminutive or arachniform cells, 407
large and medium pyramids of common type, 407
small pyramids of common type, 407
small pyramids, 404–406
stellate or fusiform cells with ascending axon divided in long horizontal branches, 407
Cortex, cerebral, layer V
arachniform and bitufted cells, 410
cells, 408–410
cells with short ascending axon, 408
cells with short axon, 408–410
fusiform or stellate cells with very long ascending axon, 410
large pyramids or Betz's cells,408
medium pyramids, 408
Cortex, cerebral, layer VI
cells, 410–412
cells with long axon, 410–412
cells with short axon, 412
fusiform cells, 412
medium pyramids, 410–411
triangular cells, 411–412
Cortex, cerebral, of lower vertebrates, 76–79
Cortex, cerebral, molecular layer
connections, 125–126
giant cells with short axon, 116–119
short axon cells, 113–127, 154
tangential thick fibers, 124
Cortex, cerebral, plexiform layer, 383–387
cells, 384–387
cells with short axon, 384–385
development, 385–386
fibers of Martinotti, 387
horizontal cells, 385–386
tufts ofpyramids, 387
Cortex, cerebral, of reptiles
deep plexiform layer, 446
homology of the superointernal cortical region, 448
layer of the pyramidal cells,446
layers, 444–445
pathways, 446–448
superficial plexiform layer, 445
white matter, 446
Cortex, cerebral, of reptiles, pathways, 446–448
contralateral association pathway or corpus callosum, 447
homolateral association pathway, 446
longitudinal association pathway, 447
Cortex, cerebral, of small mammals, 1,3, 10, 14, 23–53, 25, 33, 36, 40, 64, 148, 149, 438–441
afferent fibers, 37–38, 73–74
association areas, 440–441
association fibers, 71
callosal fibers, 42–48, 72–73, 74–75
cells of layer I, 65–66
cells of molecular layer, 27–29

cells with ascending axon, 37
cells with short axon, 70
collaterals, 7, 18, 24, 42, 52, 72
collaterals in the white matter, 17, 41
collaterals of pyramids and polymorphic cells, 33, 39, 511
connections of nerve cells, 74, 75
development, 48–51
fibers of the molecular layer, 27
fibers of the white matter, 40–42
homologies, 440–441
intrinsic fibers, 40–41
layer of the large pyramids, 33–35, 70
layer of the ovoid or polymorphic cells, 40, 70, 83
layer of polymorphic cells, 35–37
layer of the small pyramids, 32–33, 39, 69–70
layers, 64, 438
layers of the small and medium pyramids, 439
molecular layer, 26–32, 64, 65, 83
myelinated and unmyelinated fibers, 38, 39
nerve plexuses of the gray matter, 39, 40
plexiform layer, 438
projection fibers, 71
pyramidal cells, 68–69
same fundamental structure as human brain, 51
sensory cells of Golgi, 24, 36
special cells of layer I, 65–68, 203–206
terminal dendritic tufts of pyramids, 31
types of cells, 75–76
white matter, 71–73, 440
Cortex, cerebral, sensory-motor arcs, 420–422
Cortex, homotypical, 434
Cortex, inferior occipital, 55–61, 526
external sublayer, 58–59
internal sublayer, 56
layer of the large pyramids, 60–61
layer of the middle medullated fibers, 60
layer of the polymorphic cells, 61
layer of the vertical fusiform cells, 60
molecular layer, 56–60
Cortex, inferior occipital, of the small mammals, 55–61
Cortex, inferomedial, of the frontal lobe, 359–360
Cortex, insular, 281–286
fusiform cells, 283
layer of the deep stellate and fusiform cells, 284–286
layer of the fibrocellular substance, 284
layer of the granule cells, 281
layer of the medium pyramids, 281
layer of the pyramidal and large fusiform cells, 282
layer of the small fusiform and triangular cells, 283–284
layer of the small pyramids, 281
layers, 281
nervous plexuses, 286
plexiform layer, 281
Cortex, interhemispheric, 138, 325, 346–360, 415, 448
ascending axons of Martinotti, 349
ascending fascicles of the cingulum, 349
cells, 350
collaterals of the white matter of the cingulum, 348

Cortex, interhemispheric (*continued*)
  deep plexiform layer, 350
  layer of the medium and large pyramids, 351
  layer of the ovoid and triangular cells, 349–350
  layer of the polymorphic cells, 351
  layers, 348–351
  plexiform layer, 348
  structure and connection, 358–359
  terminal fibers arriving from the white matter, 348
Cortex, motor, 136, 185, 213–249. *See also* Cortex,
    motor, human
  afferent fibers, connections, 235–237
  axons of Martinotti, 213
  endogenous fibers, 245–246
  external granule formation, 221
  fibers of Martinotti, 208, 231
  fibers of S. Ramón, 232
  functional significance of axon collaterals, 211–212
  fusiform cells, 231
  granule cells, 225–226
  internal granular formation, 221
  layer of the polymorphic cells or layer of the
      fusiform and triangular cells, 229
  neurogliaform or dwarf cells, 226, 227
  parallel plexuses, 232
  pericellular arborizations, 224, 227
  pericellular nests, 213
  pyramidal cell dendrites, 227, 248n
  radial bundles, 232, 234
  sensory plexus, 234, 237
  superficial nerve net, 225
  theories of functions, 249n
Cortex, motor, human
  arborizations of the cells with short axon, 246
  association fibers, 244
  axons of the small pyramids, 210
  cells with short axon, 206–208
  cells with short axon of the third and fourth layers,
      216
  collaterals, 211
  collaterals of the white matter, 245
  eighth layer, 231
  exogenous fibers, 232
  external granular formation, 197
  fibers and nervous plexuses, 232
  granule cells, 196, 197, 221, 222
  history, 190–193
  internal granule formation, 197
  layer of the deep giant pyramids, 197
  layer of the deep large pyramids, 227–230
  layer of the external large pyramids, 213
  layer of the granule cells, 196
  layer of the medium pyramids, 196, 213
  layer of the medium pyramids and triangular cells,
      228
  layer of the small pyramids, 195, 210
  layer of the small pyramids and stellate cells, 216
  layer of the superficial large pyramids, 196
  Martinotti cells, 209–210
  myelinated fibers, 234
  plexiform layer, 195
    polymorphic cells, 197
    sensory plexus, 234–237
    stellate cells whose axon is resolved into very long
        horizontal branches, 223–225
    subcortical afferent fibers, 232–236
    superficial giant pyramids, 214–216
Cortex, motor, layer I, 198–210
  horizontal or special cells, 201–206
  short axon cells, 206–208
  terminal tufts of pyramids, 201–202
Cortex, motor, layer II
  bitufted cells, 212
  cells with short axon, 212
  dwarf cells, 213
  polygonal or stellate cells, 212
  small pyramids, 210–212
Cortex, motor, layer III, 213
Cortex, motor, layer IV
  axons, 214
  dendritic plexus, 215
Cortex, motor, layer V
  axonal collaterals, 217–219
  bitufted cells with axon resolved into small tufts of
      vertical threads, 221
Cortex, motor, layer VI
  cells with short axons, 228
  large pyramids, 227
  medium pyramids, 228
Cortex, motor, layer VII
  arachniform cell, 230
  cells with short axon, 230
  fusiform cells, 230
  medium pyramids, 229
  triangular cells, 230
Cortex, motor, of man and higher mammals, 188
Cortex, motor, of small mammals
  sensory plexus, 236–241
Cortex, motor or sensory-motor, 432–434. *See also*
    Area, motor; Cortex, motor
Cortex, motor, sensory plexus
  deep zone, 234
  middle zone, 234–235
  superficial zone, 235–236
  terminations, 234–237
Cortex, olfactory, 136, 329–330, 360–361, 363. *See also*
    Area, olfactory
  projection pathways of, 322, 414
  structure, 314
Cortex, olfactory, frontal, 326
Cortex, olfactory or limbic, 185
Cortex, olfactory, pathways originating from
  commissural pathway, 322
  internal pathway of association, 322
  projection pathway, 322
Cortex, olfactory sphenoidal, 311, 327, 373, 374
Cortex, prechiasmatic fissural, 360
Cortex, prepiriform
  fibrillar layer, 292
  molecular layer, 293
  layer of the small and medium pyramids, 293
  layer of the polymorphic cells, 293
  layer of the white matter, 293

Cortex, retrosplenial, 524–546
  areas, 526
  distinctive features, 542–544
  layers, 526–529
  localization, 528–529
  physiological significance, 544–545
  structural differences, 537–540
  structure, 529–537
Cortex, retrosplenial, of mouse
  deep plexiform layer, 541
  layer of the small fusiform cells, 541
  layer of the stellate cells, 541
  layers, 540–542
  layers V, VI, VII, 542
  plexiform layer, 541
Cortex, retrosplenial, of rabbit
  deep plexiform layer, 531–532
  layer of the large pyramids, 535
  layer of the medium pyramids, 535
  layer of the polymorphic cells, 537
  layer of the stellate cells, 530–531
  layer of the vertical fusiform cells, 531
  layers, 530
  plexiform layer, 530
  plexuses, 538
Cortex, retrosplenial of rabbit, layer IV
  fusiform neurons, 532
  nerve fibers, 535
Cortex, sensory-motor. See also Cortex, motor
  callosal fibers, 241–244
  components of layer I, 200
  functions, 235–236
  plexiform layer, 198
Cortex, sphenoidal, 228n, 251, 289–290, 312, 327, 361,
    364, 545
  dorsal-ventral association pathway, 330
  external territory, 291
  motor or projection pathway, 327–330
  projection of the, 329
Cortex, sphenoidal, olfactory, 329, 334
Cortex, spheno-occipital, 365, 366, 374
  special ganglion, 363
Cortex, suboccipital of the rabbit, 526. See also
    Cortex, retrosplenial
Cortex temporal of the dog and cat, 279
Cortex, visual, 428
  general historical idea of the structure, 429–430
  historical ideas, 428
  historical notes, 148–151
Cortex, visual, of cat, 183, 495–523
  endogenous fibers, 514
  exogenous fibers, 514
  layer of the deep large pyramids, 509
  layer of the external medium and large pyramids,
    502–503
  layer of the fibers of the white matter, 513–514
  layer of the polymorphic cells, 511
  layer of the small pyramids, 502
  layer of the stellate neurons with long axon, 503–
    509
  layers, 495–496, 498
  localization, 496

plexiform layer or molecular layer, 499
polymorphic cells, 513
pyramids with arciform axon, 512
stellate cells with long axon, 504
Cortex, visual, of cat, layer I, cells, 500
Cortex, visual, of cat, layer II
  arachniform cells, 502
  cells with short axon, 502
Cortex, visual, of cat, layer III, 502–503
Cortex, visual, of cat, layers IV and V
  cells of Golgi and cells with ascending or
    descending axon, 507–509
  dwarf or arachniform cells, 507
  granule cells, 507
  Meynert, solitary cells of, 509
  polymorphic cells, 509
  small pyramids with arciform axon, 507, 509
  stellate cells with long axon, 504–506
Cortex, visual, of cat, layer VI
  giant pyramidal cells, 509
  horizontal dendritic plexus, 510
  small pyramids with arciform axon, 511
Cortex, visual, of cat, layer VII
  sublayer of the fusiform and triangular cells, 511–
    513
  sublayer of the tightly packed neurons, 511
  superficial sublayer, 511
Cortex, visual, human, 139–186
  afferent fibers, 141–142
  arachniform cells with very short axon, 170
  bundles of dendrites and axons, 182
  cells with ascending axons, 142, 162–163, 166–167,
    181
  collaterals of the stellate cells, 182
  fusiform cell or small pyramids with short axon,
    169
  giant stellate cells, 161–162
  granule cells, 185
  large fusiform cell with ascending axon, 169
  layer of granules, 143–144
  layer of the fusiform and triangular cells, 177–178
  layer of the giant pyramids, 144, 172–174
  layer of the giant pyramids in other mammals, 176
  layer of the large stellate cells, 160–164
  layer of the medium pyramids, 155
  layer of the medium pyramids with arciform axon,
    176–177
  layer of the polymorphic cells, 144
  layer of the small pyramids, 155
  layer of the small pyramids with ascending axon,
    170–171
  layer of the small stellate cells,164–165
  layer of the stellate cells in other gyrencephalic
    mammals, 168–170
  layers, 140, 150, 152
  nerve plexuses of the gray matter, 178
  plexiform layer or molecular layer, 152–155
  pyramidal cells, 155–156, 164, 170, 172
  short axon cells, 174
  short axon cells of the layers of the small and
    medium pyramids, 156
  small pyramidal or ovoid cells with arched and

Cortex, visual, human (*continued*)
  ascending axon, 171–172, 174
  stellate cells of medium to large size, 168
  stellate cells with ascending axon, 172, 174
  stellate cells with diffusely ramified short axon, 174
  stellate cells with extensively arborized short axons, 170
  stellate cells with long axon, 165–166
  stellate cells with short axon, 163–164, 167, 168
  superficial polymorphic cells, 117, 118, 155
  white matter, 178
Cortex, visual, layers, 151–152
Croonian lecture, 83–88

Dendrites, peripheral of the pyramids, 24. *See also*
  Pyramids; *layers of individual areas*
Development of the cerebral cortex
  axons, 455–462, 620–621
  cells with long axons, 455–462
  cells with short axons, 458
  centripetal fibers, 458
  development of the myelinated fibers in human
    cerebral cortex, 193
  differentiation of the nerve cells, 455
  first phases in rodents, 453–454
  histogenetic phases in the human fetus, 454–455
  neuroglia, 15, 49–50, 462–463
Diaschisis, 486
Disc, junctional, 112
Disc, transverse, 100, 110
Double bouquet cells, 391–392, 587–589
Dreams, 476, 487n, 488n

Economy of space and protoplasm, 479
Ectostriatum, 444
Ehrlich method, 104,154, 399, 405
  limitations, 189
Embryos, study of the brain, 25
Ependyma, 14
Epispherium, 437
Epistriatum, 444
Exercise, mental, influence on growth of dendrites
  and axon collaterals, 87

Fascia dentata, 294, 320, 331, 334, 337, 338, 341, 344, 345, 441
  connections, 423
Fascicle, angular, 344
Fascicle, septomesencephalic, 442, 443
Fascicles, radial, 417
Fasciculi, radial, 39, 616
Fasciculus, arcuate, 41–44, 414
Fasciola cinerea, 338
Fibers, acoustic, second order, 264
Fibers, afferent from the thalamus, 600–601, 613, 616
Fibers, afferent to cortex, 8, 37–39, 51, 73, 74, 110, 600–601, 605, 609, 611
Fibers, alvear spheno-ammonic, 345–346
Fibers arriving from the white matter, 5, 45–48, 51, 74, 110, 124, 179

Fibers, association, 39, 41, 42, 84, 71, 72
  collaterals of projection fibers, 439
Fibers, association, centrifugal, 183
Fibers, association, contralateral, 415
Fibers, association, homolateral, 415
Fibers, association or commissural, 24
Fibers, callosal, 42,43, 51, 72–73, 75, 242, 415. *See also*
    Corpus callosum
  origins and terminations, 43, 241–244
Fibers, centripetal, development, 458
Fibers, corticothalamic, 545
Fibers, crossed spheno-ammonic, 335, 337
Fibers, exogenous of cerebral cortex
  callosal fibers, 413–415
  collaterals of the white matter, 4, 245, 414
  fibers of homolateral association, 413
  fibers of projection, 415–416
  sensory fibers, 413
Fibers, ideomotor, 185
Fibers, intrinsic of the cortex, 40
Fibers, medullated of cerebral cortex
  deep layers, 417–418
  layer I, 11, 108, 416–417
  layer II, 417
  layer III, 417
Fibers, medullated, of molecular layer, 11, 108
Fibers, moderator, 183, 185
Fibers, myelinated and unmyelinated of the cortex, 14, 25, 38–39
Fibers, oblique, 417. *See also* Fibers, afferent from thalamus
Fibers of S. Ramón, 413
Fibers of the molecular layer, 11, 21, 58, 100, 108, 416
Fibers, olfactory, 292, 329
Fibers, olfactory, second order, 293
Fibers, optic, 179–181, 184
Fibers, perforant spheno-ammonic, 331, 335, 338, 341, 344
Fibers, pericellular, 403
Fibers, projection or descending, 48, 51, 71, 415
Fibers, spheno-ammonic
  inferior perforant, 341–342
  superior perforant, 338–341, 344
Fibers, thalamocortical, 600–601, 613, 616
Fimbria, 331, 335, 338
Fissure, calcarine, 55, 139, 184
Fissure of Rolando, 197, 433
Fissure, rhinal, 291
Focus, angular, 346, 368–369
  axons, 369
  cells, 371
Focus, angular or spheno-occipital, 351, 373. *See also*
    Ganglion, spheno-occipital
  topography, 363–364
Focus, arcuate, 351
Focus of the occipital pole, 351, 355
  cells, 352
Focus, spheno-ammonic, 341, 343
Focus, spheno-occipital, 137, 341, 343, 364. *See also*
    Area, entorhinal, medial
Fornix, 325, 327, 414, 415, 546N

Fornix longus, 239, 325, 333, 352, 415, 444
Function, cerebral, histological basis of, 479

GABA, 577–607
GABA and cortical cells, 610
Ganglion, angular or spheno-occipital. *See also* Area,
    entorhinal, medial; Focus, angular
  centrifugal fibers, 371
  centripetal fibers, 371–372
  conjectures about the physiological significance,
    372–375
  deep plexiform layer, 370
  layer of the granule cells or of the small pyramids
    with arciform axons, 370
  layer of horizontal fusiform cells, 370
  layer of large stellate cells, 366–367
  layer of medium pyramids, 367–369
  layer of polymorphic and fusiform cells, 371
  layers, 364
  links with Ammon's horn and fascia dentata, 372
  as part of the visual area of rodents, 372
  plexiform layer, 364–366
  as secondary or tertiary olfactory center, 372
  as special region of unknown character, 372
  significance, 346
  white matter, 371
Ganglion of the occipital pole, 331, 367. *See also*
    Ganglion, angular or spheno-occipital
Ganglion, precallosal, 351, 353
Ganglion, spheno-occipital, 341, 360. *See also*
    Ganglion, angular or spheno-occipital
Germinal cells, 453–454
Golgi
  investigations of, 62–63
  motor cells of, 24, 36, 39, 45, 58–59, 70–71, 76, 125
  pericellular network of, 397–400
  protocol of, 26
  sensory cells of, 5, 24, 36
  theory of cortical organization, 149
  two types of cell, 24, 76
  works on cortex, 558
Golgi complex, 379
Golgi method, 24
  applicability, 189
  capriciousness, 4
  importance, 424
  improvements, 4
  particular demands of, 148
  use of neonatal or embryonic material, 4
  usefulness of, 131
Granule cells, 404, 413, 423. *See also layers of
    individual areas*
Growth cone, 86
Growth of interneuronal connections, 484–486
Growth of small terminal branches of dendrites and
    axonal collaterals, 87
Growth of the cellular elements of the cortex, 48. *See
    also* Development of the cerebral cortex
Gymnastics, cerebral, 81, 87. *See also* Connections,
    neuronal, plasticity of
Gyri, limbic, 360
Gyri, medial, inferior, and internal temporal, 252

Gyri, pre- and postcentral, differential
    cytoarchitecture, 621
Gyrus, angular, 429
Gyrus, cingulate, 347
Gyrus fornicatus, 332, 346–359
  white matter, 353–359
Gyrus, hippocampal, 137, 291, 294–322, 362n
  cells with short axon, 313
  principal (lateral) portion, 294
  stained layers, 296–303
Gyrus, marginal, 498
Gyrus, postcentral, 193, 433, 434. *See also* Cortex,
    motor
  afferent fibers, 241
  functions, 247
  granule cells, 218
  layers, 193, 214–216
  sensory plexus, 249
  structure, 246
Gyrus, precentral, 194, 433. *See also* Cortex, motor
  granule cells, 221
  layers, 195, 433
  sensory plexus, 233
  small stellate cells, 222
  structure, 246
Gyrus, superior temporal, 252

Hallucinations, 476, 487n
Hippocampal formation, connectivity of, 621
Hippocampus, external or fissural portion, 300–303
Hippocampus, fissure of, 441
Hippocampus, perforant pathways of
  direct fibers to the fascia dentata, 343–344
  fibers destined for Ammon's horn, 344
  mixed fibers, 344
  termination, 343–345
Histogenesis of the cerebral cortex, 453–464. *See also*
    Development of the cerebral cortex
Histologie du Système Nerveux de l'Homme et des
    Vertébrés
  translation, 380
Histology, cortical
  history prior to Cajal, 557–558
Histology, functional, of cerebral cortex, 465–479,
    557–621
Histology of nerve centers
  new concepts, 62
Human brain, functional superiority of, 52, 134
Human cerebral cortex, 132. *See also individual areas*
  Cajal's review of his findings, 133–138
Hyperstriatum, 444
Hypertrophy of nerve pathways, 484
Hypnosis, 487n
Hypospherium, 437

Ideas, anatomical substratum of, 181
Image, visual, 180
Impulse, principal or memory, 184
Inclusions, intranuclear, 379
Indusium, 332
Insula, 280, 283, 286
Intelligence, 87

Lamina medullaris circonvoluta, 294, 344, 345
Lateralization, cerebral, 473
Layer of the superficial polymorphic cells, 384. *See also* Cortex, cerebral, layer II; Cortex, motor, layer II
Lobe, frontal, 291, 487n
Lobe, olfactory, pedicle of, 291
Lobe, piriform, 137, 289, 291, 294–322, 326, 364, 375
  olfactory region, 300
  presubicular region, 300
  subicular region, 300
Lobule, frontal, infero-internal region of cells, 360
Lobule, sphenoidal
  layers, 307
Localization, cerebral, 428
Localization, cortical, doctrine of, 147
  three kinds of areas, 470–472
Long axon cells
  dendrites in layer I, 413

Mammals, gyrencephalic, 148, 150, 241, 327, 383
Mammals, lissencephalic 4, 7, 241, 441
Mammals, newborn, 21
Martinotti, cells of, 7, 10, 20, 24, 61, 70–71, 108, 209–210, 279, 392, 418, 421, 457, 587–590, 606
Martinotti, fibers of, 124, 125, 205, 208–210, 385, 387, 415, 608
Mechanism, ideomotor, 185
Memory, 435, 479–480
Memory areas, 474–476
Mesoglia, 510
Mesostriatum, 444
Method, of Ehrlich, 104, 154, 189, 399, 405
Method, of Ehrlich-Dogiel, 94, 98, 101, 102
Method of Golgi, 3–4, 25. *See also* Golgi method
Method, of Golgi-Cox, 94
Methylene blue, 91–92, 94–101, 104–111, 131, 206
  Cajal's methods, 101–107, 126
  vital impregnation with, 400
Meynert, solitary cells of, 149, 150–152, 172–174, 515, 520
Microglia, 510
Molecular layer, cells of, 56–58, 108. *See also* individual areas
Molecular layer, embryonic, 120. *See also* Development of the cerebral cortex
Morphology of nerve cells and neuroglial cells, 24
Movement, voluntary, incitement to, 75
Myelin sheath, 24

Neocortex, cell types, 564–565. *See also* Cells of individual layers, Cortex, cerebral
  arachniform cells, 580
  basket cells, 577
  bitufted or fusiform cells, 581–583
  cellule à double bouquet protoplasmique or dendritique, 577–580
  dendritic spines, 577
  double bouquet cells, 577
  giant cells, 577
  Martinotti cells, 565. *See also* Martinotti, cells of

morphological variants, 568–570
  neurogliaform cells, 580
  nonspiny, nonpyramidal neurons, 576–587
  pyramidal cells, definition, 565–568
  pyramidal neurons with arciform axons, 566
  short-axon cells, 7, 565
  smooth and sparsely spinous nonpyramidal cells forming local axonal plexuses, 580
  special cells of layer I, 577
  spiny neurons with arciform axon collaterals, 580–581
  spiny stellate cells, 565, 573–575, 580
  star pyramid, 579–580
  types, 568–570
Neopallium, 437
Nerves of Lancisi, 54, 322, 332, 337, 360, 414
Nerves, sensory, 24
Nests, terminal, 202, 403. *See also* Basket cells; Cells, basket
Neuroblasts, 49, 86, 154, 453, 455, 456
Neurofibrils, 379, 388, 392–396, 404, 408–411
  development, 458–462
  effects of temperature, 483
  normal and pathological alterations, 482–484
Neuroglia, 7, 15, 24, 379, 383, 384, 418–420, 462, 481, 547
  cells with long processes, 418
  cells with short processes, 418–419
  development, 15, 49–50, 462–463
  pericellular, 510
Neuroglia, radial cells in development, 49
Neurogliaform cells, 385, 590–591. *See also* Cells, arachniform
Neuroglial cells of layer I, 199
Neuron doctrine, 4, 9, 548
Neurons, cortical. *See also Cells of individual layers*
  and acetylcholine, 583
  and GABA, 576–585, 593–596
  and neuropeptides, 583, 595–597
Neurons, ideomotor, 421
Neurons, olfactory of second order, 324
Neurons, pyramidal
  intracortical collaterals, 573–576, 618
  major targets of, 572
Neuropeptides, 583
Nissl method
  limitations, 189, 524
Nucleus, angular or spheno-occipital, 375n
Nucleus rotundus, 444

Oligodendrocytes, 379
Ontogeny of the brain, 52. *See also* Development of the cerebral cortex
Organization, theories of cortical, 147

Pathway, angular or crossed spheno-ammonic lateral termination, 336–338
Pathway, ascending perforant spheno-ammonic, 339
Pathway, commissural optic, 317
Pathway, commissural spheno-ammonic, 333–336
Pathway, crossed spheno-ammonic, 335
Pathway, olfactory projection, 327

Pathway, optic alvear, 345–346
Pathway, optic, central, 181
Pathway, perforant, 137, 333
Pathway, perforant spheno-ammonic, 335
Pathway, pyramidal, 71
Pathway, reflex optic, 184
Pathway, spheno-alvear, 333, 334, 338
Pathway, spheno-ammonic, 330, 333, 375
Pathway, spheno-ammonic of the alveus, 341, 362n
Pathway, spheno-ammonic, inferior perforant, 371
Pathway, subiculo-ammonic, 332
Pathway, superior perforant spheno-ammonic of
    Ammon's horn, 371
Pathway, temporo-ammonic alvear, 362n
Pathways, olfactory, 332
Pathways, olfactory, tertiary, 360
Pathways, sensory-memory and intermemory
    association, 476–477
Peduncle, cerebral, 328
Perception, 477–478
Perception, auditory
    cortical localization, 431
Perception, visual
    cortical localization, 428–429
Plasticity of dendrites and of interneuronal
    connections, 9, 81, 87, 484–486, 621
Plexus, interstitial, 417
Plexus of Gennari, 181, 514, 516. See also Cortex,
    visual; Stria of Gennari
Plexus, sensory, 37–39, 185. See also Cortex, motor;
    Fibers arriving from the white matter
Plexuses, perineuronal, 402
Plexuses, terminal nerve, 403
Polarization, dynamic, 487n, 8, 75
Presubiculum, 138, 297–299, 300, 316, 318–322, 336–
    338, 360, 361, 545
    fibers, 321–322
    internal plexiform layer, 318–320
    layer of the medium and large pyramids, 320
    layer of the small fusiform and pyramidal cells, 318
    layer of the triangular and fusiform cells, 320–321
    layers, 318–321
    white matter, 321–322
Procedures, neurofibrillary, 424
Projection, visual, central, 478
Psalterium, 295
Psalterium, dorsal, 137, 317, 321, 333, 337, 361, 371
Pseudaxons, 121, 153
Psychic cells, 7, 79–80, 437
Psychomotor region, 55
Pulvinar, 181, 520
Purkinje cells of the cerebellum, 97
Pyramid, cerebral, 86
Pyramidal cell axons. See individual areas
Pyramidal cells
    apical dendritic tufts of, 24, 75, 100, 124–126, 200,
        608
    collaterals, 389
    neurofibrils, 379
    subcortical collaterals, 614–620
Pyramids
    intragriseal course of the axon, 415

Pyramids, dendritic tufts of, 24, 75, 100, 124–126, 200,
    608
Pyramids, differentiation of dendritic tufts of, 205. See
    also Development of the cerebral cortex
Pyramids, large and medium, 41
Pyramids of the deep layers, 412–413
Pyramids, olfactory, sphenoidal, 367
Pyramids or cells with long axons, 387

Radiation of Zuckerkandl, 330, 332, 359
Ranvier, crosses of, 110
Ranvier, nodes of, 15, 38, 110
Reflexes, ocular, 182
Region, central ammonic, external or olfactory
    portion of, 229–300
Region, olfactory, 304
Region, olfactory of the human hippocampus, 301
Region, olfactory sphenoidal, 308
Relays, secondary olfactory, 290
Reptiles, cerebral cortex of, 76, 444–448
Reticulum, pericellular, 93
Retzius, cells of, 119, 199. See also Cajal, cells of;
    Cajal-Retzius cells
Rods, small intranuclear, 396
Root, external, olfactory, 325
    collaterals, 291
Roots, olfactory, 290, 360

Sensation, anatomical site of, 185
Sensation, optic, 180
Sensation, visual, 184, 428
Septum, lucidum, 328, 330, 360
Short axon cells. See also layers of individual areas
    lack of dendrites in layer I, 413
Short-axon neurons and phylogeny, 590–600
Silver nitrate, reduced, 387, 393, 399, 411, 425n–
    426n
Sleep, 479–480
Spines, dendritic, 6, 31, 92, 94–101, 112, 116, 551,
    571–573
    plasticity, 480–482
Spongioblasts, 58, 84, 119, 125
Staining by propagation or diffusion, 96
Stains, nonneurological, 91
Strangulations, 7, 100, 405. See also Ranvier, nodes of
Stratum lacunosum, 294
Stratum lacunosum et moleculare of Ammon's horn,
    345
Stratum radiatum, 295
Stria cornea or taenia semicircularis, 326, 328–329
Stria, lateral olfactory, 294
Stria of Baillarger, second, 40
Stria of Bechterew, 200
Stria of Gennari, 136, 139, 149, 184, 178, 352, 383,
    514, 519, 614–616
    composition, 515–520
    origins of fibers, 520
Stria semicircularis
    connections, 329
Striae, supracallosal, 322, 360. See also Nerves of
    Lancisi

Structure, neurofibrillar of pyramidal cells, 379
Subiculum, 138, 294–295, 297–298, 300, 312, 314–
  316, 320, 331, 333, 334, 336, 338, 339–341, 343,
  355, 360
  cellular islets, 314–315
  fibers destined for Ammon's horn, 318
  layer of the medium and large pyramids, 315–316
  layer of the polymorphic cells, 316
  layers, 314–317
  plexiform layer, 314
  white matter, 317–318
Substantia reticularis, 294
Sulcus, central
  variations in structure, 194–195. *See also* Gyri, pre-
    and postcentral
System, central olfactory, 289

Terminations en pinceau, 41
Textura del Sistema Nervioso del Hombre y de los
  Vertebrados
  publication, 379
Thalamus, 9, 42, 413, 601, 611
Thalamus, afferent fibers, 474. *See also* Fibers arriving
  from white matter

Theories of cerebral organization
  Cajal, 470–479
  Flechsig, 465–469
  Monakow, 469–470
Theories of functional localization and sensory-motor
  interactions, 379
Theory, reticular, 87, 548
Tract, external olfactory, 136
Tract, lateral olfactory, 291–292
Tract, olfactory, 42
Transmission by contact, 40, 52, 80–87
Tuber cinereum, 333

Vacuoles, intraprotoplasmic of Golgi and Holmgren,
  396
Varicosities, dendritic, 100–101
Vertebrates, nonmammalian, 7. *See also* Batrachians;
  Birds; Reptiles
Vision, binocular, 184

Weigert method
  limitations, 524
White matter, fibers of, 13, 40, 51, 71